CONTENTS

Contributors   *vii*
Preface   *xiii*

SECTION I: BASIC PRINCIPLES AND CONSIDERATIONS OF RATIONAL CHEMOTHERAPY AND MOLECULAR TARGETED THERAPY   1

1   Biologic and Pharmacologic Basis
       of Cancer Chemotherapy   1
       Roland T. Skeel

2   Biologic Basis of Molecular Targeted Therapy   16
       Osama E. Rahma and Samir N. Khleif

3   Systematic Assessment of the Patient With
       Cancer and Consequences of Treatment   45
       Roland T. Skeel

4   Selection of Treatment for the Patient With Cancer   63
       Roland T. Skeel

SECTION II: CHEMOTHERAPY AND MOLECULAR TARGETED THERAPY OF HUMAN CANCER   69

5   Carcinomas of the Head and Neck   69
       Barbara A. Murphy

6   Carcinoma of the Lung   94
       David E. Gerber and Joan H. Schiller

7 Carcinomas of the Gastrointestinal Tract   120
Maxwell Vergo and Al B. Benson III

8 Carcinomas of the Pancreas, Liver,
Gallbladder, and Bile Ducts   151
Timothy J. Kennedy and Steven K. Libutti

9 Carcinoma of the Breast   172
Patrick Glyn Morris and Clifford A. Hudis

10 Gynecologic Cancer   199
Thomas McNally, Richard T. Penson, Chau Tran, and Michael J. Birrer

11 Urologic and Male Genital Cancers   233
Brendan D. Curti and Craig R. Nichols

12 Kidney Cancer   250
Mark T. Andolina, Colleen Darnell, and Olivier Rixe

13 Thyroid and Adrenal Carcinomas   258
Haitham S. Abu-Lebdeh, Michael E. Menefee, and Keith C. Bible

14 Melanomas and Other Cutaneous Malignancies   277
Ragini Kudchadkar and Jeffrey S. Weber

15 Primary and Metastatic Brain Tumors   297
April Fitzsimmons Eichler and Tracy T. Batchelor

16 Soft-Tissue Sarcomas   310
Robert S. Benjamin

17 Bone Sarcomas   324
Robert S. Benjamin

18 Acute Leukemias   337
Olga Frankfurt and Martin S. Tallman

19 Chronic Leukemias   394
Khaled el-Shami and Bruce D. Cheson

20   Myeloproliferative Neoplasms and
         Myelodysplastic Syndromes   418
         Elias Jabbour and Hagop Kantarjian

21   Hodgkin Lymphoma   437
         Richard S. Stein and David S. Morgan

22   Non-Hodgkin Lymphoma   451
         Mark Roschewski and Wyndham H. Wilson

23   Multiple Myeloma, Other Plasma Cell
         Disorders, and Primary Amyloidosis   491
         Rachid Baz and Mohamad A. Hussein

24   Metastatic Cancer of Unknown Origin   514
         James M. Leonardo

25   HIV-Associated Malignancies   523
         Thomas S. Uldrick, Mark N. Polizzotto, and Robert Yarchoan

**SECTION III: SUPPORTIVE CARE OF PATIENTS
WITH CANCER**   **543**

26   Side Effects of Chemotherapy and Molecular
         Targeted Therapy   543
         Janelle M. Tipton

27   Infections: Etiology, Treatment, and Prevention   566
         Thomas J. Walsh and Joan M. Duggan

28   Transfusion Therapy, Bleeding, and Clotting   596
         Mary R. Smith and NurJehan Quraishy

29   Oncology Emergencies and Critical Care Issues:
         Spinal Cord Compression, Cerebral Edema,
         Superior Vena Cava Syndrome, Anaphylaxis,
         Respiratory Failure, Tumor Lysis Syndrome,
         Hypercalcemia, and Bone Metastasis   617
         Roland T. Skeel

30 Malignant Pleural, Peritoneal, and Pericardial
Effusions and Meningeal Infiltrates   636
Rekha T. Chaudhary

31 Cancer Pain   649
Richard T. Lee and Michael J. Fisch

32 Emotional and Psychiatric Problems in
Patients with Cancer   678
Kristi Skeel Williams and Kathleen S.N. Franco-Bronson

**SECTION IV: CHEMOTHERAPEUTIC AND MOLECULAR
TARGETED AGENTS AND THEIR USE**   693

33 Classification, Use, and Toxicity of Clinically Useful
Chemotherapy and Molecular Targeted Therapy   693
Roland T. Skeel

Appendix A: Nomogram for Determining Body
Surface Area of Adults from Height and Mass   843

Appendix B: Nomogram for Determining Body
Surface Area of Children from Height and Mass   844

Index   *845*

Haitham S. Abu-Lebdeh, MD, MSc
Assistant Professor
Division of Endocrinology
Mayo Clinic
Consultant
Department of Medicine
St. Mary's Hospital–Mayo Clinic
Rochester, Minnesota

Mark T. Andolina, MD
Clinical Instructor and Fellow
Department of Hematology/
    Oncology
University Hospital Cincinnati
Cincinnati, Ohio

Tracy T. Batchelor, MD
Associate Professor
Department of Neurology
Harvard Medical School
Associate Neurologist
Department of Neurology
Massachusetts General Hospital
Boston, Massachusetts

Rachid Baz, MD
Assistant Member
Department of Malignant
    Hematology
H. Lee Moffitt Cancer Center
Assistant Professor of Oncologic
    Services
College of Medicine
University of South Florida
Tampa, Florida

Robert S. Benjamin, MD
Chairman
P.H. & Fay E. Robinson
    Distinguished Professor
Department of Sarcoma Medical
    Oncology
University of Texas Medical
    Branch Anderson Cancer Center
Houston, Texas

Al B. Benson III, MD
Professor
Division of Hematology/Oncology
Department of Medicine
Feinberg School of Medicine
Northwestern University
Professor
Division of Hematology/Oncology
Department of Medicine
Northwestern Memorial Hospital
Chicago, Illinois

Keith C. Bible, MD, PhD
Associate Professor
Division of Medical Oncology
Department of Oncology
Mayo Clinic
Consultant
Department of Oncology
St. Mary's Hospital—Mayo Clinic
Rochester, Minnesota

Michael J. Birrer, MD, PhD
Professor
Department of Medicine
Harvard Medical School
Cambridge, Massachusetts
Director
Medical Gynecologic Oncology
    and Gynecologic
    Cancer Research Program
Department of Gynecologic
    Oncology
Massachusetts General Hospital
Boston, Massachusetts

Rekha T. Chaudhary, MD
Adjunct Assistant Professor
    of Medicine
Division of Hematology and
    Oncology
University of Cincinnati
Cincinnati, Ohio

Bruce D. Cheson, MD
Head of Hematology
Professor of Medicine
Division of Hematology/Oncology
Georgetown University Hospital
Washington, District of Columbia

Brendan D. Curti, MD
Earle A. Chiles Research Institute
Providence Cancer Center
Portland, Oregon

Colleen Darnell, MD
Clinical Instructor and Resident
Department of Internal Medicine
The University of Cincinnati
Resident
Department of Internal Medicine
University Hospital of Cincinnati
Cincinnati, Ohio

**Joan M. Duggan, MD, FACP,
    AAHIVS**
Professor of Medicine and
    Physiology, Pharmacology,
    Metabolism and Cardiovascular
    Science
Program Director, Infectious
    Diseases Fellowship
Program Director/
    Medical Director, Ryan White
    Parts C and D
Department of Medicine
Division of Infectious Diseases
The University of Toledo-Health
    Science Campus,
    College of Medicine
Toledo, Ohio

**April Fitzsimmons Eichler, MD,
    MPH**
Assistant Professor
Department of Neurology
Harvard Medical School
Assistant Neurologist
Department of Neurology
Massachusetts General Hospital
Boston, Massachusetts

Khaled el-Shami, MD
Assistant Professor of Medicine
Division of Hematology and
    Oncology
Georgetown University Hospital
Washington, District of Columbia

Michael J. Fisch, MD, MPH, FACP
Chair
Department of General Oncology
MD Anderson Cancer Center
Houston, Texas

Kathleen S.N. Franco-Bronson, MD
Professor of Medicine and Psychiatry
Associate Dean of Admissions
    and Student Affairs
Cleveland Clinic Lerner
    College of Medicine
Cleveland, Ohio

Olga Frankfurt, MD
Assistant Professor of Medicine
Division of Hematology and
    Oncology
Robert H. Lurie Comprehensive
    Cancer Center
Northwestern University
Chicago, Illinois

David E. Gerber, MD
Assistant Professor
Department of Internal Medicine—
    Hematology/Oncology
University of Texas Southwestern
Simmons Comprehensive Cancer
    Center
Dallas, Texas

Clifford A. Hudis, MD
Professor
Department of Medicine
Joan & Sanford Weill Medical College
Cornell University Medical College
Chief
Breast Cancer Medicine Service
Memorial Sloan-Kettering Cancer
    Center
New York, New York

Mohamad A. Hussein, MD, MB.BCh
Professor of Medicine and
    Oncology
Division of Hematology
University of South Florida
Tampa, Florida

Elias Jabbour, MD
Assistant Professor
Department of Leukemia
MD Anderson Cancer Center
Houston, Texas

Hagop Kantarjian, MD
Professor and Chairman
Department of Leukemia
MD Anderson Cancer Center
Houston, Texas

Timothy J. Kennedy, MD, MBA
Assistant Professor
Department of Surgery
Albert Einstein College of
    Medicine
Attending Physician–Upper
    Gastrointestinal Surgical
    Oncology
Department of Surgery
Montefiore Medical Center
Bronx, New York

Samir N. Khleif, MD
Bethesda, Maryland

Ragini (Ragi) Kudchadkar, MD
Cutaneous Oncology
Assistant Member
Moffitt Cancer Center
Tampa, Florida

Richard T. Lee, MD
Assistant Professor
Department of General Oncology
Medical Director
Integrative Medicine Program
University of Texas MD Anderson
Cancer Center
Houston, Texas

James M. Leonardo, MD, PhD
Clinical Associate Professor
Department of Medicine
Columbia University of Physicians
    and Surgeons
New York, New York
Chief
Department of Hematology/
    Oncology
Bassett Cancer Institute
Bassett Healthcare
Cooperstown, New York

Steven K. Libutti, MD
Professor
Department of Surgery
Albert Einstein College of
    Medicine
Vice Chairman
Department of Surgery
Montefiore Medical Center
Bronx, New York

Michael E. Menefee, MD
Senior Associate Consultant
Division of Hematology and
    Oncology
Mayo Clinic
Jacksonville, Florida

Thomas McNally
Clinical Research Coordinator
Department of Gynecologic
    Oncology
Massachusetts General Hospital
Boston, Massachusetts

David S. Morgan, MD
Assistant Professor
Department of Medicine
Vanderbilt School of Medicine
Nashville, Tennessee

Patrick Glyn Morris, MD
Special Fellow in Breast Cancer
    Medicine
Memorial Sloan Kettering
    Cancer Center
New York, New York

Barbara A. Murphy, MD
Associate Professor of Medicine
Department of Hematology/
    Oncology
Vanderbilt University
Nashville, Tennessee

Craig R. Nichols, MD
Visiting Professor
Department of Medical Oncology
British Columbia Cancer Agency
Vancouver, British Columbia,
    Canada

Richard T. Penson, MD, MRCP
Associate Professor
Department of Medicine–
    Hematology Oncology
Harvard Medical School
Clinical Director, Medical
    Gynecologic Oncology
Department of Medicine–
    Hematology Oncology
Massachusetts General Hospital
Boston, Massachusetts

**Mark N. Polizzotto, MB, BS, FRACP,
    FRCPA**
Physician
HIV and AIDS Malignancy Branch
National Cancer Institute
Bethesda, Maryland

NurJehan Quraishy, MD
Chief Medical Officer
Ohio-Michigan Division/
    Medical Director
American Red Cross
Western Lake Erie Blood
    Services Region
Clinical Assistant Professor
    of Pathology
University of Toledo College
    of Medicine
Toledo, Ohio

Osama E. Rahma, MD
Clinical Fellow
Medical Oncology Branch
National Cancer Institute
Bethesda, Maryland

Olivier Rixe, MD, PhD
Professor of Medicine
Department of Hematology/
    Oncology
College of Medicine
University of Cincinnati
Professor of Medicine
Department of Hematology/
    Oncology
UC Cancer Institute
Cincinnati, Ohio

Mark Roschewski, MD
Assistant Director of Hematologic
    Diseases
Department of Hematology-
    Oncology
Walter Reed Army Medical Center
Washington, District of Columbia

Joan H. Schiller, MD
Professor and Chief
Department of Internal Medicine—
    Hematology/Oncology
University of Texas Southwestern
Deputy Director
Simmons Comprehensive Cancer
    Center
Dallas, Texas

Roland T. Skeel, MD
Professor of Medicine
Division of Hematology and
    Oncology
University of Toledo College of
    Medicine
Toledo, Ohio

Mary R. Smith, MD
Professor of Medicine and Pathology
Division Hematology and Oncology
Associate Dean for Graduate
    Medical Education
University of Toledo College of
    Medicine
Toledo, Ohio

Richard S. Stein, MD
Professor
Department of Medicine
Vanderbilt University School of
    Medicine
Nashville, Tennessee

Martin S. Tallman, MD
Chief, Leukemia Service
Memorial Sloan Kettering
    Cancer Center
Professor of Medicine
Weill Cornell Medical College
New York, New York

Janelle M. Tipton, MSN, RN, AOCN
Clinical Instructor
College of Nursing
University of Toledo
Oncology Clinical Nurse Specialist
Cancer Center
University of Toledo Medical Center
Toledo, Ohio

Chau D. Tran
Clinical Research Coordinator
Gillette Center for Gynecologic
    Oncology
Massachusetts General Hospital
Boston, Massachusetts

Thomas S. Uldrick, MD, MS
Staff Clinician
HIV and AIDS Malignancy
    Branch, CCR
National Cancer Institute
Bethesda, Maryland

Maxwell Vergo, MD
Medical Oncology Fellow
Division of Hematology/Oncology
Department of Medicine
Feinberg School of Medicine
Northwestern University
Medical Oncology Fellow
Division of Hematology/Oncology
Department of Medicine
Northwestern Memorial Hospital
Chicago, Illinois

**Thomas J. Walsh, MD, FACP, FCCP,
    FAAM, FIDSA**
Director, Transplantation-Oncology
    Infectious Diseases Program
Division of Infectious Diseases
Weill Cornell Medical College of
    Cornell University
New York, New York

Jeffrey S. Weber, MD, PhD
Professor
Department of Oncologic Services
University of South Florida
Senior Member
Comprehensive Melanoma
    Research Center
Moffitt Cancer Center
Tampa, Florida

Kristi Skeel Williams, MD
Associate Professor
Department of Psychiatry
The University of Toledo
Toledo, Ohio

Wyndham H. Wilson, MD, PhD
Senior Investigator
Chief, Lymphoma Therapeutics
    Section
Metabolism Branch, CCR
National Cancer Institute
Bethesda, Maryland

Robert Yarchoan, MD
Chief
HIV and AIDS Malignancy Branch
Center for Cancer Research
National Cancer Institute
Attending Physician
Center for Cancer Research
National Institutes of Health
    Clinical Center
Bethesda, Maryland

PREFACE

Advances in the systemic treatment of cancer have continued at an intense pace over the three decades since the *Handbook of Cancer Chemotherapy* was first published in 1982. This is reflected in the growth of the *Handbook* from 280 pages to over 850 pages and the expansion of the list of clinically useful antineoplastic drugs from 43 to over 125 in the current edition. As with previous editions, several new authors have been added to keep the information fresh and timely. While the number and benefit of cytotoxic agents has continued to expand in part because of the development of hematologic supportive agents that permit larger, more efficacious doses of cytotoxic medications, the greatest potential advances have been through the development of a new class of effective agents known as molecular targeted therapy. The rapid expansion of these new agents has resulted from the explosion of biologic insights into the etiology and behavior of cancer that have taken place over the last quarter century. These drugs have clearly changed the face of cancer treatment and are rapidly becoming integrated into cancer therapeutics and treatment strategies for many cancers. Because of the importance of this new class of agents, we have added a new chapter entitled "Biologic Basis of Molecular Targeted Therapy." In this chapter, we give a brief overview of the molecular basis for the activity of these agents and the relevant pathways they target in order to provide the reader with the basic knowledge and understanding of the rationale for the use of such agents in the treatment of cancer.

As with previous editions of this book, primary indications, usual dosage and schedule, special precautions, and expected toxicities have been added for new drugs and biologic agents that oncologists have begun to use in the past 5 years, and new data have been added to the information for many of the older agents. To facilitate easy access to this practical information, we have moved this section containing an alphabetical listing for all drugs used in practice to the end of the *Handbook*. In addition, each of the chapters dealing with specific cancer sites has been revised to reflect current best medical practice, including the use of molecular targeted therapy, and to point the way toward future advances.

Cure of cancer with less toxic systemic treatment has been a long-term aspiration for many people: those engaged in basic cancer research, physicians who daily are faced with anxious patients who have cancer, and others in the health profession. It has also been a fervent hope of patients and their families. Although cure is possible for some common tumors, particularly when there is only micrometastasis, and for some more advanced tumors such as lymphomas, for most patients chemotherapy remains palliative, at best. When curing and minimizing the cancer can no longer be achieved, then expert, compassionate supportive care becomes the essential and appropriate focus of the oncology team. The section on supportive care has been updated to highlight those issues and pharmacologic agents that are most essential to the daily care of patients with cancer.

The *Handbook* continues to be a practical pocket or desk reference, with a wide range of information for oncology specialists, non-oncology physicians, house officers, oncology nurses, pharmacists, and medical and pharmacy students. It can even be read and understood by many patients and their families who want to be able to find practical information about their cancer and its treatment. Unlike many other books, the *Handbook* combines in one place the most current rationale and the specific details necessary to safely administer pharmacologic therapy for most adult cancer patients.

Progress is always slower than patients, physicians, and basic scientists would like. Current research that joins the expertise and discoveries of the basic scientist, systematic investigation through clinical trials by the clinician, and their interaction in "translational" research continues to offer a realistic expectation of accelerated progress in the control of cancer in the decades ahead.

Roland T. Skeel, MD
Samir N. Khleif, MD

Biologic and Pharmacologic Basis of Cancer Chemotherapy

Roland T. Skeel

I. GENERAL MECHANISMS BY WHICH CHEMOTHERAPEUTIC AGENTS CONTROL CANCER

The purpose of treating cancer with chemotherapeutic agents is to prevent cancer cells from multiplying, invading, metastasizing, and ultimately killing the host (patient). Most traditional chemotherapeutic agents currently in use appear to exert their effect primarily on cell proliferation. Because cell multiplication is a characteristic of many normal cells as well as cancer cells, most nontargeted cancer chemotherapeutic agents also have toxic effects on normal cells, particularly those with a rapid rate of turnover, such as bone marrow and mucous membrane cells. The goal in selecting an effective drug, therefore, is to find an agent that has a marked growth-inhibitory or controlling effect on the cancer cell and a minimal toxic effect on the host. In the most effective chemotherapeutic regimens, the drugs are capable not only of inhibiting but also of completely eradicating all neoplastic cells while sufficiently preserving normal marrow and other target organs to permit the patient to return to normal, or at least satisfactory, function and quality of life.

Ideally, the cell biologist, pharmacologist, and medicinal chemist would like to look at the cancer cell, discover how it differs from the normal host cell, and then design a chemotherapeutic agent to capitalize on that difference. Until the last decade, less rational means were used for most of the chemotherapeutic agents that are now in use. The effectiveness of agents was discovered by treating either animal or human neoplasms, after which the pharmacologist attempted to discover why the agent worked as well as it did. With few exceptions, the reasons that traditional chemotherapeutic agents are more effective against cancer cells than against normal cells have been poorly understood. With the rapid expansion of information about cell biology and the factors within the neoplastic cell that control cell growth, the strictly empiric method of discovering effective new agents has changed. For example, antibodies against the protein product of the overexpressed HER2/neu oncogene have been demonstrated to be effective in controlling metastatic breast cancer and reducing recurrences after primary therapy in patients whose tumors overexpress this gene. Discovery of the constitutively activated Bcr-Abl tyrosine kinase created as a consequence of the chromosomal translocation in chronic myelogenous leukemia has led to a burgeoning era of orally administered small molecular inhibitors of antibodies targeting critical molecular changes in cancer cells and their environment. These sentinel events have presaged the development of a host of new therapeutic agents that are directed at known specific targets within and around the cancer cell. These targets have been selected because they are altered in the cancer cell and are critical for cancer cell growth, invasion, and metastasis. This increased understanding of cancer cell biology has already provided more specific and selective ways of controlling cancer cell growth in several human cancers and will continue to dominate systemic therapy drug development in the decades to come.

Inhibition of cell multiplication and tumor growth can take place at several levels within the cell and its environment:

- Macromolecular synthesis and function
- Cytoplasmic organization and signal transduction
- Cell membrane and associated cell surface receptor synthesis, expression, and function
- Environment of cancer cell growth.

A. Classic chemotherapy agents

Most agents currently in use, with the exception of immunotherapeutic agents, other biologic response modifiers, and molecular targeted therapies appear to have their primary effect on either macromolecular synthesis or function. This effect means that they interfere with the synthesis of DNA, RNA, or proteins or with the appropriate functioning of the preformed molecule. When interference in macromolecular synthesis or function in the neoplastic cell population is sufficiently great, a proportion of the cells die. Some cells die because of the direct effect of the chemotherapeutic agent. In other instances, the chemotherapy may trigger differentiation, senescence, or apoptosis, the cell's own mechanism of programmed death.

Cell death may or may not take place at the time of exposure to the drug. Often, a cell must undergo several divisions before the lethal event that took place earlier finally results in the death of the cell. Because only a proportion of the cells die as a result of a given treatment, repeated doses of chemotherapy must be used to continue to reduce the cell number (Fig. 1.1). In an ideal system, each time the dose is repeated, the same proportion of cells—not the same absolute number—is killed. In the example shown in

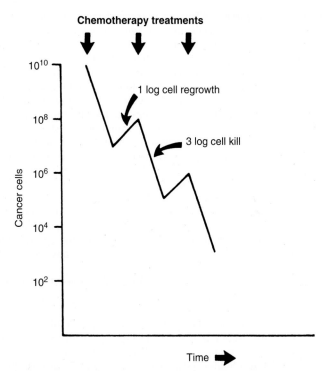

Chemotherapy treatments

1 log cell regrowth

3 log cell kill

Cancer cells

10^{10}

10^{8}

10^{6}

10^{4}

10^{2}

Time

FIGURE 1.1 The effect of chemotherapy on cancer cell numbers. In an ideal system, chemotherapy kills a constant proportion of the remaining cancer cells with each dose. Between doses, cell regrowth occurs. When therapy is successful, cell killing is greater than cell growth.

Figure 1.1, 99.9% (3 logs) of the cancer cells are killed with each treatment, and there is a 10-fold (1-log) growth between treatments, for a net reduction of 2 logs with each treatment. Starting at 10^{10} cells (about 10 g or 10 cm^3 leukemia cells), it would take five treatments to reach fewer than 10^{0}, or 1, cell. Such a model makes certain assumptions that rarely are strictly true in clinical practice:

- All cells in a tumor population are equally sensitive to a drug.
- Drug accessibility and cell sensitivity are independent of the location of the cells within the host and of local host factors such as blood supply and surrounding fibrosis.
- Cell sensitivity does not change during the course of therapy.

The lack of curability of most initially sensitive tumors is probably a reflection of the degree to which these assumptions do not hold true.

B. Biologic response modifiers and molecular targeted therapy

Within individual cells and cell populations are intricate inter-related mechanisms that promote or suppress cell proliferation, facilitate invasion or metastasis when the cell is malignant, lead to cell differentiation, promote (relative) cell immortality, or set the cell on the path to inevitable death (apoptosis). These activities are controlled in large part by normal genes and, in the case of cancer, by mutated cancer promoter genes, tumor suppressor genes, and their products. Included in these products are a host of cell growth factors that control the machinery of the cell. Some of these factors that affect normal cell growth have been biosynthesized and are now used to enhance the production of normal cells (e.g., epoetin alfa and filgrastim) and to treat cancer (e.g., interferon).

The recent expansion of our understanding of the biologic control of normal cells and tumor growth at the molecular level has only begun to offer improved therapy for cancer, though it has helped to explain differences in response among populations of patients. New discoveries in cancer cell biology have provided insights into apoptosis, cell cycling control, angiogenesis, metastasis, cell signal transduction, cell surface receptors, differentiation, and growth factor modulation. New drugs in clinical trials have been designed to block growth factor receptors, prevent oncogene activity, block the cell cycle, restore apoptosis, inhibit angiogenesis, restore lost function of tumor suppressor genes, and selectively kill tumors containing abnormal genes. Further understanding of each of these holds a great potential for providing powerful and more selective means to control neoplastic cell growth and may lead to more effective cancer treatments in the next decade. The fundamental principles related to this group of antineoplastic agents is discussed in Chapter 2.

II. TUMOR CELL KINETICS AND CHEMOTHERAPY

Cancer cells, unlike other body cells, are characterized by a growth process whereby their sensitivity to normal controlling factors has been partially or completely lost. As a result of this uncontrolled growth, it was once thought that cancer cells grew or multiplied faster than normal cells and that this growth rate was responsible for the sensitivity of cancer cells to chemotherapy. Now it is known that most cancer cells grow less rapidly than the more active normal cells such as bone marrow. Thus, although the growth rate of many cancers is faster than that of normal surrounding tissues, growth rate alone cannot explain the greater sensitivity of cancer cells to chemotherapy.

A. Tumor growth

The growth of a tumor depends on several interrelated factors.

1. **Cell cycle time,** or the average time for a cell that has just completed mitosis to grow, redivide, and again pass through mitosis, determines the maximum growth rate of a tumor but probably

does not determine drug sensitivity. The relative proportion of cell cycle time taken up by the DNA synthesis phase may relate to the drug sensitivity of some types (synthesis phase–specific) of chemotherapeutic agents.

2. **Growth fraction,** or the fraction of cells undergoing cell division, contains the portion of cells that are sensitive to drugs whose major effect is exerted on cells that are dividing actively. If the growth fraction approaches 1 and the cell death rate is low, the tumor-doubling time approximates the cell cycle time.

3. **Total number of cells in the population** (determined at some arbitrary time at which the growth measurement is started) is clinically important because it is an index of how advanced the cancer is; it frequently correlates with normal organ dysfunction. As the total number of cells increases, so does the number of resistant cells, which in turn leads to decreased curability. Large tumors may also have greater compromise of blood supply and oxygenation, which can impair drug delivery to the tumor cells as well as impair sensitivity to both chemotherapy and radiotherapy.

4. **Intrinsic cell death rate** of tumors is difficult to measure in patients but probably makes a major and positive contribution by slowing the growth rate of many solid tumors.

B. **Cell cycle**

The cell cycle of cancer cells is qualitatively the same as that of normal cells (Fig. 1.2). Each cell begins its growth during a *postmitotic period*, a phase called G_1, during which enzymes necessary for DNA production, other proteins, and RNA are produced. G_1 is followed by a period of DNA *synthesis*, in which essentially all DNA synthesis for a given cycle takes place. When DNA synthesis is complete, the cell enters a *premitotic period* (G_2), during which further protein and RNA synthesis occurs. This gap is followed immediately

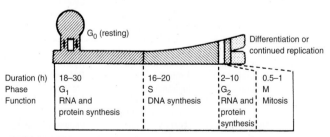

Duration (h)	18–30	16–20	2–10	0.5–1
Phase	G_1	S	G_2	M
Function	RNA and protein synthesis	DNA synthesis	RNA and protein synthesis	Mitosis

G_0 (resting)

Differentiation or continued replication

FIGURE 1.2 Cell cycle time for human tissues has a wide range (16 to 260 hours), with marked differences among normal and tumor tissues. Normal marrow and gastrointestinal lining cells have cell cycle times of 24 to 48 hours. Representative durations and the kinetic or synthetic activity are indicated for each phase.

by *mitosis*, at the end of which actual physical division takes place, two daughter cells are formed, and each cell again enters G_1. G_1 phase is in equilibrium with a *resting state* called G_0. Cells in G_0 are relatively inactive with respect to macromolecular synthesis and are consequently insensitive to many traditional chemotherapeutic agents, particularly those that affect macromolecular synthesis.

C. Phase and cell cycle specificity

Most classic chemotherapeutic agents can be grouped according to whether they depend on cells being in cycle (i.e., not in G_0) or, if they depend on the cell being in cycle, whether their activity is greater when the cell is in a specific phase of the cycle. Most agents cannot be assigned to one category exclusively. Nonetheless, these classifications can be helpful for understanding drug activity.

1. Phase-specific drugs. Agents that are most active against cells in a specific phase of the cell cycle are called *cell cycle phase–specific drugs*. A partial list of these drugs is shown in Table 1.1.

a. Implications of phase-specific drugs. Phase specificity has important implications for cancer chemotherapy.

(1) Limitation to single-exposure cell kill. With a phase-specific agent, there is a limit to the number of cells that can be killed with a single instantaneous (or very short) drug

TABLE 1.1 Examples of Cell Cycle Phase–Specific Chemotherapeutic Agents

Phase of Greatest Activity	Class	Type	Characteristic Agents
Gap 1 (G_1)	Natural product	Enzyme	Asparaginase
	Hormone	Corticosteroid	Prednisone
G_1/S junction	Antimetabolite	Purine analog	Cladribine
DNA synthesis	Antimetabolite	Pyrimidine analog	Cytarabine, fluorouracil, gemcitabine
	Antimetabolite	Folic acid analog	Methotrexate
	Antimetabolite	Purine analog	Thioguanine, fludarabine
	Natural product	Topoisomerase I inhibitor	Topotecan
	Miscellaneous	Substituted urea	Hydroxyurea
Gap 2 (G_2)	Natural product	Antibiotic	Bleomycin
	Natural product	Topoisomerase II inhibitor	Etoposide
	Natural product	Microtubule polymerization and stabilization	Paclitaxel
Mitosis	Natural product	Mitotic inhibitor	Vinblastine, vincristine, vindesine, vinorelbine
	Natural product analog of epothilone B	Mitotic inhibitor that binds to β-tubulin on microtubules	Ixabepilone

exposure because only those cells in the sensitive phase are killed. A higher dose kills no more cells.

(2) Increasing cell kill by prolonged exposure. To kill more cells requires either prolonged exposure to, or repeated doses of, the drug to allow more cells to enter the sensitive phase of the cycle. Theoretically, all cells could be killed if the blood level or, more importantly, the intracellular concentration of the drug remained sufficiently high while all cells in the target population passed through one complete cell cycle. This theory assumes that the drug does not prevent the passage of cells from one (insensitive) phase to another (sensitive) phase.

(3) Recruitment. A higher number of cells could be killed by a phase-specific drug if the proportion of cells in the sensitive phase could be increased (recruited).

b. Cytarabine. One of the best examples of a phase-specific agent is cytarabine (ara-C), which is an inhibitor of DNA synthesis and thus is active only in the synthesis phase (at standard doses). When used in doses of 100–200 mg/m^2 daily (i.e., not "high-dose ara-C"), ara-C is rapidly deaminated in vivo to an inactive compound, ara-U, and rapid injections result in very short effective levels of ara-C. As a result, single doses of ara-C are nontoxic to the normal hematopoietic system and are generally ineffective for treating leukemia. If the drug is given as a daily rapid injection, some patients with leukemia respond well but not nearly as well as when ara-C is given every 12 hours. The apparent reason for the greater effectiveness of the 12-hour schedule is that the synthesis phase (DNA synthesis) of human acute myelogenous leukemia cells lasts about 18 to 20 hours. If the drug is given every 24 hours, some cells that have not entered the synthesis phase when the drug is first administered will not be sensitive to its effect. Therefore, these cells can pass all the way through the synthesis phase before the next dose is administered and will completely escape any cytotoxic effect. However, when the drug is given every 12 hours, no cell that is "in cycle" will be able to escape exposure to ara-C because none will be able to get through one complete synthesis phase without the drug being present.

If all cells were in active cycle, that is, if none were resting in a prolonged G_1 or G_0 phase, it would be theoretically possible to kill any cells in a population by a continuous or scheduled exposure equivalent to one complete cell cycle. Experiments with patients who have acute leukemia have shown that if tritiated thymidine is used to label cells as they enter DNA synthesis, it may be 7 to 10 days before the maximum number of leukemia cells have passed through the synthesis phase. This means that, barring permutations caused by ara-C or other drugs, for ara-C to have a maximum effect on the leukemia, the repeated exposure must be continued for a 7- to 10-day period. Clinically, continuous infusion or administration of ara-C every 12 hours for 5 days or longer appears to be most effective for treating patients with newly diagnosed acute myelogenous leukemia. However, even with such prolonged exposure, it appears that a few of the cells do not pass through the synthesis phase.

2. **Cell cycle–specific drugs**. Agents that are effective while cells are actively in cycle but that are not dependent on the cell being in a particular phase are called *cell cycle–specific* (or *phase-nonspecific*) *drugs*. This group includes most of the alkylating agents, the antitumor antibiotics, and some miscellaneous agents, examples of which are shown in Table 1.2. Some agents in this group are not totally phase–nonspecific; they may have greater activity in one phase than in another, but not to the degree of the phase-specific agents. Many agents also appear to have some activity in cells that are not in cycle, although not as much as when the cells are rapidly dividing.

3. **Cell cycle–nonspecific drugs**. A third group of drugs appears to be effective whether cancer cells are in cycle or are resting. In this respect, these agents are similar to photon irradiation; that is, both types of therapy are effective irrespective of whether or not the cancer cell is in cycle. Drugs in this category are called *cell cycle–nonspecific drugs* and include mechlorethamine (nitrogen mustard) and the nitrosoureas (see Table 1.2).

D. **Changes in tumor cell kinetics and therapy implications**

As cancer cells grow from a few cells to a lethal tumor burden, certain changes occur in the growth rate of the population and affect

TABLE 1.2 Examples of Cell Cycle–Specific and Cell Cycle–Nonspecific Chemotherapeutic Agents

Class	Type	Characteristic Agents
Cell cycle–specific		
Alkylating agent	Nitrogen mustard	Chlorambucil, cyclophosphamide-melphalan
	Alkyl sulfonate	Busulfan
	Triazene	Dacarbazine
	Metal salt	Cisplatin, carboplatin
Natural product	Antibiotic	Dactinomycin, daunorubicin, doxorubicin, idarubicin
Cell cycle–nonspecific		
Alkylating agent	Nitrogen mustard	Mechlorethamine
	Nitrosourea	Carmustine, lomustine

the strategies of chemotherapy. These changes have been determined by observing the characteristics of experimental tumors in animals and neoplastic cells growing in tissue culture. Such model systems readily permit accurate cell number determinations to be made and growth rates to be determined. (Because tumor cells cannot be injected or implanted into humans and permitted to grow, studies of growth rates of intact tumors in humans must be limited largely to observing the growth rate of macroscopic tumors.)

1. **Stages of tumor growth.** Immediately after inoculation of a tissue culture or an experimental animal with tumor cells, there is a *lag phase*, during which there is little tumor growth; presumably, the cells in this phase are becoming accustomed to the new environment and are preparing to enter into cycle. The lag phase is followed by a period of rapid growth called the *log phase*, during which there are repeated doublings of the cell number. In populations in which the growth fraction approaches 100% and the cell death rate is low, the population doubles within a period approximating the cell cycle time. As the cell number or tumor size becomes macroscopic, the doubling time of the tumor cell population becomes prolonged and levels off (*plateau phase*). Most clinically measurable human cancers are probably in the plateau phase, which may account, in part, for the slow doubling time observed in many human cancers (30 to 300 days). Because the rate of change in the slope of the growth curve during the premeasurable period is unknown for most human cancers, extrapolation from two points when the mass is measurable to estimate the onset of the growth of the malignancy is subject to considerable error. The prolongation in tumor-doubling time in the plateau phase may be due to a smaller growth fraction, a change in the cell cycle time, an increased intrinsic death rate (predominantly apoptosis, which is a programmed and highly orchestrated cell death that occurs both naturally and under the influence of many types of chemotherapy), or a combination of these factors. Factors responsible for these changes include decreased nutrients or growth promotion factors, increased inhibitory metabolites or inhibitory growth factors, and inhibition of growth by other cell–cell interactions. In the intact host, new blood vessel formation is a critical determinant of these factors.

2. **Growth rate and effectiveness of chemotherapy.** Chemotherapeutic agents are most effective during the period of logarithmic growth. As might be expected, this result is particularly true for the antimetabolites, which are largely synthetic-phase specific. As a result, when human tumors become macroscopic, the effectiveness of many chemotherapeutic agents is reduced because only part of the cell population is dividing actively. Theoretically, if the cell population could be reduced sufficiently by other

means such as surgery or radiotherapy, chemotherapy would be more effective because a higher fraction of the remaining cells would be in logarithmic growth. The validity of this theoretical premise is supported by the varying degrees of success of surgery plus chemotherapy or radiotherapy plus chemotherapy in the treatment of breast cancer, colon cancer, Wilms tumor, ovarian cancer, small cell anaplastic cell carcinoma of the lung, non–small-cell carcinoma of the lung, head and neck cancers, and osteosarcomas.

III. COMBINATION CHEMOTHERAPY

Combinations of drugs are frequently more effective in producing responses and prolonging life than are the same drugs used sequentially. Combinations are likely to be more effective than single agents for several reasons.

A. Reasons for effectiveness of combinations

1. **Prevention of resistant clones.** If 1 in 10^5 cells is resistant to drug A and 1 in 10^5 cells is resistant to drug B, it is likely that treating a macroscopic tumor (which generally would have more than 10^9 cells) with either agent alone would result in several clones of cells that are resistant to that drug. If, after treatment with drug A, a resistant clone has grown to macroscopic size (if the same mutant frequency persists for drug B), resistance to that agent will also emerge. If both drugs are used at the outset of therapy or in close sequence, however, the likelihood of a cell being resistant to both drugs (excluding, for a moment, the situation of pleiotropic drug resistance) is only 1 in 10^{10}. Thus, the combination confers considerable advantage against the emergence of resistant clones. Compounding the problem of pre-existing resistant clones is the resistance that develops through spontaneous mutation in the absence of drug exposure. The use of multiple drugs with independent mechanisms of action or alternating non–cross-resistant combinations (as well as the use of surgery or radiotherapy to eliminate macroscopic tumor) theoretically minimizes the chances for outgrowth of resistant clones and increases the likelihood of remission or cure.

2. **Cytotoxicity to resting and dividing cells.** The combination of a drug that is cell cycle–specific (phase–nonspecific) or cell cycle–nonspecific with a drug that is cell cycle phase–specific can kill cells that are dividing slowly as well as those that are dividing actively. The use of cell cycle–nonspecific drugs can also help recruit cells into a more actively dividing state, which results in their being more sensitive to the cell cycle phase–specific agents.

3. **Biochemical enhancement of effect**

   a. **Combinations of individually effective drugs** that affect different biochemical pathways or steps in a single pathway can enhance each other. This may apply to some newer agents whereby blocking more than one molecular target in the interacting signal transduction pathways may magnify the interference of cell proliferation compared with that seen with either agent alone.

    b. Combinations of an active agent with an inactive agent can potentially result in beneficial effects by several mechanisms, but have limited clinical utility.

        (1) An intracellular increase in the drug or its active metabolites, by either increasing influx or decreasing efflux (e.g., calcium channel inhibitors with multiple agents affected by multidrug resistance [MDR] due to P-glycoprotein overexpression).

        (2) Reduced metabolic inactivation of the drug (e.g., inhibition of cytidine deaminase inactivation of ara-C with tetrahydrouridine).

        (3) Cooperative inhibition of a single enzyme or reaction (e.g., leucovorin enhancement of fluorouracil inhibition of thymidylate synthetase).

        (4) Enhancement of drug action by inhibition of competing metabolites (e.g., N-phosphonacetyl-L-aspartic acid inhibition of de novo pyrimidine synthesis with resultant increased incorporation of 5-fluorouridine triphosphate into RNA).

  4. Sanctuary access. Combinations can be used to provide access to sanctuary sites for reasons such as drug solubility or affinity of specific tissues for a particular drug type.

  5. Rescue. Combinations can be used in which one agent rescues the host from the toxic effects of another drug (e.g., leucovorin administration after high-dose methotrexate).

B. Principles of agent selection

When selecting appropriate agents for use in a combination, the following principles should be observed.

  1. Choose individually active drugs. Do not use a combination in which one agent is inactive when used alone unless there is a clear, specific biochemical or pharmacologic reason to do so, for example, high-dose methotrexate followed by leucovorin rescue or leucovorin followed by fluorouracil. *This principle is not applicable to the combined use of chemotherapeutic agents with biologic response modifiers or molecular targeted agents* because the cooperativity of chemotherapy and these drugs may not depend on the independent cytotoxic effect of these nonclassic agents.

  2. When possible, choose drugs in which the dose-limiting toxicities differ qualitatively or in time of occurrence. Often, however, two or more agents that have marrow toxicity must be used, and the selection of a safe dose of each is critical. As a starting point, two cytotoxic drugs in combination can usually be given at two-thirds of the dose used when the drugs are given alone. Whenever a new drug combination is tried, a careful evaluation of both expected and unanticipated toxicities must be carried out. Unexpected results such as the increased cardiotoxicity of the combination of trastuzumab with doxorubicin may occur, and this latter case has precluded the use of these agents together.

3. **Select agents for a combination for which there is a biochemical or pharmacologic rationale.** Preferably, this rationale has been tested in an animal tumor system and in the appropriate model system, and the combination has been found to be better than either agent alone.

4. **Be cautious when attempting to improve on a successful two-drug combination** by adding a third, fourth, or fifth drug simultaneously. Although this approach may be beneficial, two undesirable results may be seen, as follows:

   ▓ An intolerable level of toxicity that leads to excessive morbidity and mortality.

   ▓ Unchanged or reduced antitumor effect because of the necessity to reduce the dose of the most effective drugs to a level below which antitumor responses are not seen, despite the theoretical advantages of the combination. Therefore, the addition of each new agent to a combination must be considered carefully, the principles of combination therapy closely followed, and controlled clinical trials carried out to compare the efficacy and toxicity of any new regimen with a more established (standard) treatment program.

C. Clinical effectiveness of combinations

Combinations of drugs have been clearly demonstrated to be better than single agents for treating many, but not all, human cancers. The survival benefit of combinations of drugs compared with that of the same drugs used sequentially has been marked in diseases such as acute lymphocytic and acute nonlymphocytic leukemia, Hodgkin lymphoma, non-Hodgkin lymphomas with more aggressive behavior (intermediate- and high-grade), breast carcinoma, anaplastic small-cell carcinoma of the lung, colorectal carcinoma, ovarian carcinoma, and testicular carcinoma. The benefit is less notable in cancers such as non–small-cell carcinoma of the lung, non-Hodgkin lymphomas with favorable prognoses, head and neck carcinomas, carcinoma of the pancreas, and melanoma, although reports exist for each of these tumors in which combinations are better in one respect or another than single agents.

IV. RESISTANCE TO ANTINEOPLASTIC AGENTS

Resistance to antineoplastic chemotherapy is a combined characteristic of a specific drug, a specific tumor, and a specific host whereby the drug is ineffective in controlling the tumor without excessive toxicity. Resistance of a tumor to a drug is the reciprocal of selectivity of that drug for that tumor. The problem for the medical oncologist is not simply to find an agent that is cytotoxic but to find one that selectively kills neoplastic cells while preserving the essential host cells and their function. Were it not for the problem of resistance of human cancer to antineoplastic agents or, conversely, the lack of selectivity of those agents, cancer chemotherapy would be similar to antibacterial chemotherapy in which complete eradication of infection is regularly observed. Such a utopian state of cancer chemotherapy has not yet been achieved for most human cancers. The problem of resistance, including ways to overcome or even exploit it, remains an area of major interest for the oncologist, pharmacologist, and cell biologist. This reductionist description glosses over the fact that each of these factors is a consequence of the complex genetic characteristics and changes of the cancer cell as it evolves.

Resistance to antineoplastic chemotherapeutic agents may be either natural or acquired. *Natural resistance* refers to the initial unresponsiveness of a tumor to a given drug, and *acquired resistance* refers to the unresponsiveness that emerges after initially successful treatment. There are three basic categories of resistance to chemotherapy: kinetic, biochemical, and pharmacologic.

A. Cell kinetics and resistance

Resistance based on cell population kinetics relates to cycle and phase specificity, growth fractions and the implications of these factors for responsiveness to specific agents, and schedules of drug administration. A particular problem with many human tumors is that they are in a plateau growth phase with a small growth fraction. This factor renders many of the cells insensitive to the antimetabolites and relatively unresponsive to many of the other chemotherapeutic agents. Strategies to overcome resistance due to cell kinetics include the following:

1. Reducing tumor bulk with surgery or radiotherapy
2. Using combinations to include drugs that affect resting populations (with many G_0 cells)
3. Scheduling of drugs to prevent phase escape or to synchronize cell populations and increase cell kill.

B. Biochemical causes of resistance

Resistance can occur for biochemical reasons including the inability of a tumor to convert a drug to its active form, the ability of a tumor to inactivate a drug, or the location of a tumor at a site where substrates are present that bypass an otherwise lethal blockade. How cells become resistant is only partially understood. There can be decreased drug uptake, increased efflux, changes in the levels or structure of the intracellular target, reduced intracellular activation or increased inactivation of the drug, or increased rate of repair of damaged DNA. In one pre–B-cell leukemia cell line, bcl-2 overexpression or decreased expression of the homolog bax renders cells resistant to several chemotherapeutic agents.

Because bcl-2 blocks apoptosis, it has been proposed that its overexpression blocks chemotherapy-induced apoptosis. The interrelationship between mutations of p53, overexpression of HER2, and similar changes in a host of other oncogenes and tumor suppressor genes and resistance to the cytotoxic effects of radiotherapy and chemotherapeutic, hormonal, and biologic agents, when better understood, may further our understanding of resistance and provide new therapeutic strategies.

MDR, also called *pleiotropic drug resistance*, is a phenomenon whereby treatment with one agent confers resistance not only to that drug and others of its class but also to several other unrelated agents. MDR is commonly mediated by an enhanced energy-dependent drug efflux mechanism that results in lower intracellular drug concentrations. With this type of MDR, overexpression of a membrane transport protein called P-glycoprotein ("P" meaning pleiotropic or permeability) is observed commonly. Other MDR proteins are the MDR protein found in human lung cancer lines and the lung resistance protein. These proteins appear to have differing expression in different sets of neoplasms. Drugs that are effective in reversing resistance to P-glycoprotein do not reverse these latter MDR proteins. Combination chemotherapy can overcome biochemical resistance by increasing the amount of active drug intracellularly as a result of biochemical interactions or effects on drug transport across the cell membrane. Calcium channel blockers, antiarrhythmics, cyclosporine A analogs (e.g., PSC-833, a nonimmunosuppressive derivative of cyclosporine D), and other agents have been found to modulate the P-glycoprotein MDR effect in vitro, but limited beneficial effects have been observed clinically.

The use of a second agent to rescue normal cells may also permit the use of high doses of the first agent, which can overcome the resistance caused by a low rate of conversion to the active metabolite or a high rate of inactivation. Another way to overcome resistance is to follow marrow-lethal doses of chemotherapy by posttherapy infusion of stem cells obtained from the peripheral blood or bone marrow. This technique is effective for the treatment of some patients with lymphoma, leukemia, multiple myeloma, and a few other cancers. A more widely applicable technique is to combine higher or more frequent doses of chemotherapy with granulocyte-colony–stimulating factor or granulocyte–macrophage-colony–stimulating factor. These and other marrow-protective and marrow-stimulating agents are being used increasingly and may enhance the effectiveness of chemotherapy in the treatment of several types of cancer.

C. Pharmacologic causes of resistance

Apparent resistance to cancer chemotherapy can result from poor tumor blood supply, poor or erratic absorption, increased excretion or catabolism, and drug interactions, all leading to inadequate blood levels of the drug. Strictly speaking, this result is not true resistance; but to the degree that the insufficient blood levels are not appreciated by the clinician, resistance appears to be present. The variation from patient to patient at the highest tolerated dose has led to dose modification schemes that permit dose escalation when the toxicities of the chemotherapy regimen are minimal or nonexistent, as well as dose reduction when toxicities are great. This regulation is particularly important for some chemotherapeutic agents for which the dose–response curve is steep or for patients who have genetically altered drug metabolism, such as can occur with irinotecan. Selection of the appropriate dose on the basis of predicted pharmacologic behavior is essential for some agents not only to avoid serious toxicity but also to optimize effectiveness. This has been applied successfully to dose selection of carboplatin by predicting the time $\times$ concentration product (area under the curve) based on the individual patient's creatinine clearance.

True pharmacologic resistance is caused by the poor transport of agents into certain body tissues and tumor cells. For example, the central nervous system (CNS) is a site that many drugs do not reach well. Several drug characteristics favor transport into the CNS, including high lipid solubility and low molecular weight. For tumors that originate in the CNS or metastasize there, the drugs of choice should be those that achieve effective antitumor concentration in the brain tissue and that are also effective against the tumor cell type being treated.

D. Nonselectivity and resistance

Nonselectivity is not a mechanism for resistance but rather an acknowledgment that for most cancers and most drugs, the reasons for resistance and selectivity are only partially understood. Given a limited understanding of the biochemical differences between normal and malignant cells prior to the last 10 years, it is gratifying that chemotherapy has been as successful as frequently as it has. With the burgeoning of knowledge about the cancer cell, there is reason to hope that in 20 years, we will view current chemotherapy regimens as a fledgling—if not crude—beginning and will have found many more tumor molecular target–directed agents that have a high potential for curing the human cancers that now resist effective treatment.

Selected Readings

Adjei AA, Hidalgo M. Intracellular signal transduction pathway proteins as targets for cancer therapy. *J Clin Oncol.* 2005;23:5386–5403.

Baguley BC, Holdaway KM, Fray LM. Design of DNA intercalators to overcome topoisomerase II-mediated multi-drug resistance. *J Natl Cancer Inst.* 1990;82:398–402.

Baserga R. The cell cycle. *N Engl J Med.* 1981;304:453–459.

Clarkson B, Fried J, Strife A, et al. Studies of cellular proliferation in human leukemia. 3. Behavior of leukemic cells in three adults with acute leukemia given continuous infusions of 3H-thymidine for 8 or 10 days. *Cancer.* 1970;25:1237–1260.

Endicott JA, Ling U. The biochemistry of P-glycoprotein-mediated multidrug resistance. *Annu Rev Biochem.* 1989;58:137–171.

Friedland ML. Combination chemotherapy. In: Perry MC, ed. *The chemotherapy source book.* Baltimore: Williams & Wilkins, 1996:63–78.

Giaccone G. HER1/EGFR-targeted agents: predicting the future for patients with unpredictable outcomes to therapy. *Ann Oncol.* 2005;16:538–548.

Goldie JH, Coldman AJ. A mathematical model for relating drug sensitivity of tumors to their spontaneous mutation rate. *Cancer Treat Rep.* 1979;63:1727–1733.

Goldie JH. Drug resistance. In: Perry MC, ed. *The chemotherapy source book.* Baltimore: Williams & Wilkins, 1992:54–66.

Kinzler KW, Vogelstein B. Cancer therapy meets p53. *N Engl J Med.* 1994;331:49–50.

Quintas-Cardama A, Cortes JE. Chronic myeloid leukemia: diagnosis and treatment. *Mayo Clin Proc.* 2006;81:973–988.

Schabel FM Jr. The use of tumor growth kinetics in planning "curative" chemotherapy of advanced solid tumors. *Cancer Res.* 1969;29:2384–2398.

Sikic BI. Modulation of multidrug resistance: at the threshold. *J Clin Oncol.* 1993;11:1629–1635.

Slingerland JM, Tannock IF. Cell proliferation and cell death. In: Tannock IF, Hill RP, eds. *The basic science of oncology.* New York: McGraw-Hill, 1998:134–165.

Yarbro JW. The scientific basis of cancer chemotherapy. In: Perry MC, ed. *The chemotherapy source book.* Baltimore: Williams & Wilkins, 1996:3–18.

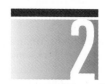

Biologic Basis of Molecular Targeted Therapy

Osama E. Rahma and Samir N. Khleif

I. INTRODUCTION

Molecular targeted therapy (MTT) is a new approach to cancer treatment that resulted from the plethora of molecular and biologic discoveries into the etiology of cancer, which took place over the last quarter of a century. Several agents have already been approved by the U.S. Food and Drug Administration (FDA) for clinical use. Many more are currently being tested in clinical trials, and their widespread integration into the mainstream for cancer treatment is expected to increase at an accelerated pace during the next decade.

Agents in this type of therapy are vastly different from the traditional chemotherapeutic agents that constitute the majority of therapy described throughout the chapters of this book. These new drugs are designed with the intention to specifically target molecules that are uniquely or abnormally expressed within cancer cells while sparing normal cells. Within this chapter, we will discuss drugs that are already available for clinical use; provide a brief description of the mechanism of action of these agents, the pathways they target, and some of their clinical uses; also address promising agents that are currently in clinical trials and may be coming soon to the clinic.

A. Characteristics of MTT

An ideal molecule for targeted therapy should have the following characteristics:

- The molecule is uniquely expressed in cancer cells; hence the therapeutic agent will specifically target the cancer and not the normal cells.
- The molecule is important for the maintenance of the malignant phenotype; therefore, once the targeted molecule has been effectively disabled, the cancer cell will not be able to develop resistance against the therapeutic agent by suppressing its function or expelling the targeted molecule from the cell.

The degree to which target molecules do not embody these characteristics coupled with nonspecificity of the therapeutic agent determines, in part, the limitations of current targets and agents.

B. Classification and type of MTT

The classification of MTT is a moving target. In this chapter, we will classify MTT based on the targeting strategy of the molecule. There are two targeting strategies for MTT:

1. **Function-directed therapy.** This therapeutic strategy is intended to restore the normal function or abrogate the abnormal function of the defective molecule or a pathway in the tumor cell. This is accomplished by:
   - Reconstituting the normal molecule
   - Inhibiting the production of a defective molecule
   - Aborting, altering, or reversing a newly acquired function by targeting the defective molecule, its function, and its downstream effect.

   Agents under this category will be classified based on the mechanism of action and subclassified based on the known affected targeted pathway.

2. **Phenotype-directed therapy.** This is a therapeutic strategy that is intended to target the unique phenotype of the cancer cell where killing the cell is more dependent on nonspecific mechanisms rather than targeting a specific pathway. Such agents include monoclonal antibodies (MoAbs)—including immune conjugates—immunotoxins, and vaccine therapy. Accordingly, agents under this category will be classified based on the type of therapy and subclassified based on the targeted pathway or molecule.

Table 2.1 summarizes the classification and FDA-approved indications of molecular-targeted agents.

TABLE 2.1	Classification and FDA-Approved Indications of Molecular-Targeted Agents				
Agent	Target	FDA Approval Cancer Type	Single Agent In Patients	Combined With	In Patients
Blocking of the Ligand-Receptor Binding					
Cetuximab	EGFR1	Metastatic colon EGFR+ Unresectable head and neck	Did not tolerate irinotecan Failed platinum	Irinotecan Radiation	Failed irinotecan Failed platinum
Panitumumab	EGFR1	Metastatic colon EGFR+	Failed chemotherapy		
Trastuzumab	HER2	Metastatic breast HER2+	Failed at least one chemo- therapy or as an adjuvant	Paclitaxel	First-line
Bevacizumab	VEGF	Advanced colon		Fluorouracil	First-line
		Locally advanced, recurrent, or metastatic NSCLC		Platinum	First-line
		Metastatic RCC		IFNα	
		Recurrent glioblastomas	Failed chemotherapy		
Inhibition of Receptor Tyrosine Kinases					
Erlotinib	EGFR	Locally advanced or metastatic NSCLC	As maintenance after four cycles of platinum, or as second- or third-line		
		Locally advanced or metastatic pancreatic		Gemcitabine	First-line
Gefitinib	EGFR	Locally advanced or metastatic NSCLC	Who demonstrated benefit from the drug		
Sunitinib	VEGFR, PDGFR, c-Kit	Advanced RCC GIST	First-line Failed or did not tolerate imatinib		
Lapatinib	HER2	Advanced, refractory breast HER2+	Failed trastuzumab	Letrozole or capecitabine	Failed trastuzumab
Pazopanib	VEGFR, PDGFR, c-Kit	Advanced RCC			

Inhibition of Intracellular Signaling Proteins and Protein Kinases

Imatinib	Bcr-Abl, PDGF, c-Kit	Newly diagnosed, blast crisis, accelerated, or chronic CML Ph+	Failed IFNα or recurrence after stem cell transplant
		Unresectable or metastatic GIST c-Kit+	
		MDS PDGFR+	
		Chronic eosinophilic leukemia	
Dasatinib	Bcr-Abl, c-Kit, PDGFR	Blast, accelerated, or chronic CML Ph+	First-line
		ALL Ph+	Failed prior therapy
Nilotinib	Bcr-Abl	Accelerated or chronic CML Ph+	First-line
Sorafenib	Raf/MEK/ERK, VEGFR-2, PDGF	Advanced RCC	First-line
		Unresectable HCC	First-line
Everolimus	mTOR	Advanced RCC	Failed sunitinib or sorafenib
Temsirolimus	mTOR	Advanced RCC	

Protein Degradation Targeted Therapy

Bortezomib	26S proteosome	MM	Refractory
		MM	Melphalan and prednisone
		Mantle cell lymphoma	Failed at least one prior therapy

Immune Modulation Targeted Therapy

Lenalidomide	Nonspecific	MM	First-line
		MDS with 5q deletion	Dexamethasone
		Transfusion dependent	Second-line

(continued)

TABLE 2.1 Classification and FDA-Approved Indications of Molecular-Targeted Agents *(continued)*

Agent	Target	FDA Approval Cancer Type	Single Agent In Patients	Combined With	In Patients
Phenotype-Directed Targeted Therapy					
Rituximab	CD20	Diffuse, large B-cell NHL CD20+	Refractory or relapsed	CHOP, or CVP	First-line
		CLL CD20+			
Alemtuzumab	CD52	B-cell CLL	Refractory or relapsed		
Ofatumumab	CD20	CLL	Failed fludarabine		
Gemtuzumab	CD33	Myeloid leukemia CD33+	Refractory		
			Older patients after the first relapse who are not candidates for chemotherapy		
Ibritumomab	CD20	B-cell follicular NHL CD20+	Refractory to rituximab		
Tositumomab	CD20	Low-grade or transformed low-grade NHL CD20+	Refractory to chemotherapy and rituximab		
Denileukin	CD25	CTCL CD25+	Persistent or recurrent		
Cancer Vaccine					
Sipuleucel-T	PAP	Metastatic prostate	Asymptomatic or minimally symptomatic hormone refractory		

ALL, acute lymphocytic leukemia; CHOP, Cytoxan, hydroxydoxorubicin, hydroxydaunorubicin, and prednisone; CML, chronic myelogenous leukemia; CTCL, cutaneous T-cell lymphoma; CVP, Cytoxan, vincristine, and prednisone; EGFR, epidermal growth factor receptor; GIST, gastrointestinal stromal tumor; HCC, hepatocellular carcinoma; IFNα, interferon-alpha; MDS, myelodysplastic syndrome; MM, multiple myeloma; mTOR, mammalian target of rapamycin; NHL, non-Hodgkin lymphoma; NSCLC, non–small-cell lung cancer; PAP, prostatic acid phosphatase; PDGFR, platelet-derived growth factor receptor; Ph+, Philadelphia chromosome–positive; RCC, renal cell carcinoma; VEGF, vascular endothelial growth factor; VEGFR, vascular endothelial growth factor receptor.

II. FUNCTION-DIRECTED THERAPY

Agents under this category target specific cellular pathways (e.g., signal transduction pathways, angiogenesis, protein degradation, and immune modulators).

A. Cell signaling targeted therapy

Signal transduction pathways are crucial for delivering messages from the extracellular environment into the nucleus and enabling the cell to carry on cellular processes including survival, cell proliferation, and differentiation. These signals are initiated from the cell surface by the interaction of molecules (ligands) such as hormones, cytokines, and growth factors with cell receptors. Cell receptors, in turn, transfer the signal through a network of molecules to the nucleus, which leads to the transcription of new molecules responsible for engineering the desired outcome.

In cancer cells, these pathways are found to be altered through the mutation of some of their components. This leads to the functional dysregulation of the affected pathways resulting in uncontrolled proliferation and inhibition of apoptosis. Accordingly, targeting the components of these pathways is a prime goal for the development of MTT. The components of these pathways include the following:

- The ligand
- The receptors for these ligands—the majority of which are kinase receptors
- The cascade of proteins that form these pathways, which are mainly protein kinases; other classes of proteins are also involved.

Accordingly, strategies targeting signal transduction pathways include the following:

- Blocking of the ligand-receptor binding. This leads to the prevention of the initiation of the signal and can be accomplished by either blocking circulating ligands or blocking ligand binding to the extracellular domain of the cellular receptor.
- Inhibition of receptor protein kinases. This leads to the prevention of phosphorylation of the intracellular kinase domain of the receptor, hence, aborting the cascade of proteins reactions in the cell signaling pathways. Blocking adenosine triphosphate (ATP) binding to the receptor is one example to achieve this inhibition.
- Inhibition of intracellular signaling proteins.

1. **Blocking of the ligand-receptor binding.** Blocking receptors and ligand-receptor interaction is currently achieved by utilizing specific MoAbs directed against the ligand or the receptor. MoAbs are biologic agents designed with the intention to specifically target soluble proteins or membrane proteins with an extracellular domain. The MoAbs can exert their antitumor effect through multiple potential mechanisms including blocking the targeted receptor or ligand and preventing its function in transmitting

signals to the nucleus, activating antibody-dependent cellular cytotoxicity, or helping to internalize the receptor and hence deliver toxic agents into the cells. The MoAb technology has been very much improved in the last decade by humanizing these agents partially in chimeric or fully humanized constructs. Substituting the murine Fc portion of the MoAb with a human equivalent leads to a significant decrease in the generation of a human antimouse antibody (HAMA) immune reaction. Although generation of human antichimera antibodies (HACAs) may still occur for those MoAbs, it does not occur with fully humanized MoAbs. This technology to humanize MoAbs has made these molecules more usable in the treatment of cancer, particularly when repetitive dosing is required. In this section, we will discuss MoAbs generated against specific membrane receptors. MoAbs that are generated against membrane nonreceptor antigens will be discussed later in the chapter (Section III.A).

a. **Epidermal growth factor receptor (EGFR) family.** The EGFRs are a small family of proteins belonging to the larger receptor tyrosine kinase (RTK) family. The EGFR family includes at least four described receptors: EGFR1, Her-2-neu (erbB2), Her3 (erbB3), and Her4 (erbB4). These receptors are glycoproteins consisting of three domains: an extracellular ligand-binding domain, a transmembrane domain, and an intracellular domain with a tyrosine kinase activity. Binding of the ligands to the receptor leads to the activation of the intracellular tyrosine kinase and the phosphorylation of the receptor, which in turn leads to activation of the downstream signal transduction pathway. The activation of this pathway promotes cell activation, proliferation, and enhanced survival. Agents have been developed against the receptors EGFR1 and Her-2-neu.

(1) **EGFR1-targeted therapy.** EGFR1 is the first member of the EGFR family to be identified. It is activated by binding to epidermal growth factor (EGF) and to transforming growth factor alpha (TGF-α). EGFR1 is found to be overexpressed in many cancers including 50% to 70% of colon, lung, and breast cancers. Several antibodies targeting EGFR have been approved by the FDA for clinical use in patients with cancer:

■ Cetuximab (Erbitux) is a humanized immunoglobulin-G (IgG1) chimeric MoAb that binds to the external ligand-binding domain of EGFR1. It also binds with much lower affinity to EGF and TGF-α. The combination of cetuximab and irinotecan can improve disease response and progression-free survival (PFS) over the use of cetuximab alone in patients with advanced colorectal carcinoma who express EGFR on their tumors and have previously failed irinotecan therapy. Recent studies have suggested that better PFS and overall survival (OS) can be achieved when cetuximab is combined with FOLFIRI (a combination made up of *fol*inic acid, *f*luorouracil, and *iri*notecan) or FOLFOX-4 (a combination made up of *fol*inic acid, *f*luorouracil, and *ox*aliplatin) in advanced colon cancer (see Chapter 7 for a definition of these regimens and further discussion). The increased response rate as a result of adding cetuximab was higher in patients with tumors expressing the wild type KRAS gene. Currently, cetuximab in combination with irinotecan is approved by the FDA to treat patients with advanced colon cancer expressing EGFR who failed irinotecan treatment or as a single agent in patients who cannot tolerate irinotecan. It is also approved in combination with radiation or as monotherapy in patients who failed prior platinum-based therapy in unresectable head and neck cancers. Recently, a phase III trial demonstrated that patients with advanced EGFR-positive non–small-cell lung cancer (NSCLC) treated with cetuximab combined with cisplatin/vinorelbine had superior survival compared to chemotherapy alone. It has also been found that, in this group of patients, KRAS mutation correlates with progressive disease and shorter median time to progression, but not with survival. Similar to other antibodies, common side effects include rash and diarrhea, and, although very uncommon, cardiac arrest and myocardial infarction (MI) were reported among the serious side effects.

▦ Panitumumab (Vectibix) is a fully humanized MoAb that has been developed against EGFR. Panitumumab binds to EGFR1 with higher affinity than cetuximab. A randomized phase III study demonstrated that patients with refractory EGFR-expressing metastatic colorectal cancer treated with panitumumab plus best supportive care had a better PFS compared to patients who received best supportive care alone. The patients who benefit from the treatment were those with tumors that did not contain KRAS mutations. Therefore, panitumumab was approved by the FDA as monotherapy for chemotherapy-refractory EGFR-expressing metastatic colon cancer. Other diseases with promising results using panitumumab include NSCLC and renal cancer. Common adverse effects include rash, peripheral edema, fatigue, and diarrhea. Serious toxicity, including bronchospasm, has been reported only rarely, and as a consequence does not require premedication for human use.

Other anti-EGFR MoAbs currently being evaluated in phase II trials include the following:

◾ Matuzumab is a humanized anti-EGFR IgG1 MoAb. The agent has been tested in a phase I trial followed by paclitaxel in EGFR-expressing advanced NSCLC with a partial response achieved in 3 of 18 patients and a complete response reported in 1 treated patient. An ongoing trial is evaluating matuzumab in combination with pemetrexed in advanced NSCLC.

◾ Nimotuzumab is a recombinant humanized IgG1 MoAb against EGFR that is approved for squamous cell carcinoma in head and neck in other countries and has been granted orphan drug status for glioma in the United States. Currently, it is being tested in combination with external radiotherapy in patients with NSCLC.

(2) Her-2-neu (HER2, erbB2)-targeted therapy. HER2 is the second member of the EGFR family. This receptor has the same basic structure as the other family members; however, no conjugate ligand has been identified for HER2. There have been no mutations identified in the HER2 gene in human cancers, yet it is overexpressed in many epithelial cancers including colon, pancreas, genitourinary, and breast cancers. HER2 signals via the phosphoinositide-3 kinase (PI3K)/Akt and mitogen-activated protein (MAP) kinase pathways, and HER2 overexpression leads to inhibition of apoptosis and increase in cell proliferation.

◾ Trastuzumab (Herceptin) was one of the first MTTs to be introduced in clinical use. It is a humanized (chimeric) MoAb that binds the HER2. While the mechanism of action of trastuzumab is not entirely clear, it is believed to act through one or more of the following mechanisms: inhibiting the tyrosine kinase signaling of the receptor; activating antibody-dependent cellular cytotoxicity; induction of apoptosis; inducing G1 arrest by modulating the cyclin-dependent kinases; inhibition of angiogenesis; and enhancing chemotherapy-induced cytotoxicity. The FDA approved trastuzumab in 1998 for use in patients with metastatic breast cancer overexpressing HER2 protein. In a large, multicenter phase III study in patients with metastatic breast cancer overexpressing HER2, it was demonstrated that trastuzumab, when used as first-line therapy in combination with chemotherapy (with either the combination of anthracyclines and cyclophosphamide or paclitaxel as a single agent), can significantly increase both the duration of response and the OS. Trastuzumab is currently used in three settings for patients with breast cancers overexpressing HER2: as a first-line therapy in combination with paclitaxel; as a second-line monotherapy in patients who have received at least one prior chemotherapy regimen; or in an adjuvant setting. Common adverse effects are asthenia, rash, and diarrhea. Serious side effects are ventricular dysrhythmia, cardiomyopathy, and thromboembolism.

▦ Pertuzumab is a fully humanized MoAb directed against the extracellular domain of HER2. When pertuzumab was added together with trastuzumab in patients with metastatic breast cancer who did not response to trastuzumab alone, the combination to the two MoAbs showed a significant efficacy. A phase III trial is currently being conducted to evaluate the efficacy of pertuzumab and trastuzumab together in combination with docetaxel in HER2 metastatic breast cancer.

▦ Ertumaxomab is a MoAb that binds HER2 and CD3. Ertumaxomab was evaluated in patients with HER2-positive metastatic breast cancer previously treated with trastuzumab and showed promising results.

b. **Vascular endothelial growth factor (VEGF).** The VEGF family of proteins is one of the specific positive regulators of angiogenesis. It is comprised of five different growth factors: VEGF-A, VEGF-B, VEGF-C, VEGF-D, and placental growth factor. Of these, VEGF-A exerts the most influence on the angiogenesis process. The VEGF proteins bind to three tyrosine-kinase receptors: VEGF receptor 1 (VEGFR1/Flt-1), VEGFR2 (kinase insult domain receptor/fetal liver kinase 1, Flk-1), and VEGFR3 (Flt-4). VEGFR2, through its interaction with VEGF, is thought to be the main mediator of tumor-associated angiogenesis and metastatic processes, while VEGFR1 plays a role in hematopoiesis. The VEGF-A is expressed or overexpressed in many tumors including lung, breast, and ovarian cancer, as well as gastrointestinal stromal tumors (GISTs) and in particular renal cell carcinoma (RCC), where the expression has been found to be high. Accordingly, targeting these molecules to abrogate their ability to stimulate tumor-associated angiogenesis constitutes a logical therapeutic strategy to control cancer. Both antibodies and small molecules have been developed as targeted therapies utilizing this pathway. Here, we will discuss the antibodies. The small molecules will be discussed later in the chapter.

▦ Bevacizumab (Avastin) is a humanized murine anti-VEGF MoAb. It functions by blocking VEGF binding to its receptors (VEGFR), thereby inhibiting the tumor-induced angiogenesis process. When combined with fluorouracil-based chemotherapy regimens in advanced colon cancer, bevacizumab demonstrated improvement of both PFS and OS. Bevacizumab has also been shown to be effective in other tumors including NSCLC (nonsquamous). When combined with paclitaxel and carboplatin, it showed higher response rates and longer disease-free survival and median survival. In untreated metastatic RCC, the addition of bevacizumab to interferon alpha resulted in an increased PFS of 5 months compared with interferon-alpha (IFNα) alone. Currently, bevacizumab is approved by the FDA for use as first-line treatment in advanced colon cancer in combination with fluorouracil-based chemotherapy; in combination with platinum-based chemotherapy as a first-line treatment in patients with locally advanced, metastatic, or recurrent NSCLC (nonsquamous); and in combination with IFNα for the treatment of patients with metastatic RCC. It is also approved as monotherapy in recurrent glioblastoma.

Bevacizumab was approved by the FDA in 2008 for use as first-line therapy in combination with paclitaxel in patients with metastatic HER2-negative breast cancer, based on an improvement in PFS of 5.9 months in patients receiving the combination compared to those receiving paclitaxel alone. However, the FDA Oncology Drugs Advisory Committee recommended that approval be withdrawn based on new trials that did not show any improvement in OS and minimal improvement in PFS. Based on the new data and the increased risk of death due to bevacizumab in the new trials (0.8% to 1.2%), the FDA is reviewing the approval of bevacizumab as first-line therapy in metastatic breast cancer.

On the other hand, while the addition of bevacizumab to gemcitabine-erlotinib did not improve OS in patients with metastatic pancreatic cancer, the PFS was significantly longer in the bevacizumab group compared with placebo. Major serious side effects include arterial thrombosis, where bevacizumab has been shown to double the incidence of this complication. The drug has also been shown to increase the incidence of hemorrhage and hypertension in certain cases. Hemoptysis seems to be a particular risk in squamous cell lung cancer.

c. **Insulin-like growth factor type I receptor (IGF1R).** IGF1R is an RTK belonging to the insulin-like growth factor (IGF) receptor family which is comprised of three transmembrane proteins and binds to the IGF-1 and IGF-2. It is overexpressed in many tumors including melanoma, colon, pancreas, prostate, and kidney cancers. IGF1R overexpression in cancer cells is an important factor for their proliferation, transformation, and metastasis. Therefore, IGF1R became an attractive target for cancer therapy.

■ Figitumumab is a new humanized MoAb against IGF1R. The combination of figitumumab, paclitaxel, and carboplatin demonstrated safety and efficacy in patients with advanced NSCLC. Other phase III trials of figitumumab in advanced NSCLC are ongoing.

2. **Inhibition of RTKs.** Kinases are enzymes that have the ability of attaching a phosphate moiety to another protein. This occurs on a side chain of a serine, threonine, or tyrosine moiety, and the side chain that becomes phosphorylated is used to classify these kinases. The phosphorylation of proteins regulates the behavior of the molecules including protein binding activity, enzymatic activity, trafficking within the cell, or degradation. As a consequence, the phosphorylation process is a crucial biochemical reaction involved with controlling the behavior of a cell. Their critical role in cancer is shown by the observation that mutations in these kinases may lead to drastic outcomes, including uncontrolled proliferation. Receptor serine/threonine kinases will be discussed in another section; here, we will discuss the RTKs. RTKs are a combination of protein families sharing several structural and functional features. These kinases are glycoprotein receptors with extracellular, transmembrane, and intracellular domains. While the transmembrane domain acts as an anchor for the receptor within the membrane of the cell, the extracellular domain contains a binding site for a specific multipeptide ligand. On receptor-ligand binding, signaling events specific to the receptor are initiated. The cytoplasmic domain contains a catalytic tyrosine kinase region and a regulatory region, which are integral to the transmission of downstream signals to the nucleus. Autophosphorylation of the receptor's kinase region initiates a signal transduction cascade leading to cell proliferation, survival/apoptosis, migration, adhesion, and promotion of angiogenesis. Some of the subfamilies in this group of RTKs include the platelet-derived growth factor receptor (PDGFR), EGFR, VEGFR, and fibroblast growth factor receptor. These RTKs are overexpressed or mutated in many human cancers. Therefore, targeting RTK activity is an attractive strategy for cancer therapy and is currently achieved by small molecules. A few small molecules have already been introduced into the clinical practice and many other are currently in clinical trials. Here we will discuss some of these molecules.

■ Erlotinib (Tarceva) is an orally available small molecule with the chemical structure of N-(-3-ethynylphenyl)-6,7-bis (2-methoxyethoxy)-4-quinazolinamine. This compound is a reversible kinase inhibitor of EGFR and acts by competing with ATP in binding the intracellular domain of the tyrosine kinase region. It blocks the signal transduction of the EGFR, leading to the inhibition of the downstream effect of the pathway including cell propagation and survival, as well as angiogenesis. Erlotinib is a highly selective inhibitor for the EGFR tyrosine kinase region, as concentrations of more than 1,000-fold are required for the inhibition of other tyrosine kinases. In phase III placebo-controlled clinical trials in patients with locally advanced or metastatic NSCLC, the efficacy of erlotinib was assessed after the failure of at least one chemotherapy regimen. Erlotinib resulted in a median survival of 6.7 months versus 4.7 months when compared to placebo. On the other hand, no major benefit was observed when erlotinib was used as a first-line therapy in combination with platinum-based chemotherapy. In a recent randomized, multinational trial, the administration of erlotinib after standard platinum-based chemotherapy resulted in improved PFS when compared to placebo. For patients with pancreatic cancer, the addition of erlotinib to gemcitabine was found to improve median survival by 13.8 days over gemcitabine alone, with an increase in 1-year survival from 17% to 24%. Accordingly, erlotinib was approved by the FDA in November 2005 for the treatment of patients with locally advanced or metastatic NSCLC as a second- or third-line therapy. The FDA has recently approved erlotinib for maintenance treatment of patients with locally advanced or metastatic NSCLC whose disease has not progressed after four cycles of platinum-based first-line chemotherapy. Erlotinib is also approved as a first-line therapy in combination with gemcitabine for locally advanced or metastatic pancreatic carcinoma. Although the trend in patients carrying the wild type RAS is to benefit more from erlotinib therapy, no significant correlation were found between KRAS mutations and outcome in patients enrolled in erlotinib trials. Clinical trials are currently being conducted to test erlotinib in combination with other agents as first-line therapy for advanced NSCLC, and as an adjuvant or neoadjuvant in patients with bladder cancer. The most common toxicities include skin rash (12%) and diarrhea (5%). MI and interstitial lung disease are reported among the serious side effects.

- Gefitinib (Iressa) is a small molecule designed to effectively inhibit the tyrosine kinase activity of the EGFR. This compound initially showed an effect in randomized phase II trials with symptomatic improvement in advanced NSCLC. However, further placebo-controlled phase III studies as frontline showed no survival benefit. Therefore, the FDA changed the labeling to limit its use to patients with locally advanced or metastatic NSCLC who have previously benefited from the drug or for patients who are already receiving the agent and have demonstrated benefit. As a first-line therapy in NSCLC, gefitinib in combination with platinum-based chemotherapy showed no benefits. Gefitinib can cause rash and diarrhea. Serious side effects include interstitial lung disease and hemorrhage.

■ Sunitinib (Sutent) is an ATP competitive inhibitor that leads to the inhibition of the phosphorylation of the kinase and inhibition of further downstream signal transduction in multiple RTKs. It functions as an inhibitor to a closely related family of RTKs including PDGFR α and β, VEGFR, stem cell factor receptor KIT, FMS-like tyrosine kinase-3 receptor, and the Ret oncoprotein. Accordingly, the sunitinib antitumor effect is multifactorial. It inhibits cell proliferation and has an antiangiogenesis effect. The antiangiogenesis effect of sunitinib is through the inhibition of both the VEGFR and PDGFR, which is important for the recruitment of pericytes. By inhibiting both VEGFR and PDGFR, sunitinib possesses a stronger inhibiting effect on angiogenesis cells than those agents targeting VEGF alone. Angiogenesis is the hallmark of RCC, and RCC has been demonstrated to overexpress VEGF and PDGF. Sunitinib would be expected to play a therapeutic role in this disease. A multinational phase III clinical trial comparing sunitinib to IFNα as a first-line treatment in advanced RCC showed a major advantage in overall survival of 11 months versus 5 months and has been approved by the FDA as first-line therapy for this indication. Kit and PDGFR play an important role in the development of the GISTs. More than 85% of GISTs possess activating mutations of the Kit kinase, and another 5% are associated with mutation in the PDGFR. Based on the mechanism of action of sunitinib, it is expected to play a role in the inhibition of such tumors and is a natural candidate for the treatment of GIST. Sunitinib showed a delay in tumor growth in patients with advanced GIST who failed imatinib compared with placebo in another phase III trial. As a result, sunitinib has been approved for patients with GIST whose disease has progressed or are unable to tolerate treatment with imatinib. Sunitinib is also currently being tested in other cancers including breast cancer and neuroendocrine tumors with promising results. Common side effects are rash, neutropenia, lymphopenia, thrombocytopenia, and increased transaminases. Serious side effects are hypertension, left ventricular dysfunction, prolonged QT, and severe hypothyroidism.

■ Lapatinib ditosylate (Tykerb) is an HER2 RTK inhibitor. It is FDA-approved for patients with advanced, refractory HER2-positive breast cancer who failed trastuzumab, as a single agent or in combination with letrozole or capecitabine. When lapatinib was combined with capecitabine, anthracyclines, taxanes, and trastuzumab in a phase III, open-label, randomized trial, patients with HER2-positive refractory locally advanced or metastatic breast cancer had a longer time to disease progression compared with capecitabine alone and a nonsignificant trend toward longer OS. On the other hand, lapatinib ditosylate showed no clinical efficacy in patients with HER2-negative metastatic breast cancer. Common side effects are diarrhea, anemia, and rash. Severe side effects are hand-foot syndrome and severe hepatotoxicity.

■ Pazopanib (Votrient) is a tyrosine kinase inhibitor of VEGFR, PDGFR, and c-Kit. Although pazopanib was found to increase PFS by 5 months compared to placebo in patients with advanced RCC who were previously untreated or who only received cytokine therapy, the increase in OS was not significant. Pazopanib is FDA-approved for patients with advanced RCC. Side effects of the drug include diarrhea, hypertension, and nausea. Noted serious side effects were hepatotoxicity, hemorrhage, MI, and QT prolongation.

■ Vandetanib (Zactima) is a multityrosine kinase inhibitor of EGFR, VEGFR2, and the RET gene, which is associated with hereditary and sporadic medullary thyroid cancer. Vandetanib demonstrated an improvement in median PFS compared to placebo in unresectable locally advanced or metastatic medullary thyroid cancer. In patients with advanced NSCLC, the addition of vandetanib to docetaxel resulted in a statistically significant improvement in PFS. Common side effects are fatigue, headache, anorexia, nausea, vomiting, diarrhea, and myelosuppression. Hypertension and corrected QT interval prolongation are occasional.

3. **Inhibition of intracellular signaling proteins and protein kinases.** This therapeutic strategy is directed against a group of proteins that function in a network of communicating cascades to transfer the signal from receptors into the nucleus to produce the intended biologic effect including cell proliferation, apoptosis, angiogenesis, etc. When mutated, these proteins produce deregulated pathways contributing to the malignant transformation of the cell. These proteins are either nonreceptor tyrosine or serine/threonine kinases. The non-RTKs are cytoplasmic kinases. Many of these are attached to and closely linked to membrane receptors. They are usually activated by the binding of ligand to their associated receptors. Some of these kinases include src, abl, and JAK. The serine/threonine kinases are intracellular kinases and some play crucial roles in carcinogenesis. These kinases include raf, kinases from the PI3K/Akt/mammalian target of rapamycin (mTOR) pathway, and the MAP kinases. Small molecules have been designed to block or reverse the effect of these pathways and some are in clinical use. In general, these molecules that inhibit the intracellular signal proteins and protein kinases can target multiple targets, including receptor kinases. They can, therefore, be classified as receptor kinase inhibitors. For the sake of simplicity, this chapter will classify these kinases based

on their primary kinases or pathway effect and will allude to their other roles within the description of the drug.

a. **Bcr-Abl tyrosine kinase.** The Bcr-Abl fusion protein is the resultant product of the translocation between the Bcr and Abl-1 genes. The Abl-1 gene encodes a nonreceptor tyrosine kinase, while the Bcr encodes a serine/threonine kinase. The product of the translocation encodes for a phosphorylated fusion protein that activates many pathways including the RAS, PI3K, and STAT pathways and results in malignant transformation. Drugs designed to target this molecule include:

   ■ Imatinib mesylate (Gleevec) was one of the first targeted therapy small molecules to enter into clinical practice. It is primarily a protein kinase inhibitor that is designed to inhibit Bcr-Abl tyrosine kinase. By inhibiting the Bcr-Abl fusion tyrosine kinase, imatinib mesylate induces apoptosis in Bcr-Abl–positive cells through binding to Abl-1 and competing with ATP, leading to inhibition of the active tyrosine kinase of the fusion protein. It is active against Bcr-Abl–positive chronic myelogenous leukemia (CML) and Bcr-Abl–positive acute lymphocytic leukemia (ALL). Imatinib mesylate produces hematologic, cytogenetic, and molecular remissions that are often long-term and sustainable. Imatinib mesylate also inhibits the receptor kinases PDGF, stem cell factor, and c-Kit. As mentioned earlier, c-Kit is mutated in 85% of GISTs. Imatinib was tested in and found to be effective in GISTs. The current FDA-approved indications for imatinib mesylate include CML that is Philadelphia chromosome–positive (Ph+) whether newly diagnosed, in chronic phase, in accelerated phase or blast crisis, after failure of IFNα therapy, or recurrence after stem cell transplant. It is also indicated in malignant c-Kit–positive GISTs that are unresectable or metastatic. Three large international phase III trials are currently ongoing to evaluate the role of imatinib mesylate in the adjuvant setting with patients with GIST. Imatinib mesylate is also FDA-approved for patients with myelodysplastic syndrome with PDGFR gene rearrangement and in patients with chronic eosinophilic leukemia. Common side effects are edema, rash, diarrhea, vomiting, and night sweats. Serious side effects are congestive heart failure (CHF), cardiogenic shock, and cardiac tamponade. Imatinib mesylate can also cause severe anemia, thrombocytopenia, and febrile neutropenia. Clinically significant resistance to imatinib mesylate is increasingly seen and has been found to occur in patients who develop mutations within the kinase domain in the Bcr-Abl proteins. Therefore, the need to develop alternative Bcr-Abl inhibitors is very important. Some of these alternative kinase inhibitors are discussed subsequently.

■ Dasatinib (Sprycel) is an oral inhibitor of multiple tyrosine kinases including Bcr-Abl, c-Kit, and PDGFR. Clinical data with dasatinib showed that 31% to 38% of imatinib-resistant and 75% of imatinib-intolerant patients with chronic phase CML reached major cytogenetic response. In addition, 30% to 59% of patients with advanced CML and Ph+ ALL showed major hematologic response. Therefore, dasatinib was initially approved for patients with chronic, accelerated, or blast phase of CML who are intolerant or resistant to prior therapy with imatinib. Subsequently, dasatinib was also approved as first-line therapy in CML based on a study that showed a superiority of dasatinib compared to imatinib in major molecular response rate and complete cytogenetic response rate at 12 months (46% versus 28% and 77% versus 66%, respectively). Dasatinib is also indicated in patients with Ph+ ALL who failed prior therapy. Ongoing trials are testing dasatinib as treatment for patients with castration-resistant progressive prostate cancer. Dasatinib can cause edema and rash. Serious side effects include CHF, prolonged QT interval, anemia, thrombocytopenia, and neutropenia.

■ Nilotinib (Tasigna) is another Abl kinase inhibitor. Similar to imatinib, it acts by competing with the ATP-binding site of Bcr-Abl. Nilotinib differs from imatinib by having a higher binding activity to the Abl kinase site with higher inhibitory activity in imatinib-sensitive cell lines. Nilotinib was found to induce both hematologic and cytogenetic responses in patients with Ph+ CML in chronic or accelerated phase who are resistant or intolerant to imatinib. Nilotinib was initially approved by the FDA in chronic- or accelerated-phase CML that is resistant or intolerant to imatinib. Similar to dasatinib, nilotinib was also subsequently approved by the FDA as first-line therapy in CML based on data demonstrating superiority over imatinib in complete cytogenetic response at 12 months (80% versus 65%) and the time of progression to accelerated phase or blast crisis. Edema, rash, nausea, diarrhea, thrombocytopenia, and anemia are among the common side effects. Prolonged QT, torsade de pointes, and sudden death are among the serious side effects.

b. **The Raf/MAP kinase pathway.** The Raf is a family of serine/threonine kinases, including A-Raf, B-Raf, and C-Raf, and is part of the RAS pathway. Raf is activated when RAS, in response to the activation of a RTK, recruits and phosphorylates Raf kinase at the membrane site. Raf, in turn, phosphorylates MEK that activates and phosphorylates ERK. Activated ERK enters the nucleus to activate other transcription factors, leading to cellular proliferation. Aberration in this pathway leads to deregulation of proliferation, resulting in transformation of the cell. B-Raf has been found to be mutated in many tumors such as melanoma, thyroid, and colorectal cancers. Therefore, inhibition of this kinase is a reasonable target in cancer treatment.

■ Sorafenib (Nexavar) is a small molecular inhibitor of C-Raf kinase that leads to the inhibition of the Raf/MEK/ERK signaling pathway. Sorafenib has also been found to be a strong inhibitor of both VEGFR2 and PDGF kinase. A large phase III study showed that sorafenib can reduce the risk of death by 23% compared to placebo in patients with advanced RCC. Therefore, sorafenib was originally approved in 2005 for patients with advanced RCC. In addition, when sorafenib was compared to IFNα-2a in untreated RCC patients, while PFS was similar in both arms, greater rates of tumor size reduction, better quality of life, and tolerability were achieved in the sorafenib arm. Sorafenib was also approved in 2007 for the treatment of patients with unresectable hepatocellular carcinoma (HCC) after it was found to prolong the median survival and the time to radiologic progression compared to placebo. Other clinical trials are ongoing to test the efficacy of sorafenib in other cancers. Common side effects are hypertension (in 9% to 17% of cases), alopecia, hypophosphatemia, and diarrhea. Severe side effects are hand-foot syndrome, chronic heart failure, and myocardial infarction.

Other RAS/RAF/MEK/ERK signaling pathway inhibitors are currently being evaluated in clinical trials:

■ GSK1120212 is an inhibitor of MAP kinase (MEK MAPK/ERK kinase). MEK 1 and 2 are upregulated in different cancers and they are involved in the activation of the RAS/RAF/MEK/ERK signaling pathway. GSK1120212 specifically inhibits MEK 1 and 2, resulting in an inhibition of growth factor-mediated cell signaling and cellular proliferation. The safety and efficacy of GSK1120212 is currently being studied in two phase II clinical trials: the first trial is being conducted in patients with BRAF mutation–positive melanoma who were previously treated with a BRAF inhibitor, and the second trial is being conducted in relapsed or refractory acute myeloid leukemia.

■ GSK2118436/SB-590885 is a selective inhibitor of RAF kinases. It has more potency toward BRAF than CRAF. SB-590885 inhibits BRAF kinase activity 100-fold more potently than sorafenib, and it may be promising in overcoming the generated resistance to inhibitors that bind to the inactive conformation of BRAF. There is also a potential of combining BRAF inhibitor (SB-590885) with a GSK MEK inhibitor (GSK1120212).

■ PLX4032/RG7204 is a selective inhibitor of the oncogenic V600E mutant BRAF kinase. PLX4032/RG7204 was studied in a phase I trial and showed 10 partial responses and 1 complete response in patients with melanoma, with 9 patients having regression of liver, lung, and bone metastases. Currently, PLX4032/RG7204 is being studied in a phase II trial in patients with V600E BRAF-mutations and a phase III randomized trial comparing PLX4032/RG7204 with dacarbazine chemotherapy in V600E-mutated melanoma.

c. **PI3K, AKT, and mTOR pathway inhibitors.** The PI3Ks are a family of lipid kinases divided into three classes based on their protein structure. Class I PI3K has been studied more closely due to the role it plays as a regulator of cell survival, proliferation, and differentiation. Class IA PI3Ks, comprised of four subunits (p110 α, β, γ, and δ), is recruited to the membrane on the activation of RTKs. This leads to a signaling cascade that activates multiple downstream signaling pathways including the AKT pathway. The mTOR pathway is downstream of the PI3K/Akt pathway and plays an important role in cell growth regulation and proliferation. The mTOR pathway is regulated by the PTEN tumor suppressor gene. The protein encoded by the PTEN gene is a phosphatase that works as an on/off switch. The switch moves to "on" position when PI3K deposits a phosphate group on the D3 position of the inositol ring; when PTEN removes the phosphate group from the same position, the switch moves to the "off" position. It has being found that genetic alterations in the PI3K pathways play an important role in different cancers including breast, colon, and ovarian cancer. Therefore, a plethora of novel agents targeting the PI3K/Akt/mTOR pathways have recently been developed for treatment of cancer. Two of these agents are already approved by the FDA and the rest are still under clinical trials and expected to reach the clinic in the next decade. They are as follows:

■ Everolimus (Afinitor) is a kinase mTOR inhibitor. It was approved by the FDA in 2009 for the treatment of advanced kidney cancer in patients who failed sunitinib or sorafenib. This was based on clinical trials that showed the median PFS of 4.0 months in patients who received everolimus versus 1.9 months in the placebo group. Common side effects include rash, edema, and diarrhea. Serious side effects include pneumonitis, anemia, leukopenia, and neutropenia.

■ Temsirolimus (Torisel) is a competitive inhibitor of mTOR kinase. It is indicated for the treatment of patients with advanced RCC based on the interim analysis of a phase III, randomized, clinical trial demonstrating temsirolimus significantly increased OS compared to IFNα-2a in patients with previously untreated advanced RCC. However, the combination therapy with IFNα-2a plus temsirolimus did not significantly improve OS as compared to IFNα-2a alone. Common side effects include anemia and hyperlipidemia. Serious anaphylaxis was also reported.

▪ XL147 is a selective inhibitor of Class I PI3K isoforms. It was studied in a phase I trial in patients with solid tumors, the majority of whom had NSCLC. The dose limiting toxicity was related to rash, and the most common side effects were rash and fatigue. XL147 is currently being studied in two phase II trials. The first trial is evaluating the safety and efficacy of XL147 in patients with advanced or recurrent endometrial cancer. The second trial is evaluating the combination of XL147 with trastuzumab or paclitaxel and trastuzumab in patients with metastatic breast cancer who have progressed on a previous trastuzumab-based regimen.

▪ XL765 is selective inhibitor of mTOR and Class I PI3K isoforms. A phase II trial is ongoing to evaluate the safety and clinical efficacy of either XL147 or XL765 in combination with letrozole in patients with breast cancer that is ER+/PGR+ and HER2 and refractory to a nonsteroidal aromatase inhibitor.

▪ GDC-0941 is another potent and selective oral inhibitor of the class I PI3K. GDC-0941 demonstrated significant efficacy in preclinical studies in breast, ovarian, lung, and prostate cancer models. It was studied in a phase I trial in solid tumors in 38 patients (10 of whom had sarcoma) and found to have good tolerability.

▪ GSK2141795 is an oral AKT inhibitor currently being studied in a phase I, open-label, two-stage study of lymphomas and solid tumors.

▪ Ridaforolimus (formerly known as deforolimus) is a novel small-molecule inhibitor of mTOR. In a multicenter phase II trial of ridaforolimus in patients with progressive advanced sarcomas, ridaforolimus more than doubled PFS when compared with historical data. It is currently being studied in endometrial, prostate, breast, and NSCLCs.

▪ AZD8055 is a selective, orally active inhibitor of mTOR kinase. It is currently in phase I/II trials in patients with advanced solid tumors.

▪ Perifosine is a synthetic alkylphospholipid that inhibits or modifies different signal transduction pathways (AKT, MAPK, and JNK). Perifosine was studied in a phase II exploratory randomized double-blind, placebo-controlled study where patients with metastatic colorectal cancer received perifosine in combination with capecitabine or placebo. Perifosine in combination with capecitabine more than doubled median time to progression over capecitabine.

B. Angiogenesis-targeted therapy

Angiogenesis is a biologic process that is crucial for the development of tumors. Tumors have exploited this physiologic process to provide the milieu to permit the growth of both primary and metastatic cancers. The process of angiogenesis starts by the release of VEGF by the tumor. VEGF binds to receptors on the blood vessels' endothelial cells, leading to their proliferation and immigration toward the source of the angiogenic signal. Although the antineoplastic effect of antiangiogenesis therapy is mediated through the effect on the environment for the cancer cell growth, the initial mechanism of current therapies is based on molecular targeting, which was previously described.

C. Protein degradation–targeted therapy

Protein degradation is one of the mechanisms by which cell function is regulated. The ubiquitin-proteosome pathway plays a very important role in this regard. The proteosome is a large complex of proteins that degrades other ubiquitinated proteins. It exerts its degradation capability through coordinated catalytic activities of its three proteolytic sites that leads to chymotryptic, tryptic, and postglutamyl peptide hydrolyticlike activities. Many key proteins in the cell cycle, apoptotic, and angiogenesis pathways are regulated by degradation, including the p53, p21, p27 (cell cycle regulatory) proteins; NF-κB, a key transcription factor that is activated by the proteosomes; and ICAM-1, VCAM, and E selectin (cell adhesion molecules). Drugs targeting degradation machinery in the cell include:

▓ Bortezomib (Velcade) is a dipeptidyl boronic acid derivative that inhibits the 26S proteosome. The 26S proteosome is the principal regulator of the intracellular protein degradation. Bortezomib is the first of its class to be approved for clinical use. Bortezomib can selectively inhibit the chymotryptic site of the proteosome. This leads to a selective inhibition of the degradation of proteins involved in cell proliferation and survival regulation; as a consequence, apoptosis is induced. Bortezomib has been found to be particularly effective in myeloma. A phase III trial that randomized patients with myeloma, who failed one to three previous therapies, to bortezomib versus high-dose dexamethasone demonstrated that bortezomib resulted in a superior outcome with respect to response frequency, time to progression, and OS. Bortezomib was approved in 2005 for the treatment of patients with refractory multiple myeloma who had received at least one prior therapy and, in 2008, as an initial treatment for patients with multiple myeloma based on the results of a phase III trial showing the superior efficacy of bortezomib plus melphalan and prednisone in delaying time to progression compared to melphalan-prednisone therapy alone. Bortezomib is also FDA-approved for patients with mantle cell lymphoma who failed at least one prior therapy. Bortezomib is currently being studied in patients with relapsed or refractory peripheral T-cell lymphoma. The observed side effects of bortezomib are asthenia, hypertension, rash, and diarrhea. Serious side effects include CHF, anemia, neutropenia, and thrombocytopenia.

- Carfilzomib is the next generation of proteasome inhibitor with higher selectivity and specificity. It binds selectively to the N-terminal threonine active sites within the proteasome and is currently being studied in phase IIb clinical trial in patients with relapsed and refractory multiple myeloma. A phase III international randomized trial will also be evaluating the efficacy of carfilzomib in combination with lenalidomide and dexamethasone versus lenalidomide and dexamethasone in patients with relapsed multiple myeloma.

D. Immune modulation–targeted therapy

1. **Specific immune modulators.** Immune homeostasis is the function of balancing the effector and inhibitory arms of the immune system. This balance prevents the overreaction of the effector immune response that can lead to the generation of harmful immune reactions against normal tissues. The inhibitory arm of the immune system is composed of cytokines/ligands (e.g., interleukin [IL]-10; TGF-β), T-cell inhibitory molecules/receptors (e.g., CTLA-4 and PD1), or immune cells (e.g., T-regulatory cells and myeloid suppressor cells). Unfortunately, the effect of the inhibitory arm of the immune system can lead to the inability of the immune system to mount a proper response against cancer. Recently, there has been significant scientific progress in the understanding of these inhibitory mechanisms and accordingly, targeting strategies against these inhibitory mechanisms have been developed with the intention of enhancing immune response against tumors. Some are aimed to interrupt the inhibitory signals of the receptors (e.g., CTLA4 or PD1) and others to neutralize the effect of inhibitory cytokines (e.g., TGF-β). Accordingly, most of the specific immune modulators are designed to target immune inhibitory molecules.

   a. **CTLA-4 inhibitors.** CTLA4 is a coinhibitory molecule that is expressed on T-cells. It is a homolog of CD28 with higher binding affinity to B7.1 (CD80) and B7.2 (CD86). CTLA4 binding to B7.1 or B7.2 ligands on antigen presenting cells sends an inhibitory signal into the T-cell leading to reduction in T-cell activation and cytokine production, creating an immunosuppressant environment. Therefore, blocking CTLA4 by using anti-CTLA4 antibodies should prevent this inhibitory signal and maintain and enhance the immune response against tumors. Currently, there are two anti-CTLA4 antibodies in clinical trials.

- Ipilimumab (MDX-010) is the first humanized anti-CTLA4 IgG1 MoAb. Ipilimumab demonstrated clinical efficacy in multiple phase II clinical trials in patients with stage III or IV unresectable melanoma. Ipilimumab was studied in patients with metastatic RCC in a phase II study: 1 of 21 patients at the lower dose and 5 of 40 patients at the higher dose had partial responses. Adverse events were mainly autoimmune toxicities in the skin and gastrointestinal tract (grade III to IV immune-related adverse effects reported in up to 33% to 40% of patients). Ipilimumab is also currently being tested in hormone-refractory prostate cancer.

- Tremelimumab is a human IgG2 antibody with high affinity for CTLA-4. Tremelimumab was evaluated in a phase II study in patients with stage III or stage IV recurrent metastatic melanoma and was found to prolong the median survival for 3 months compared to standard therapy. Similar to ipilimumab, autoimmune toxicities including dermatitis (20% to 40%), colitis (44%), uveitis (10%), and thyroiditis (3%) were reported.

b. PD1 inhibitors. PD1 is an inhibitory receptor belonging to the B7-receptor family that interacts with two known ligands: PD-L1 (B7-H1) and PDL2 (B7-DC). Tumors are known to overexpress PDL1. The interaction of PD1 with PDL1 or PDL2 results in downregulation of signals by the T-cell receptor and induction of apoptosis in activated T-lymphocytes leading to immune suppression. Accordingly, anti-PD1 antibodies are being developed in order to overcome the immunosuppression to tumor.

- CT-011 is a humanized IgG1 kappa recombinant monoclonal antibody against the PD1 receptor that blocks the interaction of PDL1 with PD1. Clinical responses were observed in six patients within 12 months after initial treatment with CT-011 in a phase I trial. One patient with follicular lymphoma had a complete remission 10 months post single dose administration. CT-011 is currently being evaluated in a number of phase II clinical studies in combination with different agents including autologous stem cell transplantation in diffused large B-cell lymphoma, FOLFOX in colorectal carcinoma, and rituximab in patients with relapsed follicular lymphoma. CT-011 is also being tested in combination with peptide vaccines.

- MDX-1106 (ONO-4538) is a fully humanized IgG4 anti-PD1 antibody. MDX-1106 was tested in a phase I trial. One patient with colorectal carcinoma experienced a partial response lasting for more than 6 months. Tumor regressions were observed in four additional patients, including two patients with melanoma, one patient with NSCLC, and one with RCC.

c. TGF-β antibodies. TGF-β is an immunosuppressive cytokine found at the site of most tumors. It inhibits T-cell proliferation and differentiation into cytotoxic or helper T-cells. In addition, it has been found that TGF-β can induce the generation of T-regulatory cells that are known to inhibit antitumor activity. As a result, antibodies targeting TGF-β have being developed for therapeutic purposes to enhance immune response against cancer.

- GC-1008 is a TGF-β neutralizing MoAb. It was evaluated in a phase I trial in patients with malignant melanoma and RCC. Five out of twenty-two patients achieved stable disease.
- AP-12009 is a TGF-β2–specific phosphorothioate. It has been studied in phase I/II in gliomas and anaplastic astrocytomas, demonstrating a significant increase in survival compared to standard temozolomide therapy.

2. Nonspecific immunomodulators. Nonspecific immunomodulators are a family of medications that are derivatives of thalidomide by minor structural modifications. These modifications lead to the enhancement of drug efficacy and the improvement in the side effect profile, including the neurologic toxicity and prothrombotic effects of thalidomide. The mechanism of action for this group of compounds is not clearly defined. Many pathways have been shown to be triggered by these medications including caspase-8, proteosome, NFκB, and the antiangiogenesis pathways.

- Lenalidomide (Revlimid) is one of the new generation of nonspecific immunomodulators. In a randomized phase III, when combined with dexamethasone, lenalidomide was found to be superior in complete response (CR), PFS, and OS to dexamethasone alone in patients with relapsed or refractory multiple myeloma. When lenalidomide is combined with dexamethasone in patients with newly diagnosed multiple myeloma, 91% of patients achieved an objective response, including 11% with CR. Lenalidomide was approved for use in combination with dexamethasone in patients with multiple myeloma who received at least one prior therapy, and in patients with myelodysplastic syndrome with 5q deletion who are transfusion dependent. Side effects of the drug were found to be tolerable and compared to thalidomide, lenalidomide ashowed no significant somnolence, constipation, or neuropathy. Common side effects are edema and rash. Serious side effects include atrial fibrillation, Stevens-Johnson syndrome, neutropenia, anemia, and thrombocytopenia.

III. PHENOTYPE DIRECTED–TARGETED THERAPY

As outlined previously, this is a therapeutic strategy that is intended to target the unique phenotype of the cancer cell where killing the cell is more dependent on direct induction of a cytotoxic effect rather than targeting a specific pathway, as discussed subsequently. Agents under this category will be classified based on the type of therapy and subclassified based on the target pathway or molecule, if applicable.

A. Nonreceptor protein–directed MoAbs

These are a group of antibodies developed to recognize specific antigens expressed on the surface of cancer cells. Their purpose is not for blocking specific pathways or receptor proteins, but rather to induce direct cytotoxic effect. These MoAbs may be used alone (unconjugated) or as a delivery system for cellular toxins, radionuclides, or chemotherapy (conjugated).

1. Unconjugated antibodies

- Rituximab (Rituxan) is an IgG1 kappa murine–human chimeric MoAb that is generated against the CD20 antigen. CD20 is expressed on the cell surface of B-cells and hence on the surface of B-cell lymphoma. Rituximab is indicated as a single agent for the treatment of relapsed or refractory B-cell non-Hodgkin lymphoma (NHL) and chronic lymphocytic leukemia (CLL) expressing the CD20 marker. Rituximab was studied in combination with CHOP (*C*ytoxan, *h*ydroxydaunorubicin, and *p*rednisone) therapy in patients with diffuse large B-cell lymphoma and resulted in better PFS and OS. Thus, rituximab was approved for patients with previously untreated diffuse large B-cell, CD20-positive NHL in combination with CHOP, or CVP (*C*ytoxan, *v*incristine, and *p*rednisone), chemotherapy (see Chapter 22). Rituximab is also used in combination with fludarabine and cyclophosphamide in previously untreated and treated patients with CD20-positive CLL. Rituximab can cause hypertension, nausea, vomiting, fever, chills, and lymphopenia. Cardiac arrhythmia, cardiogenic shock, Stevens-Johnson syndrome, toxic epidermal necrolysis, and tumor lysis syndrome are reported as serious side effects.

- Alemtuzumab (Campath) is a humanized IgG1 kappa murine–human chimeric MoAb that is directed against CD52-cell surface glycoprotein. CD52 is expressed on the surface of normal and malignant B- and T-cells, natural killer cells, monocytes, and macrophages. Alemtuzumab is indicated for the treatment of patients with B-cell CLL who have failed fludarabine based on demonstrated efficacy of the drug with 2% CR and 31% PR in this patient population. Alemtuzumab is currently being studied in combination with other agents. Common side effects are anemia, neutropenia, thrombocytopenia, rash, and diarrhea. Serious side effects are cardiac arrhythmia and cardiomyopathy. Patients who have recently been treated with this MoAb should not receive any live viral vaccines because of the immune suppression effect of the medication.

- Ofatumumab (Arzerra) is a humananized IgG1-kappa MoAb that binds to the CD20 molecule on B-lymphocytes, which leads to B-cell lysis. It is FDA-approved for refractory CLL. A recent phase II study comparing the efficacy of ofatumumab in patients with fludarabine and alemtuzumab refractory showed better overall response rates in CLL. Ofatumumab can cause rash, neutropenia, anemia, diarrhea, and sepsis.

- Epratuzumab is a humanized MoAb that binds to the CD22 glycoprotein. CD22 is expressed on the cell surface of mature B-cells in follicular NHL. An overall response rate of 54% was achieved when epratuzumab was combined with rituximab in patients with relapsed indolent NHL.

2. **Conjugated antibodies**
   a. **Cellular toxin conjugated antibodies**
      - Gemtuzumab ozogamicin (Mylotarg) is a humanized IgG4 kappa antibody directed against the CD33 antigen and conjugated with calicheamicin. Calicheamicin is a cytotoxic agent isolated from fermentation of the bacterium *Micromonospora echinospora* ssp. *calichensis*. The CD33 antigen is a sialic acid–dependent adhesion protein expressed on the surface of immature cells of the myelomonocytic lineage and on the surface of leukemic blast cells but not on the surface of normal pluripotent hematopoietic stem cells. When this fusion antibody binds to the CD33 receptors, it is internalized into the cell, and the calicheamicin is cleaved and released. Calicheamicin binds to the minor grooves of the DNA, leading to DNA breaks and apoptosis. Gemtuzumab ozogamicin is indicated for the treatment of older patients (over 60 years old) after the first relapse of myeloid leukemia expressing CD33 who are not candidates for chemotherapy. Clinical trials have shown when gemtuzumab was given as single agent, gemtuzumab may lead to 16% CR and 30% overall response with a median time to remission of 60 days. Gemtuzumab can cause fever, shivering, and nausea. Serious side effects are severe myelosuppression, hemorrhage, disseminated intravascular coagulation, and hepatotoxicity.

   b. **Radioimmunoconjugate antibodies**
      - Ibritumomab tiuxetan (Zevalin, IDEC-Y2B8) is a murine anti-CD20 MoAb conjugated to tiuxetan that chelates to pure beta-emitting yttrium-90. The mechanism of action includes antibody-mediated cytotoxicity and cellularly targeted radiotherapy (radioimmunotherapy [RIT]). It is indicated for

use in patients with rituximab CD20-positive refractory, follicular B-cell NHL. Ibritumomab tiuxetan is also being used in patients with relapsed B-cell NHL following high-dose chemotherapy and autologous stem cell transplantation with promising results. It should be used with caution in patients with 25% or greater marrow involvement with lymphoma, prior external beam radiotherapy to 25% or greater of the bone marrow, or a history of HAMAs or HACAs. Because the drug does not emit gamma radiation, hospitalization is not required. Neutropenia and thrombocytopenia are common and are related to the radionuclide dose. At the higher end of the dosing, 25% of patients will develop nadir neutrophil counts of less than $500/\mu L$. Low-grade nausea and vomiting are common. Infusion-related fever, chills, dizziness, asthenia, headache, back pain, arthralgia, and hypotension are occasional side effects.

- Iodine-131 (^{131}I)-tositumomab (Bexxar) is a murine IgG2a anti-CD20 MoAb radiolabeled with ^{131}I, an emitter of both beta and gamma radiation. The mechanism of action includes antibody-mediated cytotoxicity and cellularly targeted RIT. It is indicated as a monotherapy in patients with rituximab refractory NHL that is chemotherapy refractory, CD20-positive, low grade, or transformed low grade. Furthermore, it was found that the combination of high-dose ^{131}I-tositumomab and autologous hematopoietic stem cell transplantation is effective for relapsed B-NHL. Before dosimetric and therapeutic doses, patients are premedicated with acetaminophen 650 mg and diphenhydramine 50 mg. A saturated solution of potassium iodide, two to three drops orally three times daily, is given beginning 24 hours before the dosimetric dose and continuing for 14 days after the therapeutic dose to prevent uptake of ^{131}I by the thyroid. ^{131}I-tositumomab can cause hypertension, shivering, and diarrhea. It must be used with caution in patients with 25% marrow involvement with lymphoma, prior external beam radiotherapy to 25% of the bone marrow, or a history of HAMAs or HACAs.

B. Immunotoxins

These are recombinant proteins that are conjugated to cellular toxins and are designed to bind to specific proteins on the surface of cancer cells, internalized, and induce direct cytotoxic effect by releasing conjugated toxins intracellularly.

- Denileukin diftitox (Ontak) is a recombinant construct that includes a fragment of the IL-2 protein (Ala_1- Thr_{133}) linked to a fragment of the diphtheria toxin fragment A and B (Met_1-Thr_{387}). This construct is designed to bind to the CD25 component of the

IL-2 receptor (IL-2R) on the surface of the targeted cells expressing the receptor. The complex becomes internalized into the cytoplasm and releases the toxin to exhibit its damaging effect. The high-affinity IL-2R is normally present on the activated T- and B-lymphocytes and activated macrophages. Cutaneous T-cell lymphoma (CTCL) expresses high-affinity IL-2R and forms an appropriate target. A recent phase III randomized trial in patients with CTCL compared denileukin diftitox to placebo and showed a median PFS over 2 years, and 10% CR and 34% PR in patients who received denileukin diftitox, which is significantly better than placebo (median PFS of 124 days and overall response of 15.9%). Therefore, the indications for this agent include patients with persistent or recurrent CTCL expressing CD25. Denileukin diftitox can cause elevated liver transaminases, fever, nausea, edema, rash, and diarrhea. It can also cause serious capillary leak syndrome.

C. Cancer vaccines

This modality is a type of immunotherapy that is designed to stimulate the patient's own immune system against specific antigens expressed on the cancer cells with the intention to specifically target and destroy cancer cells with minimal side effects. Cancer vaccines are either prophylactic or therapeutic. Prophylactic vaccines are designed to prevent the causative agent of cancer. Accordingly, they generate an immune response against the infectious agent causing cancer. Four vaccines are currently available in the market: two vaccines against the human papillomavirus (Gardasil and Cervarix) and two vaccines against hepatitis B virus (Recombivax HB and Engerix-B).

The second type of cancer vaccines are therapeutic vaccines that can be used for the treatment of advanced disease or the prevention of progression of premalignant lesion or recurrence. This chapter will only be addressing therapeutic vaccines that will be used by oncologists. Therapeutic vaccines are administered to either target specific antigens that have already been identified within the tumor or to target multiple unidentified antigens. The first is usually administered in the form of peptide, protein, DNA, or RNA expressing the specific antigen, and the second is administered in the form of unfractionated whole cell lysate or intact tumor cells with the goal of eliciting T-cell responses against multiple undefined antigens expressed by the tumor. These antigens are either administered directly or pulsed on dendritic cells (antigen presenting cells). The FDA approved the first therapeutic cancer vaccine in April 2010; others are expected to be approved soon.

- Sipuleucel-T (Provenge) is an autologous, dendritic cell-based vaccine (CD54$^+$) that is pulsed with a selective prostate antigen: prostatic acid phosphatase. This antigen is expressed on 95% of prostate cancers. A phase III study in patients with metastatic, castration-resistant (hormone-refractory) prostate cancer demonstrated that sipuleucel-T increased 3-year survival by 40% compared to placebo (32.1% versus 23.0%). Based on these studies, the FDA has approved sipuleucel-T in patients with asymptomatic or minimally symptomatic metastatic hormone-refractory prostate cancer. Side effects include chills, fatigue, fever, and joint aches.

- M-Vax (DNP-VACC) consists of autologous tumor cells conjugated to a highly immunogenic hapten: dinitrophenyl. Melanoma patients who were immunized with M-Vax had a 60% survival rate over 5 years compared with a survival rate of 20% in a historical control group and a survival rate of 32% in patients treated with high-dose IFNα.

- Onco Vax is an autologous tumor cell vaccine. When given as an adjuvant to surgery, it significantly improved recurrence-free interval and recurrence-free survival compared to surgery alone in patients with melanoma.

- TroVax is a modified vaccinia Ankara that delivers the tumor antigen 5T4, which is a nonsecreted membrane glycoprotein expressed on clear and papillary RCCs. In a phase II trial, treatment of 25 patients with renal cancer (21 clear cell and 4 papillary) with the combination of high-dose IL2 and TroVax resulted in 52% of patients with stable disease with PFS of 5 months. Survival rate was 80% at 24 months, compared to the historical figure of 50% for IL2 treatment.

Selected Readings

Brachmann S, Fritsch C, Maira SM, García-Echecerría C. PI3K and mTOR inhibitors: a new generation of targeted anticancer agents. *Curr Opin Cell Biol.* 2009;21:194–198.

Coppin C, Le L, Porzsolt F, Wilt T. Targeted therapy for advanced renal cell carcinoma. *Cochrane Database Syst Rev.* 2008;2:CD006017.

Dowling RJ, Pollak M, Sonenberg N. Current status and challenges associated with targeting mTOR for cancer therapy. *BioDrugs.* 2009;23:77–91.

Durrant LG, Pudney V, Spendlove I, Metheringham RL. Vaccines as early therapeutic interventions for cancer therapy: neutralising the immunosuppressive tumour environment and increasing T cell avidity may lead to improved responses. *Expert Opin Biol Ther.* 2010;10:735–748.

Gajewski TF, Meng Y, Harlin H. Immune suppression in the tumor microenvironment. *J Immunother.* 2006;29:233–240.

Hung CF, Ma B, Monie A, Tsen SW, Wu TC. Therapeutic human papillomavirus vaccines: current clinical trials and future directions. *Expert Opin Biol Ther.* 2008;8:421–439.

Ibrahim EM, Zekri JM, Bin Sadiq BM. Cetuximab-based therapy for metastatic colorectal cancer: a meta-analysis of the effect of K-ras mutations. *Int J Colorectal Dis.* 2010;25:713–721.

Jones KL, Buzdar AU. Evolving novel anti-HER2 strategies. *Lancet Oncol.* 2009;10:1179–1187.

Liu P, Cheng H, Roberts TM, Zhao JJ. Targeting the phosphoinositide 3-kinase pathway in cancer. *Nat Rev Drug Discov.* 2009;8:627–644.

Sarnaik AA, Weber JS. Recent advances using anti-CTLA-4 for the treatment of melanoma. *Cancer J.* 2009;15:169–173.

Scagliotti G, Govindan R. Targeting angiogenesis with multitargeted tyrosine kinase inhibitors in the treatment of non-small cell lung cancer. *Oncologist.* 2010;15(5): 436–446.

Shepherd C, Puzanov I, Sosman JA. B-RAF inhibitors: an evolving role in the therapy of malignant melanoma. *Curr Oncol Rep.* 2010;12:146–152.

Tol J, Punt CJ. Monoclonal antibodies in the treatment of metastatic colorectal cancer: a review. *Clin Ther.* 2010;32:437–453.

Waldmann TA Effective cancer therapy through immunomodulation. *Annu Rev Med.* 2006;57:65–81.

Winder T, Lenz HJ. Vascular endothelial growth factor and epidermal growth factor signaling pathways as therapeutic targets for colorectal cancer. *Gastroenterology.* 2010;138:2163–2176.

Systematic Assessment of the Patient With Cancer and Consequences of Treatment

Roland T. Skeel

I. ESTABLISHING THE DIAGNOSIS

A. Pathologic diagnosis is critical

Although it might seem obvious that the diagnosis of cancer must be firmly established before chemotherapy or any other treatment is administered, the critical nature of an accurate diagnosis warrants a reminder. As a rule, there must be cytologic or histologic evidence of neoplastic cells together with a clinical picture consistent with the diagnosis of the cancer under consideration. It is rarely acceptable to initiate treatment based solely on clinical exam, radiologic evidence, and nontissue laboratory evidence, such as tumor markers. Commonly, patients present to their physician with a complaint such as a cough, bleeding, pain, or a lump; through a logical sequence of evaluation, the presence of cancer is revealed on a cytologic or histologic specimen. Less frequently, lesions are discovered fortuitously during routine examination, evaluation of an unrelated disorder, or systematic screening for cancer. With some types of cancer, pathologists can establish the diagnosis based on small amounts of material obtained from needle biopsies, aspirations, or tissue scrapings. Other cancers

require larger pieces of tissue for special staining, immunohisto-
logic evaluation, flow cytometry, examination by electron microscopy, or more sophisticated studies such as evaluation for genetic
deletions, amplifications, or other mutations.

It is often helpful to confer with the pathologist before obtaining a specimen to determine what kind and size of specimen
is adequate to establish the complete diagnosis. When a tissue
diagnosis of cancer is made by the pathologist, it is incumbent
on the clinician to review the material with the pathologist. This
practice is good medicine. It also allows the clinician to tell the
patient that he or she has actually seen the cancer and to avoid
administering chemotherapy without a firm pathologic diagnosis. In addition, the pathologist often gives a better consultation—
not just a tissue diagnosis—when the clinician shows a personal
interest.

B. Pathologic and clinical diagnosis must be consistent

Once the tissue diagnosis is established, the clinician must be
certain that the pathologic diagnosis is consistent with the clinical findings. If the two are not consistent, a search must be made
for additional information, clinical or pathologic, that allows the
clinician to make a unified diagnosis. A pathologic diagnosis, like
a clinical diagnosis, is also an opinion with varying levels of certainty. The first part of the pathologic diagnosis—and usually the
easier part—is an opinion about whether the tissue examined is
neoplastic. Because most pathologists rarely render a diagnosis
of cancer unless the degree of certainty is high, a positive diagnosis of cancer is generally reliable. The clinician must be more
cautious if the diagnosis rendered states that the tissue is "highly
suggestive of" or "consistent with the diagnosis of" cancer. Absence of definitively diagnosed cancer in a specimen does not
mean that cancer is not present, however; it means only that it
could not be diagnosed on the tissue obtained, and clinical circumstances must establish if additional tissue sampling is necessary. A second part of the pathologist's diagnosis is an opinion
about the type of cancer and the tissue of origin. This determination is not necessary in all circumstances but is usually helpful in
selecting the most appropriate therapy and making a determination of prognosis.

C. Treatment without a pathologic diagnosis

There are rare circumstances in which treatment is undertaken
before a pathologic diagnosis is established. Such circumstances
are clearly exceptions, however, and involve less than 1% of all patients with cancer. Therapy is begun without a pathologic diagnosis only when the following conditions are met:

1. The clinical features strongly suggest the diagnosis of cancer,
and the likelihood of a benign diagnosis is remote.

2. Withholding prompt treatment or carrying out the procedures required to establish the diagnosis would greatly increase a patient's morbidity or risk of mortality.

Two examples of such circumstances are (1) a primary tumor of the midbrain and (2) superior vena cava syndrome from a large mediastinal mass with no accessible supraclavicular nodes and no endobronchial disease found on bronchoscopy in the occasional patient in whom the risk of bleeding from mediastinoscopic biopsy is deemed greater than the risk of administering radiotherapy for a disease of uncertain nature.

II. STAGING

Once the diagnosis of cancer is firmly established, it is important to determine the anatomic extent or stage of the disease. The steps taken for staging vary considerably among cancers because of the differing natural histories of the tumors.

A. Staging system criteria

For most cancers, a system of staging has been established based on the following factors:

1. Natural history and mode of spread of the cancer
2. Prognostic import of the staging parameters used
3. Value of the criteria used for decisions about therapy.

B. Staging and therapy decisions

In the past, surgery and radiotherapy were used to treat patients with cancer in early stages, and chemotherapy was used when surgery and radiotherapy were no longer effective or when the disease was in an advanced stage at presentation. In such circumstances, chemotherapy was only palliative (except for gestational choriocarcinoma), and in the absence of exquisitely sensitive tumors or strikingly potent drugs, the likelihood of increasing the survival was low. As knowledge has increased about the genetic determinants of cancer growth, tumor cell kinetics, and the development of resistance, the value of early intervention with chemotherapy has been transposed from animal models to human cancers. To plan this intervention and evaluate its effectiveness, careful staging has become increasingly important. Only when the exact extent of disease has been established can the most rational plan of treatment for the individual patient be devised, whether it is surgery, radiotherapy, chemotherapy, or molecular targeted therapy alone or in combination.

Although no single staging system is universally used for all cancers, the system developed jointly by the American Joint Committee on Cancer and the TNM Committee of the International Union Against Cancer is most widely used for staging solid tumors. It is based on the status of the primary tumor (T), regional lymph nodes (N), and distant metastasis (M). For some cancers, tumor grade (G) is also taken into account. The stage of the tumor is based on a condensation of the total possible TNM and G categories to create stage groupings, usually stages 0, I, II, III, and IV, which are relatively homogeneous with respect to prognosis. When relevant to the specific cancers whose chemotherapy is discussed in Section II of this handbook, the staging system or systems most commonly used for that cancer are discussed.

III. PERFORMANCE STATUS

The performance status refers to the level of activity of which a patient is capable. It is a measure independent from the anatomic extent or histologic characteristics of the cancer and of how much the cancer or comorbid conditions have affected the patient, and a prognostic indicator of how well the patient is likely to respond to treatment.

A. Types of performance status scales

Two performance status scales are in wide use:

■ The Karnofsky Performance Status Scale (Table 3.1) has 10 levels of activity. It has the advantage of allowing discrimination over a wide scale but the disadvantages of being difficult to remember and perhaps of making discriminations that are not clinically useful.

TABLE 3.1	Karnofsky Performance Status Scale
Functional Capability	**Level of Activity**
Able to carry on normal activity; no special care needed	100%—Normal; no complaints, no evidence of disease
	90%—Able to carry on normal activity; minor signs or symptoms of disease
	80%—Normal activity with effort; some signs or symptoms of disease
Unable to work; able to live at home; cares for most personal needs; needs varying amount of assistance	70%—Cares for self; unable to carry on normal activity or to do active work
	60%—Requires occasional assistance but is able to care for most of own needs
	50%—Requires considerable assistance and frequent medical care
Unable to care for self; requires equivalent of institutional or hospital care	40%—Disabled; requires special medical care and assistance
	30%—Severely disabled; hospitalization indicated, although death not imminent
	20%—Very sick; hospitalization necessary; active supportive treatment necessary
	10%—Moribund; fatal processes progressing rapidly
	0%—Dead

TABLE 3.2	ECOG/WHO/Zubrod Performance Status Scale

Grade	Level of Activity
0	Fully active; able to carry on all predisease performance without restriction (Karnofsky 90%–100%)
1	Restricted in physically strenuous activity but ambulatory and able to carry out work of a light or sedentary nature such as light housework or officework (Karnofsky 70%–80%)
2	Ambulatory and capable of all self-care but unable to carry out any work activities; up and about >50% of waking hours (Karnofsky 50%–60%)
3	Capable of only limited self-care; confined to bed or chair >50% of waking hours (Karnofsky 30%–40%)
4	Completely disabled; cannot carry on any self-care; totally confined to bed or chair (Karnofsky 10%–20%)

■ The Eastern Cooperative Oncology Group (ECOG)/World Health Organization (WHO)/Zubrod Performance Status Scale (Table 3.2) has the advantages of being easy to remember and making discriminations that are clinically useful.

According to the criteria of each scale, patients who are fully active or have mild symptoms respond more frequently to treatment and survive longer than patients who are less active or have severe symptoms. A clear designation of the performance status distribution of patients in therapeutic clinical trials is thus critical in determining the comparability and generalizability of trials and the effectiveness of the treatments used.

B. Use of performance status for choosing treatment

In the individualization of therapy, the performance status is often a useful parameter to help the clinician decide whether the patient will benefit from treatment or will be made worse. For example, unless there is some reason to expect a dramatic response of a cancer to chemotherapy, treatment may be withheld from patients with an ECOG Performance Status Scale score of 3 or 4 because responses to therapy are infrequent and toxic effects of the treatment are likely to be great.

C. Quality of life

A related but partially independent measure of performance status can be determined based on patients' own perceptions of their quality of life (QOL). QOL evaluations have been shown to be independent predictors of tumor response and survival in some cancers, and they are important components in a comprehensive assessment of response to therapy. For some cancers, improvement in QOL measures early in the course of treatment is the most reliable predictor of survival time.

IV. RESPONSE TO THERAPY

Response to therapy may be measured by survival (with or without disease), objective change in tumor size or in tumor product (e.g., immunoglobulin in myeloma), and subjective change.

A. Survival

One goal of cancer therapy is to allow patients to live as long and with the same QOL as they would have if they did not have the cancer. If this goal is achieved, it can be said that the patient is cured of the cancer (though biologically, the cancer may still be present). From a practical standpoint, we do not wait to see if patients live a normal lifespan before saying that a given treatment is capable of achieving a cure, but we follow a cohort of patients to see if their survival within a given timespan is different from that in a comparable cohort without the cancer. For the evaluation of response to *adjuvant therapy* (additional treatment after surgery or radiotherapy that is given to treat potential nonmeasurable, micrometastatic disease), survival analysis (rather than tumor response) must be used as the definitive objective measure of antineoplastic effect. With *neoadjuvant therapy* (chemotherapy or biologic therapy given as initial treatment before surgery or radiotherapy), tumor response, and resectability are also partial determinants of effectiveness.

B. Definitions

The *overall survival rate* is used to describe the percentage of people in a cohort who are alive for a specified period of time after diagnosis or initiation of a given treatment. The *median survival time* is the time after either diagnosis or treatment at which half of the patients with a given disease are still alive. *Disease-free survival*, the length of time after treatment for a specific disease during which a patient survives with no sign of the disease, is often a useful comparator in clinical studies of adjuvant therapy, as return of disease most often represents loss of curability. *Progression-free survival* (PFS) is the length of time during and after treatment in which a patient is living with a disease that does not get worse. It is used primarily in studies of metastatic or unresectable disease.

C. Other considerations

It is, of course, possible that a patient may be cured of the cancer that was treated but dies early owing to complications associated with the treatment, including second cancers. Even with complications (unless they are acute ones such as bleeding or infection), survival of patients who have been cured of the cancer is likely to be longer than if the treatment had not been given, though shorter than if the patient had never had the cancer.

If cure is not possible, the reduced goal is to allow the patient to live longer than if the therapy under consideration were not given. It is important for physicians to know if, and with what likelihood, any given treatment will result in a longer life. Such information helps physicians to choose whether to recommend treatment and the patient to decide whether to undertake the recommended treatment program.

It is important to learn from the patient what his or her goals of therapy are and to have a frank discussion about whether those goals are realistic. This can avoid unnecessary surprises and anger at some later time, which can occur when the patient has set a goal that is not realistic and the physician has not discussed what may or may not reasonably be expected as a consequence of therapy.

D. Objective response

Although survival is important to the individual patient, it is determined not only by the initial treatment undertaken but also by biologic determinants of the patient's individual cancer and subsequent treatment; thus, survival does not give an early measurement of a given treatment effectiveness. Tumor regression, on the other hand, when measurable, frequently occurs early in the course of effective treatment and is therefore a readily used determinant of treatment benefit. Tumor regression can be determined by a decrease in size of a tumor or the reduction of tumor products.

1. Tumor size. When tumor size is measured, responses are usually classified by the Response Evaluation Criteria in Solid Tumors (RECIST) methodology first published in 2000 and revised in 2008 (RECIST 1.1), reported by Eisenhauer et al. in the European Journal of Cancer in 2009, and available online at http://www.eortc.be/recist/documents/RECISTGuidelines.pdf.

    a. Baseline lesions are characterized as "measurable" or "nonmeasurable." To be measurable, non-lymph node lesions must be 20 mm or more in longest diameter and measurable by calipers using conventional techniques, or 10 mm or more in longest diameter using computed tomography (CT). On CT scan, lymph nodes must be ≥15 mm for target lesions or 10 to 15 mm in short axis for nontarget lesions. Smaller lesions and truly nonmeasurable lesions are designated nonmeasurable. To assess response, all measurable lesions up to a maximum of two per organ and five in total are designated as "target" lesions and measured at baseline. Except for lymph nodes, only the longest diameter of each lesion is measured. The sum of the longest diameters of all target lesions is designated the "baseline sum longest diameter."

        There are a variety of lesions in cancer that cannot be measured. These include blastic and sclerotic metastatic lesions to the bone, effusions, lymphangitic disease of the lung or skin, and lesions that have necrotic or cystic centers. Bone lesions are measurable only if they include an identifiable soft-tissue component, which constitutes the measureable lesion.

b. Response categories are based on measurement of target lesions.

    (1) Complete response (CR) is the disappearance of all target lesions. If lymph nodes are included in target lesions, each node must achieve a short axis <10 mm.

    (2) Partial response (PR) is a decrease of at least 30% in sum of the longest diameters of target lesions, using as reference the baseline sum of the longest diameters.

    (3) Stable disease (SD) is when there is neither sufficient shrinkage to qualify for partial response nor sufficient increase to qualify for progressive disease.

    (4) Progressive disease (PD) is an increase of 20% or more in the sum of the longest diameters of target lesions, taking as reference the smallest sum's longest diameter recorded since the treatment started or the appearance of one or more new lesions. The sum must also demonstrate an absolute increase of at least 5 mm. While the fluorodeoxyglucose (FDG)-positron emission tomography (PET) scan cannot be used to determine measureable disease, if there is negative FDG-PET at baseline with a positive FDG-PET at follow-up, this is sign of PD, based on a new lesion.

    (5) Inevaluable for response is a category used where there is early death by reason of malignancy or toxicity, tumor assessments were not repeated, etc.

c. Time to progression based on response criteria is an additional indicator that is often used, similar to PFS. It takes into account the fact that from the patient's perspective, CR, PR, and SD may be meaningless distinctions so long as the tumor is not causing symptoms or impairment of function. It also takes into account that some agents result in disease stability for a substantial period, despite failure to produce measurable disease shrinkage. This is particularly true for biologic targeted agents where it has been shown that time to progression for some cancers is substantially prolonged, despite no measurable reduction in tumor size.

    Time to progression can also be used as an indicator of disease status when there was no measurable disease at the outset of therapy or when the therapeutic modalities were not comparable. For example, if one wanted to compare the results of surgery alone with those of chemotherapy alone, time to progression from the onset of treatment would allow a valid comparison of the effectiveness of the treatments, whereas the traditional tumor response criteria would not. Time to progression thus places each of the agents or modalities on an even basis.

d. **Survival curves.** If survival curves of patient populations having different categories of response are compared, those patients with a CR frequently survive longer than those with a lesser response. If a sizable number of CRs occur with a treatment regimen, the survival rate of patients treated with that regimen is likely to be significantly greater than that of patients who are untreated. When the number of complete responders in a population rises to about 50%, the possibility of cure for a small number of patients begins to appear. With increasing percentages of complete responders, the frequency of cures is likely to increase correspondingly.

Although patients who have partial response to a treatment usually survive longer than those who have SD or progression, it is often not easy to demonstrate that the overall survival of the treated population is better than that of a comparable untreated group. In part, this difficulty may be due to a phenomenon of small numbers. If only 15% to 20% of a population respond to therapy, the median survival rate may not change at all, and the numbers may not be high enough to demonstrate a significant difference in survival duration of the longest surviving 5% to 10% of patients (the "tail" of the curves) of the treated and untreated populations. It is also possible that the patients who achieve a PR to therapy are those who have less aggressive disease at the outset of treatment and thus will survive longer than the nonresponders, regardless of therapy. These caveats notwithstanding, most clinicians and patients welcome even a PR as a sign that offers hope for longer survival and improved QOL.

2. **Tumor products.** For many cancers, objective tumor size changes are difficult or impossible to document. For some of these neoplasms, tumor products (hormones, antigens, antibodies) may be measurable and may provide a good, objective way to evaluate tumor response. Two examples of such markers that closely reflect tumor cell mass are the abnormal immunoglobulins (M proteins) produced in multiple myeloma and the human chorionic gonadotropin produced in choriocarcinoma and testicular cancer. Other markers such as prostate-specific antigen or carcinoembryonic antigen are not quite as reliable but are nonetheless helpful measures of response of the tumor to therapy. In some cancers, reduction in the number of circulating tumor cells is also an indicator of response to therapy.

3. **Evaluable disease.** Other objective changes may occur but are not easily quantifiable. When these changes are not easily measurable, they may be termed *evaluable*. For example, neurologic changes secondary to primary brain tumors cannot be measured with a caliper, but they can be evaluated using neurologic

testing. An arbitrary system of grading the degree of severity of neurologic deficit can be devised to permit surrogate evaluation of tumor response. Evaluable disease is not a category of the RECIST criteria.

4. **Performance status changes** may also be used as a measure of objective change; although in some respects, the performance status is as representative of subjective aspects as it is of the objective status of the disease.

E. Subjective change and QOL considerations

A subjective change is one that is perceived by the patient but not necessarily by the physician or others around the patient. Subjective improvement and an acceptable QOL are often of far greater importance to the patient than objective improvement: If the cancer shrinks, but the patient feels worse than before treatment, he or she is not likely to believe that the treatment was worthwhile. It is not valid to look at subjective change in isolation, however, because temporary worsening in the perceived state of well-being may be necessary to achieve subsequent long-term improvement.

This point is particularly well illustrated by the combined modality treatment in which chemotherapy is used to treat micrometastases after surgical removal of the macroscopic tumor. In such a circumstance, the patient is likely to feel entirely well after the primary surgical procedure, but the side effects of chemotherapy increase the symptoms and make the patient feel subjectively worse for the period of treatment. The patient should be encouraged to continue treatment, however, because if the chemotherapy treatment of the micrometastases is successful, he or she will be cured of the cancer and can be expected to have a normal or near-normal life expectancy rather than dying from recurrent disease. Most patients agree that the temporary subjective worsening is not only tolerable but well worth the price if cure of the cancer is a distinct possibility. This judgment depends on the severity and duration of symptoms, functional impairment, and perceptions of illness during the acute phase of the treatment; the expected benefit (increased likelihood of survival) anticipated as a result of the treatment; and the potential long-term adverse consequences of the treatment.

In contrast, when chemotherapy is given with a palliative intent, patients (and less often physicians) may be unwilling to tolerate significant side effects or subjective worsening from treatment. Fortunately, subjective improvement often accompanies objective improvement, so those patients in whom there is measurable improvement of the cancer also feel better. The degree of subjective worsening that each patient is willing to tolerate varies, and the patient and physician together must discuss and evaluate whether the chemotherapy treatment program is worth continuing. Such discussions should include a clear presentation of the scientific facts that include objective survival and tumor response data together with whatever QOL information has been documented for the treatment proposed. Moreover, the expressed goals and desires and the social, economic, psychological, and spiritual situations of the patient and his or her family must be sensitively considered.

A word of caution about discussions of response and survival is important. Patients can more easily understand the notion of response rates than survival probabilities. For example, a 50:50 chance of the cancer shrinking helps them to understand the goals and expectations of therapy and does not lead to undue anxiety over time. On the other hand, understanding and dealing with median or expected survival estimates is more problematic intellectually and even more difficult emotionally. It is therefore usually best to give the patient a range of expected survival rather than a discrete number. For example, the physician can say, "Some patients may have progression of their disease and possibly die within 6 months, but others may go on feeling fairly well and functioning well for 2 or more years." This helps the patient and family not to focus on a single number ("They said I only had 13 months to live") and to avoid some of the feeling of impending doom.

V. TOXICITY
A. Factors affecting toxicity

One of the characteristics that distinguishes cancer chemotherapeutic agents from most other drugs is the frequency and severity of anticipated side effects at usual therapeutic doses. Because of the severity of the side effects, it is critical to monitor the patient carefully for adverse reactions so that therapy can be modified before the toxicity becomes life-threatening. Most toxicity varies according to the following factors:

1. Specific agent
2. Dose
3. Schedule of administration, including infusion rate and frequency of dose
4. Route of administration
5. Predisposing factors in the patient, including genetic variants,* that may be known and predictive for toxicity or unknown and resulting in unexpected toxic effects.

---

* An example is homozygosity for the UGT1A1*28 allele, a variation of a uridine diphosphate glucuronosyltransferase gene and its corresponding enzyme (UGT1A1), which is responsible for glucuronidation of bilirubin and involved in deactivation of Sn-38, a toxic active metabolite of irinotecan.

B. Clinical testing of new drugs for toxicity

Before the introduction of any agent into wide clinical use, the agent must undergo testing in carefully controlled clinical trials. The first set of clinical trials are called phase I trials. They are carried out with the express purpose of determining toxicity in humans and establishing the maximum tolerated dose; although with antineoplastic agents, they are done only in patients who might benefit from the drug. Such trials are undertaken only after extensive tests in animals have been completed. Much human toxicity is predicted by animal studies, but because of significant species differences, initial doses used in human studies are several times lower than doses at which toxicity is first seen in animals. Phase I trials are carried out using several schedules, and the dose is escalated in successive groups of patients once the toxicity of the prior dose has been established.

At the completion of phase I trials, there is usually a great deal of information about the spectrum and anticipated severity of acute drug effects (toxicity). However, because patients in phase I trials often do not live long enough to undergo many months of treatment, chronic or cumulative effects may not be discovered. Discovery of these toxicities may occur only after widespread use of the drug in phase II trials (to establish the spectrum of effectiveness of the drug), in phase III trials (to compare the new drug or combination with standard therapy), or from postmarketing reports (when even larger numbers and less rigorously selected patients are treated).

C. Common acute toxicities

Some toxicities are relatively common among cancer chemotherapeutic agents. Common acute toxicities include the following:
1. Myelosuppression with leukopenia, thrombocytopenia, and anemia
2. Nausea, vomiting, and other gastrointestinal effects
3. Mucous membrane ulceration and cutaneous effects, including alopecia
4. Infusion reactions.

    Some of these toxicities occur because of the cytotoxic effects of chemotherapy on rapidly dividing normal cells of the bone marrow and epithelium (e.g., mucous membranes, skin, and hair follicles) incidental to the mechanism of action of the drugs; others such as nausea and vomiting or infusion reactions are not related to the antineoplastic mechanism of action.

D. Selective toxicities

Other toxicities are less common and are specific to individual drugs or classes of drugs. Examples of drugs and their related toxicities include the following:
1. Anthracyclines and anthracenediones: irreversible cardiomyopathy
2. Asparaginase: anaphylaxis (allergic reaction), pancreatitis

3. Bleomycin: pulmonary fibrosis
4. Cisplatin: renal toxicity, neurotoxicity
5. Epidermal growth factor receptor inhibitors: acneiform rash
6. Fludarabine, cladribine, pentostatin, and temozolomide: prolonged suppression of cellular immunity with heightened risk for opportunistic infection
7. Ifosfamide and cyclophosphamide: hemorrhagic cystitis
8. Ifosfamide: central nervous system toxicity
9. Mitomycin: hemolytic-uremic syndrome and other endothelial cell injury phenomena
10. Monoclonal antibodies (e.g., rituximab, trastuzumab): hypersensitivity reactions
11. Paclitaxel: neurotoxicity, acute hypersensitivity reactions
12. Procarbazine: food and drug interactions
13. Trastuzumab: reversible cardiomyopathy
14. Vascular endothelial growth factor inhibitors: gastrointestinal perforation, impaired wound healing
15. Vinca alkaloids: neurotoxicity.

E. Recognition and evaluation of toxicity

Anyone who administers chemotherapeutic agents must be familiar with the expected and the unusual toxicities of the agent the patient is receiving, be prepared to avert severe toxicity when possible, and be able to manage toxic complications when they cannot be avoided. The specific toxicities of commonly used individual chemotherapeutic agents are detailed in Chapter 33.

For the purpose of reporting toxicity in a uniform manner, criteria are often established to grade the severity of the toxicity. For many years, a simplified set of criteria was used by several National Cancer Institute (NCI)–supported clinical trial groups for the most common toxic manifestations. Although this document was helpful, it was, in many respects, incomplete. To address this issue, a new set of more comprehensive toxicity criteria, the Common Toxicity Criteria, was developed in 1999. A revised version of these criteria (Common Terminology Criteria for Adverse Events v3.0 [CTCAE]) was published in 2003 and updated again in 2009 (CTCAE v4.0) and is available online at http://ctep.cancer.gov/protocolDevelopment/electronic_applications/ctc.htm. A host of other helpful information can be obtained online at http://ctep.cancer.gov/. All new clinical trials approved by the NCI Cancer Therapy Evaluation Program use these new toxicity criteria. Such standardization is important in the evaluation of the toxicity of cancer treatment.

F. Acute toxicity management

Prevention and treatment of bone marrow suppression can be partially achieved using filgrastim, sargramostim, epoetin alfa, and oprelvekin. Treatment of its infectious, bleeding, and anemia consequences is discussed in Chapters 27 and 28. Management of nausea and vomiting, mucositis, and alopecia as well as diarrhea, nutrition problems, and drug extravasation are discussed in Chapter 26. Other acute toxicities are discussed with the individual drugs in Chapter 33. Long-term medical problems are a special issue and are highlighted in the subsequent section.

VI. LATE PHYSICAL EFFECTS OF CANCER TREATMENT
A. Late organ toxicities

Late organ toxicities may be minimized by limiting doses when thresholds are known. In most instances, however, individual patient effects cannot be predicted. Treatment is primarily symptomatic.

1. **Cardiac toxicity** (e.g., congestive cardiomyopathy) is most commonly associated with high total doses of the anthracyclines (doxorubicin, daunorubicin, epirubicin). In addition, high-dose cyclophosphamide as used in transplantation regimens may contribute to congestive cardiomyopathy. When mediastinal irradiation is combined with these chemotherapeutic agents, cardiac toxicity may occur at lower doses. Although evaluation of ventricular ejection fraction with echocardiography or nuclear radiography studies has been useful for acutely monitoring the effects of these agents on the cardiac ejection fraction, studies have reported late onset of congestive heart failure during pregnancy or after the initiation of vigorous exercise programs in adults who were previously treated for cancer as children or young adults. The cardiac reserve in these previously treated cancer patients may be marginal. It is probable that there are some changes that take place even at low doses, and it is only because of the great reserve in cardiac function that effects are not measurable until higher doses have been used. Mediastinal irradiation also accelerates atherogenesis and may lead to premature symptomatic coronary artery disease.

   Because of the large number of women with breast cancer who are treated with doxorubicin as part of an adjuvant chemotherapy regimen, this group is of special concern and warrants ongoing clinical follow-up, although adverse cardiac effects do not appear to increase with time, up to 13 years. Trastuzumab (and perhaps other targeted agents) is also associated with cardiac toxicity, but the mechanism of toxicity is different from that of the anthracyclines and is usually reversible.

2. **Pulmonary toxicity** has been classically associated with high doses of bleomycin (more than 400 U). However, a number of other agents have been associated with pulmonary fibrosis (e.g., alkylating agents, methotrexate, nitrosoureas). Premature respiratory insufficiency, especially with exertion, may become evident with aging.

3. **Nephrotoxicity** is a potential toxicity of several agents (e.g., cisplatin, methotrexate, nitrosoureas). These agents can be associated with both acute and chronic toxicities. Other nephrotoxic agents such as amphotericin or aminoglycosides may exacerbate the problem. Even usually benign agents such as the bisphosphonates or allopurinol may be a problem. Rarely, some patients may require hemodialysis as a result of chronic toxicity.

4. **Neurotoxicity** has been particularly associated with the vinca alkaloids, cisplatin, oxaliplatin, epipodophyllotoxins, taxanes, bortezomib, and ixabepilone. Peripheral neuropathy can cause considerable sensory and motor disability. Autonomic dysfunction may produce debilitating postural hypotension. Whole-brain irradiation, with or without chemotherapy, can be a cause of progressive dementia and dysfunction in some long-term survivors. This is particularly a problem for patients with primary brain tumors and for some patients with small-cell lung cancer who have received prophylactic therapy. Survivors of childhood leukemia have developed a variety of neuropsychological abnormalities related to central nervous system prophylaxis that included whole-brain irradiation.

   It has become evident over the years that some patients (up to one in five) who have received adjuvant chemotherapy for carcinoma of the breast also have measurable cognitive deficits such as difficulties with memory or concentration. This appears to be greater for women who have received high-dose chemotherapy than for those women who have received standard-dose chemotherapy; in both groups, the incidence is higher than in control groups. It is not uncommon for patients to refer to the effects of chemotherapy with complaints about memory being worse than it was, not being able to calculate numbers in their head, or just having "chemo-brain." Rarely patients may have severe, debilitating, idiosyncratic cognitive impairment or even fatal central nervous system damage subsequent to chemotherapy.

5. **Hematologic and immunologic impairment** is usually acute and temporally related to the cancer treatment (e.g., chemotherapy or radiation therapy). In some instances, however, there can be persistent cytopenias, as with alkylating agents. Immunologic impairment is a long-term problem for patients with Hodgkin lymphoma, which may be due to the underlying disease as well as to the treatments that are used. Fludarabine, cladribine, and pentostatin, with or without rituximab, cause profound suppression of cluster of differentiation 4 (CD4) and CD8 lymphocytes and render treated patients susceptible to opportunistic infections for many months after treatment has been discontinued.

Temozolomide causes CD4 lymphopenia and also carries a risk of opportunistic infection. Complete immunologic reconstitution may take 2 years after these therapies or marrow-ablative therapy requiring stem cell reconstitution. Patients who have undergone splenectomy are also at risk of overwhelming bacterial infections.

B. Second malignancies

   1. Acute myelogenous leukemia and myelodysplasia may occur secondary to combined modality treatment (e.g., radiation therapy and chemotherapy in Hodgkin lymphoma), prolonged therapy with alkylating agents or nitrosoureas, or other chemotherapy. In general, this form of treatment-related acute leukemia arises in the setting of myelodysplasia and is refractory even to intensive treatment. Treatment with the epipodophyllotoxins also has been associated with the development of acute nonlymphocytic leukemia. This may be the result of a specific gene rearrangement between chromosome 9 and chromosome 11 that creates a new cancer-causing oncogene: ALL-1/AF-9. The peak time of occurrence of secondary acute leukemia in patients with Hodgkin lymphoma is 5 to 7 years after treatment, with an actuarial risk of 6% to 12% by 15 years. Thus, a slowly developing anemia in a survivor of Hodgkin lymphoma should alert the clinician to the possibility of a secondary myelodysplasia or leukemia.

   Fortunately, the risk of secondary leukemias in women treated with standard adjuvant therapy for breast cancer (e.g., cyclophosphamide and doxorubicin) is only modestly higher (excess absolute risk of 2 to 5 per 100,000 person years) than that in the general population.

   2. Solid tumors and other malignancies are seen with increased frequency in survivors who have been treated with chemotherapy or radiation therapy. Non-Hodgkin lymphomas have been reported as a late complication in patients treated for Hodgkin lymphoma or multiple myeloma. Patients treated with long-term cyclophosphamide are at risk of bladder cancer. Patients who have received mantle irradiation for Hodgkin lymphoma have an increased risk of breast cancer, thyroid cancer, osteosarcoma, bronchogenic carcinoma, colon cancer, and mesothelioma. In these cases, the second neoplasm is usually in the irradiated field. In general, the risk of solid tumors begins to increase during the second decade of survival after Hodgkin lymphoma. As a result, young women who have received mantle irradiation for Hodgkin lymphoma should be screened more carefully for breast cancer, starting at an age earlier than what is advised in standard screening recommendations.

C. Other sequelae

1. **Endocrine problems** may result from cancer treatment. Patients receiving radiation therapy to the head and neck region may develop subclinical or clinical hypothyroidism. This is a particular risk in patients receiving mantle irradiation for Hodgkin lymphoma. Biennial assessment of thyroid-stimulating hormone should be undertaken in these patients. Thyroid replacement therapy should be given if the thyroid-stimulating hormone level rises in order to decrease the risk of thyroid cancer. Short stature may be a result of pituitary irradiation and growth hormone deficiency.

2. **Premature menopause** may occur in women who have received certain chemotherapeutic agents (e.g., alkylating agents, procarbazine) or abdominal and pelvic irradiation. The risk is age-related, with women older than 30 years at the time of treatment having the greatest risk of treatment-induced amenorrhea and menopause. Early hormone replacement therapy should be considered in such women, if not otherwise contraindicated, to reduce the risk of accelerated osteoporosis and premature heart disease from estrogen deficiency.

3. **Gonadal failure or dysfunction** can lead to infertility in both male and female cancer survivors during their peak reproductive years. Azoospermia is common, but the condition may improve over time after the completion of therapy. Retroperitoneal lymph node dissection in testicular cancer may produce infertility due to retrograde ejaculation. Psychological counseling should be provided to these patients to help them adjust to these long-term sequelae of therapy. Cryopreservation of sperm before treatment should be considered in men. For women, there are limited means available to preserve ova or protect against ovarian failure associated with treatment. Abdominal irradiation in young girls can lead to future pregnancy loss due to decreased uterine capacity.

4. **The musculoskeletal system** can be affected by radiation therapy, especially in children and young adults. Radiation may injure the growth plates of long bones and lead to muscle atrophy. Short stature may be a result of direct injury to bone. Aromatase inhibitors increase bone loss and can contribute to pathologic osteoporotic fractures.

5. **Psychological and social concerns** can be severe as patients who have had cancer often carry an ongoing sense of vulnerability and frequent worry of the cancer returning. Changes in body image and sexual function can lead to difficulty with marriage and other relationships. Survivors may also suffer from discrimination on the job and find it difficult or impossible to get insurance, despite having been cured from their cancer.

Acknowledgments

The author is indebted to Dr. Patricia A. Ganz, who contributed to previous editions of this chapter. Most of the section on the late consequences of cancer treatment in this revision of the handbook represents Dr. Ganz's work.

Selected Readings

Cancer Therapy Evaluation Program. Common terminology criteria for adverse events (CTCAE) v4.0, 2009. Retrieved from http://ctep.cancer.gov/protocolDevelopment/electronic_applications/ctc.htm

Centers for Disease Control and Prevention. *A national action plan for cancer survivorship: advancing public health strategie*s. Atlanta: Centers for Disease Control and Prevention; 2004.

Curtis RE, Boice J-D Jr, Stovall M, et al. Risk of leukemia after chemotherapy and radiation treatment for breast cancer. *N Engl J Med.* 1992;326:1745–1751.

Eisenhauer EA, Therasse P, Bogaerts J, et al. New response evaluation criteria in solid tumours: Revised RECIST guideline (version 1.1). *Eur J Cancer.* 2009;45:228–247. Retrieved from http://www.eortc.be/recist/documents/RECISTGuidelines.pdf

Ganz PA. A teachable moment for oncologists: cancer survivors, 10 million strong and growing! *J Clin Oncol.* 2005;23:5458–5460.

Ganz PA. *Late effects of cancer in adult survivors: what are they and what is the oncologist's role in follow-up and prevention?* Alexandria: American Society of Clinical Oncology; 2005: 724–730.

Ganz PA, Hussey MA, Moinpour CM, et al. Chemotherapy in breast cancer survivors treated on Southwest Oncology Group protocol S8897. *J Clin Oncol.* 2008;26:1223–1230.

Goldhirsch A, Gelber PD, Simes RJ, et al. Costs and benefits of adjuvant therapy in breast cancer: a quality-adjusted survival analysis. *J Clin Oncol.* 1989;7:36–44.

Greene FL, Page DL, Fleming ID, et al. (Eds.) *AJCC cancer staging manual.* 6th ed. New York: Springer, 2002.

Hewitt M, Greenfield S, Stovall S. (Eds.). *From cancer patient to cancer survivor: lost in transition.* Washington: The National Academies Press; 2005.

Howard RA, Gilbert ES, Chen BE, et al. Leukemia following breast cancer: an international population based study of 376,825 women. *Breast Cancer Res Treat.* 2007;105:359–368.

Hudson MM, Mertens AC, Yasui Y, et al. Health status of adults who are long-term childhood cancer survivors: a report from the Childhood Cancer Survivor Study. *JAMA.* 2003;290:1583–1592.

Loescher LJ, Welch-McCaffrey D, Leigh SA, et al. Surviving adult cancers. Part 1: physiologic effects. *Ann Intern Med.* 1989;111:411–432.

Neglia JP, Friedman DL, Yasui Y, et al. Second malignant neoplasms in five-year survivors of childhood cancer: Childhood Cancer Survivor Study. *J Natl Cancer Inst.* 2001;93:618–629.

Nieman CL, Kazer R, Brannigan RE, et al. Cancer survivors and infertility: a review of a new problem and novel answers. *J Support Oncol.* 2006;4:171–178.

Oeffinger KC, Mertens AC, Sklar CA, et al. Prevalence and severity of chronic diseases in adult survivors of childhood cancer: a report from the Childhood Cancer Survivor Study. *J Clin Oncol.* 2005;23:3s (abstr 9).

Oken MM, Creech RH, Tormey DC, et al. Toxicity and response criteria of the Eastern Cooperative Oncology Group. *Am J Clin Oncol.* 1982;5:649–655.

Pedersen-Bjergaard J, Sigsgaard TC, Nielsen D, et al. Acute monocytic or myelomonocytic leukemia with balanced chromosome translocations to band 11q23 after therapy with 4-epidoxorubicin and cisplatin or cyclophosphamide for breast cancer. *J Clin Oncol.* 1992;10:1444–1451.

Pui CH, Ribeiro RC, Hancock ML, et al. Acute myeloid leukemia in children treated with epipodophyllotoxins for acute lymphoblastic leukemia. *N Engl J Med.* 1991;325:1682–1687.

Schagen SB, van Dam FS, Muller MJ, et al. Cognitive deficits after postoperative adjuvant chemotherapy for breast carcinoma. *Cancer.* 1999;85:640–650.

Tallman MS, Gray R, Bennett JM, et al. Leukemogenic potential of adjuvant chemotherapy for early-stage breast cancer: the Eastern Cooperative Oncology Group experience. *J Clin Oncol.* 1995;13:1557–1563.

van Leeuwen FE, Klokman JW, Hagenbeek A, et al. Second cancer risk following Hodgkin's disease: a 20-year follow-up study. *J Clin Oncol.* 1994;12:312–325.

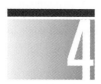

Selection of Treatment for the Patient With Cancer
Roland T. Skeel

I. SETTING TREATMENT GOALS
A. Patient perspective

Although patients most often come to the physician looking for medical perspective on what can be done about their cancer, it is critical that physicians and other health care professionals remember that unless we know what the patient's goals are, our ideas and our plans of therapy may not address the patient's needs. As a consequence, it is critical for the physician to ask the patient to share in setting treatment goals because it is the patient who must undergo the rigors of treatment and be willing to abide by its consequences. Whereas the physician's medical recommendations most commonly are accepted, some patients reject them as inappropriate for a variety of reasons. Some ask the physician for another recommendation, and others seek the opinion of a second physician. The physician must clearly present the reasons for the treatment recommendations and why those recommendations seem to be the best ways to achieve the treatment objective. The physician has the obligation to make a treatment recommendation, but the patient always has the right to reject that advice without fear that the physician will be upset, dislike the patient, or refuse to continue to give the patient care.

B. Medical perspective

Before a physician decides on a course of treatment to recommend for a patient with cancer, an achievable medical goal of treatment must be clearly defined. If the goal is to cure the patient of cancer, the strategy of therapy is likely to be different from the strategy chosen if the purpose is to prolong life or to relieve symptoms. To propose the goal of therapy, the physician must be:

- Familiar with the natural history and behavior of the cancer to be treated.
- Knowledgeable about the principles and practice of therapy for each of the treatment modalities that may be effective in that cancer.
- Well grounded in the ethical principles of the treatment of patients with cancer.
- Familiar with the theory and use of antineoplastic agents.
- Informed about the particular therapy for the cancer in question.
- Aware of the patient's individual circumstances, including stage of disease, performance status, social situation, psychological status, and concurrent illnesses.

Armed with this information and with the treatment goals in mind, the physician can develop a course of treatment and make a recommendation to the patient.

Components of the treatment plan include the following:

1. Should the cancer be treated at all? If so, is the treatment to be designed for cure, prolongation of life, or palliation of symptoms?
2. How aggressive should the therapy be to achieve the defined objective?
3. Which modalities of therapy will be used and in what sequence?
4. How will the treatment efficacy be determined?
5. What are the criteria for deciding the duration of therapy?

II. CHOICE OF CANCER TREATMENT MODALITY

A. Surgery

The oldest, most established, and still most effective way to cure most cancers is surgery. Surgery is selected as the treatment if the cancer is limited to one area and if it is anticipated that all cancer cells can be removed without unduly compromising vital structures. If it is believed that the patient can survive the operation and return to a worthwhile life, surgery is recommended. Surgery is not recommended if the risk of surgery is greater than the risk of the cancer; if metastasis always occurs despite complete removal of the primary tumor; or if the patient will be left so debilitated, disfigured, or otherwise impaired that although cured of cancer he or she feels that life is not worthwhile. If metastasis regularly (or always) occurs despite complete removal of the primary tumor, the benefits of removal of the gross tumor should be clearly defined before surgery is undertaken.

Most commonly, surgery is reserved for treatment of the primary neoplasm; at times it may be used effectively to remove isolated metastases (e.g., in lung, brain, or liver) with curative intent. Surgery is also used palliatively, such as for decompression of the brain in patients with glioma or biliary bypass in patients with carcinoma of the pancreas. In nearly all nonhematologic cancers, a surgeon should be consulted to determine the role of surgery in the optimal treatment of the patient.

B. Radiotherapy

Radiotherapy is used for the treatment of local or regional disease when surgery cannot completely remove the cancer or when it would unduly disrupt normal structures or functions. In the treatment of some cancers, radiotherapy is as effective as surgery for eradicating the tumor. In this circumstance, factors such as the anticipated side effects of the treatment, the expertise and experience of local oncologists, and the preference of the patient may influence the choice of treatment.

One determinant of the appropriateness of radiotherapy is the inherent sensitivity of the cancer to ionizing radiation. Some kinds of cancer (e.g., lymphomas and seminomas) are highly sensitive to radiotherapy. Other kinds (e.g., melanomas and sarcomas) tend to be less sensitive. Such considerations do not preclude the use of radiotherapy, however, and it is helpful to obtain the evaluation of the radiation oncologist before initiating treatment so that treatment planning can take into consideration the possible contribution of this modality.

Although radiotherapy is frequently used as the primary or curative mode of therapy, it is also well suited to palliative management of problems such as bone metastases, superior vena cava syndrome, and local nodal metastases. The use of radiotherapy in the management of spinal cord compression and superior vena cava syndrome is discussed in Chapter 29.

C. Chemotherapy

As its primary role, chemotherapy treats disease that is no longer confined to one site or region and has spread systemically. In the earliest days of chemotherapy, this interpretation directed its use to diseases that regularly presented in a disseminated form (e.g., leukemia) or after disease recurred following primary management with surgery or radiotherapy. It is now understood that widespread systemic micrometastases commonly occur early in cancer. These metastases are associated with certain predictive factors such as the axillary node metastases of carcinoma of the breast and the large tumor size and poorly differentiated histologic features of sarcomas or the genetic profile of the cancer. Therefore, chemotherapy is now applied earlier to treat systemic disease. When this treatment is used for micrometastases, the response of an individual patient cannot be measured unless the chemotherapy is used as a neoadjuvant, that is, before surgery or radiotherapy. In that case, tumor response may predict more important endpoints such as time to treatment failure and survival. More commonly, when the chemotherapy is used as an adjuvant after removal of visible disease, the effectiveness of therapy must be determined by comparing the survival (or disease-free survival) of patients who receive therapy with that of similar (control) patients who do not receive therapy for the micrometastases. Chemotherapy also has a role in the treatment of localized or regional disease. These specialized uses are discussed in Chapter 30.

D. Biologic response modifiers and molecular targeted therapy

It has long intrigued cancer biologists that cancer does not occur randomly but preferentially selects specific populations: the young, the elderly, the immunosuppressed (certain types of cancer only), and those with a strong family history of cancer. These observations have led cancer biologists to postulate that some kind of biologic control over or proclivity toward the emergence of cancer exists, which some people have and others do not, at least at the time the cancer becomes established. One prime candidate for the mechanism of biologic control of cancer has been immunity. That immunity plays some role in controlling the development of cancer has been clearly demonstrated in animal models and a few, though not most, human neoplasms. Other biologic factors, including those controlled by oncogenes and tumor suppressor genes and their protein products that affect the cancer cell directly or its environment, are becoming better defined and are even more important than classic immunity in the development of cancer.

In an attempt to exploit and enhance the biologic control that is presumed to exist to some degree in everyone, or to counteract cancer-promoting factors that facilitate cancer growth, invasion, and metastases, a variety of agents called *biologic response modifiers* and *molecular targeted therapy* have been used in the treatment of cancer. Two classes of biologic response modifiers, the interferons and lymphokines (of which interleukin-2 is an example), have been studied for many years, and there is evidence of their modest activity in some types of cancer. Related, but separate, are the molecular targeted agents discussed in Chapter 2 that inhibit the activity of abnormally expressed protein products such as the constitutively activated Bcr-Abl tyrosine kinase in chronic myelogenous leukemia or other unique components of the cancer cell. This area of intensive research (as well as Wall Street interest) has begun to reach fruition and is expected to provide an increasingly important, though expensive, contribution to effective cancer therapy.

E. Combined-modality therapy

Alone, surgery, radiotherapy, biotherapy, and chemotherapy are not appropriate for the treatment of all cancers. Frequently, patients present with cancer in which there is a bulky primary lesion, macroscopically evident regional disease, and presumed microscopic or submicroscopic systemic disease. For this reason, oncologists have turned to a multidisciplinary approach to the treatment of cancer, selecting two or more modalities of therapy for sequential or simultaneous use. This approach requires close cooperation among the surgical oncologist, radiation oncologist, and medical oncologist to provide the patient with the best overall treatment plan. Although combined-modality therapy is neither effective nor desirable for all kinds or stages of cancers, the regular practice of a multidisciplinary approach provides the best opportunity to exploit the advantages of each mode of treatment. "Tumor Boards" often serve as the format for ensuring that patients will regularly have the benefit of various treatment perspectives.

III. PALLIATIVE CARE

The medical oncologist, who is also an internist, is often seen as the coordinator of cancer treatment. In this role, although the focus is on the cancer, the broader perspective of the oncologist as a coordinator of the patient's care—in partnership with the patient—should not become obscured. Decisions about what therapy to use and how aggressively to treat the cancer are critically important to medically sound patient care. Decisions about when to stop active cancer treatment are also vitally important and may be among the most difficult responsibilities for the oncologist. It is critical that oncologists, who provide and profit from therapy, recognize the inherent conflict of interest in their dual role as caregivers and drug salespersons.

Quality of life is often enhanced in patients responding to chemotherapy and other cancer treatments; it just as surely deteriorates more rapidly when the tumor does not respond to therapy and the patient experiences the toxicity of treatment along with the pain, fatigue, cachexia, and other symptoms of the cancer. For the 50% of patients with cancer who are not cured, the decision to stop antineoplastic therapy is just as important as the selection of chemotherapy regimens earlier in the disease. There comes a time when the best advice a physician can give is for the patient to forgo additional chemotherapy or any other active cancer treatment.

The introduction and rapid acceptance of hospice programs throughout the United States during the last 35 years reflect the need for this kind of care. Hospice programs have effectively addressed the special physical, psychological, social, and spiritual needs of patients approaching the end of life and have provided the unique skills required to maintain the best possible quality of life as long as possible.

More recently, acute care hospitals have recognized that they, too, have patients who are at the end of life and need a special focus on the palliative aspects of their care. Yet too often, physicians are reluctant to "give up" and are unable to recognize or to accept when the patient will be helped more by an acknowledgment that active cancer therapy will not improve survival or enhance quality of life.

Oncologists and others caring for patients with cancer who have been trained as acute care physicians can learn specific techniques to enhance the quality of life from those who are expert in palliative care. For example, one might compare the quality of death in hospitalized patients given "maintenance" intravenous hydration with that of hospice home care patients offered oral fluids and mouth care to assuage thirst. The former method may result in an overhydrated, edematous patient who dies with an uncomfortable-sounding "death rattle" that is disconcerting to family and staff; the latter usually results in a visibly more comfortable patient who is more likely to die with less edema and without as much apparent respiratory distress.

Legitimate questions also can be raised about medical costs toward the end of life that are incurred when physicians give "futile" and "marginal" care. Development of guidelines by physicians and hospitals that define futile care, along with thoughtful consideration of when the therapy offered patients has marginal value, may enable physicians to improve the quality of life for patients and at the same time hold down one component of the rising spiral of health care costs.

Selected Readings

Brody H, Campbell ML, Faber-Langendoen K, et al. Withdrawing intensive life-sustaining treatment—recommendations for compassionate clinical management. *N Engl J Med.* 1997;336:6.

Byock I. Palliative care and oncology: growing better together. *J Clin Oncol.* 2009;27:170–171.

Drummond MF, Mason AR. European perspective on the costs and cost-effectiveness of cancer therapies. *J Clin Oncol.* 2007;25:191–195.

Emanuel EJ, Patterson WB. Ethics of randomized clinical trials. *J Clin Oncol.* 1998;16:365–366.

Ferris FD, Bruera E, Cherny N, et al. Palliative cancer care a decade later: accomplishments, the need, next steps—from the American Society of Clinical Oncology. *J Clin Oncol.* 2009;27:3052–3058.

Hillner BE, Smith TJ. Efficacy does not necessarily translate to cost effectiveness: a case study in the challenges associated with 21st-century cancer drug pricing. *J Clin Oncol.* 2009;27:2111–2113.

Jacobson M, O'Malley AJ, Earle CC, et al. Does reimbursement influence chemotherapy treatment for cancer patients? *Health Affairs.* 2006;25:437–443.

Lundberg GO. American health care system management objectives: the aura of inevitability becomes incarnate. *JAMA.* 1993;269:2254–2255.

Skeel RT. Measurement of quality of life outcomes. In Berger AM, Portnoy JL, Weissman DE (Eds.). *Principles and practice of palliative care and supportive oncology* (2nd ed.). Philadelphia: Lippincott Williams & Wilkins; 2002:1107–1122.

Carcinomas of the Head and Neck

Barbara A. Murphy

Head and neck cancers (HNCs) are defined as those arising from the upper aerodigestive system. Although a variety of histopathologic subtypes have been associated with the anatomic region, the vast majority are squamous cell carcinoma (SCA); thus, the following chapter will focus specifically on this subtype.

I. ANATOMY

Understanding HNC begins with an understanding of aerodigestive anatomy. There are five sites within the head and neck region. These include the larynx, pharynx, oral cavity, paranasal sinuses, and the major salivary glands. Each site is composed of specific subsites (Table 5.1). A cross-sectional view of the anatomic regions and the relative frequency of cancer occurring in each area are shown in Figure 5.1. Identification of the primary site and extent of disease are critical for treatment planning, as will be discussed at length subsequently. Although thyroid cancers are frequently treated by otolaryngologists, they have unique pathologic and treatment issues and are covered in Chapter 13. Skin cancers, which are also common in the head and neck region, are discussed in Chapter 14.

II. EPIDEMIOLOGY

Approximately 40,000 cases of SCAs of the head and neck are diagnosed annually within the United States. Although SCAs of the head and neck are often considered together because of their anatomic proximity, it is important to recognize that HNC is comprised of a variety of distinct disease entities that may be distinguished based on etiology, histology, epidemiology, and natural history. These include the following: (1) SCA associated with traditional risk factors of smoking and drinking, (2) nasopharyngeal carcinomas (NPCs), and

Region	Area	Site
Oral cavity	—	Lip
		Oral tongue
		Upper gum
		Lower gum
		Floor of mouth
		Hard palate
		Cheek mucosa
		Vestibule of mouth
		Retromolar area
Pharynx	Nasopharynx	Superior wall
		Posterior wall
		Lateral wall
		Anterior wall
	Oropharynx	Base of tongue
		Soft palate
		Uvula
		Tonsil, tonsillar fossa, and pillar
		Valleculae
		Lateral wall of oropharynx
	Hypopharynx	Piriform sinus
		Postcricoid region
		Hypopharyngeal aspect of aryepiglottic fold
		Posterior wall of hypopharynx
Larynx	Supraglottis	Suprahyoid epiglottis
		Infrahyoid epiglottis
		Laryngeal aspect of aryepiglottic folds
		Arytenoid
		Ventricular band (false cords)
	Glottis	True vocal cords
		Anterior commissure
		Posterior commissure
	Subglottis	Subglottis
Nasal cavity and paranasal sinuses	Nasal cavity	Septum
		Floor
		Lateral wall
		Vestibule
	Maxillary sinus	Anteroinferior
		Superoposterior
	Ethmoid sinus	
	Frontal sinus	

TABLE 5.1 Upper Aerodigestive Tract Sites and Subsites

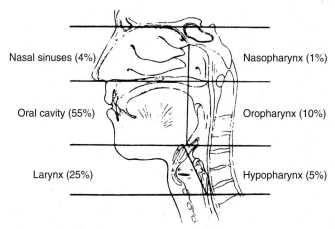

FIGURE 5.1 Anatomic divisions of the head and neck. Percentages indicate the relative frequencies of carcinoma in these regions.

(3) human papillomavirus (HPV) associated oropharyngeal cancers. The distinction between these entities is critical in order to make appropriate treatment decisions.

A. SCA with traditional risk factors

Historically, HNCs have been associated with exposure to mucosal irritants such as tobacco and alcohol. Strong epidemiologic data demonstrates that there is a dose-response relationship between cigarette use and the incidence of HNC. Of note, alcohol use interacts synergistically with tobacco use, dramatically increasing the risk of cancer. Chewing tobacco is associated with oral cavity cancers. The median age at diagnosis for tobacco-associated HNC ranges from 55 to 67 years, depending on the site. There is a marked male predominance (3:1), which is felt to reflect the patterns of prior tobacco use within the general population. Of note, there has been a decreasing incidence of HNC associated with traditional risk factors.

B. NPC

NPCs have a highly variable rate of occurrence depending on geographic region. Areas with high rates of NPC include China, Southeast Asia, and North Africa. In low-risk areas, NPC is quite uncommon. Epidemiologic studies are ongoing to identify potential differences in the etiology and behavior of NPC in low- and high-risk regions. In low-risk areas, NPC has a bimodal age distribution with peak incidence occurring between the ages of 15 and 25 years, and again between the ages of 56 and 79 years. In high-risk areas, the initial peak is lacking, and incidence rates start to decline at an earlier age.

Risk factors for the development of NPC include infection with Epstein-Barr virus (EBV), environmental factors, and genetic predisposition. In the low-risk areas, the early peak in incidence is thought to be due to genetic susceptibility in conjunction with exposure to EBV and/or other environmental contacts. EBV appears to be associated with NPC in high-risk areas; however, in the low-risk population, more traditional risk factors such as tobacco and alcohol use may play a role. Of note, the incidence of EBV infection far exceeds the rate of cancer development, thus research is ongoing to try and identify determinates that favor the development of overt cancer.

NPC is usually classified histologically using one of two systems. The first is a World Health Organization classification that breaks NPC into three subtypes: type 1, keratinizing SCA; type 2, nonkeratinizing, well differentiated SCA; and type 3, nonkeratinizing, undifferentiated SCA. Alternatively, cancers may be categorized as (1) well differentiated keratinizing SCA and (2) undifferentiated SCA. Keratinizing SCA, is most common in the low-risk and older patients, whereas undifferentiated SCA is more common in the high-risk areas.

C. HPV-associated oropharyngeal carcinomas

Over the past decade, there has been a marked increase in the incidence of oropharyngeal carcinomas, specifically tumors arising from tonsillar tissue. Data now indicates that a substantial percentage of these tumors are related to infections with HPV. The vast majority of cases within the United States are associated with serotype 16. In general, HPV-associated tonsillar cancers have a better prognosis. It should be noted, however, that a heavy smoking history mitigates the favorable outcome to a significant degree. Histologically, HPV-associated tumors are frequently described as poorly differentiated due to the immature appearance of the cells. This is a misconception as tumors cells are similar in appearance to the specialized epithelial lining of the tonsillar crypts. In addition, tumor cells are frequently basaloid in appearance. It is important to distinguish tonsillar cancers with a basaloid appearance from "basaloid SCAs," which are an aggressive subtype thought to have a poor outcome.

III. PRESENTING SYMPTOMS

The presenting symptoms of HNC vary based on the primary site; thus, a careful history may help guide the diagnostic work-up. For example, patients with hoarseness may have cancers of the larynx and should undergo endoscopic evaluation for a laryngeal mass. Common presenting complaints include pain, nonhealing ulcerative lesions, dysphagia, odynophagia, hemoptysis, epistaxis, sinus congestion, globus sensation, headaches, nonhealing dental infections, and a nonpainful neck mass. Presenting complaints of HNC are similar to symptoms associated with benign problems such as bacterial pharyngitis or sinusitis. This may lead to a protracted delay in diagnosis. Occasionally, patients may also present with complications secondary to local disease such as airway obstruction or aspiration pneumonia.

Although the bulk of patients present with symptoms related to local disease, it is important to assess systemic manifestations as well. Patients with more advanced disease may present with weight loss due to decreased oral intake and/or cancer cachexia. Other systemic manifestations of such as fatigue, neurocognitive changes, and debility should also be ascertained.

IV. STAGING AND WORK-UP
A. Initial work-up
Treatment is based on the extent of disease at presentation, so an accurate staging work-up is critical. A careful history may help point to the primary site and suggest involved structures. A thorough head and neck evaluation will include an assessment of the primary site and the extent of nodal disease. An endoscopic exam is usually performed on initial exam by an otolaryngologist to identify and/or confirm the primary site. Most patients with laryngeal or pharyngeal tumors will undergo direct laryngoscopy with biopsy to determine the extent of disease and to rule out a second primary tumor. Imaging studies are considered a standard component of the work-up in patients with locally advanced disease. The purpose of radiographic studies is to clearly define the extent of local disease, to identify nodal spread, and to rule out metastatic disease or a second primary tumor. Computed tomography scans, magnetic resonance imaging, and positron emission tomography scans may each contribute unique clinical information; it is therefore important to discuss the appropriate radiographic evaluation with the radiologist in order to optimize the staging work-up and to provide clinicians with the information needed for treatment planning.

B. TNM classification
The American Joint Committee on Cancer TNM staging system integrates clinical and pathologic information regarding size of the primary tumor (T-stage); the size, number, and location of regional lymph nodes (N-stage); and the presence of distant metastases (M-stage). Each disease site within the head and neck region has a T-staging system. However, all sites, with the exception of NPCs, share a common nodal staging system. Because NPCs are associated with extensive nodal disease, a specific N-staging system has been developed that is applicable only to this cohort of patients.

Based on the T, N, and M stages, patients are grouped into overall stages I through IV (Tables 5.2 and 5.3). In general, stage I and II

TABLE 5.2	TNM Staging System for Carcinomas of the Oral Cavity

Primary Tumor

TX	Primary tumor cannot be assessed
T0	No evidence of primary tumor
Tis	Carcinoma in situ
T1	Tumor ≤2 cm in greatest dimension
T2	Tumor >2 cm but not >4 cm
T3	Tumor >4 cm in greatest dimension
T4a	Tumor invades adjacent structures (e.g., through cortical bone) into deep extrinsic muscle of the tongue, maxillary sinus, and skin of face
T4b	Tumor invades masticator space, pterygoid plates, or skull base and/or encases internal carotid artery

Regional Nodal Status

NX	Regional lymph nodes cannot be assessed
N0	No regional lymph node metastasis
N1	Metastasis in a single ipsilateral node ≤3 cm in greatest dimension
N2a	Metastasis in a single ipsilateral node >3 cm but not >6 cm in greatest dimension
N2b	Metastasis in multiple ipsilateral nodes not >6 cm in greatest dimension
N2c	Metastasis in bilateral or contralateral lymph nodes not >6 cm in greatest dimension
N3	Metastasis in a lymph node >6 cm in greatest dimension

Distant Metastasis

M0	No distant metastasis
M1	Distant metastasis

Adapted from Edge SB, Byrd DR, Compton CA (eds). *AJCC cancer staging manual* (7th ed.). New York: Springer; 2010, p. 37.

cancers are small and do not have evidence of nodal or distant spread. Stage III includes either larger primary tumors or tumors with early regional node involvement. Stage IV lesions may be either large tumors with significant local extension, extensive nodal disease, or distant metastatic disease. The stage grouping has been developed so that advancing stage is associated with worsening prognosis. With the recognition that patients with HPV-positive disease have an improved survival despite advanced disease, changes to the TNM classification may be anticipated.

C. Assessment of comorbid disease and psychosocial issues

An initial evaluation is not complete without a detailed assessment of medical comorbidities, psychological issues, social supports, and financial status. Patients with SCA secondary to smoking and drinking frequently have comorbid diseases such as cerebrovascular disease, chronic obstructive pulmonary disease (COPD), and alcohol-related disorders. Risk stratification systems specific to HNC patients have been developed to assess long-term prognosis

	Stage Grouping for Carcinomas of the Oral Cavity, Pharynx, Hypopharynx Larynx, and Paranasal Sinuses
Stage	**Groups**
0	Tis, N0, M0
I	T1, N0, M0
II	T2, N0, M0
III	T3, N0, M0
	T1 or T2 or T3, N1, M0
IVa	T4a, N0 or N1, M0
	T1–4a, N2, M0
IVb	T4b, any N, M0
	Any T, N3, M0
IVc	Any T, any N, M1

Adapted from Edge SB, Byrd DR, Compton CA (eds). *AJCC cancer staging manual* (7th ed.). New York: Springer; 2010.

based on common comorbidities. Understanding the patient's long-term prognosis may help guide treatment decisions. A substance abuse history should be obtained from all patients, and patients with active abuse issues should be referred for appropriate counseling. Patients who are actively smoking should be advised to quit and should be referred to appropriate support services to aid in this effort. Depression and suicide are common in HNC patients, thus initial and ongoing screening for mood disorders is appropriate. Patients with the traditional risk factors of smoking and drinking may have poor support systems and lower socioeconomic status. Defining these issues at the time of initial diagnosis is important because treatment may need to be adjusted based on the patient's capacity to comply with therapy.

In addition to general considerations in the work-up of HNC as noted above, there are also specific health-related issues that may impact on the decision to use specific chemotherapy agents. Specific issues are delineated below.

1. **Bone marrow function.** Chronic alcoholism, malnutrition, and tumor-related weight loss contribute to a significant incidence of folate deficiency and decreased bone marrow reserve in many patients.

2. **Pulmonary function.** Current or distant heavy smoking increases the likelihood of COPD and chronic bronchitis, leading to an increased risk of pulmonary infection during treatment. In addition to impaired pulmonary reserve, patients have a propensity to aspirate secondary to swallowing abnormalities and may have difficulty handling their secretions.

3. **Renal function.** Platinum compounds are used as first-line agents in HNC therapy. Adequate baseline renal function and continued monitoring of renal function is needed for administration. Methotrexate is renally excreted and may accumulate in patients with renal insufficiency, leading to increased toxicity.

4. **Hepatic function.** The presence of cirrhosis, whether related to alcoholism or viral hepatitis, can complicate management as it can impair the ability to accomplish forced hydration by leading to third space accumulations of ascites or edema. Routine use of diuretics may exacerbate treatment-related electrolyte abnormalities.

5. **Neuropathy.** Platinum compounds and taxanes may cause peripheral or autonomic neuropathy. Hearing loss may develop secondary to chemotherapy or radiation therapy. Patients should be screened for baseline neuropathy or hearing loss and have their therapies adjusted accordingly. Comorbidities that may be associated with baseline neuropathy include alcoholism and diabetes.

6. **Fertility.** All chemotherapy agents may impair fertility either temporarily or permanently. For male patients who wish to ensure their reproductive capacity, sperm donation should be accomplished promptly. For female patients, induced ovulation and harvesting and preservation of ova may be considered.

7. **Concomitant drugs.** Antihypertensives, diuretics, and drugs used for glycemic control all need careful assessment, monitoring, and adjustment during therapy as patients undergo treatment. Nausea, vomiting, anorexia, and limited oral intake often lead to dehydration and weight loss, making hypotension a common occurrence during therapy. Patients may need to be weaned off antihypertensives. The use of glucocorticoids as an adjunct to antiemetics and to prevent anaphylactic reactions, coupled with irregular feeding patterns, make glycemic control difficult. It is best to emphasize careful monitoring to avoid hypoglycemia rather than focus on hyperglycemia, which is not metabolically (homeostatically) significant.

V. NATURAL HISTORY

The natural history of SCA of the head and neck can be quite variable. Tumor growth rates range from slow progression over years to rapidly expanding masses that progress measurably over days to weeks. There is a correlation between histologic grade and the rate of tumor growth, though this association is weak. The rapidity of growth may play a role in treatment decisions as surgeons may be reluctant to operate on large, rapidly expanding tumors.

Early stage cancers (stage I and II) are associated with a high cure rate. Unfortunately, the majority of patients present with locally advanced disease (T3, T4, or nodal disease). Of note, prominent nodal disease is common in patients with both NPC and HPV-associated oropharyngeal cancer. Metastatic disease at presentation is infrequent in all types of HNC, but it may develop following initial therapy. The most powerful predictor for development of metastatic disease is the extent of nodal disease at presentation. Patients who present with N0-N1 disease have a less than 5% chance of developing distant metastases, whereas patients with N2 or greater nodal disease have a 25% to 30% chance of subsequent distant spread. The most common sites of metastatic disease are lung, liver, and bone. Brain metastases are rare for patients with SCA of the head and neck.

Most recurrences appear within 18 months of primary treatment, and 90% appear within 2 years. Patients who are not cured usually die from the cancer within 3 to 4 years of diagnosis. Patients who succumb to the cancer generally experience local, regional, and distant failure in equal proportions. The manifestations of end-stage disease are typified by inanition, cachexia, aspiration, respiratory difficulty due to trouble with secretions or obstruction, fistulas, oral or neck ulceration, edema of the mucosal structures or face, and pain. Among survivors, the risk of second primary head and neck, lung, and esophagus tumors is a significant problem, thus long-term surveillance is indicated.

VI. TREATMENT: GENERAL CONSIDERATIONS

Treatment of HNC, regardless of histologic cell type or causal factors, requires a multidisciplinary approach with a team of experienced clinicians including head and neck surgeons, radiation and medical oncologists, nutritionists, speech and language pathologist, and oral health providers. Working with the patient, the treatment team must come to a consensus regarding (1) the goals of therapy, (2) treatment options that will adequately meet those goals, and (3) optimal methods for implementation and monitoring of treatment and treatment-related side effects. Although treatment paradigms are evolving rapidly, therapeutic principles for each of the major clinical entities are reviewed below.

A. SCA with traditional risk factors of tobacco and alcohol use

1. **Early-stage disease.** Small lesions without regional extension generally are treated with surgery or radiation. The choice is usually made based on the relative toxicity of therapeutic options. In addition, treatment may be determined by medical or social considerations. For example, surgery may be avoided in patients with significant comorbidities and radiation may not be an option for noncompliant patients with suboptimal social supports.

2. **Locally advanced disease.** Larger primary cancers and those with clinically detectable spread to lymph nodes (referred to as "locally advanced disease") are usually treated with a combination therapy. Combination therapy may include surgery and radiation; chemotherapy and radiation; or surgery, radiation, and chemotherapy. Often, several different treatment approaches are reasonable for any given patient. The decision as to which treatment approach to take is based on (1) biopsychosocial status of

the patient, (2) the patient's priorities and preferences regarding functionality and cosmesis, (3) the expertise and training of the treating physicians, and (4) the relative toxicities of therapy.

Locally advanced disease is usually categorized as either resectable or unresectable. Criteria for resectability are difficult to define because surgeons have differing levels of skill. Furthermore, individual surgeons differ in their opinions regarding the balance between providing patients with potentially curative surgery and the long-term morbidity of extensive resections. For those patients with locally advanced disease who undergo primary surgical resection, postoperative radiation or radiation with chemotherapy is frequently administered in order to eliminate residual disease.

In a subset of patients with resectable disease, surgery may entail loss of structures critical for speech and swallowing (e.g., larynx or base of tongue). In this cohort of patients, a radiation-based treatment approach may be preferable to surgery in order to minimize functional deficits. This is often referred to as a "function preservation" or "larynx preservation approach." Patients undergoing function preservation therapy usually receive a combination of radiation therapy and chemotherapy. Unfortunately, the optimal sequence of radiation therapy and chemotherapy has yet to be determined.

A small but significant percentage of patients present with disease that is unresectable. These patients are usually treated with a combination of radiation therapy and chemotherapy. Despite the use of aggressive chemoradiation, this group of patients does poorly.

Combined modality treatment is utilized in order to improve outcome. Outcomes of interest may include the following: (1) decreased local, regional, or distant failure rates; (2) improved survival; (3) decreased rates of second primary tumor; or (4) decreased morbidity of therapy. Over the past three decades, investigators have conducted a number of clinical trials that have helped to define current practice. Key findings from these studies include the following:

- When compared to preoperative radiation, postoperative radiation is associated with decreased complications and improved local disease control. There is no survival difference. Thus, patients undergoing surgery usually have radiation therapy postoperatively.
- There are several ways in which chemotherapy may be incorporated into treatment: (1) it may be given as induction therapy—prior to surgery or radiation; (2) it may be given as adjuvant therapy—after surgery or radiation; (3) it may be given concurrent with radiation; or (4) it may be given sequentially—induction therapy followed by concurrent chemoradiation.

- Neither induction chemotherapy followed by surgery nor adjuvant chemotherapy following surgery has improved survival.
- Postoperative chemoradiation improves local control and survival in patients at high risk for recurrence when compared to postoperative radiation therapy only.
- In patients with locally advanced disease, concurrent chemoradiation improves survival compared to radiation alone.
- In patients with laryngeal cancer, concurrent chemoradiation improves local disease control and laryngeal preservation but not survival. Improved local control is at the expense of increased late side effects.

The role of induction chemotherapy prior to concurrent chemoradiation (sequential therapy) has yet to be clearly established. Meta-analysis demonstrates a small improved survival with three cycles of aggressive induction therapy. The results of randomized phase III trials comparing concurrent chemoradiation to sequential therapy are pending.

It must be noted that the use of combined modality therapy substantially increases both the acute and late effects of treatment. Aggressive treatments push patients to their physiologic tolerance and, in some cases, well beyond. Thus, we must recognize that patients with a poor performance status and multiple comorbidities may not tolerate aggressive combined modality therapy well; it is important to tailor treatment to the patient.

3. **Metastatic disease.** Only a small percentage of patients present with metastatic disease. In this cohort of patients, treatment is directed at palliation.

B. NPCs

NPCs are exquisitely sensitive to radiation with or without chemotherapy. Thus, radiation-based treatment is the cornerstone of therapy for NPC. Furthermore, NPCs are anatomically located adjacent to the bony structures of the base of skull, making surgical excision difficult if not impossible. Patients who present with stage I or II disease are usually treated with radiation therapy alone, although there are those who would advocate for the addition of chemotherapy to the treatment of all stages of NPC. Patients with locally advanced stage III or IV disease should be treated with combined modality therapy. Data support an improvement in local control, disease-free survival, overall survival, and metastatic disease–free survival in patients treated with concurrent chemotherapy. The role of induction or adjuvant chemotherapy has yet to be clarified; however, a recent meta-analysis has confirmed a modest survival advantage for patients receiving induction therapy followed by concurrent chemoradiation.

C. HPV-associated oropharyngeal carcinomas

The optimal treatment for HPV-associated oropharyngeal carcinomas has yet to be determined. It is clear that HPV-associated tumors have an improved survival compared to non-HPV–associated tumors regardless of the type of therapy. However, smoking may mitigate the improved outcomes seen in HPV-associated tonsil cancers. Risk stratification systems that incorporate HPV and smoking status are being developed. Low-risk patients are currently being defined as those with HPV-associated tonsil cancers in nonsmokers (a history of fewer than 10 packs per year). In this population, long-term survival is over 90%; thus, in this cohort of patients, investigators are conducting and/or planning treatment trials that deescalate therapy and minimize late effects. The general consensus of the head and neck community is that a radiation-based treatment approach is preferable to a surgical approach. That being said, small tumors may be excised as a part of the initial diagnostic work-up, thus obviating the need for high doses of radiation to the pharynx.

VII. TREATMENT: CHEMOTHERAPY

The expected response of SCA to chemotherapy will vary based on well-established predictive factors. The most powerful predictive factors for antitumor response include stage, performance status, and prior treatment. Patients who present with localized disease have a substantially higher response rate than patients with metastatic disease. Patients with a good performance status are more likely to respond than those with a poor performance status. In addition, patients with a poor performance status are more likely to develop treatment-related toxicity. The more extensively treated a cancer becomes, the less likely it will respond to subsequent chemotherapy. Primarily radiation-resistant tumors or tumors that recur rapidly after radiation have also been shown to have a particularly poor outcome.

A. Single agent activity

SCA of the head and neck is modestly responsive to a number of chemotherapy agents. The phase II studies listed in Table 5.4 were largely conducted in patients with recurrent or metastatic disease. These patients tend to have been heavily pretreated and their disease is more chemoresistant than patients with previously untreated, locally advanced disease.

1. **Cisplatin.** Cisplatin is one of the most commonly used agents in HNC therapy. Response rates are similar to other single agents; however, cisplatin is associated with significant toxicity and requires aggressive supportive measures. Therefore, it is seldom used as a single agent. More commonly, it is used in combination with other agents in patients with a good performance status for whom an aggressive treatment regimen is feasible. Acute and delayed nausea and vomiting require aggressive antiemetics including 5-HT3 receptor antagonists and neurokinin-1 receptor

TABLE 5.4	Response Rate for Single Chemotherapy Agents in Recurrent HNC
Agent	**Response Rate**
Methotrexate	10%–50%
Cisplatin	9%–40%
Carboplatin	22%
Paclitaxel	40%
Docetaxel	34%
Fluorouracil	17%
Bleomycin	21%
Ifosfamide	23%
Vinorelbine	20%
Irinotecan	21%
Cetuximab	12%
Gefitinib	10%
In NPC	
Gemcitabine	13%–37%
Capecitabine	23%
Doxorubicin	39%

antagonists (aprepitant) for optimum control. A standard regimen to maintain urine output is as follows: cisplatin 60 to 100 mg/m^2 given intravenously (IV) once every 3 weeks preceded by 1 to 2 L of hydration, 12.5 to 25 g of mannitol, and 1 to 2 L of post cisplatin hydration with mannitol and/or 10 to 20 mg of furosemide. Adequate replacement of potassium, magnesium, and sodium losses is requisite, as is monitoring hydration.

2. **Carboplatin.** Carboplatin, given at an area under the curve (AUC) of 5 to 6, is easier to administer than cisplatin because there is no requirement for forced hydration and less nausea and vomiting, renal toxicity, ototoxicity, and neuropathy. Response rates comparable to single-agent cisplatin are reported but myelosuppression, in particular thrombocytopenia, can be dose-limiting. Allergic reactions may occur in patients, particularly after multiple cycles.

3. **Paclitaxel.** Paclitaxel may be given at high doses every three weeks (175–250 mg/m^2 over 3 hours) or at low doses weekly (60–120 mg/m^2). A response rate of 15% to 40% has been reported. The high-dose regimen is associated with a significant risk of neutropenia, neuropathy, and allergic reactions.

4. **Docetaxel.** Docetaxel is usually given as doses of 75 to 100 mg/m^2 IV over 1 hour every 3 weeks or as 30 to 40 mg/m^2 IV over 1 hour weekly. Neuropathy may be lower than with paclitaxel, but asthenia may be greater with the high-dose regimen. Tissue edema may occur with higher doses; thus, steroid prophylaxis is indicated.

5. **Methotrexate.** Intravenous methotrexate doses of 40 to 60 mg/m^2 IV weekly given over 15 minutes is a convenient standard single-agent treatment. Dose escalation can increase response rates but is accompanied by increased toxicity and does not improve survival. Minimal to moderate nausea and few significant acute side effects make this a well-tolerated and easily monitored treatment. Responses may occur after 1 or 2 weeks of treatment but usually require 4 to 8 weeks of treatment, so patience is needed before abandoning this regimen.

6. **Cetuximab.** Epidermal growth factor receptors are overexpressed in 90% of HNCs. Cetuximab is a monoclonal antibody that binds to epidermal growth factor receptors, thus blocking the proliferative signal. Cetuximab has been approved by the U.S. Food and Drug Administration for the treatment of metastatic disease and unresectable disease that failed prior platinum-based therapy and as a radiation-sensitizing agent. The standard regimen begins with a loading dose of cetuximab 400 mg/m^2 IV given over 2 hours followed by weekly doses of 250 mg/m^2 IV over 1 hour. Responses of up to 10% have been observed among patients with metastatic or recurrent disease. Skin rash, hypomagnesemia, and diarrhea are the common side effects. Anaphylactic reactions, although uncommon, may be severe. Of note, anaphylactic reactions are more common in areas of the southeastern United States, where rates are as high as 20%.

7. **Fluorouracil.** Fluorouracil is well tolerated and has comparable activity to cisplatin and other single agents. It is most often given as a 4- or 5-day continuous infusion. The drug is a vascular irritant at high concentrations and therefore, for prolonged infusions, a central venous catheter or access device is customary. Although suitable for use as a single agent, it is most often used in combination with other drugs.

8. **Ifosfamide.** Ifosfamide is given at doses of 1000 mg/m^2/day IV over 2 hours for 4 days every 3 to 4 weeks and yields response rates of 20% to 40%. The need for uroprotection with mesna 200 mg/m^2 before and 400 mg/m^2 after ifosfamide makes this a cumbersome single-agent regimen to administer.

9. **Bleomycin.** Bleomycin has comparable activity to other agents without associated myelosuppression or nausea. Bleomycin is dosed as 10 to 20 units/m^2 intramuscularly or IV and can be given weekly, every 2 weeks, or 5 days a month. Pulmonary toxicity is commonly seen. Responses are often very brief.

10. **Gemcitabine.** Gemcitabine, dosed at 1000 mg/m^2 weekly, has activity in NPC and is well tolerated.

11. **Anthracyclines.** Doxorubicin and mitoxantrone are useful in NPC, which is very responsive to multiple agents; many

TABLE 5.5	Response Rate for Combination Chemotherapy Agents in Recurrent HNC
Agent	**Approximate Response Rate**
Cisplatin/fluorouracil	25%–40%
Carboplatin/fluorouracil	26%
Cisplatin/paclitaxel	28%–35%
Cisplatin/docetaxel	42%
Cisplatin/cetuximab	26%
Methotrexate/bleomycin/cisplatin	48%
Paclitaxel/ifosfamide/carboplatin	55%
In NPC	
Gemcitabine/paclitaxel	41%

patients are younger with good performance status so that they often tolerate and respond to multiple sequential treatment regimens. These agents have utility in that setting.

B. **Combination chemotherapy—metastatic disease (Table 5.5)**

Similar to single agents, most novel chemotherapy regimens were initially developed in patients with metastatic or recurrent disease. Theoretically, the use of multiple agents with additive or synergistic activity and nonoverlapping toxicity should improve outcome. However, in the population of patients with HNC, confirmation of this theory proved elusive for many decades. Studies conducted in the 1980s and 1990s demonstrated that combination chemotherapy increased response rates but failed to improve survival when compared to single-agent therapy. Median survival was short (6–9 months) and was similar across treatment regimens. Only with the addition of the targeted agent cetuximab were investigators able to identify a multidrug regimen that clearly improved survival. The EXTREME trial compared cisplatin and fluorouracil to cisplatin, fluorouracil, and cetuximab. The three-drug combination was associated with a marked increase in survival. This study clearly established the critical role of cetuximab in the treatment of patients with metastatic/recurrent HNC. Other less toxic combination therapies incorporating cetuximab have been reported; however, randomized comparative trials are lacking. Several other targeted agents have been under investigation. We await the results of phase III trials to establish clinical efficacy. Because toxicity is usually greater with combination therapy, the general consensus is that these regimens are most appropriate for patients with an Eastern Cooperative Oncology Group performance status of 0 or 1. The most commonly used combination regimens used are listed below.

1. **Cisplatin and fluorouracil.** Cisplatin dosed at 75 to 100 mg/m^2 is given IV over 1 to 4 hours on day 1, and fluorouracil dosed at 600 to 1000 mg/m^2/day is given as a 96- to 120-hour

continuous infusion. Forced hydration, aggressive antiemetics, and close monitoring for electrolyte abnormalities, mucositis, dehydration, and cytopenias are needed. Recently, it has been appreciated that significant rates of neutropenia accompany this regimen and that these patients may benefit from filgrastim and prophylactic antibiotics. When this regimen is used during or after prior radiotherapy, only four days (96 hours of continuous infusion) of fluorouracil are used because of enhanced mucosal and skin toxicity in that setting.

2. **Cisplatin, fluorouracil, and cetuximab.** Cetuximab, at an initial dose of 400 mg/m^2 then 250 mg/m^2 weekly, is given with a maximum of six every 3-weeks cycles of cisplatin dosed at 100 mg/m^2 IV on day 1 and fluorouracil dosed at 1000 mg/m^2/day continuous infusion for the first 4 days of each cycle. Cetuximab is administrated until progression or unacceptable toxicity.

3. **Carboplatin and fluorouracil.** Carboplatin dosed at 300 mg/m^2 IV day 1 and fluorouracil dosed at 1000 mg/m^2/day by continuous infusion for 4 days are used for recurrent disease with responses and survival comparable to cisplatin and fluorouracil. For simultaneous chemoradiation in oropharynx cancer, carboplatin dosed at 70 mg/m^2 IV daily for 4 days and fluorouracil dosed at 600 mg/m^2 daily by continuous infusion (96 hours) for 4 days is a standard regimen. These carboplatin regimens predate the use of the Calvert formula but roughly correspond to an AUC of 5 and AUC 1.25, respectively.

4. **Cisplatin and paclitaxel.** Cisplatin dosed at 60 mg/m^2 IV and paclitaxel dosed at 135 to 175 mg/m^2 IV every 3 weeks were found to be equivalent to fluorouracil regimens in patients with recurrent disease. The lower dose of paclitaxel was better tolerated. Careful monitoring for neuropathy is needed.

5. **Carboplatin and paclitaxel—every 3 weeks.** Carboplatin AUC 6 IV and paclitaxel dosed to 175 mg/m^2 IV given every 3 weeks is a widely utilized combination regimen with similar results.

6. **Carboplatin and paclitaxel—weekly.** Carboplatin at AUC 2 IV day 1 and paclitaxel at 135 mg/m^2 IV day 1 weekly for 6 weeks or 60 mg/m^2 for 9 weeks is a simple outpatient regimen with acceptable response rate and minimal toxicity. Neutropenia is seen in 18% of patients, but febrile neutropenia is uncommon.

7. **Cisplatin and docetaxel.** Cisplatin dosed at 75 mg/m^2 IV and docetaxel dosed at 75 mg/m^2 IV each on day 1 every 3 weeks. Neutropenia is frequently seen in this regimen.

8. **Docetaxel, cisplatin, and fluorouracil.** Docetaxel dosed at 75 mg/m^2 IV on day 1, cisplatin dosed at 100 mg/m^2 IV on day 1, fluorouracil dosed at 1000 mg/m^2 IV daily on days 1 to 4 (96-hour continuous infusion) every 3 weeks for three cycles is administered. Based on the results of TAX 324, this regimen has become a widely used

treatment for patients with advanced disease and a good performance status. This regimen requires prophylactic fluoroquinolone antibiotics.

9. **Paclitaxel, ifosfamide, and cisplatin or carboplatin** is a three-drug regimen with high activity that is well tolerated but requires good performance status patients and filgrastim support.

C. Chemotherapy as a radiation sensitizer

The concurrent administration of chemotherapy and radiation has improved outcomes in a variety of clinical scenarios. These include locally advanced NPCs, advanced unresectable cancers, organ preservation in locally advanced larynx and base of tongue cancers, and in high-risk postoperative patients. Thus, concurrent chemoradiation is accepted as a standard option for these patients. Meta-analysis demonstrates that the addition of chemotherapy concurrently to radiation therapy results in up to a 4% to 8% absolute improvement in survival, which amounts to a 12% to 19% reduction in the risk of death, whether in definitive or postoperative adjuvant settings. While many regimens have been tested in these settings, high-dose cisplatin has been the most commonly studied agent. A variety of alternative single-agent and multiagent chemoradiotherapy regimens have been tested and found to be superior to radiation alone. Unfortunately, there is no comparative data to delineate the relative efficacy and toxicity of these regimens. It should be noted that the addition of chemotherapy concurrent with radiation is associated with a marked increase in both acute and late treatment effects. The dose-limiting toxicity is usually severe oral mucositis. The increased toxicity must be carefully weighed against the improved outcomes on a patient-by-patient basis. Commonly used concurrent regimens are noted below.

1. **Cisplatin** dosed at 100 mg/m^2 IV over 1 to 4 hours every 21 days during radiation.

2. **Cetuximab** dosed at 400 mg/m^2 IV on day 1 as a loading dose followed by 250 mg/m^2 IV weekly during radiation.

3. **Cisplatin and fluorouracil.** Cisplatin dosed at 60 to 75 mg/m^2 IV on day 1 and fluorouracil dosed at 600 to 1000 mg/m^2 daily for 4 days by continuous 96-hour infusion on days 1 and 29.

4. **Carboplatin and fluorouracil.** Carboplatin dosed at 70 mg/m^2 IV daily for 4 days and fluorouracil at 600 mg/m^2 daily for 4 days by continuous infusion (96 hours) is a standard regimen on days 1 and 29.

5. **Hydroxyurea and fluorouracil.** Hydroxyurea at 1000 mg orally every 12 hours for 11 doses and fluorouracil at 800 mg/m^2 daily for 5 days given as a 120-hour intravenous infusion repeated every 14 days for five cycles concomitantly with radiotherapy for 5 days every 14 days.

6. **Cisplatin and paclitaxel.** Cisplatin at 20 mg/m^2 weekly and paclitaxel at 30 mg/m^2 weekly during standard fractionated radiation.

7. **Paclitaxel** dosed at 20 to 40 mg/m^2 given over 1 hour weekly during radiotherapy.

8. **Paclitaxel, hydroxyurea, and fluorouracil** may be given on alternating weeks during simultaneous chemoradiation.

D. Combination chemotherapy—adjuvant therapy

Combination chemotherapy has also been investigated in the adjuvant setting. In patients with locally advanced NPC, a sentinel study compared radiation therapy alone to radiation with concurrent chemotherapy using cisplatin dosed at 100 mg/m^2 on days 1, 22, and 43 followed by three cycles of cisplatin and fluorouracil. The results demonstrated a marked improvement in outcome for patients treated with combined modality therapy. Critics of this trial argue that it is impossible to determine the relative contribution of the concurrent and adjuvant components of the combined treatment regimens. Furthermore, a high percentage of patients were unable to complete all three planned cycles of adjuvant therapy due to excessive toxicity. Nonetheless, this regimen remains a standard treatment option for patients undergoing therapy for locally advanced NPC. In the postoperative setting, studies have failed to demonstrate a benefit for adjuvant chemotherapy. Studies of adjuvant chemotherapy after definitive radiation therapy are limited.

E. Combination chemotherapy—induction therapy

Combination chemotherapy regimens have been extensively studied as induction therapy prior to definite treatment with either radiation or surgery. The role of induction chemotherapy is one of the most debated issues in HNC therapy and has polarized the head and neck community. It is beyond the scope of this review to provide a detailed discussion of the current status of induction chemotherapy in the treatment of HNC; however, the following is a review of critical concepts and current directions for research.

The interest in multidrug induction therapy stemmed from the observation that response rates in treatment-naïve patients is extremely high. It is clear and generally agreed on that there is no benefit to induction chemotherapy prior to surgical resection. However, the data pertaining to induction therapy prior to radiation therapy has yet to be clarified.

Induction therapy followed by radiation has been assessed in two separate populations: locally advanced disease (which can be further divided into resectable and unresectable) and larynx preservation. For patients with locally advanced disease, the primary outcome of interest is overall survival. For patients with laryngeal and hypopharyngeal tumors, the primary outcome of interest is function preservation. Unfortunately, our methods for assessing function preservation in large randomized trials are limited. Usually, function loss is defined as laryngectomy or feeding tube dependence. These are coarse and insensitive measures of functionality that fail to take into account clinically significant but less overt deficits.

Interpretation of induction trials has been complicated by three important advances in our understanding of HNC therapy: (1) the recent acceptance of concurrent chemoradiation as a standard treatment approach for improving outcomes in a variety of clinical settings; (2) the recognition that concurrent chemoradiation is associated with increased late toxicities and substantial functional deficits; and (3) the recognition that locally advanced HPV-associated oropharyngeal cancers have an excellent outcome.

VIII. SUPPORTIVE CARE

A. Support systems

Treatment of HNC is time-intensive, complex, and fraught with complications. It requires a compliant and willing patient as well as a dedicated support system. The support system is composed of the patient's caregivers, usually defined as a network of family and friends, and the healthcare team. Prior to initiating therapy, it is important to inform the patient and caregivers about anticipated treatment toxicities and their potential impact on the patient's ability to conduct routine actives of daily living. Working with the healthcare team, the patient must identify the individuals who will provide support if and when it becomes necessary. Specific issues that should be discussed include the following: (1) insurance coverage (including dental and pharmacy); (2) living situation (homeless, living alone, or living with others); (3) social supports (ability and willingness of caregivers to provided physical and emotional support); (4) financial issues (with specific discussion of ability to pay for household expenses during treatment); and (5) work issues (impact of cancer on work status of patient and caregivers). It is important to identify patients with critically limited resources in order to plan adequately for their ongoing care and to guide treatment decisions.

The healthcare team should be composed of physicians, nursing staff, nutritionists, speech and swallowing therapists, physical therapists, and social workers who are trained to deal with the unique challenges faced by HNC patients and their caregivers. Because patient support needs change dramatically over time, frequent and ongoing assessment is required.

B. Nutrition

Due to the anatomic proximity to structures critical for normal alimentation, HNC and its treatment may have a dramatic impact on oral intake. Malnutrition is associated with impaired healing, increased toxicity of treatment, and decreased survival. Therefore, it is important to identify and treat nutritional deficiencies

TABLE 5.6	Contributing Factors to Decreased Oral Intake and Weight Loss	
Problem	**Consequence**	**Intervention**
Mucositis	Pain	Analgesics
	Odynophagia	Steroids (if indicated)
	Swelling (edema)	
Xerostomia	Decreased bolus formation	Drinking sips of liquid with meals
	Lack of lubrication to facilitate swallowing	Avoidance of dry foods
Dental loss	Inability to chew food	Dietary counseling regarding soft and liquid diet
		Dentures when appropriate
Thick mucus	Gagging	Mucolytics
	Impaired swallowing	Drying agents
		Hydration
		Humidified air
		Postural maneuvers at rest
Nausea and vomiting	Decreased intake	Antiemetics
Anorexia	Decreased appetite	Appetite stimulants (e.g., megestrol acetate)
Cachexia	Metabolic alterations resulting in muscle wasting	None

in a proactive and aggressive manner. Factors contributing to decreased oral intake and weight loss are shown in Table 5.6. At the time of diagnosis and periodically thereafter, patients should undergo a nutritional assessment by a dietician who is familiar with the issues facing HNC patients. A nutritional assessment should include a weight loss history, assessment of nutrient intake, and identification of barriers to adequate nutritional intake. Treatable causes of decreased caloric intake should be identified and appropriate interventions instituted.

Ongoing monitoring and education is critical and should include routine measurement of weight, assessment of hydration, and counseling by a certified dietician. Dieticians also ensure adequate nutrition as patients transition from an enteral to oral diet.

It should also be noted that the sequelae of HNC therapy may lead to dietary adaptations that are permanent. For example, many patients experience xerostomia, which alters their ability to take in dry foods such as breads. Patients who are edentulous may have difficulty with intake of adequate protein. Dietary adaptations may predispose to long-term nutrient deficiencies that may impair overall health. Periodic dietary assessment and ongoing counseling of HNC survivors is a necessary part of health maintenance.

C. Mucositis

Radiation therapy and select chemotherapy agents cause mucositis. Mucositis is a pan-tissue inflammation of the mucosa and underlying soft tissue. The classic mucosal manifestations are erythema, ulcer, and pseudomembrane formation. Mucositis associated with systemic chemotherapy is cyclic in nature. The Common Terminology Criteria for Adverse Events v4.0 grading system for mucositis is available on the Internet at http://ctep.cancer.gov/protocolDevelopment/electronic_applications/ctc.htm. The pattern of mucositis development and resolution depends on the treatment. With chemotherapy regimens administered on a 3-week cycle, mucositis usually develops 7 to 10 days after administration and resolves 5 to 7 days later. Chemotherapy regimens administered weekly tend to have a slow escalation of mucosal symptoms over time, with resolution when chemotherapy is dose-reduced or held. Radiation-associated mucositis begins to develop 2 to 4 weeks after the initiation of therapy. Symptoms usually peak at 5 to 7 weeks, although occasionally patients will note worsening mucositis after the completion of therapy. Radiation-induced mucositis may take 4 to 12 weeks to resolve. Some patients have persistent symptomatic ulceration for protracted periods of time. It should be noted that the incidence of grade 3 to 4 mucositis increases from 25% to 35% with radiation alone to 40% to 100% with concurrent chemotherapy. Treatment of mucositis is discussed in Chapter 26.

D. Dysphasia and aspiration

Swallowing is a complex function that requires intact musculature, dentition, vasculature, and nervous system. Damage to any of these components may result in altered swallowing function. Thus, swallowing dysfunction is one of the common and devastating acute and late effects of therapy. Surgery-induced dysphagia is secondary to structural changes due to tissue extirpation and altered sensation from transected nerves. Acutely, radiation therapy–induced dysphagia is secondary to edema and painful mucositis. Over the long term, radiation therapy results in noncompliant fibrotic or contracted tissues that are unable to function normally. Of particular note, radiation may cause upper esophageal stricture formation. Stricture-induced dysphagia may be successfully treated with balloon dilation procedures.

In order to maximize swallow function, it is important to involve speech and language pathologists (SLPs) at an early point in a patient's treatment course. Healthcare providers should also be aware of signs and symptoms that may indicate aspiration, which requires rapid referral and evaluation. These include coughing or throat clearing during or after swallow. Other indications for an SLP evaluation include nasal regurgitation, drooling, pocketing food in the cheek, and food sticking in the throat. The role of the

SLP includes (1) identifying swallowing abnormalities; (2) recommending further testing; (3) developing a treatment plan (including education and swallow therapy); (4) helping dieticians develop an adequate yet safe diet; and (5) ruling out significant aspiration. Common instrumental methods to assess swallow function include the modified barium swallow and the flexible endoscopic evaluation of swallowing safety.

As noted above, dysphagia may result in dietary adaptations and/or weight loss due to inadequate caloric intake. In addition, dysphagia may result in aspiration. Aspiration puts patients at risk for acute and long-term pulmonary toxicity. Acutely, aspiration may lead to pneumonia; in patients actively undergoing myelosuppressive chemotherapy, aspiration pneumonia is associated with a high rate of morbidity and mortality. Over the long term, aspiration may lead to pulmonary fibrosis and respiratory compromise. Of note, microaspiration can simulate pulmonary metastasis.

E. Xerostomia and oral care

Poor oral health outcomes are one of the major late effects of HNC therapy. This is largely related to radiation-induced xerostomia.

Initial dental evaluation is important for all patients undergoing therapy for HNC, particularly for those who will receive radiation therapy. Patients require extensive education regarding oral hygiene and preventive strategies to avoid radiation-induced dental caries. Oral hygiene should include the use of prescription strength fluoride treatments because this agent has consistently demonstrated the ability to significantly reduce adverse late dental effects. In addition, patients undergoing radiation therapy should have extraction of nonviable teeth at least 10 to 14 days prior to initiation of therapy. This will allow adequate time for healing. As healthcare providers, our role is to assess compliance with dental hygiene regimens and to refer to oral health specialists if problems are identified.

F. Lymphedema and fibrosis

Surgery and radiation therapy can damage the soft tissues within the head and neck region with resulting lymphedema (swelling with lymphatic fluid) and fibrosis. In contemporary grading systems, lymphedema and fibrosis exist on a continuum with fibrosis, considered the end stage of tissue damage. Chronic inflammation may accompany lymphedema and fibrosis; damage may be ongoing and self-perpetuating, thus resulting in late toxicity. Generally, lymphedema and fibrosis may be characterized as involving external (neck and shoulders) or internal (pharynx and tongue) structures. Associated function loss may be severe. Early identification and treatment by certified physical therapists experienced in lymphedema and scar management is critical.

Trismus is one of the most common and problematic manifestations of fibrosis. It is caused by surgery or radiation therapy involving the mandibular joint and muscles of mastication. It is characterized by a decrease in the movement of the jaw, thus limiting the opening of the oral cavity. When trismus is severe, patients have difficulty with eating solid foods, dental hygiene, and procedures such as intubation. Trismus usually begins to develop within 1 year of the completion of therapy and is progressive in nature. Aggressive physical therapy may halt progression of symptoms; however, reversal of existing symptoms is limited.

G. Metabolic abnormalities

HNC patients are subject to a number of metabolic abnormalities. First, radiation therapy to the thyroid gland can result in gradual loss of function. Estimated to occur in 25% to 50% of patients who receive doses above 6000 cGy to the thyroid gland, hypothyroidism may develop years after the completion of therapy. Routine testing of thyroid function is recommended, particularly in patients with symptoms indicative of hypothyroidism.

Patients with late-stage HNC may develop humoral hypercalcemia of malignancy. Although estimates vary widely, up to 23% of patients with advanced recurrent HNCs will manifest hypercalcemia before death. Standard treatment with hydration, saline diuresis, and bisphosphonate therapy are used.

IX. SECONDARY CANCER PREVENTION

HNC survivors with the traditional risk factors of smoking and drinking are at risk for the development of second primary cancers. The majority of second primary tumors involve the upper aerodigestive tact. It is hypothesized that this is related in part to a field cancerization effect of tobacco and alcohol exposure. Thus, smoking cessation and abstinence from alcohol are important adjuncts to the care of these patients. Chemopreventive agents have been assessed to determine their ability to prevent second cancers from developing. Although isotretinoin (13-*cis*-retinoic acid) 1 to 2 mg/kg was shown to prevent second primary cancers in HNC patients, there was no improvement in survival, and the effect was lost when treatment was discontinued. Although data is lacking, the widespread use of vaccination against HPV infections may lead to decreases in tumors associated with this virus.

Selected Readings

Adelstein DJ, Li Y, Adams GL, et al. An intergroup phase III comparison of standard radiation therapy and two schedules of concurrent chemoradiotherapy in patients with unresectable squamous cell head and neck cancer. *J Clin Oncol.* 2003;21:92–98.

Adelstein DJ, Ridge JA, Gillison ML, et al. Head and neck squamous cell cancer and the human papillomavirus: summary of a National Cancer Institute State of the Science meeting, November 9-10, 2008, Washington DC. *Head Neck.* 2009;31:1393–1422.

Al-Sarraf M, LeBlanc M, Giri PG, et al. Chemoradiotherapy versus radiotherapy in patients with advanced nasopharyngeal cancer: phase III randomized intergroup study 0099. *J Clin Oncol.* 1998;16:1310–1317.

Bernier J, Cooper JS, Pajak TF, et al. Defining risk levels in locally advanced head and neck cancers: a comparative analysis of concurrent postoperative radiation plus chemotherapy trials of the EORTC (#22931) and RTOG (# 9501). *Head Neck.* 2005;27:843–850.

Bonner JA, Harari PM, Giralt J, et al. Radiotherapy plus cetuximab for squamous-cell carcinoma of the head and neck. *N Engl J Med.* 2006;354(6):567–578.

Brizel DM, Albers ME Fisher SR, et al. Hyperfractionated irradiation with or without concurrent chemotherapy for locally advanced head and neck cancer. *N Engl J Med.* 1998;338:1798–1804.

Brosky M. The role of saliva in oral health: strategies for prevention and management of xerostomia. *J Support Oncol.* 2007;5:215–225.

Chambers MS, Garden A, Kies MS, Martin JW. Radiation-induced xerostomia in patients with head and neck cancer: pathogenesis, impact on quality of life, and management. *Head Neck.* 2004;26:796–807.

Chan ATC. Head and neck cancer: treatment of nasopharyngeal cancer. *Annals of Oncology.* 2005;16(Supplement 2):ii265–268.

Cohen EE. Role of epidermal growth factor receptor pathway-targeted therapy in patients with recurrent and/or metastatic squamous cell carcinoma of the head and neck. *J Clin Oncol.* 2006;24:2659–2665.

Cooper JS, Pajak TF, Forastiere AA, et al. Postoperative concurrent radiotherapy and chemotherapy for high-risk squamous-cell carcinoma of the head and neck. *N Engl J Med.* 2004;350:1937–1944.

Cmelak AJ, Li S, Goldwasser MA, et al. Phase II trial of chemoradiation for organ preservation in resectable stage III or IV squamous cell carcinomas of the larynx or oropharynx: results of Eastern Cooperative Oncology Group Study E2399. *J Clin Oncol.* 2007;25(25):3971–3977.

Denis F, Garaud P, Bardet E, et al. Final results of the 94-01 French Head and Neck Oncology and Radiotherapy Group randomized trial comparing radiotherapy alone with concomitant radiochemotherapy in advanced-stage oropharynx carcinoma. *J Clin Oncol.* 2004;22:69–76.

Department of Veterans Affairs Laryngeal Cancer Study Group. Induction chemotherapy plus radiation compared with surgery plus radiation in patients with advanced laryngeal cancer. *N Engl J Med.* 1991;324:1685–1690.

Edge SE, Byrd DR, Compton CA (eds). *AJCC Cancer Staging Manual*, 7th ed. New York: Springer; 2010.

Fakhry C, Gillison ML. Clinical implications of human papillomavirus in head and neck cancers. *J Clin Oncol.* 2006;24:2606–2611.

Forastiere AA, Goepfert H, Maor M, et al. Concurrent chemotherapy and radiotherapy for organ preservation in advanced laryngeal cancer. *N Engl J Med.* 2003;349:2091–2098.

Forastiere AA, Ang K, Brizel D, et al. Head and neck cancers. *J Natl Compr Canc Netw.* 2005;3:316–391.

Forastiere AA, Metch B, Schuller DE, et al. Randomized comparison of cisplatin plus fluorouracil and carboplatin plus fluorouracil vs. methotrexate in advanced squamous-cell carcinoma of the head and neck: a Southwest Oncology Group study. *J Clin Oncol.* 1992;10:1245–1251.

Forastiere AA, Trotti A, Pfister DG, Grandis JR. Head and neck cancer: recent advances and new standards of care. *J Clin Oncol.* 2006;24:2603–2605.

Garden AS, Harris J, Vokes EE, et al. Preliminary results of Radiation Therapy Oncology Group 97-03: a randomized phase II trial of concurrent radiation and chemotherapy for advanced squamous cell carcinomas of the head and neck. *J Clin Oncol.* 2004;22:2856–2864.

Gillison M, Koch W, Carbone R. Evidence for a causal association between human papillomavirus and a subset of head and neck cancers. *J Natl Cancer Inst.* 2000; 92:709–720.

Gibson MK, Li Y, Murphy B, et al. Randomized phase III evaluation of cisplatin plus fluorouracil versus cisplatin plus paclitaxel in advanced head and neck cancer (E1395): an intergroup trial of the Eastern Cooperative Oncology Group. *J Clin Oncol.* 2005;23:3562–3567.

Hitt R, López-Pousa A, Martinez-Trufero J, et al. Phase III study comparing cisplatin plus fluorouracil to paclitaxel, cisplatin, and fluorouracil induction chemotherapy followed by chemoradiotherapy in locally advanced head and neck cancer. *J Clin Oncol.* 2005;23:8636–8645.

Kim JG, Sohn SK, Kim DH, et al. Phase II study of concurrent chemoradiotherapy with capecitabine and cisplatin in patients with locally advanced squamous cell carcinoma of the head and neck. *Br J Cancer.* 2005;93:1117–1121.

Lefebvre J-L, Chevalier D, Luboinski B, et al. Larynx preservation in pyriform sinus cancer: preliminary results of a European Organization for Research and Treatment of Cancer phase III trial. *J Natl Cancer Inst.* 1996;88:890–899.

Murphy BA. Clinical and economic consequences of mucositis induced by chemotherapy and/or radiation therapy. *J Support Oncol.* 2007;5(9 Suppl 4):13–21.

Murphy BA, Gilbert J. Dysphagia in head and neck cancer patients treated with radiation: assessment, sequelae, and rehabilitation. *Semin Radiat Oncol.* 2009; 19(1):35–42.

Murphy BA, Gilbert J, Cmelak A, Ridner SH. Symptom control issues and supportive care of patients with head and neck cancers. *Clin Adv Hematol Oncol.* 2007;5(10):807–822.

Murphy BA, Gilbert J, Ridner SH. Systemic and global toxicities of head and neck treatment. *Expert Rev Anticancer Ther.* 2007;7(7):1043–1053.

Murphy BA, Ridner S, Wells N, Dietrich M. Quality of life research in head and neck cancer: a review of the current state of the science. *Crit Rev Oncol Hematol.* 2007;62(3):251–267.

Posner MR, Hershock DM, Blajman CR, et al. Cisplatin and fluorouracil alone or with docetaxel in head and neck cancer. *N Engl J Med.* 2007;357(17):1705–1715.

Piccirillo JF, Lacy PD, Basu A, et al. Development of a new head and neck cancer-specific comorbidity index. *Arch Otolaryngol Head Neck Surg.* 2002;128: 1172–1179.

Pignon JP, Le Maitre A, Bourhis J, et al. Meta-analysis of chemotherapy in head and neck cancer (MACH-NC): an update. *Int J Radiation Oncology Biol Phys.* 2007;69(2):112–114.

Pignon J-P, le Maître A, Maillard E, Bourhis J. Meta-analysis of chemotherapy in head and neck cancer (MACH-NC): an update on 93 randomised trials and 17,346 patients. *Radiother Oncol.* 2009;92:4–14.

Pfister DG, Laurie SA, Weinstein GS, et al. American Society of Clinical Oncology clinical practice guideline for the use of larynx-preservation strategies in the treatment of laryngeal cancer. *J Clin Oncol.* 2006;24:3693–3704.

Shah KM, Young LS. Epstein-Barr virus and carcinogenesis: beyond Burkitt's lymphoma. *Clin Microbiol Infect.* 2009;15:982–988.

6 Carcinoma of the Lung

David E. Gerber and Joan H. Schiller

Carcinoma of the lung is responsible for more than 165,000 deaths each year in the United States. This represents one-third of all deaths due to cancer and more than the number of deaths due to breast, colon, and prostate cancers combined. Because early-stage lung tumors are often asymptomatic and there has been no proven approach to radiographic screening, most patients are diagnosed with advanced stage disease. Approximately 85% of cases are histologically classified as non–small-cell lung cancer (NSCLC), of which adenocarcinoma, squamous cell carcinoma, and large cell carcinoma are the primary subtypes. Small-cell lung cancer (SCLC) accounts for the remaining 15% of cases. The biology, staging, and treatment of SCLC differ substantially from NSCLC. Thus, these two groups are addressed in two separate sections.

I. ETIOLOGY

Lung cancer is predominantly a disease of smokers. Eighty-five percent of lung cancer occurs in active or former smokers, and an additional 5% of cases are estimated to occur as a consequence of passive exposure to tobacco smoke. Tobacco smoke causes an increased incidence of all four histologic types of lung cancer, although adenocarcinoma (particularly the bronchioloalveolar variant) is also found in nonsmokers. Other risk factors for lung cancer include exposure to asbestos or radon. Familial factors such as polymorphisms in carcinogen-metabolizing hepatic enzyme systems may also play a role in determining an individual's propensity to develop lung cancer.

II. MOLECULAR BIOLOGY

Numerous genetic changes have been associated with lung tumors. Most common among these include activation or overexpression of the myc family of oncogenes in SCLC and NSCLC and of the KRAS oncogene in NSCLC, particularly adenocarcinoma. Inactivation or deletion of the p53 and retinoblastoma tumor suppressor genes and a tumor suppressor gene on chromosome 3p (the FHIT gene) have been found in 50% to 90% of patients with SCLC. Abnormalities of p53 and 3p have been associated with 50% to 70% of cases of NSCLC. The KRAS mutation is more frequently found in smokers, those with adenocarcinoma, and those with poorly differentiated tumors. It is also associated with poor prognosis.

Recently, abnormalities in the epidermal growth factor receptor (EGFR) pathway have been identified, making EGFR an attractive molecular target for anticancer therapy. EGFR is expressed or overexpressed in the majority of NSCLC tumors. Binding of ligand to the extracellular domain of EGFR causes receptor dimerization, which in turn activates an intracellular tyrosine kinase domain. Autophosphorylation of the receptor induces a cascade of signal transduction events leading to cell proliferation, inhibition of apoptosis, angiogenesis, and invasion, all resulting in tumor growth and spread. Agents targeting EGFR include tyrosine kinase inhibitors (TKIs), such as gefitinib and erlotinib, and anti-EGFR monoclonal antibodies (MoAbs), such as cetuximab and panitumumab. Tumors harboring activating EGFR gene mutations, which render the cancer highly dependent on EGFR for proliferation and survival, often have dramatic and sustained responses to EGFR TKIs. KRAS and EGFR mutations are rarely found in the same tumor.

Still more recently, abnormalities in the anaplastic lymphoma kinase (ALK) gene have been identified in a subset of lung cancers. These molecular aberrations, which appear mutually exclusive with both EGFR and KRAS gene mutations, appear to render cancers highly responsive to ALK inhibitors in phase I studies. These agents are currently undergoing phase II and III testing.

III. SCREENING

Three U.S. randomized screening studies in the 1980s failed to detect an impact on mortality of screening high-risk patients with chest radiography or sputum cytology, although earlier-stage cancers were detected in the screened groups. Since then, however, low-dose spiral computed tomography (CT) has emerged as a possible new tool for lung cancer screening. Spiral CT is CT imaging in which only the pulmonary parenchyma is scanned, thus negating the use of intravenous contrast medium and the necessity of a physician having to be present. This type of scan can usually be done quickly (within one breath) and involves low doses of radiation. In a nonrandomized, controlled study from the Early Lung Cancer Action Project, low-dose CT was shown to be more sensitive than chest radiography in detecting lung nodules and lung cancer at early stages. However, despite these promising results, it is unclear whether screening with spiral CT will result in a reduction in lung cancer mortality. Potential methodologic issues pertaining to this and other screening studies include lead-time bias, length bias, and overdiagnosis. *Overdiagnosis* refers to the possibility that small tumors preferentially detected by screening would otherwise remain clinically silent until death from other causes. Furthermore, in some geographic regions, such as the midwestern United States, the incidence of benign nodules is relatively high, resulting in frequent follow-up biopsies that contribute to both the cost and morbidity of screening. To address these issues, the National Cancer Institute has recently completed a large randomized controlled trial (the Lung Screening Study) involving at least 15,000 participants over several years, and initial trial results found 20% fewer cancer deaths among the CT screened participants compared with those screened with chest radiographs.

IV. NSCLC

A. Histology

Until recently, the histologic subtype of NSCLC, while thought to influence the presentation and natural history of disease, did not affect patient management. Due to differences in both efficacy and safety, histologic designation now represents a primary consideration in treatment selection. For instance, bronchioloalveolar carcinoma, which has a predilection for younger, never-smoking women, is frequently associated with EGFR gene mutations and thus a high likelihood of response to EGFR inhibitors. Pemetrexed, a multitargeted antifolate, has greater efficacy for the treatment of nonsquamous tumors, presumably due to higher thymidylate synthase levels in squamous cell cancers. Bevacizumab, a MoAb directed against vascular endothelial growth factor (VEGF), is contraindicated in patients with squamous cell tumors due to unacceptably high rates of life-threatening hemoptysis in early phase clinical trials. These histology-dependent safety and efficacy distinctions have highlighted the importance of accurate pathologic classification.

B. Staging

The prognosis and treatment of NSCLCs are dependent primarily on stage of disease at the time of diagnosis. Major changes in the staging of lung cancer were adopted in 2009. These changes are based on an analysis of 68,463 patients with NSCLC worldwide; by contrast, the previous (1997 and 2002) editions of the TNM classification of lung cancer were based on data from 5,319 patients in North America. The 2009 TNM staging classification is shown in Tables 6.1 and 6.2; the changes are summarized in Table 6.3. Major changes include subclassification of T1 and T2 by tumor size, reclassification of additional nodule(s) in the same lobe or another ipsilateral lobe, and reclassification of malignant effusions as M1a. This reflects the similar prognosis and treatment (typically chemotherapy alone) of patients with malignant effusions and patients with distant disease. As before, a pleural or pericardial effusion is considered malignant if it has any of the following characteristics: positive cytology, exudative, or hemorrhagic. Survival based on the 2009 staging classification is shown in Table 6.4.

C. Pretreatment evaluation

The diagnosis of lung cancer is usually made by bronchial biopsy or percutaneous needle biopsy. A CT scan of the chest is necessary to evaluate the extent of the primary disease, mediastinal extension or lymphadenopathy, and the presence or absence of other parenchymal nodules in patients in whom surgical resection is a consideration. The upper abdomen is included to evaluate for hepatic or adrenal metastases. Bone scans should be obtained for the patient with bone pain or an elevated calcium or alkaline phosphatase level. Head CT or magnetic resonance imaging (MRI) is not routinely done

TNM Definitions of NSCLC	
Descriptors	**Definitions**
T	**Primary Tumor**
T0	No primary tumor
T1	Tumor ≤3 cm in the greatest dimension, surrounded by lung or visceral pleura, not more proximal than the lobar bronchus
T1a	Tumor ≤2 cm in the greatest dimension
T1b	Tumor >2 but ≤3 cm in the greatest dimension
T2	Tumor >3 but ≤7 cm in the greatest dimension or tumor with any of the following*: invades visceral pleura, involves main bronchus ≥ 2 cm distal to the carina, atelectasis/obstructive pneumonia extending to hilum but not involving the entire lung
T2a	Tumor >3 but ≤5 cm in the greatest dimension
T2b	Tumor >5 but ≤7 cm in the greatest dimension
T3	Tumor >7 cm; directly invading chest wall, diaphragm, phrenic nerve, mediastinal pleura, or parietal pericardium; tumor in the main bronchus <2 cm distal to the carina[†]; atelectasis/obstructive pneumonitis of entire lung; or separate tumor nodules in the same lobe
T4	Tumor of any size with invasion of heart, great vessels, trachea, recurrent laryngeal nerve, esophagus, vertebral body, or carina; or separate tumor nodules in a different ipsilateral lobe
N	**Regional Lymph Nodes**
N0	No regional node metastasis
N1	Metastasis in ipsilateral peribronchial and/or perihilar lymph nodes and intrapulmonary nodes, including involvement by direct extension
N2	Metastasis in ipsilateral mediastinal and/or subcarinal lymph nodes
N3	Metastasis in contralateral mediastinal, contralateral hilar, ipsilateral or contralateral scalene, or supraclavicular lymph nodes
M	**Distant Metastasis**
M0	No distant metastasis
M1a	Separate tumor nodules in a contralateral lobe; or tumor with pleural nodules or malignant pleural dissemination[‡]
M1b	Distant metastasis
Special Situations	
TX, NX, MX	T, N, or M status not able to be assessed
Tis	Focus of in situ cancer
T1[†]	Superficial spreading tumor of any size but confined to the wall of the trachea or mainstem bronchus

*T2 tumors with these features are classified as T2a if ≤5 cm.
[†]The uncommon superficial spreading tumor in central airways is classified as T1.
[‡]Pleural effusions are excluded that are cytologically negative, nonbloody, transudative, and clinically judged not to be due to cancer.
Source: Rami-Porta R, Crowley JJ, Goldstraw P. The revised TNM staging system for lung cancer. *Ann Thorac Cardiovasc Surg.* 2009;15:4–9.

TABLE 6.2   Stage Groupings by TNM Elements for NSCLC

Stage Groups	Descriptors		
	T	N	M
Ia	T1a,b	N0	M0
Ib	T2a	N0	M0
IIa	T1a,b	N1	M0
	T2a	N1	M0
	T2b	N0	M0
IIb	T2b	N1	M0
	T3	N0	M0
IIIa	T1–3	N2	M0
	T3	N1	M0
	T4	N0,1	M0
IIIb	T4	N2	M0
	T1–4	N3	M0
IV	T_{Any}	N_{Any}	M1a,b

Source: Rami-Porta R, Crowley JJ, Goldstraw P. The revised TNM staging system for lung cancer. *Ann Thorac Cardiovasc Surg.* 2009;15:4–9.

in the absence of central nervous system (CNS) signs or symptoms. Because the presence of mediastinal nodal metastases is a key factor in determining tumor resectability, lymph node sampling by mediastinoscopy, Chamberlain procedure (which samples station 5 and 6 nodes not accessible by mediastinoscopy), and/or endobronchial ultrasound is recommended in most instances when there is not clear evidence of distant disease.

Positron emission tomography (PET), a metabolic imaging scan using fluorodeoxyglucose (FDG), has emerged as a useful staging modality. PET scans are more sensitive and specific than CT scans and could thus potentially save patients with advanced disease, either within or outside of the chest, from unnecessary invasive procedures. However, it is not yet clear as to whether PET scanning can replace mediastinal lymph node sampling, as the scan can be falsely positive in inflammatory processes and falsely negative in lung tumors with low metabolic activity such as bronchioloalveolar carcinoma or carcinoid tumors. Furthermore, due to high background FDG uptake in the brain, PET-CT scans are generally not sufficient to evaluate for brain metastases, and a head CT or MRI should be performed. PET scans are frequently performed in conjunction with CT imaging (PET-CT scans) to provide enhanced anatomic detail. Randomized clinical trials have demonstrated that use of PET-CT scans decreases the total number of thoracotomies and number of futile thoracotomies performed. Population-based studies suggest that increasing use of PET-CT scans may have resulted in stage shifting.

TABLE 6.3 2009 Major Changes to TNM Classification Stage Grouping of NSCLC

Component of Classification	Changes
T	Subclassify T1 according to tumor size:
	T1a: ≤2 cm
	T1b: >2 cm but ≤3 cm
	Subclassify T2 according to tumor size:
	T2a: >3 cm but ≤5 cm (or tumor with any other T2 descriptors, but ≤5 cm)
	T2b: >5 cm but ≤7 cm
	Reclassify T2 tumors >7 cm as T3
	Reclassify T4 tumors by additional nodule(s) in the same lobe of the primary tumor as T3
	Reclassify M1 tumors by additional nodule(s) in another ipsilateral lobe as T4
	Reclassify T4 tumors by malignant pleural effusion as M1a
N	No changes
M	Subclassify M1:
	M1a: separate tumor nodule(s) in contralateral lung; tumor with pleural nodules or malignant pleural (or pericardial) effusion
	M1b: distant metastasis

Stage Grouping	Changes
Large T2 tumors (T2b) N0M0	Upstage from IB to IIA
Small T2 tumors (T2a) N1M0	Downstage from IIB to IIA
T4 tumors N0 or N1 M0	Downstage from IIIB to IIIA

Source: Rami-Porta R, Crowley JJ, Goldstraw P. The revised TNM staging system for lung cancer. *Ann Thorac Cardiovasc Surg.* 2009;15:4–9.

TABLE 6.4 Five-year Survival Rates for New Clinical Stages of NSCLC

Clinical Stage	Five-year Survival
IA	50%
IB	47%
IIA	36%
IIB	26%
IIIA	19%
IIIB	7%
IV	2%

Source: Rami-Porta R, Crowley JJ, Goldstraw P. The revised TNM staging system for lung cancer. *Ann Thorac Cardiovasc Surg.* 2009;15:4–9.

Pulmonary function testing is generally recommended before surgery and, if severe pulmonary disease is clinically apparent, before radiation therapy. Increased postoperative morbidity is associated with a predicted postoperative 1-second forced expiratory volume of less than 800 to 1000 mL, a preoperative maximum voluntary ventilation less than 35% of predicted, a carbon monoxide diffusing capacity less than 60% of predicted, and an arterial oxygen pressure of less than 60 mm Hg or a carbon dioxide pressure of more than 45 mm Hg.

D. Management of early stage NSCLC

1. Stage I disease. Surgical resection is the mainstay of treatment for stage I NSCLC, with cure rates of 60% to 80%. Lobectomy is considered superior to smaller procedures such as wedge resection. An exception may be bronchioloalveolar cancer, which spreads by lepidic (airway) growth rather than hematogenous or lymphatic spread and may be adequately treated with more focal excision. Clinical studies evaluating this approach are ongoing. If not performed preoperatively, it is recommended that mediastinal lymph nodes be sampled at the time of resection to complete staging.

In patients with medical contraindications to surgery but with adequate pulmonary function, conventional fractionated radiotherapy (e.g., 6000 cGy in 30 fractions of 200 cGy each) results in cure in about 20% of patients. Recently, advances in imaging and radiation delivery have led to the use of stereotactic radiation therapy for lung tumors. With this technology, radiation delivery to surrounding normal lung parenchyma is substantially less than that occurring with conventional radiation. Thus, it is possible to give much higher, "ablative" radiation doses over a small number of fractions (e.g., 20 Gy per fraction for three fractions). To date, outcomes with this technique appear promising, with 2-year local control rates in excess of 90%. Clinical trials of stereotactic radiation for early stage lung cancer in both medically operable and inoperable patients are ongoing.

The rationale for adjuvant chemotherapy in patients with early-stage lung cancer is based on the observation that distant metastases are the most common site of failure following potentially curative surgery. Interest in this treatment strategy grew after a 1995 meta-analysis of over 4300 patients, in which those who received cisplatin-based regimens had a survival benefit nearing statistical significance ($p = 0.07$). Since then, a number of randomized clinical trials have evaluated the role of adjuvant chemotherapy following resection of early-stage NSCLC (see Table 6.5). In a pooled analysis of five of these trials, the hazard ratio for death was 0.89 (95% confidence interval [CI], 0.82–0.96; $p = 0.005$), corresponding to a 5-year absolute benefit of 5.4% from chemotherapy. Importantly, the benefit of chemotherapy varied considerably by

TABLE 6.5

Randomized Studies of Adjuvant Chemotherapy for Resected NSCLC

Trial	Patient Population (Stage)	Number of patients	Chemotherapy regimen		Absolute overall survival benefit
CALGB 9633 (2004)	IB	344	Carboplatin	AUC 6, on day 1	12% (4-year)
			Paclitaxel	200 mg/m^2 IV on day 1 every 3 weeks for four cycles	
NCIC JBR10 (2005)	IB, II	482	Cisplatin	50 mg/m^2 IV on days 1 and 8 every 4 weeks for four cycles	15% (5-year)
			Vinorelbine	25 mg/m^2 IV on days 1, 8, 15, and 22 every 4 weeks for four cycles	
ANITA (2005)	IB, II, IIIA	840	Cisplatin	100 mg/m^2 IV on day 1 every 4 weeks for four cycles	8% (5-year)
			Vinorelbine	30 mg/m^2/wk IV on days 1, 8, 15, and 22 every 4 weeks for four cycles	
IALT (2004)	I, II, IIIA	1867	Cisplatin (options)	80 mg/m^2 IV on days 1, 22, 43, and 64 100 mg/m^2 IV on days 1, 29, and 57 100 mg/m^2 IV on days 1, 29, 57, and 85 120 mg/m^2 IV on days 1, 29, and 71	5% (4-year)
			and Vindesine	3 mg/m^2 IV weekly on days 1–29, then every 2 weeks after day 43 until last cisplatin dose	
			or Vinblastine	4 mg/m^2 IV weekly on days 1–29, then every 2 weeks after day 43 until last cisplatin dose	
			or Vinorelbine	30 mg/m^2 IV weekly on day 1 to last cisplatin dose	
			or Etoposide	100 mg/m^2 IV on days 1–3 with each cisplatin dose	

ANITA, Adjuvant Navelbine International Trialist Association; AUC, area under the curve; CALGB, Cancer and Leukemia Group B; IALT, International Adjuvant Lung Cancer Trial; IV, intravenously; NCIC, National Cancer Institute of Canada.

stage. For stage IA NSCLC, adjuvant chemotherapy resulted in a trend toward worse survival (hazard ratio [HR] for death 1.40; 95% CI, 0.95–2.06). For stage IB disease, the HR was 0.93 (95% CI, 0.78–1.10). Similarly, in the CALGB 9633 trial of patients with stage IB disease randomized to surgery alone or surgery followed by carboplatin-paclitaxel, only those patients with tumors ≥4 cm demonstrated a significant survival difference in favor of adjuvant chemotherapy (HR, 0.69; 95% CI, 0.48–0.99; $p = 0.04$). Given these data, it seems reasonable to discuss the option of adjuvant platinum-based doublet chemotherapy with good performance status (PS) patients with completely resected stage IB disease, particularly those with tumors ≥4 cm. Additional studies are needed for stage IA disease before adjuvant therapy can be routinely recommended for this group of patients.

Patients with resected stage I NSCLC are also at high risk for the development of second lung cancers (about 2% to 3% per year). To date, however, secondary prevention efforts have proven unsuccessful. Neither vitamin A nor its derivatives, β-carotene or *cis*-retinoic acid, have been found to have any benefit in chemoprevention, and contrary to predictions, they may even be deleterious. A recent phase III trial of selenium for secondary prevention was closed early when an interim analysis showed no benefit.

2. **Stage II disease.** Surgical resection is a standard component of the treatment of stage II NSCLC. Patients with peripheral chest wall invasion (T3N0) should undergo resection of the involved ribs and underlying lung. Chest wall defects are then repaired with chest wall musculature or surgical mesh and methylmethacrylate. Postoperative radiotherapy is often given. Five-year survival rates as high as 50% have been reported.

The role of adjuvant chemotherapy for resected stage II NSCLC is clearer than for stage I disease. In the Adjuvant Navelbine International Trialist Association (ANITA) trial, patients with stage IB to IIIA NSCLC were randomized to surgery alone versus surgery followed by four cycles of cisplatin plus vinorelbine. Overall survival was significantly improved at 5 years (51% versus 43%), although the survival benefit was restricted to patients with stage II and IIIA disease. In the pooled analysis of cisplatin-based adjuvant chemotherapy trials, patients with stage II NSCLC had a significant survival benefit (HR 0.83; 95% CI, 0.73–0.95). Accordingly, adjuvant chemotherapy is generally recommended following complete resection of stage II NSCLC.

Issues in the use of adjuvant therapy have also included identification of the most appropriate drugs. Given the toxicity and tolerability of cisplatin, there was an interest in substituting carboplatin for adjuvant treatment of NSCLC. Based on available data, it is generally accepted that carboplatin should not routinely be used in lieu of cisplatin, but can be considered in patients that would be considered high risk for cisplatin.

The International Adjuvant Lung Cancer, BR10, and ANITA trials all used vinca alkaloids in combination with cisplatin. Given that there is no major difference in chemotherapy doublets in advanced disease, many clinicians have extrapolated that data in advanced disease to earlier stage disease and are using other "third generation" drugs in combination with cisplatin (such as pemetrexed, docetaxel, and gemcitabine), albeit without level 1 data.

Neoadjuvant (preoperative) chemotherapy has also been studied for resectable NSCLC (see Section IV.D.3). Compared to adjuvant chemotherapy, it offers the potential advantages of reducing tumor volume before surgery (which might simplify resection), demonstrating in vivo chemosensitivity, addressing micrometastatic disease earlier, and possibly being better tolerated. Although phase III trials comparing neoadjuvant platinum-based regimens with surgery alone have demonstrated the feasibility of this approach, there is no level 1 data showing a benefit for neoadjuvant compared to adjuvant therapy. In addition, patients who undergo a pneumonectomy following induction chemoradiation have a higher incidence of treatment-related deaths.

a. **Pancoast tumors.** Pancoast tumors are upper lobe tumors that adjoin the brachial plexus and are frequently associated with Horner syndrome or shoulder and arm pain; the latter is due to rib destruction, involvement of the C8 or T1 nerve roots, or both. These tumors are often treated with preoperative chemoradiation, surgery, and then additional postoperative chemotherapy. With this approach, the preoperative chemoradiation facilitates resection in an area where neural structures might otherwise limit surgical options. Five-year survival rates range from 25% to 50%.

3. **Locally advanced (stage IIIA and IIIB) disease.** Treatment of locally advanced NSCLC is one of the most controversial issues in the management of lung cancer. Interpretation of the results of clinical trials involving patients with locally advanced disease has been clouded by a number of issues including changing diagnostic techniques, different staging systems, and heterogeneous patient populations that may have disease that ranges from "nonbulky" stage IIIA (clinical N1 nodes, with microscopic N2 nodes discovered only at the time of surgery or mediastinoscopy) to "bulky" N2 nodes (enlarged adenopathy clearly visible on chest radiographs or multiple nodal level involvement) to clearly inoperable stage IIIB disease.

a. **Nonbulky stage IIIA disease.** The optimal treatment for nonbulky stage IIIA generally consists of a local approach (surgery or radiation therapy) plus a systemic treatment (chemotherapy). Current investigational efforts are directed at identifying the optimal combined-modality approach. Possibilities include surgery followed by adjuvant chemotherapy, preoperative (neoadjuvant) chemotherapy followed by surgery, chemotherapy plus radiation therapy (either concurrent or sequential), or a trimodality approach.

The potential benefit of adding surgery to combined chemoradiation for stage IIIA NSCLC has been evaluated in a recent randomized phase III intergroup trial. In this study, 396 patients with stage T1–3N2M0 NSCLC were randomized to concurrent chemoradiation (45 Gy) with cisplatin-etoposide followed by either surgical resection or continuation of radiation therapy to 61 Gy total. Although progression-free survival was significantly longer in the surgery arm (12.8 months versus 10.5 months; $p = 0.02$), there was no significant difference in overall survival (23.6 months versus 22.2 months; $p = 0.24$). There were greater treatment-related mortalities in the surgery arm as compared to the chemoradiation alone arm (8% versus 2%), particularly for patients undergoing a pneumonectomy.

Several studies have shown, in subset analyses, that those patients receiving neoadjuvant therapy who subsequently have their N2 nodes "cleared" with preoperative therapy do better than those who do not. As of this writing, there is no level 1 evidence to recommend neoadjuvant chemotherapy over adjuvant chemotherapy, although several theoretical reasons for doing so include the fact that patients are more likely to tolerate preoperative chemotherapy over postoperative chemotherapy.

Occasionally, despite preoperative staging, patients thought to have stage I or II disease are found to have N2 nodal involvement at the time of surgery. For these stage III patients, postoperative radiation therapy (PORT; 50–54 Gy) may be considered for fit patients, preferably after completion of adjuvant chemotherapy, based on retrospective and nonrandomized studies demonstrating benefit. Currently, PORT is not recommended for patients with less than N2 nodal involvement.

b. **Bulky stage IIIA (N2) and stage IIIB.** Bulky stage IIIA and IIIB tumors are generally considered unresectable, with treatment consisting of combined chemoradiation or, in the case of malignant pleural or pericardial effusions (M1a in the new staging classification), chemotherapy alone.

(1) **Chemotherapy plus radiation therapy.** Chemotherapy plus radiotherapy is the treatment of choice for patients with bulky or inoperable stage IIIA or IIIB disease without pleural effusion. Numerous randomized studies have demonstrated an

improvement in median and long-term survival with chemotherapy plus radiation therapy versus radiation therapy alone. Active areas of investigation include choice of chemotherapy, fractionation, and treatment fields.

A randomized Japanese trial reported a 3-month survival advantage with concurrent chemoradiation over a sequential approach. Initial reports from a confirmatory randomized Radiation Therapy Oncology Group trial also showed a trend in favor of concurrent cisplatin and vinblastine with radiation over sequential chemoradiation, albeit with more toxicities, making concurrent chemoradiation therapy the treatment of choice for good PS patients.

Chemotherapy can be given in full "systemic" doses with radiotherapy, in weekly "radiosensitizing" doses, or a combination of both. One of the most commonly used chemotherapy regimens for stage III NSCLC is carboplatin in combination with paclitaxel (Table 6.6). Although single agent weekly carboplatin alone has not resulted in a survival benefit when given with radiotherapy, weekly doses of paclitaxel at 50 mg/m^2 and carboplatin area under the curve (AUC) 2 with concurrent radiation have proved promising in randomized phase II studies. Generally, concurrent therapy is followed by two cycles of full-dose carboplatin AUC 6 plus paclitaxel at 200 mg/m^2 every 21 days to treat micrometastatic disease. By contrast, with concurrent radiation therapy and commonly used cisplatin-etoposide chemotherapy regimens, drug doses during radiation therapy are considered "systemic" and may not require additional chemotherapy after radiation therapy

TABLE 6.6 Chemotherapy Regimens for Concurrent Chemoradiation for Stage III NSCLC

Induction Chemotherapy (Concurrent with Radiation)		Consolidation Chemotherapy	
Etoposide plus cisplatin			
Etoposide	50 mg/m^2 days 1–5 and 29–33	None	
Cisplatin	50 mg/m^2 days 1, 8, 29, and 36		
Carboplatin plus paclitaxel			
Carboplatin	AUC 2 weekly	Carboplatin	AUC 6, on day 1 every 3 weeks for two cycles
Paclitaxel	45 mg/m^2 over 1 hour weekly	Paclitaxel	200 mg/m^2 IV on day 1 over 3 hours every 3 weeks for two cycles

AUC, area under the curve; IV, intravenously.

is completed. No survival benefit has been shown for "consolidation" therapy.

4. **Stage IV disease.** Chemotherapy improves survival in patients with metastatic NSCLC (about 10% 1-year survival rate in untreated patients versus 30% to 35% 1-year survival rate with treatment). The principal factors predicting response to chemotherapy and survival are PS and extent of disease. Patients with a poor PS (Eastern Cooperative Oncology Group [ECOG] PS of 2–4) are less likely to respond to treatment and will tolerate the therapy poorly, although recent subset retrospective analysis has suggested that PS2 patients may also enjoy a modest benefit in survival with treatment. Favorable prognostic factors include female sex, normal serum lactic dehydrogenase level, absence of bone or liver metastases, and absence of weight loss.

a. **First-line chemotherapy.** Systemic treatment for patients with metastatic NSCLC and adequate PS (ECOG 0–1) generally includes platinum-based doublet chemotherapy. A meta-analysis of large randomized trials indicated that there is a small but significant survival advantage with platinum-based therapy compared with best supportive care. Whereas best supportive care resulted in median survival rates of 4 to 5 months and 1-year survival rates of 5% to 10%, current third-generation regimens of platins combined with paclitaxel and docetaxel, gemcitabine, vinorelbine, and pemetrexed have yielded median survivals of 8 to 9 months and 1-year survivals of 35% to 40%. In addition, randomized studies have shown an improvement in symptoms and quality of life compared with patients treated with best supportive care.

b. **Choice of chemotherapy.** The common chemotherapy regimens for advanced NSCLC are shown in Table 6.7. Historically, randomized studies have failed to show a major advantage of one new doublet regimen over another. Due to a favorable toxicity profile, carboplatin-paclitaxel was the most frequently used combination in the United States. More recently, however, certain agents have been restricted to specific histologies. For instance, pemetrexed, a multitargeted antifolate, has greater efficacy for the treatment of nonsquamous tumors, presumably due to higher thymidylate synthase levels in squamous cell cancers; pemetrexed is approved only for nonsquamous NSCLC in all settings (first-line, maintenance, and second-line). Bevacizumab, a MoAb directed against VEGF, is contraindicated in patients with squamous cell tumors due to unacceptably high rates of life-threatening hemoptysis in early phase clinical trials.

Although a direct comparison of cisplatin-based therapies and carboplatin-based therapies is limited, meta-analyses have

TABLE 6.7 Common Front-Line Regimens for Metastatic NSCLC

Cisplatin plus vinorelbine

Cisplatin	100 mg/m² IV on day 1
Vinorelbine	25 mg/m² weekly
	Repeat cycle every 4 weeks

Carboplatin-paclitaxel plus bevacizumab (nonsquamous cell histology only)

Carboplatin	AUC 6 on day 1
Paclitaxel	200 mg/m² IV on day 1 over 3 hours
	Repeat cycle every 3 weeks
Bevacizumab	15 mg/kg IV every 3 weeks until progression

Cisplatin/carboplatin plus gemcitabine

Cisplatin	100 mg/m² IV on day 1
Gemcitabine	1000 mg/m² IV on days 1, 8, and 15
	Repeat each cycle every 4 weeks

or

Cisplatin	80 mg/m² IV on day 1
Gemcitabine	1250 mg/m² IV on days 1 and 8
	Repeat each cycle every 3 weeks

or

Carboplatin	AUC 5 on day 1
Gemcitabine	1000 mg/m² IV on days 1 and 8
	Repeat each cycle every 3 weeks

Cisplatin/carboplatin plus docetaxel

Cisplatin	75 mg/m² IV on day 1
Docetaxel	75 mg/m² IV on day 1
	Repeat each cycle every 3 weeks

or

Carboplatin	AUC 6 on day 1
Docetaxel	75 mg/m² IV on day 1
	Repeat each cycle every 3 weeks

Cisplatin/carboplatin plus pemetrexed (nonsquamous cell histology only)

Cisplatin	75 mg/m² IV on day 1
Pemetrexed*	500 mg/m² on day 1
	Repeat each cycle every 3 weeks

or

Carboplatin	AUC 6 on day 1
Pemetrexed*	500 mg/m² on day 1
	Repeat each cycle every 3 weeks

Cisplatin-vinorelbine plus cetuximab

Cisplatin	80 mg/m² IV on day 1
Vinorelbine	25 mg/m² IV on days 1 and 8
	Repeat each cycle every 3 weeks
Cetuximab	400 mg/m² IV on day 1 then 250 mg/m² weekly until progression

EGFR tyrosine Kinase inhibitors

Gefitinib	250 mg by mouth daily: only in front-line therapy of patients with EGFR mutations

AUC, area under the curve; IV, intravenously.

* To reduce toxicity rates, patients treated with pemetrexed should receive (1) vitamin B_{12} 1000 μg intramuscularly every 9 weeks during treatment starting 1 week before first pemetrexed dose and (2) folic acid 400–1000 μg by mouth daily starting 1 week before first pemetrexed dose and continuing until 21 days after the last pemetrexed dose.

suggested that cisplatin may have a small benefit in terms of survival over carboplatin, albeit with a different toxicity profile. Whereas this small difference may be of limited clinical consequence for patients with metastatic disease, it may be more important in the adjuvant setting, where cure is the goal.

c. **Inhibitors of angiogenesis.** Inhibition of angiogenesis is based on the observations that neovascularization occurs in tumor tissues and rarely in other physiologic processes except wound healing. Although many antiangiogenesis agents are under investigation, such as VEGF receptor TKIs, the drug that has been shown to have survival benefit in NSCLC is the anti-VEGF MoAb bevacizumab (Avastin).

Bevacizumab has been evaluated in a randomized ECOG trial in combination with standard cytotoxic chemotherapy for advanced NSCLC, in which 878 chemonaïve patients with advanced NSCLC were randomized to receive carboplatin and paclitaxel with or without bevacizumab (15 mg/kg) every 3 weeks for six cycles. Bevacizumab was continued for up to 1 year in patients with nonprogressing disease. Patients with squamous cell histology were excluded based on phase II data showing increased hemorrhagic events as a complication with bevacizumab therapy. The study demonstrated an improvement in median survival (12.3 months versus 10.3 months; $p < 0.001$), overall response rates (35% versus 15%; $p < 0.001$), and progression-free survival (6.2 months versus 4.5 months; $p < 0.001$), favoring the bevacizumab arm. A European study showed a small improvement in progression-free survival with 7.5 mg/kg or 15 mg/kg of bevacizumab plus gemcitabine and cisplatin, compared to gemcitabine plus cisplatin alone, but no improvement in overall survival.

d. **Inhibitors of EGFR.** EGFR, also known as human epidermal growth factor receptor 1 (HER1) or ErbB1, is a transmembrane receptor tyrosine kinase. On ligand binding, receptor subunits dimerize, resulting in autophosphorylation of intracellular tyrosine residues and initiation of a signal transduction cascade resulting in cellular proliferation, resistance to apoptosis, cellular invasion, metastasis, and angiogenesis. EGFR-inhibiting drugs are classified as TKIs (also called small molecule inhibitors because of their low molecular weight) or MoAbs.

TKIs are almost always oral drugs, taken on a daily basis. They are often metabolized via the cytochrome P450 system and therefore prone to drug-drug interactions. Most of these drugs have names ending in "-ib." MoAbs are always administered intravenously and may be associated with acute infusion reactions. They have a molecular weight of approximately 150,000 daltons and have names ending in "-ab." From a mechanistic perspective, EGFR TKIs and anti-EGFR

MoAbs inhibit the activation of EGFR via direct binding to the kinase activation site or by blocking ligand-receptor binding, respectively. MoAbs may potentially also exert anticancer effects via recruitment of endogenous immune functions (e.g., antibody-dependent cellular cytotoxicity and complement-mediated cytotoxicity). The primary toxicities of EGFR TKIs are acneiform rash and diarrhea. Anti-EGFR MoAbs are also associated with acneiform rash.

Four clinical trials have randomized over 4000 total patients to platinum doublet chemotherapy with or without an EGFR TKI (two studies with gefitinib; two studies with erlotinib). None of these studies demonstrated a survival benefit. Potential explanations for these disappointing results include pharmacodynamic antagonism (EGFR TKI-induced cell-cycle arrest could reduce the efficacy of cytotoxic chemotherapy agents) and enrollment of a nonenriched population. However, in the first-line Iressa Pan-Asia Study (IPASS), in which over 1200 previously untreated nonsmokers or former light smokers in East Asia who had advanced adenocarcinoma NSCLC were randomized to gefitinib at 250 mg orally daily or carboplatin-paclitaxel, progression-free survival was superior in the gefitinib arm (HR 0.74; p <0.001), with 12-month progression-free survival rates 25% for gefitinib and 7% for carboplatin-paclitaxel. Among those patients whose tumors harbored EGFR mutations, progression-free survival was significantly longer with gefitinib (HR 0.48; p <0.001); by contrast, in the mutation-negative group, gefitinib resulted in significantly shorter progression-free survival compared with carboplatin-paclitaxel (HR 2.85; p <0.001). Although mature survival data is pending, these results suggest that single-agent gefitinib may be an appropriate first-line therapy in patients with EGFR mutations.

A phase III clinical trial of cisplatin-vinorelbine with or without the anti-EGFR antibody cetuximab in patients with EGFR-expressing NSCLC (80% to 90% of cases) demonstrated a modest but statistically significant increase in survival: 11.3 months versus 10.1 months (p = 0.04). Whether the discrepant results with EGFR TKIs or an anti-EGFR antibody combined with chemotherapy reflect differences in drug efficacy, study design, or other factors is not clear.

e. **Duration of therapy/maintenance therapy.** Four randomized studies failed to show a survival difference with "prolonged" (more than six) cycles of chemotherapy compared with a fewer (four to six) number of cycles. Thus, until recently, continuing chemotherapy until progression has not been routinely recommended.

This approach has been challenged by recent randomized clinical trials of "maintenance" chemotherapy. The term *maintenance* in this context requires clarification. In some instances, it may refer to continuation of initial therapy (as in the studies described previously). In other instances, *maintenance* refers to continuation of a component of initial therapy (as with the ongoing administration of bevacizumab or cetuximab following completion of a maximum of six cycles of combination chemotherapy). Finally, *maintenance* may refer to immediate introduction of another agent on completion of first-line chemotherapy (sometimes called "switch" maintenance). It is this concept that has been evaluated in two recent phase III studies.

In one trial, 309 patients were randomized to immediate versus delayed (instituted at time of disease progression) docetaxel at 75 mg/m^2 every 21 days on completion of four cycles of carboplatin-gemcitabine. Median progression-free survival was significantly longer in the immediate docetaxel group (5.7 months versus 2.7 months; $p = 0.0001$). Median overall survival was also longer, although the difference was not statistically significant (12.3 months versus 9.7 months; $p = 0.09$). Quality of life did not differ significantly between the two groups ($p = 0.76$). In another trial, 663 patients who had not progressed on four cycles of platinum-based chemotherapy were randomized 2:1 to maintenance pemetrexed at 500 mg/m^2 every 21 days or placebo until progression. Pemetrexed significantly improved median progression-free survival (4.3 months versus 2.6 months; $p < 0.0001$) and median overall survival (13.4 months versus 10.6 months; $p = 0.01$), benefits that were limited to nonsquamous tumors.

Although a substantial proportion of thoracic oncologists have adopted maintenance chemotherapy, a number of questions remain. First, how maintenance therapy fits into the increasingly complex overall treatment paradigm for advanced NSCLC is not clear, as some first-line regimens (such as those incorporating bevacizumab or cetuximab) continue treatment until progression. Second, it is not clear whether these studies demonstrate a benefit from early use of docetaxel or pemetrexed, or rather a benefit from exposure—regardless of timing—to these drugs.

f. **Non-platinum–based regimens.** Given the toxicities associated with platinum-based chemotherapy, particularly cisplatin, there is considerable interest in combining two nonplatinum drugs. The majority of recent randomized trials have failed to show a significant difference in survival with platinum regimens compared with non-platinum–based regimens, although the toxicity profile is different.

g. **Patients with poor performance status.** Patients with ECOG PS2 may be treated with single agent cytotoxic chemotherapy. The most commonly studied agents include vinorelbine and the taxanes. Patients with ECOG PS3–4 are generally not offered chemotherapy. A potential exception is a patient with a tumor harboring an activating EGFR mutation (see subsequent discussion). For such a patient, an EGFR TKI could result in a dramatic response without conveying substantial toxicity.

h. **Oligometastatic disease.** In certain circumstances, definitive local therapy of both thoracic disease and a metastatic site may be considered. In patients with controlled disease outside of the brain who have an isolated cerebral metastasis in a resectable area, resection followed by whole brain radiation is superior to whole brain radiotherapy alone. This oligometastatic approach appears most beneficial in patients with stage I thoracic disease, where survival approximates that of stage I patients without brain metastases. In patients with locally advanced thoracic disease, the benefit of metastasectomy is less clear. Stereotactic radiosurgery may be another option for these patients. Adrenalectomy for an isolated adrenal metastasis may be associated with up to 25% 5-year survival. Outcomes appear to be superior for patients with a metachronous rather than a synchronous metastasis.

5. **Second-line chemotherapy.** Docetaxel, pemetrexed, and erlotinib are currently approved by the U.S. Food and Drug Administration (FDA) for second-line monotherapy for patients with metastatic NSCLC.

   a. **Docetaxel.** There have been two randomized trials evaluating second-line docetaxel versus best supportive care in patients who have failed first-line therapy. Docetaxel at a dose of 75 mg/m^2 every 3 weeks significantly prolongs survival in comparison with best supportive care and, in comparison with either vinorelbine or ifosfamide, improves time to progression and 1-year survival. Moreover, it also improves quality of life. It was noted that previous paclitaxel exposure did not affect patients' response to docetaxel, suggesting no cross-resistance between the two taxane agents.

   b. **Pemetrexed.** Pemetrexed has similar antitumor activity as docetaxel in the second-line setting but with less toxicity. In a randomized trial, patients were treated with pemetrexed at 500 mg/m^2 or docetaxel at 75 mg/m^2 every 3 weeks. Overall response rates were similar (9.1% versus 8.8% for pemetrexed and docetaxel, respectively) with no differences in median survival (8.3 months versus 7.9 months for pemetrexed and docetaxel, respectively). Docetaxel was associated with higher rates of neutropenia, neutropenic fever, and hospitalization due to neutropenic events or other drug-related adverse events as compared to pemetrexed. A post hoc analysis by histology demonstrated a selective benefit for pemetrexed in nonsquamous histology.

c. **EGFR TKIs**

   (1) **Gefitinib.** Gefitinib was granted FDA approval for previously treated advanced NSCLC based on the outcomes of phase II studies. However, the subsequent phase III Iressa Survival Evaluation in Lung Cancer (ISEL) trial of over 1,600 patients failed to demonstrate a significant survival benefit compared to placebo (median 5.6 months versus 5.1 months; $p = 0.09$). A subgroup analysis showed significant benefit for patients of Asian origin and in nonsmokers (median survival 8.9 months versus 6.1 months; $p = 0.012$). Following the negative survival result, gefitinib was relabeled for use restricted to patients already receiving and benefiting from the drug or patients participating in clinical trials. This essentially removed the drug from the American and European markets, although it remained approved and widely used in Asia. Recently, interest in gefitinib has risen again in response to highly encouraging outcomes in clinically and molecularly enriched patient populations.

   (2) **Erlotinib.** Erlotinib is a similar orally available EGFR/TKI. Single-agent treatment with erlotinib for previously treated advanced NSCLC was evaluated in the National Cancer Institute of Canada BR21 trial. This study randomized 731 patients with stage IIIB or IV NSCLC who had failed one or two prior treatment regimens in a 2:1 ratio to receive erlotinib at 150 mg orally daily versus placebo. The overall response rate for erlotinib was 9% versus <1% for placebo ($p <0.001$). Stable disease was observed in 35% of patients on the erlotinib arm as compared to 27% of patients on placebo. In contrast to the results with gefitinib, there was a significant improvement in progression-free survival (2.2 months versus 1.8 months; $p <0.001$) and overall survival (6.7 months versus 4.7 months; $p <0.001$), in favor of erlotinib. While all patient subtypes in BR21 derived a survival benefit, the hazard ratio of 0.4 for never-smokers was statistically significantly different than the hazard ratio of 0.9 for smokers ($p <0.001$).

   A number of explanations for the different outcomes of the phase III ISEL (gefitinib) and BR21 (erlotinib) trials have been proposed. Erlotinib may have been administered at a more biologically effective dose, as evidenced by higher rates of rash and diarrhea in the BR21 study. The ISEL study may have selected for patients with particularly aggressive disease, as subjects were required to have disease relapse or progression within 90 days after prior platinum chemotherapy. The BR21 study did not specify timing of disease relapse or progression.

(3) Identification of the target population. Clinical parameters that appear to predict response to EGFR TKIs include never-smoking history, East Asian ethnicity, adenocarcinoma histology (particularly tumors with bronchioloalveolar features), and female gender. Molecular analysis of tumor specimens from individuals with these characteristics has revealed high rates of activating mutations in the EGFR tyrosine kinase domain. These mutations hyperactivate the EGFR tyrosine kinase, rendering cancer cells highly dependent on EGFR oncogenic pathways and thus exquisitely sensitive to EGFR inhibition. Among patients with "classic" EGFR mutations (exon 19 in-frame deletions of amino acids 747–750 and exon 21 L858R substitutions), response rates to EGFR TKIs exceed 60% and median survival exceeds 2 years. EGFR amplification and gene copy number (determined by fluorescence in situ hybridization) have also been employed to predict a survival benefit to these therapies. EGFR protein expression, determined by immunohistochemistry, is not as strongly correlated with outcomes. Additionally, development of acneiform rash has been associated with improved survival for both EGFR TKIs and anti-EGFR MoAbs in multiple disease settings, including colorectal cancer, pancreatic cancer, and NSCLC.

Clinical and molecular enrichment strategies are exemplified by the recent phase III first-line IPASS trial. In this trial, over 1200 previously untreated nonsmokers or former light smokers in East Asia who had advanced adenocarcinoma NSCLC were randomized to gefitinib at 250 mg orally daily or carboplatin-paclitaxel. Despite a highly clinically enriched population, only 60% of patients had tumors harboring EGFR mutations. Among these patients, progression-free survival was significantly longer with gefitinib (HR 0.48; $p < 0.001$); by contrast, in the mutation-negative group, gefitinib resulted in significantly shorter progression-free survival compared with carboplatin-paclitaxel (HR 2.85; $p < 0.001$). Early survival results did not show a difference between the gefitinib arm and the carboplatin-paclitaxel arm, presumably because patients were allowed to crossover to the other arm on progression. With outcomes such as these supporting EGFR mutations as strong predictors of benefit from EGFR TKIs but data from second-line trials demonstrating a survival benefit from EGFR TKIs in unselected populations, it remains debated whether and in which patients EGFR mutation testing should be routinely performed.

V. SCLC

SCLC differs from NSCLC in a number of important ways. First, it has a more rapid clinical course and natural history, with the rapid development of metastases, symptoms, and death. Untreated, the median survival time for patients with local disease is typically 12 to 15 weeks and for those with advanced disease 6 to 9 weeks. Second, it exhibits features of neuroendocrine differentiation in many patients (which may be distinguishable histopathologically) and is more commonly associated with paraneoplastic syndromes. Third, unlike NSCLC, SCLC is exquisitely sensitive to both chemotherapy and radiotherapy, although resistant disease often develops. Because of the rapid development of distant disease and its extreme sensitivity to the cytotoxic effects of chemotherapy, this mode of therapy forms the backbone of treatment for this disease, irrespective of stage.

A. Staging

Although SCLC has a propensity to metastasize quickly and micrometastatic disease is presumed to be present in all patients at the time of diagnosis, this disease is usually classified into either a local or an extensive stage. Local disease is typically defined as disease that can be encompassed within one radiation port, usually considered limited to the hemithorax and to regional nodes, including mediastinal and ipsilateral supraclavicular nodes. Extensive-stage disease is usually defined as disease that has spread outside those areas.

B. Pretreatment evaluation

Common sites of metastases for SCLC include the brain, liver, bone marrow, bone, and CNS. For this reason, a complete staging work-up has traditionally consisted of a complete blood cell count; liver function tests; CT or MRI of the brain; CT of the chest and abdomen; bone scan; and bone marrow aspiration and biopsy. As for NSCLC, PET-CT scans are now routinely employed in the initial staging of SCLC and may be considered in place of the CT chest/abdomen and bone scan. However, this complete staging work-up need not be undertaken unless the patient is a candidate for combined-modality treatment with chest radiation and chemotherapy, the patient is being evaluated for a clinical study, or the information is helpful for prognostic reasons. If the patient is not a candidate for combined-modality treatment or a clinical study, stopping the staging at the first evidence of extensive-stage disease is usually appropriate. Given that isolated bone marrow metastases are rare, bone marrow biopsies and aspirates are not usually done.

C. Prognostic factors

As in NSCLC, the major pretreatment prognostic factors are stage, performance status, and bulky disease. Hepatic metastases also confer a poorer prognosis. Due to the chemosensitivity of SCLC, if a patient's initial poor PS is due to the underlying malignancy, these symptoms often disappear quickly with treatment, resulting in a net improvement in quality of life. However, major organ dysfunction from nonmalignant causes often results in an inability of the patient to tolerate chemotherapy.

D. Therapy

1. **Combination chemotherapeutic regimens.** A number of combination chemotherapeutic regimens are available for SCLC (Table 6.8). No clear survival advantage has been consistently demonstrated for any one regimen over another. With these chemotherapy regimens, overall response rates of 75% to 90% and complete response rates of 50% for localized disease can be anticipated. For extensive-stage disease, overall response rates of about 75% and complete response rates of 25% are common. Despite these high response rates, however, the median survival time remains about 14 months for limited-stage disease and 8 to 9 months for extensive-stage disease. Less than 5% of patients with extensive-stage disease survive more than 2 years.

   At present, either cisplatin or carboplatin together with etoposide are the standard of care in North America for the treatment of SCLC. Generally, cisplatin is preferred if given with thoracic radiation for limited-stage disease. For extensive-stage disease, both cisplatin and carboplatin are widely used.

2. **Dose intensity.** A dose intensity meta-analysis of chemotherapy in SCLC, which evaluated doses not requiring bone marrow transplantation support, showed no consistent correlation between dose intensity and outcome. There have been several phase I and II clinical trials evaluating the role of marrow-ablative doses

TABLE 6.8	Chemotherapy Regimens for SCLC
Cisplatin-based	
Cisplatin	60 mg/m^2 IV on day 1
Etoposide	120 mg/m^2 IV on days 1–3 *or*
	120 mg/m^2 by mouth twice a day on days 1–3
or	
Cisplatin	25 mg/m^2 IV on days 1–3
Etoposide	100 mg/m^2 IV on days 1–3
	Repeat cycle every 3 weeks
Carboplatin-based	
Carboplatin	300 mg/m^2 IV on day 1
Etoposide	100 mg/m^2 IV on days 1–3
or	
Carboplatin	100 mg/m^2 IV on days 1–3
Etoposide	120 mg/m^2 IV on days 1–3
	Repeat cycle every 4 weeks

IV, intravenously.

of chemotherapy with subsequent progenitor cell replacement (e.g., autologous bone marrow transplantation) with disappointing survival results. In a randomized phase III study, when compared with conventional-dose chemotherapy, a high-dose regimen with stem cell support prolonged relapse-free but not overall survival.

3. **Duration of therapy.** Most randomized studies do not show a survival benefit for prolonged administration of chemotherapy. Several studies have demonstrated no survival benefit of prolonged first-line treatment over treatment on relapse. The optimal duration of treatment for SCLC is four to six cycles.

4. **Second-line therapy.** No curative regimens for patients with recurrent disease have been identified. The only drug approved for second-line therapy of SCLC is topotecan, which has a 20% to 40% response rate in patients with sensitive SCLC (those patients who relapsed 2 to 3 or more months after their first-line therapy), with a median survival of 22 to 27 weeks. Other options for patients with sensitive disease include oral etoposide, the combination of cyclophosphamide, doxorubicin, and vincristine, or a return to the first treatment regimen. For patients with refractory disease (progressed through or within 3 months of completion of first-line therapy), the response rate in phase II studies is only between 3% and 11%, and median survival is about 20 weeks.

E. **Chemotherapy plus chest irradiation**

Numerous studies combining chemotherapy and thoracic radiation therapy have been performed in patients with limited-stage SCLC. Conflicting results have been attributed to differences in chemotherapy regimens and different schedules integrating chemotherapy and thoracic radiation (concurrent, sequential, and "sandwich" approach). Two meta-analyses concluded that thoracic irradiation does result in a small but significant improvement in survival and major control of the disease in the chest, although no conclusions could be made regarding the optimal sequencing of chemotherapy and thoracic radiation. In one randomized study, twice-daily hyperfractionated radiation was compared with a once-daily schedule; both were given concurrently with four cycles of cisplatin and etoposide. Survival was significantly higher with the twice-daily regimen (median survival of 23 months versus 19 months, 5-year survival of 26% versus 16%), albeit at the expense of more grade III esophagitis. In another randomized trial, early administration of thoracic irradiation in the combined-modality therapy of limited-stage SCLC was superior to late or consolidative thoracic irradiation. These data suggest that patients with good PS and with limited disease should receive concurrent chemoradiation, preferably with twice-daily hyperfractionation.

For patients with extensive-stage disease who have complete response to chemotherapy at extrathoracic disease sites, consolidative chest radiation therapy may be considered. In a randomized study, patients who had a complete extrathoracic response and a partial or complete thoracic response after three cycles of cisplatin-etoposide were randomized to either (1) 54 Gy thoracic radiation followed by two additional cycles of cisplatin-etoposide or (2) four additional cycles of cisplatin-etoposide. Patients who received radiation had a significantly longer overall survival (17 months versus 11 months; $p = 0.04$).

F. **Prophylactic cranial irradiation**

Given the propensity of SCLC to metastasize to the brain and the resultant morbidity of this event, prophylactic cranial irradiation has been offered to patients with limited-stage disease who have an excellent response to chemoradiation. In a meta-analysis of seven trials, prophylactic cranial irradiation decreased the risk of brain metastasis, prolonged disease-free survival, and significantly increased 3-year overall survival, with a net gain of 5.4%. More recently, a randomized trial of patients with extensive stage SCLC who had had a response to chemotherapy were randomized to prophylactic cranial irradiation or observation. The trial met its primary endpoint with a reduced rate of symptomatic brain metastasis (HR 0.27; $p < 0.001$). Furthermore, prophylactic cranial irradiation significantly extended disease-free and overall survival; the 1-year survival rate was 27% in the irradiation group and 13% in the control group.

VI. PALLIATION
A. **Radiotherapy**

Palliative radiotherapy is often helpful in controlling the pain of bone metastases or neurologic function in patients with brain metastases. Chest radiotherapy may help control hemoptysis, superior vena cava syndrome, airway obstruction, laryngeal nerve compression, and other local complications. For patients with bronchial obstruction who have received maximum external-beam radiotherapy, the use of high-dose endobronchial irradiation may be of temporary benefit.

B. **Pleural effusions**

For pleurodesis, common sclerosing agents include doxycycline, talc, and bleomycin. The disadvantage of bleomycin is its cost; talc, although effective, has the disadvantage of requiring a thoracoscopy and general anesthesia for insufflation. Alternatively, an indwelling pleural drainage catheter may be placed.

C. **Colony-stimulating factors**

Filgrastim (granulocyte colony-stimulating factor) decreases the incidence of neutropenic fevers, the median duration of neutropenia, days of hospitalization, and days of antibiotic treatment in patients. However, the clinical benefit of maintaining a dose-intense approach in the treatment of patients with lung cancer has not been established. In addition, caution must be exercised when using colony-stimulating factors in patients receiving combined-modality treatment with both chemotherapy and thoracic irradiation. A randomized study by the Southwest Oncology Group found that patients receiving sargramostim (granulocyte–macrophage colony-stimulating factor) and chemotherapy with concurrent thoracic irradiation had a significant increase in thrombocytopenia over patients receiving concurrent chemotherapy and radiation therapy without growth factor.

Selected Readings

Albain KS, Swann RS, Rusch VW, et al. Radiotherapy plus chemotherapy with or without surgical resection for stage III non-small-cell lung cancer: a phase III randomized controlled trial. *Lancet.* 2009;374:379–386.

Arriagada R, Bergman B, Dunant A, et al. Cisplatin-based adjuvant chemotherapy in patients with completely resected non-small-cell lung cancer. *N Engl J Med.* 2004;350:351–360.

Cappuzzo F, Hirsch FR, Rossi E, et al. Epidermal growth factor receptor gene and protein and gefitinib sensitivity in non-small-cell lung cancer. *J Natl Cancer Inst.* 2005;97:643–655.

Ciuleanu T, Brodowicz T, Zielinski C, et al. Maintenance pemetrexed plus best supportive care versus placebo plus best supportive care for non-small-cell lung cancer: a randomised, double-blind, phase 3 study. *Lancet.* 2009.374:1432–1440.

Dillman RO, Herndon J, Seagren SL, Eaton WL Jr, Green MR. Improved survival in stage III non–small cell lung cancer: seven-year follow-up of CALGB 8433. *J Natl Cancer Inst.* 1996;88:1210–1215.

Douillard JY, Rosell R, De LM, et al. Adjuvant vinorelbine plus cisplatin versus observation in patients with completely resected stage IB-IIIA non-small-cell lung cancer (Adjuvant Navelbine International Trialist Association [ANITA]): a randomised controlled trial. *Lancet Oncol.* 2006;7:719–727.

Fidias PM, Dakhil SR, Lyss AP, et al. Phase III study of immediate compared with delayed docetaxel after front-line therapy with gemcitabine plus carboplatin in advanced non-small-cell lung cancer. *J Clin Oncol.* 2009;27:591–598.

Furuse K, Fukuoka M, Kawahara M, et al. Phase III study of concurrent versus sequential thoracic radiotherapy in combination with mitomycin, vindesine, and cisplatin in unresectable stage III non–small cell lung cancer. *J Clin Oncol.* 1999;17:2692–2699.

Gilligan D, Nicolson M, Smith I, et al. Preoperative chemotherapy in patients with resectable non-small cell lung cancer: results of the MRC LU22/NVALT 2/EORTC 08012 multicentre randomised trial and update of systematic review. *Lancet.* 2007;369:1929–1937.

Hanna N, Shepherd FA, Fossella FV, et al. Randomized phase III trial of pemetrexed versus docetaxel in patients with non-small-cell lung cancer previously treated with chemotherapy. *J Clin Oncol.* 2004;22:1589–1597.

Klasa R, Murray N, Coldman A. Dose-intensity meta-analysis of chemotherapy regimens in small-cell carcinoma of the lung. *J Clin Oncol.* 1991;9:499–508.

Lynch TJ, Bell DW, Sordella R, et al. Activating mutations in the epidermal growth factor receptor underlying responsiveness of non-small-cell lung cancer to gefitinib. *N Engl J Med.* 2004;350:2129–2139.

Mok TS, Wu YL, Thongprasert S, et al. Gefitinib or carboplatin-paclitaxel in pulmonary adenocarcinoma. *N Engl J Med.* 2009;361:947–957.

Mulshine JL, Sullivan C. Clinical practice. Lung cancer screening. *N Engl J Med.* 2005;352:2714–2720.

Murray N, Coy P, Pater J, et al. Importance of timing for thoracic irradiation in the combined modality treatment of limited-stage small-cell lung cancer. *J Clin Oncol.* 1993;11:336–344.

Neal CR, Amdur RJ, Mendenhall WM, Knauf DF, Block AJ, Million RR. Pancoast tumor: radiation therapy alone versus preoperative radiation therapy and surgery. *Int J Radiat Oncol Biol Phys.* 1991;21:651–660.

Non–Small Cell Lung Cancer Collaborative Group. Chemotherapy in non–small cell lung cancer: a meta-analysis using updated data on individual patients from 52 randomized clinical trials. *BMJ.* 1995;311:899–909.

Pignon JP, Arriagada R, Ihde DC, et al. A meta-analysis of thoracic radiotherapy for small-cell lung cancer. *N Engl J Med.* 1992;327:1618–1624.

Pignon JP, Tribodet H, Scagliotti GV, et al. Lung adjuvant cisplatin evaluation: a pooled analysis by the LACE Collaborative Group. *J Clin Oncol.* 2008;26:3552–3559.

Pirker R, Pereira JR, Szczesna A, et al. Cetuximab plus chemotherapy in patients with advanced non-small cell lung cancer (FLEX): an open-label randomized phase III trial. *Lancet.* 2009;373:1525–1531.

Rami-Porta R, Crowley JJ, Goldstraw P. The revised TNM staging system for lung cancer. *Ann Thorac Cardiovasc Surg.* 2009;15:4–9.

Rosell R, Gómez-Codina J, Camps C, et al. A randomized trial comparing preoperative chemotherapy plus surgery with surgery alone in patients with non–small-cell lung cancer. *N Engl J Med.* 1994;330:153–158.

Sandler A, Gray R, Perry MC, et al. Paclitaxel-carboplatin alone or with bevacizumab for non-small-cell lung cancer. *N Engl J Med.* 2006;355:2542–2550.

Scagliotti GV, Parikh P, von Pawel J, et al. Phase III study comparing cisplatin plus gemcitabine with cisplatin plus pemetrexed in chemotherapy-naïve patients with advanced-stage non-small-cell lung cancer. *J Clin Oncol.* 2008;26:3543–3551.

Schiller JH, Harrington D, Belani C, et al. Comparison of four chemotherapy regimens for advanced non–small cell lung cancer. *N Engl J Med.* 2002;346:92–98.

Shepherd FA, Rodrigues Pereira J, Ciuleanu T, et al. Erlotinib in previously treated non-small-cell lung cancer. *N Engl J Med.* 2005;353:123–132.

Slotman B, Faivre-Finn C, Kramer G, et al. Prophylactic cranial irradiation in extensive small-cell lung cancer. *N Engl J Med.* 2007;357:664–672.

Strauss GM, Herndon JE 2nd, Maddaus MA, et al. Adjuvant paclitaxel plus carboplatin compared with observation in stage IB non-small-cell lung cancer: CALGB 9633 with the Cancer and Leukemia Group B, Radiation Therapy Oncology Group, and North Central Cancer Treatment Group Study Groups. *J Clin Oncol.* 2008;26:5043–5051.

Thatcher N, Chang A, Parikh P, et al. Gefitinib plus best supportive care in previously treated patients with refractory advanced non-small cell lung cancer: results from a randomized, placebo-controlled multicentre study (Iressa Survival Evaluation in Lung Cancer). *Lancet.* 2005;366:1527–1537.

The PORT Meta-analysis Trialists Group. Postoperative radiotherapy in non-small-cell lung cancer: systematic review and meta-analysis of individual patient data from nine randomised controlled trials. *Lancet.* 1998;352:257–263.

Tsao MS, Sakurada A, Cutz JC, et al. Erlotinib in lung cancer—molecular and clinical predictors of outcome. *N Engl J Med.* 2005;353:133–144.

Turrisi AT, Kim K, Blum R, et al. Twice-daily compared with once-daily thoracic radiotherapy in limited small-cell lung cancer treated concurrently with cisplatin and etoposide. *N Engl J Med.* 1999;340:265–271.

Von Pawel J, Schiller JH, Shepherd FA, et al. Topotecan versus cyclophosphamide, doxorubicin, and vincristine for the treatment of recurrent small-cell lung cancer. *J Clin Oncol.* 1999;2:658–667.

Warde P, Payne D. Does thoracic irradiation improve survival and local control in limited-stage small-cell carcinoma of the lung? A meta-analysis. *J Clin Oncol.* 1992;10:890–895.

Winton T, Livingston R, Johnson D, et al. Vinorelbine plus cisplatin vs. observation in resected non-small-cell lung cancer. *N Engl J Med.* 2005;352:2589–2597.

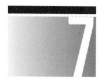

Carcinomas of the Gastrointestinal Tract

Maxwell Vergo and Al B. Benson III

Cancers of the gastrointestinal (GI) tract (esophagus, stomach, small and large intestines, and anus) account for nearly 14% of all cases of cancer in the United States and for about 20% of cancer deaths. Colon cancer is by far the most common of these malignancies, with cancer of the rectum, stomach, esophagus, small intestine, and anus occurring with decreasing frequency. Surgery continues to be the principal curative modality, but radiation and chemotherapy have increasingly important roles and, in certain adjuvant situations, improve the cure rate produced by surgery. Select patients with isolated, resectable metastatic colorectal cancer lesions also may be cured with surgical resection. Chemotherapy alone is not curative in patients with overt metastatic disease. Recent combination drug regimens have produced objective responses in up to 60% of patients, with increasing numbers of individuals obtaining stabilization of their disease. There is little question that meaningful palliation and an increase in survival can be achieved in patients who respond to chemotherapy or achieve disease stabilization. Controlled clinical trials, often by cooperative groups, have been useful in defining the natural history and therapeutic benefit of various treatment modalities. Participation in such clinical trials is encouraged.

I. CARCINOMA OF THE ESOPHAGUS

A. General considerations and aims of therapy

1. **Epidemiology.** Cancer of the esophagus is more common in men than women and occurs more often in black patients than in white patients. The average patient is in his or her 60s at presentation. Esophageal cancers are either adenocarcinoma (EAC) or squamous cell carcinoma (ESCC). Smoking and regular alcohol use are strong risk factors for ESCC and only moderate risk factors for EAC; the risk is reduced with smoking cessation in ESCC but not EAC. A unique risk factor for ESCC is other aerodigestive tract malignancies, such as head and neck or lung cancer. Risk factors associated with EAC only appear to be gastroesophageal reflux disease (GERD) and Barrett esophagitis.

   EAC tends to involve the lower third of that organ, whereas the middle third is the most common site for ESCC. Although ESCC remains the most common in Asian countries, especially East Asia, the incidence of EAC has been increasing over the past two decades in Western countries. In the United States over this time, the incidence of EAC has increased three- to eightfold. The ratio of ESCC:EAC during this time has changed from 4.7:1 in 1975 to 0.43:1 in 1998. This is believed primarily to be due to increased GERD from rising rates of obesity in these regions of the world.

   Optimal chemotherapy for the two histologic types of esophageal cancer is not known to be different in terms of overall survival (OS). There does appear to be an improved rate of response to neoadjuvant therapy with ESCC, but EAC patients who experience a response have an improved long-term prognosis compared to their ESCC counterparts, likely explaining the lack of OS difference.

2. **Clinical manifestations and pretreatment evaluation.** Carcinoma of the esophagus is usually associated with progressive and persistent dysphagia. Pain, hoarseness, weight loss, and chronic cough are unfavorable manifestations that indicate spread to regional structures (e.g., mediastinal nodes), recurrent laryngeal nerves, or fistula formation between the esophagus and the airway. The most common sites of metastasis are regional lymph nodes (which may include cervical, supraclavicular, intrathoracic, diaphragmatic, celiac axis, or periaortic lymph nodes), the liver, and the lungs.

   Diagnosis is usually made by barium swallow, endoscopy, and biopsy or lavage cytology. Staging should be based on computed tomography (CT) scan of the abdomen and chest, careful physical examination of the cervical and supraclavicular nodes, and positron emission tomography (PET)/CT imaging to rule out distant metastatic disease. In patients without metastatic disease, endoscopic esophageal ultrasound (EUS) may be useful in assessing the depth of tumor invasion, given the difference in management of T1-T2 lesions versus T3-T4 lesions. The preoperative staging of esophageal cancer with EUS is still inadequate, owing to the inability to evaluate lymph nodes accurately; PET/CT does not seem to improve this detection for locoregional nodal status. Laparoscopy has the advantage of changing management in approximately 20% of patients who have otherwise been fully staged with CT, PET/CT, and EUS. Bronchoscopy should be done for upper- and middle-third tumors to rule out a bronchoesophageal fistula. A bone scan is useful in patients with bone pain or tenderness. Survival is related to pathologic stage, which only can be defined surgically (Table 7.1).

3. **Treatment and prognosis.** The primary treatment of stage I and II carcinoma of the esophagus is surgical resection. About half of esophageal cancers are operable, and half of these are resectable. Complete surgical resection results in a median survival of approximately 18 months with 15% to 20% of patients surviving 5 years. Patients with more advanced disease (stage III) are best treated, at least initially, with nonsurgical means, usually a combination of radiation therapy and chemotherapy. In patients who respond to such treatment, the carcinoma may subsequently be operable, whereas patients with metastatic disease are best treated with systemic therapy. Palliative feeding procedures such as with a jejunostomy or gastrostomy tube may be useful if subsequent surgical resection is not to be done. For metastatic disease, the overall median survival time is less than 1 year, and the overall 5-year survival rate is 5% to 10%. The prognosis is related to the size of the lesion, the depth of penetration of the esophagus, and nodal involvement. Current controlled clinical trials are helping to evaluate the optimal chemotherapy regimen and combination with radiation in the neoadjuvant setting.

B. **Combined-modality treatment for potentially curable patients**
The poor results with immediate surgery, due in part to inadequate staging techniques, have focused attention for some years on preoperative combined-modality treatment with radiation therapy, chemotherapy, or both, followed by surgery (or, in some instances, not followed by surgery). This approach is controversial because of uncertainty of staging and conflicting results from randomized clinical trials. When this approach is used, aggressive staging including EUS, CT scanning, and laparoscopy is needed and is often combined with jejunostomy feeding tube placement for nutritional support. Despite conflicting results from randomized trials, patients with stage II and III disease are often treated in this fashion.

TNM Stages for Carcinoma of the Esophagus

Primary Tumor

Tis	HGD
T1	Invades lamina propria or submucosa
T1a	Invades lamina propria or muscularis mucosa
T1b	Invades submucosa
T2	Invades muscularis propria
T3	Invades adventitia
T4	Invades adjacent structures
T4a	Resectable tumor invading pleura, pericardium, or diaphragm
T4b	Unresectable tumor invading other adjacent structures such as aorta, vertebral body, trachea, etc.

Regional Lymph Nodes

N0	No regional nodal metastasis
N1	Metastasis in one to two regional nodes
N2	Metastasis in three to six regional nodes
N3	Metastasis in seven or more regional nodes

Distant Metastasis

M0	None
M1	Present

Stage Grouping for Squamous Cell Carcinoma* using TNM, grade (G), and tumor location[†]

0	Tis(HGD), N0, M0, G1/X, any location
IA	T1, N0, M0, G1/X, any location
IB	T1, N0, M0, G2–3, any location
	T2–3, N0, M0, G1/X, lower/X
IIA	T2–3, N0, M0, G1/X, upper/middle
	T2–3, N0, M0, G2–3, lower/X
IIB	T2–3, N0, M0, G2–3, upper/middle
	T1–2, N1, M0, any G, any location
IIIA	T1–2, N2, M0, any G, any location
	T3, N1, M0, any G, any location
	T4a, N0, M0, any G, any location
IIIB	T3, N2, M0, any G, any location
IIIC	T4a, N1–2, M0, any G, any location
	T4b, any N, M0, any G, any location
	Any, N3, M0, any G, any location
IV	Any T, any N, M1, any G

Stage Grouping for Adenocarcinoma using TNM and G

0	Tis(HGD), N0, M0, G1/X
IA	T1, N0, M0, G1–2/X
IB	T1, N0, M0, G3
	T2, N0, M0, G1–2/X
IIA	T2, N0, M0, G3
IIB	T3, N0, M0, any G
	T1–2, N1, M0, any G

(continued)

| | TNM Stages for Carcinoma of the Esophagus *(continued)* |

Stage Grouping for Adenocarcinoma using TNM and G *(continued)*

IIIA	T1–2, N2, M0, any G
	T3, N1, M0, any G
	T4a, N0, M0, any G
IIIB	T3, N2, M0, any G
IIIC	T4a, N1–2, M0, any G
	T4b, Any N, M0, any G
	Any T, N3, M0, any G
IV	Any T, Any N, M1, any G

HGD, high-grade dysplasia.
*Or mixed histology including a squamous component or not otherwise specified.
†Location of the primary cancer site defined by position of the upper (proximal) edge of the tumor in the esophagus. Upper = 10 to <25 cm, middle = 25 to <30 cm, and lower = 30 to 45 cm, esophago-gastric junction/cardia = 5 cm below esophagogastric junction.
Modified from American Joint Committee on Cancer. *AJCC cancer staging manual* (7th ed.). New York: Springer; 2010.

1. **Preoperative chemotherapy.** The National Cancer Institute Gastrointestinal Intergroup has reported a randomized trial of 440 patients with either EAC or ESCC that compared preoperative chemotherapy (cisplatin and fluorouracil [CF] for three cycles) versus surgery alone. After a median follow-up of 55.4 months, there were no median, 1-year, or 2-year survival differences between the two groups. These results differ compared with data from the Medical Research Council Clinical Trials Unit in the United Kingdom, which included 802 patients randomized to receive either two cycles of preoperative CF followed by surgery versus surgery alone. Approximately 66% of patients had adenocarcinoma. Long-term follow-up at 6 years revealed a significant difference in 5-year OS (chemotherapy versus surgery alone, 23% versus 17.1%; hazard ratio [HR] 0.84; 95% confidence interval, 0.72–0.98; $p = 0.03$) regardless of histological subtype. Different proportions of the two different histologies contribute to the difficulties in interpretation of these trials.

2. **Radiation therapy with surgery, chemotherapy, or both.** Radiation therapy, as either a preoperative or a postoperative adjunct to surgery, has not improved OS in most series, with 5-year survival rates ranging from 0% to 10%. Combined-modality treatment of radiotherapy with chemotherapy has been superior. In addition, concurrent chemotherapy and radiotherapy is superior to sequentially-administered treatment. In a randomized trial, Radiation Therapy Oncology Group (RTOG) 85-01, comparing radiotherapy alone with radiotherapy plus chemotherapy

in 121 patients, 88% of whom had squamous cell cancer, the RTOG reported a 5-year survival rate of 27% for the combined-modality group and 0% for the radiation therapy alone group, with median survival times of 14.1 months and 9.3 months, respectively. Most patients had stage T2 disease and were node negative by CT scanning.

a. **Radiation therapy plus CF**

   (1) **Radiation therapy** 180 to 200 cGy/day for 3 weeks, 5 days weekly, then 2 additional weeks to the boost field for a total of 5040 cGy, *and*

   (2) **Fluorouracil** 1000 mg/m^2/day by continuous infusion for 4 days on weeks 1, 5, 8, and 11, with cisplatin 75 mg/m^2 intravenously (IV) at 1 mg/min on the first day of each course. Reduce fluorouracil for severe diarrhea or stomatitis and cisplatin for severe neutropenia or thrombocytopenia.

   More recent phase II trials are exploring radiation with alternative chemotherapy combinations, including cisplatin with a taxane as well as the addition of a targeted agent, namely epidermal growth factor receptor (EGFR) antagonists.

   Surgery, when it can be done, is probably appropriate because most patients treated with chemotherapy and radiotherapy still have residual tumor. Even though a high proportion of patients, 25% in many series, have complete pathologic responses at surgery, the preoperative identification of these patients is not accurate. A large meta-analysis of randomized controlled trials comparing neoadjuvant chemoradiation and surgery to surgery alone included nine randomized trials with 1116 patients. The meta-analysis demonstrated that neoadjuvant chemoradiation and surgery improved the 3-year survival ($p = 0.016$) and reduced distant and local regional cancer recurrence ($p = 0.038$). There was also a higher rate of complete resection, although there was a nonsignificant trend toward increased treatment mortality with neoadjuvant chemoradiation.

   Combined chemotherapy and radiotherapy is therefore a reasonable approach for patients who refuse surgery or whose disease is unresectable for anatomic or physiologic reasons, particularly those with ESCC.

C. **Treatment of advanced (metastatic) disease**

Various agents with modest activity when used alone are available. These include cisplatin, carboplatin, fluorouracil, bleomycin, paclitaxel, docetaxel, irinotecan, gemcitabine, methotrexate, mitomycin, vinorelbine, and doxorubicin. Response rates range from 15% to 30% and are usually brief. Most data are for ESCC, the exception being paclitaxel, which appears equally effective in both histologic types. The most active drugs appear to be cisplatin, paclitaxel, and fluorouracil. Patients with no history of prior chemotherapy are more likely to respond than those who have had previous treatment. Single agents are less helpful than combination chemotherapy because of their lower response rates and brief duration of response. Cisplatin-based regimens have been most extensively tested. Among the most active are the following (for adenocarcinoma of the distal esophagus and gastroesophageal junction, see Section II).

1. **CF**
   a. **Cisplatin** 75 to 100 mg/m^2 IV on day 1.
   b. **Fluorouracil** 1000 mg/m^2/day as a continuous IV infusion on days 1 to 5. Repeat every 28 days.
2. **Paclitaxel plus cisplatin**
   a. **Paclitaxel** 175 mg/m^2 IV on day 1.
   b. **Cisplatin** 75 mg/m^2 IV on day 1. Repeat every 21 days.
3. **Carboplatin plus paclitaxel**
   a. **Carboplatin** area under the curve 5 IV on day 1.
   b. **Paclitaxel** 200 mg/m^2 IV on day 1. Repeat every 21 days.
4. **Paclitaxel plus cisplatin plus fluorouracil**
   a. **Paclitaxel** 175 mg/m^2 IV over 3 hours on day 1.
   b. **Cisplatin** 20 mg/m^2/day IV on days 1 to 5.
   c. **Fluorouracil** 750 mg/m^2/day continuous IV on days 1 to 5. Repeat every 28 days.
5. **Cisplatin plus irinotecan**
   a. **Irinotecan** 65 mg/m^2 IV on days 1, 8, 15, and 22.
   b. **Cisplatin** 30 mg/m^2 IV on days 1, 8, 15, and 22. The regimen is repeated every 6 weeks.
6. **Irinotecan plus fluorouracil plus leucovorin**
   a. **Irinotecan** 180 mg/m^2 IV over 30 minutes followed by a 30-minute break.
   b. **Leucovorin** 125 mg/m^2 IV over 15 minutes.
   c. **Fluorouracil** 400 mg/m^2 IV over 3 to 4 minutes.
   d. **Fluorouracil** 1200 mg/m^2/day continuous IV for 2 days. The regimen is repeated every 2 weeks.
7. **Cetuximab.** The addition of cetuximab to a chemotherapy backbone has yet to demonstrate a significant progression-free survival or OS advantage, but does appear to improve response rates. A large clinical trial (Eastern Cooperative Oncology Group [ECOG] 1206/Cancer and Leukemia Group B 80403) recently completed accrual and should further clarify the benefit of cetuximab in this disease.
8. **Second-line therapy** may be chosen from the list of alternative combination therapies or the single agents, including methotrexate 40 mg/m^2 IV weekly; bleomycin 15 U/m^2 IV twice weekly; vinorelbine 25 mg/m^2 IV weekly; or mitomycin 20 mg/m^2 IV

every 4 to 6 weeks. However, these therapies are not currently included in disease treatment guidelines, such as those of the National Comprehensive Cancer Network (NCCN).

D. **Supportive care**

Esophagitis during a combined-modality treatment program is nearly universal, and nutritional support frequently is required, preferably using alimentation by feeding tube placed by enterostomy. Peripheral alimentation is difficult with the continuous chemotherapy administration. Gastrostomy tubes are to be avoided in patients with potentially resectable lesions because of the usual requirement for a gastric pull-up after resection of the esophageal tumor.

E. **Follow-up studies**

For asymptomatic patients who have had potentially curative therapy, history and physical examination may be done every 3 to 6 months for years 1 to 3, every 6 months for years 3 to 5, and then annually. CT scans, endoscopy, chemistries, and complete blood count should be evaluated as clinically indicated.

II. GASTRIC CARCINOMA

A. **General considerations and aims of therapy**

1. **Epidemiology.** The incidence of stomach cancer has decreased dramatically in the United States since the beginning of the century, although it has stabilized in the last 20 years. The leading cause of cancer death in 1930, it now ranks 12th; however, worldwide it is the 4th most lethal cancer. No improvement has been seen over the last two decades though, with 5-year survival rates ranging from 45% to 71% in node-negative disease to 5% to 30% in node-positive or metastatic disease. The male-to-female ratio is nearly two to one. Stomach cancer is still the leading cause of cancer deaths among men in Japan and is also common in China, Finland, Poland, Peru, and Chile. A high rate of chronic gastritis and intestinal metaplasia of the stomach is associated with a high incidence of gastric cancer. *Helicobacter pylori* has been implicated in such changes and in gastric cancer, particularly the more distal "intestinal" type, as well as in peptic ulcer disease. Although the incidence in the United States has decreased, the location of gastric cancers has migrated proximally. Nearly half the stomach cancers occurring in white men are located proximally (gastroesophageal junction, cardia, and proximal lesser curvature).

2. **Clinical manifestations and evaluation.** The most common symptoms are weight loss, abdominal pain, nausea, vomiting, changes in bowel habits, fatigue, anorexia, and dysphagia. The diagnosis generally is made by endoscopy and biopsy, although barium swallow is frequently helpful. Endoscopic ultrasonography is

increasingly used; it is more accurate in gauging the depth of the cancer in the gastric wall than in determining nodal involvement. Laparoscopy is also helpful in improving clinical staging as it can more accurately identify peritoneal metastases and further evaluate the liver. Metastases are to the liver, pancreas, omentum, esophagus, and bile ducts by direct extension and to regional and distant lymph nodes such as those in the left supraclavicular area. Pulmonary and bone metastases are a late finding. Staging of suspected gastric cancer should initially include CT scans of the chest, abdomen, and pelvis. Tumor markers such as carcinoembryonic antigen (CEA), cancer antigen (CA) 19-9, and CA 72-4 may be useful for subsequent assessment of the response to therapy. Prognosis is reflected by accurate staging (Table 7.2). The revised staging method classifies patients according to the number of pathologically involved regional lymph nodes. The groupings are one to two (N1), three to six (N2), and seven or more involved lymph nodes (N3).

3. **Treatment and prognosis.** Most stomach cancers are adenocarcinomas. Important prognostic factors include tumor grade and gross appearance. Diffusely infiltrating lesions are less likely to be cured than sharply circumscribed, nonulcerating lesions. The presence of regional lymph node involvement or involvement of contiguous organs in the surgical specimen indicates an increased likelihood of recurrence, as does the presence of dysphagia at the time of diagnosis. Patients with proximal lesions or lesions requiring total, rather than distal subtotal, gastrectomy are also at greater risk.

There has been controversy as to the contribution of extensive lymphadenectomy (D1 versus D2 dissection) to survival benefit. Japanese surgeons have widely promoted the D2 dissection; however, randomized clinical trials including the Dutch Gastric Cancer Group and the Medical Research Council trials did not show a survival benefit of D2 over D1 lymphadenectomy. However, there was increased morbidity and mortality for those patients who underwent the D2 dissection.

B. **Treatment of advanced (metastatic, locally unresectable, or recurrent) disease**
   1. **Single agents** with activity include epirubicin, mitomycin, doxorubicin, cisplatin, etoposide, fluorouracil, irinotecan, hydroxyurea, the taxanes, and the nitrosoureas. Single agents have low response rates (15%–30%), brief durations of response, and few complete responses, and they have little impact on survival.
   2. **Combinations of drugs** are more widely used than single agents, largely because of higher response rates, more frequent complete responses, and the potential of longer survival. A large randomized phase III study (V325) enrolling mostly patients

	TNM Stages for Carcinoma of the Stomach

Primary Tumor

Tis	Carcinoma in situ
T1	Invades lamina propria, muscularis mucosa, or submucosa
T1a	Invades lamina propria or muscularis mucosa
T1b	Invades submucosa
T2	Invades muscularis propria
T3	Penetrates subserosal connective tissue without invasion of visceral peritoneum or adjacent structures*
T4	Invades serosa (visceral peritoneum) or adjacent structures*
T4a	Invades serosa (visceral peritoneum)
T4b	Invades adjacent structures*

Regional Lymph Nodes

N0	No regional nodal metastasis
N1	Metastasis in one to two regional lymph nodes
N2	Metastasis in three to six regional lymph nodes
N3	Metastasis in seven or more regional lymph nodes

Distant Metastasis

M0	None
M1	Present

Stage Grouping

0	Tis, N0, M0
IA	T1, N0, M0
IB	T1, N1, M0
	T2, N0, M0
IIA	T1, N2, M0
	T2, N1, M0
	T3, N0, M0
IIB	T1, N3, M0
	T2, N2, M0
	T3, N1, M0
	T4a, N0, M0
IIIA	T2, N3, M0
	T3, N2, M0
	T4a, N1, M0
IIIB	T3, N3, M0
	T4a, N2, M0
	T4b, N0–1, M0
IIIC	T4a, N3, M0
	T4b, N2–3, M0
IV	Any T, any N, M1

*Adjacent structures: spleen, transverse colon, liver, diaphragm, pancreas, abdominal wall, adrenal gland, kidney, small intestine, retroperitoneum.
Modified from American Joint Committee on Cancer. *AJCC cancer staging manual* (7th ed.). New York: Springer; 2010.

with metastatic gastric cancer found improved response rate (36% versus 26%), delayed time to progression (5.6 months versus 3.7 months), improved OS (18.4% versus 8.8% at 2 years), delayed decline in functionality, and delayed deterioration of quality of life with docetaxel, cisplatin, and fluorouracil (DCF) compared to CF. Significant differences in grade 3 to 4 toxicities of DCF including diarrhea (19% versus 8%), neutropenia (82% versus 57%), neutropenic fever (29% versus 12%), and neurosensory (8% versus 3%) as compared to CF have limited its use as a standard regimen. DCF as a treatment for advanced disease, therefore, represents an important proof of principle; however, the toxicity is of significant concern.

a. **DCF.** Dexamethasone 8 mg by mouth twice a day 1 day prior to chemotherapy, on the day of treatment, and the day after.

   (1) **Docetaxel** 75 mg/m^2 as a 1-hour infusion IV.

   (2) **Cisplatin** 75 mg/m^2 as a 2-hour infusion IV.

   (3) **Fluorouracil** 750 mg/m^2 daily as a continuous infusion IV on days 1 to 5. The regimen is repeated every 21 days.

b. **CF**

   (1) **Cisplatin** 100 mg/m^2 IV over 2 hours on day 1.

   (2) **Fluorouracil** 1000 mg/m^2 daily as a continuous infusion IV on days 1 to 5. The regimen is repeated every 21 days.

   A UK study randomized 274 patients to receive either epirubicin, cisplatin, and protracted infusional fluorouracil (ECF) or fluorouracil, doxorubicin, and methotrexate, which was the standard at the time. The results favored ECF with improved response rate (45% versus 20%), a 2-month improvement in median survival, and an improved 2-year OS (14% versus 5%).

c. **ECF**

   (1) **Epirubicin** 50 mg/m^2 IV bolus on day 1 followed by CF.

   (2) **Cisplatin** 60 mg/m^2 IV over 2 hours on day 1.

   (3) **Fluorouracil** 200 mg/m^2 daily as a continuous infusion IV on days 1 to 21. The regimen is repeated every 21 days.

   The REAL 2 study enrolled 1,002 patients with mostly metastatic gastric and gastroesophageal cancer and randomized patients in a two-by-two design to receive one of four anthracycline containing regimens: epirubicin and fluorouracil with either cisplatin (ECF) or oxaliplatin (EOF) as well as epirubicin and capecitabine with either cisplatin (ECX) or oxaliplatin (EOX). They concluded that capecitabine was noninferior to fluorouracil and that oxaliplatin was noninferior to cisplatin. Of note, oxaliplatin-containing regimens appeared to be better tolerated then cisplatin-containing regimens. In a secondary subset analysis, there was suggestion of a survival benefit of EOX compared with ECF.

   d. **EOF**
      (1) **Epirubicin** 50 mg/m^2 IV bolus on day 1 followed by oxaliplatin and fluorouracil.
      (2) **Oxaliplatin** 130 mg/m^2 IV over 2 hours on day 1.
      (3) **Fluorouracil** 200 mg/m^2 daily as a continuous infusion IV on days 1 to 21. The regimen is repeated every 21 days.
   e. **EOX**
      (1) **Epirubicin** 50 mg/m^2 IV bolus on day 1 followed by oxaliplatin and capecitabine.
      (2) **Oxaliplatin** 130 mg/m^2 IV over 2 hours on day 1.
      (3) **Capecitabine** 625 mg/m^2 twice daily on days 1 to 21. The regimen is repeated every 21 days.
   f. **ECX**
      (1) **Epirubicin** 50 mg/m^2 IV bolus on day 1 followed by cisplatin and capecitabine.
      (2) **Cisplatin** 60 mg/m^2 IV over 2 hours on day 1.
      (3) **Capecitabine** 625 mg/m^2 twice daily on days 1 to 21. The regimen is repeated every 21 days.

      More recently, the ToGA trial enrolled 584 patients with HER2-positive (immunohistochemistry 3+ and/or fluorescence in-situ hybridization [FISH]+) gastric cancer to receive fluorouracil or capecitabine with cisplatin and randomized to either receive trastuzumab or placebo. They found improved response rate (47.3% versus 34.5%), improved progression-free survival, and improved median OS (13.8 months versus 11.1 months). This is the first biologic agent to demonstrate a convincing survival advantage in gastric cancer.
   g. **CF or cisplatin and capecitabine with trastuzumab.** Please note that this regimen is appropriate only in HER2-positive patients, as defined by immunohistochemistry 3+ or FISH+.
      (1) **Fluorouracil** 800 mg/m^2/day continuous infusion IV on days 1 to 5 *or* capecitabine 1000 mg/m^2 orally twice daily on days 1 to 14.
      (2) **Cisplatin** 80 mg/m^2 IV over 2 hours on day 1.
      (3) **Trastuzumab** 8 mg/kg IV loading dose over 90 minutes on day 1. If tolerated, then the following cycle dose is 6 mg/kg IV over 30 to 90 minutes. The regimen is repeated every 21 days.

      After 6 cycles, if there is stable disease, then continue *only* trastuzumab maintenance until progression.

      Baseline echocardiogram every 3 months is recommended to assess for asymptomatic decline in ejection fraction seen with trastuzumab.

      Currently, the NCCN supports the use of DCF and ECF in advanced gastric cancer with a category 1 level of evidence, but other regimens including irinotecan plus cisplatin, oxaliplatin plus a fluoropyrimidine, DCF modifications, irinotecan plus a fluoropyrimidine, and paclitaxel-based regimens are supported with a category 2B level of evidence.

h. Irinotecan and fluorouracil
   (1) Irinotecan 80 mg/m^2 over 30 minutes IV days 1, 8, 15, 22, 29, 36 followed by leucovorin and fluorouracil.
   (2) Leucovorin 500 mg/m^2 over 2 hours IV on days 1, 8, 15, 22, 29, and 36 followed immediately by fluorouracil.
   (3) Fluorouracil 2000 mg/m^2 continuously over 22 hours IV on days 1, 8, 15, 22, 29, and 36. The regimen is repeated every 7 weeks (6 weeks on followed by 1 week off).

i. Irinotecan plus cisplatin
   (1) Irinotecan 65 mg/m^2 IV over 30 minutes on days 1, 8, 15, and 22.
   (2) Cisplatin 30 mg/m^2 IV over 2 hours on days 1, 8, 15, and 22. The cycle is repeated every 6 weeks.

j. Oxaliplatin plus fluorouracil
   (1) Oxaliplatin 85 mg/m^2 IV over 2 hours on day 1.
   (2) Leucovorin 200 mg/m^2 IV over 2 hours followed by fluorouracil.
   (3) Fluorouracil 2600 mg/m^2 IV continuously over 24 hours. The regimen is repeated every 2 weeks.

k. Paclitaxel plus cisplatin
   (1) Paclitaxel 100 mg/m^2 IV over 1 hour on days 1 and 8 followed by cisplatin.
   (2) Cisplatin 30 mg/m^2 IV over 30 minutes (with 2 L of normal saline) on days 1 and 8. This regimen is repeated every 21 days.

l. Fluorouracil, leucovorin, and oxaliplatin (FLO)
   (1) Oxaliplatin 85 mg/m^2 IV over 1 to 2 hours on day 1.
   (2) Leucovorin 200 mg/m^2 IV over 1 to 2 hours on day 1, followed by fluorouracil.
   (3) Fluorouracil 2600 mg/m^2 continuous IV over 24 hours. This regimen is repeated every 2 weeks.

m. FLO plus docetaxel
   (1) Oxaliplatin, leucovorin, and fluorouracil as discussed previously.
   (2) Docetaxel 50 mg/m^2 IV over 1 to 2 hours on day 1. This regimen is repeated every 2 weeks. This "modified" DCF regimen was shown to have a more acceptable adverse event profile than the DCF regimen from V325 (complicated neutropenia, 3.8% versus 29%).

n. Capecitabine plus cisplatin
   (1) Capecitabine 1000 mg/m^2 orally twice daily on days 1 to 14.
   (2) Cisplatin 80 mg/m^2 IV on day 1. This regimen is repeated every 21 days.

C. Adjuvant chemotherapy

A meta-analysis published in 2001 of over 3,658 clinical trial patients (21 comparisons) who were randomized to receive adjuvant chemotherapy versus surgery alone showed a small survival benefit for those who received adjuvant therapy (18% reduced risk of death, HR = 0.82, p <0.001).

In addition to this, in 2006 the European MAGIC trial was published accruing 503 patients with gastric cancer who were randomized to surgery alone versus three preoperative and three postoperative cycles of the ECF regimen. The patients who received chemotherapy demonstrated significant downstaging of their tumors with improved progression-free survival (19 months versus 13 months, p = 0.0001), median survival (24 months versus 20 months, p = 0.02), and 5-year survival (36% versus 23%, p = 0.009). Because only 55% of patients were able to begin postoperative therapy, it is postulated that the preoperative chemotherapy provided the most significant benefit. Other neo-adjuvant regimens, including combinations with radiation, are undergoing study.

D. Combined-modality therapy

The U.S. Gastrointestinal Intergroup has reported the results of a 556-patient randomized trial comparing surgery with or without postoperative chemotherapy (fluorouracil and leuco-vorin) and combined chemotherapy and radiation followed by two additional cycles of chemotherapy. Patients had resected stages IB through stage IV M0 adenocarcinoma of the stomach or gastroesophageal junction. Postoperative combined therapy produced a statistically significant median survival benefit (36 months versus 27 months, respectively; p = 0.005). Although the study did not show any significant difference in relapse-free survival or OS according to the extent of lymph node dissection, 54% of patients had a D0 lymphadenectomy (surgery that did not remove all of the N1 nodes), 36% had a D1 dissection, and only 10% underwent a D2 dissection (includes perigastric, celiac, splenic, hepatic artery, and cardial lymph nodes). Major toxic effects (grade 3 or higher) in the chemoradiotherapy group were predominantly hematologic (54%) and GI (33%).

E. Recommended postoperative adjuvant combined modality regimen

1. Preradiation chemotherapy (cycle 1)

a. Leucovorin 20 mg/m^2 IV bolus on days 1 to 5.

b. Fluorouracil 425 mg/m^2 IV bolus on days 1 to 5.

2. Radiotherapy and chemotherapy

a. Radiation therapy 45 Gy at 180 cGy/day to the tumor (or tumor bed) and nodal chains daily for 5 days weekly for 5 weeks (begin 28 days after initial chemotherapy).

  b. **Chemotherapy.** Started on the first day of radiotherapy and repeated during the last 3 days of radiation.
    (1) **Leucovorin** 20 mg/m^2 IV bolus followed by fluorouracil 400 mg/m^2 IV bolus on the first 4 days and last 3 days of radiation therapy.
  3. **Postradiation chemotherapy.** One month after completing chemoradiation, repeat cycle 1 for two more cycles 1 month apart.

F. Follow-up studies

Reasonable follow-up studies for patients in remission after surgery consist of history and physical examination every 3 to 6 months for years 1 to 3, every 6 months for years 3 to 5, and then annually. Complete blood cell count, chemistries, endoscopy, and radiologic imaging should be evaluated as clinically indicated. Vitamin B$_{12}$ supplementation is recommended for patients who have had proximal resections or total gastrectomy.

G. Complications

Hematologic and GI toxicities from the chemotherapy may be accentuated by concurrent radiotherapy. If the complications are sufficiently severe, chemotherapy, radiotherapy, or both should be withheld until improvement. Consideration is given to treating at reduced doses. Hematopoietic growth factors may be of benefit in preventing severe infections secondary to neutropenia, but their use has not yet resulted in improved survival.

H. Treatment of refractory disease

If the patient's disease recurs or progresses with the recommended regimens, it is reasonable to consider combinations containing drugs not previously administered.

III. CANCER OF THE SMALL INTESTINE

A. Neuroendocrine tumors (NETs)

Carcinoid tumors are the most common NET of the small intestine, often found in the appendix and ileum. They may develop in other parts of the GI tract but much less frequently. The usual histologic criteria of malignancy are not always applicable. NETs tend to be less aggressive than adenocarcinomas of the small intestine. Negative prognostic findings generally include nodal metastases, high Ki67 index (>5%), high mitotic rate, presence of clinical symptoms, tumor size (>2 cm), and elevated chromogranin A or hormonally active tumor byproducts. Five-year OS approaches about 60%, which is worse than other GI NETs. Ileal NETs tend to be more invasive then appendiceal NETs. The most common sites of metastases include lymph nodes (89.8%), liver (44.1%), lung (13.6%), peritoneum (13.6%), and pancreas (6.8%), with adjacent organs being involved due to extensive fibrosis that is characteristic of this type of tumor (Table 7.3).

TNM Stages for Neuroendocrine Tumors*

Primary Tumor

T1	Invades lamina propria or submucosa and size ≤1 cm
T2	Invades muscularis propria or size >1cm
T3	Invades through muscularis propria into subserosal tissue without penetration of overlying serosa (jejunal or ileal tumors) or invades pancreas or retroperitoneum (ampullary or duodenal tumors or into nonperitonealized structures
T4	Invades visceral peritoneum (serosa) or invades other organs

Regional Lymph Nodes

N0	No regional lymph node metastasis
N1	Regional lymph node metastasis

Distant Metastasis

M0	No distant metastasis
M1	Distant metastasis

Stage Grouping

I	T1, N0, M0
IIA	T2, N0, M0
IIB	T3, N0, M0
IIIA	T4, N0, M0
IIIB	Any T, N1, M0
IV	Any T, any N, M1

*Only for duodenum, ampulla, jejunum, and ileum.

1. **Carcinoid syndrome.** About 10% of patients with NETs have carcinoid syndrome, which includes diarrhea, abdominal cramps, malabsorption, flushing, bronchoconstriction, and cardiac valvular disease (late sequela). Approximately 90% of patients presenting with symptomatic NETs have metastatic disease to the liver, which may be under the level of detection of imaging. Serotonin is thought to be responsible for the abdominal symptoms. Its metabolite, 5-hydroxyindoleacetic acid (5-HIAA), is excreted in large quantities in the urine and is a useful marker of disease activity when measured over a 24-hour period. Other markers may be elevated, including chromogranin A, which is the most frequently-elevated carcinoid marker. The symptoms may respond to simple antidiarrheal therapy. The flushing caused by the syndrome has been attributed to bradykinin, formed by the interaction of kallikrein (produced by the tumor) with a plasma protein. If simple symptomatic measures do not suffice, the best treatment is the synthetic long-acting somatostatin analog octreotide acetate (Sandostatin). This agent, injected at a usual initial dose of 150 μg

subcutaneously (SC) every 8 hours or as the long-acting formulation (octreotide LAR depot) 20 to 30 mg intramuscularly (IM) every month, effectively decreases the secretion of serotonin and other gastroenteropancreatic peptides such as insulin or gastrin. It has been helpful in ameliorating the symptoms of carcinoid tumors (e.g., flushing and diarrhea). A common issue with octreotide treatment is fat malabsorption and therefore the addition of pancreatic enzyme replacement may be warranted. The excretion of 5-HIAA is reduced by octreotide.

2. **Treatment of advanced NETs**

   a. **Effective agents.** A recent large double-blind, randomized, phase IIIB German study (PROMID) treated patients with midgut NET either with octreotide LAR 30 mg IM every 4 weeks or placebo as first-line therapy. Median time to tumor progression was improved with octreotide treatment (14.3 months versus 6 months; HR 0.34; $p = 0.00007$). This effect persisted whether or not the tumor was active (i.e., presence of carcinoid syndrome). Of note, 95% of these patients had Ki67 indexes of less than 2% and the majority had liver tumor burden of less than or equal to 10%, which appeared to be an important prognostic factor in subset analyses. The median OS was approximately 73.7 months in the placebo group and had not been reached in the octreotide LAR group; conclusions could not be drawn given the limited number of deaths observed during the study.

      (1) **Octreotide monotherapy.** Octreotide LAR is dosed as 20 to 30 mg IM every 14 to 28 days. Consider run-in and overlap of approximately 2 weeks with octreotide acetate 150 µg SC three times a day to assess tolerability with a short-acting agent and then to allow the LAR to reach steady state. This can be continued despite progression with additional second-line agents.

      The chemotherapy agents doxorubicin, fluorouracil, dacarbazine, and streptozocin have been shown to have limited activity in this disease. ECOG E1281 randomized 249 patients with advanced carcinoid to either fluorouracil plus doxorubicin or fluorouracil plus streptozocin and found comparable response rates (16%) and progression-free survival (approximately 5 months), but they reported a significant improvement in median OS for the streptozocin group (24.3 months versus 15.7 months; $p = 0.02$). Of note, crossover to dacarbazine yielded an 8% response rate and median OS of 11.9 months. The following regimens were used.

      (2) **Streptozocin plus fluorouracil**

         (a) **Streptozocin** 500 mg/m^2/day by rapid push IV on days 1 to 5.

         (b) **Fluorouracil** 400 mg/m^2/day IV on days 1 to 5 and 36 to 40. This regimen was repeated every 10 weeks.

(3) Dacarbazine. Dacarbazine 250 mg/m^2/day by rapid push IV on days 1 to 5. This regimen was repeated every 4 weeks.

(4) Interferon-α 3 to 6 × 10^6 U/day or 10 × 10^6 U three times per week.

Targeted agents have shown promise in NETs. Some reports have indicated responses with interferon-α, including responses in combination with octreotide and in some patients previously treated with chemotherapy. A recent phase III study demonstrated no statistical difference in interferon-α versus the combination of streptozocin and fluorouracil.

(5) Sunitinib 50 mg orally daily for 4 weeks with a 2-week break (6-week cycles) was found to have activity in carcinoid tumors with a 10.2-month median time to progression.

(6) Other active agents, including bevacizumab 15 mg/kg IV every 3 weeks, showed improved progression-free survival over pegylated interferon-α-2b 0.5 mcg/kg SC every week in combination with depot octreotide in a phase II Southwest Oncology Group (SWOG) study. There is currently a phase III SWOG study (S0518) comparing bevacizumab to interferon therapy.

When the disease is confined to the liver, it is sometimes possible to achieve good palliation with hepatic artery embolization, chemoembolization, or most recently, yttrium-90 microspheres. Of note, poorly differentiated NETs or small-cell/atypical lung carcinoids are managed with a small-cell lung cancer regimen.

b. **Precautions.** Treatment of carcinoid tumors may precipitate or exacerbate the carcinoid syndrome during the first days of treatment, and the serotonin antagonists cyproheptadine and methysergide as well as octreotide should be available.

B. Adenocarcinomas

Adenocarcinomas of the small intestine are so uncommon that there is no large chemotherapy experience to report. Survival of patients with small intestinal cancer is a function of stage (Table 7.4). Radiation and infusional fluorouracil may be considered for patients with local recurrence or unresectable disease. The chemotherapy regimens employed for advanced colorectal cancer (e.g., oxaliplatin, irinotecan, fluorouracil, and leucovorin) also are generally used to treat patients with small intestine adenocarcinoma.

IV. CANCER OF THE LARGE INTESTINE

A. General considerations and aims of therapy

Taken together, cancers of the colon and rectum are by far the most frequent malignancies of the GI tract and account for the most deaths. Approximately half of patients found to have large-bowel

TABLE 7.4 TNM Stages for Carcinoma of the Small Intestine

Primary Tumor

Tis	Carcinoma in situ
T1a	Invades lamina propria
T1b	Invades submucosa*
T2	Invades muscularis propria
T3	Invades through the muscularis propria into subserosa or into non-peritonealized perimuscular tissue* with extension of ≤2 cm
T4	Perforates visceral peritoneum or directly invades other organs or structures

Regional Lymph Nodes

N0	No regional nodal metastasis
N1	Metastasis in one to three regional lymph nodes
N2	Metastasis in four or more regional lymph nodes

Distant Metastasis

M0	None
M1	Present

Stage Grouping

0	Tis, N0, M0
I	T1–2, N0, M0
IIA	T3, N0, M0
IIB	T4, N0, M0
IIIA	Any T, N1, M0
IIIB	Any T, N2, M0
IV	Any T, any N, M1

*The nonperitonealized perimuscular tissue is, for jejunum and ileum, part of the mesentery and, for the duodenum in areas where serosa is lacking, part of the interface with the pancreas. Modified from American Joint Committee on Cancer. *AJCC cancer staging manual* (7th ed.). New York: Springer; 2010.

cancers are cured by surgery, which remains the only curative modality. Local recurrence is much more common for rectal cancer (40% to 50% in nonirradiated patients). About half of large-bowel cancer recurrences are in the liver.

1. **Staging.** In the past, a commonly used staging system was the Dukes staging system, including the Astler-Coller modifications. TNM staging for colorectal cancer (Table 7.5) is currently the recommended system. The seventh edition of the *American Joint Committee on Cancer Staging Manual* modified the stage II, stage III, and stage IV disease groups by expanding the definitions of T4, N status, and M status to more accurately reflect the wide variations in survival. For example, using the Surveillance, Epidemiology and End Results database, 5-year observed survival for T4N0 patients varies by over 10% if there is a distinction

TNM Stages for Carcinoma of the Colon and Rectum

Primary Tumor

Tis	Carcinoma in situ and intramucosal (within lamina propria)
T1	Invades through muscularis mucosa into submucosa
T2	Invades muscularis propria
T3	Invades through muscularis propria into pericolorectal tissues
T4a	Penetrates to the surface of the visceral peritoneum
T4b*	Directly invades or is adherent to other organs or structures

Regional Lymph Nodes

N0	No nodal metastasis
N1	Metastasis in one to three regional nodes
N1a	Metastasis in one regional lymph node
N1b	Metastasis in two to three regional lymph nodes
N1c	Tumor deposit(s)[†] in the subserosa, mesentery, or nonperitonealized pericolic or perirectal tissues without regional lymph node metastasis
N2	Metastasis in more than four regional nodes
N2a	Metastasis in four to six regional lymph nodes
N2b	Metastasis in seven or more regional lymph nodes

Distant Metastasis

M0	None
M1a	Metastasis confined to one organ or site
M1b	Metastases in more than one organ/site or the peritoneum

Stage Grouping

0	Tis, N0, M0
I	T1–2, N0, M0
IIA	T3, N0, M0
IIB	T4a, N0, M0
IIC	T4b, N0, M0
IIIA	T1–2, N1/N1c, M0
	T1, N2a, M0
IIIB	T3–4a, N1/N1c, M0
	T2–3, N2a, M0
	T1–2, N2b, M0
IIIC	T4a, N2a, M0
	T3–T4a, N2b, M0
	T4b, N1–2, M0
IVA	Any T, any N, M1a
IVB	Any T, any N, M1b

*Adhesion secondary to inflammation and carcinoma that does not actually involve the adjacent structure or organ is not T4b disease.

[†] Discrete foci of tumor found in the pericolic and perirectal fat or in the adjacent mesentery (mesocolic fat) away from the leading edge of the tumor and showing no evidence of residual lymph node tissue but within the lymph node drainage area of the primary carcinoma with number of tumor deposits recorded.

Modified from American Joint Committee on Cancer. *AJCC cancer staging manual* (7th ed.). New York: Springer; 2010.

between penetrating to the visceral peritoneum from invading (T4a) or adhering to adjacent structures (T4b). The same is true when N1 and N2 staging is further subclassified as one involved lymph node (N1a), one to three involved lymph nodes (N1b), four to six involved lymph nodes (N2a), and finally seven or more involved lymph nodes (N2b). In addition, tumor deposits separate but adjacent to the primary tumor without evidence of lymph node tissue is N1c staging. Metastatic disease is further classified into solitary metastasis (M1a) or more than one metastasis, given the data indicating approximately 20% of patients who undergo liver resection for their metastatic colorectal cancer are disease-free at 5 years. This pathologic staging method is helpful for selecting patients who are at sufficiently high risk to justify adjuvant therapy such as chemotherapy or irradiation (rectal cancer) as well as those with metastatic disease that may still derive long-term benefit from surgical or interventional procedures. Staging is most accurately performed at the time of surgery. Abdominal, chest, and pelvic CT are helpful for preoperative assessment of extrabowel involvement, but the findings may be falsely negative when small peritoneal implants are present. Bone scans are seldom needed, except for assessment of bone pain, because bone metastases occur rather late in the course of the disease. PET scanning is considered to determine the presence of metastatic disease.

2. **Serum CEA.** CEA level may parallel disease activity, although it is not increased in all patients with colon cancer. It is worth measuring preoperatively and, if elevated, postoperatively because failure of an elevated value to return to normal may signify incomplete removal of the tumor. Likewise, a serial rise in CEA values after an initial fall to normal indicates recurrence. CEA values may also be an indicator of response during chemotherapy treatment. Patients who have a normal serum CEA level preoperatively may still demonstrate an elevated CEA value at the time of recurrence. A rising CEA level is an indication for careful re-evaluation with CT, PET, and possibly laparoscopy because some patients may have isolated, resectable, and thus potentially curable metastases, particularly involving the liver.

B. **Treatment of advanced disease**
   1. **Effective agents and combinations.** For more than 40 years, fluorouracil has been the standard agent in the treatment of advanced colorectal disease not amenable to surgical or radiotherapeutic control. Response rates have varied widely, but a generally agreed-on figure is 10% to 15%. Fluorouracil with leucovorin and bevacizumab also has activity with a median OS of 18.3 months and progression-free survival of 8.8 months.

a. **Fluorouracil plus high-dose leucovorin (weekly Roswell-Park regimen)**
   (1) **Leucovorin** 500 mg/m^2 IV given over 2 hours.
   (2) **Fluorouracil** 500 mg/m^2 IV bolus injected 1 hour after beginning the leucovorin infusion.

   The combination is administered weekly for 6 weeks followed by a 2-week rest. This regimen is now widely favored as the preferred fluorouracil plus leucovorin combination.

b. **Fluorouracil bolus weekly regimen.** Leucovorin 20 mg/m^2 IV over 2 hours followed by fluorouracil 500 mg/m^2 IV bolus injection 1 hour after leucovorin is started. Repeat weekly.

c. **Fluorouracil by 24-hour continuous infusion.** Fluorouracil 2600 mg/m^2 is given by 24-hour continuous infusion IV weekly plus leucovorin at 500 mg/m^2.

d. **Simplified biweekly infusional 5-fluorouracil/leucovorin (sLV5FU2)**
   (1) **Leucovorin** 400 mg/m^2 as a 2-hour IV infusion, followed by fluorouracil.
   (2) **Fluorouracil** 400 mg/m^2 IV bolus on day 1 *only*, then followed by fluorouracil 2.4 g/m^2 as a continuous IV infusion over 46 to 48 hours. This regimen is repeated every 2 weeks.

   Chemotherapy combinations with fluorouracil, including leucovorin, irinotecan, and oxaliplatin have demonstrated equal efficacy in both first- and second-line roles. The addition of the antivascular endothelial growth factor monoclonal antibody bevacizumab to chemotherapy as well as the use of anti-EGFR monoclonal antibodies cetuximab and panitumumab in patients who are KRAS wild-type alone or with chemotherapy has further improved response rates and survival even further to beyond 2 years. Irinotecan can be used in combination with fluorouracil or alone with or without a monoclonal antibody added. Oxaliplatin does not have efficacy in colorectal cancer without fluorouracil. Capecitabine has been shown to be noninferior to fluorouracil and therefore can be used on its own or in combination, although it should be noted that folinic acid, fluorouracil, and irinotecan (FOLFIRI) has been shown to be superior to capecitabine and irinotecan in a large phase III study (BICC-C trial), so this combination is not recommended. The fluorouracil, leucovorin, oxaliplatin, and irinotecan (FOLFOXIRI) regimen as a first-line regimen may improve response rates and survival (compared to FOLFIRI) at the cost of increased toxicity, but only one or two studies confirmed these efficacy results. The combination of bevacizumab with cetuximab or panitumumab in addition to chemotherapy in first-line therapy (CAIRO2 and PACCE studies, respectively) showed significant worsening of progression-free survival as well as increased toxicity. Therefore, this combination is not currently recommended. Lastly, the BRiTE study, which was a large observational cohort design, indicated a potential improved OS with continuation of bevacizumab beyond progression of first-line therapy (19.9 months versus 31.8 months; $p < 0.001$), but its continuation remains controversial with clinical trials currently assessing this strategy.

e. FOLFIRI

(1) **Irinotecan** 180 mg/m^2 IV over 30 to 90 minutes on day 1.

(2) **Fluorouracil** 400 mg/m^2 IV bolus on day 1.

(3) **Leucovorin** 400 mg/m^2 IV over 30 to 90 minutes on day 1, followed by fluorouracil.

(4) **Fluorouracil** 2.4 g/m^2 as a continuous infusion over 46 to 48 hours. The cycle is repeated every 2 weeks.

f. Irinotecan. Irinotecan 125 mg/m^2 as a 90-minute infusion IV is given weekly for 2 weeks with a 1-week rest *or* 180 mg/m^2 every 2 weeks *or* 300 to 350 mg/m^2 every 3 weeks.

g. Modified FOLFOX6 (mFOLFOX6)

(1) **Oxaliplatin** 85 mg/m^2 as a 120-minute infusion IV in 500 mL of 5% dextrose in water (D5W) on day 1.

(2) **Leucovorin** 400 mg/m^2 as a 120-minute infusion IV, followed by fluorouracil.

(3) **Fluorouracil** 400 mg/m^2 IV bolus on day 1.

(4) **Fluorouracil** 2.4 g/m^2 as a continuous infusion IV over 46 to 48 hours.

The cycle is repeated every 14 days. Day 1 leucovorin may be given during the same 2-hour period as the oxaliplatin, but because of the incompatibility of oxaliplatin with saline, both drugs must be in D5W.

h. FOLFOX4

(1) **Oxaliplatin** 85 mg/m^2 as a 2-hour infusion IV in 250 to 500 mL of D5W on day 1 *only* simultaneously with leucovorin.

(2) **Leucovorin** 200 mg/m^2 as a 2-hour infusion IV on days 1 and 2, followed by fluorouracil.

(3) **Fluorouracil** 400 mg/m^2 IV bolus on day 1 then fluorouracil 600 mg/m^2 as a 22-hour infusion given on days 1 and 2 every 14 days.

mFOLFOX6 is the preferred oxaliplatin-containing regimen.

i. Capecitabine. Capecitabine is dosed at 1000 to 1250 mg/m^2 administered twice daily orally on days 1 to 14 every 3 weeks (2000–2500 mg/m^2/day). In areas of the world, including the United States, where food is heavily fortified with folates, the lower dose of capecitabine has been shown to be better tolerated.

  j. Capecitabine plus oxaliplatin (XELOX)
   (1) Oxaliplatin 130 mg/m^2 IV day 1.
   (2) Capecitabine 850 to 1000 mg/m^2 by mouth twice a day for 14 days every 21 days. Again, the capecitabine dose of 1000 mg/m^2 is considered standard in Europe, but North American patients, likely due to higher dietary folate intake, have experienced greater toxicity with this starting dose and therefore are recommended to start with the lower 850 mg/m^2 dosing.

k. FOLFOXIRI
   (1) Irinotecan 165 mg/m^2 IV on day 1.
   (2) Oxaliplatin 85 mg/m^2 IV on day 1.
   (3) Leucovorin 400 mg/m^2 IV on day 1.
   (4) Fluorouracil 3200 mg/m^2 over 48-hour continuous infusion starting on day 1. Repeat this regimen every 2 weeks.

l. Bevacizumab. Bevacizumab 5 mg/kg IV over 90 minutes (first cycle), 60 minutes (second cycle), then up to 0.5 mg/kg/minute for each subsequent cycle every other week given with FOLFOX, FOLFIRI, or sLV5FU2. Bevacizumab can be used with XELOX, but the dose of 7.5 mg/kg IV every 3 weeks is recommended. Please note that the practitioner should exercise extreme caution in patients with severe bleeding or clotting issues, active coronary artery disease, or severely uncontrolled hypertension.

m. Cetuximab 400 mg/m^2 IV first infusion given over 2 hours, then 250 mg/m^2 weekly *or* 500 mg/m^2 IV every 2 weeks. This can be used alone or in combination with the listed chemotherapy regimens.

n. Panitumumab 6 mg/kg IV over 60 minutes every 2 weeks. The U.S. Food and Drug Administration has approved the use of panitumumab, another anti-EGFR monoclonal antibody, for use as a monotherapy in refractory patients with response rates of 10%, stable disease in 27%, and a 4-month improvement in progression-free survival compared to best supportive care.

Please note that only patients with KRAS wild-type mutational status derive benefit from these anti-EGFR monoclonal antibodies. It is also important to note that patients can get an acneiform rash that should be managed aggressively to prevent delays in therapy.

The current principle of treatment strategy for patients with advanced colorectal cancer encompasses a new paradigm. Treatment now represents a continuum whereby patients who are exposed to all active agents, including fluorouracil, irinotecan, oxaliplatin, bevacizumab, and anti-EGFR monoclonal antibodies (KRAS wild-type only), over the course of their illness will achieve the maximum survival advantage, now estimated as a median survival of over 2 years.

C. Adjuvant chemotherapy

1. **Colon cancer.** For patients with node-positive (stage III) resectable colon cancer, the combination of fluorouracil plus leucovorin given either by the 5-day or the weekly schedule for 6 months improves the disease-free survival (DFS) as well as the OS of patients. The recent update of the MOSAIC trial, which evaluated FOLFOX4 versus sLV5FU2 for Stage II/III colon cancer patients, found significant improvement in DFS and OS, but there was no significant difference in the subgroup of stage II colorectal cancer. In addition, the National Surgical Adjuvant Breast and Bowel Project (NSABP) trial evaluating a bolus regimen of oxaliplatin compared to weekly fluorouracil and leucovorin produced comparable 3-year DFS statistics as seen with MOSAIC for stage II and III patients, favoring the FLO regimen. Of note, increased GI toxicity has somewhat limited the use of this regimen. QUASAR has been the only large study to measure a difference in survival with adjuvant treatment for stage II colon cancer with an absolute improvement of 3.6%. Current NCCN and American Society of Clinical Oncology guidelines for high-risk stage II patients (based on clinical and histopathologic data) suggest a detailed discussion between the oncologist and patient as to the risk versus the benefit of receiving adjuvant chemotherapy for stage II disease. A current GI intergroup trial will define risk for stage II patients based on molecular markers including 18q allele deletion and microsatellite instability.

   Two large adjuvant trials for patients with stage III colon cancer comparing irinotecan with either infusional fluorouracil or bolus fluorouracil versus fluorouracil and leucovorin failed to show a DFS advantage for the combination; therefore, *irinotecan cannot be recommended as an adjuvant therapy strategy at this time.* Additional trials comparing capecitabine versus fluorouracil/leucovorin and infusional fluorouracil versus bolus fluorouracil and leucovorin have demonstrated that each of these approaches produce comparable results. For patients who are candidates for combination therapy, the FOLFOX regimen has become a standard for stage III colon cancer patients. The addition of bevacizumab has only shown transient benefit in DFS in a recent NSABP trial and did not reach its primary endpoint of DFS in the AVANT study.

   Although historic data support the use of postoperative radiotherapy for locally advanced colon cancer (Dukes B3 or C3 or any T4 lesion), a small intergroup trial did not confirm its efficacy. Combination chemotherapy should probably be incorporated into the regimen and used for a total of 6 months after radiation therapy.

The recommended colon cancer adjuvant regimens for node-positive patients (stage III) are as follows.

a. Fluorouracil plus high-dose leucovorin (weekly Roswell Park regimen) as in Section IV.B.1.a. This is given for four cycles.

b. sLV5FU2. See Section IV.B.1.d. Twelve cycles are administered.

c. Capecitabine. See Section IV.B.1.i. Eight cycles are administered.

d. mFOLFOX6. See Section IV.B.1.g. Twelve cycles are administered.

e. FOLFOX4. See Section IV.B.1.h. Twelve cycles are administered.

f. FLO

(1) Oxaliplatin 85 mg/m^2 as a 120-minute infusion IV on weeks 1, 2, and 5 of each 8-week cycle.

(2) Fluorouracil 500 mg/m^2 IV bolus weekly for 6 weeks.

(3) Leucovorin 500 mg/m^2 IV bolus weekly for 6 weeks. There are three 8-week cycles administered (total of 6 months).

2. Resected hepatic metastases. Past data have demonstrated that approximately 25% of patients with completely resected hepatic metastases secondary to colorectal cancer experience a long-term survival with more recent data approaching 50%. The goal of chemotherapy in patients with liver-only metastatic disease that is deemed unresectable is to convert them to a resectable status, called "conversion therapy." Because even a few cycles of chemotherapy can cause liver damage, the goal is to balance optimal response with that toxicity. Generally, patients receive 2 to 4 months of chemotherapy neoadjuvantly followed postoperatively with chemotherapy for a goal of approximately 6 months total if there is no evidence of residual disease. Bevacizumab can interfere with wound healing and therefore requires discontinuation 4 to 8 weeks prior to surgery.

3. Rectal cancer

a. Preoperative chemoradiation is the standard of care for patients with stage II and III rectal cancer. The NSABP R-03 showed prospectively, even though it was underpowered, that preoperative chemoradiation improved DFS with a trend toward OS compared to postoperative chemoradiation. In addition, a German group showed improved locoregional control (without survival advantage) with preoperative compared to postoperative chemoradiation, and showed significant worse acute and long-term toxic effects with postoperative chemoradiation. Currently, preoperative chemoradiation employing any of the following regimens is acceptable.

(1) Fluorouracil 225 mg/m^2 daily as a continuous infusion on the days of radiation. This regimen has become a standard in the United States and Europe.

(2) Capecitabine 825 mg/m^2 by mouth twice daily on the days of radiation. This regimen is being compared to fluorouracil in the neoadjuvant setting in a large ECOG study, but given the noninferiority in the metastatic setting, this is acceptable.

(3) Fluorouracil 400 mg/m^2 IV bolus plus leucovorin 20 mg/ m^2 IV bolus for 4 days during week 1 and week 5.

b. Postoperative chemotherapy. The European Organization for Research and Treatment of Cancer 22921 trial showed nonsignificant trends with adjuvant chemotherapy toward improved PFS and OS ($p = 0.15$ and $p = 0.12$, respectively). In a later subset analysis of patients who were downstaged from neoadjuvant therapy (cT3-T4 to pT0-T2), adjuvant chemotherapy was shown to improve OS and DFS. New adjuvant chemotherapy trials (for patients who receive preoperative chemoradiation) are investigating the use of FOLFOX with or without bevacizumab. Based on the MOSAIC trial, the addition of oxaliplatin to fluorouracil and leucovorin may be a reasonable strategy for adjuvant chemotherapy in rectal cancer.

The recommended postoperative adjuvant regimen for stage II or III rectal cancers is as follows.

(1) sLV5FU2 (see Section IV.B.1.d).

(2) Fluorouracil bolus weekly regimen (see Section IV.B.1.b).

If the patient did not receive neoadjuvant therapy, then the following regimens are recommended for adjuvant therapy:

(1) Fluorouracil plus high-dose leucovorin (weekly Roswell Park regimen), as described in Section IV.B.1.a. This regimen is given for one cycle prior to chemoradiation and then two cycles after completion of chemoradiation (see Section IV.C.3.a.1–3).

(2) mFOLFOX6, as described in Section IV.C.1.d.

(3) Capecitabine, as described in Section IV.C.1.c.

D. Follow-up

A pooled analysis of clinical trials suggests that 85% of colorectal cancer recurrences will occur within 3 years. In the asymptomatic patient, follow-up after treatment includes history and physical examination, and CEA every 3 to 6 months for 2 years, then every 6 months for 5 years. Colonoscopy often is performed 1 year after surgery and then every 3 years if no polyps are found. CT scans of the chest, abdomen, and pelvis may be considered yearly for 3 years for patients at high risk for recurrence (i.e., lymphovascular invasion or poorly differentiated tumors).

E. Complications of therapy or disease

The complications of chemotherapy are those attributable to the individual drugs. Myelosuppression, nausea, vomiting, and diarrhea are common and may require dose modification and symptomatic treatment. Radiation complications are similar and also include dysuria, tenesmus, and rectal discharge of blood or mucus. Phenazopyridine is useful in treating dysuria, and loperamide or diphenoxylate is recommended for diarrhea. If toxicity is substantial (grade 3 or 4) during radiotherapy, a treatment delay of at least

1 week is warranted. During chemotherapy with fluorouracil-based regimens, mild diarrhea (grade 1) may be treated symptomatically. Moderate diarrhea (grade 2 or 3) is an indication for dose reduction by 50%, and severe diarrhea (grade 3 or 4) is an indication for stopping chemotherapy for 1 week or longer. Dehydration is a real risk with grade 3 or 4 diarrhea, and hydration IV may be necessary. Tincture of opium or octreotide 150 μg three times a day may help to alleviate severe diarrhea.

Recent recommendations for management of irinotecan toxicity include evaluation for a GI syndrome, which can encompass diarrhea, nausea, vomiting, anorexia, abdominal cramping, dehydration, neutropenia, fever, and electrolyte abnormalities. Patients receiving irinotecan should undergo weekly assessment, at least during the first cycle, to look for concurrent toxicities. In addition to treating the diarrhea with loperamide, tincture of opium, or octreotide, oral fluoroquinolone should be initiated in any patient experiencing neutropenia, even in the absence of fever or diarrhea, or in any patient experiencing fever and diarrhea, even in the absence of neutropenia. Antibiotics should be initiated in any hospitalized patient with prolonged diarrhea regardless of granulocyte count and should be continued until resolution of diarrhea. Any patient who experiences significant treatment-related diarrhea should not receive irinotecan until diarrhea-free or at baseline bowel function for at least 24 hours without the use of antidiarrheal agents or antibiotics. In addition, abdominal cramping should be considered equivalent to diarrhea.

Oral mucositis can often be prevented on subsequent courses without dose reduction by holding ice in the mouth for 20 minutes before, during, and after the IV bolus of fluorouracil. Nausea is usually not severe with fluorouracil regimens and usually responds to prochlorperazine or dexamethasone. Hematopoietic growth factors are seldom warranted for the mild neutropenia that is observed with bolus fluorouracil therapy.

Oxaliplatin causes an acute cold sensitivity associated with distal dysesthesias or paresthesias and a chronic sensory neuropathy. Potential bevacizumab toxicities include hypertension, bleeding, delayed wound healing, arterial thrombosis, proteinuria, and GI perforation. There is also a vascular syndrome, which can include myocardial infarction, pulmonary embolus, or cerebral vascular accident. Cetuximab is associated with acneiform rash, hypersensitivity, interstitial lung disease, and infusion reactions.

V. CANCER OF THE ANAL CANAL

These cancers, constituting only 1% to 3% of all cases of large-bowel cancer, were historically treated by abdominoperineal resection with about a 50% cure rate. Major associations include a human papillomavirus infection; past receptive anal intercourse or sexually transmitted infection; past cervical, vulvar, or vaginal cancer; immunosuppression after solid organ transplantation; a human immunodeficiency virus infection; and smoking.

A. Local disease (Table 7.6)

It has been found that combined-modality treatment with chemotherapy and radiation is curative in 75% to 80% of patients and thus allows avoidance of abdominoperineal resection with retention of anal function. The following regimen is recommended.

1. Radiotherapy 4500 cGy in 25 fractions (5 weeks), concurrent with fluorouracil and mitomycin.
2. Fluorouracil 1000 mg/m^2 by continuous infusion IV daily for 4 days (days 1 to 4 and 29 to 32).
3. Mitomycin 10 mg/m^2 IV on days 1 and 29.

TABLE 7.6	TNM Staging for Carcinoma of the Anus

Primary Tumor

Tis	Carcinoma in situ (e.g., Bowen disease, high-grade squamous intraepithelial lesion, anal intraepithelial neoplasia II-III)
T1	Tumor 2 cm or less in greatest dimension
T2	Tumor >2 cm but not >5 cm in greatest dimension
T3	Tumor >5 cm in greatest dimension
T4	Tumor of any size invades adjacent organ(s)* (e.g., vagina, urethra, bladder)

Regional Lymph Nodes

N0	No regional lymph node metastasis
N1	Metastasis in perirectal lymph node(s)
N2	Metastasis in unilateral internal iliac and/or inguinal lymph node(s)
N3	Metastasis in perirectal and inguinal lymph nodes and/or bilateral internal iliac and/or inguinal lymph nodes

Distant Metastasis

M0	No distant metastasis
M1	Distant metastasis

Stage Grouping

0	Tis, N0, M0
I	T1, N0, M0
II	T2–3, N0, M0
IIIA	T1–3, N1, M0
	T4, N0, M0
IIIB	T4, N1, M0
	Any T, N2–3, M0
IV	Any T, any N, M1

*Direct invasion of the rectal wall, perirectal skin, subcutaneous tissue, or the sphincter muscle(s) is not T4.
Modified from American Joint Committee on Cancer. *AJCC cancer staging manual* (7th ed.). New York: Springer; 2010.

A biopsy should be done 8 weeks after radiation therapy only for a suspicious residual area of abnormality. If negative, no further treatment is needed. If positive, consider an additional 900 cGy (five fractions) and a 4-day course of fluorouracil 1000 mg/m^2 by continuous infusion IV on days 1 to 4 and cisplatin 100 mg/m^2 IV on day 2. If the biopsy is persistently positive, an abdominoperineal resection is appropriate.

A large U.S. Gastrointestinal Intergroup trial compared the standard regimen of mitomycin and fluorouracil versus preradiation chemotherapy followed by chemoradiotherapy using the following.

1. Cisplatin 75 mg/m^2 IV on days 1, 29, 57, and 85.
2. Fluorouracil 1000 mg/m^2 by continuous infusion IV on days 1 to 4, 29 to 32, 57 to 60, and 85 to 88.
3. Radiation 45 to 59 Gy, starting day 57.

Five-year DFS and OS were not statistically different (DFS, mitomycin-based 54% versus cisplatin-based 60%; $p = 0.17$; OS, mitomycin-based 75% versus cisplatin-based 70%; $p = 0.10$), but the cumulative colostomy rate was decreased with mitomycin-based therapy (10% versus 19%; $p = 0.02$).

B. Metastatic disease

For metastatic disease, the following regimen may be considered.

1. Fluorouracil 1000 mg/m^2/day IV continuously on days 1 to 5.
2. Cisplatin 100 mg/m^2 IV on day 2. Repeat this regimen every 4 weeks.

Cetuximab is currently under investigation in this disease.

Selected Readings

American Joint Committee on Cancer. *AJCC cancer staging manual* (7th ed.). New York: Springer; 2010.

National Comprehensive Cancer Network. NCCN guidelines and derivative information products: user guide. Retrieved from http://www.nccn.org/clinical.asp

Esophagus

Allum WH, Stenning SP, Bancewicz J. Long-term results of a randomized trial of surgery with or without preoperative chemotherapy in esophageal cancer. *J Clin Oncol.* 2009;27:5062–5067.

Cooper JS, Guo MD, Herskovic A, et al. Chemoradiotherapy of locally advanced esophageal cancer: long-term follow-up of a prospective randomized trial (RTOG 85-01). Radiation Therapy Oncology Group. *JAMA.* 1999;281:1623–1627.

Urschel JD, Vasan H. A meta-analysis of randomized controlled trials that compared neo-adjuvant chemo-radiation and surgery to surgery alone for resectable esophageal cancer. *Am J Surg.* 2003;185:538–543.

Stomach

Cunningham D, Allum WH, Stenning SP, et al. Perioperative chemotherapy versus surgery alone for resectable gastroesophageal cancer. *N Engl J Med.* 2006;355:11–20.

Hartgrink HH, van de Velde CJ, Putter H, et al. Extended lymph node dissection for gastric cancer: who may benefit? Final results of the randomized Dutch gastric cancer group trial. *J Clin Oncol.* 2004;22:2069–2077.

Macdonald JS, Smalley SR, Benedetti J, et al. Chemoradiotherapy after surgery compared with surgery alone for adenocarcinoma of the stomach or gastroesophageal junction. *N Engl J Med.* 2001;345:725–730.

Van Cutsem E, Kang Y, Chung H, et al. Efficacy results from the ToGA trial: A phase III study of trastuzumab added to standard chemotherapy (CT) in first-line human epidermal growth factor receptor 2 (HER2)-positive advanced gastric cancer (GC). *J Clin Oncol.* 2009;27:18s.

Van Cutsem E, Moiseyenko VM, Tjulandin S, et al. Phase III study of docetaxel and cisplatin plus fluorouracil compared with cisplatin and fluorouracil as first-line therapy for advanced gastric cancer: a report of the V325 Study Group. *J Clin Oncol.* 2006;24:4991–4997.

Waters JS, Norman A, Cunningham D, et al. Long-term survival after epirubicin, cisplatin and fluorouracil for gastric cancer: results of a randomized trial. 2009 ASCO Annual Meeting, abstract #LBA4509. *Br J Cancer.* 1999;80:269–272.

Small Intestine

Panzuto F, Di Fondo M, Iannicelli E, et al. Long-term clinical outcome of somatostatin analogues for treatment of progressive, metastatic, well-differentiated enteropancreatic endocrine carcinoma. *Ann Oncol.* 2006;17:461–466.

Rinke A, Muller HH, Schade-Brittinger C, et al. Placebo-controlled, double-blind, prospective, randomized study on the effect of octreotide LAR in the control of tumor growth in patients with metastatic neuroendocrine midgut tumors: a report from the PROMID study group. *J Clin Oncol.* 2009;27:4656–4663.

Large Intestine

Andre T, Boni C, Navarro M, et al. Improved overall survival with oxaliplatin, fluorouracil, and leucovorin as adjuvant treatment in stage II or III colon cancer in the MOSAIC trial. *J Clin Oncol.* 2009;27:3109–3116.

Collette L, Bossett JF, den Dulk M, et al. Patients with curative resection of cT3-4 rectal cancer after preoperative radiotherapy or radiochemotherapy: does anyone benefit from adjuvant fluorouracil-based therapy? A trial of the European Organisation for Research and Treatment of Cancer Radiation Oncology Group. *J Clin Oncol.* 2007;25:4379–4386.

Grothey A, Sugrue MM, Purdie DM, et al. Bevacizumab beyond first progression is associated with prolonged overall survival in metastatic colorectal cancer: results from a large observational cohort study (BRiTE). *J Clin Oncol.* 2008;26:5326–5334.

Roh MS, Colangelo LH, O'Connell MJ, et al. Preoperative multimodality therapy improves disease-free survival in patients with carcinoma of the rectum: NSABP R-03. *J Clin Oncol.* 2009;27:5124–5130.

Tournigand C, Andre T, Achille E, et al. FOLFIRI followed by FOLFOX6 or the reverse sequence in advanced colorectal cancer: a randomized GERCOR study. *J Clin Oncol.* 2004;22:229–237.

QUASAR Collaborative Group, Gray R, Barnwell J, et al. Adjuvant chemotherapy versus observation in patients with colorectal cancer: a randomized study. *Lancet.* 2007;370:2020–2029.

Van Cutsem E, Nowacki E, Lang I, et al. The CRYSTAL trial: efficacy and safety of irinotecan and 5-FU/LV with and without cetuximab in the first-line treatment of metastatic colorectal cancer. 2007 ASCO Annual Meeting Proceedings Part 1. *J Clin Oncol.* 2007;25(18S):4000.
Van Cutsem E, Peeters M, Siena S. Open label phase III trial of panitumumab plus best supportive care versus best supportive care alone in patients with chemotherapy-refractory metastatic colorectal cancer. *J Clin Oncol.* 2007;25:1658–1664.

Anus

Ajani JA, Winter KA, Gunderson LL, et al. Fluorouracil, mitomycin, and radiotherapy vs fluorouracil, cisplatin, and radiotherapy for carcinoma of the anal canal: a randomized controlled trial. *JAMA.* 2008;299:1914–1921.

Carcinomas of the Pancreas, Liver, Gallbladder, and Bile Ducts

Timothy J. Kennedy and Steven K. Libutti

I. ADENOCARCINOMA OF THE PANCREAS

A. Epidemiology

Pancreatic cancer is the eighth most common cancer for both genders combined but is the fourth leading cause of cancer death and is responsible for approximately 5% of cancer-related deaths. Recent estimates are that 42,000 individuals were diagnosed with pancreatic adenocarcinoma in the United States in 2009. The overall 5-year survival rate of all patients diagnosed with pancreatic adenocarcinoma remains less than 5%. For the majority of patients, the disease is either locally advanced and unresectable or metastatic at the time of diagnosis, and the median survival in these patients is 3 to 18 months. Approximately 15% of patients present with localized disease that is amenable to surgical resection; even in the most selective patient subgroups, however, median survival is only 2 years and anticipated 5-year survival rates are only 12% to 20%.

B. Etiology

Risk factors for pancreatic cancer include age, sex, and race. The disease is more common in the elderly, with the median age at diagnosis for pancreatic cancer being 72 years of age. Men and African-Americans have a higher risk than others. Cigarette smoking, alcohol consumption, obesity, *Helicobacter pylori* infection, and exposure to chemicals such as beta-naphthylamine and benzidine are also associated with an increased risk. Chronic pancreatitis and diabetes have been commonly associated with carcinoma of the pancreas but whether this association is causal is uncertain. The risk of pancreatic cancer is also increased in patients with certain familial cancer syndromes, but hereditary pancreatic cancer makes up less than 5% of cases. Hereditary pancreatic cancer has been observed in rare families with an autosomal site-specific pattern, in families with BRCA2 mutations, and in families with hereditary nonpolyposis colorectal cancer. Likewise, families with p16 germline mutations may be at higher risk of developing pancreatic cancer. Greater than 80% of resected pancreatic cancers harbor either activating point mutations in KRAS or inactivating mutations of the tumor suppressor genes p16, p53, and DPC4.

C. Presenting signs and symptoms

Pancreatic cancer–associated symptoms are not specific and usually occur when the disease is already incurable. Pain is the most common presenting symptom. It occurs in three-fourths of patients with carcinoma of the head of the pancreas and in virtually all patients with carcinoma of the body or tail. Usually, the pain is a dull ache in the epigastrium that radiates to the right upper quadrant when the tumor is in the head of the pancreas or to the left upper quadrant when the tumor is in the body or tail; the pain may radiate to the lumbar region of the back. Weight loss can be significant and is associated with anorexia, steatorrhea, nausea, diarrhea, and early satiety, which are other symptoms related to cancer of the pancreas. The nonspecific, vague nature of these complaints may delay diagnosis for several months. Seventy percent of patients with carcinoma of the head of the pancreas have jaundice, whereas fewer than 15% of patients with carcinoma of the pancreatic body have jaundice. Depression and diabetes commonly precede pancreatic cancer and can be early symptoms. Of patients aged 50 years and older with recent onset of diabetes, about 1% are diagnosed with pancreatic cancer within 3 years. Physical findings are generally associated with advanced carcinomas and include weight loss, hepatomegaly, and an abdominal mass. A palpable gallbladder in the absence of cholecystitis or cholangitis suggests malignant obstruction of the common bile duct (Courvoisier sign), and it is present in about 25% of all patients with pancreatic cancer. Other physical findings, which can be indicative of distant metastases, include Trousseau syndrome (migratory superficial phlebitis), ascites, Virchow node (left supraclavicular lymph node), a periumbilical mass (Sister Mary Joseph node), or a palpable pelvic shelf on rectal examination (Blumer shelf).

D. Diagnostic evaluation

Accurate diagnostic imaging is used to determine whether a patient with pancreatic cancer is a candidate for surgical resection or has an incurable disease. Computed tomography (CT) is the most commonly used study and is very effective when performed according to a standard pancreatic protocol with thin slices and triphasic cross-sectional imaging. CT scans can demonstrate masses in the pancreas or dilatation of the pancreatic duct or the common bile duct. Sensitivity and specificity of CT are about 90%, but CT can miss tumors less than 2 cm in size. Endoscopic retrograde cholangiopancreatography demonstrates subtle ductal abnormalities; sensitivity and specificity are in excess of 90% with biopsies detecting tumors smaller than 1 to 2 cm in diameter. Endoscopic ultrasound (EUS) may be useful for staging (i.e., nodal status), determination of major vessel invasion, and at times for fine needle aspiration (FNA) for pathologic determination of tumor. To determine vascular invasion, there are three options: helical CT, magnetic resonance arteriography, or EUS. Percutaneous FNA of suspicious abnormalities identified on CT scan can confirm the diagnosis of pancreatic cancer with 80% to 90% sensitivity and 100% specificity. A common histologic hallmark of pancreatic adenocarcinoma is an associated desmoplastic reaction that, in a given tumor mass, can vastly overestimate the malignant cell mass. Furthermore, pancreatic cancer may be associated with varying degrees of acute or chronic pancreatitis or cyst formation, which may make it difficult to make a diagnosis with FNA and may lead to false-negative results.

E. Laboratory tests

The majority of tumor markers have not proven to be specific or sensitive enough for pancreatic cancer. Cancer antigen (CA) 19-9 is a cell surface glycoprotein that is associated with pancreatic cancer and has been shown to be elevated in 90% of patients with pancreatic cancer. A 20% or greater fall in the serum marker following treatment is a good prognostic indicator and is associated with improved survival. Rising serum levels may be a useful early indicator of recurrent or progressive disease once a diagnosis has been established, but because of low specificity it is not used as a screening method. However, there are data to support the obtaining of a CA19-9 level in all patients in whom pancreatic cancer is suspected.

F. Staging and preoperative evaluation

   1. Staging. The primary tumor, regional lymph nodes, and potential sites of metastatic disease must be carefully assessed (Table 8.1). The staging system has been modified to better take into account "resectability" of disease. *Resectable disease* is loosely defined as disease confined to the pancreas without involvement of the celiac axis or major vessels. A surgeon experienced in pancreatic surgery should evaluate each case individually when determining resectability as there are numerous clinical caveats.

TABLE 8.1	TNM Staging for Pancreatic Cancer

Stage	Definition
0	Tis, N0, M0
Ia	T1 (tumor ≤2 cm, confined to pancreas), N0, M0
Ib	T2 (tumor >2 cm, confined to pancreas), N0, M0
IIa	T3 (extrapancreatic extension but no celiac axis or mesenteric artery involvement), N0, M0
IIb	T1–3, N1, M0
III	T4 (involvement of celiac axis or superior mesenteric artery; unresectable primary tumor), any N, M0
IV	Any T, any N, M1

N1, any nodal metastases; M1, any distant metastases.
From American Joint Committee on Cancer. *AJCC cancer staging manual* (7th ed.). New York: Springer; 2010.

2. **Preoperative evaluation.** Preoperative evaluation should be performed stepwise from least invasive to most invasive as indicated by the clinical situation. Preoperative evaluation can be stopped when metastatic disease or definite evidence for unresectable locoregional spread is identified. All patients should undergo triphasic helical CT of the abdomen for detection of pancreatic masses and evaluation of vessel encasement. If there is no evidence of metastatic disease and no major blood vessel involvement is identified, then laparoscopy can be used to identify small metastases in the liver or peritoneum. The use of positron emission tomography with 2-[^{18}F]fluoro-2-deoxy-D-glucose in the preoperative evaluation of patients with pancreatic cancer is still controversial and not routinely used.

G. **Primary therapy**

1. **Surgery.** Three-fourths of patients with pancreatic cancer are operative candidates, but only 15% to 20% have resectable tumors. Patients without evident metastatic cancer or major blood vessel involvement and whose performance status permits operative intervention are candidates for curative surgery.

2. **Radiation therapy.** External-beam radiation therapy can palliate locally advanced unresectable carcinomas. It may also be used as a surgical adjuvant in combination with chemotherapy. Great care and expertise must be exercised to plan the radiation fields. These fields must encompass known disease without excessive involvement of adjacent normal tissue. Surgical clips placed during laparotomy or laparoscopy can guide treatment. Intraoperative external-beam radiotherapy has been successful in placing a high dose on the local tumor while protecting the surrounding normal tissues but has not increased the cure rate of pancreatic cancer.

3. Combined-modality therapy

a. Resected carcinomas.
Local and distant recurrence continues to be a common problem after complete resection of pancreatic cancer. Options for the adjuvant treatment for pancreatic cancer continue to be in evolution. A prospective randomized study by the Gastrointestinal Tumor Study Group (GITSG) compared observation to postoperative chemoradiation with bolus fluorouracil (5-FU). The study showed an overall survival benefit (median survival: 20 months versus 11 months, $p = 0.03$) and a 2-year survival benefit (42% versus 15%), but this study is criticized for small patient numbers, low radiation doses, long accrual time, and early termination. The European Organization for Research and Treatment of Cancer performed a similar trial that showed a trend toward improved outcome in the treatment group (median survival: 17.1 months versus 12.6 months, $p = 0.099$). This study is also criticized for low radiation doses and underpowering of the study. A complicated trial in a 2×2 design was completed by the European Group for Pancreatic Cancer (ESPAC-1); it is difficult to interpret and has some trial design concerns including selection bias and treatment variability. An intriguing outcome of the analysis is that the chemotherapy group seemed to have a survival benefit over observation (median survival: 20.1 months versus 15.5 months, $p = 0.009$); however, the chemoradiotherapy group seemed to do worse than the controls. The Radiation Therapy Oncology Group trial 97-04 had the benefit of modern radiation doses and the addition of gemcitabine to the chemotherapy regimen. However, a survival benefit of gemcitabine over 5-FU (18.8 months versus 16.7 months, $p = 0.047$) was seen only in pancreatic head adenocarcinomas. Most recently, the Charite Onkologie (CONKO-001) was the first trial showing that gemcitabine alone in the adjuvant setting can prolong disease-free and overall survival without significant toxicities compared to observation alone (median survival 22.8 months versus 20.2 months, $p = 0.005$, and 5-year survival of 21% versus 9%). All of these trials show that in an acceptable candidate, chemotherapy improves survival; however, the addition of radiotherapy is still controversial. A prospective randomized trial of bolus 5-FU/leucovorin versus gemcitabine versus observation following surgery (ESPAC-3) is currently in progress and should provide more definitive results on the use of chemotherapy without chemoradiation in the adjuvant setting. At this time, no standardized regimen has been established for the adjuvant treatment of resected pancreatic cancer. 5-FU–based chemoradiation with additional gemcitabine

chemotherapy as well as chemotherapy alone with gemcitabine, 5-FU, or capecitabine are listed in the guidelines for the adjuvant treatment of pancreatic cancer. Alternative adjuvant chemotherapy regimens (with or without radiotherapy) include the following:

1. Gemcitabine alone (1000 mg/m^2 on days 1, 8, and 15 with a 1-week break) *or*

2. 5-FU 225 mg/m^2 by continuous intravenous (IV) infusion throughout radiation therapy followed by four to six courses of bolus 5-FU weekly, or gemcitabine (1000 mg/m^2 on days 1, 8, and 15 with a 1-week break) *or*

3. 5-FU 425 mg/m^2 by IV push 1 hour after leucovorin 20 mg/m^2 by IV push daily for 4 days during the first week of radiation therapy and for 3 days during the fifth week of radiation therapy followed by four to six courses of bolus 5-FU weekly or gemcitabine (1000 mg/m^2 on days 1, 8, and 15 with a 1-week break) *or*

4. Capecitabine 1500 mg/m^2 daily in divided doses with radiation therapy followed by four to six courses of bolus 5-FU weekly or gemcitabine (1000 mg/m^2 on days 1, 8, and 15 with a 1-week break). Capecitabine can be used in the chemotherapy only part of the regimen as well, but there is no phase III data to confirm capecitabine in this setting.

b. **Borderline resectable pancreatic cancer.** Management of borderline resectable pancreatic cancer remains a challenging field without a defined approach and requires a multidisciplinary effort. This subgroup of patients with pancreatic cancer is potentially resectable if they have a good response with preoperative chemotherapy or combined chemotherapy with radiation. There are a number of phase II studies looking at gemcitabine-based chemotherapy regimens and chemoradiation regimens for the neoadjuvant treatment of borderline resectable or resectable pancreatic cancer. However, there have been no phase III studies and there is no consensus among groups as to the preferred chemotherapeutic regimen or whether radiation should be utilized in the neoadjuvant setting.

c. **Localized unresectable carcinoma.** A series of randomized trials conducted by the GITSG demonstrated superior survival of patients with localized but unresectable pancreatic cancer when treated with combined-modality therapy compared with patients treated with radiation therapy or chemotherapy alone. These clinical trials utilized split-course radiation therapy, which most contemporary studies no longer use. Current clinical trials do not support a specific combined-modality treatment program; however, most studies utilize doses of 50 to 60 Gy with concomitant 5-FU. Other radiation sensitizers being utilized in studies are gemcitabine, paclitaxel, and cisplatin. There is evidence to suggest that concurrent gemcitabine and radiation can yield similar results to 5-FU–based chemoradiation, although this has not been assessed in any randomized trials. Most recommend that an additional course of gemcitabine-based chemotherapy be considered for patients with locally advanced pancreatic cancer who are receiving chemoradiation therapy. Other options for locally advanced disease are systemic chemotherapy without radiotherapy or chemotherapy followed by consolidated chemoradiation.

H. Chemotherapy of metastatic disease

Patients with pancreatic cancer are often poor candidates for chemotherapy because of severe weight loss, poor performance status, severe pain, lack of measurable or evaluable disease, and presence of jaundice or hepatic involvement, which may interfere with clearance of therapeutic agents. The primary goals for advanced pancreatic cancer are palliation and improved survival. Randomized clinical trials have demonstrated survival and quality-of-life benefits to chemotherapy in selected patients with advanced pancreatic cancer compared to best supportive care alone.

1. Single agents. A number of single agents have demonstrated clinical activity; however, no agent has demonstrated consistent complete or partial response rates greater than 20%. Gemcitabine has been accepted as first-line therapy for metastatic pancreatic cancer in patients with adequate performance status based on a phase III trial that compared bolus 5-FU and gemcitabine with a primary endpoint being the "clinical benefit score." Clinical benefit was defined as sustained (more than 4 weeks) improvement of one of the following parameters without worsening of any of the others: performance status, composite pain measurement (average pain intensity and narcotic analgesic use), and weight. The improvement in clinical benefit score in the gemcitabine and 5-FU arms were 23.8% and 4.8%, respectively ($p = 0.0022$). In addition, there was a significant improvement in median survival (5.65 months versus 4.41 months, $p = 0.0025$) and in survival at 12 months (18% versus 2%). Therapy was generally well tolerated with a low incidence of grade 3 or 4 toxicities. The toxicities with gemcitabine include bone marrow suppression, lethargy, flulike syndrome, nausea and vomiting, and peripheral edema.

2. Combination chemotherapy. Despite promising phase II studies, the combination of gemcitabine with other cytotoxic drugs, including 5-FU, cisplatin, oxaliplatin, and irinotecan, has not been proven to be superior to gemcitabine alone in demonstrating a survival benefit. A recently reported U.K. Phase III trial (U.K. National

Cancer Research Institute study) utilizing higher doses of gemcitabine and capecitabine identified a trend toward improved median overall survival (7.1 months versus 6.2 months, $p = 0.077$). When this group performed a meta-analysis of their study with two additional studies, they identified a significant survival benefit in favor of the gemcitabine combination ($p = 0.02$). Furthermore, a meta-analysis of five platinum-based randomized trials did reveal a significant improvement in median overall survival ($p = 0.01$) for the combination over gemcitabine alone. The results of a randomized phase II trial of three different regimens in patients with advanced pancreatic cancer suggested that capecitabine plus oxaliplatin is comparable to gemcitabine combined with either capecitabine or oxaliplatin. Gemcitabine has also been investigated in multidrug combination chemotherapy regimens. Two regimens, which have shown promising activity but are associated with higher rates of toxicity, are a combination of cisplatin, epirubicin, 5-FU, and gemcitabine and a combination of gemcitabine, docetaxel, and capecitabine.

3. **Novel targeted agents.** A better understanding of the biology of cancer has led to the development of novel agents targeting pathways of cancer cell survival. Clinical trials have explored the combination of gemcitabine with a variety of biological "targeted" agents such as bevacizumab, cetuximab, and erlotinib over the past decade. Despite their promise in preclinical studies, most of these studies have not shown a survival advantage over standard monotherapy gemcitabine. Results of the Cancer and Leukemia Group B phase III trial, which evaluated gemcitabine plus bevacizumab (antivascular endothelial growth factor [VEGF] antibody) compared with gemcitabine plus placebo, and the Southwest Oncology Group phase III trial, which assessed gemcitabine plus cetuximab (targets epidermal growth factor receptor [EGFR]) versus gemcitabine alone, did not reveal any improvement in survival with the addition of the biologic agent. However, in a phase III trial of patients with advanced or metastatic pancreatic cancer randomly assigned to receive either erlotinib (inhibitor of EGFR tyrosine kinase) plus gemcitabine or gemcitabine alone, patients in the erlotinib arm showed statistically significant improvement in median and 1-year survival (6.24 months versus 5.91 months, $p = 0.038$, and 23% versus 17%, respectively). There was a slight increase in incidence of grade 3 to 4 skin rash and diarrhea in the group receiving erlotinib, although there was no overall difference in quality of life between the two groups. The U.S. Food and Drug Administration has approved erlotinib in combination with gemcitabine for first-line treatment of patients with locally advanced or metastatic pancreatic cancer.

4. **Current recommendations**
   a. **Erlotinib** 100 mg by mouth daily plus gemcitabine 1000 mg/m^2 weekly for 3 weeks with a 1-week break.
   b. **Single-agent therapy with gemcitabine** 1000 mg/m^2 IV of 4-week cycles of three weekly doses followed by a 1-week rest is recommended for patients with metastatic pancreatic cancer and with an Eastern Cooperative Oncology Group performance status of 0 to 2, who are not eligible for clinical trials.
   c. **Patients with a very good performance status** can use a doublet such as gemcitabine and oxaliplatin (GemOx) with gemcitabine 1000 mg/m^2 on days 1 and 8 plus oxaliplatin 130 mg/m^2 over 2 hours on day 8 every 3 weeks *or*
   d. **Capecitabine and gemcitabine.** Capecitabine at 1500 mg/m^2 daily in twice-daily divided doses on days 1 to 14 and gemcitabine 1000 mg/m^2 on days 1 and 8 every 3 weeks *or*
   e. **Capecitabine and oxaliplatin.** Capecitabine at 1500 mg/m^2 daily in twice daily divided doses on days 1 to 14 plus oxaliplatin 130 mg/m^2 on day 1 every 3 weeks.
5. **Second-line chemotherapy.** There is no standard second-line regimen for advanced pancreatic cancer after gemcitabine failure, and there is a paucity of trials in this setting. Current recommendations encourage treatment in a clinical trial but when an investigational therapy is not available there are other alternatives. Gemcitabine may offer palliative benefits in the second-line setting in patients who have not been treated with gemcitabine previously. Results from a phase II study suggest that fixed-dose–rate GemOx may have activity in patients who become resistant to standard gemcitabine therapy. Other treatment options include 5-FU or capecitabine with or without oxaliplatin. The CONKO-3 study randomized 168 gemcitabine refractory patients with pancreatic cancer to 5-FU and leucovorin or 5-FU, leucovorin, and oxaliplatin. This study revealed an improved overall survival of 2 months in the arm containing oxaliplatin (4.8 months versus 2.3 months, $p = 0.0077$).

II. PANCREATIC NEUROENDOCRINE TUMORS (PNETs)
A. Epidemiology
PNETs are rare malignancies with an overall incidence of 1 to 2 cases/100,000 people per year. They account for less than 2% of all digestive malignant tumors and 1% of all endocrine tumors. These tumors cover a spectrum of neoplasms, many, but not all, of which originate from the pancreatic islets of Langerhans and are therefore known as "islet cell tumors." Although the peak incidence of occurrence is between 40 and 60 years of age, a significant number of patients diagnosed are under 35 years of age. PNETs are broadly categorized into those with and those without a clinical syndrome

and therefore have been termed "functional" or "nonfunctional." Approximately 50% of these tumors secrete one or more hormones excessively, which may cause clinical symptoms of excessive hormone release: most commonly insulin or gastrin; less commonly glucagon, serotonin, or adrenocorticotropic hormone; and rarely vasoactive intestinal peptides (VIPs), growth hormone–releasing hormone, or somatostatin. The other 50% are nonfunctional and are generally discovered through symptoms related to tumor burden itself or as incidental findings. Most neuroendocrine tumors (with the exception of insulinomas, of which 90% are benign) are malignant and have the ability to metastasize, most commonly to lymph nodes or the liver and less commonly to bone, lung, brain, or other organs. However, these tumors are usually slow growing with low mitotic activity and often have an insidious presentation. Management of PNETs depends on the pathologic differentiation, stage at diagnosis, and presence of symptoms related to hormone secretion.

B. Presentation

Islet cell tumors may occur with the multiple endocrine neoplasia type I (MEN-I) syndrome. In families with this autosomal dominant syndrome, 80% of affected members develop islet cell tumors, most commonly gastrinoma (54%), insulinoma (21%), glucagonoma (3%), or VIPoma (1%). Gastrinoma is often suspected in patients with recurrent peptic ulcers and associated diarrhea and steatorrhea. Evaluation includes measuring gastrin levels (basal and stimulated) and gastric acidity. The frequent use of proton pump inhibitors (PPIs) can be responsible for false positive tests and therefore PPIs must be discontinued 1 week prior. About one-fourth of gastrinomas are associated with MEN-I and tend to be multicentric. Eighty percent to ninety percent of gastrinomas occur in the duodenum and head of the pancreas and the majority of gastrinomas (60% to 90%) are malignant. Insulinomas are typically single, small, benign lesions equally distributed in the head, body, and tail of the pancreas that present with symptoms of fasting hypoglycemia. The diagnosis of insulinoma may be established by a supervised 48- to 72-hour fasting of the patient followed by insulin and glucose testing. Patients with insulinoma have elevated C-peptide. An insulin level greater than 3 μU/mL when blood glucose is less than 40 mg/dL with an insulin to glucose ratio of 0.3 or less reflects an inappropriate secretion of insulin at the time of hypoglycemia and is used to document these tumors. Classically, glucagonomas are associated with necrolytic migratory erythema, mild diabetes, diarrhea, severe muscle wasting, and marked hyperaminoaciduria. VIPomas are associated with episodic severe secretory diarrhea with hypokalemia, hypochlorhydria, and metabolic acidosis.

C. Primary treatment

Surgical resection is the optimal treatment for pancreatic endocrine tumors. Before resection, the first goal of treatment must be to control endocrine syndromes.

1. **Gastric acid suppression.** The H^+/K^+-adenosine triphosphatase inhibitors omeprazole and lansoprazole successfully control gastric acid secretion in patients with gastrinoma. Optimal doses must be individualized and periodically re-evaluated. Gastric acid secretion in the hour preceding the next dose of omeprazole or lansoprazole should be less than 10 mEq in patients who have had no previous gastric surgery and less than 5 mEq in those who have had an acid-reducing procedure. The starting dose is 60 mg/day with both agents. Doses greater than 80 mg/day should be divided. Similar, newer agents in the same class of PPIs are equally as efficacious.

2. **Insulin suppression.** Diazoxide, an insulin release inhibitor, when given at 3 to 8 mg/kg/day by mouth divided in three doses (e.g., 50 to 150 mg by mouth three times a day), is the therapy of choice for hypoglycemia associated with insulinoma when dietary measures fail. A diuretic should be given with diazoxide to prevent water retention.

3. **Octreotide acetate** is a somatostatin analog that inhibits gut hormone secretion. It is generally useful for carcinoid and VIPoma syndromes and is possibly useful for controlling symptoms in patients with glucagonomas, gonadotrophic hormone–releasing tumors, and gastrinomas. In patients with unresectable insulinoma, it can reduce insulin secretion by 50% and return blood glucose levels to normal. However, it must be initiated cautiously in patients in the hospital because profound hypoglycemia may occur. The usual starting dose of octreotide is 50 μg subcutaneously twice a day; thereafter, the dose and frequency of injections can be increased to 100 μg three times a day. More recently, a long-acting preparation (octreotide LAR) has become available. The dose should be 20 to 30 mg intramuscularly monthly, depending on doses that the patient was requiring of the short-acting preparation. It is designed to provide the convenience of once-a-month or twice-a-month injections once a stable dose of the shorter-acting preparation is established.

D. Management of locally advanced or metastatic islet cell tumors

Surgical resection is recommended for resectable locoregional recurrence. For patients with unresectable locoregional recurrence, radiation therapy for symptom control or participation in a clinical trial is recommended. Patients with metastatic disease to the liver should be considered for surgical resection as well. However, for patients who are found to be unresectable and have symptomatic or clinically significant tumor burden, somatostatin analogs can be helpful in the management of symptomatic disease related to hormonal secretion. The most commonly utilized somatostatin analogs in clinical studies for PNETs are octreotide, lanreotide, and pasireotide. A recent phase III placebo–controlled randomized study comparing long-acting octreotide to placebo for the treatment of midgut neuroendocrine tumors demonstrated a 66% reduction in risk of disease progression. The PROMID study showed antitumor benefit in patients with functioning and nonfunctioning tumors treated with octreotide LAR. In an analysis of patients with nonfunctioning tumors, time to tumor progression for patients receiving octreotide LAR was 28.8 months versus 5.9 months for those on placebo (hazard ratio [HR] = 0.25). For patients with functioning tumors, time to tumor progression for patients receiving octreotide LAR was 14.3 months and 5.5 months for those on placebo (HR = 0.23). Current studies are being conducted to compare pasireotide to placebo for the management of symptoms and lanreotide to placebo for evaluation of impact on progression-free survival.

The systemic chemotherapeutic agents that have shown most benefit in PNETs are streptozocin, doxorubicin, 5-FU, and temozolomide. Streptozocin is the most active single agent, with a 50% response rate. The addition of other agents such as 5-FU and doxorubicin was associated with even higher response rates. The combination of streptozocin and doxorubicin was demonstrated to have a superior response rate (69%), median survival (26.5 months), and time to tumor progression (20 months) than the combination of streptozocin and 5-FU or single agent chlorozotocin in a North Central Cancer Treatment Group study. The dosing of this regimen was streptozocin 500 mg/m^2 IV on days 1 to 5 and doxorubicin 50 mg/m^2 IV on days 1 and 22; this regimen was repeated every 6 weeks. Toxicity from this regimen was common, with renal impairment occurring in about 30% of patients receiving a streptozocin-based regimen; nausea and vomiting in about 60% of patients; and leukopenia in about 75%, but only 10% with a white blood cell count of less than 1000 μL. A more recent phase III study comparing streptozotocin and 5-FU to doxorubicin and 5-FU demonstrated improved median survival in the streptozotocin/5-FU arm (24.3 months versus 15.7 months, $p = 0.03$). Another agent that has demonstrated some efficacy against PNETs in phase II trials is temozolomide, which has been used in combination with other agents such as thalidomide and bevacizumab.

Recent investigations in PNETs have identified attractive potential molecular targets such as EGFR, VEGF and its receptor (VEGFR), and insulinlike growth factor receptor (IGFR). Multiple studies have demonstrated overexpression of VEGF and VEGFR in PNETs and that this overexpression correlates with decreased progression-free survival. Phase II studies of bevacizumab, sorafenib, and sunitinib have been promising and have demonstrated response rates of 10% to 20% and improvements in progression-free survival. Recently, an international phase III trial comparing sunitinib (37.5 mg once a day) to placebo in the treatment of PNETs was closed prematurely after accruing 171 patients. Interim analysis revealed a significant difference in progression-free survival (11.4 months versus 5.5 months).

Another potentially promising target in PNETs is the mTOR pathway. mTOR is a conserved serine/threonine kinase that regulates cell growth and metabolism in response to environmental factors and signaling downstream of receptor tyrosine kinases, such as IGFR, VEGFR, and EGFR. Two mTOR inhibitors that have been studied in PNETs are temsirolimus and everolimus. Temsirolimus was found to have modest clinical activity, with a response rate of 5.6% and median time to progression of 6 months. Everolimus in combination with octreotide LAR demonstrated a response rate of 27% and a progression-free survival of 63 weeks. Based on these encouraging results, RADIANT 3, a randomized double-blind, placebo-controlled, multicenter phase III study of everolimus or best supportive care in patients with advanced islet cell carcinoma, was developed and is currently accruing.

Locoregional therapies are also available and include ablative therapies such as radiofrequency ablation (RFA), microwave ablation, cryoablation, or embolization therapies such as bland embolization, chemoembolization, drug-eluting beads, and radioembolization. Newer experimental techniques such as percutaneous hepatic perfusion (PHP) may also have a role in this setting.

III. CARCINOMA OF THE BILE DUCTS (CHOLANGIOCARCINOMA) AND GALLBLADDER CARCINOMA

A. Introduction

Biliary tract cancers are invasive adenocarcinomas that arise from the epithelial lining of the gallbladder and intrahepatic (peripheral) and extrahepatic (hilar and distal biliary tree) bile ducts. Biliary tract cancers affect approximately 12,000 people in the United States annually. In 2009, there were an estimated 9760 new cases and 3370 deaths in the United States. However, this figure does not include cases of intrahepatic biliary cancers, which are included with primary liver cancers in national databases. Although the incidence of extrahepatic cholangiocarcinoma has remained constant, the incidence of intrahepatic cholangiocarcinoma has increased markedly over the past two decades.

B. Epidemiology and presentation

The development of biliary tract cancers appears to be related to chronic inflammatory conditions, autoimmune disease, biliary calculi, several infectious agents, and certain carcinogens. Risk factors for gallbladder cancer, of which cholelithiasis is the most prevalent, are associated with the presence of chronic inflammation. Calcification of the gallbladder (porcelain gallbladder), a result of chronic inflammation, has also been associated with gallbladder cancer. No predisposing factors have been found in most patients diagnosed with cholangiocarcinoma, although there is evidence that particular risk factors may be associated with the disease in some patients. These risk factors are associated with chronic inflammation and include cholelithiasis, ulcerative colitis, liver flukes, exposure to thorium oxide (Thorotrast), primary sclerosing cholangitis, and congenital anomalies such as choledochal cysts. Recently, intrahepatic cholangiocarcinoma has been associated with hepatitis C viral infection and may be partly responsible for an increased incidence of intrahepatic cholangiocarcinoma. Biliary tract cancers are usually diagnosed at a late stage due to the aggressive nature and rapid spreading of these tumors. Patients with gallbladder cancer can present with a clinical presentation that mimics biliary colic or chronic cholecystitis. Primary gallbladder malignancy is incidentally found in 0.4% to 2% of laparoscopic cholecystectomy specimens. Carcinoma of the gallbladder most commonly presents with pain, nausea and vomiting, and weight loss. Other possible clinical presentations of gallbladder cancer include a suspicious mass detected on ultrasound or jaundice. About one-third of patients present with jaundice, which is typically associated with advanced disease not amenable to surgical resection. Patients with intrahepatic cholangiocarcinoma are likely to present with nonspecific symptoms such as fever, weight loss, or abdominal pain; symptoms of biliary obstruction are uncommon. Alternatively, intrahepatic cholangiocarcinoma may be detected incidentally as an isolated intrahepatic mass on imaging. In contrast, patients with extrahepatic cholangiocarcinoma are more likely to present with jaundice with evidence of biliary obstruction on subsequent imaging.

C. Natural history and pathogenesis

Biliary tract malignancies are related anatomically and are characterized by local invasion, regional lymph node metastasis, vascular encasement, and distant metastasis. The only chance for cure of biliary tract cancers is complete surgical resection; however, only 10% of patients present with early stage disease and are considered surgical candidates. The key prognostic factors are completeness of resection, lymph node status, and tumor differentiation. However, recurrence rates even in this group of resectable patients remains quite high and thus systemic chemotherapy in either the adjuvant or palliative setting is the mainstay of the treatment plan for almost all patients. Median overall survival in patients with unresectable or metastatic biliary tract cancer is less than 1 year. Gallbladder cancer appears to be the most aggressive of biliary tract cancers and has the shortest median survival. Although biliary tract cancers are similar in their aggressive course and resistance to chemotherapy, gallbladder cancer, intrahepatic cholangiocarcinoma, and extrahepatic cholangiocarcinoma have different molecular profiles and ideally should be studied independently. However, due to a relatively small number of patients, these diseases have been combined in most clinical trials analyzing systemic chemotherapy. Despite a paucity of randomized phase III studies, consensus first-line systemic therapy is emerging from the results of smaller phase II trials.

D. Chemotherapy

The advantage of systemic chemotherapy over supportive care alone in improving survival and quality of life was first suggested in an evaluation of 5-FU plus leucovorin and etoposide therapy versus best supportive care among a group of patients with pancreatic and biliary tract cancer. The overall survival in the chemotherapy group was 6 months versus 2.5 months for the supportive care group but only 37/90 patients had biliary tract cancers. Despite limitations of this study, because of ethical considerations, this will likely represent the only trial comparing benefits of chemotherapy to best supportive care in advanced biliary tract cancer.

5-FU–based regimens have been the most tested regimens in a randomized fashion in biliary tract cancer. 5-FU plus leucovorin has demonstrated response rates of 32% and overall survival of 6 months. Combination therapy with cisplatin consistently yields response rates of 10% to 40% and median survival times somewhat better than 5-FU alone. 5-FU combinations with taxanes, etoposide, streptozotocin, and irinotecan have not shown superiority over 5-FU alone. Similar to the experience with 5-FU plus cisplatin combinations, capecitabine plus cisplatin demonstrated somewhat higher response rates and overall survival. The fluoropyrimidines uracil-tegafur and S-1 (a fluoropyrimidine mixture) have also been evaluated in biliary tract cancers and results have been similar to the experiences with 5-FU and capecitabine, and slightly better with the addition of cisplatin.

Gemcitabine, a nucleotide analogue determined to be active against advanced pancreatic cancer, has been extensively studied in patients with advanced or metastatic biliary tract cancer. Response rates with single-agent gemcitabine are in the range of 0% to 30% with median overall survival of 5 to 14 months. Gemcitabine and cisplatin or oxaliplatin combinations have been extensively studied in biliary tract cancers. Studies have demonstrated response rates of 21% to 53% and median overall survival of 5 to 15 months; these results are somewhat better than the results from single-agent gemcitabine. Gemcitabine in combination with capecitabine demonstrated response rates of 30% and median overall survival of 14 months, suggesting a benefit similar to the gemcitabine-based platinum combinations. A recent pooled analysis of 104 chemotherapy trials involving 1368 biliary tract cancer patients from 1999 to 2006 pointed toward gemcitabine as the most active agent and that gemcitabine-based platinum regimens offer a slight advantage over other regimens. Among gemcitabine-cisplatin or GemOx combinations, which have similar response rates and median overall survival rates, the toxicity and tolerability data tend to favor GemOx combinations.

Recent studies utilizing molecular features of biliary tract cancers and targeted therapies have been published. The most promising of these appears to be a multicenter phase II trial looking at bevacizumab, a humanized monoclonal antibody against VEGF, being tested in combination with gemcitabine and oxaliplatin.

E. Current recommendations
   1. **5-FU** 500 mg/m^2 IV push on days 1 to 5 every 4 weeks or 500 mg/m^2 IV weekly.
   2. **5-FU** 400 mg/m^2 IV on days 1 to 5 and streptozocin 500 mg/m^2 IV on days 1 to 5.
   3. **Patients with a very good performance status** can use a doublet such as GemOx with gemcitabine 1000 mg/m^2 on day 1 and 8 plus oxaliplatin 130 mg/m^2 over 2 hours on day 8 every 3 weeks *or*
   4. **Gemcitabine** 1000 mg/m^2, 5-FU 600 mg/m^2, and leucovorin 20 mg/m^2 IV on days 1, 8, and 15 every 4 weeks.
   5. **Capecitabine** 1500 mg/m^2 daily in twice-daily divided doses on days 1 to 14 and gemcitabine 1000 mg/m^2 on days 1 and 8 every 3 weeks *or*
   6. **Capecitabine** 1500 mg/m^2 daily in twice-daily divided doses on days 1 to 14 plus oxaliplatin 130 mg/m^2 on day 1 every 3 weeks.

IV. PRIMARY CARCINOMA OF THE LIVER
   A. Epidemiology
   Hepatocellular carcinoma (HCC) accounts for 80% to 90% of primary liver cancer. HCC is a major health problem worldwide with well over 500,000 cases diagnosed each year. It is the fifth most common cancer worldwide and the third most common cause of cancer-related death, with most cases occurring in Asia. Although less common in the United States, the incidence is rising with approximately 20,000 cases diagnosed in 2009. The latest statistics for 2009 estimated 22,620 cases, but this number also includes

intrahepatic bile duct cancer as well. Ninety percent of primary cancers of the liver are HCC or hepatoma; the remaining cancers include cholangiocarcinomas (about 7%), hepatoblastomas, angiosarcomas, and other sarcomas. In the United States, the peak incidence is in the sixth decade of life, whereas in Asia and Africa it occurs much earlier in life.

B. **Etiology and risk factors**

The rates of HCC are two to four times higher in males than females. Eighty to ninety percent of cases of HCC develop in a cirrhotic liver, and cirrhosis is the strongest predisposing factor for HCC. Overall, 80% of cases of HCC are attributable to chronic infections with either hepatitis B or hepatitis C virus. Chronic hepatitis B viral infection is common in Asian and African countries and accounts for most cases of HCC. Chronic carriers of hepatitis B have a 100-fold relative risk for developing HCC with an annual incidence rate of 2% to 6% in cirrhotic patients. In contrast, chronic hepatitis C viral infection is more common in Western countries. Other causes of HCC include alcoholic liver cirrhosis, aflatoxin (a natural product of the *Aspergillus* fungus found in various grains), hereditary hemochromatosis, autoimmune hepatitis, α1-antitrypsin deficiency, and Wilson disease.

The incidence of HCC is increasing in the United States, particularly among the population infected with the hepatitis C virus. Approximately 4 million people in the United States are chronically infected with hepatitis C virus, and the annual incidence among hepatitis C patients with hepatitis C–related cirrhosis is estimated to be between 2% and 8%. Approximately 1.5 million people are chronically infected with hepatitis B in the United States; the annual incidence of HCC in patients with hepatitis B–induced cirrhosis is 2.5%. In those carriers without cirrhosis, the annual incidence is 0.5%.

C. **Presenting signs and symptoms**

Patients with primary carcinoma of the liver commonly complain of right upper quadrant pain, abdominal distention, or weight loss. The pain is usually dull or aching but may be acute and radiate to the right shoulder. Fatigue, loss of appetite, and unexplained fever may occur. Patients with underlying cirrhosis may present with hepatic decompensation: new ascites, variceal bleeding, jaundice, or encephalopathy. Rarely, patients present with paraneoplastic syndromes. Erythrocytosis is the most common; hypercalcemia, hyperthyroidism, and carcinoid syndrome have also been described. Physical findings include nodular hepatomegaly with an arterial bruit and hepatic rub. Extrahepatic spread occurs in about 50% of patients during the course of the illness. Twenty percent of patients have lung metastases.

D. Diagnostic evaluation and screening

There are several published studies that have demonstrated reduction in HCC mortality with the utilization of screening programs for high-risk individuals such as those with cirrhosis or chronic hepatitis viral infections. Serum α-fetoprotein (AFP) and liver ultrasound are the most widely used methods for screening for HCC. Most groups recommend periodic testing with AFP and ultrasonography every 6 to 12 months. Additional imaging is recommended in the setting of a rising serum AFP or following identification of a liver nodule on liver ultrasound. HCC lesions are characterized by arterial hypervascularity, deriving most of their blood supply from the hepatic artery. This is in contrast to surrounding liver, which receives most of its blood supply from the portal venous system. Therefore, the most commonly utilized tests for diagnostic imaging of HCC are triphasic helical CT or triphasic dynamic contrast-enhanced magnetic resonance imaging (MRI). CT or MRI for lesions greater than 2 cm demonstrating classic arterial enhancement is diagnostic for HCC. For lesions 1 to 2 cm in size, a classic arterial enhancement pattern on both CT and MRI is considered diagnostic for HCC. Liver lesions less than 1 cm should be followed closely with periodic repeat imaging. Liver lesions greater than 1 cm that do not demonstrate classic arterial enhancement should undergo tissue biopsy to confirm the diagnosis.

E. Laboratory tests

AFP is a tumor marker that is elevated in 60% to 70% of patients with HCC. Serum AFP is not a sensitive or specific test for HCC. However, results of AFP testing can be used in conjunction with imaging to guide management of patients with suspected AFP. An AFP greater than 200 in a patient with a liver lesion greater than 2 cm has a high predictive value for HCC and can be considered diagnostic even without the classic enhancement pattern on imaging.

F. Staging and preoperative evaluation

1. **Staging.** Patients diagnosed with HCC should undergo an extensive work-up that includes determination of the etiology of underlying liver disease including hepatitis panel, assessment of other comorbidities, imaging studies to evaluate for metastatic disease (chest imaging and bone scan as most common sites for metastases are lung, bone, and abdominal lymph nodes), and evaluation of underlying hepatic function, including a determination of any evidence of portal hypertension. An effective staging system should incorporate tumor characteristics (AJCC TNM classification, Table 8.2) and underlying liver disease (Child-Pugh classification), as both of these factors impact choice of treatment and patient survival. A number of staging systems for patients with HCC have been devised. Some of the

TABLE 8.2	TNM Staging for HCC
Stage	**Definition**
I	T1 (solitary tumor any size without vascular invasion), N0, M0
II	T2 (solitary tumor any size with vascular invasion; or multiple tumors, none >5 cm) N0, M0
IIIA	T3a (multiple tumors >5 cm), N0, M0
IIIB	T3b (single or multiple tumors of any size involving a major branch of the portal vein or hepatic vein), N0, M0
IIIC	T4 (direct invasion of adjacent organ other than gallbladder, or with perforation of visceral peritoneum), N0, M0
IVA	Any T, N1, M0
IVB	Any T, any N, M1

From American Joint Committee on Cancer. *AJCC cancer staging manual* (7th ed.). New York: Springer; 2010.

most commonly utilized include the Okuda staging system, Cancer of the Liver Italian Program score, Japanese Integrated Staging score, Chinese University Prognostic Index, simplified (Vauthey) staging for HCC, Izumi TNM modification, French classification system, and the Barcelona Clinic Liver Cancer staging classification. Each of these scoring systems has limitations, and therefore no one staging system has been universally accepted. Following work-up, patients are stratified into one of the following groups: metastatic disease, locally advanced unresectable disease not amenable to transplantation, resectable or transplantable but performance status precludes operation, and resectable or transplantable with appropriate performance status.

2. **Preoperative evaluation.** The selection of patients with HCC for surgical resection incorporates information regarding tumor extent, severity of underlying liver disease, assessment of liver functional reserve, and general medical condition of the patient. The general criteria for unresectability of HCC includes large size of tumor with insufficient hepatic remnant after liver resection, multifocal bilobar lesions, extrahepatic tumor metastases, and tumor with main portal vein or hepatic vein/inferior vena cava involvement. In addition, resection is generally recommended only in the presence of preserved liver function with no evidence of portal hypertension.

G. Primary therapy

At presentation, only 25% of patients with HCC have potentially resectable lesions. Results of large retrospective studies have demonstrated 5-year survival of 50% to 70% in select patients undergoing liver resection for HCC in the setting of preserved liver function.

However, the number of patients with HCC considered good candidates for resection in the United States is quite low because the majority of patients have underling Child grade B or C cirrhosis. In addition, recurrence rates at 5 years following liver resection for HCC are quite high and approach 70%. Liver transplantation may permit resection of small tumors in patients with advanced cirrhosis, and survival is similar to or better than that seen after resection without transplantation. Patients with HCC who meet the Milan criteria for transplantation are those patients with one nodule less than 5 cm or two to three nodules that are less than 3 cm and no evidence of macrovascular involvement or extrahepatic disease. These select patients treated with liver transplantation have low recurrence rates with 5-year survival rates of greater than 75%. The main problem with transplantation is timely organ availability. Patients with localized disease who are not candidates for either resection or transplantation should be considered for ablative therapies or embolization. In addition, for patients awaiting liver transplantation, a number of studies have investigated the role of locoregional therapies in controlling disease as a bridge to transplantation. The locoregional therapies available include ablative therapies such as RFA, microwave ablation, cryoablation, or percutaneous ethanol injection and embolization therapies such as bland embolization, chemoembolization, drug-eluting beads, and radioembolization. Newer experimental techniques such as PHP may also have a role in this setting.

H. Therapy of advanced HCC

The majority of patients diagnosed with HCC have advanced disease at presentation and are not candidates for surgery or locoregional therapies. Unfortunately, HCC is a relatively chemoresistant tumor and is highly resistant to cytotoxic chemotherapy. Clinical studies evaluating the use of chemotherapy such as doxorubicin have reported low response rates to therapy and evidence for a favorable impact on survival is lacking. However, two recent phase III studies have found sorafenib to be beneficial in the treatment of patients with metastatic or locally advanced HCC. Sorafenib is an oral multikinase inhibitor that suppresses tumor cell proliferation and angiogenesis. In a large multicenter, randomized, placebo-controlled phase III trial (SHARP), the efficacy of sorafenib versus placebo in patients with advanced HCC was evaluated. In this study, 602 patients with advanced measurable HCC, no prior systemic therapy, good performance status, and preserved liver function were randomized to either sorafenib 400 mg twice a day or placebo with best supportive care. Median survival was significantly longer in the sorafenib arm (10.7 months versus 7.9 months, HR = 0.69, $p < 0.001$). Another phase III trial with similar design, the Asia-Pacific study, randomized 226 patients in a 2:1 fashion to either sorafenib or placebo. Patients in this study were Asian and tended to be younger with underlying hepatitis B and a higher number of tumor sites compared to the SHARP trial. This study also demonstrated improved median survival in the sorafenib arm (6.5 months versus 4.2 months, HR = 0.68, p = 0.014). Overall, sorafenib is well tolerated with limited side effects, the most common being diarrhea, weight loss, and hand-foot skin reaction. As a result of these studies, sorafenib is now considered the standard of care for patients with advanced and metastatic HCC who are not candidates for curative or locoregional therapies, but at present only patients with good liver function have been rigorously studied.

Selected Readings

Burris HA, Moore MJ, Andersen J, et al. Improvements in survival and clinical benefit with gemcitabine as first-line therapy for patients with advanced pancreas cancer: a randomized trial. *J Clin Oncol.* 1997;15:2403–2413.

Eckel F, Schmid RM. Chemotherapy in advanced biliary tract carcinoma: a pooled analysis of clinical trials. *Br J Cancer.* 2007;96:896–902.

Gastrointestinal Tumor Study Group. Further evidence of effective adjuvant combined radiation and chemotherapy following curative resection of pancreatic cancer. *Cancer.* 1987;59:2006–2010.

Glimelius B, Hoffman K, Sjoden PO, et al. Chemotherapy improves survival and quality of life in advanced pancreatic and biliary cancer. *Ann Oncol.* 1996;7:593–600.

Klinkenbijl JH, Jeekel J, Shamoud T, et al. Adjuvant radiotherapy and 5-fluorouracil after curative resection of cancer of the pancreas and periampullary region: phase III trial of the EORTC gastrointestinal tract cancer cooperative group. *Annals of Surgery.* 1999;230(6):776–782.

Kvols LK, Moertel CG, O'Connell MJ, et al. Treatment of the malignant carcinoid syndrome: evaluation of a long-acting somatostatin analogue. *N Engl J Med.* 1986;315:663–666.

Llovet JM, Ricci S, Mazzaferro V, et al. Sorafenib in advanced hepatocellular carcinoma. *N Engl J Med.* 2008;359:378–390.

Louvet C, Labianca R, Hammel P, et al. Gemcitabine in combination with oxaliplatin compared with gemcitabine alone in locally advanced or metastatic pancreatic cancer: results of a GERCOR and GISCAD phase III trial. *J Clin Oncol.* 2005;23(15):3509–3516.

Moertel CG, Frytak S, Hahn RG, et al. Therapy of locally unresectable pancreatic carcinoma: a randomized comparison of high dose (6000 rads) radiation alone, moderate dose radiation (4000 rads–5-fluorouracil), and high dose radiation–5-fluorouracil. Gastrointestinal Tumor Study Group. *Cancer.* 1981;48:1705–1710.

Moertel CG, Lefkopoulo M, Lipsitz S, et al. Streptozocin–doxorubicin, streptozocin–fluorouracil, or chlorozotocin in the treatment of advanced islet-cell carcinoma. *N Engl J Med.* 1992;326:519–523.

Moore MJ, Golstein D, Hamm J. et al. Erlotinib plus gemcitabine compared with gemcitabine alone in patients with advanced pancreatic cancer; a phase III trial of the National Institute of Cancer Clinical Trials Group. *J Clin Oncol.* 2007;25:1960–1966.

Neoptolemos JP, Stocken DD, Friess H, et al. A randomized trial of chemoradiotherapy and chemotherapy after resection of pancreatic cancer. *N Engl J Med.* 2004; 350:1200–1210.

Oberg K, Kvols L, Caplin M, et al. Consensus report on the use of somatostatin analogs for the management of neuroendocrine tumors of the gastroenteropancreatic system. *Ann Oncol.* 2004;15:966–973.

Oettle H, Post S, Neuhaus P, et al. Adjuvant chemotherapy with gemcitabine vs. observation in patients undergoing curative-intent resection of pancreatic cancer; a randomized controlled trial. *JAMA.* 2007;297:267–277.

Safford SD, Coleman RE, Gockerman JP, et al. Iodine-131 metaiodobenzylguanidine treatment for metastatic carcinoid. Results in 98 patients. *Cancer.* 2004;101(9):1987–1993.

Takada T, Amano H, Yasuda H, et al. Is postoperative adjuvant chemotherapy useful for gallbladder carcinoma? A phase III multicenter prospective randomized controlled trial in patients with resected pancreaticobiliary carcinoma. *Cancer.* 2002;95:1685–1695.

Tsukuma H, Hiyama T, Tanaka S, et al. Risk factors for HCC among patients with chronic liver disease. *N Engl J Med.* 1993;328:1797–1801.

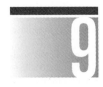

Carcinoma of the Breast

Patrick Glyn Morris and Clifford A. Hudis

I. NATURAL HISTORY, EVALUATION, AND MODES OF TREATMENT

A. Epidemiology and risk factors

Carcinoma of the breast gave way to carcinoma of the lung as the most common cause of cancer deaths among women in the United States in 1986. Despite a decline in incidence since 2003, in 2009, more than 192,000 new cases of breast cancer were diagnosed, and there were about 40,000 women who died from this disease. Currently, more women survive due to earlier diagnosis and better therapy, and the absolute number of deaths per year has been declining since about 1990 with a disease-specific mortality decrease of 2.2% per year since then.

The incidence of breast cancer varies widely among different populations. Women in Western Europe and the United States have a higher incidence than women in most other parts of the world, possibly in part because of the high intake of animal protein, fat, and probably linked to total caloric intake and increased rates of obesity. Caucasian women in the United States are more likely to develop breast cancer compared with African-American women. Mortality from breast cancer, however, is higher in

African-American women than other ethnic or racial groups, although this is confounded by the general increase in cancer-related mortality for lower socioeconomic groups regardless of specific ethnicity. While discrete causes of breast cancer cannot be identified in most individual women, many factors increase a woman's risk of developing the disease. Among the strongest of the risk factors is family history, particularly if more than one family member has developed breast cancer at an early age. More precisely, genetic linkage analysis led to the discovery of dominant germ-line mutations in two tumor-suppressor genes, BRCA1 and BRCA2, localized to chromosomes 17 and 13, respectively, which are associated with a high risk of female breast cancer as well as ovarian cancer (BRCA1 and BRCA2), male breast cancer (BRCA2), and other cancers. Although these mutations account for less than 10% of all cases of breast cancer, together they may account for over 70% of inherited cases in high-risk populations. It is important to note that most patients with a family history of breast cancer do not have a defined inherited mutation and other, less common, causative mutations are sometimes seen. However, if a woman with breast cancer is under the age of 50 years and has any relative who developed breast cancer before she was 50 years old, her chance of having a mutation in BRCA1 or BRCA2 rises to as much as 25%. Other factors that increase her probability of a mutation include any relative with ovarian cancer or a personal history of bilateral breast cancer or ovarian cancer. Carriers of these mutations have up to a 70% lifetime risk of breast cancer, depending on familial history, perhaps the specific mutation, and other cellular genes that may modify penetrance. The 5-year survival rate of patients with either of the BRCA mutations is not significantly less than for other patients with breast cancer after adjusting for the specific subtypes of breast cancer carriers tend to develop. Additional factors that increase breast cancer risk are early menarche, late age at birth of first child, and prior benign breast disease (particularly if there is a high degree of benign epithelial atypia). Present use of birth control pills appears to have a small effect on the risk of developing breast cancer (relative risk, 1.24); risk from prior use diminishes over time. Although breast cancer may occur among men, such cases represent less than 1% of all breast cancers and are infrequently seen in most hospitals. Male carriers of BRCA2 mutations have a 6% lifetime risk of breast cancer, significantly increasing their risk in comparison to the general population.

Hormone replacement therapy (HRT) can increase the risk of breast cancer. In the Women Health Initiative study, researchers found an increased breast cancer risk of about 10% for every 5 years of HRT use. There was a greater risk with combined estrogen/progesterone products than with estrogen therapy alone; following the publication of this report, there was a marked decrease in the use of HRT followed in short order by a decline in the incidence of postmenopausal hormone-receptor–positive breast cancer.

B. Prevention

The risk of hormone-receptor–positive breast cancer can be reduced. At least three trials using selective estrogen receptor modulators (SERMs) have demonstrated that 3 to 5 years of preventive treatment with these agents reduces the rate of breast cancer development over the short term. Women at increased risk because of family history, age, and other risk factors, who are treated with the SERM tamoxifen, 20 mg/day, were found to have a 45% reduction in the rate of occurrence of invasive breast cancer compared with women treated with placebo. Noninvasive disease and preneoplastic breast lesions were also decreased. Raloxifene, 60 or 120 mg/day, also appears to reduce the risk of breast cancer in postmenopausal women (who had osteoporosis and a standard or reduced risk of breast cancer), with a relative risk of 0.26. Despite these benefits, SERMs are associated with an increased risk of both venous thromboembolism and endometrial cancer, although the risks with raloxifene appear to be lower than tamoxifen, which has been associated with an increased risk for endometrial cancer of 1.5 to 2 times that of untreated women. In addition, neither of these agents has demonstrated an improvement in survival when used for breast cancer prevention. In the Study of Tamoxifen against Raloxifene trial, these agents were compared and raloxifene was found not to decrease the incidence of preinvasive carcinomas despite a seemingly better outcome than tamoxifen for prevention of invasive cancers. Lasofoxifene, in a trial addressing osteoporosis, similarly reduced the incidence of breast cancer. These agents have similar but not identical toxicity profiles that may guide clinical decisions.

There are several options in the management of women at very high risk because of family history or known gene mutations. Increased surveillance, through the addition of magnetic resonance imaging (MRI) screening on a yearly basis as a supplement to standard mammography, was effective in a high-risk population. In mutation carriers who are at risk for both breast and ovarian cancer, bilateral oophorectomy after childbearing age has been recommended because of the inadequacy of screening tests for ovarian cancer and because it reduces the risk of primary breast cancer. Risk-reducing mastectomy is an effective option with a relative risk reduction of about 90%. Note that despite risk-reducing mastectomy, there is always a small risk of breast cancer in residual breast glandular tissue. SERMs may be useful in patients with BRCA1 and BRCA2 mutations as well. Analysis of blood samples of women who participated in the P-01 (tamoxifen) trial showed that mutation carriers also had a 47% lower risk of breast cancer.

C. Detection, diagnosis, and pretreatment evaluation

1. **Screening.** Because more lives can be saved if breast cancer is diagnosed at an early stage, many screening programs have been designed to detect small, early cancers. Monthly breast self-examination for all women after puberty and yearly breast examinations by a physician or other trained professional after a woman is 20 years of age is generally recommended, although evidence of effectiveness is limited. Mammography reduces breast cancer mortality by 25% to 30% in women older than 50 years. The benefit for women aged 40 to 50 years has been more difficult to demonstrate because the incidence of breast cancer is lower. Hence, more examinations are needed to find a cancer and save a life. However, additional benefits of early detection via mammography include the option for less disfiguring surgery, reduced utilization of radiation therapy, and decreased need for chemotherapy and other systemic treatments. Therefore, the absolute benefits extend beyond the simple endpoint of survival. As a result, mammography is recommended at age 40 years as a baseline, once every 1 to 2 years between the ages of 40 and 50 years (depending on risk factors and the recommending organization), and yearly after 50 years of age. An upper age of effectiveness is not established. For high-risk women and in family members of mutation-positive patients, annual mammography should be initiated 10 years earlier than the youngest diagnosed relative. Patients with Hodgkin lymphoma (regardless of a history of mantle field irradiation) should have a baseline mammogram by age 25. In BRCA1/BRCA2 mutation carriers, MRI of the breast has recently been approved for screening in addition to annual mammography. Mammography has clearly led to the discovery of many earlier cancers and sharply increased the discovery of preinvasive cancers (ductal carcinoma in situ). These latter are not (yet) invasive and their treatment can be far less complicated than that of invasive breast cancer. Other screening modalities can include ultrasound, but it is more typically used diagnostically to evaluate palpable lesions.

2. **Presenting signs and symptoms.** Although a large number of nonpalpable cancers are found by mammography, invasive breast cancer is still often discovered by a woman herself as an isolated, painless lump in the breast. If the mass has gone unnoticed, ignored, or neglected for a time (or if it is particularly rapidly growing or aggressive), there may be fixation to the skin or underlying chest wall, ulceration, pain, or inflammation. Some early lesions present with discharge or bleeding from the nipple. Occasionally, the primary lesion is not discovered, and the woman presents with symptoms of metastatic disease, such as pleural effusion,

nodal disease, or bony metastases. About half of all lesions are in the upper outer quadrant of the breast (where most of the glandular tissue of the breast is). About 20% are central masses and 10% are in each of the other quadrants. Up to one-quarter of all women with breast cancer have axillary node metastasis at the time of diagnosis, although this is less common when the primary tumor has been detected by screening.

3. **Staging.** Carcinoma of the breast is staged according to the size and characteristics of the primary tumor (T), the involvement of regional lymph nodes (N), and the presence of metastatic disease (M). An abridged version of the commonly used TNM classification of breast cancer is shown in Table 9.1, and the stage grouping is outlined in Table 9.2. In 2010, the revised American Joint Commission on Cancer staging system for breast cancer was published. Although preliminary staging is commonly done before surgery, definitive staging that can be used for prognostic and further treatment planning purposes usually must await postsurgical pathologic evaluation when the primary tumor size and the histologic involvement of the lymph nodes are established. In up to 30% of patients with palpable breast masses (not found by mammography) but without clinical evidence of axillary lymph node involvement, the histologic evaluation of the nodes reveals cancer. In patients with negative nodes by routine histologic evaluation, serial sectioning may reveal microscopic cancer deposits in additional patients. The principal changes in the new staging system take into consideration the widespread use of immunohistochemical (IHC) and molecular biologic techniques that afford pathologists the ability to detect microscopic metastatic lesions down to the level of isolated tumor cells. It is not clear that there is prognostic value if cancer cells in nodes are detected by enhanced examination, and the current staging system designates nodes as pathologically negative if cells are identified by IHC alone and are in clusters of less than 0.2 mm. The identifier "(i)" is used to indicate isolated tumor cells such that pN0(i+) indicates node-negative disease but the presence of such cells in the node. Similarly, "(mol +)" indicates that a molecular examination such as polymerase chain reaction has found evidence of malignant cells. These changes are included in Table 9.1.

D. **Diagnostic evaluation**

1. **Before biopsy** the woman should have a careful history, during which attention should be paid to risk factors, and a physical examination, with a focus not only on the involved breast but also on the opposite breast, all regional lymph node areas, the lungs, bone, and liver. This examination should be followed by bilateral mammography to help assess the extent of involvement and to look for additional ipsilateral or contralateral disease.

TABLE 9.1 TNM Classification of Breast Cancer

Primary Tumor (T)

TX	Primary tumor cannot be assessed
T0	No evidence of primary tumor
Tis	Carcinoma in situ
Tis (DCIS)	Ductal carcinoma in situ
Tis (LCIS)	Lobular carcinoma in situ
Tis (Paget)	Paget disease of the nipple with no tumor (Paget disease associated with a tumor is classified according to the size of the tumor)
T1	Tumor $\leq$2 cm in greatest dimension
T1mic	Microinvasion <0.1 cm in greatest dimension
T1a	Tumor >0.1 cm but not >0.5 cm in greatest dimension
T1b	Tumor >0.5 cm but not >1 cm in greatest dimension
T1c	Tumor >1 cm but not >2 cm in greatest dimension
T2	Tumor >2 cm but not >5 cm in greatest dimension
T3	Tumor >5 cm in greatest dimension
T4	Tumor of any size with direct extension to chest wall or skin, only as described subsequently
T4a	Extension to chest wall, not including pectoralis muscle
T4b	Edema (including peau d'orange) or ulceration of the skin of the breast, or satellite skin nodules confined to the same breast
T4c	Both T4a and T4b
T4d	Inflammatory carcinoma

Regional Lymph Nodes (N): Clinical Classification

NX	Regional lymph nodes cannot be assessed (e.g., previously removed)
N0	No regional lymph node metastasis
N1	Metastasis in movable ipsilateral axillary lymph node(s)
N2	Metastases in ipsilateral axillary lymph nodes fixed or matted, or in clinically apparent ipsilateral internal mammary nodes in the absence of clinically evident axillary lymph node metastasis
N2a	Metastasis in ipsilateral axillary lymph nodes fixed to one another (matted) or to other structures
N2b	Metastasis only in clinically apparent ipsilateral internal mammary nodes and in the absence of clinically evident axillary lymph node metastasis
N3	Metastasis in ipsilateral infraclavicular lymph node(s), or in clinically apparent ipsilateral internal mammary lymph node(s) and in the presence of clinically evident axillary lymph node metastasis; or metastasis in ipsilateral supraclavicular lymph node(s) with or without axillary or internal mammary lymph node involvement
N3a	Metastasis in ipsilateral infraclavicular lymph node(s) and axillary lymph node(s)
N3b	Metastasis in ipsilateral internal mammary lymph node(s) and axillary lymph node(s)
N3c	Metastasis in ipsilateral supraclavicular lymph node(s)

(continued)

TNM Classification of Breast Cancer *(continued)*

Regional Lymph Nodes (pN) Pathologic Classification

pNX	Regional lymph nodes cannot be assessed (e.g., previously removed or not removed for pathologic study)
pN0	No regional lymph node metastasis histologically, no additional examination for isolated tumor cells
pN0(i−)	No regional lymph node metastasis histologically, negative IHC staining
pN0(i+)	Isolated tumor cells identified histologically or by positive IHC staining, no cluster >0.2 mm
pN0(mol−)	No regional lymph node metastasis histologically, negative molecular findings (RT-PCR)
pN0(mol +)	No regional lymph node metastasis histologically, positive molecular findings (RT-PCR)
pN1	Metastasis in one to three axillary lymph nodes and/or in internal mammary nodes with microscopic disease detected by sentinel lymph node dissection but not clinically apparent
pN1mi	Micrometastasis (>0.2 mm, none >2.0 mm)
pN1a	Metastasis in one to three axillary lymph nodes
pN1b	Metastasis in internal mammary nodes with microscopic disease detected by sentinel lymph node dissection but not clinically apparent
pN1c	Metastasis in one to three axillary lymph nodes and in internal mammary lymph nodes with microscopic disease detected by sentinel lymph node dissection but not clinically apparent
pN2	Metastasis in four to nine axillary lymph nodes or in clinically apparent internal mammary lymph nodes in the absence of axillary lymph node metastasis
pN2a	Metastasis in four to nine axillary lymph nodes (at least one tumor deposit >2.0 mm)
pN2b	Metastasis in clinically apparent internal mammary lymph nodes in the absence of axillary lymph node metastasis
pN3	Metastasis in 10 or more axillary lymph nodes, in infraclavicular lymph nodes, or in clinically apparent ipsilateral internal mammary lymph nodes in the presence of one or more positive axillary lymph nodes; or in more than three axillary lymph nodes with clinically negative microscopic metastasis in internal mammary lymph nodes; or in ipsilateral supraclavicular lymph nodes
pN3a	Metastasis in 10 or more axillary lymph nodes (at least one tumor deposit >2.0 mm) or metastasis to the infraclavicular lymph nodes
pN3b	Metastasis in clinically apparent ipsilateral internal mammary lymph nodes in the presence of one or more positive axillary lymph nodes; or in more than three axillary lymph nodes and in internal mammary lymph nodes with microscopic disease detected by sentinel lymph node dissection but not clinically apparent
pN3c	Metastasis in ipsilateral supraclavicular lymph nodes

Distant Metastasis (M)

MX	Distant metastasis cannot be assessed
M0	No distant metastasis
M1	Distant metastasis

RT-PCR, reverse transcriptase-polymerase chain reaction.
Modified from the American Joint Committee on Cancer Staging. *AJCC cancer staging manual* (7th ed.) New York: Springer; 2010.

TABLE 9.2	Stage Grouping of Breast Cancer*
Stage	**Description**
0	Tis, N0, M0
I	T1, N0 or Nmi, M0
IIA	T2, N0, Mo
	T0–1, N1, M0
IIB	T2, N1, M0
	T3, N0, M0
IIIA	T0–2, N2, M0
	T3, N1–2, M0
IIIB	T4, any N, M0
IIIC	Any T, N3, M0
IV	Any T, any N, M1

*Patients are staged in the highest group possible for their composite TNM. For example, a patient with T1a, N2, M0 would have stage IIIA disease because of the N2 status.

2. **Excisional or core needle biopsy of the primary lesion** is performed, and the specimen is given intact (not in formalin) to the pathologist, who can divide the specimen for histologic examination, hormone receptor assays, and HER2 testing (by immunohistochemistry examination or fluorescence in-situ hybridization [FISH]).

3. **After confirmation of the histology,** the patient is evaluated for possible metastatic disease. It is important to emphasize that history and physical examination are the most critical components of this assessment.

   a. **Typical studies** include a chest radiograph, complete blood count, and blood chemistry profile.

   b. **Other studies,** including radionuclide scan of the bones, skeletal survey (usually obtained only if the radionuclide scan is positive), and computed tomography (CT) scan of the liver (abdomen), are optional unless the history, physical examination, or blood studies suggest a poor prognosis or point to specific organ involvement. There is continued evolution in imaging recommendations, and recent data suggest that integrated positron emission tomography-CT may replace most or all other imaging tests.

   c. **Histology.** About 75% to 90% of all breast cancers are infiltrating ductal carcinomas, and up to 10% are infiltrating lobular carcinomas; these two types have similar overall behavior but the latter tend to be hormone responsive and HER2-negative. In addition, their patterns of metastatic spread can vary even if the overall risks of metastases are similar. The remainder of the histologic types of invasive breast carcinoma may have a somewhat better prognosis but are usually managed more according to the stage than to the histologic type. Microarray technology has added nuance to the traditional, histology-based categorization of breast cancer and supports the view that this is a disease with distinct subtypes. About 15% of breast cancers are basal-like (basal epithelial subtype) with a relatively high concordance with the conventionally defined "triple negative" (hormone-receptor and HER2-negative) subset. Luminal tumors are generally hormone receptor–positive, but it is the luminal A subtype that is most clearly hormone responsive. Triple negative tumors are seen in association with BRCA1 mutations and in women of lower socioeconomic status. Each of these subtypes (luminal A, B, basal-like, HER2-positive, etc.) is associated with a distinct typical natural history in terms of time to develop distant metastases.

E. Approach to therapy

Many institutions have established multidisciplinary teams or centers to facilitate coordinated treatment planning. It may be useful in some settings to pursue this particular clinical care structure, but there are other reasonable strategies to employ in the development of an optimal care plan for individual patients.

1. **Consultation** with a surgeon, radiotherapist, and medical oncologist is generally required once the diagnosis of carcinoma is suspected or histologically confirmed or after definitive surgery has been accomplished. Multimodal therapy has had a profound impact on the outcome of breast cancer as it has allowed for organ preservation and improved disease-free survival (DFS) and overall survival. Any clinician treating patients for breast cancer should be very familiar with the roles and interventions offered by the other members of the team. It is also critical to have the patient (and her family if she desires) share in the therapy decisions after hearing the options, the relative advantages and disadvantages of each approach, and the recommendations of the consultants. The patient should be given an opportunity to hear why the recommended treatment is thought by the physicians to be best and to decide whether the treatment is appropriate for her.

2. **Goals of therapy** differ depending on the stage of disease being treated.

   a. **For early-stage invasive disease,** the goal of therapy is to eradicate the primary tumor and to suppress the growth of or eliminate micrometastases, thereby preventing recurrence and death. In the postoperative setting, this is called *adjuvant therapy*. There are three broad classes of systemic adjuvant therapy: hormone therapy (tamoxifen or, in postmenopausal women, an aromatase inhibitor), chemotherapy (any of a large number of standard combination regimens), and immunotherapy (trastuzumab for patients with HER2-positive tumors). These options are weighed and combined on an individualized basis based on careful risk-benefit analyses. Of course, while treating postoperative patients who may be cured by their surgery (and radiation therapy), we seek to avoid unnecessary short- and long-term drug-induced toxicities. Of particular concern is the increased incidence of second cancers (myelodysplasia and leukemias in particular with chemotherapy, and uterine cancer with tamoxifen) arising years after the completion of therapy. Other risks can include osteoporosis with aromatase inhibitors (AIs) and cardiac dysfunction following anthracycline or trastuzumab use. It is important to emphasize that despite these toxicities, overall survival has generally been improved in the patient populations treated with these modalities. However, one goal of ongoing investigational studies is to determine the minimum therapy that is effective for preventing the maximum number of recurrences in any given clinical situation.

b. **For locally advanced disease,** defined as stage IIIA or T3–4 disease or more, including inflammatory breast cancer, the goal of systemic therapy changes somewhat. In addition to critically important systemic control, there is the added potential benefit of local response facilitating less disfiguring surgery and, in some cases, any surgery. This is referred to as *neoadjuvant* or *preoperative systemic therapy*, and it specifically can reduce the size of an initially unresectable tumor or convert the planned surgical intervention from mastectomy to breast conservation. In the research setting, preoperative administration of systemic therapy allows the opportunity to test both the therapeutic efficacy of novel drugs and regimens as well as the ability to conduct correlative science studies, thereby potentially optimizing drug development.

c. **For advanced (metastatic) disease,** the goal of therapy is to lengthen survival when possible and to palliate or limit symptoms and signs of the disease using therapy with an acceptable toxicity profile. In this setting, long-term toxicity is not usually of great importance, but short-term toxicity is a major focus for both physician and patient because the aim of therapy is to improve how the patient feels (quality of life) as well as to prolong survival. The general approach is to use hormone therapy if possible, anti-HER2 therapies when HER2 is amplified or overexpressed in the tumor, and chemotherapy as sequential single agents. There are myriad novel targeted therapies in development and an increasing number of treatments with proven impact on overall survival.

3. **Surgery** remains the most frequently used mode of primary therapy for the vast majority of women with breast cancer. Over the past half century, the extent of surgery has evolved toward less disfiguring procedures. Hence, breast conservation (lumpectomy) with radiation therapy and an examination of the sentinel nodes (or in some cases, an axillary node dissection) is now routine. Surgical margins should be free of tumor, but an exact definition of the safe width is not uniformly accepted. Complete axillary node dissection is unnecessary in most cases when a sentinel node procedure, performed by an experienced surgeon, reveals no cancer. Following breast conservation (and generally after the completion of chemotherapy), radiotherapy is delivered to control any microscopic cancer remaining in the breast. The decision to radiate nodal fields varies with the stage of the cancer. In terms of distant DFS and overall survival, appropriate candidates for breast conservation have the same outcomes as if they were treated with mastectomy. Therefore, many patients opt for breast conserving surgery and radiotherapy over mastectomy. Apart from patient preference, mastectomy is indicated when the tumor is too large or locally advanced to allow breast conservation (although preoperative systemic therapy can facilitate breast conservation in this situation), if the tumor is multicentric/multifocal, when the patient has a contraindication to radiation therapy, if it is an ipsilateral recurrence in a previously radiated breast (again, a contraindication to additional radiation therapy), or when margins free of tumor cannot be obtained.

   There remain wide geographic variations in the use of breast-conserving surgery throughout the United States and without obvious medical justification. For patients who have had mastectomy, reconstruction can be accomplished by several approaches and requires a skilled plastic surgeon. It may be done at the time of mastectomy or delayed for a period (usually 1 to 2 years). There is no evidence that any (or no) reconstructive approach has any impact on the natural history of breast cancer.

4. **Radiation therapy.** The role of radiation therapy in the management of carcinoma of the breast has been expanded since the early 1970s. Radiotherapy is now commonly used in conjunction with breast conservation as part of the primary therapy. In this circumstance, the radiotherapy is commonly delivered to the entire breast with a boost of therapy to the tumor bed using external-beam therapy. More recently, shorter courses of external-beam radiation may be considered for treating the breast only. In addition, radiation therapy to only the affected part of

the breast is now used in early-stage disease. Partial breast irradiation may be delivered by brachytherapy or focused external-beam treatment. Radiotherapy may also be employed following mastectomy in women who have a particularly high likelihood of local recurrence. When the risk of local recurrence is high, radiation therapy is associated with improved overall survival. Typically, postmastectomy radiation is indicated if the primary tumor is larger than 5 cm or if four or more positive lymph nodes were found in the axilla, although there is potential benefit on survival even in lower risk patients, such as those with one to three positive axillary lymph nodes. Following breast conservation, radiation may be omitted in patients older than 70 years of age with estrogen receptor–positive tumors smaller than 2 cm if they are treated with antiestrogen therapy. However, with longer follow-up, an increase in breast recurrences is found without radiation, but with no detectable impact on survival. Radiation therapy is generally administered after completion of cytotoxic therapy (when indicated). Radiation therapy is also helpful as adjunctive therapy for metastatic or locally advanced and unresectable disease. Local recurrences and isolated or specific (e.g., painful bone lesions particularly with impending fracture) distant metastases also are frequently treated successfully with radiotherapy.

5. **Systemic therapy** is used to reduce the likelihood of recurrence after local therapy for early-stage disease and to treat more advanced disease with or without distant metastasis. For operable (curable) breast cancer, The Early Breast Cancer Trialists' Collaborative Group (EBCTCG) analysis of adjuvant therapy demonstrates a clear benefit of postoperative chemotherapy or hormonal therapy (including ovarian ablation in premenopausal women). Although the precise estimates of benefit vary with each half-decade review and update, in very general terms systemic therapy reduces the risk of recurrence by as much as 50%. Similarly, the odds of death are also reduced by as much as 30%. Similar proportional risk reductions are seen in node-positive as well as node-negative disease with the proviso that lower risk disease yields proportionately smaller absolute benefits for therapy. Historically, medical oncologists relied on node status, tumor size, hormone receptor status, HER2 status, and perhaps DNA synthesis rate (percentage of cells in the synthesis phase), as well as any of a number of other factors to aid in determining risk for individual patients so that the oncologists could then estimate the benefits of specific systemic therapies and guide patients. More recently, commercially available tests that provide prognosis, or more importantly, prediction of benefit for specific systemic therapies, have become available. As always,

physiologic age of the patient and comorbid conditions are also important considerations in adjuvant therapy decisions.

6. **Endocrine therapy** includes surgical, radiotherapeutic, or drug-induced ablation or inhibition of ovarian function. It also includes antiestrogens (typically SERMs), aromatase inhibitors, progestins, androgens, and even corticosteroids. Tumors with no expression of either the estrogen or the progesterone receptor will generally not respond to hormone therapies, and the greater the expression of these receptors the greater the probability of benefit. However, there is no clear threshold (above zero) below which one can be certain that endocrine therapy will be ineffective. Similarly, when the estrogen receptor is detected, it is not clear that the level of the progesterone receptor is important. Variations in test quality and results remain important challenges in this area.

F. Prognosis

Breast cancer can vary from aggressive and rapidly fatal to relatively indolent disease with late-appearing metastasis. Molecular studies increasingly support the view that breast cancer is a collection of diseases rather than one single entity. At present, clinicians can use the following factors to provide crude estimates of the likelihood of relapse and survival, but this is an area where newer diagnostics may rapidly improve our current approach.

1. **Stage.** Axillary node involvement and the size of the primary tumor are major determinants of the likelihood of survival.

   a. **Nodes.** In one large National Surgical Adjuvant Breast and Bowel Project (NSABP) study, before the use of modern adjuvant therapy, 65% of all patients who underwent radical mastectomy survived 5 years, and 45% survived 10 years. When no axillary nodes were positive, the 5-year survival rate was nearly 80% and the 10-year survival rate 65%. If any axillary nodes were positive, the 5-year survival rate was less than 50% and the 10-year survival rate 25%. If four or more nodes were positive, the 5-year survival rate was 30% and the 10-year survival rate less than 15%. Since that time (1975), there has been improvement, with 5-year survival rates of 87% for stage I, 75% for stage II, 45% for stage III, and 13% for stage IV breast cancer. Lymph node involvement by conventional light microscopy remains the single most important prognostic factor in making survival predictions and treatment decisions. It is important to distinguish modern cases in which malignant cells are detected in lymph nodes using higher sensitivity techniques. Their prognosis is not as clearly established.

   b. **Primary tumor.** Patients with large primary tumors generally face higher risks of relapse and death compared to patients with small tumors, irrespective of the nodal status, although patients with large primary tumors are more likely to have node involvement. Tumors that are fixed to the skin or to the chest wall have worsened prognoses compared to those that are not. Patients with inflammatory carcinomas have a particularly poor prognosis, with a median survival time of less than 2 years and a 5-year survival rate of less than 10% in some series. Neoadjuvant systemic therapy has improved the outcome significantly for this subset of patients by enabling local control surgery and improving long-term rates of relapse and death.

2. **Estrogen and progesterone receptors.** Although stage of disease is critical in determining the risk of recurrence, the timing of events is heavily influenced by tumor biology, particularly hormone receptor status. Patients with tumors that do not express estrogen or progesterone receptors (or do so at only very low levels) are much more likely to experience recurrence during the first few years after diagnosis than those who have receptor-positive disease. This observation is true for both premenopausal and postmenopausal patients within each major node group (zero, one to three, and four or more). Over decades, the risk of relapse and death is approximately the same but the distribution of these events is more even with hormone receptor–positive disease and skewed to the earlier years when the receptors are absent.

3. **Her-2/neu gene** amplification and overexpression of its transmembrane receptor is associated with impaired survival in early-stage breast cancer. Amplification (as is seen in 20% to 30% of early breast cancer) results in worse prognosis with earlier appearance of metastatic disease. However, it is now clear that this gene and receptor are predictive factors for response to trastuzumab and with that therapy the outcome for patients with HER2-positive disease may be superior to that of other subtypes.

4. **Gene profiling.** There are several tools and assays using divergent technologies to provide more precise individualized estimates of the risk of relapse ("prognosis") and the benefits of specific treatments ("prediction"). The MammaPrint test (Agendia, Inc., Huntington Beach, CA) provides prognosis for node-negative breast cancer regardless of receptor status. The OncotypeDx (Genomic Health, Inc., Redwood City, CA) provides prognosis for node-negative, hormone receptor–positive breast cancer treated with tamoxifen and predicts the benefits of conventional combination chemotherapy as an additional treatment for this cohort. It may be similarly useful in hormone receptor-positive, node-positive disease. These technologies are based on our ability to determine gene expression on fresh frozen or paraffin embedded tissues.

With regard to the OncotypeDx, the following are some considerations:

- Patients with a result (recurrence score [RS]) of less than 18 (about 50% of patients in most series) are considered low risk and will probably not benefit from the addition of cytotoxic therapy to their hormonal manipulation.
- Patients with an RS of greater than 30 have a high risk of systemic disease and will obtain the maximum benefit from chemotherapy.
- Patients with an intermediate score (18 to 30) currently represent a decision-making dilemma and a large trial is under way to better define the value of chemotherapy in this patient population.

5. **Other prognostic factors** are still undergoing study as to whether they can provide information as independent prognostic factors, particularly for node-negative cancers. In all cases, the key is whether or not they are reliable, validated, reproducible, and additive or supplemental in a meaningful way to the existing tools.

6. **Adjuvant! Online** is a web-based decision-making tool (see www .adjuvantonline.com) that allows clinicians and patients to input key individual variables, model the impact of specific treatments, and display the benefits both numerically and graphically. There are well-recognized limits to this approach, but it can be very useful in providing easily interpretable information.

II. SYSTEMIC THERAPY OF BREAST CANCER

A. Cytotoxic therapy

As with other cancers, the basis for the effectiveness of cytotoxic drugs in the treatment of carcinoma of the breast is not completely understood. In general, a combination of two or more drugs is more effective in the adjuvant setting than single agents, and nearly all treatment programs use a variety of drugs either in concurrent combination or sequentially. In addition to their cytotoxic effects, chemotherapeutic agents may induce menopause in premenopausal women and this may represent an additional anticancer effect.

1. **Response to therapy.** In the adjuvant setting, it is impossible to determine whether individual patients have responded to treatment for micrometastatic disease unless they relapse as there are no parameters to measure. Relapse means that treatment did not eradicate all disease, did not prevent the development of new disease, or only slowed the growth of microscopic metastases. Determination of the appropriate adjuvant therapy option for individuals must therefore depend on extrapolations from large randomized studies.

2. **Treatment of early disease (adjuvant therapy).** As discussed previously, standard treatment of early disease depends on a variety of factors; there is not yet a single agreed-on optimal chemotherapy regimen for any subset of women with breast cancer. Therefore, as a first priority, patients should be encouraged to participate in clinical trials. If none is available or the patient declines, Table 9.3 can be used as a guide for assessing risk.

   a. **Choice of therapy.** Cytotoxic therapy is recommended for most otherwise healthy patients with hormone receptor–negative tumors that are 0.5 to 1 cm in size or greater regardless of node status. Patients with HER2 overexpression or gene amplification generally receive chemotherapy and trastuzumab. Regardless of whether they receive cytotoxic therapy, most patients with hormone receptor–positive invasive cancer of

TABLE 9.3	Prognostic Factors for Assessing Risk of Recurrence of Breast Cancer
Value	**Parameter**
Nodal status	Risk increases with presence of metastasis and numbers of nodes involved
Tumor size	Risk increases with tumor size independent of nodal status
Estrogen and progesterone receptors	Positive receptors confer better prognosis
Age	Complex factor (biology chronology): Women aged 45 to 49 years have best prognosis, with increasing likelihood of deaths from their breast cancer in older and younger age groups
Morphology	Higher nuclear grade, higher histologic grade, tumor necrosis, peritumoral lymphatic vessel invasion, increased microvessel density tumors have worse prognosis
DNA content and proliferative capacity	Tumors that are diploid and have low synthesis-phase fraction do better than those that are aneuploid or have a high synthesis-phase fraction (by flow cytometry)
HER2/neu (c-erbB-2)	Amplification is associated with earlier relapse and shorter survival. HER2/neu (c-erbB-2) testing by either FISH expressed as molecules/gene copy ratio (2.0 or more copies) or by IHC staining expressed as 0–3+, where 3+ correlates best with FISH positivity.
OncotypeDx Recurrence Score	Provides risk of recurrence ("prognosis") and benefit of combination chemotherapy with CMF (and possibly cyclophosphamide, doxorubicin, and fluorouracil) ("prediction") for hormone receptor–positive tumors
Mammaprint	Provides prognosis regardless of hormone receptor status

CMF, cyclophosphamide, methotrexate, and 5-fluorouracil; FISH, fluorescent in situ hybridization; IHC, immunohistochemistry.

any size should be treated with hormone therapy (tamoxifen if premenopausal and an aromatase inhibitor—alone or after tamoxifen—if postmenopausal). The goal of adjuvant chemotherapy is to decrease the risk of death and systemic disease. Due to the risks of competing causes of death, cytotoxic therapy is less commonly recommended in the adjuvant treatment of older women (based on physiologic and not solely on absolute chronologic age). The value of cytotoxic therapy when added to antiestrogen therapy in low-risk node-negative, hormone receptor–positive patients is partially addressed by the OncotypeDx discussed previously, although a number of additional tests may become available for this purpose.

b. **Traditional chemotherapy options.** Currently, a wide range of chemotherapy options exists, which generally developed as sequential experimental arms in lineages of clinical research. Cyclophosphamide, methotrexate, and 5-fluorouracil (CMF) remains an option for some low- risk patients and may actually be a superior regimen for the basal-like subtype of triple-negative disease. Four cycles of doxorubicin (Adriamycin) and cyclophosphamide (AC) is a standard regimen, which has been improved with the addition of taxanes and every other week ("dose-dense") scheduling. With regard to the anthracyclines, the Oxford overview and the EBCTCG update showed a 3% absolute survival and recurrence benefit with anthracycline-based regimens compared with CMF at 5 years and 4% survival benefit at 10 years notwithstanding the special toxicities (cardiac in particular and leukemia) these regimens may cause. We highly recommend reviewing the EBCTCG update in *Lancet* 2005 (included in our list of "Selected Readings") for a better understanding of the evolution of breast cancer therapy.

c. **Addition of taxanes.** Multiple phase III trials have evaluated the addition of taxanes (paclitaxel or docetaxel) to chemotherapy regimens for early-stage breast cancer. Both the pivotal Cancer and Leukemia Group B protocol 9344 and the NSABP B28 trial supported the use of paclitaxel after AC for node-positive breast cancer regardless of receptor status, tamoxifen use, patient age, or the number of positive lymph nodes. Retrospective analysis suggests that the benefit is limited in patients with hormone receptor–positive, HER2-negative disease, but other studies have not been consistent in this regard. A slightly differently designed trial (Breast Cancer International Research Group 001) addressed the same question. In this trial, six cycles of concurrent docetaxel, doxorubicin, and cyclophosphamide (TAC) were compared to six cycles of fluorouracil, doxorubicin, and cyclophosphamide as adjuvant therapy for node-positive patients. The study showed superiority of TAC in all patient groups. Similar findings were noted when epirubicin was used instead of doxorubicin. Three cycles of fluorouracil, epirubicin, and cyclophosphamide (FEC) followed by three cycles of docetaxel were found to be superior to six cycles of FEC in node-positive patients by the French Adjuvant Study Group. (Selected readings includes an overview [meta-analysis] of the available taxane studies by DeLaurentiis et al.)

d. **Use of trastuzumab in the adjuvant setting.** HER-neu–positive breast cancer accounts for 20% to 30% of all cases of breast cancer. In the absence of treatment, these patients have a higher risk of recurrence and earlier death. Trastuzumab prolongs survival in the metastatic setting and prevents recurrence and death in the adjuvant setting as well. The use of trastuzumab along with chemotherapy (a taxane was included in most of these trials) in high-risk node-negative as well as node-positive patients was associated with a 39% to 52% reduction in the risk of recurrence and significant improvements in survival. Trastuzumab does not cross the blood-brain barrier, and the rates of recurrence in the brain, as opposed to all other sites, may not be reduced in the adjuvant setting. There are many active anti-HER2 agents in development for metastatic disease and one small molecule tyrosine kinase inhibitor (lapatinib) has been approved. Lapatinib is currently being tested as adjuvant therapy in randomized control trials. Additional agents with activity in the metastatic setting include trastuzumab-DM1, pertuzumab, neratinib, and several heat shock protein-90 inhibitors. These drugs may be tested in the adjuvant setting in the future.

e. **High-dose chemotherapy.** Dose escalation beyond "standard" dose levels, including those that require support with autologous bone marrow or peripheral blood progenitor cell reinfusion, has not been shown to offer advantage over conventional therapy and should not be offered. Dose-dense therapy was developed in recognition of the lack of benefit for higher dose regimens and instead relies on the increased cytotoxicity of more frequent standard doses. This approach requires growth factor support and has been shown to be superior in several randomized trials. For AC and paclitaxel, this is now a standard approach.

f. **Some commonly used regimens (refer to previous discussion about choice of regimen based on nodal status) are as follows.**
   - Cyclophosphamide, doxorubicin, and fluorouracil:
     - Cyclophosphamide 100 mg/m^2 by mouth on days 1 to 14.
     - Doxorubicin 30 mg/m^2 intravenously (IV) on days 1 and 8.

- Fluorouracil 500 mg/m^2 IV on days 1 and 8. Repeat the cycle every 4 weeks.
- Docetaxel and cyclophosphamide:
  - Docetaxel 75 mg/m^2 IV push through a rapidly running intravenous line.
  - Cyclophosphamide 600 mg/m^2 IV. Repeat every 3 weeks.
- AC plus taxane (dose-dense)
  - Doxorubicin 60 mg/m^2 IV push through a rapidly running intravenous line.
  - Cyclophosphamide 600 mg/m^2 IV. Repeat every 2 weeks with growth factor support. After four cycles, switch to paclitaxel 175 mg/m^2 IV 3-hour infusion every 2 weeks for four cycles.
- FEC
  - Fluorouracil 500 mg/m^2 IV on day 1.
  - Epirubicin 100 mg/m^2 IV on day 1.
  - Cyclophosphamide 500 mg/m^2 IV on day 1. Repeat cycle every 21 days.
- TAC
  - Docetaxel 75 mg/m^2 on day 1.
  - Doxorubicin 50 mg/m^2 on day 1.
  - Cyclophosphamide 500 mg/m^2 on day 1. Repeat cycle every 21 days.

For patients with HER2-positive disease, trastuzumab may be added to a taxane after completion of four cycles of AC. Options include the following:

- Paclitaxel 80 mg/m^2 weekly for 12 weeks given concurrently with
- Trastuzumab 4 mg/m^2 as an initial loading dose, followed by 2 mg/m^2 weekly, which is continued for 52 weeks or
- During the paclitaxel component of the dose-dense therapy using the same schedule of trastuzumab as previously mentioned or
- Conventionally administered docetaxel (100 mg/m^2 every 3 weeks for four cycles) with trastuzumab.

Alternatively, adjunctive therapy for positive patients may begin with docetaxel 100 mg/m^2 with carboplatin (area under the curve = 6) once every 3 weeks for six cycles with trastuzumab.

In all cases, trastuzumab is generally administered with and after chemotherapy for 1 full year, although the optimum duration of trastuzumab is the subject of ongoing clinical trials.

g. **Tips**

(1) Limit the number of cycles of doxorubicin in any combination regimen to six (300 to 360 mg/m^2 or less) to limit enhanced cardiotoxicity from the combination.

(2) Avoid concurrent administration of trastuzumab in combination with anthracyclines.

(3) Monitor for peripheral neuropathy with taxanes, especially in diabetics and older patients.

3. **Cytotoxic therapy of advanced (metastatic) disease.** Among the cytotoxic drugs, the most commonly used agents include doxorubicin, cyclophosphamide, methotrexate, fluorouracil, paclitaxel, docetaxel, albumin-bound paclitaxel, gemcitabine, capecitabine, vinorelbine, and ixabepilone. Each of these agents has a response rate of 15% to 40% when used as a single agent (depending on the prior therapies and patient population). With very few exceptions, the data have not supported a survival advantage in the metastatic setting with combination chemotherapy, and toxicity is generally greater so most patients are best palliated with sequential single agents.

Cytotoxic chemotherapy is used as first-line treatment for advanced disease in patients with hormone receptor–negative disease. Its use in lieu of hormone therapy in patients with hormone receptor–positive disease when multiple organ systems are involved is controversial, as some clinicians believe it offers more rapid responses whereas endocrine therapy may offer longer disease stabilization.

Cytotoxic chemotherapy produces clinical benefit (response and disease stabilization) in 60% to 80% of patients regardless of their estrogen receptor status. The responses to therapy at times are durable, but the median duration of treatment in most studies is less than 1 year. Clearly, improved survival is desirable, but the impact of many regimens on survival is modest. However, for patients with HER2-positive metastatic breast cancer, trastuzumab has improved survival, demonstrating that translational science can lead to therapeutic advances once the appropriate biological target is identified. In support of this, the benefits of trastuzumab are limited to patients who are HER2 3+ positive by immunohistochemistry or those who are FISH positive. Second-line chemotherapy is dependent on the specific prior treatments received by an individual patient. If the patient relapses while on treatment or within 6 months after finishing treatment for micrometastatic disease (adjuvant therapy), it is not likely that these drugs used in combination can be helpful in achieving a second remission. In addition, in selecting appropriate therapeutic approaches, the side-effect profiles of the multiple treatment options should be considered in conjunction with patient-related considerations such as symptoms and residual toxicities from prior treatments.

Bevacizumab is a humanized monoclonal antibody targeting vascular endothelial factor. Its use in combination with a variety of chemotherapy agents is associated with higher response rates and longer time to progression, but it has not had an impact on overall survival. Additional antiangiogenic agents are currently in clinical trials, and bevacizumab is being studied in the adjuvant setting. Other novel therapeutics include the poly(ADP-ribose) polymerase inhibitors, one of which has been associated with a survival advantage in combination with conventional combination therapy in triple-negative breast cancer in a randomized phase II study. Effective individual drugs and regimens in addition to those used in the adjuvant setting include the following (note: This is by no means an all-inclusive list. Regimens listed are commonly used in clinical practice):

- Paclitaxel 150 to 175 mg/m^2 IV over 3 hours every 3 weeks, *or* 80 mg/m^2 over 1 hour weekly.
- Docetaxel 60 to 100 mg/m^2 IV over 1 hour every 3 weeks (premedication with oral corticosteroids such as dexamethasone 8 mg twice a day for 5 days starting 1 day prior to starting docetaxel is necessary to reduce the severity of fluid retention and hypersensitivity reactions).
- Vinorelbine 20 to 30 mg/m^2 IV over 6 to 10 minutes weekly.
- Capecitabine 1250 mg/m^2 orally twice daily on days 1 to 14 followed by a 1-week rest. Repeat cycle every 3 weeks.
- Gemcitabine/paclitaxel
    - Gemcitabine 1250 mg/m^2 IV days 1 and 8 followed by a 1-week rest, *plus*
    - Paclitaxel 175 mg/m^2 IV on day 1. Repeat every 3 weeks.
- Nab-paclitaxel 260 mg/m^2 IV over 30 minutes given every 3 weeks or 100 to 130 mg/m^2 over 30 minutes weekly.
- Weekly trastuzumab and paclitaxel (for HER2-positive disease)
    - Trastuzumab 4 mg/m^2 IV as an initial loading dose, followed by 2 mg/m^2 weekly *with*
    - Paclitaxel 200 mg/m^2 IV every 3 weeks, or Nab-paclitaxel as discussed previously.
- Bevacizumab may be given with first- or second-line chemotherapy typically at a dose of 15 mg/kg every third week or 10 mg/kg every other week. It is not clear that there is only one appropriate chemotherapy "partner" for bevacizumab.
- Lapatinib may be given at a dose of 1250 mg orally once a day on days 1 to 21 continuously in combination with capecitabine 2,000 mg/m^2/day on days 1 to 14 in patients with advanced, refractory HER2-positive breast cancer who have failed prior therapies including anthracyclines, taxanes, or trastuzumab. Lapatinib can also be given in combination with letrozole (2.5 mg daily) in postmenopausal, HER2-positive, hormone receptor–positive breast cancer at a dose of 1500 mg.

4. **Dose modifications** are regimen-specific. Readers must review the original source references for any regimen they administer.

B. **Endocrine (hormonal) therapy**

This therapy is effective because breast cancers retain hormone dependence. In premenopausal women, if the breast cancer growth is supported by estrogen production from the ovary, antiestrogen therapy, removal of endogenous estrogen by oophorectomy, or suppression of estrogen production using a leuteinizing hormone–releasing hormone (LHRH) agonist, regression of the cancer can result. Complicating the anticipated actions of SERMS are the presence of different classes of estrogen receptors, different ligands, many receptor-interacting proteins, a host of transcription-activating factors, and several response elements. In some tissues, this class of "antiestrogen" has estrogenic effects (i.e., bone).

1. **Treatment of early disease (adjuvant therapy)**. Among the antihormonal drugs, the most commonly used agents are tamoxifen (a SERM), anastrozole, and letrozole and exemestane (aromatase inhibitors). Toremifene is an alternative to tamoxifen, but raloxifene is used for the treatment of osteopenia and as a chemopreventative and not as adjuvant therapy. The AIs (anastrozole, letrozole, and exemestane) block estrogen production at the cellular level by inhibiting reversibly or irreversibly to the aromatase enzyme (responsible for conversion of male hormones and other precursors to estrogen). Aromatase inhibition has not been shown to be effective in premenopausal patients and therefore tamoxifen is the hormone therapy of first choice. In postmenopausal women, AIs offer additional benefit to what was observed with 5 years of tamoxifen, including a survival advantage in patients with node-positive, receptor-positive tumors. Both the ATAC trial and the BIG 1–98 trials demonstrated an advantage to upfront use of an AI (anastrozole and letrozole, respectively) over tamoxifen therapy. Results of the IES study demonstrated a superior DFS with sequential therapy using exemestane following 2 to 3 years of tamoxifen to 5 years of tamoxifen alone. Fewer side effects are seen in this population with the use of AIs in comparison to tamoxifen. Letrozole after about 5 years of tamoxifen was effective, and a clinical trial is now evaluating a third 5-year period of treatment (i.e., 10 years versus 5 years of letrozole following 5 years of tamoxifen). Importantly, the AIs offer lower incidence of venous thromboembolic events and endometrial carcinoma compared to tamoxifen but are associated with a higher incidence of osteoporosis and musculoskeletal complaints.

Tamoxifen, 20 mg daily, is recommended in premenopausal women with hormone receptor–positive disease. It should be continued for 5 years. Longer durations do not improve survival.

In receptor-positive patients, its benefits are additive to those of chemotherapy (when used), and it is not clear whether ovarian suppression adds to chemotherapy and tamoxifen. It has a relatively low risk in the adjuvant setting, and our current recommendations generally include tamoxifen where it is indicated in addition to chemotherapy in Table 9.4.

Tamoxifen and AIs (for postmenopausal patients) improve DFS and overall survival in most patients with estrogen receptor–positive tumors. Although the proportional reduction (about 25%) in death rate is similar for both high- and low-risk patients (e.g., node-positive and node-negative), the absolute benefit is greater for those at higher risk of recurrence and death. The improvement in DFS is superior with all AIs, and there is an associated more significant reduction in contralateral breast cancer with these drugs in comparison to tamoxifen.

Tamoxifen is metabolized by CYP2D6, and this activity can be inhibited by certain selective serotonin reuptake inhibitor antidepressants and by inherited variations in single nucleotide polymorphisms (SNPs). However, there is no prospective evidence that SNP testing can yet guide individual patients to better selection of hormone therapy and improved outcomes.

2. **Treatment of advanced (metastatic) disease.** Hormonal therapy is indicated in women who have had a positive test for estrogen or progesterone receptors in their tumor tissue. This approach is not generally recommended for women who have previously been shown to be unresponsive to hormonal manipulation. It is also not appropriate therapy for women with visceral crises. For premenopausal women, oophorectomy still may be the treatment of choice. The LHRH analogs goserelin and leuprolide can achieve the equivalent of a medical oophorectomy. This treatment may then be combined with an AI or tamoxifen in such patients. For postmenopausal women, an AI should be used as the initial hormonal therapy. Responses to endocrine therapy tend to last longer than responses to cytotoxic chemotherapy, frequently lasting 12 to 24 months. Second-line hormonal manipulation (e.g., using fulvestrant, a selective estrogen receptor down-regulator) is a reasonable option if the tempo of disease progression allows such. Sequential hormone manipulation may be most appropriate for patients with indolent hormone receptor–positive breast cancer, such as those with bone-dominant disease.

Doses of commonly used drugs are the following:
- Tamoxifen 20 mg by mouth daily
- Anastrozole 1 mg by mouth daily
- Letrozole 2.5 mg by mouth daily
- Exemestane 25 mg by mouth daily

- Fulvestrant 250 to 500 mg intramuscularly (into buttock) monthly after loading with 500 mg on days 1 and 15
- Megestrol acetate 40 mg by mouth four times a day.

C. Complications of therapy

A large range of possible side effects have been associated with treatments for breast cancer and vary extensively between agents and individuals. Acute toxicities are primarily hematologic and gastrointestinal. Subacute toxicities include alopecia, hemorrhagic cystitis, hypertension, edema, and neurologic abnormalities. Chronic or long-term toxicities may be cardiac, neoplastic, or neurologic. Premenopausal women need to be aware of menstrual irregularities, early menopause, and infertility as a consequence of chemotherapy and should be referred for consideration of fertility preservation when desired. Dose modifications for specific regimens must be based on the original sources. Readers are urged to review the original reports for any regimen they prescribe. In addition, because of individual differences, toxicities that are worse than expected may occur, and the responsible physician must always be alert to special circumstances that dictate further attenuation of the drug doses. The drug data listed in Chapter 33 should be consulted for the individual toxicities, precautions, and toxicity prevention measures for each drug.

Like all therapeutic interventions, adjuvant tamoxifen therapy also has consequences. These include a twofold to fourfold increase in endometrial cancer, an increase in cataracts, and an increase in thromboembolic disease. Hot flashes are common but can be ameliorated in some women with venlafaxine 25 to 50 mg daily. While there is also reduction in the hot flashes from using a progestin, such as megestrol, 20 mg twice a day, the effect of the progestin on the risk of recurrence is not known. Adverse effects on vaginal mucosa may be ameliorated with minimal systemic estrogen effect by the estradiol vaginal ring or by an estradiol tablet administered intravaginally (Vagifem). While fractures related to osteoporosis decrease with tamoxifen, there does not appear to be any reduction in cardiovascular events. AIs, on the other hand, may worsen osteoporosis despite an absence of increased fracture incidence in many trials. Caution and possibly anticoagulation should be exercised in treating women with Factor V Leiden who begin treatment with tamoxifen in the prevention or adjuvant setting.

Bisphosphonates are commonly administered IV to all patients with bone metastases due to their role in reduction of skeletal events. Recently, randomized studies in the adjuvant setting have demonstrated reductions in the risk of bone and other metastases but no impact on survival. These agents may become part of standard adjuvant therapy if additional trials are positive.

IV bisphosphonate options include zoledronic acid 4 mg over 15 minutes *or* pamidronate 60 to 90 mg over 1 to 2 hours.

Acknowledgments

The authors are indebted to Dr. Iman Mohamed, who contributed to previous editions of this chapter. Several sections in this revision of the handbook represent her work.

Selected Readings

Albain KS, Nag SM, Calderillo-Ruiz G, et al. Gemcitabine plus paclitaxel versus paclitaxel monotherapy in patients with metastatic breast cancer and prior anthracycline treatment. *J Clin Oncol.* 2008;26(24):3950–3957.

Buchholz TA. Radiation therapy for early-stage breast cancer after breast-conserving surgery. *N Engl J Med.* 2009;360(1):63–70.

Chia S, Gradishar W, Mauriac L, et al. Double-blind, randomized placebo controlled trial of fulvestrant compared with exemestane after prior nonsteroidal aromatase inhibitor therapy in postmenopausal women with hormone receptor-positive, advanced breast cancer: results from EFECT. *J Clin Oncol.* 2008;26(10):1664–1670.

Chlebowski RT, Kuller LH, Prentice RL, et al. Breast cancer after use of estrogen plus progestin in postmenopausal women. *N Engl J Med.* 2009;360(6):573–587.

Citron ML, Berry DA, Cirrincione C, et al. Randomized trial of dose-dense versus conventionally scheduled and sequential versus concurrent combination chemotherapy as postoperative adjuvant treatment of node-positive primary breast cancer: first report of Intergroup Trial C9741/Cancer and Leukemia Group B Trial 9741. *J Clin Oncol.* 2003;21(8):1431–1439.

Cleator S, Heller W, Coombes RC. Triple-negative breast cancer: therapeutic options. *Lancet Oncol.* 2007;8(3):235–244.

de Boer M, van Deurzen CH, van Dijck JA, et al. Micrometastases or isolated tumor cells and the outcome of breast cancer. *N Engl J Med.* 2009;361(7):653–663.

De Laurentiis M, Cancello G, D'Agostino D, et al. Taxane-based combinations as adjuvant chemotherapy of early breast cancer: a meta-analysis of randomized trials. *J Clin Oncol.* 2008;26(1):44–53.

Dowsett M, Cuzick J, Ingle J, et al. Meta-analysis of breast cancer outcomes in adjuvant trials of aromatase inhibitors versus tamoxifen. *J Clin Oncol.* 2010;28(3):509–518.

Early Breast Cancer Trialists' Collaborative Group. Effects of chemotherapy and hormonal therapy for early breast cancer on recurrence and 15-year survival: an overview of the randomised trials. *Lancet.* 2005;365:1687–1717.

Early Breast Cancer Trialists' Collaborative Group, Clarke M, Coates AS, et al. Adjuvant chemotherapy in oestrogen-receptor-poor breast cancer: patient-level meta-analysis of randomised trials. *Lancet.* 2008;371(9606):29–40.

Fisher B, Land S, Mamounas E, Dignam J, Fisher ER, Wolmark N. Prevention of invasive breast cancer in women with ductal carcinoma in situ: an update of the national surgical adjuvant breast and bowel project experience. *Semin Oncol.* 2004;28(4):400–418.

Geyer CE, Forster J, Lindquist D, et al. Lapatinib plus capecitabine for HER2-positive advanced breast cancer. *N Engl J Med.* 2006;355(26):2733–2743.

Gianni L, Norton L, Wolmark N, et al. Role of anthracyclines in the treatment of early breast cancer. *J Clin Oncol.* 2009;27(28):4798–4808.

Gnant M, Mlineritsch B, Schippinger W, et al. Endocrine therapy plus zoledronic acid in premenopausal breast cancer. *N Engl J Med.* 2009;360(7):679–691.

Gradishar WJ, Krasnojon D, Cheporov S, et al. Significantly longer progression-free survival with nab-paclitaxel compared with docetaxel as first-line therapy for metastatic breast cancer. *J Clin Oncol.* 2009;27(22):3611–3619.

Henderson IC, Berry DA, Demetri GD, et al. Improved outcomes from adding sequential paclitaxel but not from escalating doxorubicin dose in an adjuvant chemotherapy regimen for patients with node-positive primary breast cancer. *J Clin Oncol.* 2003;21(6):976–983.

Hillner BE, Ingle JN, Berenson JR, et al. American Society of Clinical Oncology guideline on the role of bisphosphonates in breast cancer. *J Clin Oncol.* 2000;18(6): 1378–1391.

Hudis CA. Trastuzumab—mechanism of action and use in clinical practice. *N Engl J Med.* 2007;357(1):39–51.

Jones S, Holmes FA, O'Shaughnessy J, et al. Docetaxel with cyclophosphamide is associated with an overall survival benefit compared with doxorubicin and cyclophosphamide: 7-year follow-up of US Oncology Research Trial 9735. *J Clin Oncol.* 2009;27(8):1177–1183.

Lee SJ, Schover LR, Partridge AH, et al. American Society of Clinical Oncology recommendations on fertility preservation in cancer patients. *J Clin Oncol.* 2006; 24(18):2917–2931.

Lyman GH, Giuliano AE, Somerfield MR et al. American Society of Clinical Oncology Guideline recommendations for sentinel lymph node biopsy in early-stage breast cancer. *J Clin Oncol.* 2005;23(30):7703–7720.

Mamounas EP, Bryant J, Lembersky B, et al. Paclitaxel after doxorubicin plus cyclophosphamide as adjuvant chemotherapy for node-positive breast cancer: results from NSABP B-28. *J Clin Oncol.* 2005;23(16):3686–3696.

Miller K, Wang M, Gralow J, et al. Paclitaxel plus bevacizumab versus paclitaxel alone for metastatic breast cancer. *N Engl J Med.* 2007;357(26):2666–2676.

Mook S, Schmidt MK, Weigelt B, et al. The 70-gene prognosis signature predicts early metastasis in breast cancer patients between 55 and 70 years of age. *Ann Oncol.* 2010;21(4):717–722.

Muss HB, Berry DA, Cirrincione CT, et al. Adjuvant chemotherapy in older women with early-stage breast cancer. *N Engl J Med.* 2009;360(20):2055–2065.

Nabholtz J, Pienkowski T, Mackey J, et al. Phase III trial comparing TAC (docetaxel, doxorubicin, cyclophosphamide) with FAC (5-fluorouracil, doxorubicin, cyclophosphamide) in the adjuvant treatment of node positive breast cancer (BC) patients: interim analysis of the BCIRG 001 study. *Proc Am Soc Clin Oncol.* 2002;21:abstr# 141.

Paik S, Shak S, Tang G, et al. A multigene assay to predict recurrence of tamoxifen-treated, node-negative breast cancer. *N Engl J Med.* 2004;351(27):2817–2826.

Paik S, Tang G, Shak S, et al. Gene expression and benefit of chemotherapy in women with node-negative, estrogen receptor-positive breast cancer. *J Clin Oncol.* 2006; 24(23):3726–3734.

Partridge AH, Winer EP. On mammography — more agreement than disagreement. *N Engl J Med.* 2009;361(26):2499–2501.

Piccart-Gebhart M, Procter M, Leyland-Jones B, et al. Trastuzumab after adjuvant chemotherapy in HER2-positive breast cancer. *N Engl J Med.* 2005;353(16):659–672.

Recht A, Edge SB, Solin LJ, et al. Postmastectomy radiotherapy: clinical practice guidelines of the American Society of Clinical Oncology. *J Clin Oncol.* 2001;19(5): 1539–1569.

Robson M, Offit K. Management of an inherited predisposition to breast cancer. *N Engl J Med.* 2007;357(2):154–162.

Romond EH, Perez EA, Bryant J, et al. Trastuzumab plus adjuvant chemotherapy for operable HER2-positive breast cancer. *N Engl J Med.* 2005;353(16):1673–1684.

Seidman AD, Berry D, Cirrincione C, et al. Randomized phase III trial of weekly compared with every-3-weeks paclitaxel for metastatic breast cancer, with trastuzumab for all HER-2 overexpressors and random assignment to trastuzumab or not in HER-2 nonoverexpressors: final results of Cancer and Leukemia Group B protocol 9840. *J Clin Oncol.* 2008;26(10):1642–1649.

Slamon DJ, Leyland-Jones B, Shak S, et al. Use of chemotherapy plus a monoclonal antibody against HER2 for metastatic breast cancer that overexpresses HER2. *N Engl J Med.* 2001;344(11):783–792.

Sledge GW, Neuberg D, Bernado P, et al. Phase III trial of doxorubicin, paclitaxel, and the combination of doxorubicin and paclitaxel as front-line chemotherapy for metastatic breast cancer: an intergroup trial (E1193). *J Clin Oncol.* 2003;21(4):588–592.

Sørlie T, Perou CM, Tibshirani R, et al. Gene expression patterns of breast carcinomas distinguish tumor subclasses with clinical implications. *Proc Natl Acad Sci USA.* 2001;98(19):10869–10874.

Sparano JA, Wang M, Martino S, et al. Weekly paclitaxel in the adjuvant treatment of breast cancer. *N Engl J Med.* 2008;358(16):1663–1671.

Thomas ES, Gomez HL, Li RK, et al. Ixabepilone plus capecitabine for metastatic breast cancer progressing after anthracycline and taxane treatment. *J Clin Oncol.* 2007;25(33):5210–5217.

Veronesi U, Cascinelli N, Mariani L, et al. Twenty-year follow-up of a randomized study comparing breast-conserving surgery with radical mastectomy for early breast cancer. *N Engl J Med.* 2002;347(16):1227–1232.

Visvanathan K, Chlebowski RT, Hurley P, et al. American Society of Clinical Oncology clinical practice guideline update on the use of pharmacologic interventions including tamoxifen, raloxifene, and aromatase inhibition for breast cancer risk reduction. *J Clin Oncol.* 2009;27(19):3235–3258.

Vogel VG, Costantino JP, Wickerham DL, et al. Effects of tamoxifen vs raloxifene on the risk of developing invasive breast cancer and other disease outcomes: the NSABP study of tamoxifen and raloxifene (STAR) P-2 trial. *JAMA.* 2006;295(23): 2727–2741.

von Minckwitz G, Kümmel S, Vogel P, et al. Neoadjuvant vinorelbine-capecitabine versus docetaxel-doxorubicin-cyclophosphamide in early nonresponsive breast cancer: phase III randomized GeparTrio trial. *J Natl Cancer Inst.* 2008;100(8):542–551.

Whelan TJ, Pignol JP, Levine MN, et al. Long-term results of hypofractionated radiation therapy for breast cancer. *N Engl J Med.* 2010;362(6):513–520.

Winer EP, Hudis C, Burstein HJ, et al. American Society of Clinical Oncology technology assessment on the use of aromatase inhibitors as adjuvant therapy for postmenopausal women with hormone receptor-positive breast cancer: status report 2004. *J Clin Oncol.* 2005;23(3):619–629.

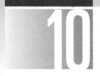

Gynecologic Cancer

Thomas McNally, Richard T. Penson, Chau Tran, and Michael J. Birrer

I. CERVICAL CANCER

In 2009, the American Cancer Society (ACS) reported an estimated 11,270 new cases of cervical cancer in the United States, with 4,070 deaths attributable to the disease. Historically a common disease, cervical cancer has become relatively rare in the developed world, thanks to successful screening with the Papanicolaou (Pap) test, which has allowed for early detection and therefore drastically reduced mortality rates. In developing countries, however, where access to effective and regular screening is not always available, the incidence of disease is much higher. As many as 300,000 women die globally each year as a result of cervical cancer.

The vast majority of cervical cancers are caused by human papillomavirus (HPV) infection. The development of an effective HPV vaccine has made the disease all the more preventable, and the mortality associated with cervical cancer in developed countries should decrease further in the coming decades. Still, global rates will remain high until both the vaccine and Pap test are readily and consistently available in both poor and developed countries.

A. Histology

Cervical cancer is classified as squamous cell carcinoma (keratinizing, nonkeratinizing, verrucous: 80% to 85%; endometrioid and adenocarcinoma,15%; and adenosquamous: 3% to 5%).

B. Screening

Early-stage disease is asymptomatic, and preinvasive lesions are found only after abnormal routine screening Pap smear of the ecto-/endocervix (transformation zone) junction. Cervical cancer mortality has decreased in the United States by over 70% since the Pap test was introduced in 1941.

Cervical cancer in the absence of demonstrable HPV infection is extremely rare, and HPV testing appears to be more sensitive and superior to standard Pap screening. Conventional cytology screening is reported to be 60% (30% to 87%) sensitive for dysplasia. Newer techniques using an ethanol medium (Sure-Path, BD Diagnostics, Franklin Lakes, NJ; Thin-Prep, Hologic, Bedford, MA; MonoPrep, MonoGen, Lincolnshire, IL) are as effective as conventional methods, are easier to read, and allow for sexually transmitted infection and HPV testing.

The Pap test is simple, safe, inexpensive, and well validated. Screening should start within 3 years of initiating sexual intercourse, or from age 21, and be repeated every 1 to 3 years. Approximately 3.5 million women have an abnormal Pap smear every year in the United States. The American Congress of Obstetricians and Gynecologists (ACOG) and ACS recommend that if a patient is exposed to diethylstilbestrol or is immunosuppressed (e.g., due to human immunodeficiency virus [HIV] infection), screening should be indefinite. HPV-negative women over the age of 30 years with normal Pap tests can decrease their screening interval to every 3 years and stop at the age of 70, at which point the risk of having significant dysplasia is about 1 in 1000.

The older terminology (mild, moderate, severe dysplasia) was replaced with cervical intraepithelial neoplasia I to III, based on the replacement of each third of the epithelium. This has since been replaced by the present system of "abnormal squamous cells of unknown significance" (ASCUS), which represents two-thirds of all abnormal Pap smears, and squamous intraepithelial lesions (SILs), which can be further classified as low-grade SIL or high-grade SIL.

An ASCUS Pap should trigger HPV testing. If positive, the patient should be referred for colposcopy. Women older than 40 years with normal endometrial cells on Pap smear require endometrial biopsy. There is a clear correlation between cytologic diagnosis and histologic diagnosis at colposcopy in approximately half of patients.

C. Clinical disease and staging

1. **Clinical presentation.** The most common symptoms of invasive cervical cancer are abnormal vaginal bleeding, either postcoital or intramenstrual, and vaginal discharge. Larger tumors may also interfere with urination and defecation, and may be accompanied by pelvic pain. Once the disease has metastasized to the regional lymph nodes, unilateral leg swelling, back pain, neuropathic pain, and postobstructive renal failure are also common symptoms. It should be noted that many women with cervical cancer do not present with any symptoms, but rather with disease detected during pelvic examination or screening procedures. The most common clinical sign of cervical cancer is an abnormal lesion on the cervix, usually detected by a physician during a pelvic exam. The exophytic lesion often presents as necrotic and friable. Involvement of surrounding tissues should be assessed, including the parametria, sidewalls, and uterosacral ligaments, as well as the superficial groin and femoral lymph nodes and the supraclavicular region. Infiltration of surrounding tissues is the most common reason to consider chemotherapy over surgery.

2. **Diagnosis.** Once an abnormal cervical lesion has been assessed by a physician, a tissue biopsy should be performed to either

confirm or rule out malignancy. The physician should make sure the biopsy is deep enough so as to include non-necrotic tissue, thus ensuring a diagnostically relevant sample.

3. **Prognostic factors.** Stage, histologic grade and type, tumor size, depth of stromal invasion, involvement of parametrium, and lymphovascular space invasion all influence prognosis. Pelvic lymph node metastasis significantly decreases the survival rate of patients.

4. **Staging (Table 10.1).** Cervical cancer is staged clinically and includes palpation, colposcopy, cystoscopy, endocervical curettage, proctoscopy, hysteroscopy, intravenous (IV) urography, and radiograph. Many centers also use magnetic resonance imaging (MRI) to define the local extent of disease and positron emission tomography (PET)/computed tomography (CT) to determine if there is any metastatic spread. Postoperatively, pathologic staging does not change clinical International Federation of Gynecology and Obstetrics (FIGO) staging.

	2009 FIGO Staging for Carcinoma of the Cervix Uteri

FIGO Stages

I	Cervical carcinoma confined to the uterus (extension to corpus should be disregarded)
IA	Invasive carcinoma diagnosed only by microscopy. All macroscopically visible lesions—even with superficial invasion—are stage IB.
IA1	Stromal invasion ≤3.0 mm in depth and extension ≤7.0 mm
IA2	Stromal invasion >3.0 mm but ≤5.0 mm in depth with extension ≤7.0 mm
IB	Clinically visible lesion confined to the cervix uteri or preclinical cancers greater than stage IA
IB1	Clinically visible lesion ≤4.0 cm in greatest dimension
IB2	Clinically visible lesion >4 cm in greatest dimension
II	Tumor invades beyond the uterus, but not to pelvic wall or lower third of the vagina
IIA	Without parametrial invasion
IIA1	Clinically visible lesion ≤4.0 cm in greatest dimension
IIA2	Clinically visible lesion >4 cm in greatest dimension
IIB	With obvious parametrial invasion
III	Tumor extends to pelvic wall and/or involves lower third of vagina and/or causes hydronephrosis or nonfunctioning kidney
IIIA	Tumor involves lower third of vagina with no extension to pelvic wall
IIIB	Tumor extends to pelvic wall and/or causes hydronephrosis or nonfunctioning kidney
IV	Carcinoma has extended beyond true pelvis or has involved (biopsy proven) the mucosa of the bladder or rectum. A bullous edema, as such, does not permit a case to be allotted stage IV.
IVA	Spread of growth to adjacent organs
IVB	Spread to distant organs

D. Treatment

Over the last century, management of cervical cancer has changed significantly: (1) more precancerous disease is managed through colposcopy, (2) there is now a preference for surgery over primary radiation, and (3) there is new evidence in the last 10 years that chemoradiation is significantly superior to radiation as primary or adjuvant therapy.

1. **Dysplasia and in situ carcinoma.** Options for treatment include conization (loop diathermy or cold knife), loop electrosurgical excision procedure, or hysterectomy. Lymphadenectomy is not required if stage IA-1 disease is demonstrated, as risk of metastases is very small (1%). If margins are positive, completion of hysterectomy or chemoradiation is needed. With negative margins, careful follow-up is adequate.

2. **Early-stage disease.** Early-stage disease can be treated with either chemoradiation or surgery, both of which have similar survival rates but different morbidity. Surgery may better preserve sexual function, although this has not been confirmed in well-controlled studies. Surgery should also be considered in premenopausal women where ovarian function can be preserved, in patients with an undiagnosed pelvic mass, in patients with more risk of bowel toxicity from radiotherapy (RT; adhesions because of pelvic inflammatory disease, endometriosis, inflammatory bowel disease, or in very thin women), or when compliance with the RT schedule may be difficult (with socially disadvantaged patients, for example).

   The only randomized controlled trial (RCT) to compare RT with surgery for treatment of stage IB cervical cancers reported equivalent survival (83%) and similar recurrence rates (surgery 25%; RT 26%). However, surgery was associated with more serious adverse events (28% versus 12%), and 64% of the surgical patients required postoperative radiation, likely associated with increased morbidity. An important goal is to identify patients who would likely need RT and then avoid surgery; most clinicians now use PET/CT scans to screen for metastatic disease and MRI to evaluate the extent of local disease. This allows patients with more advanced disease to be triaged and treated with primary chemotherapy.

   Morbidly obese patients are typically not considered for standard surgery because of high surgical risk, though robotically assisted surgery may prove safer. Age does not appear to be a significant contraindication to radical hysterectomy. Treatment should be appropriately tailored in unusual circumstances such as pregnancy or patients with HIV.

   Lymphadenectomy is a standard part of surgical management of any early-stage disease being treated with radical hysterectomy. Sentinel node biopsy is still investigational. Retrospective analysis of lymph-node debulking of palpable nodes prior to RT suggests a survival advantage in the prechemoradiation era, but is now more controversial and obsolete with modern imaging (MRI and PET/CT) and chemotherapy.

Adjuvant chemotherapy is necessary for women who have high-risk features after radical hysterectomy (positive lymph nodes, margins, or parametrium). A Southwest Oncology Group RCT in 243 women revealed that chemoradiation with cisplatin and 5-fluorouracil (5-FU) was significantly superior to RT alone (overall survival [OS] at 4 years of 81% with chemoradiation versus 71% with RT), though it had more toxicity.

If preservation of fertility is desired, vaginal radical trachelectomy (removal of only the cervix) with lymphadenectomy for small (less than 2 cm) tumors appears to be associated with an increased fertility (with up to 50% of patients becoming pregnant postradical trachelectomy) along with acceptable risk of recurrence in carefully selected patients. Tumor size is the single most important criterion in considering fertility-preserving surgery, but other criteria, including grade, canal involvement, lymphovascular space invasion, and MRI, are increasingly considered.

3. **Locally advanced disease (stage IIB–IVA).** In 1999, the National Cancer Institute (NCI) released a clinical alert about the large survival advantage in five NCI-sponsored clinical trials of the administration of concurrent chemotherapy with RT. A systematic review of 18 randomized trials revealed absolute benefit in progression-free survival (PFS) and OS of 16% (95% confidence interval 13 to 19) and 12% (8% to 16%), respectively, but with twice the gastrointestinal (GI) toxicity. Late toxicity is anticipated to be less with concurrent chemotherapy because of the total lower dose of RT.

Weekly cisplatin 40 mg/m^2 during RT has become the popular strategy because of its more favorable toxicity profile compared to cisplatin and 5-FU. There has not been a direct comparison of cisplatin versus cisplatin and 5-FU, though many extrapolate their equivalence from Gynecologic Oncology Group (GOG)-120, which compared RT with cisplatin versus the combination of cisplatin, 5-FU, and hydroxyurea versus hydroxyurea alone in 526 patients with stages IIB, III, IVA cancer. In both groups who received radiation and cisplatin, the 3-year survival rate was 65% compared to 47% for women receiving radiation and hydroxyurea.

Combining cisplatin with another agent improves response at the expense of considerably worse toxicity, but many clinicians suspect that two drugs are better than one. A provocative RCT presented at the 2009 meeting of the American Society of Clinical Oncology suggested a 32% improvement in OS for cisplatin 40 mg/m^2 and gemcitabine 124 mg/m^2 (both weekly for 6 weeks) over cisplatin alone 40 mg/m^2 weekly for 6 weeks as chemotherapy ($p = 0.0220$). Typically half of the operative specimens from bulky tumors contain residual carcinoma after chemoradiation, and an adjuvant extrafascial hysterectomy is typically recommended.

4. **Adenocarcinoma.** Adenocarcinoma is associated with a worse prognosis, with no clear data that a more aggressive approach results in a better outcome. Treatment is typically the same as that for squamous cell carcinomas.

5. **Neoadjuvant and adjuvant chemotherapy.** Primary chemotherapy (neoadjuvant) with combination platinum-based chemotherapy (cisplatin, vincristine, bleomycin) can have a very high response rate (90% in stage IB2) with consolidative adjuvant radiation. However, early positive results could not be confirmed and this approach has fallen out of favor.

6. **Palliative chemotherapy.** For recurrent tumors, the ultimate goals of treatment are palliative, and the most active single agents are cisplatin, ifosfamide, paclitaxel, vinorelbine, and topotecan with response rates of 15% to 23%. Response rates of tumors located within a radiation field are typically halved; in the chemotherapy era, palliative chemotherapy is less effective. Combination platinum-based therapy with ifosfamide, paclitaxel, or topotecan is associated with higher response rates for all three agents, but cisplatin 50 mg/m^2 on day 1 with topotecan 0.75 mg/m^2 on days 1 to 3 is the only combination associated with an OS advantage (9.4 months versus 6.5 months). Despite this, the standard of care is cisplatin 50 mg/m^2 on day 2 and paclitaxel 135 mg/m^2 on day 1 as a 3- or 24-hour infusion because of its better toxicity profile. Single-agent, nonplatinum combination or paclitaxel and carboplatin are reasonable options. A newer study (GOG-240) compares cisplatin and paclitaxel with topotecan and paclitaxel, with and without bevacizumab, because with cisplatin as the standard in chemotherapy, response rates to platinum combination regimens has fallen.

7. **Novel biologics.** There is a desperate need for more effective therapy for recurrent cervical cancer. Agents that target the vascular endothelial growth factor, epidermal growth factor, and HER2/neu receptors are currently in clinical trial and look promising.

8. **Palliative care.** Supportive care, which addresses physical, psychological, social, and spiritual issues, is an essential part of the holistic care of patients as they approach the end of their life. Common medical problems include pain, nausea and vomiting, lymphedema, obstruction (genitourinary and GI), and fistulae, and require multiprofessional care.

II. ENDOMETRIAL CANCER

Endometrial cancer is the most common gynecologic malignancy. The ACS estimates that there were 42,160 new cases in 2009 in the United States, with 7780 deaths attributable to the disease. The cancer typically presents at an early stage with vaginal bleeding in postmenopausal women. Because it usually presents while still confined to the uterus, it is often readily cured with surgery alone. Prior treatment with tamoxifen is a significant risk factor for developing endometrial cancer. As tamoxifen has been used in the prevention and treatment of all stages of breast cancer, a significant population of women has been exposed to this drug and is therefore at increased risk of developing endometrial cancer.

A. Histology

Endometrial cancer includes endometrial carcinomas (95%) and mesenchymal tumors (5%). Mesenchymal tumors are comprised of uterine sarcomas (leiomyosarcomas and endometrial stromal sarcoma) and mixed epithelial/stromal tumors (carcinosarcomas and adenosarcomas). Histologic subtypes of endometrial carcinomas include endometrioid (75% to 80%), serous (5% to 10%), clear cell (1% to 5%), and other rare carcinomas (less than 2%), such as mucinous, squamous cell, transitional cell, and small-cell cancers. Endometrial carcinomas are also designated as types I and II, with type I being an estrogen-driven, endometrioid tumor occurring in obese women, and type II referring to all other, more aggressive histologic subtypes.

B. Screening

Screening is not necessary for endometrial cancer as the disease typically presents early with postmenopausal vaginal (PMV) bleeding and has a good prognosis with effective treatment (surgery). Although screening patients by ultrasound for thickened endometrial stripe has been advocated for patients who are on tamoxifen and are at increased risk of endometrial cancer, there is no clear survival advantage over clinical surveillance for PMV bleeding. Therefore, the role of ultrasound is probably limited to surveillance of pre-existing benign lesions. By contrast, in patients at higher than average risk of endometrial cancer because of a family history of colorectal cancer (Lynch II syndrome), prophylactic hysterectomy and bilateral salpingo-oophorectomy (BSO) prevents all (100%) uterine cancers.

C. Clinical disease

1. **Clinical presentation.** The most common symptoms of invasive endometrial cancer are abnormal vaginal bleeding and discharge. Because such bleeding can be caused by disorders other than cancer, special attention should be paid to women with abnormal bleeding who are either postmenopausal or who are at high risk for endometrial cancer and are over the age

of 40 years. Metastatic intraperitoneal disease may also cause symptoms similar to ovarian cancer, including abdominal distension, pelvic pressure, and pelvic pain. On pelvic ultrasound, a thickened endometrium is a sign of possible endometrial cancer and should be followed up by a gynecologic oncologist.

2. **Diagnosis.** For a definitive diagnosis of endometrial cancer, a tissue biopsy must be performed, usually through an endometrial biopsy (EMB) or fractional dilation and curettage (D&C). Today, EMB is the preferred method of evaluating abnormal uterine bleeding. It should be noted that EMB has proven more effective in postmenopausal, rather than premenopausal, women and is better at confirming the presence of cancer rather than its absence. In cases where outpatient EMB is not possible, or if abnormal bleeding persists despite negative biopsy, fractional D&C should be performed. Tissue samples from either diagnostic method allow for pathologic evaluation of the endometrium, which can help determine the cause of the patient's symptoms, even if they are not the result of cancer.

3. **Prognostic factors.** The 5-year survival rate for endometrial cancer is 83%, and tumor-related prognostic factors at diagnosis include histologic subtype, stage, grade, depth of myometrial invasion, and lymphovascular space invasion. The prognosis of type I carcinomas is more favorable than that of type II because of their lower grade and sensitivity to hormone therapy.

   The presence of certain molecular abnormalities also contributes to poor prognosis. One such abnormality is the overexpression of the epidermal growth factor receptor (EGFR). In endometrioid adenocarcinomas, overexpression of EGFR decreases the overall 5-year survival rate from 89% to 69%; in serous and clear cell, the presence of EGFR overexpression decreases the survival rate from 86% to 27%.

4. **Staging (Table 10.2).** Endometrial cancer is surgically staged. As per FIGO recommendation, the surgery is done via an abdominal incision, followed by parametrial washings along with examination and palpation of omentum, liver, adnexal surfaces, peritoneal cul-de-sac, and enlarged aortic and pelvic nodes. Total abdominal hysterectomy (TAH) with BSO and complete lymphadenectomy are also standard in the United States. It should be noted, however, that the benefits of complete lymphadenectomy have been challenged with two negative randomized studies and are not standard in Europe. Further pathologic examination and frozen section assessment also contribute to accurate staging.

D. Treatment

1. **Surgery.** Surgery is most commonly all that is needed to cure endometrial cancer. Although ACOG recommends at least a

| 2009 FIGO Staging for Carcinoma of the Epithelium of the Corpus Uteri

FIGO Stages

I	Tumor confined to the corpus uteri
IA	No invasion of or invasion is less than half of myometrium
IB	Invasion equal to or more than half of myometrium
II	Tumor invades cervical stroma but does not extend beyond uterus (endocervical glandular involvement only is considered stage I)
III	Local and/or regional spread of tumor
IIIA	Tumor involves serosa of corpus and/or adnexa
IIIB	Vaginal and/or parametrial involvement
IIIC	Metastases to pelvic and/or para-aortic lymph nodes
IIIC-1	Positive pelvic nodes
IIIC-2	Positive para-aortic lymph nodes with or without positive pelvic lymph nodes
IV	Tumor invades bladder mucosa and/or bowel mucosa and/or distant metastases
IVA	Tumor invades bladder mucosa and/or bowel mucosa
IVB	Distant metastases, including intra-abdominal metastases and/or inguinal lymph nodes

TAH-BSO and node dissection, the role of nodal dissection is increasingly controversial. Laparoscopic surgery is associated with significantly shorter hospital stays and better quality of life. The use of robotically-assisted laparoscopic hysterectomy has increased dramatically, especially in the obese patient population, and has resulted in significantly lower perioperative complications (4% versus 21%, $p = 0.007$).

Debulking involved lymph node metastases (greater than 8 mm) may have an impact on prognosis, but lymphadenectomy for patients with stage I and II disease is not associated with a survival advantage in a recent RCT, and a growing consensus appears to support less aggressive surgical approaches in women with grade 1 or 2 endometrioid tumors with less than 50% myometrial invasion, less than 2 cm in tumor length, and no obvious other macroscopic disease.

Prophylactic TAH-BSO has been reported to prevent 100% of uterine cancers of women undergoing risk-reducing surgery for hereditary nonpolyposis colon cancer.

2. **RT.** Radiation is given adjuvantly to reduce the risk of local recurrence (brachytherapy to the vaginal vault postoperatively). External-beam RT (EBRT) is indicated for completely resected, node-positive disease (stage IIIC) and is also considered for higher risk patients (poor grade, or adverse histology, deep invasion, advanced age) with early-stage disease. However, this is increasingly controversial as there is no proven survival

advantage. RT in the form of brachytherapy is administered to the vaginal vault for high-risk tumors and tumors involving the lower uterine segment. More extensive RT (extended field) may be indicated in carefully selected patients with small volume residual disease, but the benefit has to be weighed against the risk of late complications.

Medically unfit patients with serious comorbidities can be treated with primary RT with good clinical benefit, and radiation is very good palliation of symptomatic metastases (brain or bone metastases, pelvic pain, or bleeding).

3. **Hormonal therapy.** Hormonal therapy is recommended only for patients with recurrent or inoperable tumor that is estrogen receptor (ER)/progesterone receptor (PR) positive. Adjuvant progestin therapy is not recommended because of excess cardiovascular mortality. Clinical responses to progestins (such as medroxyprogesterone acetate 80 mg twice a day) are consistently reported in approximately one-third of patients (15% to 34%), similar to other agents, such as tamoxifen, and probably no better than the highest reported response rate with tamoxifen alternating with a progestin. Aromatase inhibitors and gonadotropin-releasing hormone agonists are reasonable alternatives.

4. **Chemotherapy (Table 10.3).** The role of systemic therapy for endometrial cancer is changing and controversial. Adjuvant chemotherapy has been reported to increase 5-year survival rates (from 78% to 88%, hazard ratio [HR] 0.51, $p = 0.02$) in high-risk early-stage disease and is commonly recommended for deep penetrative, node-positive, poor-grade tumors. Although one

---

TABLE 10.3   Chemotherapy Regimens for Endometrial Cancer

1. **Doxorubicin and cisplatin:**
   Doxorubicin 60 mg/m^2 IV every 3 weeks
   Cisplatin 50 mg/m^2 IV every 3 weeks
2. **Megestrol acetate** 80 mg twice a day
3. **Topotecan** 1.2–1.5 mg/m^2/d IV on days 1–5 every 3 weeks
4. **TC:**
   Carboplatin AUC 6 IV on day 1
   Paclitaxel 175 mg/m^2 IV on day 1 every 4 weeks
5. **TAP:**
   Doxorubicin 45 mg/m^2 IV on day 1
   Cisplatin 50 mg/m^2 IV on day 1
   Paclitaxel 160 mg/m^2 IV on day 2

AUC, area under the curve; IV, intravenous; TAP, paclitaxel, doxorubicin, and cisplatin; TC, carboplatin and paclitaxel.

standard combination is paclitaxel, doxorubicin, and cisplatin, paclitaxel and carboplatin is the most popular choice because of a better toxicity profile. These are being compared in GOG-209.

Recurrent disease (especially ER/PR-negative disease) is often treated with further palliative chemotherapy such as weekly paclitaxel, liposomally encapsulated doxorubicin, topotecan, low-dose gemcitabine, and cisplatin. However, response rates are very low and benefit is rarely durable.

5. **Uterine papillary serous carcinoma.** All uterine papillary serous carcinomas, except those limited to a polyp, are typically treated with chemotherapy after initial surgery. Although they more commonly have HER2/neu overexpression or amplification, trastuzumab has no proven role.

6. **Novel biologics.** The role of mTOR, AKT inhibitors, and PI3 kinase inhibitors looks promising for endometrioid tumors, but remains investigational. One report suggests that with a 16% response rate, bevacizumab is worthy of further study.

7. **Multimodality therapy.** GOG-122 (doxorubicin-cisplatin versus whole-abdominal irradiation [WAI]) changed the landscape of endometrial cancer treatment with proof that chemotherapy improved survival compared to radiation alone for stage III and IV disease, with 50% compared to 38% of patients alive at 5 years (HR 0.68, $p < 0.01$). These patients need tailored multimodality therapy; however, the sequence and schedule are not optimally defined. Therapy most commonly consists of surgery, followed by chemotherapy and tailored RT. Paclitaxel, doxorubicin, and cisplatin (TAP) is thought to be more toxic than the more popular regimen of paclitaxel and carboplatin.

8. **Follow-up.** Surveillance requires a pelvic exam every 3 months in the first 2 years to detect a potentially curable local recurrence, and supportive care should address functional, psychological, social, and spiritual issues.

III. UTERINE SARCOMAS
A. Histology
Endometrial stromal sarcomas (ESSs) and undifferentiated endometrial sarcomas are rare forms of uterine sarcomas. ESSs, whose cells resemble endometrial stromal cells, are low-grade. Other uterine sarcomas include malignant mixed müllerian tumor (MMMT) and leiomyosarcomas.

B. Clinical disease
1. **Clinical presentation and diagnosis.** ESSs are a specific histologic subtype within the larger group of mesenchymal tumors of the uterine corpus. The most common symptom experienced by women with ESS is abnormal vaginal bleeding. ESS tumors

are almost always low-grade and on gross examination usually present as a single mass. They can occur in sites other than the uterus, including the ovary, fallopian tube, cervix, vagina, vulva, pelvis, abdomen, retroperitoneum, placenta, sciatic nerve, or round ligament. ESS can be mistaken for endometrial stromal nodules; two distinguishing characteristics are infiltrating margins with or without angioinvasion, both of which are found in sarcomas but are absent in nodules. A definitive diagnosis of ESS is not possible from endometrial curettage specimens alone, and a full hysterectomy is required.

Undifferentiated endometrial sarcomas are marked by extensive cytologic atypia to the point where they can no longer be recognized as arising from the endometrial stroma. Grossly, these tumors resemble undifferentiated mesenchymal tumors and mimic high-grade sarcomas in behavior.

2. **Prognostic factors.** Stage and grade for all three types are important when considering a patient's prognosis. ESS has a good prognosis, in part due to its low-grade characteristics, and most are cured surgically. However, low-grade ESS behaves aggressively if the following characteristics are present: high expression of androgen receptors or low expression of estrogen receptors. The relapse rate for ESS is 62%. Recurrence commonly includes pulmonary metastases and responds to hormonal therapy (progestins or aromatase inhibitors). MMMTs, which behave in a manner similar to high-grade sarcomas, are often fatal and have a relapse rate of 85%.

3. **Staging** is according to FIGO criteria.

C. **Treatment**

ESS is typically treated with surgery and possible hormonal therapy, including progestins or aromatase inhibitors. Leiomyosarcoma is treated with surgery, RT, and palliative chemotherapies. These include gemcitabine with docetaxel and occasionally hormonal therapy, as with ESS. MMMT is treated with surgery followed by multimodal therapies, including RT and chemotherapy. Chemotherapy includes carboplatin with paclitaxel or ifosfamide with cisplatin, although the latter combination is much more toxic. Chemotherapy (cisplatin-ifosfamide and mesna) may be superior to other regimens as postsurgical therapy in stage I to IV carcinosarcoma (MMMT) of the uterus (52% versus 58% [WAI], HR 0.789, $p = 0.245$).

IV. OVARIAN CANCER

Ovarian cancer is a relatively rare disease, with an incidence of about 1 in 70 women. In the United States, there were 21,550 new cases of ovarian cancer and 14,600 deaths attributable to the disease in 2009, according to the ACS. As early-stage ovarian cancer is rarely symptomatic, and due to the fact that there are no effective screening protocols, ovarian cancer patients typically present with advanced stage disease (stages II to IV). Although the tumors are very responsive to chemotherapy, thus enabling the majority of patients to live for years with their disease (overall 5-year survival rate is 45.6%), the patients are rarely cured. The cause of epithelial ovarian cancer remains unknown, but theories relate it to incessant ovulation or abnormalities in the fallopian tube fimbria.

A. Histology

Epithelial ovarian carcinomas are classified as serous (70%), endometrioid (20%), clear cell (<10%), and more rare types including Brenner and undifferentiated or mixed epithelial tumors. Seventy-five percent of papillary serous carcinomas of the ovary are diagnosed in the advanced stages, while only 40% of mucinous, endometrioid, and clear cell carcinomas are diagnosed in the advanced stages. Gene profiling studies suggest that treatment will be tailored to genotype or histology. However, these studies are only in the planning stages.

B. Screening

Screening for ovarian cancer would be an important benefit because most patients present with advanced, and therefore incurable, disease. Screening tests (ultrasound and cancer antigen [CA]-125) appear sensitive, but there are no data that suggest that screening improves survival. The challenges of developing an effective screening regimen are considerable: (1) there is no clear premalignant precursor, (2) serous carcinoma appears to develop rapidly, and (3) the morbidity from the diagnostic procedure (laparotomy) requires that the screening tests be very specific. The serum marker CA-125 is elevated in only 50% of patients with stage I disease, but is elevated in 90% of stage II to IV ovarian cancers. CA-125 testing typically has a specificity of 97% to 99%, but with a 1 in 70 lifetime risk of ovarian cancer, occult disease is present in only 1 of 2,300 postmenopausal women. As a result, a false positive rate of 1% to 3% is unacceptably high.

The largest CA-125 based screening study reported to date included 21,935 postmenopausal healthy women in the United Kingdom. In the study, a positive CA-125 test was followed by ultrasound, and the death rate was apparently halved by screening (18 of 10,977 versus 9 of 10,958, $p = 0.083$). The definitive UK Collaborative Trial of Ovarian Cancer Screening in 200,000 postmenopausal normal-risk women is expected to report by 2014. In contrast to previous studies, the CA-125 arm of the trial uses Risk of Ovarian Cancer Algorithm (ROCA), which examines previous CA-125 values from a screened subject to interpret her latest CA-125 test and decide whether to refer for ultrasound. In preliminary data, ROCA resulted in only 100 surgeries to find 41 cancers (positive predictive value [PPV] 41%) compared with 855 surgeries to find 44 cancers when using ultrasound alone (PPV 5%). The US study (Prostate, Lung, Colorectal, and Ovary Cancer Screening Trial) has enrolled 150,000 subjects: 75,000 women screened for lung, colorectal, and ovarian cancer, and 75,000 men screened for prostate, lung, and colorectal cancer. In the first analysis, 89 cancers were diagnosed, with 60 from screening (PPV 1% to 1.3%), and the surgery-to-cancer ratio was greater than 20:1 with 72% stage III or IV. There continues to be speculation about whether the sensitivity of screening can be improved by the use of other biomarkers. Screening with six monthly CA-125 and transvaginal ultrasound is recommended in high-risk populations (positive family history, BRCA-mutation carrier). However, risk-reducing salpingo-oophorectomy reduces the risk of subsequent cancer by 90% to 95% and is a safer strategy once a woman has finished bearing children.

C. Clinical disease

1. **Clinical presentation and diagnosis.** The most common symptoms experienced by women with ovarian cancer include persistent bloating, pelvic or abdominal pain, early satiety, and urinary urgency or frequency. While these symptoms are common and not specific to women with cancer, they have been found to be much more common and severe in women with an ovarian malignancy. Other symptoms reported include fatigue, indigestion, back pain, pain during intercourse, constipation, and menstrual irregularities, although these do not appear to be any more common in women with cancer. The most common clinical sign of ovarian cancer is an adnexal mass as found on a pelvic ultrasonography (ultrasound) or through manual palpation during a pelvic exam. Most masses do not prove malignant in premenopausal women. As such, a simple cyst less than 8 cm in diameter in a premenopausal woman can be followed up by the treating physician in 1 to 3 months. Adnexal masses in premenarchal or postmenopausal women, however, are much more concerning for malignancy, especially if they are large and complex. Physical features of an adnexal mass commonly associated with malignancy, as seen on a pelvic ultrasound, include irregular borders, multiple echogenic patterns due to presence of solid elements, multiple irregular septa, and bilateral tumors. A serum CA-125 level greater than 35 U/mL in nonpregnant women should also be cause for concern for ovarian cancer. Typically, a conclusive diagnosis is not possible until after surgery, followed by an assessment of the surgical specimen by a pathologist.

2. **Prognostic factors.** Prognostic factors for epithelial ovarian cancer include stage, volume of residual disease, grade, and histologic subtype. With respect to stage, the 5-year survival

is directly correlated. Stage I disease has a 90% 5-year survival, while stage II disease has an 80% 5-year survival. The percentage decreases dramatically for stage III (15% to 20% 5-year survival) and stage IV (less than 5% 5-year survival). Optimally cytoreduced patients (<1 cm) have a higher median survival than suboptimally cytoreduced patients.

Epithelial ovarian cancer subtypes have different overall patient survivals with respect to both histology and stage at diagnosis. Among early stage (I and II) ovarian carcinomas, patients with endometrioid and mucinous tumors have a 10-year survival rate of 85% and 79%, respectively, while those patients with clear cell and high-grade serous tumors have a 10-year survival rate of 70% and 57%, respectively. However, compared to endometrioid and serous tumors, clear cell and mucinous tumors have a dramatically poorer prognosis in late stage (III and IV) disease. The overall 10-year survival rate for all stages is 39%.

Low-grade and low malignant potential (LMP) cancers have better survival rates than high-grade cancers, but are more likely to be refractory for chemotherapy. The grade of the ovarian cancer affects the overall patient survival due to differences in the gene expression of proliferative markers. Late-stage high-grade tumors express high levels of genes involved in cell proliferation and metastasis, such as PDCD4, E2F3, MCM4, CDC20, and PCNA. LMPs and low-grade serous tumors exhibit low expression of proliferation markers such as CDC2, KIF11, TOP2A, CCNB1, and MKI67, as well as activation of wild-type p53.

3. **Staging (Table 10.4).** Staging for ovarian cancer occurs at surgery. Per FIGO, complete exploration of the abdomen and pelvis with resection of all gross disease as well TAH-BSO and pelvic and para-aortic lymphadenectomy are recommended. If desired, fertility-conserving surgery may be performed on patients with low-stage, low-grade lesions.

D. Treatment

1. **Cytoreductive surgery.** Ovarian cancer is one of the only cancers where resection of metastatic disease is a standard part of initial management. Laparotomy is often both the diagnostic procedure and initial therapeutic intervention, and the key to cure.

Griffiths was one of the first to pioneer the concept that successful surgical debulking to a residual tumor size of ≤1.5 cm (now 1 cm) maximum diameter results in superior survival. Surgical cytoreduction (debulking) has several purposes: (1) it removes some or all of the tumor, (2) it improves physiology (GI obstruction and protein loss to ascites), (3) it removes de novo chemotherapy-resistant clones, and (4) it facilitates drug delivery by removing tumor with a compromised blood supply. Patients are stratified into "optimally" (<1 cm residual disease)

TABLE 10.4	2000 FIGO Staging for Carcinoma of the Ovary

FIGO Stages

I	Tumor limited to the ovaries
IA	Tumor limited to one ovary; capsule intact, no tumor on ovarian surface; no malignant cells in ascites or peritoneal washings
IB	Tumor limited to both ovaries; capsule intact, no tumor on ovarian surface; no malignant cells in ascites or peritoneal washings
IC	Tumor limited to one or both ovaries with any of the following: capsule ruptured, tumor on ovarian surface, malignant cells in ascites or peritoneal washings
II	Tumor involves one or both ovaries with pelvic extension
IIA	Extension and/or implants on uterus and/or tube(s); no malignant cells in ascites or peritoneal washings
IIB	Extension to other pelvic tissues; no malignant cells in ascites or peritoneal washings
IIC	Extension to other pelvic tissues; with malignant cells in ascites or peritoneal washings
III	Tumor involves one or both ovaries with microscopically confirmed peritoneal metastasis outside the pelvis and/or regional lymph node metastasis
IIIA	Microscopic peritoneal metastasis beyond pelvis
IIIB	Macroscopic peritoneal metastasis beyond pelvis ≤2 cm in greatest dimension
IIIC	Peritoneal metastasis beyond pelvis ≥2 cm in greatest dimension and/or regional lymph node metastasis
IV	Distant metastasis (excluding peritoneal metastasis)

or "suboptimally" cytoreduced; it is the second most powerful predictor of outcome after stage.

Primary or "neoadjuvant" chemotherapy has gained popularity with preliminary data from European Organization for the Research and Treatment of Cancer (EORTC) 55971, an RCT of initial chemotherapy or initial surgery in a poorer prognosis group (median PFS 12 months and OS 30 months) of 718 women. There were equivalent outcomes, with a 2% mortality after upfront debulking surgery, suggesting that neoadjuvant chemotherapy may be safer in patients that have disease that is difficult to resect, significant comorbidities, or are older in age, and that it may also get more patients to have an optimal surgical procedure at some point in their clinical course.

Follow-up for patients should include a pelvic examination and CA-125, initially every 3 months, though early detection of recurrence does not appear to improve survival.

2. **Early-stage ovarian cancer.** Although only 15% of ovarian cancers present as early-stage disease, one-third to one-half of all cured patients are from this group. Formal staging is required

by a surgeon with subspecialty training with an exploratory laparotomy, TAH-BSO, omentectomy, complete examination of the peritoneal surfaces, multiple biopsies, peritoneal washings, and para-aortic and pelvic lymph node sampling. Patients diagnosed with apparently early-stage ovarian cancer without adequate staging should undergo a second exploratory surgery for definitive staging. Approximately one-quarter will be upstaged by positive nodes.

The 5-year survival of patients with stage I epithelial cancer is ≥90%. Patients with stage IA and IB disease of low-grade do not need adjuvant chemotherapy. All other patients require adjuvant platinum-based chemotherapy based on the joint International Collaboration in Ovarian Neoplasia (ICON I) and EORTC's ACTION study for an 8% improvement in OS.

GOG-157 compared three with six cycles of carboplatin and paclitaxel (TC) in early-stage disease. While more cycles were associated with more toxicity, there is also a significant superior survival outcome (in serous tumors), and most patients receive six cycles of chemotherapy if they can tolerate it.

3. **Advanced-stage ovarian cancer.** The principles of treatment for patients with advanced ovarian cancer are to (1) surgically cytoreduce, or debulk, tumor with surgery, followed by (2) chemotherapy (Table 10.5). A remission (normal CA-125 and CT scan) only translates into cure for a minority, but 5-year survival rates for patients treated with platinum-based regimens are >40%. Even after a complete response to first-line chemotherapy, only approximately half of patients with negative second-look operations are eventually cured.

4. **Platinum-based first-line chemotherapy.** Chemotherapy has improved through the last 40 years from single-agent alkylators (melphalan and cyclophosphamide) to anthracycline combinations and finally platinum- and taxane-based therapy. Cisplatin and carboplatin (less GI toxicity but more heme toxicity), nonclassic alkylators, were demonstrated to have a significant survival advantage, and meta-analysis of randomized trials before 1991 concluded that cisplatin combinations were superior to single-agent or noncisplatin therapy, and that cisplatin and carboplatin were equally effective. Paclitaxel inhibits microtubule depolymerization and demonstrated significant activity in patients with ovarian cancer refractory to platinum chemotherapy, once hypersensitivity reactions to the diluent ethoxylated castor oil in paclitaxel were overcome by dexamethasone premedication. GOG-111 reported a substantial survival advantage replacing cyclophosphamide with paclitaxel in 410 randomly assigned women with suboptimally debulked advanced ovarian cancer. Cisplatin 75 mg/m^2 and paclitaxel 135 mg/m^2 over 24 hours

TABLE 10.5   Chemotherapy Regimens for Ovarian Cancer

First-line Therapy:

1. **Paclitaxel and carboplatin:**
   Carboplatin AUC 5–7.5 IV on day 1
   Paclitaxel 175 mg/m^2 IV over 3 hours on day 1 every 3 weeks for six cycles.

2. **Paclitaxel and cisplatin:**
   Paclitaxel 135 mg/m^2 IV over 24 hours on day 1
   Carboplatin 75–100 mg/m^2 in normal saline IP on day 2
   Paclitaxel 60 mg/m^2 in normal saline IP on day 8 every 3 weeks for six cycles.

3. **Dose-dense paclitaxel and carboplatin:**
   Cisplatin AUC 6 IV on day 1
   Paclitaxel 80 mg/m^2 IV over 1 hour on days 1, 8, and 15 every 3 weeks for six cycles.

Platinum-sensitive Therapy:

1. **Paclitaxel and carboplatin:**
   Carboplatin AUC 5–7.5 IV on day 1
   Paclitaxel 175 mg/m^2 IV over 3 hours on day 1 every 3 weeks for six cycles.

2. **Gemcitabine carboplatin:**
   Gemcitabine 1000 mg/m^2 IV over 30 minutes on days 1 and 8
   Carboplatin AUC 4 IV on day 1 every 3 weeks for six cycles.

3. **PLD and carboplatin:**
   PLD 30 mg/m^2 on day 1
   Carboplatin AUC 5 IV on day 1 every 3 weeks for six cycles.

Platinum-resistant Therapy:

1. **PLD** 40 mg/m^2 IV over 1 hour every 4 weeks

2. **Paclitaxel** 80 mg/m^2 over 1 hour weekly (FDA-approved regimen is every 21 days)

3. **Bevacizumab** 15 mg/kg IV every 3 weeks (NCCN preferred drug—not FDA-approved)

4. **Topotecan**
   Regimen 1 (every 21 days): 1–1.5 mg/m^2/d IV over 30 minutes on days 1–5 (often 1.25 mg/m^2 on days 1–4) every 3 weeks
   Regimen 2: 3.75–4 mg/m^2 IV over 30 minutes on days 1, 8, and 15 every 4 weeks.

5. **Gemcitabine** 800–1000 mg/m^2 IV on days 1 and 8 every 3 weeks for six cycles

6. **Etoposide** 50 mg PO twice a day on days 1–10 or 14 every 21 days (related to WCC tolerance).

AUC, area under the curve; FDA, U.S. Food and Drug Administration; IP, intraperitoneal; IV, intravenously; NCCN, National Comprehensive Cancer Network; PLD, pegylated liposomally encapsulated doxorubicin; PO, by mouth; WCC, white cell count.

was associated with more alopecia, neutropenia, fever, and allergic reactions, but improved median OS from 24 to 38 months (p <0.001). Standard of care was defined in GOG-158, which compared cisplatin and paclitaxel with TC. Six cycles of carboplatin area under the curve (AUC) 7.5 and paclitaxel 175 mg/m^2 over 3 hours was a convenient outpatient regimen that produced less GI, renal, and metabolic toxicity, and had a similar degree of peripheral neuropathy with a median OS of 57 months.

5. **Promising strategies.** A number of different strategies have been pursued to try and improve survival outcomes, but moderate increases in platinum dose or density, alternate cytotoxics that are active in recurrent disease (such as gemcitabine, pegylated liposomally-encapsulated doxorubicin [PLD], and topotecan-based triplets), have not impacted survival.

Four strategies appear promising but await confirmatory studies: (1) intraperitoneal administration, (2) the addition of bevacizumab, (3) maintenance therapy, and (4) dose-dense paclitaxel. A better appreciation of the biologic mechanisms underpinning the behavior of ovarian cancer is anticipated to herald the rational integration of novel targeted therapeutics, personalized to particular subsets of cancer genotype [such as BRCA-defective serous tumors, poly-(ADP-ribose) polymerase [PARP] inhibitors, or BRAF overexpressing low-grade tumors].

6. **Intraperitoneal chemotherapy.** Delivering regional chemotherapy with the highest possible concentration of drug at the tumor appears rational. Ovarian cancer invites intraperitoneal (IP) infusion with a high ratio of IP to systemic drug concentration (cisplatin $10\times$, paclitaxel $1000\times$). Three randomized studies have suggested a substantial survival advantage. However, unacceptable toxicity has been a barrier to utilization of IP which is not considered standard therapy.

GOG-104 was a randomized trial of IV cyclophosphamide with either IP or IV cisplatin and associated with an 8-month median survival advantage. GOG-114 included IV paclitaxel with IP cisplatin and two initial cycles of moderate dose carboplatin and an 11-month survival advantage. The third study (GOG-172) led to an NCI alert about the potential advantage of IP therapy in patients with optimally debulked ovarian cancer because of an unprecedented 16-month survival advantage. The Armstrong regimen of paclitaxel 135 mg/m^2 over a 24-hour period (to reduce neurotoxicity) followed by IP cisplatin 100 mg/m^2 on day 2 with IP paclitaxel 60 mg/m^2 on day 8 given every 3 weeks for six cycles was associated with more fatigue and hematologic, GI, metabolic, and neurologic toxicity, with significantly worse quality of life, but an improvement in median duration of OS from 50 to 66 months ($p = 0.03$).

The GOG recommends trying to put the IP catheter in at the time of original laparotomy if possible, but if a bowel resection is required, a first cycle of IV chemotherapy followed by a laparoscopically placed IP catheter may reduce complications. BardPort (Bard Access System, Salt Lake City, UT) silicone peritoneal catheter 14.3 Fr with no Dacron cuff (U.S. Food and Drug Administration [FDA]-approved for use in IP therapy) and silicone 9.6 Fr single-lumen IV access devices are most commonly used.

Concerns remain that IP chemotherapy may not reach subperitoneal disease, lymph nodes, or areas walled off by adhesions. However, the biggest concerns are about catheter complications (infection, pain, and blockage), which are serious in a quarter of patients and prevented 58% of patients from completing IP therapy in GOG-172. Technical challenges remain a barrier to its use in some settings, and a further study (GOG-252) will explore IP carboplatin, dose-dense paclitaxel, and the role of bevacizumab.

7. **Bevacizumab.** GOG-218 investigated the integration of bevacizumab in the upfront treatment of advanced ovarian cancer with TC. A preliminary report suggested that maintenance, not just concurrent bevacizumab, is associated with a statistically significant PFS advantage. Bevacizumab is a particularly promising agent as the response rate is highest in ovarian cancer compared with any other solid tumor. Toxicities in patients with recurrent disease have included hypertension, proteinuria, and arterial thromboses. One study was halted with 5 of 44 patients developing bowel perforations, two of which proved fatal.

8. **Maintenance therapy.** In patients with suboptimally debulked disease, who are destined to have relapse, maintenance therapy is a rational strategy. GOG-178 compared 1 year of single-agent paclitaxel with only 3 months, and it appeared to delay the time to recurrence by an additional 7 months. Though it is not a standard of care, it provoked GOG-212, which investigates a potentially less neurotoxic agent, polyglutamated paclitaxel (Xyotax).

9. **Dose-dense (weekly) paclitaxel.** Weekly paclitaxel in the recurrent setting is associated with more peripheral neuropathy but less overall toxicity, both hematologic and nonhematologic, and has become a popular option. A recent RCT of AUC 6 carboplatin with either paclitaxel 180 mg/m^2 every 21 days or 80 mg/m^2 every 7 days (dose-dense paclitaxel [Taxol] and carboplatin [dd-TC]) in 631 Japanese patients reported better median PFS (28 months versus 17 months), and OS at 2 years (84% versus 78%, $p = 0.05$). Grade 3 and 4 anemia was reported more frequently in the dd-TC group, and other toxicities were similar in both groups. This strategy is being tested in GOG-262.

10. **PARP inhibition.** Possibly the most promising area of investigation is the inhibition of PARP. PARP adds nicotinamide adenine dinucleotide polymers to histones and other nuclear proteins, thereby improving cell survival after DNA damage. If this system is inhibited, PARP-1 activation cannot lead to DNA repair through the base excision repair pathway. If there is no other repair system, such as when a patient carries a BRCA-1 or -2 mutation, or has functional impairment in the repair pathways,

which has been reported in up to nearly half of serous ovarian tumors (synthetic lethality), apoptosis results. The oral agent olaparib (AZD-2281) is well tolerated with responses in a third of heavily pretreated patients with BRCA mutations, and the IV PARP inhibitor BSI-201 (iniparib) has improved response rates, PFS, and OS in triple negative breast cancer, which has a similar genotype. Other agents such as ABT-888 (veliparib) are in development.

11. **Docetaxel and carboplatin.** The SCOTROC study demonstrated that docetaxel was significantly less neurotoxic than paclitaxel and equally effective in combination with carboplatin, and is a valid but less used alternate to paclitaxel.

12. **Recurrent disease.** Most patients develop recurrent disease, initially with subsequent remission, then continual treatment, and finally palliation, most commonly of bowel obstruction. Ovarian cancer is sometimes considered a chronic disease, as treatment with palliative chemotherapy allows patients to live for years with their disease and with good quality of life.

 Recurrent ovarian cancer is triaged by the predictive factor, platinum-free interval, and divided into potentially platinum sensitive (more than 6 months since prior platinum) with a median survival measured in years and platinum-resistant disease with survival measured in months.

 The definition of relapse is important as a rising CA-125 typically has a lead time of 2 to 6 months before symptoms develop. Patients with an asymptomatic rising marker can be managed expectantly, as palliative chemotherapy has toxicities and OV05/55955 clearly demonstrated that treating women with an asymptomatic rising CA-125 adversely affected quality of life and did not impact survival. The study was designed to detect a 10% improvement in 2-year OS and randomized 1,442 patients to (1) immediate chemotherapy if CA-125 levels rose to greater than twice the upper limit of normal (a median of 5 months earlier), or (2) patient and clinician were blinded to the CA-125, and then got treatment at symptomatic progression of disease.

13. **Platinum-sensitive disease.** Rechallenge with a platinum combination is appropriate with a platinum-free interval of at least 6 months and standard combinations include (1) paclitaxel and carboplatin, (2) gemcitabine and carboplatin, and (3) PLD and carboplatin.

 ICON 4 demonstrated an absolute improvement in the 1-year PFS of 10% and 18% reduction in risk of death ($p = 0.02$) for paclitaxel and carboplatin over conventional platinum-based chemotherapy. The AGO (German) study led to the FDA approval of the combination for platinum-sensitive recurrent ovarian cancer with a 28% improvement in PFS for carboplatin and gemcitabine over carboplatin ($p = 0.0031$). Lastly, CALYPSO, reported only in abstract form, suggests that PLD carboplatin may be associated with a significant superior PFS (11.3 months versus 9.4 months, $p = 0.005$), and less alopecia and neurotoxicity.

14. **Platinum-resistant disease**. When disease becomes resistant to platinum, the goals are maximum time without symptoms from cancer or toxicity from treatment. Chemotherapy is chosen as much on the convenience and side effect profile as potency, and response rates are consistently poor (15% to 20%). Continual, sequential, single-agent palliative chemotherapy has been the mainstay of treatment for recurrent disease. CA-125 may better predict response to treatment and outcome than CT scans. PLD, topotecan, a different taxane schedule (e.g., a weekly paclitaxel), rechallenge with platinum, gemcitabine, altretamine, pemetrexed, or oral etoposide are all reasonable options. Hormonal therapy, often tamoxifen, can be effective in ER-positive tumors. The role of surgery is controversial. Many patients are appropriate for clinical trials, and an exciting number of agents are being investigated.

15. **Palliative care**. Obstructive symptoms typically herald the last months of patients' lives and require intense and multiprofessional care. Surgery should be limited to patients with chemotherapy-responsive disease, and for others a gastric venting tube alleviates vomiting. Total parenteral nutrition does not substantially alter the clinical course, and attending to end-of-life issues is an essential part of compassionate care.

V. VULVAR CANCER

Vulvar cancer is rare, representing 4% of all gynecologic malignancies and 0.6% of all cancers in women. The ACS estimates that 3,580 women were diagnosed with vulvar cancer in 2009, with 900 deaths attributable to the disease. Older women are at increased risk, with less than 20% of cases occurring in women under the age of 50, and roughly half occurring in women 70 years and older. Vulvar cancer in younger women tends to be associated with HPV infection. The disease usually presents with symptoms at an early stage, making it a highly treatable disease. However, due to its very personal nature, as well as its relative rarity, symptoms may often go unaddressed for some time, allowing the disease to progress beyond the early stages.

A. Histology

Carcinoma of the vulva is classified as squamous (80% to 90%), melanoma (9%), and Bartholin gland cancer and sarcomas (1% to 11%).

B. Screening

There are no routine screening protocols for the detection of vulvar cancer, and clinical presentation is the earliest detection point for the disease. However, patients should be encouraged to be vigilant about their genital health, and clinicians should be proactive in examining and performing biopsies on vulvar abnormalities.

C. Clinical disease

1. Clinical presentation and diagnosis. The majority of women who present with early-stage vulvar cancer have a recognizable lesion on the vulva, along with local symptoms, including soreness and itching. The treating clinician should proceed directly to tissue biopsy in order to avoid delay in diagnosis. The biopsy should include both the cutaneous lesion in question and the underlying stroma in order to determine the depth of invasion, if any. If left untreated for a long period of time, advanced-stage disease may result, and the patient will often present with local pain, bleeding, and surface drainage. Advanced disease can also metastasize to the regional lymph nodes and eventually more distant tissues.

2. Prognostic factors. Age of patient, clinical stage, nuclear grade, depth of tumor invasion, and presence of lymph node metastasis are significant prognostic parameters, with depth of tumor invasion being an independent factor. Patients with metastasis to the inguinal lymph nodes will experience recurrences within 2 years of first-line therapy, and the long-term survival is reduced by 50%. In addition, the overexpression of p53 has been linked to tumor aggressiveness.

3. Staging (Table 10.6). The method of staging vulva cancer is surgery with histologic findings.

D. Treatment

1. Early-stage disease. Vulvar cancer is surgically staged. Early-stage tumors (microinvasive, stage I and II) are treated with surgical approaches. Microinvasive tumors can usually be successfully treated with local resection, but multifocal disease remains a problem. All patients should be carefully followed.

a. Stage IA. Stage I disease is subdivided based on depth of stromal invasion. For stage IA lesions, invading less than 1 mm into the stroma, the treatment of choice is radical local excision without lymph node dissection, as the risk of nodal invasion for these lesions is less than 1%.

b. Stage IB. Stage IB lesions have ≥1 mm stromal invasion. As the risk of inguinofemoral node involvement is ≥8%, it is recommended that patients undergo inguinofemoral lymph node dissection. Whether patients need a unilateral or bilateral lymph node dissection (for midline lesions) depends on the location of the lesion.

c. Stage II. Surgical resection of stage II lesions needs to procure a ≥1 cm circumferential tumor-free margin around the primary lesion. In order to achieve this goal, the excision may

TABLE 10.6	2009 FIGO Staging for Carcinoma of the Vulva

FIGO Stages

	Primary tumor cannot be assessed
	No evidence of primary tumor
0	Carcinoma in situ (preinvasive carcinoma)
I	Tumor confined to vulva or vulva and perineum, with negative nodes
IA	Lesions ≤2 cm in greatest dimension and with stromal invasion ≤1.0 mm
IB	Lesions ≤2 cm in greatest dimension and with stromal invasion >1.0 mm
II	Tumor of any size with extension to adjacent perineal structures (one-third lower urethra, one-third lower vagina, anus), with negative nodes
III	Tumor of any size with or without extension to adjacent perineal structures (one-third lower urethra, one-third lower vagina, anus), with positive inguinofemoral lymph nodes
IIIA	With one lymph node metastasis (≥5 mm), or one to two lymph node metastasis(es) (<5 mm)
IIIB	With two or more lymph node metastases (≥5 mm), or three or more lymph node metastases (<5 mm)
IIIB	With positive nodes with extracapsular spread
IV	Tumor invades other regional (two-thirds upper urethra, two-thirds upper vagina) or distant structures
IVA	Tumor invades any of the following: (i) upper urethral and/or vaginal mucosa, bladder mucosa, rectal mucosa, or fixed to pelvic bone (ii) fixed or ulcerated inguinofemoral lymph nodes
IVB	Any distant metastasis including pelvic lymph nodes

involve a radical local excision, a partial radical vulvectomy, an excision using a three-incision technique, or the involvement of plastic surgery and skin flaps.

In general, given the long-term side effects and morbidity of RT, this treatment modality is avoided in the management of early-stage disease. For patients whose tumors have a positive margin, following initial surgical excision, the recommendation is for surgical re-excision unless this is anatomically not feasible or the patient is not an appropriate surgical candidate for re-excision. Re-excision is favored over RT given the toxicity associated with RT.

RT is usually recommended for patients with two or more microscopically positive groin nodes, one or more macroscopically positive lymph nodes, evidence of extracapsular nodal involvement, or in some aggressive cases where only a small number of lymph nodes were retrieved.

2. **Advanced-stage disease**
   a. **Stage III and IV.** In general, the treatment of advanced-stage disease is individualized. Although many of these lesions can be

resected surgically, this treatment modality may significantly impair quality of life. For example, for tumors involving the urethra, anus, bladder, or pelvic bone, surgical resection would require removing vital structures or pelvic exenteration with creation of a urinary conduit and colostomy. Given the morbidity of this surgical procedure, for these patients, the favored treatment modality is chemo-RT. In these cases, chemo-RT can be given preoperatively in order to reduce tumor volume and allow for a less radical surgical resection. For tumors that completely respond to chemo-RT, surgical resection can be omitted. In general, these patients are treated with RT and concurrent cisplatin and 5-FU chemotherapy as radiation sensitizers.

b. **Palliative chemotherapy.** In patients with advanced-stage disease, those too medically infirm for surgery, or those with inoperable disease, palliative chemotherapy may be appropriate as treatment when curative intent is not feasible. Therapeutic options are limited and agents active in other squamous cancers, such as cisplatin, 5-FU, doxorubicin, methotrexate, mitomycin C, bleomycin, cisplatin, and paclitaxel, are associated with low response rates in vulvar cancer. Novel targeted therapies with promise in the treatment of vulvar cancer include anti-EGFR tyrosine kinase inhibitors (TKIs) such as erlotinib and monoclonal antibodies such as cetuximab, either as single-agent therapy or in combination with chemotherapeutic drugs such as cisplatin.

VI. OVARIAN GERM CELL TUMORS

Germ cell tumors represent a rare subset of ovarian cancer. They usually present in a younger age group (median age 30 years) compared with epithelial ovarian cancers. The etiology of these tumors remains unknown. They are highly chemosensitive, and as such, are usually highly curable.

A. Histology

Germ cell tumors account for 2% to 3% of ovarian cases and are comprised of the following subtypes: dysgerminoma, yolk sac tumor, embryonal carcinoma, polyembryoma, nongestational choriocarcinoma, mixed germ cell tumor, and teratoma. The majority of patients (50% to 75%) are diagnosed in the early stages (I and II).

B. Screening

Because these tumors are so rare, there is currently no screening strategy. However, diagnosis should be considered preoperatively in the young, and markers should be drawn so that treatment can be planned accordingly (especially for fertility-sparing surgery).

C. Clinical disease

1. **Clinical presentation and diagnosis.** Malignant ovarian germ cell tumors usually occur in women much younger than with

epithelial ovarian cancer, with a median age between 16 and 20 years, depending on the specific histologic type. Common signs and symptoms of the disease include a pelvic mass, usually detected during a pelvic exam, and abdominal pain, often resulting from ovarian rupture, hemorrhage, or torsion. Other symptoms include abdominal distension, fever, and vaginal bleeding, although these are less common. Many germ cell tumors will produce biologic markers, which are useful in the diagnosis and observation of the disease. The two most common are human chorionic gonadotropin (hCG) and α-fetoprotein (AFP). Elevated AFP suggests a teratoma rather than dysgerminoma, the most common histologic subtype. As with epithelial ovarian cancer, CA-125 may also be elevated in patients with germ cell tumors.

2. **Prognostic factors.** Patients diagnosed with germ cell tumors have a relatively good prognosis due to sensitivity to chemotherapy. A combination of complete resection of tumors, proper surgical staging, and effective therapy ensures a high survival rate. Long-term survivorship can be achieved even without complete tumor resection or with advanced tumors at presentation.

3. **Staging.** Per FIGO recommendation, staging follows the same principles as for epithelial ovarian tumors (see Table 10.4).

D. **Treatment**

Surgery is the first step in managing malignant ovarian germ cell tumors. Because the patient population is fairly young, it is not unreasonable to attempt fertility-sparing surgery while attempting to optimally resect the tumor bulk. If only one ovary is involved, then a unilateral salpingo-oophorectomy is performed while the contralateral ovary and uterus is preserved. For management of stages II to IV, dysgerminoma is more commonly bilateral and at least a biopsy is required from the contralateral ovary. However, as chemotherapy is so effective, BSO is often not required. Debulking of advanced disease, however, is important. Second-look surgery may be advantageous for patients whose primary tumor was incompletely resected and contained a teratoma.

Most patients are candidates for platinum-based chemotherapy following surgery, except patients whose tumor was stage IA dysgerminoma or immature, grade I teratoma, in which surveillance is appropriate. Three courses of bleomycin 30 units weekly IV, etoposide 100 mg/m^2 on days 1 to 5, and cisplatin, 20 mg/m^2 on days 1 to 5 (BEP) is the standard treatment for completely resected disease; four courses of BEP are necessary for residual disease. In the recurrent setting, patients are initially treated with one cycle of standard vinblastine, ifosfamide, and cisplatin (see Chapter 11, Section III.E) followed by two cycles of high-dose carboplatin and etoposide. Alternate agents include taxanes, gemcitabine, and ifosfamide.

VII. STROMAL OR GRANULOSA CELL TUMORS

Stromal or granulosa cell tumors (GCTs) are very rare, hormone-secreting tumors that can cause precocious puberty in young girls.

A. Histology

GCTs account for 70% of malignant sex-cord stromal tumors but only 5% of malignant ovarian tumors. GCTs are comprised of adult-type (AGCT; 95%) and juvenile-type (JGCT; 5%).

B. Clinical disease

1. **Clinical presentation.** The most common symptoms of AGCT are abnormal vaginal bleeding, abdominal distension, and abdominal pain. The pain and distension are due to the usually large size of the tumor at diagnosis. Some patients may have ascites, and premenopausal women may experience menometrorrhagia, oligomenorrhea, or amenorrhea. Because GCTs are estrogen-secreting, breast tenderness, uterine myohypertrophy, and endometrial hyperplasia are also common signs and symptoms. In JGCT, prepubertal patients commonly present with isosexual precocious pseudopuberty. Patients will also almost always present with increasing abdominal girth, and a palpable mass will be found during abdominal, pelvic, or rectal exam. Finally, abdominal pain, dysuria, and constipation are common.

2. **Prognostic factors.** Stage at diagnosis, increasing tumor size, rupture and nuclear grade in stage I patients, nuclear atypia, and increased mitotic activity all contribute to poorer prognosis for patients with AGCTs. For JGCTs, however, surgical stage and mitotic activity are the most significant prognostic factors.

3. **Staging.** Per FIGO recommendation, the staging system used for GCTs is the same as that used for epithelial ovarian cancer.

C. Treatment

Standard treatment for GCTs includes hysterectomy with BSO followed by platinum-based chemotherapy along the lines derived from experience with epithelial ovarian tumors. Chemotherapy for GCTs also frequently includes taxanes. Some studies have shown that a conservative surgical approach without hysterectomy may be appropriate for some patients with JGCT. Studies of the use of TKIs, including imatinib, have shown some promise in treating GCTs. Further research, however, is required.

VIII. GESTATIONAL TROPHOBLASTIC NEOPLASM (GTN)

A. Histology

The histologic patterns of GTNs depend on the state of the preceding pregnancy. After molar pregnancy, GTN presents with the histologic pattern of either molar tissue or choriocarcinoma (CCA). Following a miscarriage or term pregnancy, GTN presents with the histologic pattern of CCA. Following ectopic pregnancy, the histologic pattern is either of molar tissue or CCA. Placental-site trophoblastic tumor is a rare form of CCA.

B. Screening

Following either a partial or complete molar pregnancy, patients should have weekly hCG serum level measurements until they are normal for 3 weeks, followed by monthly hCG screening for 6 months. If nondetectable hCG levels are reached, the risk of developing GTN approaches zero.

C. Clinical disease

1. Clinical presentation. The signs and symptoms for GTNs vary depending on the extent of disease. Locally invasive disease usually presents with IP bleeding or vaginal hemorrhage resulting from the tumor perforating the myometrium or uterine blood vessels. Metastatic disease is usually found in the lungs, vagina, brain, and liver, and is usually hemorrhagic, causing hemoptysis, IP bleeding, and acute neurologic deficits. GTN can cause various radiologic patterns in the lungs, including pleural effusion, alveolar or snowstorm pattern, discrete rounded densities, or embolic pattern. Vaginal lesions may also be present and are highly hemorrhagic; biopsy of these lesions should be completely avoided. Patients with cerebral metastases have a high rate of fatal hemorrhage during the first week of treatment and may need RT first (standard in United States) or low-dose chemotherapy to "cool off" (standard in the United Kingdom). Finally, patients with liver metastases usually present with jaundice, intra-abdominal pain, or epigastric pain.

2. Diagnosis. During diagnostic workup, all patients should have a base-line hCG taken and hepatic, thyroid, and renal function tests. If chest radiography is negative for metastatic disease, a chest CT scan should also be performed. It is unlikely that asymptomatic patients with normal pelvic exam and negative chest CT scan would have brain or liver metastasis. However, if vaginal or lung metastases are present, a head or abdominal CT should be obtained to rule out brain or liver metastases.

3. Prognostic factors. Site of involvement, tumor volume (hCG level, size and number of metastases), prior chemotherapy, and duration of disease all contribute to poor prognosis. Delayed diagnosis, high levels of hCG, and brain or liver metastases could lead to resistance to single-agent chemotherapy. The development of choriocarcinoma following term pregnancy also has poor prognosis.

4. Staging (Table 10.7). Per FIGO recommendation, an anatomic staging system is used in the case of GTN.

D. Treatment

1. Stage I or low-risk metastatic GTN. For patients with early-stage or low-risk GTN, the choice of treatment plan is based on whether the patient desires to preserve fertility. If the ability to conceive is no longer a concern, management should include hysterectomy with single-agent adjuvant chemotherapy. The chemotherapy is necessary as a precaution against tumor

FIGO Anatomic Staging for Gestational Trophoblastic Neoplasia

FIGO Stages

I	Disease confined to the uterus
II	GTN extends outside of the uterus, but is limited to the genital structures (adnexa, vagina, broad ligament)
III	GTN extends to the lungs, with or without known genital tract involvement
IV	All other metastatic sites

GTN, gestational trophoblastic neoplasm.

cells spread to locations outside the primary site and to treat occult metastases. If the patient wishes to preserve fertility, single-agent chemotherapy should be administered with methotrexate or actinomycin D (ACT-D). Both treatments are well tolerated, but patients on ACT-D do have a higher instance of side effects. These include nausea (61% versus 50%), emesis (33% versus 14%), and alopecia (26% versus 14%). Currently, the preferred regimen is methotrexate 100 mg/m^2 by IV bolus and 200 mg/m^2 by IV infusion over 12 hours, followed by folinic acid 15 mg intramuscularly or orally every 12 hours for four doses starting 24 hours after the start of methotrexate. If the patient is resistant to methotrexate, ACT-D should be used. If resistance to single-agent therapy develops, patients should be treated with combination therapy, including methotrexate, ACT-D, and cyclophosphamide or etoposide, methotrexate, ACT-D, cyclophosphamide, and vincristine (EMA-CO; Table 10.8).

TABLE 10.8　Multiagent Chemotherapy Regimens for Gestational Trophoblastic Disease

Regimen	Schedule and Doses	Regimen	Repeated
EMA-CO	Etoposide	100 mg/m^2 IV days 1–2	Every 2 wks
	Actinomycin	0.5 mg IV push days 1–2	
	Methotrexate	100 mg/m^2 IV push, then 200 mg/m^2 IV over 12h day 1	
	Leucovorin	15 mg IM or PO q 12 h × 24 h after MTX	
	Vincristine	1 mg/m^2 IV push day 8	
	Cyclophosphamide	600 mg/m^2 IV push day 8	
EMA-EP	Etoposide*	100 mg/m^2 IV push day 8	
	Cisplatin*	80 mg/m^2 IV day 8	

EMA-CO, etoposide, methotrexate, ACT-D, cyclophosphamide, and vincristine; EMA-EP, etoposide, methotrexate, actinomycin, and cisplatin.
*Same as EMA-CO, except substitute etoposide/cisplatin for vincristine/cyclophosphamide.

Patients with low-risk stage II and III disease can also be treated with single-agent chemotherapy, similar to stage I. If patients have high-risk stage II or III disease, they should be treated with EMA-CO. If resistance occurs, etoposide can be substituted with cisplatin on day 8, and the methotrexate dose can be elevated to $1 \ g/m^2$.

Patients with stage IV disease should be treated with rigorous combination chemotherapy (EMA-CO) and selective RT and surgery. If the patient has cerebral metastases, the dose of methotrexate should be increased to $1 \ g/m^2$ and RT should be applied.

After the first line of chemotherapy, additional treatment is withheld as long as the patient's hCG levels continue to fall. Patients with stage I, II, or III disease should be followed up after treatment with weekly hCG tests until levels reach normal for 3 consecutive weeks, then monthly for 12 months. Patients with stage IV disease should have weekly hCG tests until normal for 3 weeks, followed by monthly tests for 24 months. Risk of recurrence after initial remission varies by stage of disease: 2.9% for stage I disease, 8.3% for stage II, 4.2% for stage III, and 9.1% for stage IV.

Selected Readings

Cervical Cancer

Bergmark K, Avall-Lundqvist E, Dickman PW, Henningsohn L, Steineck G. Vaginal changes and sexuality in women with a history of cervical cancer. *N Engl J Med.* 1999;340:1383–1389.

Classe JM, Rauch P, Rodier JF, et al. Surgery after concurrent chemoradiotherapy and brachytherapy for the treatment of advanced cervical cancer: morbidity and outcome: results of a multicenter study of the GCCLCC (Groupe des Chirurgiens de Centre de Lutte Contre le Cancer). *Gynecol Oncol.* 2006;102:523–529.

Cosin JA, Fowler JM, Chen MD, Paley PJ, Carson LF, Twiggs LB. Pretreatment surgical staging of patients with cervical carcinoma: the case for lymph node debulking. *Cancer.* 1998;82:2241–2248.

Dueñas-González A, Zarba JJ, Alcedo JC, et al. A phase III study comparing concurrent gemcitabine (Gem) plus cisplatin (Cis) and radiation followed by adjuvant Gem plus Cis versus concurrent Cis and radiation in patients with stage IIB to IVA carcinoma of the cervix. *J Clin Oncol.* 2009;27:18s.

Green JA, Kirwan JM, Tierney JF, et al. Survival and recurrence after concomitant chemotherapy and radiotherapy for cancer of the uterine cervix: a systematic review and meta-analysis. *Lancet.* 2001;358:781–786.

Koliopoulos G, Sotiriadis A, Kyrgiou M, Martin-Hirsch P, Makrydimas G, Paraskevaidis E. Conservative surgical methods for FIGO stage IA2 squamous cervical carcinoma and their role in preserving women's fertility. *Gynecol Oncol.* 2004;93:469–473.

Landoni F, Maneo A, Colombo A, et al. Randomised study of radical surgery versus radiotherapy for stage Ib-IIa cervical cancer. *Lancet.* 1997;350:535–540.

Long HJ 3rd, Bundy BN, Grendys EC Jr, et al. Randomized phase III trial of cisplatin with or without topotecan in carcinoma of the uterine cervix: a Gynecologic Oncology Group Study. *J Clin Oncol.* 2005;23:4626–4633.

Mayrand MH, Duarte-Franco E, Rodrigues I, et al. Human papillomavirus DNA versus Papanicolaou screening tests for cervical cancer. *N Engl J Med.* 2007;357:1579–1588.

Moore DH, Blessing JA, McQuellon RP, et al. Phase III study of cisplatin with or without paclitaxel in stage IVB, recurrent, or persistent squamous cell carcinoma of the cervix: a gynecologic oncology group study. *J Clin Oncol.* 2004;22:3113–3119.

Peters WA 3rd, Liu PY, Barrett RJ 2nd, et al. Concurrent chemotherapy and pelvic radiation therapy compared with pelvic radiation therapy alone as adjuvant therapy after radical surgery in high-risk early-stage cancer of the cervix. *J Clin Oncol.* 2000;18:1606–1613.

Rose PG, Ali S, Watkins E, et al. Long-term follow-up of a randomized trial comparing concurrent single agent cisplatin, cisplatin-based combination chemotherapy, or hydroxyurea during pelvic irradiation for locally advanced cervical cancer: a gynecologic oncology group study. *J Clin Oncol.* 2007;25:2804–2810.

Rose PG, Bundy BN, Watkins EB, et al. Concurrent cisplatin-based radiotherapy and chemotherapy for locally advanced cervical cancer. *N Engl J Med.* 1999;340:1144–1153.

Sardi JE, Giaroli A, Sananes C, et al. Long-term follow-up of the first randomized trial using neoadjuvant chemotherapy in stage Ib squamous carcinoma of the cervix: the final results. *Gynecol Oncol.* 1997;67:61–69.

Sit AS, Kelley JL, Gallion HH, Kunschner AJ, Edwards RP. Paclitaxel and carboplatin for recurrent or persistent cancer of the cervix. *Cancer Invest.* 2004;22:368–373.

Smith AE, Sherman ME, Scott DR, et al. Review of the Bethesda system atlas does not improve reproducibility or accuracy in the classification of atypical squamous cells of undetermined significance smears. *Cancer.* 2000;90:201–206.

Thigpen T. The role of chemotherapy in the management of carcinoma of the cervix. *Cancer J.* 2003;9:425–432.

Wright TC Jr. Cervical cancer screening in the 21st century: is it time to retire the PAP smear? *Clin Obstet Gynecol.* 2007;50:313–323.

Ovarian Germ Cell Tumors

Gershenson DM, Morris M, Cangir A, et al. Treatment of malignant germ cell tumors of the ovary with bleomycin, etoposide and cisplatin. *J Clin Oncol.* 1990;8:715–720.

Pectasides D, Pectasides E, Kassanos D. Germ cell tumors of the ovary. *Cancer Treat Rev.* 2008;34:427–441.

Williams S, Blessings J, Liao SY, Ball H, Hanjani P. Adjuvant therapy of ovarian germ cell tumors with cisplatin, etoposide and bleomycin: a trial of the Gynecologic Oncology Group. *J Clin Oncol.* 1994;12:701–706.

Endometrial Cancer

Amant F, Moerman P, Neven P, Timmerman D, Van Limbergen E, Vergote I. Endometrial cancer. *Lancet.* 2005;366:491–505.

Benedet JL, Bender H, Jones H 3rd, Ngan HY, Pecorelli S. FIGO staging classifications and clinical practice guidelines in the management of gynecologic cancers. *Int J Gynaecol Obstet.* 2000;70:209–262.

Benedetti-Panici P, Maneschi F, Cutillo G, D'Andrea G, Manci N, Rabitti C. Anatomical and pathological study of retroperitoneal nodes in endometrial cancer. *Int J Gyncol Cancer.* 1998;8:1837–1842.

ASTEC/EN.5 Study Group, Blake P, Swart AM, et al. Adjuvant external beam radiotherapy in the treatment of endometrial cancer (MRC ASTEC and NCIC CTG EN.5 randomised trials): pooled trial results, systematic review, and meta-analysis. *Lancet.* 2009;373(9658):137–146.

Carey MS, Gawlik C, Fung-Kee-Fung M, et al. Systematic review of systemic therapy for advanced or recurrent endometrial cancer. *Gynecol Oncol.* 2006;101:158–167.

Creutzberg CL, van Putten WL, Koper PC, et al. Surgery and postoperative radiotherapy versus surgery alone for patients with stage-1 endometrial carcinoma: multicentre randomised trial. PORTEC Study Group. Post operative radiation therapy in endometrial carcinoma. *Lancet.* 2000;355:1404–1411.

DeNardis SA, Holloway RW, Bigsby GE 4th, Pikaart DP, Ahmad S, Finkler NJ. Robotically assisted laparoscopic hysterectomy versus total abdominal hysterectomy and lymphadenectomy for endometrial cancer. *Gynecol Oncol.* 2008;111(3):412–417.

Dizon DS. Treatment options of advanced endometrial carcinoma. *Gynecol Oncol.* 2010;117:373–381.

Fiorica JV, Brunetto VL, Hanjani P, et al. Phase II trial of alternating courses of megestrol acetate and tamoxifen in advanced endometrial carcinoma: a Gynecologic Oncology Group study. *Gynecol Oncol.* 2004;92:10–14.

Fleming GF, Brunetto VL, Cella D, et al. Phase III trial of doxorubicin plus cisplatin with or without paclitaxel plus filgrastim in advanced endometrial carcinoma: a Gynecologic Oncology Group Study. *J Clin Oncol.* 2004;22:2159–2166.

Hogberg T. Adjuvant chemotherapy in endometrial carcinoma: overview of randomised trials. *Clin Oncol.* 2008;20(6):463–469.

Khalifa MA, Mannel RS, Haraway SD, Walker J, Min KW. Expression of EGFR, HER-2/neu, P53, and PCNA in endometrioid, serous papillary, and clear cell endometrial adenocarcinomas. *Gynecol Oncol.* 1994;53:84–92.

Kornblith AB, Huang HQ, Walker JL, Spirtos NM, Rotmensch J, Cella D. Quality of life of patients with endometrial cancer undergoing laparoscopic international federation of gynecology and obstetrics staging compared with laparotomy: a Gynecologic Oncology Group study. *J Clin Oncol.* 2009;27(32):5337–5342.

Lentz SS. Endocrine therapy of endometrial cancer. *Cancer Treat Res.* 1998;94:89–106.

Mariani A, Webb M, Galli L, Podratz K. Potential therapeutic role of para-aortic lymphadenectomy in node-positive endometrial cancer. *Gynecol Oncol.* 2000;76:348–356.

Mundt AJ, Murphy KT, Rotmensch J, Waggoner SE, Yamada SD, Connell PP. Surgery and postoperative radiation therapy in FIGO Stage IIIC endometrial carcinoma. *Int J Radiat Oncol Biol Phys.* 2001;50:1154–1160.

Neven P, De Muylder X, Van Belle Y, Van Hooff I, Vanderick G. Longitudinal hysteroscopic follow-up during tamoxifen treatment. *Lancet.* 1998;351:36.

Nout RA, Putter H, Jürgenliemk-Schulz IM, et al. Vaginal brachytherapy versus external beam pelvic radiotherapy for high-intermediate risk endometrial cancer: results of the randomized PORTEC-2 trial. 2008 ASCO Annual Meeting. *J Clin Oncol.* 2008;26.

Pecorelli S. Revised FIGO staging for carcinoma of the vulva, cervix and endometrium. *Int J Gynaecol Obstet.* 2009;105:103–104.

Randall ME, Filiaci VL, Muss H, et al. Randomized phase III trial of whole-abdominal irradiation versus doxorubicin and cisplatin chemotherapy in advanced endometrial carcinoma: a Gynecologic Oncology Group Study. *J Clin Oncol.* 2006;24:36–44.

Schmeler KM, Lynch HT, Chen LM, et al. Prophylactic surgery to reduce the risk of gynecologic cancers in the Lynch syndrome. *N Engl J Med.* 2006;354:261–269.

Thigpen JT, Brady MF, Alvarez RD, et al. Oral medroxyprogesterone acetate in the treatment of advanced or recurrent endometrial carcinoma: a dose-response study by the Gynecologic Oncology Group. *J Clin Oncol.* 1999;17:1736–1744.

Wolfson AH, Brady MF, Rocereto T, et al. A gynecologic oncology group randomized phase III trial of whole abdominal irradiation (WAI) vs. cisplatin-ifosfamide and mesna (CIM) as post-surgical therapy in stage I-IV carcinosarcoma (CS) of the uterus. *Gynecol Oncol.* 2007;107(2):177–185.

Ovarian Cancer

Armstrong DK, Bundy B, Wenzel L, et al. Intraperitoneal cisplatin and paclitaxel in ovarian cancer. *N Engl J Med.* 2006;354:34–43.

Bristow RE, Eisenhauer EL, Santillan A, Chi DS. Delaying the primary surgical effort for advanced ovarian cancer: a systematic review of neoadjuvant chemotherapy and interval cytoreduction. *Gynecol Oncol.* 2007;104(2):480–490.

Cannistra SA. Cancer of the ovary. *N Engl J Med.* 2004;351:2519–2529.

Cannistra SA, Matulonis U, Penson R, et al. Bevacizumab in patients with advanced platinum-resistant ovarian cancer. *J Clin Oncol.* 2007;25:5180–5186.

Chan JK, Tian C, Fleming GF, et al. The potential benefit of 6 vs. 3 cycles of chemotherapy in subsets of women with early-stage high-risk epithelial ovarian cancer: an exploratory analysis of a Gynecologic Oncology Group study. *Gynecol Oncol.* 2010;116(3):301–306.

Colombo N, Guthrie D, Chiari S, et al. International Collaborative Ovarian Neoplasm trial 1: a randomized trial of adjuvant chemotherapy in women with early-stage ovarian cancer. *J Natl Cancer Inst.* 2003;95:125–132.

du Bois A, Quinn M, Thigpen T, et al. 2004 consensus statements on the management of ovarian cancer: final document of the 3rd International Gynecologic Cancer Intergroup Ovarian Cancer Consensus Conference (GCIG OCCC 2004). *Ann Oncol.* 2005;16(Suppl 8):viii7–vii12.

Goff BA, Mandel LS, Drescher CW, et al. Development of an ovarian cancer symptom index: possibilities for earlier detection. *Cancer.* 2007;109:221–227.

Fong PC, Boss DS, Yap TA, et al. Inhibition of poly(ADP-ribose) polymerase in tumors from BRCA mutation carriers. *N Engl J Med.* 2009;361(2):123–134.

Harter PA, Hahmann M, Lueck HJ, et al. Surgery for recurrent ovarian cancer: role of peritoneal carcinomatosis: exploratory analysis of the DESKTOP I trial about risk factors, surgical implications, and prognostic value of peritoneal carcinomatosis. *Ann Surg Oncol.* 2009;16:1324–1330.

Jacobs IJ, Skates SJ, MacDonald N, et al. Screening for ovarian cancer: a pilot randomised controlled trial. *Lancet.* 1999;353:1207–1210.

Kaku T, Ogawa S, Kawano Y, et al. Histological classification of ovarian cancer. *Med Electron Microsc.* 2003;36:9–17.

Katsumata N, Yasuda M, Takahashi F, et al. Dose-dense paclitaxel once a week in combination with carboplatin every 3 weeks for advanced ovarian cancer: a phase 3, open-label, randomised controlled trial. *Lancet.* 2009;17:1331–1338.

Kauff ND, Satagopan JM, Robson ME, et al. Risk-reducing salpingo-oophorectomy in women with a BRCA1 or BRCA2 mutation. *N Engl J Med.* 2002;346:1609–1615.

Köbel M, Kalloger S, Santos J, Huntsman DG, Gilks CB, Swenerton KD. Tumor type and substage predict survival in stage I and II ovarian carcinoma: insights and implications. *Gynecol Oncol.* 2010;116(1):50–56.

Markman M, Rothman R, Hakes T, et al. Second-line platinum therapy in patients with ovarian cancer previously treated with cisplatin. *J Clin Oncol.* 1991;9(3):389–393.

McGuire WP, Hoskins WJ, Brady MF, et al. Cyclophosphamide and cisplatin compared with paclitaxel and cisplatin in patients with stage III and stage IV ovarian cancer. *N Engl J Med.* 1996;334:1–6.

Parmar MK, Ledermann JA, Colombo N, et al. Paclitaxel plus platinum-based chemotherapy versus conventional platinum-based chemotherapy in women with relapsed ovarian cancer: the ICON4/AGO-OVAR-2.2 trial. *Lancet.* 2003;361:2099–2106.

Partridge E, Kreimer AR, Greenlee RT, et al. Results from four rounds of ovarian cancer screening in a randomized trial. *Obstet Gynecol.* 2009;113(4):775–782.

Pfisterer J, Plante M, Vergote I, et al. Gemcitabine plus carboplatin compared with carboplatin in patients with platinum-sensitive recurrent ovarian cancer: an intergroup trial of the AGO-OVAR, the NCIC CTG, and the EORTC GCG. *J Clin Oncol.* 2006;24(29):4699–4707.

Pujade-Lauraine E, Mahner S, Kaern J, et al. A randomized, phase III study of carboplatin and pegylated liposomal doxorubicin versus carboplatin and paclitaxel in relapsed platinum-sensitive ovarian cancer (OC): CALYPSO study of the Gynecologic Cancer Intergroup (GCIG). *J Clin Oncol.* 2009;27:18s.

O'Shaughnessy J, Osborne C, Pippen J, et al. Efficacy of BSI-201, a poly (ADP-ribose) polymerase-1 (PARP1) inhibitor, in combination with gemcitabine/carboplatin (G/C) in patients with metastatic triple-negative breast cancer (TNBC): Results of a randomized phase II trial. *J Clin Oncol.* 2009;27:18s.

Ozols RF, Bundy BN, Greer BE, et al. Phase III trial of carboplatin and paclitaxel compared with cisplatin and paclitaxel in patients with optimally resected stage III ovarian cancer: a Gynecologic Oncology Group study. *J Clin Oncol.* 2003;21(17): 3194–3200.

Rose PG, Nerenstone S, Brady MF, et al. Secondary surgical cytoreduction for advanced ovarian carcinoma. *N Engl J Med.* 2004;351:2489–2497.

Rustin GJ, van der Burg ME, on behalf of MRC and EORTC. A randomized trial in ovarian cancer (OC) of early treatment of relapse based on CA125 level alone versus delayed treatment based on conventional clinical indicators (MRC OV05/EORTC 55955 trials). *J Clin Oncol.* 2009;27:18s.

Vasey PA, Jayson GC, Gordon A, et al. Phase III randomized trial of docetaxel-carboplatin versus paclitaxel-carboplatin as first-line chemotherapy for ovarian carcinoma. *J Natl Cancer Inst.* 2004;96(22):1682–1691.

Vergote I. Randomized trial comparing primary debulking (PDS) with neoadjuvant chemotherapy (NACT) followed by interval debulking (IDS) in stage IIIC-IV ovarian, fallopian tube, and peritoneal cancer. IGCS Bangkok, October 25th 2008.

Visintin I, Feng Z, Longton G, et al. Diagnostic markers for early detection of ovarian cancer. *Clin Cancer Res.* 2008;14:1065–1072.

Zorn KK, Bonome T, Gangi L, et al. Gene expression profiles of serous, endometrioid, and clear cell subtypes of ovarian and endometrial cancer. *Clin Cancer Res.* 2005;11(18):6422–6430.

Gestational Trophoblastic Neoplasm

Horowitz NS, Goldstein DP, Berkowitz RS. Management of gestational trophoblastic neoplasia. *Semin Oncol.* 2009;36:181–189.

Stromal or Granulosa Cell Tumor

Jamieson S, Fuller PJ. Management of granulosa cell tumour of the ovary. *Curr Opin Onc.* 2008;20:560–564.

11 Urologic and Male Genital Cancers

Brendan D. Curti and Craig R. Nichols

I. BLADDER CANCER

A. General considerations and staging

More than 90% of patients with bladder cancer have transitional cell carcinoma (TCC). Other histologies include squamous cell neuroendocrine and adenocarcinoma. TCC falls into two major groups: superficial and invasive. The biology and natural history of these two groups differ markedly. The major factors that influence treatment choice and prognosis in bladder cancer are stage (0 to IV), histological grade (1 to 3), and location of the tumor within the bladder. Nuclear over expression of the tumor suppressor gene p53 and the Lewis-x blood group are associated with poorer prognosis in TCC.

The standard evaluation of a patient with invasive bladder cancer should include cystoscopy under anesthesia, computed tomography (CT) imaging of the abdomen and pelvis, chest radiograph, complete blood cell count (CBC), and serum chemistry profile. Chest CT and bone scan may also be helpful when stage IV disease is suspected. The TNM staging system is summarized in Table 11.1.

B. General approach to therapy

1. **Superficial-stage, low-grade tumors.** Patients with stage 0 or I tumors are usually treated by transurethral resection (TUR) and fulguration to achieve local control. Over 80% of patients will have recurrent bladder cancer despite initial complete resection. The risk of local recurrence may be reduced by administration of intravesical therapy, with the strongest benefit conferred by Bacillus Calmette-Guérin (BCG) vaccine. Diffuse carcinoma in situ may also be treated with intravesical therapy or cystectomy.

2. **Deep-stage, high-grade tumors.** Patients with muscle-invasive disease (stage II or III) are usually managed by radical cystectomy. Partial cystectomy may be used in highly selected patients with small and ideally located focal disease. Definitive radiation therapy can also be considered, although there has never been a direct comparison of the outcomes of radical cystectomy to radiation. Several randomized studies have shown a survival

TABLE 11.1   TNM Staging of Bladder Cancer

TX: Primary tumor cannot be assessed
T0: No evidence of primary tumor
Ta: Noninvasive papillary carcinoma
Tis: Carcinoma in situ
T1: Tumor invades subepithelial connective tissue
T2: Tumor invades muscle
T2a: Superficial (inner half)
T2b: Deep (outer half)
T3: Tumor invades perivesical fat
T3a: Microscopically
T3b: Macroscopically (extravesical mass)
T4: Tumor invades any of the following: prostate, uterus, vagina, pelvic wall, or abdominal wall
T4a: Tumor invades the prostate, uterus, or vagina
T4b: Tumor invades the pelvic wall or abdominal wall

Stage groupings are as follows:
Stage 0: Ta or Tis, N0, M0
Stage I: T1, N0, M0
Stage II: T2, N0, M0
Stage III: T3 or T4a, N0, M0
Stage IV: T4b, N0, M0; any T, N1 to 3, M0 to 1

Modified from Edge SB, Byrd DR, Compton CC, et al (Eds.). *AJCC cancer staging manual* (7th ed.). New York: Springer; 2010.

benefit with platinum-containing combination administered before radical cystectomy. A meta-analysis of 10 randomized studies also showed a statistically significant 5-year survival benefit for platinum-containing combinations, but not for cisplatin monotherapy. Several smaller studies suggest a benefit of postsurgical adjuvant therapy comparable to neoadjuvant treatment, but there are no randomized comparisons to determine the optimal timing for chemotherapy.

3. **Advanced and metastatic tumors.** The prognosis for locally advanced and metastatic disease is poor. Patients with locally advanced disease or local recurrences can be considered for radiation therapy. Patients with advanced or metastatic disease can be offered systemic chemotherapy or clinical trial participation. There is evidence that chemotherapy can prolong survival and that combination chemotherapy is superior to single agents.

C. **Treatment regimens and evaluation of response**
   1. **Intravesical chemotherapy**
      a. **Method of administration and follow-up.** Intravesical therapy is usually administered in a volume of 40 to 60 mL through a Foley catheter. The catheter is then clamped and the agent

retained for 2 hours. This procedure delivers a high local concentration to the tumor area while usually avoiding systemic effects. Patients with superficial bladder cancers require lifelong surveillance with cystoscopy (initially every 3 months, then every 6 months, then annually) because of the high probability of recurrence even with intravesical therapy. Patients with diffuse carcinoma in situ should have biopsy confirmation of response after intravesical therapy and lifelong cystoscopic surveillance. Patients with persistent or recurrent cancer may require cystectomy.

  b. **Selection of patients for intravesical therapy.** The indications for intravesical therapy are as follows:

   (1) Prevention of relapse in patients with high grade Ta and stage I lesions after TUR.

   (2) Prevent recurrence or progression in patients with two or more previously resected bladder tumors.

   (3) Treatment of carcinoma in situ. A course of instillation therapy is usually given, followed by repeat biopsies. Persistence of carcinoma in situ is an indication for more aggressive local management with cystectomy or definitive radiation.

   Intravesical therapy is not indicated for muscle-invasive TCC.

  c. **Specific intravesical therapeutic regimens**
   BCG 120 mg weekly for 6 to 8 weeks, *or*
   Thiotepa 30 to 60 mg weekly for 4 to 6 weeks, *or*
   Mitomycin 20 to 40 mg weekly for 6 to 8 weeks, *or*
   Doxorubicin 50 to 60 mg weekly for 6 to 8 weeks

  d. **Selection of therapy.** BCG is the agent of choice for intravesical therapy. Two separate studies have shown BCG to be superior to thiotepa and doxorubicin in preventing recurrence. Two published meta-analyses suggest significantly less tumor recurrence with BCG compared to mitomycin. In addition, BCG demonstrates higher rates of response in carcinoma in situ.

  e. **Response to therapy.** Intravesical BCG decreases tumor recurrence by approximately 50% in patients with Ta or T1 disease. The complete response rate with BCG in carcinoma in situ is approximately 70% to 80%. Despite these favorable response rates, the benefit of maintenance BCG therapy is controversial and the benefit of intravesical therapy in preventing progression to invasive or metastatic bladder cancer is still unclear.

  f. **Complications of therapy.** All of the agents mentioned can cause symptoms of bladder irritation (pain, urgency, hematuria) and allergic reactions. Thiotepa is systemically absorbed and can occasionally cause myelosuppression. This is rare with mitomycin and doxorubicin. Patients receiving thiotepa should have their CBC monitored closely. Mitomycin can cause dermatitis in the perineal area and hands. BCG is occasionally associated with systemic symptoms including fever, chills, malaise, arthralgias, and skin rash. Septic reactions and disseminated BCG infections are rare.

2. **Neoadjuvant chemotherapy**. Platinum-containing neoadjuvant combination chemotherapy can increase resectability and can confer a survival benefit compared to radical cystectomy in patients with muscle-invasive TCC. Adjuvant chemotherapy is preferred at some centers because it does not delay possible curative surgery. There are few prospective randomized studies of adjuvant chemotherapy after cystectomy and no large studies comparing neoadjuvant with adjuvant chemotherapy.

3. **Bladder-sparing therapy**. Combination chemotherapy and radiation can be offered to patients with muscle-invasive bladder cancer who desire bladder preservation or are not candidates for radical cystectomy. Cisplatin chemotherapy concurrent with radiation increases local control. Approximately 30% of patients are free of recurrence 5 years after combined modality therapy for muscle-invasive disease. Salvage cystectomy has been used in some patients who do not achieve a complete response or recur after a bladder-sparing approach. There have been no randomized trials comparing bladder preservation therapy with radical cystectomy. Local symptoms from radiation including urinary frequency, incontinence, and proctitis usually resolve, but can persist in some patients. Candidates for a bladder-sparing approach are patients with favorable tumors (e.g., no involvement of the trigone or ureter) or patients who are unfit for radical cystectomy due to comorbidities.

4. **Systemic chemotherapy for advanced disease**.
   a. **Specific chemotherapy drugs and regimens**. Drugs active against bladder cancer include cisplatin, gemcitabine, doxorubicin, vinblastine, methotrexate, pemetrexed cyclophosphamide, ifosfamide, carboplatin, paclitaxel, and docetaxel. Cisplatin is the most active drug single agent in TCC. The MVAC regimen (methotrexate, vinblastine, doxorubicin, and cisplatin) is considered by many genitourinary oncologists to be a "gold standard" in advanced bladder cancer because of the number of studies confirming response. A study comparing gemcitabine and cisplatin (GC) to MVAC showed comparable efficacy, duration of response, and less toxicity with GC. Specific regimens are shown in Table 11.2.
   b. **Response to therapy**. MVAC induces complete response in approximately 15% of patients and partial response in 35%, for an overall response rate of 50% in patients with metastatic disease. The median survival is 14 months. The toxicity of

Regimen or Single Agent	Doses and Schedules
Methotrexate/ vinblastine/ doxorubicin/ cisplatin	Methotrexate 30 mg/m^2 IV on day 1
	Vinblastine 3 mg/m^2 IV on day 2
	Doxorubicin 30 mg/m^2 IV on day 2
	Cisplatin 70 mg/m^2 IV on day 2 (with adequate pre- and posthydration)
	Repeat methotrexate and vinblastine on day 15 and 22 if white blood cell count >2000/μL and platelet count >50,000/μL.
	Cycles should be repeated every 28 days.
Gemcitabine/ cisplatin	Gemcitabine 1000 mg/m^2 day 1
	Cisplatin 70 mg/m^2 on day 2
	Repeat gemcitabine on day 8 and 15 if white blood cell count >2000/μL and platelet count >50,000/μL. Cycles should be repeated every 28 days.
Carboplatin/ gemcitabine	Carboplatin AUC 5 day 1
	Gemcitabine 1000 mg/m^2 day 1 and day 8
	Cycles repeated every 21 days
Carboplatin/ paclitaxel	Carboplatin AUC 6
	Paclitaxel 225 mg/m^2
	Cycles repeated every 21 days
Paclitaxel	250 mg/m^2 IV over 24 hours every 21 days

TABLE 11.2 Combination Chemotherapy and Active Single Agents for Cancer of the Bladder

AUC, area under the curve; IV, intravenously.

the regimen is substantial and patient selection in regard to medical comorbidities and performance status is important. Response to chemotherapy is monitored by periodic measurement of tumor masses with the expectation that most patients who will respond will do so within the first one or two cycles of treatment.

Patients who cannot tolerate cisplatin-based chemotherapy because of poor performance status or renal insufficiency may be considered for carboplatin-based therapy. Combinations containing carboplatin, gemcitabine, docetaxel, or paclitaxel have all shown activity.

Management of the non-TCC histologies arising from the bladder is difficult. Local therapies should be identical to TCC, but the role of chemotherapy is limited. Non-TCC histologies respond poorly to chemotherapy with the exception of neuroendocrine tumors. Neuroendocrine tumors of the bladder are usually treated similarly to small-cell lung cancer with cisplatin and etoposide chemotherapy and local radiation for those with bladder-confined disease. Although the initial response rate is high with neuroendocrine histology, the incidence of recurrence and death from metastatic disease is also high.

c. **Complications of systemic therapy.** The major dose-limiting toxicity of MVAC is myelosuppression, which often precludes the administration of chemotherapy on days 15 and 22. GC produces significantly less neutropenia and mucositis but more thrombocytopenia. Cisplatin can cause renal tubular injury, but this can usually be prevented by vigorous hydration and repletion of electrolytes. Cisplatin is also highly emetogenic and requires aggressive management to minimize nausea and vomiting.

d. **Follow-up.** Patients with advanced disease can be followed every few months for symptomatic progression. Serial x-ray studies or bone scans are costly and are of minimal value.

II. PROSTATE CANCER

A. Background

Carcinoma of the prostate is the second most common cancer in the United States after nonmelanoma skin cancer. An elevated prostate-specific antigen (PSA) is the most common finding leading to a diagnosis of prostate cancer. There are considerable controversies about the value of PSA screening because aggressive prostate cancer can be present with a normal PSA and, conversely, many men with an elevated PSA and biopsy-proven prostate cancer can have indolent disease that does not change life span. The number of new prostate cancer diagnoses is estimated at 192,000 in 2009 with over 27,000 deaths. However, the median survival of patients with early prostate cancer exceeds 10 years. The benefit of aggressive surgical or radiotherapeutic management of these patients may be largely dependent on individual patient comorbidities and the biology of the tumor.

B. Staging

Accurate staging in prostate cancer is often difficult before definitive surgery. There are many published prostate nomograms that can be helpful in predicting pathologic stage, determining patient outcome, and guiding treatment. These nomograms use PSA, clinical stage (based on physical exam including digital rectal exam), the Gleason score, and the number of positive biopsy cores to determine the probability of organ-confined disease, seminal vesicle invasion, and lymph node involvement. The 5-year progression-free and overall survival of radical prostatectomy or external beam radiation is also estimated by the nomogram.

Initial staging of prostate cancer may also include abdominal and pelvic CT scans, chest radiographs, bone scan, liver function tests, and acid phosphatase measurements depending on the initial PSA, the clinical suspicion for metastatic disease, and the patient's goals for therapy. The most commonly used staging is the

TNM Staging of Prostate Cancer

T-Stage

TX: Primary tumor cannot be assessed

T0: No evidence of primary tumor

T1: Clinically inapparent tumor not palpable or visible by imaging

T1a: Tumor incidental histologic finding in 5% or less of tissue resected

T1b: Tumor incidental histologic finding in more than 5% of tissue resected

T1c: Tumor identified by needle biopsy (e.g., because of elevated PSA)

T2: Tumor confined within prostate

T3: Tumor extends through the prostatic capsule

T4: Tumor is fixed or invades adjacent structures other than seminal vesicles

Stage groupings are as follows:

Stage I: T1a, N0, M0, G1

Stage II: T1a, N0, M0, G2 to 4

T1b, c, N0, M0, any G

T2, N0, M0, any G

Stage III: T3, N0, M0, any G

Stage IV: T4, N0, M0, any G

Any T, N1 to 3, M0, any G

Any T, any N, M1, any G

TNM system shown in Table 11.3. The modified Whitmore-Jewett or American Urologic Association system is also used. In the American Urologic Association system, stages A, B, C, and D correspond closely to stages I, II, III, and IV in the TNM system.

C. General considerations and goals of therapy

Selection of therapy for prostate cancer is complex and based on the extent of disease as well as the age and general medical condition of the patient. Although many biases exist, there are no prospective randomized trials comparing treatment modalities in patients with organ-confined disease.

With the possible exception of young patients (less than 65 years of age), T1a prostate cancer may be followed without further therapy because few patients will have disease progression. For other patients with organ-confined disease (T1b, T1c, T2), several treatment options exist. Radical prostatectomy (using the traditional perineal or retropubic approach, or using laparoscopy and/or robotic-assisted techniques) and external beam radiation therapy (using intensity-modulated radiation therapy [IMRT], proton beam or other modern image-guided treatment planning) probably offer equivalent disease-free and overall survival when PSA and Gleason score are taken into account. Observation or active surveillance should also be considered for patients with low-grade, organ-confined tumors. The choice of primary therapy should be based on the patient's performance status, goals for treatment, and toxicities of each modality. Toxicities of radical prostatectomy include the risks of anesthesia, bleeding, urinary leakage, and erectile dysfunction. Diarrhea, tenesmus, and rectal bleeding are more common with radiation. In general, younger men are more likely to receive radical prostatectomy whereas older men are more likely to receive radiation therapy. Lastly, brachytherapy and cryosurgery may also be alternatives for management of localized disease.

Patients with stage III tumors are often treated with radiation therapy. However, elderly patients or patients in poor general health may be followed with observation because the natural history of prostate cancer can be slow with progression over years rather than months. The addition of early hormonal therapy to radiation therapy may be considered in higher stage disease or in patients with Gleason grade 7 or greater. The addition of docetaxel-based chemotherapy in high-risk localized prostate cancer is being studied, but has not yet shown a survival benefit.

D. Treatment of metastatic disease

The initial treatment of choice in patients with metastatic disease is androgen ablation. Radiation for symptomatic localized metastasis may also be considered.

1. Androgen ablation. Surgical or medical castration is associated with an overall response of 75% of patients with metastatic prostate cancer, lasting a median of 18 months. Luteinizing hormone-releasing hormone (LHRH) analogs or orchiectomy are the primary initial treatment options and have equivalent PSA and radiographic response rates. Patient preference, existing medical conditions, and cost influence treatment choice. There are currently no good predictive markers for response in clinical practice although some data suggest circulating tumor cell (CTC) assays may be superior to PSA in assessing response and prognosis.

a. Orchiectomy is still a standard treatment for metastatic disease because it is relatively inexpensive and obviates the need for injections or daily medications. This procedure can often be done on an outpatient basis. However, most men choose a nonsurgical method of androgen ablation.

b. LHRH analogs are synthetic peptides administered by parenteral injection. These agents occupy the receptors for LHRH in the pituitary gland. Initially the release of LH is increased, causing a rise in the serum testosterone level (and possible tumor flare). The presence of super-physiologic LHRH analog blocks the physiologic pulsatile LH release from the pituitary, causing a fall in the serum testosterone to castration levels, usually within 2 weeks. The most commonly used LHRH agonists are:

- ▪ Leuprolide 7.5 mg intramuscular (IM) depot monthly or 22.5 mg IM depot every 3 months or 30 mg IM depot every 4 months.
- ▪ Goserelin 3.6 mg subcutaneous (SC) depot monthly or 10.8 mg SC every 3 months.

    Tumor flare can usually be avoided by the concurrent use of antiandrogens. Disadvantages of LHRH agonists compared to surgical castration are the potential for poor patient compliance and the high cost of treatment. The possible benefit of intermittent hormonal therapy is currently being studied in randomized trials. Small studies suggest equivalent cancer outcomes and enhanced tolerance using intermittent dosing.

c. **LHRH analogs and antiandrogens** (total androgen blockade) have also been studied. Synthetic antiandrogens such as flutamide, bicalutamide, and nilutamide act by competing with testosterone at the level of the cellular receptor. A large randomized trial of flutamide given after orchiectomy did not show improvement in survival. Because of the lack of consistent evidence of benefit as well as added cost and toxicity, total androgen blockade is not considered standard initial treatment in patients with metastatic disease.

d. **Estrogens.** DES (diethylstilbestrol) is effective but not frequently used because of concern about potential cardiotoxicity and thrombophlebitis. Historically 3 to 5 mg/day of DES has been given; however, 1 mg/day produces fewer side effects without shortening survival. Painful gynecomastia can be prevented by superficial radiation (5 Gy) to the breast tissue before starting DES.

e. **Second-line hormonal therapies** have low response rates (less than 20%) and the median duration of response is 4 months. Initial hormone therapy should be continued to maintain castration levels of testosterone. Second-line therapies include addition of antiandrogens, estrogens, ketoconazole, and progestins. Patients who were initially treated with combined modality therapy occasionally respond to withdrawal of the antiandrogen. This should be considered before proceeding to more toxic therapies.

2. **Cytotoxic chemotherapy.** Patients who relapse from or fail to respond to androgen ablation can be considered for cytotoxic chemotherapy. Trials of chemotherapy before 2000 did not show any convincing benefit and induced significant toxicity in men who had impaired bone marrow reserve due to multiple courses of palliative radiation. More recent studies of mitoxantrone and docetaxel chemotherapy have shown some clinical benefit.

a. Mitoxantrone

▪ Mitoxantrone 12 mg/m^2 every 3 weeks and

▪ Prednisone 5 mg twice a day.

This regimen demonstrated improved pain control and reduced need for analgesic medications compared to patients treated with prednisone alone in a randomized trial with no improvement in overall survival. This regimen is still used and has a relatively low toxicity profile.

b. Docetaxel chemotherapy. Two large randomized trials of docetaxel-based chemotherapy were the first to demonstrate a survival benefit over mitoxantrone and prednisone. The median survival benefit is modest (approximately 3 months); however, a greater proportion of patients are alive at 1, 2, and 3 years after docetaxel chemotherapy compared to mitoxantrone or best-supportive care.

▪ Docetaxel 75 mg/m^2 every 3 weeks and prednisone 5 mg twice a day *or*

▪ Docetaxel 60 mg/m^2 intravenously (IV) day 2 and estramustine 280 mg twice a day by mouth days 1 to 5 and prednisone 5 mg twice a day during 3 week cycles.

Docetaxel monotherapy is now the most common regimen for castration-resistant prostate cancer in men with good functional status. There are many phase II and III studies looking at docetaxel in combination with other biologic agents like atrasentan, dasatinib, and AT-101. There is no standard salvage regimen after docetaxel chemotherapy. Clinical trials should be offered to patients with good functional status.

3. Vaccine therapy. The U.S. Food and Drug Administration (FDA) has recently approved the first therapeutic vaccine in prostate cancer, sipuleucel-T. Sipuleucel-T is indicated in patients with symptomatic or minimally symptomatic metastatic hormone refractory prostate cancer. The drug is an autologous dendritic (DC) cell vaccine that is derived from the patient's own cells and pulsed with the prostatic acid phosphatase antigen in the presence of granulocyte-macrophage colony stimulating factor. It is administered at a dose that contains a minimum of 50 million pulsed DCs in 3 doses at approximately 2 weeks apart.

4. Evaluation of response. PSA, palliation of bone pain, and radiographic response can be used to assess treatment response. Care must be taken in the interpretation of bone scans to distinguish between healing bone (which can show increased radiotracer uptake) and progressive cancer.

5. Complications of therapy. All androgen ablation therapies will cause sexual dysfunction, including impotence and decreased libido. Orchiectomy can rarely be complicated by local infection or hematoma. LHRH analogs can cause an initial flare of the disease and are frequently associated with vasomotor symptoms ("hot flashes"). Androgen ablation can also cause diarrhea, osteoporosis, and hepatic dysfunction. Estrogens are associated with thromboembolic disease, fluid retention, and cardiac disease. Chemotherapy side effects include nausea and vomiting, mucositis, marrow suppression, peripheral neuropathy, integumentary changes, infusion reactions, and alopecia.

6. **Follow-up.** Patients treated with radical prostatectomy can be followed with PSA measurements every 3 to 6 months. Patients with a rising PSA level, evidence of local recurrence, and no evidence of metastatic disease can be considered for salvage radiation therapy to the prostatic bed. Some patients can be considered for bisphosphonate therapy. Osteoporosis is a complication of androgen deprivation therapy and may benefit from treatment. Monthly IV bisphosphonate therapy with zoledronic acid may decrease the incidence of skeletal related complications such as pathologic fractures in patients with bone metastases from prostate cancer.

III. TESTICULAR CANCER (GERM CELL TUMORS)

A. Overview

Although primary neoplasms of the testis can arise from Leydig or Sertoli cells, more than 95% of testicular cancers are of spermatogenic or germ cell origin. Germ cell tumors (GCTs) are rare, accounting for 1% of all malignancies in men. However, they are important malignancies because they represent the most common solid tumor in young men and because of their high degree of curability. With the advent of cisplatin-based chemotherapy, accurate tumor markers, and aggressive surgical approaches, overall cure rates for patients with disseminated disease exceed 90% and patients with early-stage disease are nearly always cured. GCT is also one of the few solid tumors for which salvage chemotherapy can be curative.

B. Histology

GCTs are categorized as either seminomatous or nonseminomatous (which includes a variety of other histologies such as embryonal cell carcinoma, choriocarcinoma, and yolk sac tumors). Pure seminoma accounts for 40% of patients with GCTs. Although mild elevations of the β-subunit of human chorionic gonadotropin (hCG) may be seen, pure seminoma is never associated with an elevation of α-fetoprotein (AFP). Nonseminomatous GCT can cause elevations of hCG, AFP, or both.

C. **Staging**

Pretreatment staging should include serum tumor markers (AFP, hCG) and CT of the abdomen and chest. Other radiographic procedures should be undertaken only if symptoms or physical examination dictate.

1. **Stage I.** Tumor confined to the testis with or without involvement of the spermatic cord or epididymis.
2. **Stage II.** Tumor with metastasis limited to retroperitoneal lymph nodes (IIA, 5 or fewer nodes, all ≤2 cm; IIB, more than 5 nodes or any node >2–5 cm; IIC, any node mass >5 cm).
3. **Stage III.** Tumor spread beyond retroperitoneal lymph nodes.

D. **Treatment strategies and management of specific situations**

The therapeutic approach to the patient with testicular cancer depends on the histology of the tumor and the clinical or pathologic stage of the disease.

1. **Seminoma**
    a. **Clinical stage I.** Over 75% of patients with testicular seminoma present with early-stage disease and are often cured with orchiectomy alone. The former paradigm of adjuvant radiation therapy is rapidly being replaced by active surveillance for clinical stage I disease. Both the European and Canadian consensus guidelines list active surveillance as the primary option for clinical stage I disease and this practice is being rapidly adopted in the United States. Precise guidelines for surveillance imaging guidelines are in evolution, but current recommendations range to as low as two CTs over the first 2 years to much more intensive schedules that have frequent and prolonged imaging. The imaging schedules being developed in the Oregon/British Columbia Testicular Cancer Consortium include four CTs (6 months, 1 year, 18 months, and 30 months) based in part on the median time to relapse (13 months). Adjuvant radiation therapy or consideration of adjuvant carboplatin should be reserved for uncommon circumstances.
    b. **Stage II.** Traditional management of the small fraction of patients with stage II disease has been allocated by tumor volumes. Patients with small volume retroperitoneal disease (stage II A disease) have often been given therapeutic radiation at doses slightly higher than the doses given as adjuvant therapy (3000–3500 cGy) and chemotherapy reserved for the 20% or so of patients who recurred after therapeutic radiation therapy. Patients with bulky disease (>5 cm) are given combination chemotherapy (usually bleomycin, etoposide, and cisplatin [BEP] × 3 or etoposide and cisplatin [EP] × 4 as described below for nonseminoma) with a very high expectation of cure.

2. **Nonseminoma**

   a. **Stage I disease**. The currently preferred option for patients is surveillance without a retroperitoneal lymph node dissection (RPLND). Because 30% of these patients eventually experience relapse, they must be followed closely with serum markers, exam, and interspersed CT scans of the abdomen. Most patients who recur will do so within the first 2 years. Historically these patients had been pathologically staged and treated with a RPLND. Patients with pathologically confirmed stage I disease do not need any further therapy because only approximately 10% show relapse. In about 25% of patients, clinical stage I disease is found to be stage II pathologically at RPLND and treatment for these patients is discussed in the following section. The major complication of RPLND has been retrograde ejaculation with subsequent infertility, although this is rare in experienced centers using nerve-sparing procedures.

   b. **Stage II disease**. Patients with clear-cut radiographic evidence of stage II disease and elevated serum markers should be treated primarily with chemotherapy. If the lymph nodes are equivocal and markers are negative, an RPLND can be considered or close observation with repeat CT to document growth. Patients with pathologically confirmed and completely resected stage II disease have a relapse rate of about 30%. Patients with fully resected pathologic stage II disease either can be treated with two cycles of adjuvant chemotherapy after RPLND or can be followed closely and treated with standard chemotherapy if they show relapse.

   c. **Stage III disease**. About 30% of patients present with stage III disease. The most common site of involvement is the lungs, but liver, bone, and brain can also be involved with metastatic disease. These patients are further categorized as good, intermediate, or poor risk based on the primary site, level of marker elevation, and involvement of brain, liver, or bone. An international germ cell prognostic classification has been developed based on a retrospective analysis of more than 5,000 patients with metastatic GCTs. Poor risk (poor prognosis) patients according to the International Germ Cell Cancer Consensus Classification System include those with the following:

   ▪ Mediastinal primary site *or*

   ▪ Nonpulmonary visceral metastasis (e.g., liver, bone, and brain) *or*

   ▪ Elevation of AFP >10,000 ng/mL, hCG >10,000 ng/mL, or LDH >10 × upper limit of normal (ULN)

Patients with nonseminoma without mediastinal primary or nonpulmonary visceral metastasis
- Have a good prognosis with the AFP <1000 ng/mL, hCG <1000 ng/mL, and LDH <1.5 × UNL;
- Have an intermediate prognosis if any of the markers is in the intermediate range (AFP 1000–10,000 ng/mL, hCG 1000–10,000 ng/mL, and LDH 1.5–10 × UNL).

d. **Recommended therapy.** All patients with stage II or III disease who require chemotherapy should receive cisplatin-based chemotherapy, as follows:
BEP
- Cisplatin 20 mg/m^2 IV over 30 minutes on days 1 to 5, *and*
- Etoposide 100 mg/m^2 IV on days 1 to 5, *and*
- Bleomycin 30 U IV push weekly on days 1, 8, and 15
- Repeat every 21 days regardless of blood cell counts for two (adjuvant therapy), three (good risk patients), or four (intermediate or poor risk) cycles.

If the patient has fever associated with granulocytopenia, give the next cycle at the same doses, followed by daily SC injections of granulocyte colony-stimulating factor (filgrastim) or a single dose of pegfilgrastim. Other chemotherapy regimens such as VIP (etoposide, ifosfamide, cisplatin) have not improved outcome and are more toxic. Substitution of carboplatin for cisplatin is inferior therapy and should not be used.

e. **Surgery for residual disease.** Patients who have a complete response with chemotherapy should be followed and do not require any further treatment. Patients whose marker levels normalize but who have not achieved a radiographic complete response should undergo complete surgical resection of residual disease. If the resected material reveals only teratoma, necrosis, or fibrosis, then no further therapy is necessary and the patient should be followed. If there is carcinoma in the resected specimen, the patient should receive two more cycles of cisplatin-based chemotherapy (cisplatin and etoposide).

f. **Follow-up.** Most patients who experience relapse do so within the first 2 years, although late relapses do occur. In general, patients should be followed with every 2 month physical examination, chest x-ray studies, and serum marker measurements during the first year and every 4 months during the second year. Patients should then be followed about every 6 months for the third and fourth year and yearly thereafter. Because tumors can arise in the contralateral testis, patients should be taught to do testicular self-examination.

E. Salvage chemotherapy

1. **Standard-dose therapy**. Patients who respond to first-line chemotherapy and then relapse are still curable with salvage regimens such as VIP or TIP:

VIP

- Vinblastine 0.11 mg/kg (4.1 mg/m^2) IV push on days 1 and 2, *and*
- Ifosfamide 1.2 g/m^2 IV over 30 minutes on days 1 to 5, *and*
- Cisplatin 20 mg/m^2 IV over 30 minutes on days 1 to 5

TIP

- Paclitaxel 250 mg/m^2 CI over 24 hours day 1
- Ifosfamide 1.5 gm/m^2 IV days 2 to 5
- Cisplatin 25 mg/m^2 IV days 2 to 5

Repeat every 21 days for four cycles. Any radiographic abnormalities that persist after salvage chemotherapy should be considered for surgical resection.

2. **High-dose chemotherapy with autologous stem cell transplantation**. High-dose chemotherapy with carboplatin and etoposide with or without cyclophosphamide or ifosfamide followed by autologous stem cell transplantation (ASCT) should be considered for patients requiring salvage chemotherapy. Overall, about 15% to 25% of these patients are long-term survivors. The role of ASCT in the initial salvage setting is still under evaluation. Patients with incomplete response, high markers, high disease volume, and late relapse may be best candidates for initial salvage ASCT.

F. Prognosis

With these strategies, the overall cure rate for patients with stage I disease is more than 98%, stage II disease more than 95%, and stage III disease more than 80%.

G. Complications of therapy

Because patients are cured, the short- and long-term toxicities are of considerable importance. The short-term toxicities of the described chemotherapy regimens include nausea and vomiting, myelosuppression, renal toxicity, and hemorrhagic cystitis. The major long-term morbidities include infertility, pulmonary fibrosis, and a small but definite risk of secondary leukemia.

H. Mediastinal and other midline germ cell tumors

GCTs can arise in several midline structures including the retroperitoneum, mediastinum, and pineal gland. All patients with GCTs at these sites should have a testicular ultrasound examination to exclude an occult primary tumor. Mediastinal nonseminomatous GCTs are associated with Klinefelter syndrome and with rare hematologic malignancies (particularly acute megakaryocytic leukemia). Small mediastinal seminomas can be treated with radiation therapy alone. Widespread tumors or nonseminomatous tumors should be treated with four cycles of BEP chemotherapy. Salvage chemotherapy (including autologous bone marrow transplantation) in patients with nonseminomatous mediastinal GCT is ineffective.

IV. CANCER OF THE PENIS
A. General considerations

Penile cancer is rare in North America but is a significant health problem in many developing countries. These tumors are nearly always squamous cell in origin and are associated with the presence of a foreskin and poor hygiene. Typically, these tumors present as a nonhealing ulcer or mass on the foreskin or glans. The most common treatment is wide surgical excision or penectomy, depending on the size and location of the lesion. Prophylactic inguinal lymph node dissection is indicated in certain subgroups of patients. Radiation therapy can also provide local control, especially with small tumors. However, local relapse may be up to 30% and surgery is still considered standard management, especially for larger tumors.

B. Chemotherapy for systemic disease

Active single agents include bleomycin, cisplatin, and methotrexate, with response rates of 20% to 50%. Combination chemotherapy results in high response rates, but whether survival is improved over that with single agents is unknown. A reasonable regimen is cisplatin 100 mg/m^2 on day 1, with fluorouracil 1000 mg/m^2/day given by continuous infusion on days 1 to 4. Cycles can be repeated every 21 days.

Selected Readings

Testis

Bhatia S, Abonour R, Porcu P, et al. High-dose chemotherapy as initial salvage chemotherapy in patients with relapsed testicular cancer. *J Clin Oncol.* 2000;18(19): 3346–3351.

Bosl GJ, Motzer RJ Testicular germ-cell cancer. *N Engl J Med.* 1997;337:242–254.

International Germ Cell Consensus Classification: a prognostic factor-based staging system for metastatic germ cell cancer. *J Clin Oncol.* 1997;15:594–603.

Loehrer PJ Sr, Gonin R, Nichols CR, et al. Vinblastine plus ifosfamide plus cisplatin as initial salvage therapy in recurrent germ cell tumor. *J Clin Oncol.* 1998;16: 2500–2504.

Saxman SB, Finch D, Gonin R, et al. Long-term follow-up of a phase III study of three versus four cycles of bleomycin, etoposide, and cisplatin in favorable-prognosis germ-cell tumors: the Indiana University experience. *J Clin Oncol.* 1998;16(2): 702–706.

Williams SD, Birch R, Einhorn LH, et al. Treatment of disseminated germ-cell tumors with cisplatin, bleomycin, and either vinblastine or etoposide. *N Engl J Med.* 1987;316:1435–1440.

Bladder

Advanced Bladder Cancer Meta-analysis Collaboration: Neoadjuvant chemotherapy in invasive bladder cancer: a systematic review and meta-analysis. *Lancet.* 2003;361:1927–1934.

Grossman HG, Natale RB, Tangen CM, et al. Neoadjuvant chemotherapy plus cystectomy compared with cystectomy alone for locally advanced bladder cancer. *N Engl J Med.* 2003;349:859–866.

Herr HW, Schwalb DM, Zhang ZF, et al. Intravesical bacillus Calmette–Guérin therapy prevents tumor progression and death from superficial bladder cancer: ten-year follow-up of a prospective randomized trial. *J Clin Oncol.* 1995;13:1404–1408.

Lamm DL, Blumenstein BA, Crawford ED, et al. A randomized trial of intravesical doxorubicin and immunotherapy with bacille Calmette–Guérin for transitional-cell carcinoma of the bladder. *N Engl J Med.* 1991;325:1205–1209.

Loehrer PJ Sr, Einhorn LH, Elson PJ, et al. A randomized comparison of cisplatin alone or in combination with methotrexate, vinblastine, and doxorubicin in patients with metastatic urothelial carcinoma: a cooperative group study. *J Clin Oncol.* 1992;10:1066–1073.

Okeke AA, Probert JL, Gillatt DA, et al. Is intravesical chemotherapy for superficial bladder cancer still justified? *BJU Int.* 2005;96:763–767.

von der Maase H, Hansen SW, Roberts JT, et al. Gemcitabine and cisplatin versus methotrexate, vinblastine, doxorubicin, and cisplatin in advanced or metastatic bladder cancer: results of a large, randomized, multinational, multicenter, phase III study. *J Clin Oncol.* 2000;17:3068–3077.

Prostate

Bill-Axelson A, Holmberg L, Ruutu M, et al. Radical prostatectomy versus watchful waiting in early prostate cancer. *N Engl J Med.* 2005;352:1977–1984.

Eisenberger MA, Blumenstein BA, Crawford ED, et al. Bilateral orchiectomy with or without flutamide for metastatic prostate cancer. *N Engl J Med.* 1998;339(15):1036–1042.

Messing EM, Manola J, Sarosdy M, et al. Immediate hormonal therapy compared with observation after radical prostatectomy and pelvic lymphadenectomy in men with node-positive prostate cancer. *N Engl J Med.* 1999;341:1781–1788.

Partin AW, Kattan MW, Subong ENP, et al. Combination of PSA clinical stage and Gleason score to predict pathology in men with localized prostate cancer: a multiinstitutional update. *JAMA.* 1997;277:1445–1451.

Tannock IF, Osoba D, Stockler MR, et al. Chemotherapy with mitoxantrone plus prednisone or prednisone alone for symptomatic hormone-resistant prostate cancer: a Canadian randomized trial with palliative end points. *J Clin Oncol.* 1996;14:1756–1764.

Tannock IF, de Wit R, Berry WR, et al. Docetaxel plus prednisone or mitoxantrone plus prednisone for advanced prostate cancer. *N Eng J Med.* 2004;351:1502–1512.

Penile Cancer

Culkin DJ, Beer TM. Advanced penile carcinoma. *J Urol.* 2003;170:359–365.

Kroon BK, Horenblas S, Nieweg O. Contemporary management of penile squamous cell carcinoma. *J Surg Oncol.* 2005;89:43–50.

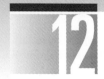

12 Kidney Cancer

Mark T. Andolina, Colleen Darnell, and Olivier Rixe

I. RENAL CELL CARCINOMA (RCC)

An enhanced understanding of RCC has led to advances in both medical management and innovations in surgical management. Small tumors less than 4 cm and selected tumors 4 to 7 cm, formerly treated with open radical nephrectomy, are now treated with laparoscopic partial nephrectomy with similar oncologic outcomes. In addition to surgical advances, the past 5 years have seen a wealth of new biologic and targeted drugs that have activity in RCC.

A. Histopathology

Clear cell carcinoma of the kidney, an adenocarcinoma arising from the proximal convoluted tubules (PCTs), accounts for 85% of primary renal neoplasms. The inactivation or deletion of the Von Hippel-Lindau (VHL) gene on chromosome 3p is associated with an enhanced production of vascular endothelial growth factor (VEGF), and is found in 50% to 60% of sporadic clear cell renal carcinomas. VEGF is believed to augment the growth of new blood vessels typically seen with clear cell kidney cancer and its metastases.

Papillary carcinomas account for 10% and also arise from the PCTs but are distinct from clear cell carcinomas, are often multifocal, and are often with multiple genetic abnormalities. Papillary carcinomas are further divided into two subtypes depending on pathology, gene expression, and prognosis. Type I tend to be a lower grade at diagnosis and carry a better prognosis, while Type II tend to be a higher grade with a poorer prognosis. The remaining 5% of renal carcinomas include oncocytomas (well-differentiated adenocarcinomas) and chromophobic and transitional carcinomas. Wilms tumor (nephroblastoma) is seen predominantly in childhood.

The most widely used and most predictive grading system for renal cell cancer is the Fuhrman Nuclear Grade.

B. Epidemiology

Kidney cancer is listed among the world's 10 most common cancers. More than 57,000 Americans were diagnosed with kidney cancer in 2009, an increase from approximately 36,000 in 2006. Males account for 60% of diagnoses and African-Americans have the highest rate of any racial or ethnic group. Nearly 13,000 patients will die in 2010 from kidney cancer.

C. Risk factors

In general, cigarette smoking roughly doubles the risk of kidney cancer with an increased dose-dependent risk in heavy smokers. Approximately 30% of males and 25% of females with renal cancer have a history of tobacco use. Industrial exposure to cadmium, asbestos, petroleum byproducts, and ingestion of the drug phenacetin (analgesic nephropathy) has been associated with a higher risk. Lesser risk factors include acquired multicystic kidney disease, patients with end-stage renal disease who are on hemodialysis, obesity, and hypertension. Several hereditary conditions predispose patients to renal cell cancers. Notably, VHL disease, an autosomal dominant hereditary condition involving the inactivation of the tumor-suppressor VHL gene, predisposes patients to a variety of neoplasms including clear cell histology renal carcinoma. Inactivation of the VHL gene stimulates angiogenesis through VEGF and its receptor targets in new therapeutic agents. The VHL gene is also mutated in a high number of sporadic or nonhereditary RCCs.

Birt-Hogg-Dubé (BHD) syndrome is an autosomal dominant disorder associated with fibrofolliculomas (benign hair follicle tumors), pulmonary cysts, and renal cancers most commonly of the chromophobe, oncocytoma histology, or a hybrid of the two subtypes. BHD syndrome is caused by a germline mutation in the tumor-suppressor BHD gene, which encodes a novel protein folliculin that has an unknown function.

D. Clinical characteristics

The most common clinical signs and symptoms of renal cancer include hematuria (56% of patients), flank pain (38%), abdominal mass (36%), weight loss (27%), and fever (11%). However, the classic triad of hematuria, flank pain, and abdominal mass occurs in less than 20% of patients and many are asymptomatic until the disease is advanced. Twenty-five percent of renal cancers are found incidentally in radiographic imaging, and 30% of patients will have metastatic disease at diagnosis. Common metastatic sites are lung (75%), soft tissues (36%), bone (20%), and liver (18%); brain metastases are often a late manifestation. Hypercalcemia is present in up to 20% of patients despite the absence of bony metastases and is related to ectopic production of parathyroid hormone–related protein, osteoclast activating factor, or tumor necrosis factor. Erythrocytosis due to excess erythropoietin production has been described in 3% of patients. Ectopic production of other hormones including renin and glucagon produce clinical manifestations of hypertension

TABLE 12.1 Staging and Prognosis of Kidney Cancer

Stage	Clinical Characteristic(s)	TNM	Five-Year Survival
I	Tumor ≤7 cm confined to the kidney	T1, N0, M0	81%
II	Tumor >7 cm confined to the kidney	T2, N0, M0	74%
III	Tumor extending into major veins or perinephric tissues but not into the ipsilateral adrenal gland and not beyond Gerota fascia, or with regional node metastasis	T3, N0, M0 or T1–3, N1, M0	53%
IV	Tumor invading beyond Gerota fascia including into the ipsilateral adrenal gland or distant metastatic disease	T4, any N, M0 or any T, any N, M1	10%

Modified from Edge SB, Byrd DR, Compton CC. *AJCC cancer staging manual* (7th ed.). New York: Springer; 2010.

and hyperglycemia, respectively. Stauffer syndrome, identified in up to 20% of patients, is a hepatic dysfunction associated with elevated alkaline phosphatase, transaminases, activated partial thromboplastin time, and hepatomegaly in the absence of liver metastases.

E. Staging

RCCs are traditionally staged using the TNM staging system (Table 12.1). Newer prognostic systems include the University of California, Los Angeles, integrated staging system (UISS) and the Memorial Sloan-Kettering Cancer Center (MSKCC) system. The UISS (Table 12.2), more predictive for localized tumors, factors in TNM staging, Fuhrman grade, and Eastern Cooperative Oncology

TABLE 12.2 UISS Staging for Patients with Localized Disease

UISS Risk	T Stage	Fuhrman Grade	ECOG PS	Two-Year Survival
Low (I)	T1	1–2	0	96%
Intermediate (III)		Not Low or High		66%
High (V)	T3	2–4	≥1	9%
	T4	1–4	Any	

ECOG, Eastern Cooperative Oncology Group; PS, performance status.
Risk of recurrence after nephrectomy. Recommendation is to perform computed tomography scan of the chest and abdomen more frequently in the intermediate- and high-risk groups. There are also two intermediary categories: II and IV.

TABLE 12.3	MSKCC Risk Stratification for Metastatic Disease	
Risk Factors	**Number of Risks**	**Two-Year Survival**
No prior nephrectomy KPS <80	0	45%
Hgb < normal Calcium > normal	1–2	17%
LDH > normal	3–5	3%

Hgb, hemoglobin; LDH, lactate dehydrogenase; KPS, Karnofsky Performance Scale.

Group performance status and stratifies patients into low-, intermediate-, or high-risk categories. The MSKCC system (Table 12.3) for advanced disease includes Karnofsky performance status, elevated lactate dehydrogenase levels, anemia, hypercalcemia, and the absence of prior nephrectomy, and predicts favorable, intermediate, or poor risk groups.

F. **Treatment considerations**

1. **Localized disease**. The majority of patients present with localized disease. The preferred treatment has become laparoscopic partial nephrectomy. First performed in 1990, it is associated with less postoperative pain, a shorter recovery time, and less overall morbidity. A radical nephrectomy, which includes removal of the perinephric fat and regional lymph nodes, is indicated for tumors that are greater than 7 cm and involve the renal pelvis. Most surgical patients with limited disease are cured. There is no current recommendation for adjuvant therapy, although there are open clinical trials investigating the role for adjuvant medical therapies (see subsequent discussion). Adjuvant radiation therapy does not improve survival as RCC is relatively radioresistant.

2. **Metastatic disease**. For patients with a solitary metastatic lesion at presentation, or on relapse, surgical removal of the metastatic foci can occasionally be curative. Cytoreductive nephrectomy has been shown to improve survival and is indicated in patients with good performance status, no brain metastases, and without rapidly progressing extrarenal disease. Inoperable, metastatic RCC is treated with molecular targeted therapy, antiangiogenic therapy, and immunotherapy (see subsequent discussion). Neither hormonal therapy nor chemotherapy has been shown to improve survival in patients with metastatic clear cell histology renal cancer. Some patients with non-clear cell renal carcinoma respond to chemotherapy.

G. Treatment regimens

1. Immunotherapy

a. Interleukin-2 (IL-2; aldesleukin [Proleukin]) mediates its antitumor effects through activation of a patient's lymphocytes, particularly those that are CD56+, converting them into lymphokine-activated killer cells. IL-2 alone results in overall response rates of up to 20% that include long-term survivors. There is a wide range of IL-2 doses and schedules, but recent randomized data shows high-dose bolus therapy (see Chapter 33) is more likely to lead to complete responses and long-term remissions than outpatient subcutaneously administered therapy. High-dose bolus therapy is highly toxic and is associated with a capillary leak syndrome (including hypotension, fluid retention, renal and hepatic hypoperfusion, and pulmonary edema), and it requires inpatient care by experienced personnel. High-dose bolus IL-2 is still an option for selected good-risk patients.

b. Interferon yields response rates of approximately 10%. Numerous treatment doses and schedules have been utilized. A representative one is 5 million IU/m^2 subcutaneously three times per week. The median response durations range between studies from 6 to 12 months. Response correlates with Karnofsky performance status greater than 80% and prior nephrectomy. It is rarely used now, owing to the demonstrated efficacy of several molecular targeted agents.

2. Molecular targeted agents—VEGF inhibitors

a. Sunitinib is a multikinase inhibitor that interferes with all receptors for platelet-derived growth factor receptor (PDGFR) and vascular endothelial growth factor receptor (VEGFR). Typical dosing is 50 mg orally per day for 4 weeks followed by a 2-week rest. Partial response rates of up to 40% with median time to disease progression greater than 8 months have been reported. Overall survival using sunitinib as a first-line agent is 26.4 months.

b. Sorafenib is another tyrosine kinase inhibitor, which at doses of 400 mg orally twice per day has been shown to improve progression-free survival versus placebo (24 weeks versus 12 weeks) after cytokine failure.

c. Bevacizumab, an antibody to VEGF, has response rates of 10% with some patients having progression-free intervals as long as 5 years. Doses of up to 10 mg/kg intravenously every 2 weeks have been utilized. Trials were performed in combination with interferon and showed improved overall survival. The activity of bevacizumab as a single agent is not well known, which led to approval by the U.S. Food and Drug

Administration (FDA) of the combination in patients with metastatic RCC.

   d. Pazopanib is a multi-VEGF inhibitor and PDGFR inhibitor that is the latest biologic compound to show activity in RCC. It is the latest FDA approved biologic agent for advanced RCC. The usual dosage is as follows:

   1. 800 mg by mouth daily without food
   2. 200 mg by mouth daily without food, if moderate hepatic impairment
   3. 400 mg or less by mouth if strong inhibitors of CYP3A4 cannot be avoided, as it is metabolized primarily by enzyme.

   Overall response rate is 30% and progression-free survival increased from 2.8 months for placebo to 11.1 months for pazopanib. Overall survival data are not yet available.

3. **Molecular targeted agents—mammalian target of rapamycin (mTOR) inhibitors**

   a. Temsirolimus is a novel kinase inhibitor that is a derivative of rapamycin. After temsirolimus complexes with the immunophilin FKBP12, the complex inhibits mTOR kinase activity. mTOR, as a master regulator of cell physiology, is involved in regulation of cell growth and angiogenesis, and changes that are induced downstream from mTOR as a consequence of the temsirolimus inhibition lead to cell cycle arrest at the G1 phase. In a randomized trial comparing interferon with temsirolimus in poor-risk patients with advanced RCC, overall survival was statistically better in the temsirolimus arm (10.9 months versus 7.3 months). The usual dosage and schedule is 25 mg intravenously weekly.

   b. Everolimus is a serine-threonine kinase inhibitor of mTOR. Everolimus is indicated for patients with advanced RCC who failed sorafenib or sunitinib based on a 2008 study in which progression-free survival doubled compared to placebo. The usual dosage and schedule is as follows:

   1. 10 mg by mouth once daily
   2. Reduce dose to 5 mg by mouth once daily for patients with Child-Pugh class B hepatic impairment or as needed to manage adverse drug reactions
   3. If strong inducers of CYP3A4 are required, increase daily dose in 5 mg increments to a maximum of 20 mg once daily.

4. **Cytotoxic chemotherapy/hormonal therapy.** Of historic note, vinblastine, medroxyprogesterone acetate, and tamoxifen, at best, produce responses in fewer than 5% of patients and therefore cannot be recommended.

5. **Adjuvant therapy.** No adjuvant therapy has been proven to improve survival after resection. However, there are ongoing trials with both sunitinib and sorafenib in the adjuvant setting for resected RCC at high risk of relapse.

6. **Combination therapy.** Newer doublets including bevacizumab and erlotinib (a tyrosine kinase receptor inhibitor that targets epidermal growth factor receptor), sunitinib and interferon, and sorafenib plus interferon do not demonstrate higher activity compared to single agents.

H. **Treatment strategies in the metastatic setting**

IL-2 is the treatment of choice for those who can tolerate its toxicities. Sunitinib or sorafenib should be considered in patients who are not candidates for intensive IL-2 therapy. Patients who progress after one of the active agents in RCC can be tried on another. The optimal sequence of drugs is not yet known. Whenever possible, after first-line therapy, participation in a clinical trial is recommended.

Selected Readings

Overviews

Mandell JS, McLaughlin JK, Schlehofer B, et al. International renal-cell study. IV. Occupation. *Int J Cancer.* 1995;61:601–605.

Motzer RJ, Mazumdar M, Bacik J, Berg W, Amsterdam A, Ferrara J. Survival and prognostic stratification of 670 patients with advanced renal cell carcinoma. *J Clin Oncol.* 1999;17(8):2530–2540.

Pancuck AJ, Zisman A, Belldegrun AS. The changing natural history of renal cell carcinoma. *J Urol.* 2001;166:1611.

Rini BI, Campbell SC, Escudier B. Renal cell carcinoma. *Lancet.* 2009;373(9669):1119–1132.

Rini BI. Metastatic renal cell carcinoma: many treatment options, one patient. *J Clin Oncol.* 2009;27(19):3225–3234.

Zisman A, Pantuck AJ, Wieder J, et al. Risk group assessment and clinical outcome algorithm to predict the natural history of patients with surgically resected renal cell carcinoma. *J Clin Oncol.* 2002;20:4559–4566.

Surgery

Chin AI, Lam JS, Figlin RA, Belldegrun AS. Surveillance strategies for renal cell carcinoma patients following nephrectomy. *Rev Urol.* 2006;8(1):1–7.

Biswas S, Kelly J, Eisen T. Cytoreductive nephrectomy in metastatic clear-cell renal cell carcinoma: perspectives in the tyrosine kinase inhibitor era. *Oncologist.* 2009; 14(1):52–59.

Figlin RA, Pierce WC, Kaboo R, et al. Treatment of metastatic renal cell carcinoma with nephrectomy, interleukin-2, and cytokine-primed or CD8(+) selected tumor infiltrating lymphocytes from primary tumor. *J Urol.* 1997;158(3):740–745.

Policari AJ, Gorbonos A, Milner JE, Flanigan RC. The role of cytoreductive nephrectomy in the era of molecular targeted therapies. *Int J Urol.* 2009;16(3): 227–233.

Immunotherapy/Targeted Agents

Escudier B, Szczylik C, Eisen T, et al. Randomized phase III trial of the raf kinase and VEGF inhibitor sorafenib (BAy 43-9006) in patients with advanced renal cell carcinoma (RCC). *J Clin Oncol.* 2005;23:380.

Fisher RI, Rosenberg SA, Fyfe G. Long-term survival update for high-dose recombinant Interleukin-2 therapy in patients with renal cell carcinoma. *Cancer J Sci Am.* 2000;6(Suppl 1):S55–S57.

Gollob J, Richmond T, Jones J, et al. Phase II trial of sorafenib plus interferon alpha 2b as first or second-line therapy in patients with metastatic renal cell cancer. *J Clin Oncol.* 2006;24(Suppl 18S):226s.

Hainsworth JD, Sosman JA, Spigel DR, Edwards DL, Baughman C, Greco A. Treatment of metastatic renal cell carcinoma with a combination of bevacizumab and erlotinib. *J Clin Oncol.* 2005;23(31):7889–7896.

Hudes G, Carducci M, Tomczak P, et al. A phase 3, randomized, 3-arm study of temsirolimus (TEMSR) or interferon-alpha (IFN) or the combination of TEMSR + IFN in the treatment of first-line, poor-risk patients with advanced renal cell carcinoma (adv RCC). *J Clin Oncol (Meeting Abstracts).* 2006;24(18S):LBA4.

McDermott DF, Regan MM, Clark JI, et al. Randomized phase III trial of high-dose interleukin-2 versus subcutaneous interleukin-2 and interferon in patients with metastatic renal cell carcinoma. *J Clin Oncol.* 2005;23(1):133–141.

Motzer RJ, Escudier B, Oudard S, et al. Efficacy of everolimus in advanced renal cell carcinoma: a double-blind, randomized, placebo-controlled phase III trial. *Lancet.* 2008;372(9637):449–456.

Motzer RJ, Michaelson MD, Redman BG, et al. Activity of SU11248, a multitargeted inhibitor of vascular endothelial growth factor receptor and platelet-derived growth factor receptor, in patients with metastatic renal cell carcinoma. *J Clin Oncol.* 2006;24:16–24.

Rini BI, Small EJ. Biology and clinical development of vascular endothelial growth factor- targeted therapy in renal cell carcinoma. *J Clin Oncol.* 2005;23: 1028–1043.

Rosenberg SA, Lotze MT, Yang JC, et al. Prospective randomized trial of high-dose interleukin-2 alone or in conjunction with lymphokine-activated killer cells for the treatment of patients with advanced cancer. *J Natl Cancer Inst.* 1993;85: 622–632.

Ryan CW, Goldman BH, Lara PN Jr, et al. Sorafenib plus interferon-a2b as first-line therapy for advanced renal cell carcinoma: SWOG 0412. *J Clin Oncol.* 2006;24(Suppl 18S):223s.

Schwartzentruber D. Guidelines for the safe administration of high-dose interleukin-2. *J Immunother.* 2001;24:287–292.

Sternberg CN, Davis ID, Mardiak J, et al. Pazopanib in locally advanced or metastatic renal cell carcinoma; results of a randomized phase III trial. *J Clin Oncol.* 2010;28(6):1061–1068.

Yang JC. Bevacizumab for patients with metastatic renal cancer: an update. *Clin Cancer Res.* 2004;10(18 Pt 2):6367S–6370S.

13

Thyroid and Adrenal Carcinomas

Haitham S. Abu-Lebdeh, Michael E. Menefee, and Keith C. Bible

Endocrine cancers account for 2.7% of all newly diagnosed cancers but only 0.44% of cancer deaths in the United States, largely due to the overall good prognosis of the most common endocrine malignancy, differentiated thyroid cancer. Thyroid cancers account for almost 95% of endocrine cancers and for two-thirds of the deaths from this group of diseases. Although the efficacy of cytotoxic chemotherapy is limited in differentiated thyroid cancers, it has an established role in anaplastic thyroid cancer, adrenocortical cancer, and pheochromocytoma/paraganglioma. Moreover, novel therapeutics—in particular tyrosine kinase inhibitors (TKIs)—have emerged as promising approaches to treating several endocrine cancers. Here, thyroid and adrenal neoplasms are discussed with emphasis on individualizing therapy for patients afflicted with these diseases. Neuroendocrine cancers, in particular pancreatic islet cell carcinomas (as well as other pancreatic malignancies), are discussed separately in Chapter 8.

I. THYROID CARCINOMA
A. Background
1. **Incidence.** About 37,000 new cases of thyroid carcinoma are diagnosed in the United States annually, accounting for approximately 1600 deaths. The incidence of thyroid carcinoma is now about 9 per 100,000, with approximately 2.7 times as many women as men affected. The peak incidence is at age 40 for women and age 60 for men. Thyroid cancers are increasing—in women at >5% per year; mortality is also up by one-third in the last decade, suggesting that the increasing incidence is real and not due to better screening/detection. Thyroid carcinoma is now over twice as common in the United States as it was 10 years ago, and it is now the seventh most common cancer in U.S. women.

2. **Etiology and prevention.** In most patients, the cause of thyroid carcinoma is unknown, but prior remote head and neck radiation exposure, hereditary factors, and/or preceding autoimmune thyroid disease are implicated in some patients. Radiation to the neck during childhood for diseases including Hodgkin lymphoma, enlarged thymus, or even skin diseases such as acne can

be causative. Thyroid cancer has been observed 20 to 25 years after radiation exposure among atomic bomb survivors, and in some regions of Japan the incidence of thyroid cancer in screened populations is as high as 0.1%—10-fold greater than expected based on U.S. incidence rates. In cases of accidental radioisotope exposure, expeditious use of potassium iodide can block the thyroid uptake of radioactive iodine (RAI).

Some cases of thyroid carcinoma are familial. Medullary thyroid cancer (MTC) is seen in multiple endocrine neoplasia (MEN) syndrome types 2A and 2B and in the familial MTC (FMTC) syndrome associated with germline mutation of the RET proto-oncogene. In these syndromes, prophylactic thyroidectomy should be undertaken in at-risk individuals at young ages. Furthermore, there are kindreds of patients with increased heritable risk of differentiated thyroid cancers, known as familial non-MTC, but such kindreds are uncommon.

Prolonged stimulation by thyroid-stimulating hormone (TSH), as seen in endemic goiter and autoimmune thyroid disease, may also lead to the development of thyroid carcinoma. As autoimmune thyroid disease is more prevalent in women, this may in part explain why thyroid cancer is so much more common in women than men. Further, this may also help explain why many patients with thyroid cancer relate a family history of autoimmune thyroid disease and suffer from autoimmune thyroid disease themselves.

3. **Histologic types**. The most common types of thyroid carcinoma are as follows.

a. **Differentiated thyroid cancer (DTC; 88%)**. DTC includes papillary thyroid cancer (PTC; 85%), follicular thyroid cancer (FTC; 12%), and Hürthle cell (3%) subtypes. DTCs are derived from thyroglobulin-producing follicular cells (thyrocytes) and are typically initially RAI responsive. Hürthle cell carcinoma, a histological variant of FTC often of more aggressive behavior, has variously been subsumed under the FTC classification rather than being considered a unique histotype. RET/PTC gene rearrangements or RAS, BRAF, or MEK-ERK pathway mutations are present in 70% of PTCs, and upregulation of vascular endothelial growth factor (VEGF) signaling is also common in metastatic disease. FTC may be associated with RAS mutations and mutations on chromosome 3 (pax8-PPAR mutations). DTCs most often secrete thyroglobulin; hence, it can be used as a tumor marker in antithyroglobulin antibody–negative patients.

b. **Medullary thyroid cancer (UTC; 4%)**. MTCs are derived from thyroid parafollicular or C cells, the source of the hormone calcitonin. Activating mutations of the RET proto-oncogene are characteristic, with germ line activating RET mutations as seen in FMTC and MEN2 a predisposing factor. MTC most often produces both immunoreactive calcitonin and carcinoembryonic antigen, which can be used as tumor markers.

c. **Anaplastic thyroid cancer (ATC; 2%).** ATC is the most aggressive of all thyroid cancers, with only about 10% historical 1-year survival from diagnosis. ATC can arise de novo, but is generally thought to result from thyrocytes via dedifferentiation in DTC tumors. ATC (grade 4 thyroid cancer) is distinguished from the undifferentiated histotype (grade 3) in part by loss of TTF-1 expression, and abnormalities in p53 signaling are also common.

d. **Thyroid lymphoma (5%).** Thyroid lymphomas are uncommon and represent cancers of lymphoid tissues, as discussed in Chapters 21 and 22.

e. **Thyroid sarcoma (<1%).** Thyroid sarcomas are also rare, and they should be treated in accordance with their underlying histology, as discussed in Chapter 16.

f. **Squamous cell carcinoma of the thyroid (<1%).** Rarely, squamous cell cancers arise in the thyroid; they are best treated as in head and neck primary squamous cell carcinoma (see Chapter 5).

4. **Prognosis**

a. **Cell types/histology.** PTCs and mixed PTC/FTCs have similar, generally favorable biologic and prognostic behaviors. Most DTCs grow slowly, with recurrence risk 0.5% to 1.6% per year, and with less than 15% mortality at 20 years. Even patients with lung metastases have a 20-year survival rate exceeding 50%.

Pure FTCs have a somewhat worse prognosis than cancers with papillary elements, with 10-year survival in FTC and PTC at 85% and 93%, respectively. Recent studies have shown that FTCs with vascular invasion have a relatively worse prognosis, whereas FTC patients without vascular invasion do almost as well as PTC patients.

About 25% of MTCs are familial, as part of three clinical syndromes (MEN-IIa, MEN-IIb, and familial non-MEN MTC). Regional nodal and distant metastases are more common and occur in early stages of the disease in MTC, with 10-year survival after surgical resection of MTC at 40% to 60%.

Patients with ATC have an abysmal prognosis, with a median survival of only 4 months and a historical 10% survival 1 year from diagnosis.

b. **Other factors.** Prognosis is worse if tumor size is >4 cm, patient age >40 years of age and/or male gender, distant metastases are present, and/or DNA content is aneuploid. DTC tends to metastasize first to lymph nodes, then to lung, and somewhat less commonly bone—with 5-, 10-, and 15-year survivals of 53%, 38%, and 30%, respectively. Other sites of metastases in DTC include subcutaneous structures, liver, and also brain. In contrast to most other cancers, limited regional lymph node metastasis of DTC does not influence survival substantially, and radiation-induced DTC is not associated with a worse prognosis.

Several systems are used to predict outcomes in DTC, including for example, the MACIS scoring system (*m*etastases, $+3$ if metastases; *a*ge, ≤ 39 years of age $= 3.1$, $>40 =$ age in years $\times 0.08$; *c*ompleteness of resection, $+1$ if primary resection is incomplete; *i*nvasion, $+1$ if pathologically invasive; and *s*ize, $0.3 \times$ largest dimension in centimeters) with median prognosis estimated based on the total score as indicated in Table 13.1.

B. Diagnosis and staging

Although physical examination is the primary screening modality for the detection of thyroid cancer, in populations at increased risk, neck ultrasound is an important supplemental approach. Any solitary thyroid nodule should be considered malignant until proved otherwise. Although toxic nodular goiters are less likely to contain carcinoma, a nodule in the setting of hyperthyroidism does not preclude malignancy.

Because most thyroid tumors spread primarily by local extension and regional nodal metastasis, assessment of the extent of disease in the neck is critical. In recent years, ultrasound has become integrated into endocrinology practices and is very helpful in assessing risk of cancer, and in facilitating expeditious outpatient fine needle aspiration (FNA) of suspicious thyroid nodules. FNA does not require local anesthesia and is considered safer and easier to perform than core biopsy, with accuracy between 50% and 97%, depending on the type of cancer, the experience of the pathologist, and the institution; however, there are times when formal core biopsies are required, including when lymphoma is suspected.

TABLE 13.1	MACIS Prognostic Scoring System for Thyroid Cancer
Total MACIS Score	**Twenty-Year Survival**
<6	99%
6	89%
7–8	56%
>8	24%

Modified from Edge SB, Byrd DR, Compton CC. *AJCC cancer staging manual* (7th ed.). New York: Springer; 2010.

Diagnostic RAI imaging is not now commonly used in the primary assessment of thyroid nodules, but remains a mainstay of assessment in patients with high-risk disease or with metastatic radioiodine-avid DTC after primary surgery. Chest radiography should be performed before surgery to rule out macroscopic pulmonary metastasis. If there is any clinical or laboratory suggestion of bone or other metastases, skeletal radiographs, computed tomography (CT) scan, positron emission tomography (PET) scan, and/or a radionuclide bone scan should be considered on a case-by-case basis.

Several issues should also be kept in mind in assessing disease extent and response to therapy. First, iodinated contrast materials should not be used in any DTC patients who may be candidates for therapeutic radioiodine, as the iodine load can saturate tumor binding sites and thereby render therapeutic RAI ineffective. In general, a 2-month delay of RAI is preferred after any iodinated contrast. Second, anatomic imaging in surveillance of patients and in following disease course is important. In DTC for instance, a negative iodine/thyroid scan does not exclude the possibility of metastatic disease, as small pulmonary nodules often escape detection using this modality. Further, some DTCs will become radioiodine refractory and will not image even in the presence of bulky metastases. Third, although tumor markers can be very helpful in patient surveillance in the postoperative setting in DTC and MTC, they must be used judiciously. Thyroglobulin can be neutralized by patient antithyroglobulin antibodies, and therefore the two tests should always be measured in tandem. If antithyroglobulin antibody is elevated, thyroglobulin levels are uninterpretable. Moreover, with time and interval therapies, thyroglobulin production by DTCs diminishes concordant with tumor dedifferentiation, thereby yielding misleading results—and again emphasizing the importance of anatomic imaging in high-risk patients or those with advanced disease. Thyroglobulin levels are also less predictable in estimating disease extent in patients receiving novel therapies.

Also worthy of comment is that PET imaging should be used judiciously in thyroid cancer. In ATC, PET can be very helpful; however, some DTCs do not image well via PET. In DTC, PET avidity tends to correlate with more aggressive tumor behavior.

Patients with thyroid carcinoma are typically euthyroid; however, elevated TSH with increased thyroid peroxidase antibodies may be seen with Hashimoto thyroiditis, which may coexist in 20% of patients with thyroid lymphoma and also sometimes in DTC.

The most widely accepted tumor staging system, TNM, uses tumor size and extent, presence of lymph node spread, and distant metastasis (Table 13.2). Any ATC is considered stage IV (A, B, or C),

	Pathologic TNM Staging System for Thyroid Cancer		
Stage	**Papillary or Follicular, Age <45**	**Papillary or Follicular, Age >45; Medullary Any Age**	**Anaplastic, Any Age**
I	M0	T1, N0, M0	—
II	M1	T2, N0, M0	—
III	—	T3, N0, M0 T1–3, N1a, M0	—
IV	—	T4, Any N, M0 T1–3, N1b, M0 Any T, Any N, M1	Any

M1, distant metastasis; N1a, metastasis to central lymph node compartment; N1b, metastasis to other lymph nodes; T1, <2 cm; T2, 2–4 cm; T3, >4 cm; T4, any tumor invading tissue beyond thyroid capsule.

and there are no TNM stage III or IV patients with DTC who are younger than 45 years. This staging system is suboptimal in thyroid cancer, prompting use of algorithms such as the MACIS system discussed above.

C. Treatment

Therapeutic approach in thyroid cancer depends considerably on the histologic type, extent of disease, patient symptoms, and rate of disease progression. Careful management of disease residing in the neck so as to protect airway, esophagus, and other critical structures is also of paramount importance.

1. Differentiated thyroid cancer (DTC)

a. Surgery. Bilateral near-total or total thyroidectomy is the best initial approach in thyroid cancer, taking into consideration that with DTC the incidence of disease in the contralateral lobe is 20% to 87%. Further, total thyroidectomy is conducive to RAI surveillance, and simplifies follow-up in patients with high-risk disease. Limited lymph node involvement does not influence survival but is associated with an increase in local recurrence risk; therefore, routine central compartment neck dissection should be considered. Total thyroidectomy with modified neck dissection is often preferred for those who have lateral cervical lymph node involvement. Mortality consequent to thyroidectomy in DTC is extremely low. Complications include recurrent laryngeal nerve damage that is permanent in 2% of patients and hypoparathyroidism that is lifelong in 1% to 2% of patients.

b. TSH suppression. TSH suppression via administration of "supratherapeutic" levothyroxine is an essential component in the treatment of high-risk DTC, as residual cancer cells are usually initially responsive to TSH growth stimulation. Levothyroxine (T_4, usual dosage range 125 to 200 μg by mouth daily) is administered to keep the TSH level suppressed below 0.1 mIU/L in high-risk patients, including those with systemic metastases and/or residual disease following surgery. However, suppression of TSH below 0.1 mIU/L imposes long-term adverse effects on bone and can negatively impact quality of life, sometimes producing symptoms of thyrotoxicosis. Angina can also be provoked by suppressive dosage levothyroxine, as can tachycardia or sometimes even frank cardiac arrhythmia, so care must be used in the selection of patients in whom the risks of aggressive TSH suppression is justified.

c. **Radiotherapy—RAI.** Radiation can be applied in two general ways in the treatment of DTC: systemic RAI versus focal external beam or stereotactic radiotherapy. Destruction of residual normal thyroid tissue after thyroidectomy with RAI (^{131}I) is termed radioactive remnant ablation (RRA). RRA is different from "RAI therapy"; in RAI therapy, larger doses of RAI are used to attempt to destroy persistent cancer, whereas RRA is used to eliminate residual normal thyroid tissue remaining after primary surgery. RRA is widely used in practice in the United States following thyroidectomy, but there has recently been increased scrutiny of the prudence of RRA in patients with anticipated excellent long-term prognosis as estimated using the prognostic algorithms (e.g., MACIS).

When ablation is carried out postoperatively, it is usually done 4 to 6 weeks after thyroidectomy. RRA allows for better subsequent imaging with RAI when looking for metastasis and also improves the utility of thyroglobulin in the detection of residual thyroid cancer (as remnant thyroid tissue is destroyed). An RRA dose of 30 mCi (1110 MBq) to 150 mCi (5550 MBq) is commonly used, with the lower dose of 30 mCi more typical, with an estimated 6 rem whole body exposure. For patients who are at a low risk of tumor recurrence, remnant ablation is controversial.

Treatment with RAI (^{131}I) is usually recommended for patients with DTC and known postoperative residual disease, patients with distant metastases, and/or patients with locally invasive lesions. For patients with nodal metastases that are not large enough to excise, a dose of 100 to 175 mCi of RAI is commonly given (3700 to 6475 MBq). Locally invasive cancer that is not completely resected is alternatively often treated with 150 to 200 mCi of RAI (5550 to 7400 MBq), while patients with distant metastasis are treated with 200 to 250 or even 300 mCi (7400 MBq). The potential exception to this schema is lung metastasis; a dose of up to 80 mCi of RAI (2960 MBq) whole body retention by dosimetry at 48 hours is generally used to avoid radiation-induced pulmonary fibrosis.

Effective and safe use of RAI treatment requires that tumor cells that are capable of concentrating iodide (i.e., DTC), and appropriate patient preparation to bring TSH levels up by either temporarily withholding thyroid hormone administration or via administration of recombinant TSH is necessary. In the former situation, due to its long half life, T_4 is discontinued and T_3 is initiated for a period of 6 weeks prior to the scan, with all thyroid medication withheld in the 2-week period prior to RAI administration. Ideally, TSH of 25 to 30 $\mu m/mL$ is required for successful ablation or radiotherapy. Alternatively, recombinant TSH can be used to stimulate thyroid cell uptake of RAI in the absence of T_4 withdrawal; this approach maintains better quality of life but adds considerably to expense. A low iodine diet is also required for RAI efficacy, as dietary iodine can compete with RAI for uptake in normal thyrocytes and tumor and thereby reduce RAI therapeutic efficacy. Compliance with a low iodine diet is assessed via measurement of 24-hour urinary iodine excretion.

Patients receiving high dose RAI (150 to 300 mCi) must be treated at centers with special lead-lined containment rooms, with monitoring of treated patients to assure compliance with environmental radiation safety regulations and patient and population safety. The duration of hospitalization depends on the dose given, posttherapy method of transportation home, and contact of patient with the general public. Potential side effects of RAI include temporary bone marrow suppression (this can last weeks or even months with repeated high RAI dosage), transient nausea, sialoadenitis/dry mouth (with possible permanent cessation of salivary flow), skin reaction over the tissue concentrating the radioiodine, and pulmonary fibrosis. The use of very high cumulative RAI doses (usually when approaching 1000 mCi) have also rarely been associated with acute myelogenous leukemia, as well as rarely with bladder and breast cancers. Scintigraphy should be performed 4 to 10 days after RAI therapy to assess uptake of RAI by tumor and to detect residual carcinoma perhaps not otherwise seen using other imaging approaches.

d. **Radiotherapy—focal approaches including external beam radiotherapy.** The role of external radiation therapy in DTC is limited to treating progressive residual locoregional tumor in the neck that does not concentrate iodine and that is otherwise not amenable to effective surgery. External beam radiotherapy is also used for localized painful bony metastasis or other locally threatening disease. Stereotactic radiosurgical approaches

(Gamma Knife, Elekta, Stockholm, Sweden; CyberKnife, Accuray, Sunnyvale, CA) are also used in patients with recurrent cancer at previously irradiated sites and when tumors are proximal to critical radiation-sensitive tumors.

e. **Systemic therapies.** Systemic cytotoxic chemotherapy has produced disappointing results in DTC. Recently, VEGF-receptor-inhibitory TKIs (e.g., sunitinib, sorafenib, pazopanib) have shown promise in phase II clinical trials. Although partial response rates as assessed by Response Evaluation Criteria in Solid Tumors criteria range from 20% to 50% using these agents, no survival advantage from use of TKIs in DTC patients has yet been demonstrated. Expert consensus nevertheless presently favors selective use of TKIs in treating patients with imminently threatening rapidly progressive metastatic DTC, and it is best in conjunction with a clinical trial.

2. **Medullary thyroid cancer (MTC)**

   a. **Surgery.** MTC, like DTC, is best treated initially with surgery—with the caveat that patients with FMTC syndromes should be subject to early prophylactic thyroidectomy.

   b. **Radiotherapy.** As MTC does not uptake iodine, RAI has no role. Locoregional radiation therapy, however, is useful in some patients as palliative therapy, as discussed previously.

   c. **Systemic therapies.** Suppressive levothyroxine therapy is of no benefit in MTC. As MTC most often harbors receptors for somatostatin, somatostatin analogues such as octreotide have been preliminarily tested as therapeutic in MTC. The precise extent of benefit to be attained from the use of therapeutic octreotide in MTC remains uncertain; however, some patients appear to gain benefit.

   Recently, orally bioavailable TKIs (e.g., vandetanib, sunitinib, sorafenib, pazopanib) that inhibit RET have been tested in phase II and III clinical trials in MTC, with promising initial results. Prolonged disease stabilization as well as impressive clinical responses have been reported, but impact on survival has not yet been established. Expert consensus supports the selective application of TKIs in patients with rapidly progressive imminently threatening MTC, and it is best in conjunction with ongoing clinical trials.

3. **Anaplastic thyroid cancer (ATC)** has been historically associated with only 10% overall survival 1 year from diagnosis. As a result, improved therapies are sorely needed. Although locoregional recurrence is a major issue, most deaths result primarily from systemic disease.

   a. **Surgery.** Surgery alone is seldom curative in ATC, and when undertaken should be followed at least by locoregional radiotherapy. Surgery also has an uncertain role in treating patients with stage 4C (metastatic) disease. In locoregionally confined disease (stage 4A/B), surgery has the potential to protect vital structures within the neck otherwise imminently threatened by tumor invasion and should be considered.

b. **Radiotherapy.** Radiotherapy has an established role in the locoregional treatment of ATC. In stage 4C ATC, where no possibility of cure is anticipated, radiotherapy represents an attractive alternative to surgery, and it is best to use an accelerated regimen.

In stage 4A and 4B disease where a "curative intent" approach is elected, a more protracted radiation therapy course best utilizing intensity modulated radiation therapy (IMRT) should be strongly considered. In this latter circumstance, administration of concomitant radiosensitizing chemotherapy should be considered, as chemotherapy has the potential also to treat occult systemic disease.

c. **Systemic therapies for ATC.** Discouragingly, ATC is almost universally disseminated when diagnosed, accounting for its dire prognosis even when apparently only regionally spread. Most (about 60%) of all ATCs are unresectable or metastatic at the time of presentation.

(1) **Single-agent chemotherapy.** The two classes of cytotoxic agents with the greatest evidence in support of efficacy in ATC are anthracyclines (e.g., doxorubicin) and taxanes (e.g., paclitaxel), each with response rates in advanced disease as high as 50%. Improved survival may be achieved in patients with advanced disease who respond to these agents. Furthermore, there is accumulating rationale that the use of these agents in combination with IMRT in the adjuvant setting may also extend survival.

■ **Doxorubicin** at a dosage of 60 to 75 mg/m^2 intravenously (IV) every 3 weeks has resulted in objective responses in 20% to 45% (median, 34%) in patients with advanced ATC. Alternatively, weekly doxorubicin at a dosage of 20 mg/m^2 IV is similarly or perhaps even slightly more effective—and preferred in debilitated patients.

■ Taxanes (paclitaxel and docetaxel) also have activity in ATC, with paclitaxel (60 to 90 mg/m^2/week) shown to have a transient response rate of 53%.

■ Novel agents including combretastatin and TKIs (e.g., sunitinib, sorafenib, pazopanib) have also produced anecdotal responses in phase II ATC trials, and are currently under active evaluation as candidate ATC therapeutics, especially combined with cytotoxins. In particular, TKIs produce frequent clinical responses in DTC and are considered emerging therapeutics in these cancers.

(2) **Combination chemotherapy.** Combination chemotherapy has been used in ATC, but it is uncertain whether multiagent therapy impacts survival more than single-agent therapies.

- Cisplatin 50 mg/m^2 IV plus doxorubicin 50 mg/m^2 IV every 3 weeks is sometimes used in ATC but has not yet been shown to improve survival over single agents.
- Doxorubicin 50 mg/m^2 IV combined with docetaxel 50 mg/m^2 IV (with growth factor support) administered every 3 weeks has also been used in advanced ATC, as has doxorubicin 50 mg/m^2 IV combined with paclitaxel 220 mg/m^2 IV administered every 3 weeks. However, combination therapy carries higher risk and side effects than monotherapy, and has not yet been shown to have a survival advantage in ATC.

At present, even if a patient with advanced ATC responds to chemotherapy, a prolongation of the median survival time by several months is generally all that can be achieved. Therefore, novel therapies should be strongly considered, with particular interest presently in combination regimens involving either TKIs or combretastatin. For a list of active trials visit www.clinicaltrials.gov.

II. ADRENAL CARCINOMA

A. Adrenal cortical carcinoma (ACC)

1. **Incidence and etiology.** ACC is a rare tumor, with approximately 300 new cases occurring annually in the United States. It accounts for 0.05% to 0.2% of all cancers and for 0.2% of cancer deaths. It has a prevalence of 0.5 to 2 per 1 million of the population worldwide. There is a bimodal distribution with the overwhelming majority of patients being affected during the fourth and fifth decades of life. However, a second peak can be seen in the pediatric population in children under the age of 5 years, and adults of any age can be affected. The incidence in women is slightly higher than in men (1.2:1.0). Tumors can be either functional (hormone-producing) or nonfunctional. Functional tumors are more common in women, but also occur commonly in men. The overwhelming majority of ACC cases are sporadic; however, this malignancy can occur more frequently in certain genetic syndromes including Li-Fraumeni syndrome, Beckwith-Wiedemann syndrome, MEN-1, and familial adenomatous polyposis. There have been no clear and consistent, modifiable lifestyle risk factors that have been identified that influence the risk of developing ACC.

2. **Clinical manifestations**. Adrenal carcinoma may present in several modes.
   a. **Hormonal excess**. Forty to sixty percent of patients present with a functioning tumor, with signs and symptoms of hypercortisolism (20% to 40%), and virilization (40% to 50%) being the most common with feminization (<10%) and hyperaldosteronism (<1%) occurring much less frequently. Many ACC patients may have elevated adrenal hormones without overt clinical signs of excess.
   b. **Abdominal mass**. An adrenal mass may present as a palpable or, more rarely, visible lesion in a patient with a large mass and a thin body habitus. More often, the mass is either detected during an evaluation for the presence of unexplained abdominal pain or due to signs or symptoms of hormonal excess or constitutional symptoms (weight loss, anorexia, malaise, fatigue) that are suggestive of an underlying malignancy. An adrenal mass may also be detected as an incidental finding when abdominal imaging for some other purpose is being performed.
3. **Pathology and diagnosis**. Most malignant adrenal masses represent metastatic lesions from another primary cancer. The greater diagnostic dilemma is created by the presence of a solitary adrenal nodule or mass. While there are radiographic criteria that can help distinguish benign adrenal lesions from malignant ones, these are not absolute. Furthermore, it can be very difficult to discern an adrenal adenoma from ACC based on tumor histology alone. CT scans and magnetic resonance imaging (MRI) are helpful in diagnosing ACC. A CT scan finding of a large unilateral adrenal mass with irregular borders and a heterogeneous and hypervascular interior is almost always an indication of adrenal cancer. On MRI, adrenal cancer has intermediate to high signal intensity on T2-weighted images in contrast to benign lesions, which have low signal intensity. Furthermore, MRI is a helpful tool in detecting vascular invasion. PET scans have demonstrated some promise in the staging and follow-up of patients with ACC. Other nuclear traces, such as (11)C-metomidate, also are very sensitive and specific for the identification of adrenal cortical tumors, but are not routinely available for clinical use.

   Histologically, differentiating ACC from clear cell renal cell carcinoma can also prove challenging without the appropriate clinical background. The molecular pathogenesis is not as well defined for ACC as it is with other solid tumors, in part due to its rarity. Nonetheless, some studies have detected genetic alterations in patients with familial ACC which may also be relevant in sporadic forms of ACC. In particular, mutations in beta catenin, the insulinlike growth factor pathways, and p53 have been identified as mutated and overexpressed in ACC, and to a lesser degree, adrenal adenomas.

4. **Staging and prognosis.** The most commonly used staging system (derived from the TNM classification system) for ACC is presented in Table 13.3.

   Metastases of ACC most commonly occur in the lung (60%), lymph nodes (43%), liver (53%), and bone (10%). The median survival time of patients with well-differentiated carcinoma is 40 months, whereas patients with anaplastic ACC have a more dismal median survival time of 5 months. The median survival time of patients with stage I, II, or III disease is 24 to 28 months and for stage IV disease 12 months. Intratumoral hemorrhage, number of mitotic figures per high-power field, and tumor size correlate with survival rates.

5. **Treatment.** Due to the extremely low incidence of this disease, few clinicians or medical centers have sufficient experience treating it, and an effort should be made to refer these patients to centers that have clinical trials pertaining to this disease. This caveat notwithstanding, several guidelines regarding its treatment can be given.

   a. **Surgery.** Surgical resection provides the best opportunity for cure or prolonged survival for patients who have localized disease. Furthermore, patients who have metastatic disease that is amenable to surgical resection and who undergo successful metastasectomy have improved survivals compared to those receiving systemic therapy. This is a paradigm shift from the typical oncology patient with metastatic disease for whom surgery is usually not a consideration. That said, many patients have either local invasion that is too extensive or metastases that cannot be resected who will require systemic therapy.

      Surgery for the primary tumor should be performed, ideally, by a surgeon with a great deal of experience resecting

TABLE 13.3	MacFarlane/TNM Staging System for Adrenal Cortical Cancer		
Stage	**Tumor**	**Nodes**	**Metastasis**
I	T1 (≤5 cm)	N0	M0
II	T2 (>5 cm)	N0	M0
III	T3 (local invasion)	N0	M0
	T1/T2	N1 (mobile)	M0
IV	Any T (and N2)	N2 (fixed)	M1
	T4 (gross invasion of adjacent organs)		

ACCs. An area of evolving controversy is the role of laparoscopic resection for adrenal masses. Until data mature from
ongoing trials evaluating open versus laparoscopic adrenalectomy, open should remain the standard of care.

b. Radiotherapy. Radiation therapy provides symptomatic relief
from pain due to local or metastatic disease, especially bony
metastases. It has also been used to prevent local recurrence
after surgical resection (40 to 55 Gy over 4 weeks), but the
benefit is uncertain, and there is no proof that it improves
survival.

c. Systemic therapy. Systemic therapy for ACC consists of controlling excessive hormonal production, in appropriate patients,
and treating the carcinoma with cytotoxic therapy. ACC has
historically been refractory to many chemotherapeutics, in
part due to its high expression of drug-resistance proteins.
Nevertheless, progress has been made with the use of combination chemotherapy. Indications for chemotherapy include
recurrent, metastatic, and nonresectable ACC. Agents used
are the following.

(1) Adrenal cortical suppressants

(a) Mitotane (*o,p′*-DDD; Lysodren) has been used to treat
ACC since 1960. It inhibits steroid biosynthesis and,
with prolonged use, destroys adrenal cells. The cytotoxic effects of mitotane against ACC are not well established. Much of the benefit derived from mitotane
is primarily due to its adrenolytic effects and subsequent reduction in excessive hormone production.
Now that many ACC patients are diagnosed at earlier
stages, the effects of mitotane for advanced disease
are less certain and cytotoxic agents are usually warranted, although often mitotane remains a part of the
therapeutic strategy. The drug is highly lipid soluble
and is subsequently concentrated in both normal and
malignant adrenal cortical cells. Reports of its plasma
half-life range from 18 to 159 days.

(i) Dosage and administration. Treatment with mitotane is started at 2 to 6 g/day by mouth in three
divided doses, then gradually increased monthly
by 1 g/day until 9 to 10 g/day is reached or until the
maximum tolerated dose is achieved with no side
effects. Blood levels of *o,p′*-DDD should be maintained between 14 and 20 μg/mL to demonstrate
a therapeutic response. Mitotane serum level was
shown in a retrospective study to be the only significant prognostic factor for tumor response. Levels
of more than 20 μg/mL have a higher incidence of

toxicity. Starting at a small dose and increasing it gradually may delay achieving adequate plasma levels; frequently, starting at a higher dose of 6 to 9 grams may be tolerated and may shorten the time required to achieve therapeutic effect.

(ii) **Side effects.** Nausea and vomiting occur in 80% of patients. Severe neurotoxicity, which may occur during long-term treatment, presents as somnolence, depression, ataxia, and weakness in 40% of patients. Reversible diffuse electroencephalographic changes may also occur. Adrenal insufficiency occurs in 50% of patients (without replacement), and dermatitis develops in 20% of patients. Because the maximal dosage is often limited by the severity of and the patient's tolerance to the side effects, the total dose may range widely from patient to patient.

(iii) **Glucocorticoid replacement.** During mitotane treatment, it is necessary to provide replacement therapy for the adrenal insufficiency that is induced by mitotane. Therapy will often need to be maintained for several weeks to months after mitotane is discontinued until adrenal function returns. Replacement can be achieved by administering the equivalent of hydrocortisone 20 mg orally in the morning and 10 mg in the evening. Plasma cortisol should be used to monitor adrenal function during mitotane use. If severe trauma or shock develops, mitotane should be discontinued immediately and larger doses of corticosteroids (e.g., hydrocortisone 100 mg three times a day) should be administered. Fludrocortisone may also be required to maintain adequate mineralocorticoid homeostasis.

(b) **Alternative adrenal cortical suppressants.** Many patients cannot tolerate mitotane at a dose sufficient to achieve therapeutic levels. These patients can be treated with other adrenal cortical suppressants including metyrapone (750 mg by mouth every 4 hours), which reduces cortisol production by inhibiting 11β-hydroxylase. However, this results in accumulation of deoxycorticosterone and can induce hypertension and hypokalemic alkalosis.

Another agent is aminoglutethimide (250 mg by mouth every 6 hours initially, with a stepwise increase in dosage to a total of 2 g/day or until limiting side effects that resemble those of mitotane appear). Aminoglutethimide inhibits conversion of cholesterol to pregnenolone. Neither of these medications has antitumor effects, but they are effective in relieving the signs and symptoms of excessive hormonal secretion. Combining both in smaller doses might reduce the side effects seen in taking higher doses of either agent alone. Another medication that can be used is ketoconazole up to 800 mg/day. It is a potent adrenal inhibitor that produces clinical alleviation of the signs and symptoms within 4 to 6 weeks.

(2) Cytotoxic chemotherapy. Very few patients will have a sustained, objective response to single-agent mitotane. More commonly, cytotoxic drugs are being used in patients who show no response to mitotane or in combination with mitotane in the first-line setting. The optimal regimen has not clearly been identified; however, cisplatin-containing regimens have consistently demonstrated the greatest activity.

The most commonly used regimen is etoposide 100 mg/m^2 IV on days 5 to 7, doxorubicin 20 mg/m^2 on days 1 and 8, and cisplatin 40 mg/m^2 on days 1 and 9 every 4 weeks, combined with mitotane 4 gm/day for 3 to 8 months. This resulted in objective response in almost 50% of patients treated during a phase II clinical trial; an international, randomized, phase II study is ongoing to confirm this benefit. For patients with marginal performance status who may not be a candidate for triple therapy or doxorubicin, single-agent cisplatin or a platinum doublet, most commonly with etoposide, or an agent such gemcitabine, can be considered.

- Cisplatin 75 to 100 mg/m^2 was combined with mitotane 4 g by mouth daily. This resulted in a 30% objective response that lasted for 7.9 months. The survival duration in this study was 11.8 months.
- Etoposide 100 mg/m^2 IV on days 1 to 3 plus cisplatin 100 mg/m^2 IV given in cycles every 4 weeks plus mitotane led to partial remission in 33% of 18 patients with ACC.

Another regimen that was used frequently in the past and still can be considered for refractory patients is a combination of streptozocin 1 gm/day by mouth for 5 days then 2 gm every 3 weeks combined with mitotane 1 to 4 gm by mouth daily. Clinical trials are of high priority in this patient population due to a lack of durable, effective regimens.

d. Alternative modalities

(1) Arterial embolization. Another modality used for palliation of ACC is arterial embolization. It is used to decrease the bulk of the tumor, suppress tumor function, and relieve pain. Embolic agents used include polyvinyl alcohol foam and surgical gelatin.

(2) **Thermal ablation.** Both cryoablation and radiofrequency ablation have been used to palliate patients with oligome-tastasis. These procedures can be limited by the location and size of the tumors.

III. PHEOCHROMOCYTOMA AND PARAGANGLIOMA

A. Description and diagnosis

Pheochromocytomas arises from chromaffin cells mainly in the adrenal medulla (90% of cases), whereas paraganglias are histologi-cally indistinguishable tumors that arise at other sites (e.g., carotid body/skull base, urinary bladder, heart, and organ of Zuckerkandl). About 800 cases are diagnosed in the United States every year, and although it is found in up to 0.3% of autopsy subjects, it is respon-sible for less than 0.5% of all cases of hypertension. Pheochromo-cytoma can be hereditary, as part of the MEN syndrome (MEN-IIa, MEN-IIb), or familial with no other manifestation of the MEN syndrome. When part of the MEN syndrome, it is almost always benign. It may also occur in conjunction with Von Hippel-Lindau disease, tuberous sclerosis, Sturge-Weber syndrome, and Carney syndrome. Patients with pheochromocytoma can present with sus-tained or episodic hypertension, but hypertension does not usually correlate with the amount of catecholamine production. The diag-nosis of pheochromocytoma relies on a thorough history and phys-ical examination, increased catecholamine levels in the plasma and the urine (including epinephrine, norepinephrine, dopamine, and total metanephrines), cross-sectional imaging such as CT or MRI, and/or [131I]metaiodobenzylguanidine (MIBG) scintigraphy. Although pheochromocytoma is a rare tumor, early detection and treatment are crucial, owing to its high morbidity and potential mortality (stroke, myocardial infarction). The incidence of ma-lignancy is about 10%, with the only definite proof of malignancy being metastatic disease, as there are no definitive histopathologic criteria for malignancy. The overall 5-year survival rate for patients with malignant pheochromocytoma is 36% to 44%.

B. Treatment

1. **Surgery.** Surgery, the only definitive therapy for pheochromo-cytoma, requires careful preoperative preparation to achieve control of blood pressure and prevent hypertensive crisis and potentially fatal outcome from surgery. Phenoxybenzamine, an α-adrenergic receptor blocker, is started 1 to 2 weeks before sur-gery in a dose of 10 to 20 mg by mouth three or four times daily. Many patients require the addition of β-blockers, which are in-dicated for persistent tachycardia; however, *to prevent hyperten-sive crisis secondary to unopposed vasoconstriction, β-blockers*

should not be given before α-antagonists. Other α-adrenergic blockers including prazosin, a selective α_1-antagonist, have also been used successfully for preoperative preparation of pheochromocytoma. Metyrosine 250 mg 4 times daily (maximum 4 gm/day) can also be used but is associated with frequent side effects. Intraoperatively, blood pressure can be controlled by titration with nitroprusside. Surgical isolation of unperturbed primary tumors is also critical; therefore, referral to expert surgeons commonly treating this neoplasm should be made if pheochromocytoma or paraganglioma is suspected. Contralateral adrenalectomy of a normal gland is generally not recommended in patients with a high incidence of bilateral disease (e.g., MEN-II), despite the high risk of subsequent involvement. In patients with metastatic disease, there is no evidence to support improved survival after local debulking. Catecholamine and metanephrine levels should be measured 1 week after surgery to confirm total removal of the tumor. Surgical mortality is estimated around 2% and usually correlates with the severity of hypertension. Patients whose localized benign disease is fully resected should have normal life expectancy; however, close postoperative follow-up is mandatory because of the possibility of residual tumor and as 10% of patients have metastasis with another 10% with multiple primary tumors at the time of diagnosis. Follow-up should include history, physical, catecholamine and metanephrine measurements, and CT imaging initially at 3-month intervals then yearly thereafter.

2. **Chemotherapy.** Chemotherapy is reserved for inoperable metastatic, imminently threatening disease, as its efficacy is limited.
   - Cyclophosphamide 750 mg/m^2 IV plus vincristine 1.4 mg/m^2 IV on day 1 and dacarbazine 600 mg/m^2 IV on days 1 and 2 repeated in 3 to 4 weeks resulted in objective response in 61% of patients, with catecholamine/metanephrine levels decreasing in 74% of patients, and with median response duration averaging 28 months and minimal overall toxicity.
   - Streptozocin alone and in combination with other chemotherapeutics has yielded favorable results in the treatment of neuroendocrine tumor in the gastrointestinal tract, and has also sometimes been used in pheochromocytoma.

     Emerging approaches to treating recurrent malignant pheochromocytoma and paraganglioma include TKIs (e.g., sunitinib, pazopanib), currently being evaluated in multicenter phase II trials based on encouraging anecdotal experience with these agents.

3. **Radiation therapy.** [^{131}I]MIBG is generally actively taken up and concentrated by pheochromocytoma cells with high sensitivity and specificity. Consequently, high-dose radiotherapeutic [^{131}I] MIBG has been historically used to treat pheochromocytoma

in metastatic MIBG-avid tumors. However, this approach has considerable bone marrow toxicity and is unfortunately of limited palliative benefit, so it is best used in conjunction with clinical trials. External beam radiotherapy, Gamma Knife, and CyberKnife stereotactic approaches can provide local control in focally symptomatic or threatening metastases.

Selected Readings

Thyroid Carcinoma

AACE/AME Task Force on Thyroid Nodules. American Association of Clinical Endocrinologists and Associazione Medici Endocrinologi medical guidelines for clinical practice for the diagnosis and management of thyroid nodule. *Endocr Pract.* 2006;12(1):63–102.

Cooper DS, Doherty GM, Haugen BR, et al. Revised American Thyroid Association management guidelines for patients with thyroid nodules and differentiated thyroid cancer. American Thyroid Association (ATA) Guidelines Taskforce on Thyroid Nodules and Differentiated Thyroid Cancer. *Thyroid.* 2009;19:1167–1214.

Kloos RT, Eng C, Evans DB, et al. Medullary thyroid cancer: management guidelines of the American Thyroid Association. American Thyroid Association Guidelines Task Force. *Thyroid.* 2009;19:565–612. Review. Erratum in: *Thyroid.* 2009;19:1295.

Smallridge RC, Marlow LA, Copland JA. Anaplastic thyroid cancer: molecular pathogenesis and emerging therapies. *Endocr Relat Cancer.* 2009;16:17–44.

Adrenal Cortical Carcinoma

Bornstein SR. Stratakis CA. Chrousos GP. Adrenal cortical tumors: recent advances in basic concepts and clinical management. *Ann Intern Med.* 1999;130:759–771.

Berruti A, Terzolo M, Sperone P, et al. Etoposide, doxorubicin and cisplatin plus mitotane in the treatment of advanced adrenal cortical carcinoma: a large prospective phase II trial. *Endocr Relat Cancer.* 2005;12(3):657–666.

Mansmann G, Lau J, Balk E, Rothberg M, Miyachi R, Bornstein SR. The clinically inapparent adrenal mass: update in diagnosis and management. *Endocr Rev.* 2004;25(2):309–340.

Strosberg JR, Hammer GD, Doherty GM. Management of adrenocortical carcinoma. *J Natl Compr Canc Netw.* 2009;7:752–758.

Tabarin A, Bardet S, Bertherat J, et al. Exploration and management of adrenal incidentalomas. French Society of Endocrinology Consensus. *Ann Endocrinol (Paris).* 2008;69:487–500.

Terzolo M, Angeli A, Fassnacht M, et al. Adjuvant mitotane treatment for adrenocortical carcinoma. *N Engl J Med.* 2007;356:2372–2380.

Pheochromocytoma

Averbuch SD, Steakley CS, Young RC, et al. Malignant pheochromocytoma: effective treatment with a combination of cyclophosphamide, vincristine, and dacarbazine. *Ann Intern Med.* 1988;109:267–273.

Carling T. Multiple endocrine neoplasia syndrome: genetic basis for clinical management. *Curr Opin Oncol.* 2005;17:7–12.

Pacak K, Eisenhofer G, Ahlman H, et al. Pheochromocytoma: recommendations for clinical practice from the First International Symposium. October 2005. *Nat. Clin Pract Endocrinol Metab.* 2007;3:92–102.

Vanderveen KA, Thompson SM, Callstrom MR, et al. Biopsy of pheochromocytomas and paragangliomas: potential for disaster. *Surgery.* 2009;146:1158–1166.

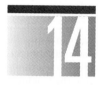

Melanomas and Other Cutaneous Malignancies

Ragini Kudchadkar and Jeffrey S. Weber

More than 1 million Americans were diagnosed with skin cancer in 2009, making it the most common malignancy in the United States and accounting for considerable morbidity. Melanoma accounted for approximately 68,720 cases and was responsible for an estimated 8650 deaths in 2009, which far surpasses the number of deaths due to all other skin malignancies combined. Melanoma continues to increase in incidence at a higher rate than any other cancer in the United States, except for non–small-cell lung cancer in women. Approximately 5890 cases of nonepithelial skin cancer cases were diagnosed in 2009. These less common tumors of the skin include Merkel cell cancer, Kaposi sarcoma (see Chapter 25), and mycosis fungoides (MF).

I. MELANOMA
A. Natural history
   1. **Etiology and epidemiology.** Melanoma arises from pigment-producing melanocytes that migrate to the skin and eye from the neural crest during embryologic development. Approximately 5% of melanoma occurs in noncutaneous sites such as the eye and mucous membranes of the oropharynx, sinuses, vagina, and anus. Patients can present with regional lymph node involvement or distant metastatic disease without any primary being identified. This occurs in approximately 5% of patients. Melanoma occurs more commonly in men than women and has a peak age at incidence of approximately 50 years. Owing to the young age of many melanoma patients, this disease takes a striking toll in terms of the average number of years of life lost per patient in the United States. The incidence of the disease has increased in the United States to the point where melanoma is now the sixth most common cancer in men or women. The substantial increase in incidence is presumably due to increased

exposure to sunlight (primarily ultraviolet B radiation), with the greatest risk of melanoma felt to be in those who have intermittent intense sun exposure, particularly in fair-skinned, light-haired individuals with red and blonde hair, and blue or green eyes. The cultural emphasis on sun-tanned skin as an indicator of physical health and beauty has played a major role in this increase. Depletion of the ozone layer may contribute as well. Sunny parts of the United States have the highest incidence of the disease, especially California, Florida, Arizona, and Texas, which include three of the four most populous states in the United States. One particular melanoma subtype, lentigo maligna melanoma, which often occurs on the face, may be more closely associated with long-term occupational sun exposure and is seen in farmers and other outdoor workers. Patient education in prevention, including use of sun-protective clothing, performing outdoor activities at times other than the brightest sunlit hours of the day, use of topical sunscreens, refraining from use of sun-tan parlors, use of skin self-examination, and avoiding sun-tanning ("tanned skin = damaged skin"), should be emphasized. Individuals with xeroderma pigmentosa, an autosomal recessive disorder, typically incur multiple basal and squamous skin cancers and melanoma because their skin lacks the ability to repair damage induced by ultraviolet radiation.

2. **Precursor lesions, genetics, and familial melanoma.** Melanomas arise not only from sporadic or familial atypical nevi but also from other congenital and acquired nevi; however, approximately half of cutaneous melanomas arise without a clear cut precursor lesion. Individuals who have more than 20 benign nevi are at increased risk for melanoma. Approximately 10% of patients with melanoma have a family history of this cancer. Careful surveillance should be carried out in patients with these risk factors. Suspicious-appearing lesions or lesions that appear to have changed coloration, shape, height, or have bled should be excised. The familial atypical multiple mole melanoma syndrome is characterized by a young mean age at diagnosis (34 years) and multiple lesions. The most common germline mutation seen in familial melanoma occurs in the tumor suppressor gene CDKN2A. CDKN2A, PTEN, NRAS, and BRAF mutations have also been seen in nonfamilial melanoma.

3. **Types and appearance of primary lesions.** Clinical features, classically known as "ABCD," that raise suspicion for melanoma include:
   - *A*symmetry of a lesion
   - *B*orders that are irregular
   - *C*olor that is multihued
   - *D*iameter greater than 6 mm (i.e., "larger than the diameter of a pencil eraser").

Other characteristics of concern include history of recent growth, change in pigmentation, ulceration, itching, or bleeding. Any pigmented lesion that returns after excision should be re-evaluated with biopsy. Nonpigmented skin lesions that behave like melanoma should be examined with immunohistochemical stains S-100 and HMB-45 as 1% to 2% of melanomas are amelanotic.

There are four clinical types of primary cutaneous melanoma. Superficial spreading melanoma is the most common type, accounting for 70% of melanomas. It is commonly found on the trunks of men and lower extremities of women. Nodular melanoma comprises 10% to 15% of melanomas and has an early vertical growth phase. It is commonly found on the trunks of men. Those lesions associated with intermittent sun exposure are often (50% to 60%) B-RAF mutated but C-KIT wild-type. Lentigo malignant melanoma accounts for approximately 10% of cases. It is characterized by flat, large (1- to 5-cm) lesions located on the arms, hands, and face of the elderly (median age 70 years) in particular and is known for a relatively longer radial phase. Acral lentiginous melanoma is seen in approximately 3% to 5% of cases and occurs primarily on the palmar surfaces of the hands, plantar surfaces of the feet, and under nails on the digits. This melanoma subtype is most commonly seen in individuals with darker-pigmented skin and is felt not to be as closely related to sun exposure as the other subtypes. Mutations in exons 9 and 11 of the C-KIT gene are more commonly observed in acral lentiginous and mucosal melanomas than other subtypes, but still only occur in about 20% to 30% of these cases.

In general, melanoma is felt to show two distinct growth phases: an initial radial phase during which the melanoma enlarges in a horizontal/superficial pattern above the basal lamina of the skin, followed eventually by a vertical growth phase characterized by invasion deeply with exposure to lymphatic vessels and the vasculature. It is during the vertical growth phase that metastases are felt to be most likely to occur.

4. **Patterns of metastases**. Melanoma has a proclivity for direct nodal spread presumably through the lymphatics, but a significant proportion of lesions exhibit hematogenous spread as well. Common sites of metastases include lung, liver, bone, subcutaneous areas, and, primarily in late stages, brain. However, melanoma can spread to virtually any site and can imitate virtually any solid malignancy in its pattern of spread. Following diagnosis, approximately 25% of patients will develop visceral metastases. An additional 15% may develop disease limited to lymph nodes. Patients who present with lymph

nodal or metastatic involvement without any obvious primary site may have undergone spontaneous remission of the primary, a phenomenon that may be attributable to some degree of immune system involvement. Interestingly, those patients may have a better outcome than similarly staged patients with known primaries. Patients with "cancer of unknown primary" should have their biopsy material analyzed with the immuno-histochemical stains S-100 and HMB-45 to consider the possibility of melanoma.

5. **Ocular melanoma.** Ocular melanoma is the most common malignancy of the eye in adults. It may occur in any eye structure that contains melanocytes, although uveal tract sites predominate, followed by choroid, ciliary body, and iris in decreasing frequency. Standard therapy may consist of either enucleation (often utilizing a "no touch" technique) or brachytherapy with radioisotopes such as iodine-125. A recently published large randomized study of those two treatments revealed that for primary uveal tumors less than 5 mm in depth, the outcome for survival was identical. This tumor metastasizes most frequently to the liver and appears to be no less sensitive to both biologic agents and chemotherapy than is cutaneous melanoma.

B. Staging

Melanoma is staged according to the American Joint Committee on Cancer staging system (see Tables 14.1 to 14.3). All patients should have a careful history and physical examination with special attention to the skin including scalp, mucous membranes, and regional lymph nodes. Laboratory studies should include complete blood count, blood urea nitrogen, serum creatinine, liver panel, alkaline phosphatase, and serum lactate dehydrogenase at baseline. A baseline chest radiograph is obtained to evaluate for pulmonary lesions. A computed tomography (CT) scan can be considered if clinically warranted. Elevation of liver function tests warrants further imaging of the liver, most typically with CT. Unexplained bone pain should also be evaluated with CT or magnetic resonance imaging. Primary lesions equal to or thicker than 1.0 mm are at higher risk of regional lymph node involvement; therefore, the use of sentinel node mapping is recommended for lesions between 0.76 and 1 mm and above.

C. Surgical treatment

The standard treatment for skin lesions suspected of being melanoma is excisional biopsy rather than incisional or "shave" biopsies. A subsequent wide and deep excision is required to provide adequate tumor-free margins as melanoma has a known propensity for local recurrences. While there is some variation in recommendations, most experts would advocate a 1-cm tumor-free margin for melanomas less than 1 mm in thickness

TABLE 14.1	TNM Classification for Melanoma	
T Status Classification	**Thickness (mm)**	**Ulceration**
T1	≤1.0	a = no ulceration *and* mitosis <1/mm^2
		b = with ulceration *or* mitosis ≥1/mm^2
T2	1.01–2.0	a = no ulceration
		b = with ulceration
T3	2.01–4.0	a = no ulceration
		b = with ulceration
T4	>4.0	a = no ulceration
		b = with ulceration
N Status Classification	**Number of Lymph Nodes**	**Involvement**
N1	1	a = microscopic
		b = macroscopic
N2	2–3	a = microscopic
		b = macroscopic
		c = "in-transit" or "satellite" present but no lymph nodes involved
N3	≥4	This classification applies also if "in-transit" or "satellite" lesions present *with* metastatic nodes.
M Status Classification	**Metastatic Site**	**Serum LDH**
M1a	Distant subcutaneous, skin, or node	Not elevated
M1b	Lung	Not elevated
M1c	All other visceral sites	Not elevated
M1c	Any	Elevated

LDH, lactate dehydrogenase.
From Edge SB, Byrd DR, Compton CC. *AJCC cancer staging manual* (7th ed.). New York: Springer; 2010.

TABLE 14.2	Clark Levels of Invasion
Level	**Description**
I	Limited to the epidermis
II	Invades papillary dermis
III	Extends to papillary–reticular dermal junction
IV	Invades reticular dermis
V	Invades subcutaneous fat

Stage	TNM (Pathologic)	Five-Year Survival (%)
IA	T1a	95
IB	T1b	90
	T2a	89
IIA	T2b	77
	T3a	
IIB	T3b	65
	T4a	
IIC	T4b	45
IIIA	N1a	53
	N2a	49
IIIB	N1b	51
	N2b	46
IIIC	N3	27
IV	M1a	19
All others	M	<10

TABLE 14.3 Approximate Survival in Melanoma Based on Stage Grouping

From Balch CM, Gershenwal JE, Soong SJ, et al. Final version of 2009 AJCC melanoma staging and classification. *J Clin Oncol.* 2009;27:2199–2206.

and 1- to 2-cm margins for deeper primary lesions if technically possible, following current National Comprehensive Cancer Network guidelines. Additionally, for primary lesions of at least 1 mm, sentinel node mapping is recommended. Lymph node "drainage areas" are assessed via a specific lymph node (sentinel node(s)—sometimes more than one) into which lymphborne metastases generally first occur. The absence of tumor involvement in the lymph node is associated with a reduced risk of nodal spread and relapse in general and eliminates the need for subsequent dissection of that nodal basin. In the recent Multi-Center Sentinel Lymph Node Trials 1, 1347 patients with primary melanomas of 1.2 to 3.5 mm, felt to be at intermediate risk of recurrence, were randomly allocated to receive either observation or a sentinel node biopsy, with completion lymphadenectomy if the sentinel node was positive and observation only if negative. A delayed lymph node dissection was performed in case of nodal recurrence in either group. Preliminary results from that trial suggest that there was no survival advantage for the performance of a sentinel lymph node biopsy in this risk group, although it reduced the relative risk of recurrence at any site by 26%, reduced the absolute chance of recurrence locoregionally from 15.6% to 3.4%, and confirmed that those with a positive sentinel node had a worse outcome than those with a negative sentinel node biopsy.

D. Adjuvant therapy

Eastern Cooperative Oncology Group (ECOG) protocol E1684 was a large randomized adjuvant trial of interferon (IFN)-α_{2b} in patients with deep primary lesions (>4 mm thick) or regional lymph node involvement that showed statistically significant improvement in overall survival in the treated group compared to the observation group. The regimen used was IFN 20 million IU/m^2 intravenously (IV) 5 days/week for 4 weeks (as a "loading phase") followed by 10 million IU/m^2 subcutaneously (SC) 3 days/week for 48 weeks as a maintenance phase. Toxicity was significant, but quality-of-life analysis demonstrated overall benefit. The follow-up study of observation versus the same IFN regimen versus a lower dose regimen, ECOG 1690, also showed a significant disease-free survival advantage over the observation arm but not a benefit in overall survival for the high-dose regimen. The difference between these two studies may be that patients on the observation arm in the subsequent trial (1690) may have been treated with immunotherapy (including IFN or interleukin [IL]-2) at the time of relapse. Several recent meta-analyses of randomized trials of high-dose IFN have shown that while there is a statistically significant and consistent advantage in relapse-free survival, the benefit for overall survival is very modest, at 2% to 3%. Nonetheless, given that patients with deep cutaneous primaries and/or lymph node involvement are at high risk for metastatic recurrence and that the majority of patients who suffer metastatic relapse will die of their disease, it is reasonable to treat such high-risk patients with either adjuvant high-dose IFN or to consider entrance into a clinical trial.

Chemotherapy as a single adjuvant modality has not been shown to be more beneficial than observation alone, and high-dose IFN with chemotherapy confers no difference in relapse-free or overall survival between the single agent and combined therapy arms. Peginterferon, which prolongs the half-life of the drug, allowing it to be delivered weekly, has been tested in several adjuvant trials in resected melanoma. Only in patients whose lesions were detected at sentinel node biopsy was there an advantage in disease-free survival for peginterferon.

E. Therapy of metastases

1. General considerations about systemic therapy

a. Patient selection. While melanoma is considered relatively resistant to chemotherapy, certain favorable prognostic factors do lend themselves to longer survivals with single-agent or multiagent chemotherapy, or even high-dose IL-2. These include ECOG performance status 0 or 1; subcutaneous, lymph node, or pulmonary metastasis with normal lactate dehydrogenase (M1a or M1b disease); no prior chemotherapy; normal marrow, renal, and hepatic function; and absence of central nervous system (CNS) metastases. The biologic basis for these findings has not been fully elucidated. When reviewing potential therapy for stage IV melanoma patients, patient characteristics as well as the natural history of their metastatic disease must be considered. Surgical resection should be considered for one or even two sites of metastases that are resectable with a reasonable surgical procedure associated with modest morbidity. Failing that, for unresectable disease, an evaluation should be made whether the patient has indolent disease, suggesting that immunotherapy might be useful, or more aggressive disease, indicating that other approaches are warranted. While a clinical trial should be a first consideration for patients with metastatic disease, high-dose IL-2 should be considered for the subset of patients that qualify for that rigorous therapy.

2. **Biologic agents**. This class of agents has been extensively tested in melanoma, a histology where they have met with some success.

   a. **Interleukin-2 (IL-2)** appears to be the most active, currently approved single agent for patients with visceral metastases. It is most commonly used in a high-dose regimen of IL-2 at 600,000 IU/kg given in 15-minute infusions IV every 8 hours for a maximum of 14 doses on a day 1 and day 15 schedule every 6 to 8 weeks. This schedule produces responses in 15% to 20% of patients, with 5% to 6% complete response, many of long duration. A review of National Cancer Institute data with high-dose IL-2 showed a response rate of 50% in patients with disease limited to cutaneous/subcutaneous sites only (i.e., M1a disease). Because this drug is associated with a capillary leak syndrome that can include hypotension, fluid retention, renal and hepatic hypoperfusion, and pulmonary edema, the previously discussed dose and schedule require inpatient care in a monitored setting with nursing staff and physicians that are experienced and skilled in its use. Given these effects, patients must be in relatively good health, and a cardiac stress test should be performed prior to treatment in anyone above 50 years of age or any patient with multiple cardiac risk factors. It should be noted that the older literature may express IL-2 dosing in other than international units. Therefore, when comparing various studies, a rule of thumb for conversions is $1 \text{ mg} = 3 \times 10^6$ Cetus Units $= 6 \times 10^6$ Roche Units $= 18 \times 10^6$ IU.

   b. **Interferon (IFN) (alfa$_{2b}$ and alfa$_{2a}$)** has been examined with a wide range of doses, schedules, and routes from 3 to 50×10^6 IU/m^2 given SC, intramuscularly, or IV, administered three to five times per week. These agents have been found to have response rates of approximately 10% to 15% in a variety of studies. Additionally, some patients may have stable disease lasting many months or longer. In regards to dosing, some investigators believe that higher doses of IFN (20 MIU/m^2 IV, such as those given in adjuvant therapy) act more by inhibiting tumor cell proliferation, while lower doses of IFN ($\leq$5 MIU/m^2 SC) may be more immunostimulatory. IFN is in general not commonly used in the metastatic setting, though a select population of patients with limited disease may benefit from this treatment.

c. **Ipilimumab** is a human immunoglobulin G1 antibody directed against the immune checkpoint protein cytotoxic T-lymphocyte antigen-4, expressed on activated T-cells. It has been extensively tested in stage IV melanoma and is an active drug, with objective response rates of 7% to 20%. Many responses are sustained over time, and ipilimumab has been shown to induce novel patterns of response, with slow regression over 6 to 12 months, progression followed by regression, and new lesions appearing while other baseline lesions continue to regress. This drug has also demonstrated unique side effects that are directly related to its immune mechanism of action, called immune-related adverse events, consisting of rashes, colitis with diarrhea, hepatitis, pancreatitis, and hypophysitis leading to pituitary insufficiency. In relapsed/refractory melanoma at 3 mg/kg, ipilimumab plus a peptide vaccine has been reported in a 670-patient trial to have superior overall survival compared to the peptide vaccine alone, which is the first positive controlled randomized trial in stage IV melanoma ever conducted, and establishes a new standard of care.

d. **Tyrosine kinase/signal transduction inhibitors**. These "small molecule" inhibitors, including pan-tyrosine kinase inhibitors sorafenib and sunitinib which likely inhibit tumor-related angiogenesis, have been investigated and have little activity as single agents or when added to chemotherapy in stage IV melanoma. Clinical trials have been conducted with carboplatin and paclitaxel with sorafenib based on promising phase II single center data. Unfortunately, the PRISM trial sponsored by Bayer did not show a median or overall survival difference between carboplatin and paclitaxel with or without sorafenib administered to patients as second-line therapy.

The recent discovery that up to 50% of melanomas have a common activating mutation in the B-RAF gene, at the V600E position, has provoked the testing of a number of small molecule RAF inhibitors in stage IV melanoma. Very promising early data, from a phase II trial of 30 patients with the oral B-RAF inhibitor PLX-4032 from Plexxicon-Roche, resulted in a 70% objective response rate in mostly refractory melanoma patients with a V600E mutation. This drug is now being evaluated in a second-line phase II and a front-line randomized phase III trial, the latter in comparison to dacarbazine alone.

Approximately 20% of patients with mucosal melanoma have been shown to harbor an activating C-KIT mutation in exons 9, 11, or both. This also can lead to amplification of C-KIT. In a small pilot trial, and in a number of anecdotal publications, blockade of C-KIT with the oral inhibitor imatinib induced rapid and dramatic regression in patients with C-KIT mutated mucosal melanoma; however, the duration of these responses are yet to be known.

   e. **Combinations of biologic agents.** The role of combinations of biologic agents remains an area of ongoing study, but they have thus far not shown demonstrable advantage.

3. **Chemotherapy**
   a. **Single-agent chemotherapy.** Most cytotoxic agents commonly used in other tumor types are inactive in this disease. Several agents possess modest activity in melanoma with responses obtained primarily in lung and nonvisceral sites and typically in ambulatory patients with few or no symptoms of their disease.

   (1) **Dacarbazine** has historically been the most widely utilized single agent for the treatment of metastatic melanoma. The most commonly used doses are 200 mg/m^2 IV on days 1 to 5 every 3 weeks or 750 to 800 mg/m^2 IV on day 1 every 4 to 6 weeks. Most responses to this agent occur in subcutaneous or lymph node sites. Response rates are between 10% to 20% and the median time to progression is 2 to 3 months.

   (2) **Platinum-containing drugs.** Cisplatin 100 mg/m^2 IV every 3 weeks *or* carboplatin 400 mg/m^2 IV every 3 weeks appears to have similar efficacy.

   (3) **Taxanes.** Docetaxel 60 to 100 mg/m^2 is given in 1-hour infusions IV every 3 weeks, *or* paclitaxel 135 to 215 mg/m^2 is given in 3-hour infusions IV every 3 weeks.

   (4) **Temozolomide** is an oral imidazole agent that is biochemically converted to the active (dacarbazine) intermediate monomethyl triazeno imidazole carboxamide in an acid environment with significant CNS penetrance and therefore the potential for clinical responses in the difficult subpopulation of patients with CNS metastases. Typical doses are 150 to 200 mg/m^2 by mouth daily for 5 days every 28 days, or continuous administration for 6 of 8 weeks at 75 mg/m^2, both with equivalent efficacy.

   (5) **Vinca alkaloids** such as vinblastine and **nitrosoureas** such as carmustine have been used primarily in combinations and have modest single-agent activity in melanoma.

b. Multiagent chemotherapy. Despite decades of trials, no combination chemotherapy has emerged as a standard therapy. While multiple regimens have shown high response rates in single arm phase II or nonrandomized trials, there are no convincing data from randomized trials to show both statistically significant improvements in response rate and median survival compared with single-agent therapy (usually dacarbazine). While a phase II study of the "Dartmouth Regimen" suggested a higher response rate than dacarbazine alone, a phase III trial demonstrated no significant difference in progression-free or overall survival compared to dacarbazine alone. Cisplatin, vinblastine, and dacarbazine/temozolomide are currently an acceptable off-protocol combination regimen (Table 14.4). Carboplatin combined with paclitaxel every 3 weeks is emerging as the most common combination treatment used off protocol based on the results of the PRISM trial control arm discussed above (see Section I.E.2.d).

4. Biochemotherapy. Three randomized studies have compared the combination of polychemotherapy (cisplatin, vinblastine, and dacarbazine) with the biologic agents IL-2 and IFN versus the chemotherapy regimen alone. The first published randomized

TABLE 14.4 Multiagent Systemic Therapy for Melanoma

Regimen	Drug Dosages
BCDT ("Dartmouth regimen")	Carmustine 150 mg/m²/day on day 1 every 6 weeks Cisplatin 25 mg/m²/day on days 1–3 every 3 weeks Dacarbazine 220 mg/m²/day on days 1–3 every 3 weeks Tamoxifen 20 mg by mouth daily
CVD	Cisplatin 20 mg/m²/day on days 1–4 every 3 weeks Vinblastine 1.6 mg/m²/day on days 1–4 every 3 weeks Dacarbazine 800 mg/m² on day 1 only every 3 weeks
Biochemotherapy*	CVD as above, *together with:* IL-2 9 MIU/m²/once a day by continuous infusion IV on days 1–4 (96 hours)* IFN-α_{2b} 5 MU/m² SC on days 1–5, 7, 9, 11, and 13 G-CSF 5 μg/kg SC once a day on days 7–16 Repeat cycle every 21 days for maximum of four cycles.
Cyclophosphamide and moderate-dose IL-2	Cyclophosphamide 350 mg/m² IVPB on day 1 IL-2 22 MIU/m² IVPB on days 4–8 and 11–15 Repeat cycle every 21 days for three cycles. Thereafter give every 28–42 days.

G-CSF, granulocyte colony-stimulating factor; IFN, interferon; IL, interleukin; IV, intravenously; IVPB, intravenously (piggy-back); SC, subcutaneously.
*On day 1, begin IL-2 2–3 hours after chemotherapy.

comparison showed improved response rate and median time to progression (4.9 months versus 2.4 months) in favor of the combined chemotherapy with biotherapy. Unfortunately, confirmatory studies have shown no difference in median time to disease progression or median survival. A recently published phase II study of biochemotherapy delivered with IL-2 in a decrescendo regimen, followed in stable or responding patients by maintenance IL-2, resulted in a favorable median survival of over 12 months. While patient selection may have played a role in this favorable outcome, the high response rates seen with that regimen suggest that it is a reasonable alternative for untreated patients with rapidly growing disease, or as a neoadjuvant regimen prior to a planned resection of bulky stage III locoregional disease.

F. Regional therapy

1. **Local perfusion.** For patients with subcutaneous metastases limited to a single extremity, arteriovenous cannulation and perfusion of that limb with agents such as melphalan, cisplatin, or tumor necrosis factor-α, often with hyperthermia, yield higher tissue concentrations of the drugs than are achievable by intravenous administration. Phase II studies often show impressive response rates. Whether there is any survival advantage to this therapy compared with systemic treatment remains controversial. Because of issues such as cost, the equipment required, and the physician training needed to implement this approach, its practicality is limited. Hepatic arterial infusion therapy is theoretically appealing for ocular melanoma metastatic only to the liver; ongoing studies are being conducted currently to further evaluate this treatment modality. This therapy looks more active than systemic chemotherapy in ocular melanoma, although it is unclear that such an approach improves median survival.

2. **Intralesional therapy** with Bacillus Calmette-Guérin (BCG), IFN-α, granulocyte-macrophage colony-stimulating factor, IL-2, and other agents has also been used with varying degrees of success in treatment of very small dermal metastases.

3. **Treatment of central nervous system metastases.** Dexamethasone 10 mg IV followed by 6 mg every 6 hours IV or by mouth is given to reduce cerebral edema. As soon as possible, radiation should be started by either stereotactic, gamma knife, or three-dimensional conformal techniques. For solitary lesions, surgical resection followed by radiotherapy may yield a significant group of survivors over 1 year who experience good quality of life. The role of temozolomide needs to be further explored in this group of patients.

4. **Radiotherapy** is of variable efficacy in the treatment of symptomatic regional or bony metastases but sometimes may yield symptomatic benefit. We routinely add daily temozolomide at

75 mg/m^2 to whole brain radiation to augment its antitumor activity when administered to patients with multiple CNS metastases.

5. **Surgery,** when utilized judiciously, can result in long-term disease-free survivals of up to 20% in individuals with isolated metastatic sites. The median survival for those patients is 30 to 36 months. Indications for surgical resection of metastases include gastrointestinal metastases that are chronically bleeding or if there is impending bowel obstruction or perforation and single brain metastases, especially if bleeding prior to the start of biologic therapy (as long-term steroid use, which is frequently needed in the setting of brain metastasis, is antagonistic with biologic agents). The role of adjuvant therapy in patients who have undergone and are clinically free of disease is being evaluated in several trials, and such metastasectomy patients should always be considered for vaccine or other adjuvant trials when available. An alternative approach is to treat such patients with IFN as described previously.

G. Experimental and future therapies

Experimental and future therapies are of great importance in this disease. Only a few salient approaches will be discussed here. A variety of references are available for further reading (see "Selected Readings").

1. **Therapeutic vaccines** remain an area of intense interest, and much potential is expected in the coming years, although current clinical results have shown limited activity. In general, toxicity from vaccine therapy tends to be quite low, usually limited to local reactions to the vaccine or the immunologic adjuvant that may be combined with the antigenic stimulus. Most vaccine studies have dealt primarily with patients who have been rendered surgically free of all macroscopic disease but thus far have been without significant benefit. A polyvalent melanoma cell vaccine and Melacine (GlaxoSmithKline, Middlesex, UK), a vaccine derived from allogeneic melanoma cell lines (approved for use in metastatic disease in Canada), are example of vaccines that have achieved objective responses in patients with metastatic tumors. Vaccination with peptides derived from tumor-associated antigens specifically designed to associate with T-cells in the context of major histocompatibility complex class I or II molecules and vaccines based on vaccinia-infected melanoma cell lysates are examples of other approaches of note. Potential advantages to vaccine-based therapy include relatively little toxicity, the possibility of long-term disease stabilization, and an immunologic effect that may continue long after dose administration.

2. **Cellular therapy.** The administration of ex vivo activated cells such as cytotoxic T-cells theoretically specific for melanoma continues to be of interest. Currently, there is no randomized

evidence that the addition of cultured T-cells to IL-2 therapy, for instance, is superior to IL-2 alone. A significant advance may be the development of tumor infiltrating lymphocyte (TIL) therapy. These effector T-cells are grown from enzyme-digested tumors and are expanded in tissue culture over 3 to 6 weeks, often resulting in an oligoclonal population of highly tumor-specific T-cells. On adoptive transfer with high-dose IL-2, response rates of up to 50% were seen. Newer approaches include the use of lymphoid depletion prior to adoptive transfer of TIL, which allows the effectors to proliferate during the process of homeostatic lymphoid proliferation. During that time, many memory effector cells will populate the T-cell pool, resulting in long-lasting tumor specific T-cells in the peripheral circulation. The addition of total body irradiation to TIL therapy with high-dose IL-2 results in even higher response rates of up to 72%, with favorable median survivals of greater than 12 months in recurrent melanoma patients who have failed IL-2 and chemotherapy.

II. NONMELANOMA SKIN CANCER
A. Etiology and epidemiology

The American Cancer Society estimates there were nearly 1 million new cases of basal cell carcinoma (BCC) and squamous cell carcinoma (SCC) in the United States in 2009. These lesions occur twice as frequently in men than in women. BCC occurs 4 times more commonly than SCC (70% to 80% versus 10% to 30%). Both are seen predominantly in the elderly. Risk factors for these two lesions include age greater than 60 years, prior heavy sun exposure, fair complexion, and light colored eyes or hair. Sun exposure, especially sunburns early in life, is the most important risk factor for development of these lesions, similar to melanoma. Other etiologic factors include prior irradiation to the skin for benign disorders, chronic inflammation, scarring or burns, and arsenic exposure. Patients who are chronically immunosuppressed such as those with chronic lymphocytic leukemia and prior organ transplant are also at increased risk, as are individuals with genetic disorders including xeroderma pigmentosum. There is evidence that human immunodeficiency virus infection may predispose to a clinically more aggressive SCC or BCC. Multiple BCCs or SCCs frequently occur in 30% to 50% of individuals.

B. Diagnosis and clinical features

1. **Diagnosis of both SCC and BCC is made by biopsy,** including incisional, excisional, or sometimes "shave," depending on the clinical situation. Staging systems are not typically utilized for these tumors as both have generally low potential for metastases. BCC originates in the basal layer of the epidermis and often presents as a nodular, ulcerative lesion ("rodent ulcer") with pearly or

translucent edges and central ulceration. Approximately 30% of BCCs are found on the nose. Only about 0.1% of BCCs metastasize. Metastases typically occur when a long-standing lesion has been neglected. Lymph node metastases are the most common site (60%), with lung and bone metastases occurring less frequently. Despite being uncommon, once metastases occur, survival is significantly decreased to 8 to 10 months. SCCs often arise from crusty-appearing sun-damaged skin areas and demonstrate a higher rate of metastases (2%) than BCCs. Patients whose SCC arises from causes other than actinic damage (e.g., immunosuppression) may display a more rapid course with higher rates of metastases (20% to 50%). Neglected lesions, large ulcerated lesions, and poorly differentiated histology are risk factors for metastases. The great majority of metastases initially occur in lymph nodes (90%), with approximately 50% of patients developing metastases to other sites such as lung and bone. SCCs may begin as premalignant lesions called actinic keratoses (AKs) that are rough, pink or flesh-colored areas on sun-exposed skin. In situ SCC, known as Bowen disease, exists prior to dermal invasion and appears as red-colored patches and is larger than AKs.

2. **Local treatment.** Surgical excision, electrodesiccation, curettage, Mohs micrographic surgery, radiation therapy, and cryotherapy all result in similar cure rates of approximately 95% when lesions are identified early. Treatment options are typically based on individual factors including the area involved, available treatment facilities, and physician skill. Surgical excision to attain margins of at least 3 to 10 mm is the preferred treatment in SCC because of the higher metastatic potential. BCC, which has a lower metastatic potential, can be treated with any of the above techniques as well as cryotherapy. Radiation therapy is the treatment of choice for areas where extensive surgical resection would result in poor cosmetic outcome, such as near eyelids, ear lobes, or the tip of the nose.

   Mohs micrographic surgery is an involved procedure in which thin layers are meticulously removed, chemically fixed, and immediately reviewed microscopically to be assured of clear margins. Although this therapy is highly operator dependent, Mohs surgery currently has the highest 5-year cure rate and has become the standard of care for local primary or recurrent BCC and SCC lesions.

   Topical treatment delivery of fluorouracil is used for AK and SCC in situ and is applied directly to the involved skin. It is generally not systemically absorbed, therefore almost no systemic toxicity is seen. Local side effects include red discoloration of the skin and photosensitivity. Imiquimod is approved by the U.S. Food and Drug Administration for local therapy of AKs and some small BCCs. Both agents are applied locally daily for up to 3 weeks.

3. **Treatment of metastatic disease.** Metastases from either BCC or SCC may be treated with cisplatin-containing chemotherapy regimens. Despite response rates as high as 70% with chemotherapy, once metastases have occurred, cure is no longer possible and survival is typically less than 1 year. Hedgehog signal transduction inhibitors are showing early promise in the treatment of metastatic BCCs. Clinical trials with these agents are ongoing.

C. **Merkel cell carcinoma**

1. **Etiology and epidemiology.** Merkel cell cancer is a rare cutaneous neuroendocrine tumor that arises in the basal layer of the epidermis. Approximately 500 cases are diagnosed yearly in the United States. Its microscopic appearance is that of small blue cells with scant cytoplasm and hyperchromatic nuclei ("small cell cancer of the skin"). Merkel cell cancer is 20 times more likely to occur in Caucasians than non-Caucasians, occurs more frequently in males than females, and affects persons at a median age of 65 to 70 years. Sun exposure is felt to be the major risk factor. Recent studies have identified a polyomavirus in Merkel cell tumors.

2. **Clinical features.** Initially, it may be seen as a blue or bluish red, nontender, firm skin lesion, starting as a nodule but increasing in size rapidly over weeks to months. The most commonly involved sites are the face and neck (50%) and the extremities (40%). There is no universally accepted staging system for this uncommon tumor; however, stage I is considered localized disease, stage II is involvement of regional lymph nodes, and stage III represents systemic metastases. In general, Merkel cell cancer has a tendency toward an aggressive, recurrent course similar in some ways to small-cell lung cancer or melanoma. Most patients experience recurrence within 12 months of initial treatment. Fifty percent of patients experience local and regional nodal recurrences and one-third later develop metastatic disease. The most frequent distant metastatic sites are liver, lung, and bones. The overall 5-year survival rate for all stages is 50%.

3. **Treatment.** The rarity of this tumor precludes any prospective randomized treatment data. Standard therapy for this disease includes surgical resection with 2-cm margins when possible, followed by lymph node dissection. Sentinel lymph node surgery has become the preferred technique as a negative lymph node precludes more extensive surgery.

Because of the risk of local recurrence, radiation therapy to the primary site and to the site of pathologically involved lymph nodes should be considered, especially in stage I disease. There has been no established role for adjuvant chemotherapy. High-risk patients may be offered chemotherapy; however, there is no data that it offers a survival advantage. For metastatic disease, the two most common regimens used have been cyclophosphamide, doxorubicin, and vincristine or cisplatin and etoposide at doses utilized for small-cell lung cancer. Response rates for these regimens are about 60%.

D. Mycosis fungoides (MF)

1. **Etiology and epidemiology.** MF is a cutaneous T-cell–derived lymphoma with a CD4 T-helper cell immunophenotype. It is an uncommon lymphoma, with just over 500 new cases diagnosed in the United States per year. It is seen predominantly in males with a median age of approximately 60 years. The lymphocytic infiltrate seen in this disease is present in the upper aspect of the dermis, obscures the junction between the dermis and epidermis, and characteristically infiltrates the epidermis in clusters of cells that are called Pautrier microabscesses. Involved lymph nodes have similar histologic findings. Biopsies early in the course of the disease (the "premycotic phase") may show nonspecific, nondiagnostic skin changes.

2. **Clinical features.** Patients with this disorder tend to display a skin rash that is erythematous, somewhat scaling, and pruritic. Over time, patches, plaques, and even ulcers can be seen. Patients may exhibit erythroderma and lymphadenopathy. Sézary syndrome is a leukemic phase of MF with circulating lymphoma cells noted on peripheral smear. The course of MF can be variable, with a minority of patients having "skin-only" involvement to patients having extensive visceral metastases to the liver, lungs, spleen, and gastrointestinal tract. Staging is according to the TMN (B) system (Tables 14.5 and 14.6) and is based on the amount of skin involved and the presence of patches, plaques, or tumors. Patients with stage IA to IIA MF have an excellent prognosis with median survival greater than 11 years. Individuals

TABLE 14.5	**TNMB Classes for Mycosis Fungoides**
T1	Limited patch/plaque lesions <10% of total skin surface
T2	Generalized patch/plaque lesion ≥10% of total skin surface
T3	Tumors
T4	Erythroderma, generalized skin involvement
N0	No clinically palpable lymph nodes
N1	Enlarged lymph nodes but microscopically negative
N2	Nonpalpable lymph nodes but microscopically involved
N3	Clinically palpable lymph nodes that are microscopically involved
M0	No visceral involvement
M1	Visceral involvement
B0	Absence of peripheral blood involvement
B1	Peripheral blood involvement

	TABLE 14.6 Clinical Stages for Mycosis Fungoides		
Stage	**T**	**N**	**M**
IA	T1	N0	M0
IB	T2	N0	M0
IIA	T1–2	N1	M0
IIB	T3	N0–1	M0
IIIA	T4	N0	M0
IIIB	T4	N1	M0
IVA	T1–4	N2–3	M0
IVB	Any	Any	M1

Note: B symptoms have no specific bearing on this staging system.

with stage IIB to III disease have median survival of 3 to 4 years. Among patients with T4 lesions, a subgroup characterized by younger age (less than 65 years), less advanced stage (III), and no evidence of blood involvement, has been shown to have a favorable prognosis with a median survival of approximately 10 years. Stage IVA/IVB has a poor prognosis with a median survival of less than 1.5 years. A subgroup of MF cases may undergo transformation to a large-cell lymphoma characterized by CD30 positivity, which also heralds a poor prognosis.

3. **Treatment.** For individuals whose disease is confined only to the skin, electron beam radiation, the combination of a photosensitizing substance such as psoralen and ultraviolet radiation (PUVA), extracorporeal photopheresis, bexarotene gel, or topical application of nitrogen mustard or carmustine can lead to complete response of disease and potential for cure. Thick plaque disease may be better treated with electron beam therapy because PUVA and topical nitrogen mustard may be less able to penetrate the deep lesions. Imiquimod is being evaluated for this use as well. Patients who fail one of the local/topical therapies can be treated with a different type of local therapy and still have good control of the disease. For visceral disease or Sézary syndrome, systemic therapy such as interferon-α 3 million units SC three times a week given continuously or gradually escalated to a cumulative weekly dose of 18 million units can yield response rates of over 60%. Combined regimens of IFN-α and retinoids such as bexarotene (150 mg per day) are being evaluated for enhanced immune modulation. "Traditional" antilymphoma chemotherapy agents such as cyclophosphamide, doxorubicin, vincristine, and prednisone appear less active in this type of lymphoma than in other non-Hodgkin lymphomas and are typically reserved for those cases of MF that transform

to large B-cell lymphomas or when disease becomes refractory to other systemic or local agents. Purine analogs such as fludarabine and pentostatin have some activity with response rates of 20% to 70%. Novel uses of gemcitabine (1200 mg/m^2 weekly $\times$ 3 every 28 days) and liposomal doxorubicin (20 to 40 mg/m^2 every 2 to 4 weeks) used as single agents are being studied with reports of overall response rates of approximately 80% in refractory patients. Another agent, denileukin diftitox, has been approved for refractory disease with response rates of 30% to 70%.

Acknowledgments

The authors are indebted to Drs. Karen S. Milligan and Walter D.Y. Quan, Jr., who contributed to previous editions of this chapter. Several sections in this revision of the handbook represent their work.

Selected Readings

Melanoma

Atkins MB, Lee S, Flaherty LE, et al. A prospective randomized phase III trial of concurrent biochemotherapy with cisplatin, vinblastine, dacarbazine, IL-2 and interferon alpha-2b versus CVD alone in patients with metastatic melanoma (E3695): an ECOG-coordinated Intergroup trial. *Proc Am Soc Clin Oncol.* 2003;2847.

Atkins MB, Lotze MT, Dutcher JP, et al. High-dose recombinant interleukin 2 therapy for patients with metastatic melanoma: analysis of 270 patients treated between 1985–1993. *J Clin Oncol.* 1999;17:2105–2116.

Bajetta E, Del Vecchio M, Nova P, et al. Multicenter phase III randomized trial of polychemotherapy (CVD regimen) versus the same chemotherapy (CT) plus subcutaneous interleukin-2 and interferon a-2b in metastatic melanoma. *Ann Oncol.* 2006;17:571–577.

Balch CM, Gershenwal JE, Soong SJ, et al. Final version of 2009 AJCC melanoma staging and classification. *J Clin Oncol.* 2009;27:2199–2206.

Brinkman JA, Fausch SC, Weber JS, Kast WM. Peptide-based vaccines for cancer immunotherapy. *Expert Opin Biol Ther.* 2004;4(2):181–198.

Chapman PB, Einhorn LH, Meyers ML, et al Phase III multicenter randomized trial of the Dartmouth regimen versus dacarbazine in patients with metastatic melanoma. *J Clin Oncol.* 1999;17:2745–2751.

Curtin JA, Fridlyand J, Kageshita T, et al. Distinct sets of genetic alterations in melanoma. *New Engl J Med.* 2005;353:2135–2147.

Eggermont AMM, Suciu S, Santinami M, et al. Adjuvant therapy with pegylated interferon alfa-2B versus observation alone in resected stage III melanoma: final results of EORTC 18991, a randomized phase III trial. *Lancet.* 2008;372:117–126.

Fecher LA, Cummings SD, Keefe MJ, et al. Toward a molecular classification of melanoma. *J Clin Oncol.* 2007;25:1606–1620.

Fong L, Small EJ. Anti-cytotoxic T-lymphocyte antigen-4 antibody: the first in an emerging class of immunomodulatory antibody for cancer treatment. *J Clin Oncol.* 2008;26:5275–5283.

Gogas H, Ioannovich J, Dafni U, et al. Prognostic significance of autoimmunity during treatment of melanoma with interferon. *New Engl J Med.* 2006;254:709–718.

Haluska FG, Hodi FS. Molecular genetics of familial melanoma. *J Clin Oncol.* 1998;16:670.

Ives NJ, Stow RL, Lorigan P, Wheatley K. Chemotherapy compared with biochemotherapy for treatment of metastatic melanoma: a meta-analysis of 18 trials involving 2621 patients. *J Clin Oncol.* 2007;25:5426–5434.

Kim KS, Legha SS, Gonzalez R, et al. A phase III randomized trial of adjuvant biochemotherapy versus interferon alfa-2b in patients with high risk for melanoma recurrence. *J Clin Oncol.* 2006;24(18s):453s.

Kirkwood JM, Ibrahim JG, Sosman JA, et al. High-dose interferon alfa-2b significantly prolongs relapse-free and overall survival compared with the GM2-KLH/QS-21 vaccine in patients with resected stage IIb–III melanoma: results of Intergroup Trial E1694/S9512/C509801. *J Clin Oncol.* 2001;19:2370–2380.

Kirkwood JM, Manola J, Ibrahim J, et al. A pooled analysis of Eastern Cooperative Oncology Group and Intergroup Trials of adjuvant high-dose interferon for melanoma. *Clin Can Res.* 2004;10:1670–1677.

Lee CC, Faries MB, Wanek LA, Morton DL. Improved survival after lymphadenectomy for nodal metastasis from an unknown primary melanoma. *J Clin Oncol.* 2008;26:535–541.

Middleton MR, Grob JJ, Aaronson N, et al. Randomized phase III study of temozolomide vs. dacarbazine in the treatment of patients with advanced metastatic malignant melanoma. *J Clin Oncol.* 2000;18:158–166.

Morton DL, Thompson JF, Cochran AJ, et al. Sentinel-node biopsy or nodal observation in melanoma. *New Engl J Med.* 2006;355:1307–1317.

Morton DL, Wen DR, Wong JH, et al. Technical details of intraoperative lymphatic mapping for early stage melanoma. *Arch Surg.* 1992;127:392.

Nonmelanoma Skin Cancer

Aasi S, Leffell D. Cancer of the skin. In: DeVita VT, Hellman S, Rosenberg SA (eds.). *Cancer: principles and practice of oncology* (7th ed.). Philadelphia: Lippincott Williams & Wilkins; 2005:1717–1744.

Feng H, Shuda M, Chang Y, Moore PS. Clonal integration of polyomavirus in human Merkel cell carcinoma. *Science.* 2008;319:1096–1100.

Fleming ID, Amonette R, Monaghan T, et al. Principles of management of basal and squamous carcinoma of the skin. *Cancer.* 1995;75:699.

Foss F. Mycosis fungoides and the Sézary's syndrome. *Curr Opin Oncol.* 2004;16(5): 421–428.

Goessling W, McKee PH, Mayer RJ. Merkel cell carcinoma. *J Clin Oncol.* 2002;20: 588–598.

Guthrie TH Jr, Porubsky ES, Luxenberg MN, et al. Cisplatin-based chemotherapy in advanced basal and squamous cell carcinomas of the skin: results in 28 patients including 13 patients receiving multimodality therapy. *J Clin Oncol.* 1990;8:342–346.

Marmur ES, Schmults CD, Goldberg DJ. A review of laser and photodynamic therapy for the treatment of nonmelanoma skin cancer. *Dermatol Surg.* 2004; 30(2):264–271.

Preston DS, Stern RS. Non-melanoma cancers of the skin. *N Engl J Med.* 1992;327:1649.

Rupoli S, Barulli B, Guiducci B, et al. Low-dose interferon-alpha 2b combined with PUVA is an effective treatment of early stage mycosis fungoides: results of a multicenter study. Cutaneous-T Cell Lymphoma Multicenter Study Group. *Haematologica.* 1999;84:809–813.

Siegel RS, Pandolfino T, Guitart J, et al. Primary cutaneous T-cell lymphoma: review and current concepts. *J Clin Oncol.* 2000;18:2908–2925.

Von Hoff DD, LoRusso PM, Rudin CM, et al. Inhibition of the Hedgehog Pathway I advanced basal-cell carcinoma. *New Engl J Med.* 2009;361:1–9.

Primary and Metastatic Brain Tumors

April Fitzsimmons Eichler and Tracy T. Batchelor

I. PRIMARY BRAIN TUMORS

A. Incidence

According to the Central Brain Tumor Registry of the United States (CBTRUS), there were an estimated 51,510 cases of new malignant and nonmalignant primary brain tumors (PBTs) diagnosed in the United States in 2007. This includes an estimated 20,500 new cases of malignant brain and central nervous system (CNS) tumors, representing 1.42% of all malignant cancers and accounting for 12,740 deaths in the same year. The age-adjusted 5-year relative survival from 1999 to 2005 for all malignant PBTs—including lymphomas, leukemias, tumors of the pituitary and pineal glands, and olfactory tumors of the nasal cavity—was 35%. The only established risk factor for PBT is ionizing radiation at high doses, which has been associated with an increased incidence of nerve sheath tumors, meningiomas, and gliomas. However, radiation-associated tumors account for only a small percentage of PBTs.

B. Gliomas

Gliomas account for 36% of all PBTs and include astrocytic, oligodendroglial, and ependymal tumors. Astrocytomas are the most frequent type and these tumors manifest a wide spectrum of clinical behavior. Malignant gliomas—including anaplastic oligodendroglioma, anaplastic astrocytoma, and glioblastoma (GBM; the most common malignant PBT)—are not curable, although each may respond to radiation and chemotherapy. Astrocytomas are graded based on the presence or absence of the following histologic features: nuclear atypia, mitoses, endothelial proliferation, and necrosis.

1. **Grades I and II astrocytoma.** Pilocytic astrocytomas are World Health Organization (WHO) grade I tumors that most commonly arise in the posterior fossa. These tumors are most common in the pediatric population and can be cured if a total resection is achieved. WHO grade II astrocytomas (low-grade astrocytomas) are most commonly observed in the third and fourth decades of life. This tumor typically appears as a nonenhancing, diffuse, hypointense mass on T1-weighted magnetic resonance imaging (MRI). Even with a characteristic appearance, biopsy is necessary to determine the histologic subtype and because up to 30% of nonenhancing tumors are shown to be anaplastic (WHO grade III) at the time of surgery. Median survival for low-grade gliomas (LGGs)—which includes low-grade astrocytoma, oligoastrocytoma, and low-grade oligodendroglioma—ranges from 7 to 9 years with a 5-year survival of 60% to 70%. Important prognostic factors for survival include age, performance status, preoperative tumor size, extent of resection, and histology, with astrocytic tumors fairing worse than oligodendroglial tumors.

   If feasible, a maximal safe resection should be performed and then the patient should be followed regularly with serial MRI studies and clinical examinations. Data from four prospective randomized clinical trials in adults with LGG indicate that (1) postoperative radiation therapy compared with observation is associated with improved progression-free survival but not overall survival and (2) radiation doses of 45 to 54 Gy result in similar outcomes to higher doses (59 to 65 Gy) and are associated with improved tolerability. Based on these data, postoperative radiation therapy is often recommended for patients after a subtotal resection or biopsy, particularly if there are additional "high risk" features such as advanced age (>40 years), elevated MIB-1 labeling index (>3% to 5%), or pure astrocytoma histology. Even in low-risk LGG patients, defined in one recent prospective observation study as adults <40 years of age with neurosurgeon-determined gross-total resection, the risk of tumor progression at 5 years may be as high as 50%.

   In the event of tumor progression on computed tomography (CT) or MRI, further surgery, if possible, may be performed and involved field radiation (IFR) or chemotherapy is recommended, depending on the histologic subtype. If, at the time of the recurrence, the histopathology demonstrates a higher grade astrocytoma, chemotherapy can be initiated, which will be discussed in the following section.

2. **Grades III and IV astrocytoma.** Anaplastic astrocytoma (WHO grade III) occurs most commonly in the fourth and fifth decades, whereas glioblastoma (WHO grade IV) occurs most commonly in the fifth and sixth decades. Median survival times are

24 to 36 months and 12 to 15 months, respectively. These two types of tumors may be indistinguishable by MRI because both often appear as diffuse hypointense lesions on T1-weighted images and both readily enhance after administration of intravenous contrast. These tumors are most commonly observed in the cerebral hemispheres and can have cystic or hemorrhagic components.

Histologic diagnosis is made by stereotactic biopsy or resection. Surgical debulking is the preferred initial treatment to minimize neurologic morbidity. Retrospective studies and the adjusted analysis of a prospective randomized trial of fluorescence-guided resection have suggested that gross total resection is associated with longer survival. Resection also relieves mass effect, which allows a patient to better tolerate subsequent IFR and often allows discontinuation of corticosteroids. Following surgery, standard therapy includes IFR up to 60 Gy, given in combination with temozolomide for grade IV tumors (see later). Management of anaplastic astrocytoma remains controversial because of a lack of randomized prospective data, but postoperative IFR or IFR with concurrent temozolomide are the most common treatment approaches. Positive prognostic factors include high Karnofsky performance score, gross total resection, and younger age. In addition, multiple studies have now shown that methylation of the O^6-methylguanine-DNA methyltransferase (MGMT) promoter is prognostic of improved survival and may be predictive of increased responsiveness to temozolomide chemotherapy in GBM.

a. **Chemotherapy.** Chemotherapy is now considered the standard of care for newly diagnosed glioblastoma based on the results of a European Organization for Research and Treatment of Cancer (EORTC) and National Cancer Institute of Canada (NCIC) randomized, multicenter trial of 573 patients comparing IFR (radiation arm) with IFR plus concurrent temozolomide (TMZ) followed by 6 months of postradiation, monthly TMZ (chemoradiation arm). Patients treated with chemoradiation had a median survival of 14.6 months, compared with 12.1 months in the radiation arm. In addition, the 2- and 5-year survival rates were 27% and 10% in the chemoradiation group compared with 11% and 2% in the radiation group, respectively.

In 2009, the U.S. Food and Drug Administration (FDA) approved bevacizumab (Avastin), a monoclonal antibody against vascular endothelial growth factor (VEGF), as a single agent for use in treatment of recurrent glioblastoma. Approval was based on two prospective studies showing a 20% to 30% objective response rate and a median response duration of approximately 4 months. In addition, bevacizumab was associated with decreased steroid use over time. The most frequent adverse events were infection, fatigue, headache, hypertension, epistaxis, and diarrhea. Grade 3 or higher adverse events were similar to those seen in other primary cancer types and included bleeding/hemorrhage, CNS hemorrhage, hypertension, venous and arterial thrombosis, wound-healing complications, proteinuria, gastrointestinal perforation, and reversible posterior leukoencephalopathy. There is also a large experience with bevacizumab in combination with irinotecan (CPT-11) for recurrent malignant glioma. However, in a randomized noncomparative trial, median progression-free survival and overall survival were not significantly different in the combination arm (5.6 months and 8.7 months, respectively) compared with the bevacizumab monotherapy arm (4.2 months and 9.2 months) and toxicity was higher with combination therapy. Several large randomized placebo controlled trials are investigating the efficacy of bevacizumab in combination with chemoradiation for newly diagnosed glioblastoma.

Recurrent glioblastoma may also be treated by surgical debulking with or without carmustine (BCNU) wafers, radiosurgery, nitrosoureas such as BCNU or lomustine (CCNU), or other single agent therapies such as carboplatin. A wide range of targeted agents are also in clinical trials. The following are regimens that have been used both in the adjuvant setting and for patients who have recurrence after surgery, IFR, or both.

b. **Regimens for newly diagnosed malignant glioma**

(1) **Temozolomide** (TMZ) is administered differently depending upon whether it is being used in combination with IFR or not.

    ▪ TMZ is dosed at 75 mg/m^2 daily, 7 days per week, when given concurrently with IFR, for the entire duration of radiation. Trimethoprim-sulfamethoxazole should be administered thrice weekly with the daily temozolomide as prophylaxis against *Pneumocystis jiroveci* pneumonia.

    ▪ TMZ is dosed at 150 to 200 mg/m^2 by mouth daily for 5 consecutive days in a 28-day treatment cycle when given alone.

    Administration of TMZ using a 21-day on followed by 7-day off schedule, a strategy aimed at overcoming resistance by depleting MGMT, has been compared with standard 5 days on, 23 days off TMZ in the postradiation setting for newly diagnosed GBM in a randomized study of 1153 patients but results are not yet available. Until then, 5-day per month TMZ remains the standard of care, regardless of a patient's MGMT methylation status.

(2) PCV is a combination of three antineoplastic agents given in a 6-week cycle:

- Lomustine 110 mg/m^2 by mouth on day 1
- Vincristine 1.4 mg/m^2 (maximum 2 mg) intravenously (IV) on days 8 and 29
- Procarbazine 60 mg/m^2 by mouth days 8 through 21 of the 42-day cycle

PCV is typically administered for 6 to 12 months or until tumor progression. PCV is associated with more myelotoxicity and neurotoxicity than other commonly prescribed chemotherapeutic drugs for malignant glioma.

c. Regimens for recurrent GBM

(1) Bevacizumab is administered at a dose of 10 mg/kg IV every 2 weeks. Dose reductions may be required, most commonly for hypertension or proteinuria. When given in combination with irinotecan, the dose of bevacizumab remains the same and irinotecan is dosed at 340 mg/m^2 for patients on enzyme-inducing anticonvulsants and 125 mg/m^2 for patients not on enzyme-inducing anticonvulsants.

(2) BCNU may be administered as monotherapy and is given in either one dose or in two to three divided consecutive daily doses for a total of 150 to 200 mg/m^2 IV every 6 weeks.

(3) BCNU wafers are a depot source of BCNU that can be surgically implanted at the time of resection. The FDA approved the 3.85% BCNU wafer for recurrent GBM after a phase III, double-blind, placebo-controlled clinical study involving 222 patients undergoing surgery for recurrent malignant glioma showed that BCNU wafers increased median survival from 20 to 28 weeks. A second randomized trial was conducted using BCNU wafers at the time of initial diagnosis of malignant glioma and led to FDA approval for newly diagnosed malignant glioma. This study showed a median survival of 13.9 months in the BCNU wafer group versus 11.6 months in the placebo arm. However, when anaplastic and nonglial histologies were excluded from the analysis, a survival advantage for patients with GBM was not observed.

3. Oligodendroglioma (WHO grades II and III)

a. Characteristics. Low-grade (WHO grade II) oligodendroglioma (LGO) and anaplastic (WHO grade III) oligodendrogliomas (AO) are glial tumors that are found almost exclusively in the cerebral hemispheres and represent 4% to 15% of all gliomas. The peak incidence occurs in the fourth through sixth decades of life. Oligodendrogliomas have increased cellularity with homogeneous, hyperchromatic nuclei surrounded by clear cytoplasm: the classic "fried-egg" appearance. Allelic loss of the short arm of chromosome 1p and the long arm of chromosome 19q occurs in 50% to 70% of both AO and LGO and predicts better response to chemotherapy and longer survival. These tumors are hypointense on T1-weighted MRI scans and hyperintense on T2-weighted images and are located in the deep white matter. The median survival for WHO grade II oligodendrogliomas and WHO grade III oligodendrogliomas has been reported as 9.8 to 16.7 years and 3.5 to 5 years, respectively. However, these estimates do not stratify patients based on the underlying status of chromosomes 1p and 19q and patients with codeleted anaplastic oligodendroglioma have a median survival of 10 to 13 years in some series.

b. **Treatment**. Although the optimal treatment for these tumors remains controversial, the general approach is similar to that for astrocytomas. In all cases, if a tumor is suspected, a stereotactic biopsy should be performed or confirmed tumors should be resected, if feasible. Residual or unresectable LGOs can be followed with serial MRI studies and clinical examinations. As with low-grade astrocytomas, oligodendrogliomas with elevated MIB-1 labeling ($>3\%$ to 5%) are considered higher risk and, therefore, are often treated like grade III tumors. Following the initial resection of an AO, radiation has been a standard recommendation. However, because grade III tumors have shown 60% to 100% response rates to PCV, this form of chemotherapy or temozolomide may be administered either prior to IFR or in the postradiation period. PCV has been shown to prolong disease-free survival but not overall survival in two randomized phase III trials in patients with AO. Temozolomide has shown a 31% objective response rate as initial therapy for LGO in patients with clinical and/or radiographic progression and no prior therapy other than surgery and a recent randomized study by Wick et al. in patients with anaplastic gliomas suggests that TMZ has comparable efficacy to PCV and is better tolerated.

C. **Medulloblastoma (WHO grade IV)**

1. **Characteristics**. Medulloblastomas are malignant embryonal tumors of the posterior fossa. Eighty percent are found in children under the age of 15 and this neoplasm accounts for 20% of all pediatric brain tumors. Medulloblastomas represent 1% of tumors in patients older than 20 years. Histologically, the tumor is characterized by poorly differentiated, densely packed, hyperchromatic, nucleated, small, round, blue cells. Medulloblastomas are invasive and tend to metastasize through the cerebral spinal fluid (CSF) to the rest of the CNS. The staging evaluation for these patients should include contrast-enhanced MRI of the entire neuraxis (brain and spinal cord) and lumbar puncture for

CSF cytopathology if the latter can be safely performed. If disseminated disease is found at the time of the diagnosis (poor risk category), radical tumor resection confers little to no survival benefit.

2. **Treatment**. Treatment for local disease involves surgical resection, followed by craniospinal radiation (CSR) in adults to a dose of 36 Gy with a boost to the tumor bed to 54 Gy. In the average risk patient, this treatment approach is associated with a 60% 5-year progression-free survival. In an attempt to minimize the long-term side effects of radiation in children, one study reported acceptable results with 23.4 Gy of CSR given, with a boost to the tumor bed to 55.8 Gy, followed by cisplatin-based chemotherapy. This approach resulted in a 5-year progression-free survival of 79%.

There are multiple chemotherapy regimens for medulloblastomas, all of which were developed in the pediatric population. A common approach involves the use of the following drugs in combination: etoposide, cisplatin, cyclophosphamide or CCNU, and vincristine. In patients with recurrent medulloblastoma, high-dose chemotherapy with autologous stem cell rescue may be beneficial.

D. **Primary central nervous system lymphoma in immunocompetent patients**
Primary CNS lymphoma (PCNSL) is a diffuse large B-cell lymphoma arising within the CNS. This tumor accounts for 3.1% of all PBTs and the median age at diagnosis is 60. Ocular involvement is seen in 5% to 20% of cases and leptomeningeal spread in 20% to 40% of cases. Sixty percent of tumors are supratentorial and commonly involve the periventricular regions and corpus callosum. Twenty-five percent to fifty percent of cases have multifocal disease at the time of diagnosis. The lesions are hypointense to isointense on T1-weighted MRI and enhance homogeneously on postgadolinium images. The tumors are responsive to corticosteroids and, as a result, these drugs should be avoided until a diagnosis has been established. The only role for surgery in PCNSL is to establish the diagnosis by biopsy. These tumors should not be resected except in the rare circumstance of brain herniation from mass effect.

Extent of disease evaluations for patients with PCNSL should include gadolinium-enhanced MRI of the brain and spine; positron emission tomography-CT scan of chest, abdomen and pelvis; ophthalmologic evaluation with slit lamp examination; lumbar puncture for CSF cytopathology, flow cytometry, and immunoglobulin heavy gene rearrangement testing; serum lactate dehydrogenase level; and a bone marrow biopsy. Patients should also be tested for the human immunodeficiency virus.

Whole-brain radiation therapy (WBRT) results in a 90% response rate, but the median survival with WBRT alone is less than

12 months. PCNSL is sensitive to many types of chemotherapy, with all successful regimens involving the use of high-dose methotrexate (3.5 to 8 g/m^2). Either alone or in combination with other chemotherapeutic drugs, methotrexate-based treatment is associated with radiographic response rates of 50% to 100% and survival durations of 40 to 90 months with or without the use of WBRT. The use of combination therapy is supported by a recent randomized phase 2 study of 79 patients with PCNSL showing significantly higher response rates with four courses of the combination of high-dose methotrexate and high-dose cytarabine compared with methotrexate alone (46% versus 18%, respectively).

■ Methotrexate 3.5 g/m^2 day 1 and cytarabine 2 g/m^2 every 12 hours on days 2 and 3. The first 0.5 g/m^2 of the methotrexate is given over 15 minutes and the remaining 3 g/m^2 is given over 3 hours with attention to alkalinization of the urine and maintenance of urine output of at least 100 mL/hour for the first 24 hours. Twenty-four hours after the start of the methotrexate infusion, leucovorin 25 mg is administered every 6 hours IV × 4, the oral for a total of 10 doses. Serum methotrexate levels should be followed and should fall by approximately 1 log per day. When the serum methotrexate concentration falls below 0.5×10^{-7} M (0.05 μM), the leucovorin may be discontinued. Each cytarabine dose is given over 1 hour. The regimen is repeated every 3 weeks for four courses.

■ Methotrexate is associated with potentially severe nephrotoxicity so renal function must be closely monitored during methotrexate treatment. Autologous stem cell transplantation may have a role for patients with chemosensitive disease either at first remission or at first relapse, but randomized trials are needed to determine whether survival is better than with standard-dose chemotherapy.

II. BRAIN METASTASES
A. Incidence
Brain metastases are much more common than PBT in adults. The incidence is approximately 2.8 to 11.1 per 100,000 person-years in the United States. It is suspected that 20% to 25% of patients dying of cancer each year have brain metastases. Most commonly, cerebral metastases arise from cancer of the lung, breast, skin (melanoma), kidney, and colon.

B. Treatment
1. **Surgery**. Because metastatic cancers often do not extensively infiltrate the surrounding normal brain parenchyma, these tumors can usually be resected without significant neurologic morbidity. However, this approach should be attempted only when the tumors are accessible and few in number, as revealed

by CT or MRI, and when the patient's cancer is under good control systemically. In the 25% of all brain metastasis patients who have single or solitary lesions, surgery followed by WBRT results in longer survival than WBRT alone (40 versus 15 weeks for cerebral metastases from lung cancer).

2. **Radiation therapy.** WBRT is recommended for patients with brain metastases because micrometastatic disease is often present. Small brain metastases (generally <4 cm in diameter) that are solitary or persistent after WBRT may be treated with stereotactic radiosurgery (linear accelerator, cobalt source/gamma knife, proton radiosurgery). This technique uses a stereotactic frame and specialized external-beam focusing. It permits a high dose of radiation to be delivered to a small region in a single fraction. However, cerebral radiation necrosis is a potential complication and may necessitate either surgery or prolonged use of corticosteroids. The decision to proceed with either radiosurgery or resection should be individually tailored and based on status of the primary tumor, performance status, location of the tumor, and number of tumors. A randomized trial has shown that the addition of stereotactic radiosurgery (SRS) to WBRT increases survival in patients with single brain metastasis and achieves effective palliation in patients with one to three brain metastases. More recently, a randomized trial has shown that for patients with four or fewer brain metastases, the addition of WBRT to SRS improves intracranial disease control but does not alter overall survival compared with SRS alone. Limited neurocognitive testing in that trial suggested that intracranial disease progression rather than receipt of WBRT was the most important predictor of neurocognitive decline.

3. **Chemotherapy.** Chemotherapy has a limited role in the treatment of brain metastases. However, there are exceptions, because metastases from breast cancer occasionally respond well to the usual regimens for breast tumors. Lymphomatous brain masses may also respond to methotrexate-based chemotherapy.

III. LEPTOMENINGEAL METASTASES

The treatment of leptomeningeal metastases includes radiation therapy to symptomatic areas of the CNS (e.g., to the base of the brain for cranial nerve dysfunction or lumbosacral spine for cauda equina disease) and intrathecal (IT) chemotherapy with methotrexate, cytarabine (ara-C), or thiotepa.

A. Chemotherapy regimens

1. **Methotrexate** 12 to 15 mg per dose is the most commonly used IT chemotherapeutic agent. It is generally administered twice a week until the cytologic examination shows clearance of malignant cells from the CSF, then once a month as maintenance.

2. **Cytarabine-liposomal** 50 mg is a sustained-delivery form (De-poCyt, DepoFoam, Pacira Pharmaceuticals, San Diego, CA) of cytarabine for IT administration that allows treatment every 2 weeks. This is an advantage over conventional IT drugs, which must be delivered two to three times each week. Concurrent administration of oral corticosteroids (dexamethasone 4 mg twice a day on days 1 to 5) is required with the sustained-release form of cytarabine as the main side effect from this medication is arachnoiditis. Nonliposomal cytarabine can also be delivered intrathecally. The most common dose is 30 mg/m^2 given every 4 days until normalization of spinal fluid.

3. **Thiotepa** 12 mg is a third IT chemotherapeutic agent that may be used if there is no response to methotrexate or cytarabine. However, the short CSF half-life of this agent may compromise its efficacy.

B. Administration

All chemotherapeutic agents for IT administration should be freshly prepared in preservative-free diluent. Because drugs that are administered into the lumbar subarachnoid space result in lower concentrations of the drugs in the upper spine and brain, it is advisable to administer these drugs through an Ommaya reservoir, a device that is implanted under the scalp and connected by a catheter, through a burr hole, to the frontal horn of the lateral ventricle. This method allows more reliable delivery of drug to the CSF and better distribution of drug along CSF pathways and avoids the necessity of repeated lumbar punctures for the patient.

C. Complications

Complications of IT chemotherapy include arachnoiditis and leukoencephalopathy. The latter is more likely to occur if the perforated tubing of the Ommaya catheter becomes lodged in brain tissue rather than the lateral ventricle. Myelosuppression is not usually significant unless the patient undergoes spinal irradiation or systemic chemotherapy as well. Oral leucovorin is generally given after IT methotrexate (10 mg leucovorin by mouth every 6 hours for six to eight doses, starting 24 hours after the methotrexate) to prevent bone marrow or mucous membrane toxicity.

IV. TREATMENT OF CEREBRAL EDEMA
A. Corticosteroids

These drugs are usually started soon after the diagnosis of a brain tumor is established. However, if PCNSL is suspected on the basis of the CT or MRI, then corticosteroids should be withheld until after a biopsy has been done. In the rare patient with PCNSL who requires emergent antiedema measures, mannitol may be administered (see later). Dexamethasone 10 mg IV followed by 4 mg every 6 hours by mouth or IV reduces or eliminates the lethargy, headaches, visual blurring, and nausea caused by cerebral edema and also often reduces some of the focal neurologic signs and symptoms such as hemiparesis. The corticosteroid dose should be tapered and discontinued after a complete surgical resection has been performed or after radiation therapy has been completed and resumed if symptoms recur. The dose should be held at the lowest dose that maximizes therapeutic benefit and minimizes side effects (e.g., gastric irritation, insomnia, mood swings, cushingoid body features, increased appetite, and myopathy).

B. Treatment of refractory cerebral edema

1. Increase dexamethasone. When moderate doses of dexamethasone do not effectively control cerebral edema, the dose may be increased transiently up to 10 to 24 mg IV every 4 to 6 hours. This dose should usually not be maintained for longer than 48 to 72 hours.

2. An osmotic diuretic in an urgent situation may act more rapidly than a corticosteroid. Mannitol 75 to 100 g IV (as a 15%–25% solution) is given by rapid infusion over 20 to 30 minutes and repeated at 6 to 8 hours intervals as needed. Careful monitoring of electrolytes, serum osmolarity, fluid intake and output, and body weight is essential to avoid dehydration. The osmotic diuresis may be discontinued when there is improvement in the signs and symptoms from cerebral edema and when the corticosteroids or other measures to reduce cerebral edema have taken effect.

V. TREATMENT OF SEIZURES

A. Seizures

Seizures are a common presenting feature in patients with brain tumors, with an incidence of approximately 20%. Prophylactic treatment for patients with brain tumors who have not had a seizure is not beneficial. However, it is common practice to administer a prophylactic anticonvulsant for a period of time after a biopsy or a craniotomy. If the patient has not had a seizure and has undergone only an uncomplicated biopsy or resection, the anticonvulsant may be discontinued after 4 to 8 weeks. If a patient does have a seizure and is to be placed on an anticonvulsant, levetiracetam is often recommended because is does not have cytochrome P-450 enzyme-inducing properties that can influence chemotherapy metabolism. Alternative monotherapies include phenytoin, carbamazepine, oxcarbazepine, and valproic acid. If the patient has further seizures despite having sufficient serum levels of an anticonvulsant, then a second agent may be added. For those on long-term anticonvulsant therapy, it is important to check drug levels at intervals, especially after dosages of other medications have been changed or new medications have been added.

B. Common side effects

Common side effects of anticonvulsant treatment include sedation, nausea, rash, diplopia, dysmetria, ataxia, and hepatic dysfunction. A rare but serious toxicity is Stevens-Johnson syndrome, which is an immune complex–mediated hypersensitivity disorder. There may be an

TABLE 15.1 Antiepileptic Drugs: Enzyme-Inducing versus Non–Enzyme-Inducing	
Enzyme-Inducing	**Non–Enzyme-Inducing**
Carbamazepine (Tegretol)	Felbamate (Felbatol)
Oxcarbazepine (Trileptal)*	Gabapentin (Neurontin)
Phenobarbital	Lacosamide (VIMPAT)
Phenytoin (Dilantin)	Lamotrigine (Lamictal)
Primidone (Mysoline)	Levetiracetam (Keppra)
	Pregabalin (Lyrica)
	Tiagabine (Gabitril)
	Topiramate (Topamax)
	Valproic acid (Depakote)
	Zonisamide (Zonegran)

*Weakly enzyme-inducing.

increased risk of this complication in patients undergoing simultaneous cranial irradiation and corticosteroid taper. This may present as a rash beginning as macules that may develop into papules, vesicles, bullae, urticarial plaques, or confluent erythema. A fever is present in 85% of cases.

C. Cytochrome P-450 induction

Several commonly used anticonvulsants (phenytoin, phenobarbital, and carbamazepine) may induce the hepatic cytochrome P-450 enzyme system with potentially important clinical implications. This may result in increased metabolism and reduced plasma levels of chemotherapeutic drugs that undergo hepatic metabolism. This has been demonstrated in a trial of the topoisomerase I inhibitor irinotecan (CPT-11) in patients with recurrent malignant gliomas. It was found that the maximum tolerated dose of CPT-11 was approximately fourfold higher in patients taking cytochrome P-450–inducing anticonvulsants than in patients not on these drugs. This emphasizes the importance of using anticonvulsants only when clearly indicated. Non-enzyme–inducing antiepileptic drugs include valproic acid, gabapentin, lamotrigine, levetiracetam, topiramate, and zonisamide (Table 15.1).

Selected Readings

Abrey LE, Batchelor TT, Ferreri AJ, et al. Report of an international workshop to standardize baseline evaluation and response criteria for primary CNS lymphoma. *J Clin Oncol.* 2005;23:5034–5043.

Andrews D, Scott C, Sperduto P, et al. Whole brain radiation therapy with or without stereotactic radiosurgery boost for patients with one to three brain metastases: Phase III results of the RTOG 9508 randomised trial. *Lancet.* 2004;363:1665–1672.

Aoyama H, Shirato H, Tago M, et al. Stereotactic radiosurgery plus whole-brain radiation therapy vs stereotactic radiosurgery alone for treatment of brain metastases: A randomized controlled trial. *JAMA.* 2006;295:2483–2491.

Batchelor TT, Leoffler JS. Primary CNS lymphoma. *J Clin Oncol*. 2006;24:1281–1288.

Brem H, Piantadosi S, Burger PC, et al. Placebo-controlled trial of safety and efficacy of intraoperative controlled delivery by biodegradable polymers of chemotherapy for recurrent gliomas. The Polymer– Brain Tumor Treatment Group. *Lancet*. 1995; 345:1008–1012.

Cairncross J, Seiferheld W, Shaw E, et al. An intergroup randomized controlled clinical trial (RCT) of chemotherapy plus radiation (RT) versus RT alone for pure and mixed anaplastic oligodendrogliomas: initial report of RTOG 94-02. *J Clin Oncol*. 2004;22:107s.

Chamberlain MC. Neoplastic meningitis. *Oncologist*. 2008;13:967–977.

Eichler AF, Loeffler JS. Multidisciplinary management of brain metastases. *Oncologist*. 2007;12:884–898.

Ferreri A, Reni M, Foppoli M, et al. High-dose cytarabine plus high-dose methotrexate versus high-dose methotrexate alone in patients with primary CNS lymphoma: a randomised phase 2 trial. *Lancet*. 2009;374:1512–1520.

Friedman HS, Prados MD, Wen PY, et al. Bevacizumab alone and in combination with irinotecan in recurrent glioblastoma. *J Clin Oncol*. 2009;27:4733–4740.

Glantz MJ, Cole BF, Forsyth PA, et al. Practice parameter: anticonvulsant prophylaxis in patients with newly diagnosed brain tumors— report of the Quality Standards Subcommittee of the American Academy of Neurology. *Neurology*. 2000;54:1886–1893.

Hegi ME, Diserens AC, Gorlia T. et al. MGMT gene silencing and benefit from temozolomide in glioblastoma. *N Engl J Med*. 2005;352:997–1003.

Hoang-Xuan K, Capelle L, Kujas S, et al. Temozolomide as initial treatment for adults with low-grade oligodendrogliomas or oligoastrocytomas and correlation with chromosome 1p deletions. *J Clin Oncol*. 2004;22:3133–3138.

Illerhaus G, Marks R, Ihorst G, et al. High-dose cheomtherapy with autologous stem-cell transplantation and hyperfractionated radiotherapy as first-line treatment of primary CNS lymphoma. *J Clin Oncol*. 2006;24:3865–3870.

Johannessen AL, Torp SH. The clinical value of Ki-67/MIB-1 Labeling Index in Human Astrocytomas. *Pathol Oncol Res*. 2006;12:143–147.

Louis DN, Ohgaki H, Wiestler OD, et al. *WHO classification of tumours of the central nervous system*. Lyon: IARC Press; 2007.

Packer RJ, Gajjar A, Vezina G, et al. Phase III study of craniospinal radiation therapy followed by adjuvant chemotherapy for newly diagnosed average-risk medulloblastoma. *J Clin Oncol*. 2006;24:4202–4208.

Patchell RA, Tibbs PA, Walsh JW, et al. A randomized trial of surgery in the treatment of single metastases to the brain. *N Engl J Med*. 1990;322:494–500.

Shaw EG, Berkey B, Coons SW, et al. Recurrence following neurosurgeon-determined gross-total resection of adult supratentorial low-grade glioma: results of a prospective clinical trial. *J Neurosurg*. 2008;109:835–841.

Stummer W, Reulen HJ, Meinel T, et al. Extent of resection and survival in glioblastoma multiforme: identification of and adjustment for bias. *Neurosurgery*. 2008;62: 564–576.

Stupp R, Mason WP, van den Bent MJ, et al. Radiotherapy plus concomitant and adjuvant temozolomide for glioblastoma. *N Engl J Med*. 2005;352:987–996.

van den Bent M, Taphoorn M, Brandes A, et al. Phase II study of first-line chemotherapy with temozolomide in recurrent oligodendroglial tumors: the European Organization for Research and Treatment of Cancer Brain Tumor Study Group 26971. *J Clin Oncol*. 2003;21:2525–2528.

Van den Bent M, Afra D, de Witte O, et al. Long-term efficacy of early versus delayed radiotherapy for low-grade astrocytoma and oligodendroglioma in adults: the EORTC 22845 randomised trial. *Lancet*. 2005;366:985–990.

Westphal M, Hilt D, Bortey E, et al. A phase 3 trial of local chemotherapy with bio-degradable carmustine (BCNU) wafers (Gliadel wafers) in patients with primary malignant glioma. *Neuro-Oncology.* 2003;5:79–88.

Wick W, Hartmann C, Engel C, et al. NOA-04 Randomized phase III trial of sequential radiochemotherapy of anaplastic glioma with procarbazine, lomustine, and vin-cristine or temozolomide. *J Clin Oncol.* 2009;27:5874–5880.

Yung WKA, Prados M, Yaya-Tur R, et al. Multicenter phase II trial of temozolomide in patients with anaplastic astrocytoma or anaplastic oligoastrocytoma at first relapse. *J Clin Oncol.* 1999;17:2762–2771.

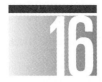

Soft-Tissue Sarcomas

Robert S. Benjamin

I. CLASSIFICATION AND APPROACH TO TREATMENT

A. Types of soft-tissue sarcomas

The soft-tissue sarcomas are a group of diseases characterized by neoplastic proliferation of tissue of mesenchymal origin. Thus, they differ from the more common carcinomas, which arise from epithelial tissue. Sarcomas can arise in any area of the body and from any origin; however, they most commonly arise in the soft tissue of the extremities, trunk, retroperitoneum, or head and neck area. There are more than 50 different types of sarcomas, classified according to lines of differentiation toward normal tissue. For example, rhabdomyosarcoma shows evidence of skeletal muscle fibers with cross-striations, liposarcoma shows fat production, and angiosarcoma shows vessel formation, and there are several types within each of these groups. Precise characterization of the types of sarcoma is often impossible, and these tumors are called *unclassified sarcomas.* All of the primary bone sarcomas may arise in soft tissue, leading to such diagnoses as extraskeletal osteosarcoma, extraskeletal Ewing sarcoma, and extraskeletal chondrosarcoma. A common diagnosis in the recent past was malignant fibrous histiocytoma (MFH). This tumor is characterized by a mixture of spindle (or fibrous) cells and round (or histiocytic) cells arranged in a storiform pattern with frequent areas of pleomorphic appearance and frequent giant cells. There is no evidence of differentiation toward any particular tissue type. Many tumors previously called pleomorphic fibrosarcoma, pleomorphic rhabdomyosarcoma, and so forth were classified as MFH. As immunohistochemistry and molecular diagnostic techniques have improved, many of the tumors previously classified as MFH have been reclassified as pleomorphic something else. Furthermore, there are strong opponents of the term MFH because there is no evidence that the tumors have either fibrous or histiocytic origin, and pleomorphic tumors previously classified as MFH are frequently now referred to as unclassified high-grade pleomorphic sarcomas.

B. Metastases

Metastatic spread of all sarcomas tends to be through the blood rather than through the lymphatic system. The lungs are by far the most frequent site of metastatic disease. Local sites of metastasis by direct invasion are the second most common area of involvement, followed by bone and liver. (Liver metastases are common with intra-abdominal sarcomas, especially gastrointestinal stromal tumors [GISTs]; however, metastases to soft tissue are common with myxoid liposarcomas.) Central nervous system (CNS) metastases are extraordinarily rare except in alveolar soft-part sarcoma.

C. Staging

Staging of sarcomas is complex and demands an expert sarcoma pathologist. Tumors have been staged according to two systems: the American Joint Committee on Cancer (AJCC) staging system and the Musculoskeletal Tumor Society staging system. The new International Union Against Cancer (UICC)/AJCC staging system, with international acceptance, takes portions from each of the older systems and more appropriately identifies patients at increased risk of metastatic disease. Further revisions to this system are still under way, and a final, widely accepted system is still not universally accepted. As current and older publications still refer to the older systems, however, all will be included.

1. **The old AJCC staging system**
   a. **Tumor grade.** The primary determinant of stage is tumor grade. Grade 1 tumors are stage I; grade 2 tumors are stage II; and grade 3 tumors are stage III. Any tumor with lymph node metastases is automatically stage III. Any tumor with gross invasion of bone, major vessel, or major nerve is stage IV.
   b. **Stage.** Further divisions of stages I to III into A and B are based on tumor size.
      - A: Tumor smaller than 5 cm
      - B: Tumor size 5 cm or larger.
         In stage III, lymph node metastases are classified as IIIC. In stage IV, local invasion is called IVA, and IVB represents distant metastases.
2. **The Musculoskeletal Tumor Society staging system.** The Musculoskeletal Tumor Society stages sarcomas according to grade and compartmental localization. The Roman numeral reflects the tumor grade.
   - Stage I: Low grade
   - Stage II: High grade

■ Stage III: Any-grade tumor with distant metastasis.

The letter reflects compartmental localization. Compartments are defined by fascial planes.

■ Stage A: Intracompartmental (i.e., confined to the same soft-tissue compartment as the initial tumor)

■ Stage B: Extracompartmental (i.e., extending outside of the initial soft-tissue compartment into the adjacent soft-tissue compartment or bone).

A stage IA tumor is a low-grade tumor confined to its initial compartment, a stage IB tumor is a low-grade tumor extending outside the initial compartment, and so forth.

3. **The new AJCC staging system**. The stage is determined by tumor grade, tumor size, and tumor location relative to the muscular fascia. There are now four tumor grades.

■ Grade 1: Well differentiated
■ Grade 2: Moderately differentiated
■ Grade 3: Poorly differentiated
■ Grade 4: Undifferentiated.

Tumor size is now divided at less than or equal to 5 cm or more than 5 cm (in the old AJCC system, it was less than 5 cm or more than or equal to 5 cm).

■ T1: ≤5 cm
■ T2: >5 cm.

Tumor status is subdivided by location relative to the muscular fascia.

■ Ta: Superficial to the muscular fascia
■ Tb: Deep to the muscular fascia.

The AJCC stage grouping is as follows.

Stage I	T1a, 1b, 2a, 2b	N0	M0	G1–2
Stage II	T1a, 1b, 2a	N0	M0	G3–4
Stage III	T2b	N0	M0	G3–4
Stage IV	Any T	N1	M0	Any G
	Any T	N0	M1	Any G

The new staging system divides patients according to necessary therapy.

■ Stage I patients are adequately treated by surgery alone.
■ Stage II patients require adjuvant radiation therapy.
■ Stage III patients require adjuvant chemotherapy.
■ Stage IV patients are managed primarily with chemotherapy, with or without other modalities.

D. Evaluation

Patients are evaluated and followed according to the plan in Table 16.1.

Soft-Tissue Sarcoma Evaluation

Tests*	Initial	During Treatment	Follow-Up (If No Evidence of Disease)
History and physical examination	X	Before each treatment	Year 1: every 2 months Years 2 and 3: every 3 months Year 4: every 4 months Year 5: every 6 months Then yearly
CBC, differential, and platelet counts†	X	Twice weekly	Yearly
Electrolytes†	X	Before each treatment	—
Chemistry profile†	X	Before each treatment	Every 4 months
Urinalysis	If giving ifosfamide	As indicated by symptoms	—
PT, APTT, fibrinogen	X	—	—
Chest radiograph	X	Before each treatment	Same as for history and physical examination
CT scan chest	If chest radiograph appears normal	To confirm chest radiograph findings (if initially abnormal) or for surgical planning	If chest radiograph becomes equivocal
MRI primary (if not intra-abdominal)	X	Preoperatively	—
Ultrasound primary	—	—	Year 1: every 4 months Years 2 and 3: every 6 months
PET-CT	X	Every 2–3 cycles if preoperative therapy is given	
CT of abdomen and pelvis	If myxoid liposarcoma or retroperitoneal or pelvic primary tumor	If baseline, every third cycle	If baseline: Year 1: every 4 months Years 2 and 3: every 6 months
ECG	If cardiac history	—	—
Cardiac nuclear scan (for ejection fraction)	If cardiac history	If doxorubicin dose is to exceed standard limits for schedule	Yearly for 2 years, then as clinically indicated

(continued)

Tests*	Initial	During Treatment	Follow-Up (If No Evidence of Disease)
Central venous catheter	X	—	—
Bone marrow or screening MRI of spine and pelvis	If small cell tumor	—	—
Bone scan	If indicated by history	—	—
Plain film	If indicated by history	—	—

APTT, activated partial thromboplastin time; CBC, complete blood count; CT, computed tomography; ECG, electrocardiogram; MRI, magnetic resonance imaging; PET, positron emission tomography; PT, prothrombin time.
*May be ordered more frequently if patient is on a medical treatment program.
†Often required more frequently if patient is on a medical treatment program.

E. Primary treatment

1. **Surgery and radiotherapy.** Treatment of the primary tumor involves surgery with or without radiation therapy. If radiation therapy is not used, surgery must be radical. Although this may often involve amputation or complete excision of the involved muscle group from origin to insertion, more and more frequently, wide local resection is performed, with or without adjuvant radiation, depending on stage and extent of negative margins.

2. **Adjuvant chemotherapy.** The role of adjuvant chemotherapy remains controversial, with both positive and negative results reported. A meta-analysis of individual patient data indicated a highly significant decrease in the risk of disease recurrence (either local or distant) and death in patients treated with adjuvant chemotherapy; thus, *some investigators believe that adjuvant therapy is clearly indicated for patients whose histologic type, grade, or location is known to convey a poor prognosis.* The meta-analysis confirms a survival benefit for patients with primary sarcomas of the extremities as well as increased local or distant disease-free interval for all patients treated with doxorubicin (Adriamycin)-based adjuvant chemotherapy. The Italian Cooperative Study Group using epirubicin and ifosfamide for patients with current stage III disease also demonstrated overall survival and disease-free survival advantage for patients treated with chemotherapy; however, the statistical significance of the survival advantage was lost with further follow-up. An updated meta-analysis, including

studies combining ifosfamide with anthracyclines, shows a survival advantage, but the largest, modern study from the European
Organization for the Research and Treatment of Cancer is negative; thus the controversies continue.

F. Prognosis

Prognosis is related to stage, with a 5-year survival rate of 99%
for new AJCC/UICC stage I, 82% for stage II, and 52% for stage III.
Corresponding rates of disease-free survival at 5 years are 78% for
stage I, 64% for stage II, and 36% for stage III. Long-term results
are still worse. The survival rate for stage IV disease is less than
10%; however, a definite fraction of patients in this category can
be cured. Most patients with stage IV disease, if left untreated, die
within 6 to 12 months; however, there is great variation in actual
survival, and patients may go on with slowly progressive disease
for many years.

G. Treatment response

Response to treatment is measured in the standard fashion for
solid tumors with the addition of tumor necrosis, both radiologi-
cally and pathologically, but there are increasing examples where
good responses are missed by standard criteria, and newer approaches to computed tomography (CT) and magnetic resonance
imaging (MRI) evaluation and use of positron emission tomography is becoming more frequent.

1. **Complete remission**. This implies complete disappearance of all
   signs and symptoms of disease.
2. **Partial remission**. Standard Response Evaluation Criteria in Solid
   Tumors (RECIST) (see Chapter 3, Section IV.D.1) are generally
   employed. This requires a 30% or greater decrease in measurable disease, calculated by comparing the sum of the longest
   diameters of all lesions before and after therapy. When disease
   can be followed objectively by MRI or CT, marked tumor necrosis attributable to chemotherapy demonstrated by imaging or
   pathology is at least the equivalent of a partial response by RE-
   CIST criteria. For GIST, Choi criteria—a 10% decrease in size or
   a 15% decrease in tumor density—are more predictive of time to
   progression or disease-specific survival than RECIST response,
   and Choi criteria or minor modifications thereof are under
   study in other sarcomas.
3. **Stable disease or improvement**. Lesser degrees of tumor shrinkage are categorized by some physicians as stable disease and by
   others as improvement or minor response. Stable disease implies a smaller than 20% increase in disease for at least 8 weeks.
   There is increasing recognition that stable disease or improvement that persists for at least 4 months is at least as meaningful
   for ultimate patient benefit as partial response. For all response
   categories, no new disease must appear during response. Many

investigators consider absence of progressive disease by RECIST, especially if maintained for more than 24 weeks, to be as good as response.

4. **Progression.** New disease in any area or a 20% or more increase in measurable disease constitutes progressive disease.

5. **Survival.** All patients whose disease responds objectively to chemotherapy survive longer than do patients with progressive disease, and the degree of prolongation of survival is directly proportional to the degree of antitumor response that can be measured.

II. CHEMOTHERAPY

A. General considerations and aims of therapy

Although there are numerous types of soft-tissue sarcomas, there are few differences among them regarding responsiveness to a standard soft-tissue sarcoma regimen. GISTs and alveolar soft-part sarcomas and, to a lesser extent, solitary fibrous tumors (also called hemangiopericytomas), clear cell sarcomas, and epithelioid sarcomas respond less frequently to standard regimens than do the other soft-tissue sarcomas. GISTs, in particular, should not be treated with doxorubicin- and ifosfamide-based chemotherapy. GISTs are usually characterized by mutated c-Kit and have a high response rate with prolonged remissions after treatment with imatinib at 400 mg daily. Patients who do not respond or who relapse after initial therapy may respond to higher doses up to 800 mg in divided doses daily or to sunitinib. Patients with GIST and exon 9 mutations respond more frequently and for longer to 800 mg of imatinib than to 400 mg. There is increasing suggestion that alveolar soft-part sarcomas should be treated with vascular endothelial growth factor inhibitors, and that solitary fibrous tumors are best treated with a combination of antiangiogenic agents and chemotherapy (e.g., bevacizumab-temozolomide). Angiosarcomas, especially those primary in the skin, can respond to paclitaxel, while other sarcomas do not. Two tumors—Ewing sarcoma and rhabdomyosarcoma—particularly in children, are responsive to dactinomycin, vincristine, or etoposide. The other tumors are not. The goal of therapy for patients with advanced disease is primarily palliative, although a small fraction (about 20%) of patients who achieve complete remission are, in fact, cured. The first aim, therefore, is to achieve complete remission. Several investigators, including the author, have shown that the prognosis is the same whether complete remission is obtained by chemotherapy alone or by chemotherapy with adjuvant surgery, that is, surgical removal of all residual disease. Short of complete remission, partial remission causes some palliation, with relief of symptoms and prolongation of survival by about 1 year. Any degree of improvement or stabilization of previously advancing disease likewise increases survival.

B. Effective drugs

The most important chemotherapeutic agent is doxorubicin, which forms the backbone of all combination chemotherapy regimens. Ifosfamide, an analog of cyclophosphamide that has documented activity even in patients who are refractory to combinations containing cyclophosphamide, is usually included in frontline chemotherapy combinations. It is always given together with the uroprotective agent mesna to prevent hemorrhagic cystitis. Dacarbazine, a marginal agent by itself, adds significantly to doxorubicin in prolonging remission duration and survival as well as increasing the response rate. Cyclophosphamide adds marginally, if at all, but is included in some effective regimens. Gemcitabine is an active agent, more so when combined with docetaxel, but with exceptions of uterine leiomyosarcoma and some angiosarcomas, these agents are usually reserved for second-line therapy. Trabectedin, approved in most countries outside of the United States, is also an active agent.

The key to effective sarcoma chemotherapy is the steep dose–response curve for doxorubicin. At a dose of 45 mg/m^2, the response rate is lower than 20% compared with a 37% response rate at a dose of 75 mg/m^2. A similar dose–response relationship exists for ifosfamide and for combination chemotherapy, and the regimens with the best reported results are those using the highest doses.

C. Primary chemotherapy regimen (adjuvant or advanced)

The most effective primary chemotherapy regimens include doxorubicin and ifosfamide (high-dose AI) or doxorubicin and dacarbazine (ADIC), with or without the addition of cyclophosphamide (CyADIC) or ifosfamide and mesna (MAID). The CyADIC regimen is a modification of the standard CyVADIC regimen, which includes vincristine. Because analysis has shown that vincristine makes no significant contribution and produces neurotoxicity, its addition at a dose of 2 mg maximum or 1.4 mg/m^2 weekly for 6 weeks and then once every 3 to 4 weeks is recommended only for treatment of rhabdomyosarcoma and Ewing sarcoma.

By giving doxorubicin and dacarbazine by continuous 72- or 96-hour infusion, with the two drugs mixed in the same infusion pump, nausea and vomiting are markedly reduced, and the chemotherapy can be continued until a cumulative doxorubicin dose of 600 to 800 mg/m^2 is reached, with less cardiac toxicity than with standard doxorubicin administration and a cumulative dose of 450 mg/m^2.

1. **The high-dose AI regimen** is as follows:
   - Doxorubicin by continuous 72-hour infusion at 75 mg/m^2 IV (25 mg/m^2/day for 3 days), *and*
   - Ifosfamide 2.5 g/m^2 intravenously (IV) over 2 to 3 hours daily for 4 days.

- Vincristine 2 mg total dose is added on day 1 for small-cell tumors such as rhabdomyosarcoma and Ewing sarcoma (high-dose AI with vincristine).
- Mesna 500 mg/m^2 is mixed with the first ifosfamide dose, and 1500 mg/m^2 is given as a continuous infusion over 24 hours for 4 days in 2 L of alkaline fluid.
- Filgrastim (granulocyte colony-stimulating factor) 5 μg/kg subcutaneously (SC) is given on days 5 to 15 or until granulocyte recovery to 1500/μL. Alternatively, pegfilgrastim at a dose of 6 mg is given on day 5.
- Repeat cycle every 3 weeks.

2. **The continuous-infusion CyADIC regimen** is as follows:
   - Cyclophosphamide 600 mg/m^2 IV on day 1, *and*
   - Doxorubicin, by continuous 96-hour infusion at 60 mg/m^2 IV (15 mg/m^2/day for 4 days), *and*
   - Dacarbazine by continuous 96-hour infusion at 1000 mg/m^2 IV (250 mg/m^2/day for 4 days) mixed in the same bag or pump as the doxorubicin. Doses should be divided into four consecutive 24-hour infusions.
   - Repeat cycle every 3 to 4 weeks.

3. **The continuous-infusion ADIC regimen** is as follows:
   - Doxorubicin by continuous 96-hour infusion at 90 mg/m^2 IV (22.5 mg/m^2/day for 4 days), *and*
   - Dacarbazine by continuous 96-hour infusion at 900 mg/m^2 IV (225 mg/m^2/day for 4 days) mixed in the same bag or pump as the doxorubicin. Doses should be divided into four consecutive 24-hour infusions.
   - Repeat cycle every 3 to 4 weeks.

4. **The MAID regimen** is as follows:
   - Mesna by continuous 96-hour infusion at 8000 mg/m^2 IV (2000 mg/m^2/day for 4 days).
   - Doxorubicin by continuous 72-hour infusion at 60 mg/m^2 IV (20 mg/m^2/day for 3 days).
   - Ifosfamide by continuous 72-hour infusion at 6000 mg/m^2 IV (2000 mg/m^2/day for 3 days). Doses should be divided into three consecutive 24-hour infusions. (Some investigators prefer to infuse ifosfamide over 2 hours rather than 24 hours because of higher single-agent activity with the shorter infusions.)
   - Dacarbazine by continuous 72-hour infusion at 900 mg/m^2 IV (300 mg/m^2/day for 3 days) mixed in the same bag or pump as the doxorubicin. Doses should be divided into three consecutive 24-hour infusions.
   - Repeat cycle every 3 to 4 weeks.

5. **Dose modification.** Doses of doxorubicin, cyclophosphamide, ifosfamide, and mesna should be increased by 25% and may be decreased by 20% for each course of therapy to achieve a lowest

absolute granulocyte count of about 500/µL if growth factors are not used. *The maximum doxorubicin dose is limited to 600 to 800 mg/m²*, depending on the duration (48 to 96 hours) of infusion, at which point therapy should be discontinued unless cardiac biopsy specimens indicate that it is safe to continue. With Ewing sarcoma and rhabdomyosarcoma, therapy may be continued, and dactinomycin 2 mg/m² in a single dose or 0.5 mg/m² daily for 5 days may be substituted for the doxorubicin, with continuation of the regimen for a total of 18 months.

6. **An alternative regimen for children with rhabdomyosarcoma** is an alternating regimen, using ifosfamide and etoposide alternating with the so-called vincristine, Adriamycin, and cyclophosphamide (VAdriaC) regimen.

   ■ Vincristine 1.5 mg/m² is given weekly × 3 for the first two cycles of VAdriaC and then on day 1 only.

   ■ Doxorubicin is given at a dose of 60 to 75 mg/m² as a 48-hour continuous infusion, *and*

   ■ Cyclophosphamide 600 mg/m² is given daily for 2 days (with mesna).

   After 3 weeks,

   ■ Ifosfamide is given at a dose of 1800 mg/m² daily for 5 days (with mesna), *and*

   ■ Etoposide is given at a dose of 100 mg/m² daily for 5 days.

   Chemotherapy cycles are alternated every 3 weeks for 39 weeks.

7. **Vincristine, dactinomycin, and cyclophosphamide (VAC).** A less-intensive, older, but still effective regimen for children with good-prognosis rhabdomyosarcoma is the so-called pulse VAC regimen. Dactinomycin is given at a total dose of 2 to 2.5 mg/m² by divided daily injection over 5 to 7 days (e.g., 0.5 mg/m² daily for 5 days) repeated every 3 months for a total of five courses. Cyclophosphamide pulses of 275 to 330 mg/m² daily for 7 days are begun at the same time but are given every 6 weeks with vincristine 2 mg/m² on days 1 and 8 of each cyclophosphamide cycle. Cyclophosphamide cycles are terminated prematurely if the white blood cell counts fall below 1500/µL. Chemotherapy continues for 2 years. (The necessity of the 2-year duration of the chemotherapy program is not certain.)

D. **Secondary chemotherapy**

Secondary chemotherapy for patients with sarcoma is relatively unrewarding, with response rates lower than 10% for almost all conventional drugs or regimens tested. The best commercially available drug is ifosfamide, which, if not used in primary treatment, produces a response in about 20% of patients. High-dose ifosfamide (12 g/m² or higher) may produce responses in patients resistant to lower doses in combination. Gemcitabine in the author's experience has a response rate of 18% and has become the standard drug for salvage therapy. Recent data indicates that the combination of gemcitabine and docetaxel (the Gem-Tax regimen) improves response rate, time to progression, and survival in a randomized comparison with gemcitabine alone; thus the Gem-Tax regimen should be considered as the secondary treatment of choice for most soft-tissue sarcomas. Exceptions are myxoid liposarcoma and synovial sarcoma, where the regimen has minimal activity. In contrast, at least for myxoid liposarcoma, trabectedin is highly active and should be considered the secondary treatment of choice.

The Gem-Tax regimen is as follows:

- Gemcitabine 900 mg/m^2 over 90 minutes on days 1 and 8.
- Docetaxel 100 mg/m^2 on day 8 only.
- Filgrastim (granulocyte colony-stimulating factor) 5 μg/kg SC is given on days 9 to 15 or until granulocyte recovery to 1500/μL. Alternatively, pegfilgrastim at a dose of 6 mg is given on day 9.

The duration of gemcitabine infusion is critical, as it can only be converted to its active metabolite, gemcitabine triphosphate, at a rate of 10 mg/m^2/min. Doses are reduced 25% to 675 mg/m^2 and 75 mg/m^2, respectively, for patients with extensive prior therapy or pelvic radiation. Dexamethasone 8 mg by mouth twice a day should be given for 3 days starting 1 day prior to docetaxel.

Trabectedin has a response rate of no more than 10% to 20% overall but can cause prolonged stability in previously progressing patients, dramatic tumor regressions in a few, and frequent responses in those with myxoid liposarcoma. For patients with this subtype, RECIST responses are seen in about 40% of patients, Choi responses in about 80% of patients, and progressive disease in just over 10%.

Trabectedin is administered as follows:

- Trabectedin 1.5 mg/m^2 over 24 hours IV day 1 only. Premedicate on day 0 with dexamethasone 8 mg by mouth.
- Pegfilgrastim 6 mg SC on day 3.

Patients who do not respond to doxorubicin, ifosfamide, Gem-Tax, or trabectedin should be entered in a phase II study of a new agent to see if some activity can be established because other reasonably good alternatives do not exist.

E. Complications of chemotherapy

Side effects of sarcoma chemotherapy can be classified into three categories: life threatening, potentially dangerous, and unpleasant.

1. **Life-threatening complications of chemotherapy are infection or bleeding.** Thrombocytopenia lower than 20,000/μL occurs with this type of chemotherapy when growth factors are used to maintain dose intensity, but bleeding is rare and can be minimized by transfusing platelets at 10,000/μL. Approximately 20% to 40% of patients have documented or suspected infection related to drug-induced neutropenia at some time during their

treatment course. These infections are rarely fatal if treated promptly with broad-spectrum, bactericidal antibiotics at the onset of the febrile neutropenia episode.

2. **Potentially dangerous side effects of chemotherapy** include the following.

   a. **Mucositis,** which occurs in fewer than 25% of patients, may interfere with oral intake or may act as a source of infection.

   b. **Granulocytopenia** predisposes the patient to infection but, because of its brevity, rarely causes infection.

   c. **Cardiac damage** from doxorubicin rarely causes clinical problems at the doses recommended, with usually reversible congestive heart failure occurring in fewer than 5% of patients.

   d. **Renal insufficiency** is a rare complication of ifosfamide. Fanconi syndrome, particularly manifested by a significant loss of bicarbonate, is a dose-related complication of ifosfamide, occurring in 10% to 30% of patients at standard ifosfamide doses and in close to 100% with high-dose regimens, the morbidity of which can be minimized by the routine use of alkaline infusions and correction of electrolyte levels with intravenous or oral replacement therapy. Only rarely does the nephrotoxicity progress to renal failure, often precipitated by dehydration or administration of minimally nephrotoxic drugs such as nonsteroidal anti-inflammatory drugs (NSAIDs). Patients treated with ifosfamide should be instructed to avoid NSAIDs, even years after chemotherapy!

   e. **CNS toxicity** of ifosfamide is rarely a serious complication. Patients frequently demonstrate minor confusion, disorientation, or difficulty with fine movements. Somnolence and coma are rarely seen in patients without hypoalbuminemia and/or acidosis.

   f. **Hemorrhagic cystitis,** a rare complication of cyclophosphamide therapy, used to be the dose-limiting toxicity of ifosfamide. It can be prevented in most cases by administration of another agent, mesna, before and after each ifosfamide dose, allowing higher doses of ifosfamide to be used.

   g. **Pulmonary toxicity,** manifested by increasing dyspnea, is seen in less than 10% of patients treated with the Gem-Tax combination, but occurs with about twice the frequency of that seen with gemcitabine alone. Careful attention to the possible occurrence of this problem and prompt treatment with high doses of corticosteroids can be life-saving.

   h. **Hepatic toxicity** is the limiting toxicity of trabectedin. If the drug is withheld when alkaline phosphatase is elevated, serious hepatitis is rarely a problem, and the incidence of this effect is less than 5% when dexamethasone premedication is utilized.

3. **Unpleasant but rarely serious problems** include nausea and vomiting (primarily from dacarbazine, ifosfamide, and docetaxel) and alopecia (from doxorubicin, cyclophosphamide, ifosfamide, and docetaxel). Gemcitabine, and to a greater extent, the Gem-Tax combination, can cause profound fatigue. Gemcitabine can also cause drug fever and a rash (often confused for cellulitis) that can respond to corticosteroids.

F. **Special precautions**
   1. **Ifosfamide.** Patients must be kept well hydrated with an alkaline pH to prevent CNS toxicity and minimize nephrotoxicity. Sodium bicarbonate or sodium acetate should be added to IV fluids at an initial concentration of 100 to 150 mEq/L, and fluid administration should be adjusted to produce a urine output of at least 2 L/day and to maintain the serum bicarbonate concentration at 25 mEq/L or higher. Other electrolytes should be adjusted as needed on a daily basis. Serum albumin should be kept within normal limits.
   2. **Doxorubicin.** Avoid extravasation. Continuous infusions must (and short infusions should) be administered through a central venous catheter. Attention to cumulative dose administered (varying according to the schedule of administration) is critical to minimize the risk of cardiac toxicity.
   3. **Trabectedin.** Avoid extravasation. Continuous infusions must (and short infusions should) be administered through a central venous catheter.

Selected Readings

Antman KH, Crowley J, Balcerzak SP, et al. An intergroup phase III randomized study of doxorubicin and dacarbazine with or without ifosfamide and mesna in advanced soft tissue and bone sarcomas. *J Clin Oncol.* 1993;11:1276–1285.

Antman KH, Montella D, Rosenbaum C, Schwen M. Phase II trial of ifosfamide with mesna in previously treated metastatic sarcoma. *Cancer Treat Rep.* 1985;69:499–504.

Benjamin RS, Legha SS, Patel RS, Nicaise C. Single agent ifosfamide studies in sarcomas of soft tissue and bone: the M.D. Anderson experience. *Cancer Chemother Pharmacol.* 1993;31:S174–S179.

Demetri GD, von Mehren M, Blanke CD, et al. Efficacy and safety of imatinib mesylate in advanced gastrointestinal stromal tumors. *N Engl J Med.* 2002;347:472–480.

Elias A, Ryan L, Sulkes A, et al. Response to mesna, doxorubicin, ifosfamide, and dacarbazine in 108 patients with metastatic or unresectable sarcoma and no prior chemotherapy. *J Clin Oncol.* 1989;7:1208–1216.

Fata F, O'Rielly E, Ilson D, et al. Paclitaxel in the treatment of patients with angiosarcoma of the scalp or face. *Cancer.* 1999;86:2034–2037.

Frustaci S, Gherlinzoni F, De Paoli A, et al. Adjuvant chemotherapy for adult soft tissue sarcomas of the extremities and girdles: results of the Italian Randomized Cooperative Trial. *J Clin Oncol.* 2001;19:1238–1247.

Grosso F, Jones RL, Demetri GD, et al. Efficacy of trabectedin (ecteinascidin-743) in advanced pretreated myxoid liposarcomas: a retrospective study. *Lancet Oncol.* 2007;8:595–602.

Harrison L, Franzese F, Gaynor J, Brennan MF. Long-term results of a prospective randomized trial of adjuvant brachytherapy in the management of completely resected soft tissue sarcomas of the extremity and superficial trunk. *Int J Radiat Oncol Biol Phys.* 1993;27:259–265.

Joensuu H, Roberts PJ, Sarlomo-Rikala M, et al. Effect of the tyrosine kinase inhibitor STI571 in a patient with a metastatic gastrointestinal stromal tumor. *N Engl J Med.* 2001;344:1052–1056.

Le Cesne A, Blay JY, Judson I, et al. Phase II study of ET-743 in advanced soft tissue sarcomas: a European Organisation for the Research and Treatment of Cancer (EORTC) soft tissue and bone sarcoma group trial. *J Clin Oncol.* 2005;23:576–584.

Lindberg RD, Martin RG, Romsdahl MM, et al. Conservative surgery and radiation therapy for soft tissue sarcomas. In: Martin RG, Ayala AG, eds. *Management of primary bone and soft tissue tumors.* Chicago: Year Book; 1977:289–298.

Maki RG, Wathen JK, Patel SR et al. An adaptively randomized phase 2 study of gemcitabine and docetaxel vs. gemcitabine alone in patients with metastatic soft-tissue sarcomas. *J Clin Oncol.* 2007;25:2755–2763.

Patel SR, Benjamin RS. Sarcomas: part I and II. *Hematol Oncol Clin North Am.* 1995;9:513–942.

Patel SR, Gandhi V, Jenkins J, et al. Phase II clinical investigation of gemcitabine in advanced soft tissue sarcomas and window evaluation of dose-rate on gemcitabine triphosphate accumulation. *J Clin Oncol.* 2001;19:3483–3489.

Patel SR, Vadhan-Raj S, Burgess MA, et al. Results of two consecutive trials of dose-intensive chemotherapy with doxorubicin and ifosfamide in patients with soft-tissue sarcomas. *Am J Clin Oncol.* 1998;21:317–321.

Patel SR, Vadhan-Raj S, Papadopoulos N, et al. High-dose ifosfamide in bone and soft-tissue sarcomas: results of phase II and pilot studies—dose response and schedule dependence. *J Clin Oncol.* 1997;15:2378–2384.

Pisters P, Leung D, Woodruff J, Shi W, Brennan MF. Analysis of prognostic factors in 1,041 patients with localized soft tissue sarcomas of the extremities. *J Clin Oncol.* 1996;14:1679–1689.

Soft tissue sarcoma. In: Greene FL, Page DL, Fleming ID, et al. (eds.) *AJCC cancer staging manual* (6th ed.). New York, NY: Springer-Verlag; 2002:193–197.

Sarcoma Meta-analysis Collaboration. Adjuvant chemotherapy for localised resectable soft-tissue sarcoma of adults: meta-analysis of individual data. *Lancet.* 1997; 350:1647–1654.

Therasse P, Arbuck SG, Eisenhauer EA, et al. New guidelines to evaluate the response to treatment in solid tumors. *J Natl Cancer Inst.* 2000;92:205–216.

van Oosterom AT, Judson I, Verweij J, et al. Safety and efficacy of imatinib (STI571) in metastatic gastrointestinal stromal tumours: a phase I study. *Lancet.* 2001; 358:1421–1423.

Verweij J, Casali PG, Zalcberg J, et al. Progression-free survival in gastrointestinal stromal tumours with high-dose imatinib: randomised trial. *Lancet.* 2004;364:1127–1134.

Wunder J, Healey J, Davis A, Brennan MF. A comparison of staging systems for localized extremity soft tissue sarcoma. *Cancer.* 2000;88:2721–2730.

Zalupski MM, Ryan J, Hussein M, et al. Defining the role of adjuvant chemotherapy for patients with soft tissue sarcoma of the extremities. In: Salmon SE, ed. *Adjuvant therapy of cancer VII.* Philadelphia: Lippincott; 1993:385–392.

Bone Sarcomas
Robert S. Benjamin

There are four major sarcomas of bone, each differing somewhat in clinical behavior, chemotherapy responsiveness, and prognosis. All present as painful bony lesions, and all metastasize preferentially to lung and then to other bones. The prognosis of untreated sarcomas of the bone is inversely proportional to their chemotherapy responsiveness. The sarcomas are considered in order of greatest to least chemotherapeutic responsiveness: Ewing sarcoma, osteosarcoma, malignant fibrous histiocytoma of bone, and chondrosarcoma.

Response to treatment is evaluated according to the usual criteria used for solid tumors and identical to that reported in Chapter 16 for soft-tissue sarcomas. It is often difficult to assess the response of primary bone tumors to chemotherapy prior to surgery, and the response on positron emission tomography-computed tomography correlates best with pathologic tumor destruction. Magnetic resonance imaging can be very misleading. Complete resection and examination of the total specimen often are required to determine response to therapy in a primary or even a metastatic lesion and to confirm complete remission.

I. STAGING
Bone tumors are staged according to American Joint Committee on Cancer (AJCC) criteria as well as the criteria of the Musculoskeletal Tumor Society.

A. The AJCC staging system
The stage is determined by tumor grade, tumor size, and presence and sites of metastases. There are four tumor grades:
- Grade 1: Well differentiated—low grade
- Grade 2: Moderately differentiated—low grade
- Grade 3: Poorly differentiated—high grade
- Grade 4: Undifferentiated—high grade.

Ewing sarcoma is classified as G4.

Tumor size is divided at less than or equal to 8 cm. Tumor size determines A and B, substages of stages I and II, and stage III:
- T1 = ≤8 cm
- T2 = >8 cm
- T3 = Discontinuous tumors in the primary bone site.

Metastatic status is subdivided by presence and location of metastases:
- M0 = No distant metastases
- M1 = Distant metastases

- M1a = Lung
- M1b = Other distant sites, including lymph nodes.

The AJCC stage grouping is as follows:

Stage IA	G1–2	T1	N0	M0
Stage IA	G1–2	T2	N0	M0
Stage IIA	G3–4	T1	N0	M0
Stage IIB	G1–2	T2	N0	M0
Stage III	Any G	T3	N0	M0
Stage IVA	Any G	Any T	N0	M1a
Stage IVB	Any G	Any T	Any N	M1b (includes N1)

B. The Musculoskeletal Tumor Society staging system

The Musculoskeletal Tumor Society stages sarcomas according to grade and compartmental localization. The Roman numeral reflects the tumor grade:

- Stage I: Low grade
- Stage II: High grade
- Stage III: Any-grade tumor with distant metastasis.

The companion letter reflects tumor compartmentalization.

- Stage A: Confined to bone
- Stage B: Extending into adjacent soft tissue.

C. Evaluation of staging

Thus, a stage IA tumor is a low-grade tumor confined to bone, and a stage IB tumor is a low-grade tumor extending into soft tissue, and so forth. Patients are evaluated and followed according to the plan in Table 17.1.

II. EWING SARCOMA

A. General considerations and aims of therapy

1. Tumor characteristics. Ewing sarcoma is a highly malignant, small, round-cell tumor of bone. Together with other members of the Ewing Family of Tumors (EFT), most notably primitive neuroectodermal tumor, Ewing sarcoma is characterized by a specific t(11;22) chromosome translocation that results most commonly in the EWS-FLI-1 gene rearrangement. It is now believed that all members of the EFT should be considered as the same tumor. It occurs most commonly in the second decade of life, and 90% of patients are younger than 30 years. There is a slight male predominance. The most common locations are the pelvis or the diaphysis of long tubular bones of the extremities. Often, systemic symptoms of fever and leukocytosis suggest infection. Radiographically, the predominant feature is osteolysis, although sclerosis does occur. Frequently, the periosteal reaction has the so-called onion skin pattern with layering of subperiosteal new bone, frequently with spicules radiating out from

TABLE 17-1 Primary Bone Sarcoma Evaluation

Tests*	Before Therapy	On Initial Treatment	Preoperative	On Subsequent Treatment	Follow-Up
History and physical examination	X	Before each treatment	X	Before each treatment	Year 1: every 2 months Years 2 and 3: every 3–4 months Year 4: every 4 months Year 5: every 6 months Then yearly
CBC, differential, and platelet counts†	X	Twice weekly	X	Twice weekly	Yearly
Chemistry profile†	X	Before each treatment	X	Before each treatment	Year 1: every 4–6 months Then yearly
Calculated creatinine clearance	X	For methotrexate	—	For methotrexate	—
Electrolytes, mg†	X	Before each treatment	X	Before each treatment	—
Urinalysis	If ifosfamide is given	As indicated by symptoms	X	Before each treatment	—
PT, APTT, fibrinogen	X	Before each IA treatment and every day while on IA treatment	X	—	—
Plain films of primary tumor	X	Every two cycles	X	Every 3 months	Year 1: every 4–6 months Then yearly
CT of primary tumor	X	After two to four cycles	X	—	At end of treatment for head and neck or pelvic primaries
MRI of primary tumor	—	For surgical planning only	—	—	—
Bone scan	X				
PET-CT‡	X	After two to four cycles	If needed to assess response	—	—

Chest radiograph	X	Before each treatment	X	Year 1: every 2 months; Years 2 and 3: every 3–4 months; Year 4: every 4 months; Year 5: every 6 months; Then yearly
Chest CT	X	If chest radiograph is equivocal, to assess response, or for surgical planning	If chest radiograph is equivocal, to assess response, or for surgical planning	If chest radiograph is equivocal or for surgical planning
Angiogram	—	Before each preoperative treatment	—	—
Bone marrow	Only for small cell tumors with metastases	—	—	—
ECG	If cardiac history	—	If cardiac history	—
Cardiac scan	If cardiac history	—	If doxorubicin dose exceeds standard limits for schedule	—
Central venous catheter	X	—	—	—
Bone tumor conference	X	—	—	If further multidisciplinary decisions are required

APTT, activated partial thromboplastin time; CBC, complete blood cell count; CT, computed tomography; ECG, electrocardiogram; IA, intra-arterial; MRI, magnetic resonance imaging; PET, positron emission tomography; PT, prothrombin time.

*Tests may be ordered more frequently based on clinical indications.

†Required more frequently if patient is on a medical treatment program.

‡Procedure is strongly suggested but optional.

the cortex. Prognosis, until the era of modern chemotherapy, was extremely poor, with a 5-year survival rate lower than 10% and almost half of patients dying within 1 year of diagnosis. Because Ewing sarcoma is a high-grade tumor and, by definition, is almost always accompanied by a soft-tissue mass, it usually is staged as AJCC stage IIB or IV depending on the demonstration of metastatic disease in lung (IVA), bone (IVB), or both. Bone metastases confer a markedly worse prognosis.

2. **Primary treatment.** Because of the poor prognosis and because of the mutilative surgery involved in resection of the primary lesion, radiotherapy has been the primary modality for local tumor control. As techniques for limb salvage surgery have become more widely practiced, attempts to use surgery rather than radiation therapy are again increasing. There are indications that the use of surgery not only increases the rate of local control but also may improve overall prognosis. While this may, in fact, be the case, conclusions need to be tempered by the fact that patients with the worst prognosis are not offered surgical resection.

B. Chemotherapy

The most effective primary chemotherapy regimens include vincristine, doxorubicin, and ifosfamide (high-dose VAI) or cyclophosphamide (VAdriaC), with or without the addition of dacarbazine (CyVADIC). In most cases where ifosfamide is not used in the primary treatment, ifosfamide and etoposide are added in rotating fashion or after completion of the doxorubicin-based regimen.

1. **The high-dose VAI regimen** is as follows:
   - ▓ Vincristine 2 mg total dose on day 1.
   - ▓ Doxorubicin (Adriamycin) by continuous 72-hour infusion at 75 mg/m^2 intravenously (IV) (25 mg/m^2/day for 3 days), *and*
   - ▓ Ifosfamide 2.5 g/m^2 IV over 2 to 3 hours daily for 4 days.
   - ▓ Mesna 500 mg/m^2 is mixed with the first ifosfamide dose, and 1500 mg/m^2 is given as a continuous infusion over 24 hours for 4 days in 2 L of alkaline fluid.
   - ▓ Filgrastim (granulocyte colony-stimulating factor) 5 μg/kg subcutaneously is given on days 5 to 15 or until granulocyte recovery to 1500/μL. Alternatively, pegfilgrastim at a dose of 6 mg is given on day 5.
   - ▓ Repeat cycle every 3 weeks.

2. **CyVADIC regimen.** Another good chemotherapeutic regimen for Ewing sarcoma, particularly in adult patients, is the continuous-infusion CyVADIC regimen, which is mentioned in Chapter 16 (see Section II.C).
   - ▓ Cyclophosphamide 600 mg/m^2 IV on day 1.
   - ▓ Vincristine 1.4 mg/m^2 (2 mg maximum) IV weekly for 6 weeks, then on day 1 of each cycle.

- Doxorubicin (Adriamycin) 60 mg/m^2 IV by 96-hour continuous infusion through a central venous catheter (15 mg/m^2/day for 4 days).
- Dacarbazine 1000 mg/m^2 IV by 96-hour continuous infusion (250 mg/m^2/day for 4 days) mixed in the same bag or pump as the doxorubicin. Doses should be divided into four consecutive 24-hour infusions.
- Repeat cycle every 3 to 4 weeks.

3. **Dose modifications.** Courses are repeated with a 25% increase or decrease in the doses of cyclophosphamide and doxorubicin, depending on morbidity. Courses are repeated in 3 to 4 weeks as soon as recovery to 1500 granulocytes/μL and 100,000 platelets/μL occurs. Complications are as described in Chapter 16 (see Section II.E), with the addition of peripheral neuropathy from vincristine. When the cumulative dose of doxorubicin has reached 800 mg/m^2, therapy is discontinued.

4. **Alternative regimens.** Alternative regimens omit dacarbazine; vary doses of cyclophosphamide up to 4200 mg/m^2; give dactinomycin with, or in place of, doxorubicin; and in some patients, add other drugs. The most common pediatric regimen at present alternates two regimens every 2 to 3 weeks: ifosfamide plus etoposide; and vincristine and doxorubicin plus cyclophosphamide, with dactinomycin substituted for doxorubicin after a cumulative (bolus) dose of 375 mg/m^2 (VAdCA). In a recent intergroup study, this regimen was superior to VAdCA alone. The schedule of drug administration is as follows.

   a. **Initial combination** is as follows:
      - Ifosfamide 1800 mg/m^2 IV daily × 5 (with mesna), *and*
      - Etoposide 100 mg/m^2 IV daily × 5.

   b. **Three weeks later, start** is as follows:
      - Vincristine 1.5 mg/m^2 IV on day 1, *and*
      - Doxorubicin 75 mg/m^2 IV on day 1, *and*
      - Cyclophosphamide 1200 mg/m^2 IV on day 1.

   c. **Two to three weeks later,** return to the first regimen, and repeat. At a cumulative doxorubicin dose of 375 mg/m^2, substitute dactinomycin 1.25 mg/m^2. Chemotherapy continues for a total of 1 year for the 3-week regimen, but, especially for pediatric patients, the more intensive but shorter 2-week regimen is preferred.

   d. **Another version** of the alternating regimen starts with an intensive VAdriaC regimen with the doxorubicin and vincristine given by 72-hour continuous infusion and the cyclophosphamide dose increased to 4200 mg/m^2 divided into two equal doses on days 1 and 2.

5. **Responses.** Most patients with metastatic disease obtain complete remission; however, almost all patients, especially those

with bone metastases, experience relapse and ultimately die of disease. When chemotherapy is used in the therapy of primary disease with surgery or radiation therapy, prognosis depends on the size and location of the primary tumor. Patients with large flat-bone lesions have a lower than 30% cure rate compared with a 60% to 70% cure rate for those patients with long-bone lesions, which are generally smaller. An alarming complication of the chemotherapy and radiation therapy combination is a high frequency of second malignancies in cured patients, with 4 of 10 patients in one series developing secondary sarcomas within the radiated fields. This complication is another reason for considering surgical intervention rather than radiation because chemotherapy is required for cure whether or not the primary lesion can be controlled with radiation.

6. **Secondary chemotherapy**. Occasional responses have been seen with etoposide (VP-16), topoisomerase I inhibitors, other alkylating agents (especially ifosfamide), the nitrosoureas, and cisplatin. A combination of etoposide and ifosfamide is now frequently used in patients for whom those drugs were not used in initial therapy. High-dose ifosfamide (14 g/m^2 divided over 3 to 7 days, either as a 2-hour infusion with each dose or as a continuous infusion) with mesna or high-dose doxorubicin (90 mg/m^2) plus dacarbazine (900 mg/m^2) as a 96-hour continuous infusion is occasionally effective in producing brief remissions in patients for whom these agents were not used or were used at substantially lower doses during initial therapy. For patients receiving the five most active drugs in primary treatment, second-line therapy consists of a topoisomerase I inhibitor plus an alkylating agent. The most commonly studied regimen is cyclophosphamide plus topotecan, but increasingly in the United States the combination of vincristine, irinotecan, and temozolomide is gaining favor. Secondary responses are extremely poor, and the survival of a relapsed patient with Ewing sarcoma is measured in weeks unless the relapse occurs after a disease-free interval of more than 2 years.

7. **High-dose chemotherapy**. The standard chemotherapy used for Ewing sarcoma is accompanied by severe but transient myelosuppression. The availability of hematopoietic growth factors to reduce infectious complications provides an added measure of safety but is not routinely required. The author's policy has been to use growth factors for regimens known to cause febrile neutropenia in at least 30% of patients or in patients who have had febrile–neutropenic episodes during a previous course of chemotherapy rather than to reduce the doses of the myelosuppressive drugs.

Bone marrow transplantation or peripheral stem cell rescue programs are still being investigated in patients presenting with poor prognostic features (large pelvic primary tumors, metastatic disease, poor response to induction chemotherapy) but have not yet been demonstrated to improve prognosis. Such regimens have been tried with negative results in patients relapsing after standard chemotherapy and have been demonstrated to have no significant benefit. Clearly, this approach should not be used in patients with relapse.

III. OSTEOSARCOMA

A. General considerations

Osteosarcoma is a tumor with a poor prognosis in the absence of effective chemotherapy. It is the most common primary bone sarcoma. Frequently, it affects patients 10 to 25 years old and tends to be located around the knee in about two-thirds of patients, with two-thirds of those tumors involving the distal aspect of the femur. As with other sarcomas of bone, pulmonary metastases are most common, followed by bone metastases. Because conventional osteosarcoma is a high-grade tumor by definition and is accompanied by a soft-tissue mass in 90% or more of patients, it is usually staged as IIB or IIIB, depending on the demonstration of metastatic disease in lung or bone.

B. Role of chemotherapy

Chemotherapy is usually employed in the neoadjuvant or adjuvant situation, and its value preoperatively has been conclusively demonstrated. Patients who show a complete response to preoperative chemotherapy with tumor destruction of at least 90% have significantly improved survival. Response rates in evaluable tumors range from 30% to 80%. Cure of primary disease with adjuvant chemotherapy is 50% to 80%.

C. Effective agents

The four major standard single agents in the treatment of osteosarcoma are cisplatin, doxorubicin, ifosfamide, and high-dose methotrexate.

D. Recommended regimen

A variety of regimens may be recommended based on preliminary or more extensive evaluation.

1. Doxorubicin and cisplatin

- Doxorubicin 90 mg/m^2 IV by 96-hour continuous infusion through a central venous catheter, *and*
- Cisplatin 120 mg/m^2 intra-arterially (for primary tumor) or IV on day 6.
- Repeat every 4 weeks.

Three to four courses of therapy should be administered preoperatively. Postoperative therapy depends on the response of the primary tumor. Patients with tumor necrosis of 90% or more should continue on the same regimen for three to six postoperative courses or until a cumulative doxorubicin dose of 800 mg/m^2 is reached. If cisplatin must be discontinued earlier, decrease the doxorubicin dose to 75 mg/m^2 IV by 72-hour continuous infusion and substitute ifosfamide 2500 mg/m^2 IV over 3 hours daily for 4 days (the dose-intensive doxorubicin and ifosfamide regimen for soft-tissue sarcoma; see Chapter 16, Section II.C.1).

2. **Alternative regimen.** After primary chemotherapy, if there is less than 90% tumor necrosis at surgery, switch to the alternative regimen as follows.

   a. High-dose methotrexate 12 g/m^2 IV every 2 weeks for 8 weeks with leucovorin rescue (see Section III.E.2).

   b. Three weeks later, administer ifosfamide 2 g/m^2 IV over 2 hours for 5 consecutive days, with mesna 1200 mg/m^2 IV in three divided doses each day (i.e., 400 mg/m^2 IV every 4 hours × 3) or by continuous infusion after a loading dose of 400 mg/m^2 mixed with the first ifosfamide dose plus doxorubicin 75 mg/m^2 IV by 72-hour continuous infusion. Three weeks later, repeat the course.

   c. Three to four weeks later, repeat the entire cycle of four courses of methotrexate and two courses of ifosfamide-doxorubicin. End with four more courses of high-dose methotrexate.

3. **There are many alternative approaches to chemotherapy, such as** adding high-dose methotrexate and/or ifosfamide to the induction regimen and continuing with the same three to four drugs postoperatively. The combination of bleomycin, cyclophosphamide, and dactinomycin (BCD) is rarely, if ever, used anymore.

E. **Special precautions in administration**

1. **Cisplatin.** Prehydration is necessary, with overnight infusion of IV fluids at 150 mL/h or 1 L of fluid over 2 hours (for adults), followed by at least 6 L of fluid containing potassium chloride (at least 20 mEq/L) and magnesium sulfate (at least 4 mEq/L) for the first 1 or 2 days or after cisplatin administration. The addition of mannitol (66 mL of a 15% solution) before cisplatin, followed by 266 mL of a 15% solution mixed with normal saline in a total volume of 1 L to run simultaneously with the cisplatin over 2 to 3 hours, is preferred by many investigators. Particular care in electrolyte balance, including frequent determinations of magnesium levels, is necessary. In the presence of severe hypomagnesemia, magnesium sulfate up to 1 to 2 mEq/kg may be infused over 4 hours.

2. **High-dose methotrexate.** The pretreatment-calculated creatinine clearance rate should be at least 70 mL/min.

   a. Methotrexate administration and alkalization of urine. Before administration of high-dose methotrexate, 0.5 mEq/kg of sodium bicarbonate is infused IV over 15 to 30 minutes in an attempt to create an alkaline urine. Allopurinol 300 mg/day for 3 days is given starting 1 day before the methotrexate infusion. Methotrexate is dissolved in no more than 1000 mL of 5% dextrose in water, with a final concentration of about 2 g/100 mL. The total dose ranges from 8 g/m^2 for patients over 40 years old to 12 g/m^2 for children and young adults. The dose should be increased on subsequent courses if an immediate postinfusion methotrexate level is less than 10^{-3} M. Sodium bicarbonate 50 mEq is added per liter of methotrexate solution, which is infused over 4 hours. After completion of the methotrexate infusion, 10 mL/kg of an IV infusion of 5% dextrose in water with 50 mEq/L of bicarbonate is given over 2 hours if the patient is unable to drink or if the 24-hour methotrexate levels of the previous high-dose methotrexate treatment have been higher than 1.5×10^{-5} M. The IV infusion is then discontinued, and the patient is encouraged to drink sufficient fluid to produce about 1600 mL/m^2 of alkaline urine for the first 24 hours and 1900 mL/m^2 daily for the next 3 days. Sodium bicarbonate 14 to 28 mEq by mouth every 6 hours is administered to ensure alkaline urine. The pH of the urine is measured, and if it is less than 7, an extra dose of bicarbonate is administered.

   b. Leucovorin rescue. Twenty-four hours after the start of the methotrexate infusion, leucovorin 15 to 25 mg is administered by mouth every 6 hours for at least 10 doses or intramuscularly if the oral medication is not tolerated.

   c. Serum methotrexate levels. These levels should be followed and should fall at approximately 1 log/day. When methotrexate concentration falls below 10^{-7} M, leucovorin may be safely discontinued. IV hydration is required whenever oral intake is inadequate to produce sufficient urine output as previously defined, for abnormal serum methotrexate concentration, for persistent vomiting, or for early toxicity.

3. Ifosfamide. Patients must be kept well hydrated with an alkaline pH to prevent central nervous system (CNS) toxicity and minimize nephrotoxicity. Sodium bicarbonate or sodium acetate should be added to IV fluids at an initial concentration of 100 to 150 mEq/L and fluid administration adjusted to produce a urine output of at least 2 L/day and maintain the serum bicarbonate concentration at 25 mEq/L or higher. Other electrolytes should be adjusted as needed on a daily basis. Serum albumin should be kept within normal limits.

F. Complications

Complications of chemotherapy depend on the drugs. For doxorubicin, the major complication is infection owing to neutropenia.

Other complications include stomatitis, nausea and vomiting, and delayed cardiac toxicity, as discussed in the management of soft-tissue sarcomas (see Chapter 16, Section II.E). Ifosfamide produces myelosuppression, nausea and vomiting, and alopecia, similar to doxorubicin. Hemorrhagic cystitis, once the dose-limiting toxicity, is rarely seen because the use of mesna has become routine. The most serious toxicities of ifosfamide are nephrotoxicity and CNS toxicity. Nephrotoxicity in the form of Fanconi syndrome is a frequent problem, the morbidity of which can be minimized by the routine use of alkaline infusions and correction of electrolyte levels with intravenous or oral replacement therapy. Only rarely does the nephrotoxicity progress to renal failure, often precipitated by dehydration or administration of minimally nephrotoxic drugs such as nonsteroidal anti-inflammatory drugs (NSAIDs). Patients treated with ifosfamide should be instructed to avoid NSAIDs, even years after chemotherapy. Correction of acid–base balance and hypoalbuminemia can essentially prevent the CNS toxicity (see Chapter 16, Section II.E). Dactinomycin causes similar side effects to those of doxorubicin, but not cardiac toxicity. Methotrexate predominantly causes stomatitis, but it may cause myelosuppression and renal, hepatic, and CNS abnormalities. Cisplatin and dacarbazine cause severe nausea and vomiting. In addition, cisplatin nephrotoxicity is primarily a tubular defect, with hypomagnesemia as the most prominent manifestation, but hypocalcemia, hypokalemia, and hyponatremia also occur. Delayed cumulative nephrotoxicity can cause impaired glomerular function as well. Ototoxicity may occur but is less common. Delayed neurotoxicity also occurs. Both cisplatin and methotrexate can, by causing renal toxicity, exacerbate their other side effects.

G. Recurrence and treatment of refractory disease

Patients with osteosarcoma who are refractory to a combination of doxorubicin and cisplatin may respond to high-dose methotrexate; patients refractory to high-dose methotrexate may respond to doxorubicin plus cisplatin; and patients refractory to both may respond to ifosfamide or, rarely, to BCD. However, treatment of refractory disease is usually disappointing, and participation in studies of new agents is indicated for patients whose disease cannot be resected. Surgical resection of pulmonary metastases remains the only viable secondary therapy for most patients. For this reason, careful follow-up for detection of metastases while they are still at the stage of resectability is indicated.

H. High-dose chemotherapy

The standard chemotherapy used for osteosarcoma is accompanied by severe but transient myelosuppression. The availability of hematopoietic growth factors to reduce infectious complications provides an added measure of safety but is not routinely required. Our policy has been to use growth factors only for regimens known to cause febrile neutropenia in at least 30% of patients or in patients who have had febrile–neutropenic episodes during a previous course of chemotherapy rather than to reduce the doses of the myelosuppressive drugs.

Bone marrow transplantation or peripheral stem cell rescue programs have not been demonstrated to improve prognosis.

IV. MALIGNANT FIBROUS HISTIOCYTOMA OF BONE

This entity, characterized by a purely lytic lesion in bone, has an exceptionally poor prognosis when treated with surgery alone, although the number of reported patients is small. It may be extremely difficult to distinguish from fibroblastic osteosarcoma and may be best considered as a fibroblastic osteosarcoma with minimal (i.e., no detectable) osteoid production. The tumor responds well to the CyADIC regimen for soft-tissue sarcomas, with more than half of patients obtaining at least partial remission. In addition, cisplatin at a dose of 120 mg/m^2 every 4 weeks has caused remissions, even in patients who did not respond to primary therapy. A particularly attractive approach for patients with large, unresectable primary tumors is the administration of cisplatin by the intra-arterial route. Complete tumor destruction in one patient and a good partial remission in a second patient are the reported results among three patients so treated. Systemic doxorubicin may be added, as for osteosarcomas (see Section III.D.1). Alternatively, responses have been seen after high-dose methotrexate-based regimens for osteosarcomas (see Section III.D.2). After local tumor destruction, surgery may be employed to remove residual disease. Because of the poor prognosis, adjuvant chemotherapy with the continuous-infusion CyADIC regimen is recommended until an 800 mg/m^2 cumulative doxorubicin dose has been reached.

V. CHONDROSARCOMA

The chemotherapy for chondrosarcoma is totally inadequate, and no regimen can be recommended except for the rare patients with mesenchymal chondrosarcoma, a subtype that may respond to CyADIC chemotherapy or cisplatin, or with dedifferentiated chondrosarcoma, which should be treated the same way as osteosarcoma. Most patients have conventional chondrosarcoma and are candidates only for surgical management. Metastatic disease should be treated with phase II protocols in an attempt to determine some effective type of chemotherapy that may be recommended in the future.

Selected Readings

Bacci G, Briccoli A, Ferrari S, et al. Neoadjuvant chemotherapy for osteosarcoma of the extremity: long-term results of the Rizzoli's 4th protocol. *Eur J Cancer.* 2001;37:2030–2039.

Bacci G, Ferrari S, Bertoni F, et al. Neoadjuvant chemotherapy for peripheral malignant neuroectodermal tumor of bone: recent experience at the Istituto Rizzoli. *J Clin Oncol.* 2000;18:885–892.

Bacci G, Ferrari S, Bertoni F, et al. Prognostic factors in nonmetastatic Ewing's sarcoma of bone treated with adjuvant chemotherapy: analysis of 359 patients at the Istituto Ortopedico Rizzoli. *J Clin Oncol.* 2000;18:4–11.

Bacci G, Ferrari S, Longhi A, et al. Neoadjuvant chemotherapy for high grade osteosarcoma of the extremities: long-term results for patients treated according to the Rizzoli IOR/OS-3b protocol. *J Chemother.* 2001;13:93–99.

Benjamin RS, Murray JA, Carrasco CH, et al. Preoperative chemotherapy for osteosarcoma: a treatment approach facilitating limb salvage with major prognostic implications. In: Jones SE, Salmon SE, eds. *Adjuvant therapy of cancer, vol IV.* New York: Grune & Stratton; 1984:601–610.

Bone sarcoma. In: Greene FL, Page DL, Fleming ID, et al. (eds.) *AJCC cancer staging manual* (6th ed.). New York, NY: Springer-Verlag; 2002:187–192.

Chawla SP, Benjamin RS, Abdul-Karim FW, et al. Adjuvant chemotherapy of primary malignant fibrous histiocytoma of bone: prolongation of disease free and overall survival. In: Jones SE, Salmon SE, eds. *Adjuvant therapy of cancer, vol IV.* New York: Grune & Stratton; 1984:621–629.

Gehan EA, Sutow WW, Uribe-Botero G, et al. Osteosarcoma: the M. D. Anderson experience, 1950–1974. In: Terry WD, Windhorst D, eds. *Immunotherapy of cancer: present status of trials in man.* New York: Raven Press; 1978.

Grier H, Krailo M, Link M, et al. Improved outcome in non-metastatic Ewing's sarcoma (EWS) and PNET of bone with the addition of ifosfamide (D) and etoposide (E) to vincristine (W), Adriamycin (Ad), cyclophosphamide (C), and actinomycin (A): a Children's Cancer Group (CCG) and Pediatric Oncology Group (POG) report. *Proc Am Soc Clin Oncol.* 1994;13:A1443.

Kushner BH, Meyers PA, Gerald WL, et al. Very-high-dose short-term chemotherapy for poor-risk peripheral primitive neuroectodermal tumors, including Ewing's sarcoma in children and young adults. *J Clin Oncol.* 1995;13:2796–2804.

Rosen G, Caparros B, Nirenberg A. The successful management of metastatic osteogenic sarcoma: a model for the treatment of primary osteogenic sarcoma. In: van Oosterom AT, Muggia FM, Cleton FJ, eds. *Therapeutic progress in ovarian cancer, testicular cancer and the sarcomas.* Hingham; New Zealand: Leiden University Press; 1980:244–265.

Acute Leukemias
Olga Frankfurt and Martin S. Tallman

I. GENERAL FEATURES OF ACUTE LEUKEMIAS

The acute leukemias are a heterogeneous group of disorders characterized by clonal proliferation and abnormal differentiation of neoplastic hematopoietic progenitor cells. Accumulation of immature hematopoietic cells, or blasts, in the bone marrow and peripheral blood ultimately leads to inhibition of normal hematopoiesis. If left untreated, acute leukemias are rapidly fatal.

Over the last 40 years, significant therapeutic advances have been made and many patients can now be cured of their disease. The general treatment approach for most patients with acute leukemia includes eradication of the leukemic clone with intensive systemic chemotherapy, followed by some form of consolidation and, in certain cases, maintenance therapy. Despite this strategy, most patients under the age of 55 and the vast majority of older adults die from their disease.

Numerous questions regarding optimal therapeutic strategies for patients with acute leukemia remain unanswered. Hence, all patients with acute leukemia should be considered candidates for clinical trials and treated in centers where appropriate intensive and comprehensive care can be provided.

A. Epidemiology

The incidence of acute myeloid leukemia (AML) and acute lymphoblastic leukemia (ALL) is 2.7 and 1.5 per 100,000 of the population, respectively, and is slightly higher in males than in females. Sixty percent of patients with ALL are children, with a peak incidence in the first 5 years of life. The second peak emerges after the age of 60 years. The incidence of AML rises exponentially after the age of 40 years with the median age of disease presentation at 68 years. The median age of patients diagnosed with acute promyelocytic leukemia (APL), a distinct subtype of AML, is 40 years, and the incidence of the disease does not increase with advanced age. While in general the incidence of acute leukemias is slightly higher in the populations of European descent, the incidence of APL may be higher among patients of Hispanic origin.

B. Etiology and risk factors of acute leukemias

Although the association of the acute leukemias with various infectious, genetic, environmental, and socioeconomic factors has been evaluated extensively, the etiology remains obscure in most cases.

1. **Infection.** There is a strong association between Epstein-Barr virus, a DNA virus causing infectious mononucleosis, and Burkitt lymphoma/leukemia.

2. **Genetic factors** have been implicated in the pathogenesis of acute leukemia based on epidemiologic studies, showing the 25% increased risk of ALL within 1 year in a monozygotic twin of an affected infant. There is also a fourfold increase in risk of developing leukemia in dizygotic siblings. The risk of developing acute leukemia is significantly higher in patients with Down and Klinefelter syndromes, and conditions with excessive chromosome fragility such as Fanconi anemia, ataxia telangiectasia, and Bloom syndrome.

3. **Exposures to chemotherapy and radiation** significantly increase the risk of developing acute leukemias. AML with chromosome 5 and/or 7 abnormality has been reported to occur 2 to 9 years after therapy with alkylating agents. Topoisomerase inhibitors have been linked to the development of AML and ALL with 11q23 aberration, characteristically 1 to 3 years after the exposure. An increased incidence of acute leukemias has been reported after radiation exposure such as atomic bomb explosion, the Chernobyl accident, and therapeutic radiation. Increased incidence of leukemia has been linked to the exposure to gasoline, benzene, tobacco, diesel, motor exhaust, and electromagnetic fields.

C. **Clinical and laboratory features**

Clinical and laboratory features of acute leukemias and their associated signs and symptoms are shown in Table 18.1.

D. **Diagnosis, classification, and prognostic features in acute leukemias**

The acute leukemias are divided into AML and ALL, based on the morphologic, immunohistochemical, and immunophenotypic characteristics of the stem cell of origin. Although the peripheral blood smear may be highly suggestive of the diagnosis, examination of the bone marrow aspirate and core biopsy is essential to confirm the diagnosis and to determine the extent of the disease. Cytogenetic analysis and molecular studies may aid in establishing an accurate diagnosis, estimate prognosis, and guide therapy.

1. **AML classification.** Currently, two pathologic classifications are used to define AML. The morphology-based French-American-British (FAB) classification, devised in 1976, utilizes cytochemical stains and, more recently, immunophenotyping by flow cytometry to differentiate myeloid from lymphoid blasts (Tables 18.2 and 18.3). According to FAB classification, eight subcategories of AML are established based on the type of the cell involved and the degree of differentiation (Table 18.4). A more recent World Health Organization (WHO) classification created in 1999 and updated in 2008 generated 17 subclassifications of AML, based on presence of dysplasia, chromosomal translocations, and molecular markers (see Table 18.4). Additional changes included

Clinical and Laboratory Features of Acute Leukemia

Clinical and Laboratory Findings	Signs and Symptoms
Anemia	Pallor, fatigue, exertional dyspnea, CHF
Neutropenia	Fever, infection
Thrombocytopenia	Petechiae, ecchymosis, retinal hemorrhages
Leukocytosis (10% of patients with WBC >100,000)	Hepatomegaly, splenomegaly, lymphadenopathy (more common in ALL)
	Bone pain (40%–50% of children with ALL, 5%–10% of adults)
	Gingival hypertrophy (particularly when derived from monocytic lineage)
	Leukemia cutis
	Solitary mass or "granulocytic sarcoma" (<5% of AML at presentation), composed of leukemia myeloid cells, in any organ, including bones, breast, skin, small bowel, mesentery, obstruction lesions of genitourinary and hepatobiliary tracts)
Leukostasis	Dyspnea, hypoxia, mental status changes
Mediastinal Mass (80% of patients with T-cell ALL, rare in AML)	Cough, dyspnea, chest pain
CNS involvement (<1% in AML at presentation, 3%–5% of adult ALL)	Headache, diplopia, cranial neuropathies, particularly CN VI, VIII, papilledema, nausea, vomiting
Elevated PT, PTT, low fibrinogen	Intracranial bleeding, DIC (particularly in APL)
Acute renal failure (uncommon), acidosis, hyperkalemia, hyperphosphatemia, hypocalcemia, elevated LDH and uric acid level	Tumor lysis syndrome

ALL, acute lymphoblastic leukemia; AML, acute myeloid leukemia; APL, acute promyelocytic leukemia; CHF, congestive heart failure; CN, cranial nerve; CNS, central nervous system; DIC, disseminated intravascular coagulation; LDH, lactate dehydrogenase; PT, prothrombin time; PTT, partial thromboplastin time; WBC, white blood cell.

the decrease of the diagnostic threshold to 20% blasts (from the original classification of 30%, hence eliminating the refractory anemia with excess blasts transformation category of myelodysplastic syndrome [MDS]) and the diagnosis of AML regardless of the percent of marrow blasts in marrows with evidence of

 Common Histochemical Stains That Characterize the Nonlymphoid Cells

Sudan black B (myeloblasts, promyelocytes)
Peroxidase (myeloblasts, promyelocytes)
Nonspecific esterases that are inhibited by sodium fluoride (monoblasts)
Periodic acid–Schiff (pronormoblasts in erythroleukemia)

18.3	Antigens Commonly Demonstrated by Flow Cytometry Techniques	
Cell Lineage	**Antigens**	
Lymphoid B	CD19, CD20, cytoplasmic CD22, CD23, CD79a	
Lymphoid T	CD1, CD2, cytoplasmic CD3, CD4, CD5, CD7, CD8	
Myelomonocytic	Myeloperoxidase, CD11c, CD13, CD14, CD33, CD117 (c-kit)	
Erythrocytic	Glycophorin A	
Megakaryocytic	Von Willebrand factor, GPIIb (CD41), GPIIIa(CD61)	
Natural killer cells	CD16, CD56	
Nonlineage–specific	TdT, HLD-DR	

T A B L E 18.4	WHO Classification of AML (Simplified)

AMLs with recurrent cytogenetic translocations
- AML with t(8;21) (q22;22); RUNX1-RUNX1T1
- AML with inv(16)(p13q22) or t(16;16)(p13;q22); CBFβ/MYH11
- APL (FAB M-3; t(15;17)(q22;q12) (*PML/RAR*-α) and variants
- AML with t(9;11)(p23q23); MLLT3-MLL
- AML with t(6;9)(p23;q34); DEK-NUP214
- AML with inv(3)(q21q26.2) or t(3;3)(q21;q26.2); RPN-EVI1
- AML (megakaryoblastic) with t(1;22)(p13;q13); PBM15-MKL1
- *Provisional entity:* AML with mutated NPM1
- *Provisional entity:* AML with mutated CEBPA1

AML with myelodysplasia-related changes

Therapy-related myeloid neoplasms

AML, not otherwise specified (correlated with FAB subtype)
- AML minimally differentiated (FAB M0)
- AML without maturation (FAB M1)
- AML with maturation (FAB M2)
- Acute myelomonocytic leukemia (FAB M4)
- Acute monocytic leukemia (FAB M5)
- Acute erythroid leukemia (FAB M6)
- Acute megakaryocytic leukemia (FAB M7)
- Acute basophilic leukemia
- Acute panmyelosis with myelofibrosis

Acute leukemias of ambiguous lineage
- AUL
- Mixed phenotype acute leukemia with t(9;22)(q34;q11.2); BCR-ABL1
- Mixed phenotype acute leukemia with t(v;11q23); MLL rearranged
- Mixed phenotype acute leukemia, B/myeloid, NOS
- Mixed phenotype acute leukemia T/myeloid, NOS
- *Provisional entry: Natural killer–cell lymphoblastic leukemia/lymphoma*

AML, acute myeloid leukemia; APL, acute promyelocytic leukemia; AUL, acute undifferentiated leukemia.

abnormal hematopoiesis and clonal cytogenetic abnormalities such as t(8;21), t(15;17), and t(16;16) or inv(16).

2. **Prognostic factors in AML.** Prognostic factors in AML could be viewed as patient-related characteristics (age, performance status [PS]) and leukemic clone–related characteristics. Advanced age is an adverse prognostic factor. Even after accounting for risk factors such as cytogenetics, molecular genetics, presence of antecedent hematologic disorder, and PS, older patients have worse outcome than younger patients: 40% to 60% complete response (CR) rates, and only 5% to 16% are alive at 5 years.

However, chronologic age alone should not be the only determinant of whether patients should receive potentially curative chemotherapy because age is not the most important prognostic factor for either treatment-related mortality (TRM) or resistance to therapy (see Section IV.G.1).

AML-related prognostic characteristics include WBC count at presentation, presence of antecedent hematologic disorder, prior exposure to the cytotoxic therapy, as well as cytogenetic and molecular changes. In fact, cytogenetic and molecular genetic changes in leukemia cells at diagnosis are the most important prognostic characteristic for predicting the rate of remission, relapse, and overall survival (OS). Younger adult patients are commonly separated into three risk groups: favorable, intermediate, or adverse (Table 18.5).

Based on the recent analysis of 1213 patients with AML treated on Cancer and Leukemia Group B (CALGB) protocols, the 5-year survival for patients with favorable, intermediate, and poor-risk cytogenetics was 55%, 24%, and 5%, respectively.

Complex karyotype, defined by the presence of three or more (in some studies five or more) chromosomal abnormalities, occurs in 10% to 12% of patients and is associated with very poor outcome. Monosomal karyotype, a recently proposed cytogenetic category, has a particularly poor survival (5-year OS of 4%). It is defined by presence of a single monosomy (excluding isolated loss of X and Y) in association with at least one additional monosomy or structural chromosome abnormality (excluding core binding factor [CBF] AML).

Cytogenetically normal (CN)-AML patients harboring internal tandem duplication (ITD) of the FLT-3 gene have an inferior outcome compared to those without FLT-3-ITD. In the recent series, 5-year survival of patients with a normal karyotype and the presence of FLT3 mutations was 20% compared to that of 42% for patients with normal karyotype without FLT3 mutation. In a clinical trial, the information regarding FLT3 status is unlikely to change the initial therapy; however, this may change, as FLT3 inhibitors become part of the armamentarium of agents active against AML.

	AML Prognostic Groups Based on Cytogenetic and Molecular Data at Presentation*

Favorable
- t(15;17)—with any other abnormality
- inv(16) or t(16;16)[†] or del(16q)—with any other abnormality or c-KIT
- t(8;21)[†]—without del(9q) or complex karyotype or c-KIT
- Mutated NPM1 without FLT3-ITD (normal karyotype)
- Double-mutated CEBPA (normal karyotype)

Intermediate
- +8,[‡] +6, del(12p)
- Mutated NPM1 and FLT3-ITD (normal karyotype)
- Wild-type NPM1 and FLT3-ITD (normal karyotype)
- Wild-type NPM1 without FLT3-ITD (normal karyotype)
- t(9;11)(p22;q23); MLLT3-MLL

Unfavorable
- −5 or del(5q)
- −7 or del(7q)
- inv(3q)(q21q26.2) or t(3;3)
- t(6;9)(p23;q34)
- t(v;11)(v;q23); MLL rearranged
- Complex karyotype (three or more abnormalities)
- Inv(16) with c-KIT or t(8;21) with c-KIT

Unknown
- All other clonal chromosomal aberrations with fewer than three abnormalities

CEBPA, CCAAT enhancer binding protein alpha.
*Determined by conventional cytogenetic techniques, fluorescent in situ hybridization, or polymerase chain reaction.
[†] Karyotypes in these two groups are part of "core-binding factor–type" acute leukemia.
[‡] Some evidence suggests that trisomy 8 confers an unfavorable prognosis

In several, but not all, studies, presence of nucleophosmin (NPM) mutation (and the absence of a FLT3 ITD mutation) in CN-AML confers an improved outcome with higher CR, relapse-free survival (RFS), and event-free survival (EFS) rates. NPM1+/FLT3− genotype demonstrate rates of CR and OS similar to those of the CBF leukemias.

Double mutation (biallelic) in the CCAAT enhancer binding protein alpha (CEBPA) gene in CN-AML patients predicts a favorable outcome. It remains to be established whether presence of FLT3 negates the positive effect of CEBPA. Among the cytogenetically favorable CBF-AML, presence of the c-KIT mutation exerts a negative influence of outcome in retrospective studies. Internal tandem duplication of the MLL gene has also been associated with poor prognosis in patients with normal karyotype.

WHO 2008 Classification of ALL

Precursor B lymphoblastic leukemia/lymphoma NOS
Precursor B lymphoblastic leukemia/lymphoma with recurrent genetic abnormalities
    t(9; 22) (q34; q11.2); BCR-ABL1
    t(v; 11q23); MLL rearranged
    t(12;21)(p13;q22); TEL/AML 1 (ETV6-RUNX1)
    B-ALL with hyperdiploidy
    B-ALL with hypodiploidy
    t(5;14)(q31;q32); IL3-IGH
    t(1;19)(q23;p13.3); E2A-PBX1 (TCF-PBX1)
Precursor T-cell acute lymphoblastic leukemia

3. **ALL classification.** The diagnosis and classification of ALL is based on cell morphology, immunohistochemistry, as well as immunophenotypic and cytogenetic features. Marrow involvement of more than 25% lymphoblasts is used to differentiate ALL from lymphoblastic lymphoma, in which the preponderance of tumor bulk is in nodal structures. Approximately 70% to 75% of adult ALL cases are of precursor B-cell origin; 20% to 25% are of T-cell origin (Tables 18.6 and 18.7).

Immunophenotypes of ALL

Type and Subtype	Characteristic Markers	Frequency in Adult ALL
B-cell precursors	**CD19$^+$, CD22$^+$, CD79a$^+$, cIg$^{+/-}$, PAX5, sIgμ$^-$, HLA-DR$^+$** **CD20, CD34–variable expression** **CD45–may be absent**	~70%–75%
Early precursor (pre–pre- or pro-) B cell	CD19$^+$, cCD79a$^+$, cCD22$^+$, TdT$^+$, CD10$^-$	11%
Common (early pre-) B cell	CD10$^+$	52%
Pre-B cell	CD10$^{+/-}$, c-μ$^+$	9%
Mature B cells	**CD19$^+$, CD22$^+$, CD79a$^+$, cIg$^+$, sIgμ$^+$, sIgλκ$^+$, sIgλ$^+$**	~5%
T lineage	**Most common: CD7$^+$, cCD3$^+$ (lineage specific)**	~20%–25%
Precursor T-cell	TdT$^+$, HLA-DR$^{+/-}$, CD2$^-$, CD1$^-$, CD4$^-$, CD8$^-$	6%
T-cell	TdT$^{+/-}$, HLA-DR$^-$, CD2$^+$, CD1$^{+/-}$, CD4$^{+/-}$, CD8$^{+/-}$	18%

cCD3, cytoplasmic CD3; c-μ$^+$, cytoplasmic chains; cIg, cytoplasmic immunoglobulin; sIg, surface immunoglobulin; PAX5, paired box 5; TdT, terminal deoxynucleotidyl transferase.

4. **Prognostic factors in ALL**. Although modern intensive chemotherapy regimens have abolished multiple prognostic factors identified in the past, several biologic and clinical features of ALL still predict response to therapy, remission duration, disease-free survival (DFS), and help to determine the intensity of the induction and postremission therapy. Similar to the patients with AML, the outcome of therapy for patients with ALL worsens with increasing age. In multivariate analysis, age over 60 years is associated with a particularly poor prognosis, with shorter remission durations and worse survival. Presenting WBC of greater than 30,000/μL is an adverse prognostic factor predicting shorter remission durations that pertains more to precursor B-lineage ALL. (Threshold WBC greater than 100,000/μL may be important for T-cell ALL.) The time required to achieve CR (more than 4 weeks) following induction chemotherapy has been demonstrated to be an adverse prognostic factor in several, but not all, clinical trials. A report from the GIMEMA ALL group demonstrated that response (defined as peripheral blast count of 0 to 1000/μL on day 10) to 7 days of initial prednisone treatment prior to induction was prognostic in predicting disease outcome in adult patients with ALL. A recently published study demonstrated that presence of minimal residual disease (MRD), defined as greater than or equal to a 10^{-4} reduction in the leukemic cell burden detected at diagnosis at weeks 16 to 22 (detected by leukemia-specific reverse transcription [RT]-polymerase chain reaction [PCR] probes), was a very strong predictor of relapse.

   Similar to AML, cytogenetic abnormalities are one of the most important factors predicting outcome in ALL. Approximately half of the patients with ALL have cytogenetic abnormalities, which usually take the form of translocation rather than deletion, as seen more commonly in AML. The landmark International ALL trial (UKALLXII/ Eastern Cooperative Oncology Group [ECOG] E2993) conducted by the Medical Research Council (MRC; now the National Cancer Research Institute) in the United Kingdom and the ECOG in the United States identified in a very large number of patients the incidence and clinical associations of more than 20 specific cytogenetic abnormalities. The t(4;11), t(8;14), complex karyotype (five or more abnormalities), and hypodiploid/near triploidy abnormalities all were associated with a poorer EFS and OS compared to patients with other abnormalities. Other adverse cytogenetic abnormalities include t(9;22), t(1;19), 9p21, and 11q23. Alternatively, patients with high hyperdiploidy or a del(9p) were associated with an improved outcome.

E. **Acute leukemias of ambiguous lineage**
   With the expansion of immunophenotyping panels, use of electron microscopy, and gene rearrangement studies for the

characterization of acute leukemia, increasing degrees of infidelity of myeloid and lymphoid markers is demonstrated. Cases in which differentiation between AML and ALL is difficult are described by the WHO as "acute leukemia of ambiguous lineage" and comprise those cases that show no evidence of lineage differentiation (i.e., acute undifferentiated leukemia [AUL]) or those with blasts that express markers of more than one lineage (mixed phenotype acute leukemia [MPAL]; see Table 18.4). AUL often expresses human leukocyte antigen (HLA)-DR, CD34, and/or CD38, but by definition lacks lineage-specific markers. MPAL can either contain a distinct blast population of different lineages, one blast population with markers of different lineages on the same cell, or a combination of both.

II. INITIAL SUPPORT

Once the diagnosis of acute leukemia has been established, the next 24 to 48 hours are spent preparing the patient for the initiation of cytotoxic chemotherapy. The following issues need to be addressed in almost all individuals facing induction chemotherapy.

A. Hyperleukocytosis, leukostasis, and leukapheresis

Hyperleukocytosis, defined as an absolute blast count of more than 100,000/μL, predisposes to rheologic problems and is associated with increased induction mortality in AML. Leukostasis, manifesting as cerebral and cardiopulmonary dysfunction due to vascular obstruction and/or vessel wall necrosis with hemorrhage, occurs almost exclusively in AML and represents an oncologic emergency. Given the increased risk of early death with hyperleukocytosis, steps to rapidly reduce the blast counts should be undertaken as soon as the diagnosis is made. In the hemodynamically stable patient, leukapheresis is the most rapid way to lower the blast count; however, no impact on long-term outcome has been shown. With very high blast counts (more than 200,000/μL), decreasing the blast count by 50% may have to be the initial goal because mathematic modeling suggests that prolonged leukapheresis after a "3-L exchange" does not significantly decrease the blast count further. Leukapheresis may be repeated daily. Systemic chemotherapy should be initiated immediately after emergent leukapheresis or if leukapheresis cannot be performed. Hydroxyurea 3 to 5 g/m^2/day split into three doses daily until WBC are less than 10,000 to 20,000/μL is commonly used. In patients presenting with hyperleukocytosis, an allopurinol dose of 600 mg twice a day is well tolerated for the first 2 days, followed by 300 mg twice a day for 2 to 3 days. Emergent cranial radiation for hyperleukocytosis and cranial nerve palsies (or other severe neurologic deficit) is another treatment modality that may be used.

Blood transfusions in the anemic patient with hyperleukocytosis should be undertaken with great care as an aggressive packed red blood cell transfusion in such patients may precipitate symptoms of hyperviscosity. Unless the patient has symptoms due to anemia, a packed cell volume (hematocrit) of 20% to 25% is a reasonable goal.

B. Hydration and correction of electrolyte imbalance

Dehydration needs to be corrected and adequate urine output maintained to prevent renal failure due to the deposition of cellular breakdown products resulting from the tumor lysis syndrome. In the absence of cardiac disease, normal saline with or without 5% dextrose (D5W) is infused to maintain the urine output at more than 100 mL/h. The concomitant use of loop diuretics may be necessary in patients with congestive heart failure.

A variety of electrolyte abnormalities, such as hypocalcemia, hyperphosphatemia, and hyperkalemia, may occur in patients with acute leukemia. Hypocalcemia may cause potentially lethal cardiac (ventricular arrhythmias, heart block) and neurologic (hallucination, seizures, coma) complications. In an asymptomatic patient with laboratory evidence of hypocalcemia and hyperphosphatemia, calcium replacement is not recommended as it may precipitate metastatic calcifications. However, in a patient with symptomatic hypocalcemia, calcium gluconate may be carefully administered to correct the clinical symptoms. Hyperkalemia, defined by a potassium level of greater than 6 mmol/L, caused by massive cellular degradation, may precipitate significant neuromuscular (muscle weakness, cramps, paresthesias) and potentially life-threatening cardiac (asystole, ventricular tachycardia, and ventricular fibrillation) abnormalities. Patients should be treated with oral sodium-potassium exchange resin, such as sodium polystyrene 15 to 30 g every 6 hours and/or combined glucose/insulin therapy.

Serum electrolytes, uric acid, phosphorus, calcium, and creatinine should be monitored several times a day, depending on the severity of the clinical condition and degree of metabolic abnormality. Early hemodialysis may be required in patients who develop oliguric renal failure or recalcitrant electrolyte disturbances. The electrocardiogram should be obtained and cardiac rhythm monitored while these abnormalities are corrected.

C. Prevention of uric acid nephropathy

Hyperuricemia is common at presentation and may also occur with the tumor lysis caused by chemotherapy. Allopurinol is the mainstay of prevention of uric acid nephropathy. The usual initial adult dose is 300 mg (150 mg/m^2) twice per day for 2 to 3 days, which is then decreased to 300 mg once a day. Allopurinol should be stopped after 10 to 14 days to lessen the risk of rash and hepatic dysfunction. If chemotherapy needs to be initiated urgently, allopurinol at a dose of 600 mg twice per day is well tolerated for 1 to 2 days. With the advent of allopurinol, the role of urine alkalinization has become less clear. Although urine alkalinization increases uric acid solubility, it decreases the solubility of urinary phosphates and may promote phosphate deposition in patients susceptible to the tumor lysis syndrome (e.g., B-cell ALL and T-cell lymphoblastic leukemia). A commonly employed method of urine alkalinization is to hydrate the patient with D5W to which two syringes of sodium bicarbonate (44 mEq of $NaHCO_3$ per syringe) have been added per liter.

Rasburicase, a recombinant urate oxidase, is a safe and effective alternative to allopurinol. Although the recommended dose of rasburicase is 0.15 to 0.2 mg/kg/day for 5 days, at our institution an excellent control of hyperuricemia was achieved with a lower dose of 3 mg/day. Administration of 3 mg of rasburicase to 18 patients with hyperuricemia secondary to leukemia/lymphoma resulted in the normalization of the uric acid in 11 patients with just a single dose of rasburicase, in 6 patients with two doses, and in 1 patient with three doses.

D. Correction of coagulopathy

Hemostatic defect secondary to thrombocytopenia may be potentiated by the presence of consumption coagulopathy (disseminated intravascular coagulation [DIC]). Life-threatening bleeding complications are particularly common in patients with APL due to the presence of DIC and primary fibrinolysis (see APL management, Section VII). Lysozyme released from monoblasts in M4 and M5 subtypes of AML may trigger a clotting cascade leading to consumption coagulopathy. In ALL, therapy with L-asparaginase (L-Asp) may lead to DIC. Additionally, sepsis may contribute to coagulopathy in newly diagnosed patients with acute leukemias. Frequent monitoring of coagulation parameters and adequate replacement with cryoprecipitate or fresh frozen plasma products in appropriate patients is critical.

E. Blood product support (see Chapter 28)

Most patients with acute leukemia present with evidence of bone marrow failure. Symptomatic anemia, hemoglobin less than 8 g/dL, thrombocytopenia less than 10,000/μL, as well as signs of bleeding, must be corrected. The threshold below which platelet transfusion is needed may be higher (e.g., 20,000/μL) if conditions known to increase the risk of bleeding such as severe mucositis, fever, anemia, and coagulopathy are present. Blood products should be leukoreduced to decrease the risk of febrile nonhemolytic transfusion reaction; alloimmunization to HLAs, which may lead to subsequent refractoriness to platelet transfusion; and transmission of cytomegalovirus (CMV). Additionally, blood products should be gamma irradiated to reduce the risk of transfusion-related graft-versus-host disease

(GVHD). Patients who are potential candidates for stem cell transplant (SCT) should be screened for CMV and receive CMV-negative blood until CMV status is determined.

F. HLA typing

Patients who are candidates for SCT should be HLA typed prior to the initiation of therapy because chemotherapy-induced severe myelosuppression will not leave enough lymphocytes for HLA typing. However, occasionally an inadequate number of circulating lymphocytes and the presence of blast cells preclude the ability to carry out HLA typing prior to initial therapy. HLA-matched platelet transfusions may need to be administered to patients who develop alloimmunization and become refractory to pooled or single-donor platelets.

G. Fever or infection (see Chapter 27)

Patients frequently have a fever or an infection at initial diagnosis. The cardinal rule is that all patients with acute leukemia and fever are presumed to have an infection until proved otherwise. Given the additional myelosuppressive and immunosuppressive effects of chemotherapy, severe infections should be treated aggressively before initiating chemotherapy. However, the antibiotic treatment frequently needs to be administered concurrently with induction chemotherapy. Patients with acute leukemia need a careful physical examination daily. There should be close attention toward potential sites of infection, including the fundi, sinuses, oral cavity, intertriginous areas, perineum (attempts are made to avoid internal rectal examination during neutropenia), and catheter sites. A dental consultation at the time of diagnosis is often useful.

H. Vascular access

Because of the need for several sites of venous access for at least 1 month, a multiple-lumen implantable catheter (e.g., Hickman catheter or peripherally inserted central catheter line) must be placed as soon as possible (except in patients suspected to have APL). An implantable port is not recommended for patients with leukemia because there is higher risk of infection and hematoma at the access site. Because of the coagulopathy in patients with APL, the placement of a long indwelling catheter is avoided altogether if at all possible and certainly until the coagulopathy has been completely corrected and the patient is in a CR. A risk of life-threatening bleeding in patients with APL is present even when most or all of the routine coagulation studies are normal.

I. Suppression of menses

A serum human chorionic gonadotropin (β-hCG) assay (pregnancy test) should be done in all premenopausal women prior to initiation of chemotherapy. It may be desirable to prevent menses during chemotherapy to avoid the severe menorrhagia due to the thrombocytopenia. Medroxyprogesterone (Provera)

10 mg twice per day may be started 5 to 7 days before the expected starting time of the next menstrual period. It may be increased to 10 mg three times per day or higher if breakthrough bleeding occurs. Medroxyprogesterone acetate IM (Depo-Provera) is contraindicated in the thrombocytopenic and neutropenic patient.

J. Birth control and fertility

Given the potential teratogenic effects of cytotoxic chemotherapy, appropriate measures for preventing conception must be addressed with women of reproductive age undergoing chemotherapy. Although there are no clear data linking chemotherapy in the male partner to teratogenic effects in the fetus, it is prudent to suggest that appropriate birth control measures be undertaken in this situation as well.

Late effects of chemotherapy, such as infertility, need to be considered in younger patients. Sperm cryopreservation should be offered to men of reproductive age prior to initiation of chemotherapy.

Gonadal function in women seems to be less affected by cytotoxic chemotherapy. Cryopreservation of *fertilized* eggs is currently available, while cryopreservation of *unfertilized* eggs may be conducted on the investigational basis.

K. Psychosocial support

Patients with acute leukemia are usually previously healthy individuals who have suddenly had to accept the possibility of their own imminent mortality. Intensive psychological and spiritual support by the healthcare team, family, and religious leaders is critical for maintaining the patient's sense of well-being.

III. THERAPEUTIC PRINCIPLES AND APPROACH TO THERAPY OF ACUTE LEUKEMIA

A. Therapeutic aim

The goals of chemotherapy are to eradicate the leukemic clone and re-establish normal hematopoiesis in the bone marrow. Long-term survival is seen only in patients in whom a CR is attained. Although leukemia therapy is toxic and infection is the major cause of death during therapy, the median survival time of untreated (or unresponsive) acute leukemia is 2 to 3 months, and most untreated patients die of bone marrow failure and its complications. The doses of chemotherapy are never reduced because of cytopenia, because lowered doses still produce the unwanted side effects (further marrow suppression) without having as great a potential for eradicating the leukemic clone and ultimately improving marrow function.

B. Forms of chemotherapy and response criteria

1. Induction chemotherapy is initial intensive chemotherapy given in an attempt to eradicate the leukemic clone and to induce a CR. The term *complete response* depicts patients who achieve recovery of normal peripheral blood counts with recovery of bone marrow cellularity, including the presence of less than 5% blast cells, in the absence of extramedullary disease. The aim of induction chemotherapy is to reduce the leukemia cell population by several logs from the clinically evident total body tumor burden of 10^{12} leukemia cells (about 1 kg), commonly seen at diagnosis, to below the cytologically detectable level of 10^9 cells. It is important to note that because achievement of initial CR represents only a 3- to 6-log leukemia cell reduction, a substantial leukemia cell burden persists, and patients usually relapse within months if further therapy is not administered. Induction therapy is typically initiated as soon as diagnostic work-up has been completed, as there retrospective data suggesting that treatment outcome might be adversely impacted when treatment is delayed by more than 5 days from the diagnosis.

2. **Postremission chemotherapy** is administered subsequently to achievement of a CR in a further attempt to eradicate the residual, but often undetectable, leukemic clone. In a younger patient population, considering the relatively high rate of CR after the induction, future advances are likely to be made through improved postremission therapy. Patients older than 60 years tend to achieve suboptimal CR rates of 40% to 60% and poor 5-year OS of approximately 10%, and should be enrolled in investigational protocols aimed at improving induction and consolidation therapy.

   ▪ *Consolidation therapy* involves repeated courses of the same drugs at similar or higher doses as those used to induce the remission, which are given soon after the remission has been achieved (2 to 3 weeks after the recovery of blood counts). Consolidation often requires further hospitalization.

   ▪ *Maintenance therapy* pertains primarily to ALL and includes low doses of drugs designed to be administered on an outpatient basis for up to 2 years. In AML, this strategy applies only to APL.

3. **The definition of response** is based on the peripheral blood counts and the status of the recovered bone marrow. If the marrow is hypoplastic, it is imperative to repeat the bone marrow biopsy to document remission on recovery.

   ▪ *CR* is the return of the complete blood count to a "normal" absolute neutrophil count (ANC) of more than $1500/\mu L$ and to a platelet count of more than $100,000/\mu L$ in conjunction with a normal bone marrow (i.e., normal cellularity, less than 5% blasts or promyelocytes and promonocytes, an absence of obvious leukemic cells, and absence of extramedullary disease). Presence of minimal residual disease (MRD) as determined by flow cytometry or PCR analysis is a predictor of the relapse. Relapse rates range from 0% in patients with a reduction to less than 10^{-4} leukemic cells detected at the completion of the induction (compared to leukemia cell burden at diagnosis) to 14% in those with 10^{-3} to 10^{-4} to 89% in patients with 1% residual disease.

■ *Partial response* is the persistence of morphologically identifiable residual leukemia (5% to 15% leukemic cells in the bone marrow).

IV. THERAPY FOR ADULT AML (OTHER THAN APL)

The day that induction chemotherapy is started is arbitrarily called day 1. Bone marrow aspiration and biopsy are typically repeated on day 14. If the bone marrow is severely hypoplastic with fewer than 5% residual blasts or if the bone marrow is aplastic, no further chemotherapy is given, and the patient is supported until bone marrow recovery occurs (usually 1 to 3 weeks more). A bone marrow examination is repeated 2 weeks later (about days 26 to 28). Once a CR has been documented, the potential benefit of further consolidation therapy should be determined on an individual basis.

A. Induction therapy

Factors that influence the choice of the initial chemotherapeutic agents include the patient's age, cardiac function, and PS. An age of 60 years has traditionally been considered a cut-off point to recommending induction chemotherapy due to higher prevalence of unfavorable cytogenetics, antecedent myelodysplasia, expression of multidrug resistant protein, as well as frequency and severity of comorbid conditions affecting the ability to tolerate intensive chemotherapy. The initial drug doses outlined below are based on the presence of normal hepatic and renal function and do not require modification for depressed (or elevated) peripheral blood counts.

1. **"3 + 7."** During the last 35 years, a series of clinical trials have identified an induction regimen of 3 days of anthracycline (daunorubicin [DNR] 60 to 90 mg/m^2/day, idarubicin 10 to 12 mg/m^2/day, or mitoxantrone, and anthracenedione, 12 mg/m^2/day) and 7 days of cytarabine (Ara-C) 100 to 200 mg/m^2, which is considered standard (Table 18.8). With such regimens, the anticipated rate of CR in younger patients (younger than 55 to 60 years) is 60% to 80%. No other intervention has been convincingly demonstrated to be better. Several randomized trials have compared DNR at 45 to 60 mg/m^2 with idarubicin, mitoxantrone, aclarubicin, and amsacrine; with respect to OS, none of the agents appeared to be superior to DNR at the equivalent doses. In younger patients, idarubicin, which attains a higher intracellular drug concentration, was shown to induce higher remission rates, longer response duration, and improved OS. In older adults, however, a randomized trial showed no benefit of one anthracycline/anthracenedione over

TABLE 18.8	Commonly Administered Induction Regimens in AML

"3 + 7": For patients able to withstand rigorous therapy
Cytarabine 100 mg/m^2/24-hour continuous IV infusion on days 1 to 7 *and*
- DNR 60–90 mg/m^2 IV bolus on days 1 to 3 *or*
- Idarubicin 12 mg/m^2 IV bolus on days 1 to 3 *or*
- Mitoxantrone 12 mg/m^2 IV bolus on days 1 to 3.

HDAC for patients with cardiac disease
Cytarabine 2 to 3 g/m^2 IV infusion over 1–2 hours every 12 hours for 12 doses, *or*
Cytarabine 2 to 3 g/m^2 IV infusion over 2 hours every 12 hours on days 1, 3, and 5

HDAC, high-dose cytarabine; IV, intravenous.

the other. In a recently published randomized clinical trial, a higher dose of DNR (90 mg/m^2/day) resulted in a higher rate of CR (70.6 versus 57.3, p <0.001) and improved OS (23.7 versus 15.7 months, p = 0.003) as compared with a lower (than standard) dose (45 mg/m^2/day). Although 60 mg/m^2/day was never formally compared to 90 mg/m^2/day, doses that exceed 45 mg/m^2/day for induction are now considered standard. Several nuances will require further clarification, particularly in patients older than 50 years; for example, those with unfavorable cytogenetic profile, FLT3-ITD+ and MLL-PTD mutation did not benefit from the higher doses of DNR.

2. **Cytarabine dose intensification.** The merit of cytarabine dose intensification has been explored in several clinical trials. Based on the results, the rate of CR was not affected by the administration of high-dose cytarabine (HDAC) compared to the standard dose.

In a Southwest Oncology Group (SWOG) study, patients received DNR (45 m/m^2 for 3 days) and were randomized to receive either standard-dose cytarabine (SDAC) (200 mg/m^2 continuous infusion for 7 days) or HDAC (2 g/m^2 every 12 hours for 6 days for a total dose of 24 g/m^2). The CR rates were equivalent. Subsequently, complete responders in the HDAC arm were given another HDAC plus DNR cycle for consolidation, whereas complete responders in the SDAC group were randomized to receive two additional courses of SDAC plus DNR or one course of HDAC plus DNR. With the median follow-up of 51 months, survival was not significantly better in the HDAC arm. However, the RFS was somewhat better following the HDAC induction compared to those with SDAC induction (33% versus 21% for the younger group and 21% versus 9% for the older group).

In conclusion, induction therapy with HDAC plus DNR is associated with greater toxicity than SDAC plus DNR, but *without* improvement in CR rate or survival. Following CR induction with SDAC, consolidation with HDAC increases the toxicity but not survival or DFS. Hence, the use of HDAC induction outside the clinical trial is not recommended.

3. **Other regimens**. Many permutations to the standard "7 + 3" regimen have been studied over the years in attempts to improve the CR rate of induction therapy and prolong survival. The addition of other agents such as 6-thioguanine and etoposide (3 + 7 + 3) to the "7 + 3" regimen have improved the CR rate and response duration in some studies, but these regimens produce increased toxicity without improvement in OS. The SWOG trial comparing a combination of SDAC and DNR with mitoxantrone and etoposide in patients older than 55 years showed similar CR rates (43% versus 34%) and therapy-related toxicity (16% versus 22%), respectively. Furthermore, the risk of secondary acute leukemia from topoisomerase inhibitors needs to be considered in patients who are potentially long-term survivors. HDAC has been examined through a protocol that contained a second induction course on day 16 of TAD (6-thioguanine, cytarabine, and DNR) or HAM (HDAC plus mitoxantrone) for double induction (TAD-TAD versus TAD-HAM). CR and OS rates were similar in these two treatment groups. However, TAD-HAM was associated with a higher CR rates (65% versus 49%) and 5-year survival (25% versus 18%) in the unfavorable subgroup of patients defined by lactate dehydrogenase (LDH) higher than 700 U/L, greater than 40% blasts in the day 16 bone marrow, and unfavorable cytogenetics.

Addition of modulators of multidrug resistance did not provide additional benefits. Sensitization of leukemic cells to chemotherapy with hematopoietic growth factors, such as granulocyte colony-stimulating factor (G-CSF) and granulocyte/macrophage colony-stimulating factor (GM-CSF), have brought conflicting results, with most studies demonstrating lack of benefits; hence, it is not recommended in the absence of the clinical trial. Addition of gemtuzumab ozogamicin (GO) to conventional chemotherapy did not improve CR rates or DFS. As a consequence, the U.S. Food and Drug Administration (FDA) accelerated approval from 2000 has been withdrawn and drug availability limited to currently treated patients or trials conducted through an investigational new drug application only.

The use of an anthracycline or an anthracenedione is contraindicated in patients with severe underlying cardiac disease, particularly if the patient has had a recent myocardial infarction or has an ejection fraction of less than 50%. The choice of therapy in this situation is HDAC, although the optimum dose and schedule of HDAC therapy are not known (i.e., number of doses, dosage, infusion rate; see Table 18.8).

B. Residual disease

Patients who have residual disease at day 28 should be considered primary treatment failures and have alternative therapy initiated. If a significant response has been demonstrated at the day 10 to 14 marrow examination (greater than 50% to 60% reduction in leukemic infiltration) but residual leukemia persists, a second course of similar chemotherapy is given (or an alternative regimen such as HDAC). Patients with significant involvement of leukemia on day 10 to 14 (less than 40% to 50% leukemic reduction) should receive an alternative chemotherapy regimen. There is no dose modification for the second course based on blood cell counts. The doses of drugs may be decreased for the second cycle if the total dose of anthracycline would be cardiotoxic or hepatic dysfunction attributed to the chemotherapy develops.

C. Common HDAC toxicities

Neurotoxicity (cerebellar dysfunction, somnolence) occurs more frequently in older patients and as the number of doses of HDAC increases. Renal and hepatic dysfunction contributes to the development of neurotoxicity. One- to two-hour infusions are generally recommended as opposed to the original infusion rate over two to three hours, as the neurotoxicity appears to be decreased with shorter infusion times.

Reducing the dose of cytarabine in the face of renal dysfunction may decrease the risk of neurotoxicity. The following schema has been suggested to decrease neurotoxicity in the face of renal dysfunction. For a baseline serum creatinine level of 1.5 to 1.9 mg/dL or an increase in serum creatinine of 0.5 to 1.2 mg/dL from baseline, reduce the cytarabine to 1 g/m^2 per dose. For a baseline serum creatinine of more than 2 mg/dL or an increase of serum creatinine of greater than 1.2 mg/dL from baseline, reduce the cytarabine dose to 100 mg/m^2/day.

Because cytarabine is secreted in tears, ulcerative keratitis can be prevented by instilling eye drops (saline, methylcellulose, or steroid) every 4 hours while awake and Lacri-Lube ophthalmic ointment (Allergan, Inc., Irvine, CA) at bedtime, starting at the time HDAC is initiated and continuing for 2 to 3 days after the last dose of HDAC.

D. Postremission therapy

Despite attaining a CR, the majority of patients with AML relapse, necessitating further therapy aimed at eradication of the residual yet undetected leukemic clone. There are three general treatment strategies for postremission therapy: consolidation chemotherapy, autologous hematopoietic stem cell transplantation (auto-HSCT), or allogeneic (allo-) HSCT. Although the optimum postremission strategy remains to be defined, almost all younger adults with AML benefit from further therapy. The type of postremission therapy should be determined based on prognostic factors, particularly age, cytogenetic, and molecular genetic findings at diagnosis. Patients with AML in first CR should be considered candidates for investigational protocols examining postremission therapy options. For patients who cannot be enrolled in protocol studies, the approach to postinduction therapy used as a guide at Northwestern University is shown in Table 18.9. Consolidation should be initiated when the peripheral blood counts have returned to normal (ANC more than 1500/μL and platelet count more than 100,000/μL), marrow cellularity is normal, infections have resolved, and mucositis has cleared.

Current data suggest that HDAC offers a distinct advantage over SDAC consolidation in patients younger than 55 to 60 years of age. A landmark study conducted by CALGB demonstrated that four cycles of HDAC (3 g/m^2 every 12 hours on days 1, 3, and 5) are superior to four courses of intermediate cytarabine (400 mg/m^2 continuous intravenously (IV) on days 1 to 5) or SDAC (100 mg/m^2 continuous IV on days 1 to 5). More than 40% to 50% of patients will be in a continuous CR 5 years after consolidation with HDAC. The beneficial effect of cytarabine dose intensification, however, was restricted to patients with CBF-AML and, to a lesser extent, to patients with CN-AML, whereas outcome of patients with other cytogenetic abnormalities was not affected by the cytarabine dose.

The addition of other agents such as DNR or amsacrine to HDAC consolidation therapy failed to show improvements in long-term outcomes.

1. **Favorable-risk AML.** Postremission therapy with three to four cycles of HDAC or other intensive cytotoxic regimen is considered standard for younger adults with CBF-AML, NPM1+/FLT3-ITD−, and double-mutated CEBPA (see Table 18.9). A retrospective study conducted by CALGB demonstrated that three

TABLE 18.9	**HDAC Consolidation Regimens**

■ Cytarabine 3 g/m^2 IV infusion over 1–3 hours every 12 hours on days 1, 3, and 5 for two to four monthly courses, *or*

■ Cytarabine 3 g/m^2 IV infusion over 2 hours every 12 hours on days 1 to 6 for one to three monthly courses (most patients cannot tolerate more than one or two courses of standard HDAC), *or*

■ *For patients over age 60* and/or *patients with renal dysfunction (including creatinine less than 2.0 mg/dL):* Cytarabine 1.5 g/m^2 IV infusion over 1–3 hours every 12 hours on days 1, 3, and 5 for two to three monthly courses in younger patients, but for only one course for patients >60 years as there is no evidence that any postremission therapy is effective in prolonging CR in older adults compared to induction therapy alone.

HDAC, high-dose cytarabine; IV, intravenous.

or more cycles of HDAC (cumulative dose: 54 to 72 g/m^2) are superior to a single cycle (18 g/m^2); however, in a joint collaboration between the M.D. Anderson Cancer Center, SWOG, and ECOG, reporting a large number of patients with CBF-AML, the outcome even among patients treated with HDAC or any post-remission therapy was not as favorable as previously reported in earlier series with many fewer patients. Neither auto- nor allo-HSCT showed advantage over consolidation therapy in first remission.

However, several subsets of CBF-AML, such as t(8;21) with high WBC, CBF-AML with c-kit mutation, or persistence of MRD, do poorly with the conventional therapy and may benefit from the allo-HSCT.

2. **Intermediate-risk AML.** Long-term survival for patients presenting with intermediate cytogenetics is 40% to 45%. For patients younger than age 60, with the intermediate cytogenetics in general and CN-AML with unfavorable molecular markers (lack of mutated NPM1, double CEBPA, as well as presence of FLT3-ITD mutation), data (although not all prospective) support the use of allo-HSCT. The largest collection of prospective cohort data in this subgroup by the MRC documented superior 3-year relapse rates of 18% for allo-HSCT, 35% for auto-HSCT, and 55% for chemotherapy consolidation, and 3-year survival rates of 65%, 56%, and 48%, respectively. The U.S. Intergroup Study did not demonstrate advantage for allo-HSCT, although analysis was based on a much smaller cohort of patients. The optimal timing of allo-HSCT is yet to be established, although retrospective data collected from the Center for Blood and Marrow Transplant Research demonstrated lack of additional benefit from receiving consolidation chemotherapy prior to matched-sibling HSCT in first CR. In other words, patients in postinduction CR may proceed immediately to allo-HSCT.

Auto-HSCT has been studied in this subgroup of patients but has not been shown to represent an advantage over consolidation chemotherapy alone in randomized studies conducted during the last decade.

3. **Adverse-risk AML.** Despite the CR rates of up to 60%, this group of patients with AML has a 5-year OS of 11% (ranging from 3% to 20%) depending on the specific cytogenetic abnormality at diagnosis (e.g., 4% of patients with monosomal karyotype are alive at 4 years). The U.S. Intergroup Study demonstrated a significant long-term survival advantage for patients with unfavorable cytogenetics who received allo-HSCT for consolidation as compared to auto-HSCT or conventional chemotherapy. Although the total number of patients analyzed in this and similar trials has been small, matched-sibling allo-HSCT likely represents the

therapy with the best potential to prevent relapse. Data from the European Organisation for Research and Treatment of Cancer GIMEMA AML-10 trial and from three consecutive studies of the Hemato-Oncology Cooperative Group and the Swiss Group for Clinical Cancer Research (HOVON-SAKK) group demonstrated an advantage of the allo-HSCT among younger patients with adverse cytogenetics. The outcome after allo-HSCT from fully matched unrelated donor (MUD), based on molecular high-resolution HLA typing, appear to be similar to that of allo-HSCT from matched siblings. The Center for International Blood and Marrow Transplant Research reported a long-term survival probability of 30% for patients with AML with adverse cytogenetics transplanted in first CR from MUD.

Given the dismal outcome of high-risk AML patients treated with the conventional therapy, allo-HSCT from either matched related or unrelated donors in first CR is considered a reasonable treatment option.

E. Primary refractory AML

Several studies have shown that lack of early blast clearance or lack of response to the first induction cycle are major predictors for poor survival, and conventional therapy offers almost no chance of cure for these patients. Even with the allo-HSCT, the most aggressive approach available, the rates of relapse and mortality are high, yielding OS of 20% to 30%. Alternative conditioning regimens are being studied in this setting. Patients with induction failure, who are not eligible for allo-HSCT, should be considered for clinical trial evaluating novel agents.

F. Relapsed AML

1. Prognostic factors. A significant number of patients with AML who achieve a remission will ultimately relapse. Unfortunately, the prognosis of patients with relapsed disease is poor and treatment options remain unsatisfactory. The long-term survival depends on the ability to achieve a remission and receive consolidation with allo-HSCT. Initial remission duration, cytogenetics, and age determine which therapeutic approach should be undertaken: curative, palliative, or in the context of a clinical trial (Table 18.10).

2. Interventions on relapse include intensive chemotherapy with conventional agents, investigational therapies on a clinical trial including the immunoconjugate agent GO, palliative intent chemotherapy, or best supportive care. Individuals who relapsed after allo-HSCT may be eligible for immunosuppression withdrawal and/or donor lymphocyte infusions as an immunologic maneuver to generate a graft-versus-leukemia (GVL) effect.

a. Standard chemotherapy. The selection of conventional salvage therapy, the optimal dose of cytarabine, and the benefits of

TABLE 18.10 Prognostic Index for Younger Adults With AML in Relapse

		Survival Probability, %	
Risk	Index Score in Points	At 1 Year	At 5 Years
Favorable (9% of patients)	0–6	70	46
Intermediate (25% of patients)	7–9	49	18
Unfavorable (66% of patients)	10–14	16	4

Score, in patients 15–60 years of age (acute promyelocytic leukemia excluded), is estimated based on the following factors:
- Duration of remission prior to relapse: >18 months—0 points; 7–17 months—3 points; ≤6 months—5 points
- Cytogenetics at the initial diagnosis: inv(16) or t(16;16)—0 points; t(8;21)—3 points; other—5 points
- Prior hematopoietic stem cell transplant: no—0 points; yes—2 points
- Age at time of relapse: ≤35 years—0 points; 36–45 years—1 point; >45 years—2 points.

the addition of an anthracycline or other agents all remain important unanswered questions. HDAC (2 to 3 g/m^2 for 8 to 12 doses) paired with mitoxantrone, etoposide, methotrexate (MTX), and fludarabine have produced short-lived (4 to 6 month) CRs in 40% to 60% of patients with relapsed AML. A randomized trial conducted by SWOG failed to demonstrate a significant benefit to the addition of mitoxantrone to cytarabine 3 g/m^2 every 12 hours for six doses. The German AML Cooperative Group trial compared cytarabine 3 g/m^2 versus cytarabine 1 g/m^2 administered twice daily on days 1, 2, 8, and 9 in patients younger than 60 years of age. All patients received mitoxantrone. There was no substantial difference in CR rate or median OS. Thus, dose-intense cytarabine should probably be viewed as an essential component of a conventional salvage program, but escalation to 3 g/m^2 is probably not justified given the increased toxicity. There appears to be no value to adding standard-dose anthracyclines. However, there are multiple single-arm trials using escalated doses of anthracyclines that may present a reasonable alternative. A combination of topotecan and cytarabine induced CR in 35% to 70% of patients with AML and high-risk MDS. Nucleoside analogs, such as cladribine and fludarabine, showed activity in pediatric and adult AML. A recent study reported a 61% CR rate and 7-month CR duration in patients with AML treated with a combination of fludarabine, Ara-C, G-CSF, and idarubicin.

(1) **"7 + 3."** Up to half of patients who undergo induction with the "7 + 3" regimen respond to a repeat course of "7 + 3." Patients who relapse within 6 to 12 months of the last chemotherapy are unlikely to respond to the same regimen again. Thus, a different regimen should be considered.

(2) HDAC regimens. Fifty to seventy percent of patients respond to HDAC. Although HDAC combination regimens may have a slightly higher response rate, their increased toxicity may not make them significantly better than single-agent HDAC. Patients who relapse within 6 to 12 months of HDAC intensification are unlikely to have a significant response to further HDAC. The doses given for the HDAC are those originally described for each regimen. Options include the following:

- HDAC plus anthracycline
  - HDAC 3 g/m^2 IV infusion over 2 hours every 12 hours on days 1 to 4, *plus*
  - Mitoxantrone 10 mg/m^2/day IV on days 2 to 5 or 2 to 6.
- Cyclophosphamide, topotecan, and cytarabine
  - Cyclophosphamide 500 mg/m^2 IV every 12 hours on days 1 to 3, *and*
  - Topotecan 1.25 mg/m^2/day by continuous infusion on days 2 to 6, *and*
  - Cytarabine 2 g/m^2 IV over 4 hours daily for 5 days on days 2 to 6.
- Mitoxantrone, etoposide, and cytarabine (MEC) may produce significant gastrointestinal and cardiac toxicity. It is not recommended for patients older than 60 years of age or those with borderline cardiac function. A variation of MEC currently used by the ECOG is as follows:
  - Etoposide 40 mg/m^2/day IV infusion over 1 hour on days 1 to 5, *followed immediately by*
  - Cytarabine 1 g/m^2/day IV infusion over 1 hour on days 1 to 5, *and*
  - Mitoxantrone 4 mg/m^2/day IV on days 1 to 5, given after completion of HDAC each day.
- Fludarabine, cytarabine, G-CSF, and idarubicin (FLAG-IDA)
  - Fludarabine 30 mg/m^2/day IV over 30 minutes on days 1 to 5, *and*
  - Cytarabine 2 g/m^2/day IV over 4 hours on days 1 to 5, *and*
  - Idarubicin 10 mg/m^2/day on days 1 to 3, *and*
  - G-CSF 5 µg/kg subcutaneously (SC) 24 hours after the completion of chemotherapy and until neutrophil regeneration.
- Fludarabine, cytarabine, idarubicin, plus GO
  - Fludarabine 25 mg/m^2/day IV over 30 minutes on days 1 to 5, *and*
  - Cytarabine 2 g/m^2/day IV over 4 hours on days 1 to 5, *and*

■ Idarubicin 10 mg/m²/day on days 1 to 3, *and*

■ GO 3 mg/m² on day 6 *(if available)*

■ G-CSF 5 μg/kg SC 24 hours after the completion of chemotherapy as medically indicated.

(3) Non-HDAC regimens

■ Etoposide 100 mg/m²/day IV on days 1 to 5 and mitoxantrone 10 mg/m²/day IV on days 1 to 5 represents an active and well-tolerated combination that is commonly used for relapsed or refractory leukemia.

■ High-dose etoposide 70 mg/m²/h continuous IV infusion for 60 hours and high-dose cyclophosphamide 50 mg/kg (1850 mg/m²)/day IV infusion over 2 hours on days 1 to 4 is a highly toxic but active regimen that does not require bone marrow support. It is active against HDAC-resistant AML (30% CR). This regimen may be useful for young patients who are good candidates for allo-HSCT while waiting for an unrelated donor search to be completed. This regimen may also be associated with substantial toxicity.

b. Salvage consolidation with HSCT. Allo-HSCT is the preferred consolidation therapy once salvage remission has been achieved. The source of the stem cells include HLA identical sibling, MUD, umbilical cord (UCB) unit (typically use two), or a haploidentical donor. HSCT with reduced-intensity conditioning (RIC) regimen is associated with increased risk of relapse compared to that of standard conditioning regimen and is being evaluated prospectively. If allo-HSCT is not possible, auto-HSCT could be considered. Although retrospective studies in selected patients demonstrate a 20% to 50% probability of long-term survival, it is often impossible to collect leukemia-free stem cells at this phase of the disease.

Patients who sustain a relapse after allo-HSCT can be managed with withdrawal of immunoprophylaxis with or without donor lymphocyte infusions. Such interventions would not be possible in patients who already suffer from GVHD. Transplant recipients who relapse a year or longer after undergoing HSCT may be offered a second HSCT.

c. Investigational strategies and novel agents. Improved understanding of the molecular pathogenesis of AML has led to the development of molecularly targeted approaches. However, as the AML phenotype (aside from APL) results from multiple genetic/epigenetic lesions affecting differentiation, proliferation, and apoptosis, it is likely that eradication of the leukemic clone will require a combination of multiple agents.

(1) Several FLT3 inhibitors demonstrated in vitro cytotoxicity in leukemic cells. Although first-generating of FLT-3 inhibitors showed minimal activity in patients with AML, some of the newer ones are active as a single agent and are currently investigated in combination with chemotherapy in salvage as well as in front-line settings.

(2) Hypomethylating agents. 5-azacitidine (5-Aza) and decitabine have received FDA approval for patients with MDS. Approximately a third of patients ($n = 113$) participating in clinical trials demonstrating survival advantage of 5-Aza were classified as having AML by current WHO criteria (20% to 30% of bone marrow blasts). Among those patients, 2-year OS was 50% in the 5-Aza arm compared with 16% in the conventional treatment regimen arm.

(3) Clofarabine. In phase I/II studies, a novel nucleoside analog clofarabine induced a 16% CR rate in patients with relapsed AML. When clofarabine was combined with cytarabine, the overall response rate was 32%, with a CR rate of 22%. When clofarabine was administered to previously untreated older patients with AML, the CR was 60%. Randomized clinical trials comparing a combination of clofarabine and cytarabine with "7 + 3" are ongoing.

d. Central nervous system (CNS) prophylaxis may be considered in patients at high risk of CNS recurrence such as patients with WBC greater than 50,000/μL or those with myelomonocytic (FAB M4) or monocytic (FAB M5) differentiation. Patients treated with HDAC (greater than 7.2 g/m^2) do not require intrathecal (IT) therapy as they achieve therapeutic drug level in the cerebrospinal fluid (CSF). If required, IT therapy with MTX 12 mg or Ara-C 30 mg is used. For patients with CNS involvement (uncommon on presentation), chemotherapy should be administered via Ommaya catheter together with 30 mg of hydrocortisone.

G. AML in older adults

1. **Background.** AML is a disease of older adults, as the median age of diagnosis is 68 years. Despite the refinements in supportive care and chemotherapy programs, the long-term survival rates have improved little over the last 35 years for patients over age 55. Standard remission-induction and postremission therapy results in median DFS of 10 months and rare long-term survival. Because of the effects of comorbid disease and age on normal physiology, older adults are less able to withstand the inherent toxicity of induction chemotherapy than young adults. There are also intrinsic differences in the biology of older adults with AML: a higher percentage of the leukemic cells express Pgp at diagnosis (71% versus 35% in younger patients) and existence of an overt or covert antecedent hematologic disorder that predisposes to drug resistance. Moreover,

AML in older adults is associated with a greater number of high-risk cytogenetic abnormalities (i.e., abnormalities of chromosomes 5 and 7 and complex karyotypes). As reported by the MRC, the favorable cytogenetic risk group was less common in patients over age 55 (7% versus 26% in patients younger than 55), while complex karyotypes were more common (13% versus 6%). Furthermore, patients over age 55 with complex karyotype predicted a poor outcome with OS of 2% at 5 years. The MRC recognized a predictive hierarchical cytogenetic classification for older adults similar to previous analysis for younger patients, although 5-year OS for favorable cytogenetic group patients over age 55 was 34% compared with 65% for younger patients (and 13% and 41%, respectively, for intermediate cytogenetic risk).

The decision to forgo therapy in an older patient with AML should not be made a priori based solely on age; rather, the decision to treat or not to treat should be based on more substantive factors such as the presence of comorbid disease, PS before diagnosis, quality of life before diagnosis, and projected long-term survival. Studies suggest that remission-induction chemotherapy provides better quality of life and longer survival compared to supportive care only.

2. **Induction therapy**. Older patients with excellent PS and a lack of comorbidities may expect a CR rate of 50% and mortality under 15% from the standard induction therapy. Patients with similar PS but adverse cytogenetics may expect CR rates of only 20% to 30% and dismal long-term survival.

Although attenuated doses of "7 + 3" have been recommended in the past, full-dose therapy is now generally recommended in older adults without significant comorbidities, in part owing to improvements in supportive care. In fact, the AML Study Group (AMLSG) has been using 60 mg/m^2 of DNR in the elderly patient population without unexpected morbidity and mortality and recently, HOVON-SAKK/AMLSG demonstrated that the dose of 90 mg/m^2 was safe in patients up to 65 years of age.

Continuous attempts have been made to improve the efficacy of this regimen by varying the doses of Ara-C; comparing one anthracycline or anthracenedione with another; combining with other chemotherapeutic agents; using growth factors as priming agents; or as supportive care. Improved CR rates in many of the phase II studies were not confirmed in the randomized phase III trials.

Although karyotype may be unknown at diagnosis, delays in initiating therapy may not be harmful in older patients, thus allowing an individual approach to care.

- Standard "7 + 3": Cytarabine 100 mg/m^2/day or 200 mg/m^2/day IV continuous infusion on days 1 to 7, *and either*
  - DNR 60 to 90 mg/m^2/day for 3 days *or*
  - Idarubicin 8 to 12 mg/m^2/day IV bolus on days 1 to 5.
- Modified HDAC decreases the cytarabine dose to try to diminish the neurotoxicity that is dose-limiting in older adults. Modified HDAC is generally believed to be more toxic than the "7 + 3" regimen. We do not routinely recommend the use of HDAC for induction in older patients given the lack of data to support a higher CR rate and the significantly increased morbidity and mortality associated with HDAC during the induction period. In selected older patients with excellent PS and a decreased ejection fraction, one can consider using modified HDAC. Although the optimum dose and schedule are not known, 1.5 to 2 g/m^2 IV over 2 hours every 12 hours for 8 to 12 doses is commonly used.

  For older patients with suboptimal PS and several comorbidities and organ dysfunctions, low-dose cytarabine (20 mg twice a day SC for 10 days) was demonstrated to be superior in terms of OS compared to that of hydroxyurea in a randomized trial. However, the magnitude of improvement was not so dramatic to make hydroxyurea and supportive care an unreasonable option. Even with this low-intensity therapy, the 30-day mortality was 26% and patients with adverse cytogenetics did not derive any benefit at all. Any discussion regarding therapeutic intervention should refer to the observation that 74% of older patients estimated their chance of cure with "7 + 3" to be 50% or more, whereas 85% of their physicians estimated this chance to be less than 10%. Considering the poor outcome of older patients with AML with standard therapy, serious consideration ought to be given to the enrollment of patients in clinical trials evaluating novel agents.

3. **Postremission therapy.** Older patients may tolerate one or two cycles of lower doses of HDAC (1.5 g/m^2 every 12 hours on days 1, 3, and 5) than is usually given for younger adults, although a beneficial impact of HDAC consolidation chemotherapy on long-term outcome is not proven. The CALGB trial of varying doses of cytarabine (100 mg/m^2/day, 400 mg/m^2/day, and 3 g/m^2) reported similar 5-year DFS and OS within each arm (each less than 15% and 8%, respectively). Other reports have demonstrated that prolonged consolidation courses (over four cycles) will likely not benefit long-term outcomes. Recent data suggest that CBF-AML and NPM1+/FLT3/ITD-AML patients may benefit from dose escalation of consolidation. A recently published randomized clinical trial compared four cycles of GO postinduction therapy (6 mg/m^2 every 4 weeks) with observation in older patients with AML. There were no significant differences between the groups with regard to

rate of relapse, nonrelapse mortality, and OS and DFS at 5 years (17% versus 16%). Novel therapeutic approaches are needed. Current strategies include incorporation of less intensive therapy, such as incorporation of agents such as GO, FTIs, and bcl-2 antisense oligonucleotides into consolidation (and induction) therapy. Auto-HSCT may be considered for fit patients, although, as in younger patients, the exact integration of this therapy is not known. RIC allo-HSCTs have allowed allo-HSCT in older patients, but this modality should still be considered experimental in this setting. Current treatment options include the following:

- HDAC 1.5 g/m^2 IV infusion over 3 hours every 12 hours on days 1, 3, and 5 (better tolerated) for one course (with careful attention to cerebellar toxicity and to renal function; if either is noted to be apparent, HDAC should be immediately discontinued).
- Cytarabine 100 mg/m^2/day for 5 days per course.

However, there are not definitive data showing that postremission therapy benefits older adults.

4. **Other therapeutic approaches**

   a. **Gemtuzumab ozogomycin (GO),** a recombinant humanized monoclonal anti-CD33 antibody conjugated to a highly potent antitumor antibiotic calicheamicin, was approved by the FDA for the treatment of patients older than 60 years with CD33+ AML in first relapse who are not candidates for cytotoxic therapy. The majority of AML blast cells (80% to 90%) express the CD33 surface antigen, while pluripotent hematopoietic stem cells/tissues and nonhematopoietic cells do not. After administration, GO is believed to be internalized into lysosomes, where the calicheamicin dissociates form the antibody, migrates to the nucleus, and causes double-stranded DNA breaks. With the FDA withdrawal of prior "accelerated" approval and removal from the market, it will be available only on clinical trial.

   GO has been administered at a dose of 9 mg/m^2 as a 2-hour IV infusion on days 1 and 15. Leukoreduction with leukapheresis or hydroxyurea to lower the WBC below 30,000/μL prior to GO therapy is recommended. No dose adjustments for anemia or thrombocytopenia should be made. Benadryl may be administered prior to infusion. Acetaminophen has the potential to contribute to hepatotoxicity (increased free radicals) and theoretically should be avoided.

   GO was voluntarily removed from the market and is not readily available in routine clinical practice.

   b. **Reduced intensity conditioning (RIC) (mini)-HSCT.** Older adults are increasingly offered an option of undergoing nonmyeloablative or mini-HSCT as a postremission therapy. Although most of the studies evaluating mini-HSCT are limited to a single institution experience, they show feasibility of this potentially curative approach in the older patient population. A retrospective study from the Cooperative German Transplant Study Group of 368 patients demonstrated that survival is comparable between patients receiving stem cells from the sibling donor or MUD.

c. **Other investigational therapies** include FLT-3 inhibitors, clofarabine, cloretazine, azacitidine/decitabine with histone deacetylase inhibitors or GO, or chemotherapy with GO.

V. THERAPY-RELATED AML
A. Background

Therapy-related AML (t-AML) is a recognized clinical syndrome occurring after exposure to cytotoxic and/or radiation therapy. AML that develops after the exposure to the alkylating agent is characterized by the cytogenetic abnormalities involving chromosomes 5 and/or 7, a long latency (7 to 10 years), and, frequently, an antecedent MDS. Patients who develop AML following exposure to topoisomerase II inhibitors have a rearrangement of chromosome 11q23 (MLL) or 21q22 (RUNX1), a relatively short latency period (2 to 3 years), and myelomonocytic or monocytic differentiation. High-dose chemotherapy with auto-HSCT has been increasingly implicated in the pathogenesis of secondary leukemias. In one study, the estimated cumulative probability of developing therapy-related MDS or AML was approximately 8.6% ± 2.1% at 6 years among 612 patients undergoing high-dose chemotherapy and HSCT for Hodgkin lymphoma and non-Hodgkin lymphoma. The most important risk factor appears to be large cumulative doses of alkylating agents. However, patient age and previous radiotherapy, particularly total-body irradiation as part of the conditioning regimen, are additional risk factors.

B. Therapy

Although up to 50% of patients with t-AML may achieve a CR with chemotherapy, the median remission duration is approximately 5 months. Therapeutic options include supportive care, "7 + 3," HDAC, or other chemotherapy regimens. Amonafide, a topoisomerase II inhibitor, has shown promising activity in patients with AML, particularly AML arising on the background of MDS, and is being evaluated in combination with Ara-C in clinical trials.

Younger patients with t-AML should be considered for allo-HSCT in first remission. Nonmyeloablative allo-HSCT is under investigation for those who are not eligible to undergo standard HSCT. The European Group for Blood and Marrow Transplantation Registry reported 35% 3-year OS in 65 patients with t-AML treated with auto-HSCT.

The main considerations for patients with t-AML include the status of primary malignancy, the patient's PS, age, and the leukemic karyotype. All patients should be treated on a clinical trial if at all possible, and those eligible should be transplanted.

VI. AML DURING PREGNANCY

The outcomes of both the mother and the fetus must be considered when discussing the therapeutic options for a pregnant woman who develops AML. Pregnancy does not appear to alter the course of AML, with more than 75% of patients achieving a CR after standard chemotherapy. Therapeutic abortion must be considered if AML develops during the first trimester. If therapeutic abortion is not an option or if AML develops during the second or third trimester, induction chemotherapy may be undertaken. Although there is a slightly increased risk of premature labor and fetal death, in most cases "7 + 3" appears to be well tolerated by both the patient and the fetus. Idarubicin is more lipophilic, favoring an increased placental transfer and had a higher DNA affinity, compared to other anthracyclines; hence, DNR should be offered instead.

VII. ACUTE PROMYELOCYTIC LEUKEMIA (APL)

APL is a distinct subtype of AML, designated M3 by the FAB classification. It accounts for 10% to 15% of cases of adult AML in the general population and perhaps 20% to 25% of AML cases in Latin America. The median age at presentation (40 years) is significantly lower than that of patients diagnosed with other AML subtypes (68 years). Due to the remarkable sensitivity of APL to anthracyclines, all-*trans*-retinoic acid (ATRA), and arsenic trioxide (ATO; As_2O_3), it has become the most curable acute leukemia in adults, with cure rates exceeding 80% with contemporary therapeutic strategies.

A. Cytogenetic abnormalities and prognostic factors

The characteristic molecular genetic abnormality in APL is a balanced reciprocal translocation between the gene for retinoic acid receptor α (RARα) located on chromosome 17 and the gene for promyelocytic leukemia (PML) located in chromosome 15, resulting in two hybrid gene products: PML-RARα and RARα-PML. PML-RARα fusion protein, detectable by the PCR technique, is essential for the diagnosis and identification of MRD. Four alternative chromosomal translocations have been identified (PLZF-RARα, NPM-RARα, NuMA-RARα, and STAT5b-RARα). Prognostic factors are listed in Table 18.11.

TABLE 18.11 Adverse Prognostic Features in APL

- Age (>50–60 years)
- Male gender
- High WBC (>10,000/μL)
- Low platelet count (<40,000/μL)

WBC, white blood count.

TABLE 18.12 Management of Coagulopathy in APL

- Initiate ATRA therapy at the first suspicion of the diagnosis
- Monitor DIC panel at least twice daily
- Maintain fibrinogen level at 100–150 mg/dL with cryoprecipitate transfusions
- Maintain platelet count at 30,000–50,000/μL with platelet transfusions three or four times a day if necessary
- Avoid central line placement
- Avoid aminocaproic acid

ATRA, all-*trans*-retinoic acid; DIC, disseminated intravascular coagulation.

B. Management of coagulopathy in APL

Coagulopathy, a peculiar presenting feature of APL, must be managed aggressively at the suspicion of APL diagnosis, as it results in a high rate of spontaneous and potentially fatal hemorrhage. Pooled data through the late 1980s suggested that under the best of circumstances with cytotoxic induction chemotherapy, 5% of APL patients would die of CNS hemorrhage within the first 24 hours of hospitalization and another 20% to 25% would die of CNS hemorrhage during induction chemotherapy. With intensive supportive care and the introduction of ATRA therapy, the most recent studies suggest that less than 5% of patients will die of hemorrhage during induction chemotherapy, while overall induction mortality in APL remains approximately 10% reported in clinical trials (likely higher when all patients are considered). Regardless of clinical manifestations, essentially all patients with APL have laboratory features of DIC. Table 18.12 outlines the general management plan to minimize complications of the coagulopathy in APL.

C. APL therapy (Table 18.13)

Based on cumulative experience of multiple cooperative groups, therapy for APL should include simultaneous administration of ATRA and anthracycline-based chemotherapy for induction and consolidation and a combination of ATRA and chemotherapy for maintenance (particularly for high-risk subgroups of patients). ATRA, a vitamin A derivative, is able to induce a high rate (85%) of short-lived clinical remissions by promoting cell maturation, differentiation, and apoptosis without producing marrow hypoplasia.

1. **Induction.** Simultaneous administration of ATRA and anthracycline-based chemotherapy results in 95% CR rates. Development of primary resistance has been reported in a few anecdotal cases only and essentially does not exist in true APL. Several randomized clinical trials demonstrated not only that addition of ATRA to chemotherapy leads to the improved EFS and OS compared to chemotherapy alone, but that a *simultaneous* administration of ATRA and chemotherapy is superior to a *sequential* one in

TABLE 18.13 Therapeutic Recommendations for APL

Induction recommendations
- Induction therapy should consist of the administration of concomitant ATRA and anthracycline-based chemotherapy
- Based on the available data, induction therapy should not be modified due to the presence of features such as secondary chromosomal abnormalities, FLT3 mutations, CD56 expression, and BCR3 PML-RARA isoform.
- ATRA 45 mg/m^2/day by mouth is divided into two doses with food given every day until CR (no longer then 90 days) plus an anthracycline, either DNR 50–60 mg/m^2/day for 3 days or idarubicin 12 mg/m^2 every other day for 4 doses. In the modified regimen used by the PETHEMA group, the fourth dose of idarubicin was omitted in patients older than 70 years of age.
- It appears reasonable to initiate treatment with ATRA first for 2 to 3 days in patients with clinical evidence of bleeding to ameliorate the coagulopathy before initiating anthracycline-based therapy, provided the WBC count is not high (<10,000/μL). Otherwise, concurrent ATRA plus anthracycline-based therapy has been routine practice and may have the advantage of decreasing the incidence of retinoic acid syndrome (now referred to as the APL differentiation syndrome; see subsequent discussion).
- Treatment with ATRA should be continued until occurrence of terminal differentiation of blasts and achievement of the CR, which occurs in virtually all patients after the conventional ATRA + anthracycline induction schedules.
- No therapeutic modifications should be made based on the presence of incomplete blast maturation (differentiation) detected up to 90 days after the start of therapy, as demonstrated by morphology, cytogenetics, or molecular studies.
- Presence of MRD (demonstrated in up to 50%) after induction, as determined by RT-PCR, does not have prognostic implications and does not warrant change in therapeutic approach.
- The role of cytarabine in induction among patients with low and intermediate risk remains unclear; however, cytarabine plays a major role in patients with high-risk disease.

Consolidation recommendations
- The goal of consolidation therapy is an achievement of molecular remission as determined by the RT-PCR, as it has been convincingly correlated with the improved outcome.
- Addition of ATRA to chemotherapy in consolidation seems to provide a clinical benefit; typically given 45 mg/m^2/day in two divided doses for 7–15 days.
- Two to three cycles of anthracycline-based chemotherapy are considered standard:
  - DNR 50–60 mg/m^2/day IV for 3 days, *or*
  - Idarubicin 5 mg/m^2/day on days 1 to 4 (consolidation #1), mitoxantrone 10 mg/m^2/day on days 1 (consolidation #2), *and* idarubicin 12 mg/m^2 on day 1 only (consolidation #3), as in PETHEMA regimen, *or*
  - DNR 60 mg/m^2/day IV for 3 days and Ara-C 200 mg/m^2/day IV for 7 days, as in European APL 93 regimen
- High-risk patients (WBC >10 × 10^9/L) younger than 60 years should receive at least one cycle of intermediate- and high-dose cytarabine:
  - Idarubicin 5 mg/m^2/day × 4; Ara-C 1000 mg/m^2/day × 4; ATRA 45 mg/m^2/day × 15 (consolidation #1)
  - Mitoxantrone 10 mg/m^2/day × 5; ATRA 45 mg/m^2/day × 15 (consolidation #2)
  - Idarubicin 12 mg/m^2/day × 1; Ara-C 150 mg/m^2/day/8 hours × 4; ATRA 45 mg/m^2/day × 15 (consolidation #3)

(continued)

TABLE 18.13 Therapeutic Recommendations for APL *(continued)*

Arsenic can be considered for two cycles as an early consolidation followed by two courses of anthracycline and ATRA as given in the North American C9710 Intergroup trial
■ Arsenic therapy should be considered in the context of a clinical trial or for the patients not fit to receive chemotherapy.

Maintenance recommendations
■ ATRA 45 mg/m^2/day by mouth, divided into two doses with food for 15 days every 3 months (or 7 days on/7 days off *plus* 6-mercaptopurine 90–100 mg/m^2/day *plus* MTX 10–15 mg/m^2/week all for 2 years), *or*
■ ATRA 45 mg/m^2/day by mouth divided into two doses with food for 1 year, *or*
■ ATRA 45 mg/m^2/day divided into two doses with food for 15 days every 3 months for 2 years.
■ Because early treatment intervention in patients with evidence of MRD results in better outcome than treatment in hematologic relapse, follow-up of PCR for PML-RARα every 3 months for up to 3 years is recommended for high-risk patients. Patients with low- and intermediate-risk disease can be monitored much less frequently or perhaps not at all (low-risk disease).

APL, acute promyelocytic leukemia; Ara-C, cytarabine; ATRA, all-*trans*-retinoic acid; CR, complete response; DNR, daunorubicin; MRD, minimal residual disease; PCR, polymerase chain reaction; RT, reverse transcription; WBC, white blood cell.

terms of CR rates (87% versus 70%), 4-year relapse rate (RR; 20% versus 36%), and 4-year OS (71% versus 52%). The choice of anthracycline is still debated; in the ATRA era, idarubicin is more frequently used as a monotherapy, while DNR is mainly used in combination with other drugs (typically cytarabine).

The role of cytarabine in the induction regimens for APL remains controversial, as comparable CR rates have been reported using ATRA/DNR/cytarabine and ATRA/idarubicin regimens. In a randomized trial reported by the European APL group, patients treated with ATRA/DNR had higher rates of CR, but demonstrated increased rates of relapse compared to those of patients treated with ATRA/DNR/cytarabine. Another randomized trial demonstrated similar rates of CR, RR, and OS between ATRA/idarubicin and ATRA/DNR/cytarabine arms; additionally, a small increase in mortality in remission was noted in the group receiving cytarabine.

ATO-based therapy may be considered in patients for whom an anthracycline-based regimen is contraindicated. After the demonstration of impressive outcomes in the treatment of patients with relapsed APL pioneered in China and replicated in the Western populations, at least four clinical trials addressed the role of ATO in the front-line setting. The CR rates in these studies were 86% to 95%; however, arsenic was combined with ATRA and/or chemotherapy and/or GO in some patients, particularly those presenting with leukocytosis.

2. **Consolidation.** High rates of molecular remissions (approximately 95%) after at least two cycles of postinduction anthracycline-based chemotherapy have led to the adoption of this strategy as the standard for consolidation. The benefit of ATRA addition to consolidation chemotherapy has not been demonstrated in randomized trials. However, historical comparison of consecutive trials carried independently by GIMEMA and PETHEMA groups showed statistically significant improvement in outcome with the addition of ATRA to chemotherapy.

The role of cytarabine in consolidation has remained controversial, as several retrospective analysis conducted in the pre-ATRA era failed to show the difference in outcome with its addition. In ATRA-containing regimens, the role of cytarabine remains unresolved. However, there is a definitive role for intermediate-dose cytarabine or HDAC in patients who present with high-risk disease (high risk for relapse) with a WBC greater than 10,000/uL. As already mentioned, a recent randomized study by the European APL group reported an increased risk of relapse with the omission of cytarabine from the induction and consolidation. However, such results might have been attributed to the type and dose of anthracycline and the lack of ATRA given in consolidation. The joint analysis of European APL and PETHEMA groups demonstrated a significantly reduced cumulative incidence of relapse in younger patients (younger than 65 years) with lower risk APL (WBC less than 10×10^9/L) treated with anthracycline monotherapy in the PETHEMA LPA99 trial compared to that of patients treated with a regimen including cytarabine in the European APL 2000 trial. However, a trend in favor of cytarabine administration was observed in high-risk patients (WBC greater than 10×10^9/L). Similarly, results of a recently published Italian study suggested an advantage of adding cytarabine to the ATRA-based therapy in high-risk patients.

Based on the available data, it has been our practice to add at least one cycle of cytarabine therapy for patients younger than 60 years who present with elevated WBC (greater than 10×10^9/L) and provide an anthracycline–ATRA combination for patients with low- and intermediate-risk disease.

Recently, the use of ATO administered in combination with ATRA and chemotherapy has been supported by the results of the large randomized North American Intergroup study. In this study, two cycles of ATO, 25 days each (5 days per week for 5 weeks) administered on achievement of CR and before the standard postremission therapy with two courses of DNR and ATRA, resulted in significantly better EFS and OS compared to that of patients receiving chemo-ATRA consolidation alone. However, the outcomes of the control arm (chemo-ATRA alone) was significantly worse than those reported by other groups using ATRA and anthracycline-based chemotherapy. Consequently, some consider the use of ATO in front-line consolidation restricted to clinical trials. In addition, more patients are being treated with ATO in induction and consolidation with minimal chemotherapy.

3. **The role of HSCT.** Because of the high cure rates with ATRA and chemotherapy combinations, there is no role for a routine use of HSCT for patients with APL in molecular remission after consolidation chemotherapy. Given the poor prognosis of those very few patients who have evidence of MRD after completion of consolidation therapy, allo-HSCT should be considered. Due to the rapid progression from positive MRD to overt hematologic relapse, additional therapy (such as ATO) should be administered to reduce the tumor burden and hopefully achieve a molecular remission prior to transplantation. If an HLA-matched donor is not available or a patient's PS precludes the allo-HSCT, therapy with ATO, GO, or both might be considered. For patients who achieve a molecular remission, subsequent auto-HSCT may be considered as part of consolidation therapy. Although such approaches lead to good clinical results, it is also possible that similar rates of long-term remission could be obtained with multiple courses of ATO and/or GO.

4. **Maintenance.** In the pre-ATRA era, several studies showed a definitive benefit of maintenance chemotherapy. Because the ATRA became standard therapy, a combination of ATRA and low-dose chemotherapy was superior to ATRA alone, chemotherapy alone, and observation in terms of RR and DFS. However, the results of two recent studies showed no advantage of maintenance therapy in patients who achieved a molecular remission after the third cycle of consolidation. The optimal schedule, dose, duration of maintenance therapy, as well as a targeted patient population, are still under investigation. Therapeutic recommendations for APL outside of clinical trials are given in Table 18.13.

D. **APL differentiation syndrome (DS)**

APL DS (formerly retinoic acid syndrome [RAS]) is a complication of ATRA therapy that manifests by unexplained fever, weight gain, respiratory distress, pericardial and pleural effusion, periodic hypotension, and acute renal failure. Typically, RAS occurs between the second day and the third week of ATRA therapy, with the incidence between 5% and 27% and a mortality rate (for those who develop RAS) between 5% and 29%. Although a rising WBC count may be a risk factor for RAS, it may occur with a WBC count below 5000/μL. If the WBC count is greater than 5000 to 10,000/μL on presentation, ATRA and chemotherapy should be given concurrently. If the WBC count rises to more than 10,000/μL during ATRA monotherapy, induction chemotherapy should be added. Regardless of the WBC count or the risk of neutropenic sepsis, at the first sign of RAS, dexamethasone (10 mg IV twice per day) should be initiated. If the symptoms are mild, ATRA may be continued concomitantly with steroids under careful observation. However, if the symptoms are severe or do not respond to steroid therapy, ATRA should be temporarily discontinued. Several uncontrolled trials reported a very low mortality rate with the prophylactic corticosteroid therapy in patients with leukocytosis; however, no prospective randomized studies were conducted to address this issue.

E. Relapsed APL

Two studies conducted in the pre-ATO era suggested a benefit for preemptive therapy at the development of the molecular relapse compared with treatment initiated at the time of frank hematologic relapse. Although the benefit of early intervention with the ATO-based therapy remains to be proven, the high risk of hemorrhagic death and development of APL MDS associated with overt disease argues strongly in favor of an early intervention. Hence, molecular monitoring of MDS every 3 months for 3 years is recommended (see Table 18.13).

1. **Arsenic trioxide (ATO).** Approximately 10% to 20% of patients treated with a combination of ATRA and chemotherapy eventually relapse. Although second remissions with standard therapy are common, particularly if the last exposure to ATRA occurred more than 6 to 12 months prior to relapse, they are not durable. Several clinical trials show that ATO has remarkable activity in this patient population, leading to its FDA approval in this setting. Preclinical mechanisms of action of ATO include apoptosis and APL cell differentiation. Chinese investigators demonstrated CR rates of at least 85% and 2-year DFS of 40% in patients with relapsed APL. A U.S. multicenter study of ATO for induction and consolidation therapy for relapsed APL confirmed the high CR and long-term survival rates, and most importantly, 85% rate of molecular remission after the completion of the consolidation therapy. Combination of ATO with other active agents (ATRA, chemotherapy, GO) for relapsed APL (induction and consolidation phases) are actively being studied.

   ATO either alone or in combination with ATRA results in remission rates in excess of 90% in previously untreated patients. Incorporation of ATO into the consolidation regimen if first CR has been evaluated by the North American C9710 Intergroup APL trial. The most significant toxicities associated with ATO therapy include ventricular arrhythmia caused by the prolongation of QT interval, hyperleukocytosis, and APL differentiation syndrome.

2. **Gemtuzumab ozogomycin (GO).** A high rate of CD33 expression on the promyelocytes and in vitro activity of GO in ATRA- and ATO-resistant leukemia cell lines provided a rationale for the GO therapy in patients with APL. In patients with evidence of molecular relapse, single-agent GO reinstated the molecular remission in

14 of 16 patients, while 2 patients suffered from the disease progression. Combination of GO and ATRA in previously untreated patients resulted in an 88% CR rate. The optimal role of GO for the therapy of APL are currently explored in clinical trials.

GO was voluntarily removed from the market and is not readily available in routine clinical practice.

3. **HSCT in relapsed APL.** Despite the high initial CR rates in relapsed disease, many patients relapse following ATO-based treatment. Results of retrospective studies have demonstrated that HSCT may be an effective option at this point or on achievement of second CR following ATO therapy. Auto-HSCT is associated with lower transplant-related mortality and is a reasonable option for patients in molecular remission and prolonged (greater than 1 year) first CR. Allo-HSCT is associated with a higher rate of transplant-related mortality but offers greater antileukemic activity due to the GVL effect. It could be recommended for patients who fail to achieve a complete molecular remission or those with short CR duration. Table 18.14 gives recommendations for treatment of relapsed APL.

TABLE 18.14 Recommendations for Relapsed APL

- For patients with confirmed molecular relapse (two successive PCR-positive results, demonstrating stable or rising PML-RARA transcript levels), pre-emptive therapy must be initiated to prevent frank relapse.
- ATRA and chemotherapy combination may be used as a salvage regimen; however, ATO-based regimens are considered the first option in the setting of relapsed APL.
- ATO
  - Induction: 0.15 mg/kg IV over 2 hours daily until bone marrow remission occurs, up to cumulative maximum of 60 doses. Bone marrow biopsy should be obtained on or before day 28 of therapy, and subsequently weekly until CR.
  - Consolidation: start 3–4 weeks after completing the induction therapy at 0.15 mg/kg IV over 2 hours daily or 5/7 days, for a cumulative total of 25 doses.
  - Maintain potassium >4 mEq/L and magnesium >1.8 mg/dL.
  - Frequent EKG monitoring. If QTc interval remains normal, may reduce frequency to once every 2 weeks.
  - Monitor WBC count and for signs of APL syndrome. Institute steroids (dexamethasone 10 mg IV twice a day) at the earliest suggestion of the APL syndrome.
- HSCT. Patient should be referred for the evaluation for the HSCT
  - Allogeneic-HSCT if fail to achieve a molecular remission
  - Autologous-HSCT if in the molecular remission.
- For patients in whom HSCT is not feasible, repeated cycles of ATO with or without ATRA with or without chemotherapy should be considered.

APL, acute promyelocytic leukemia; ATO, arsenic trioxide; ATRA, all-*trans*-retinoic acid; CR, complete response; EKG, electrocardiogram; HSCT, hematopoietic stem cell transplantation; IV, intravenously; PCR, polymerase chain reaction; WBC, white blood cell.

VIII. THERAPY FOR ADULT ALL

Over the last 35 years, significant advances have been made in the management of adult ALL. Current therapeutic strategies incorporate a more intensive induction and postremission regimens and take into account biologic and clinical features of the disease. Despite an excellent initial response to therapy (CR 80% to 90%), the overall long-term DFS is 35% to 50% in adult patients with ALL. Most chemotherapeutic regimens for ALL have been developed as complete programs without testing the contributions of the individual components, and they had not been compared to one another in a rigorous prospective randomized fashion. All patients undergoing therapy for ALL should be enrolled in clinical trials.

The goals of intensified therapy are to eliminate leukemia cells, as determined by light microscopy and flow cytometry, prior to the emergence of drug-resistant clones, to restore normal hematopoiesis, and to provide adequate chemoprophylaxis for the sanctuary sites such as the CNS. A typical ALL regimen consists of induction, consolidation/intensification, and maintenance; CNS prophylaxis is usually administered during induction and consolidation.

Recent data from phase II trials demonstrate that young adults who were treated on adult protocols fared significantly worse than the same age group treated on pediatric protocols. This superior outcome has been attributed to the more intensive treatment on pediatric protocols, which include high-dose steroids and L-Asp as well as better adherence to the therapy by patients, parents, and doctors. Currently, clinical trials evaluating the pediatric-type therapy in adult patients up to the age of 40 years are ongoing.

A. Induction

The addition of an anthracycline to the standard pediatric ALL induction regimen of vincristine, prednisone, and L-Asp increased CR rates in adults from 50% to 60% to 70% to 90% and median duration of the disease remission to approximately 18 months. In some studies, dexamethasone has been substituted for prednisolone due to its higher in vitro activity and better CNS penetration. However, findings of a small, randomized study showed that an augmented dose of prednisolone produced results comparable to those achieved with dexamethasone in the context of intensive chemotherapy. Although L-Asp proved to be of value in the preanthracycline era, and in pediatric trials produced better survival when administered during induction and/or postinduction phases, its role in anthracycline-based adult programs is evolving. Given the significant toxicity of L-Asp, many investigators do not recommend its use in older patients; however, incorporation of L-Asp in intensive regimens for young adults is actively investigated. The newer pegylated form of L-Asp (peg-asp) has a prolonged half-life and has been FDA-approved for pediatric ALL. The

CALGB 9511 trial substituted peg-asp for native asparaginase and demonstrated CR rate of 76%, median OS of 22 months, and DFS at 7.5 years of 21%.

Attempts to further improve the outcome of patients with ALL led to the incorporation of agents such as cytarabine, cyclophosphamide, etoposide, mitoxantrone, and MTX in induction and postinduction therapy. It is unclear whether intensification with additional agents or using multiple phases of induction therapy improved CR rates in the unselected patients; however, it may benefit certain subgroups. The use of growth factors during induction may alleviate complications of prolonged bone marrow suppression and avoid delays in delivering dose-intensive chemotherapy. In a double-blind, randomized trial conducted by CALGB, administration of G-CSF shortened the duration of neutropenia from 29 days in the placebo group to 16 days in G-CSF group. The CR rates were higher with G-CSF (90% versus 81%), whereas induction mortality was higher in the placebo group (11% versus 4%).

B. Consolidation (intensification) therapy

This typically includes three to eight cycles of non–cross-resistant drugs administered after the remission induction. As mentioned previously, no randomized studies have compared the plethora of existing regimens (Linker trial, French LALA-94 trial, CALGB 8811 study, the MRC UKALL XA, GIMEMA ALL 0288 trial, the PETHEMA ALL-89 randomized trial, hyper-cyclophosphamide, vincristine, doxorubicin, and dexamethasone [CVAD], or R-hyper-CVAD).

C. Maintenance

The benefit of maintenance therapy in adult patients with ALL is unclear. In patients with low-risk disease, who enjoy outcomes similar to pediatric patients, maintenance therapy appears to be justified. Considering that more than half of the high-risk patients relapse while undergoing maintenance therapy, alternative strategies of eradicating MRD are urgently needed. The utility of maintenance therapy has been questioned for patients with T-cell ALL, and it is not given for patients with mature B-cell ALL or those with Philadelphia (Ph1) chromosome–positive disease.

The traditional maintenance regimen is given for approximately 2 years and includes daily doses of 6-mercaptopurine, weekly doses of MTX, and monthly doses of vincristine and prednisone. Dose intensification or extension of maintenance beyond 3 years does not appear to be of benefit, whereas its omission has been associated with shorter DFS.

D. Recommendations for the therapeutic regimens for pre-B– and T-cell lineage ALL

Although T-cell ALL previously had a poor prognosis with standard induction and maintenance chemotherapy, with the advent of more intensive chemotherapy regimens, response rates and long-term DFS are comparable with those for precursor B-cell ALL. A response rate of 100% and a projected long-term DFS of 59% was demonstrated by the regimen devised by Linker and colleagues[1] in 2002 for T-cell ALL. The CALGB 8811 protocol produced a 100% CR rate with a 63% 3-year RFS for a similar group of patients. Precursor B-cell and T-cell ALL are treated with similar regimens in most contemporary protocols.

1. **Berlin-Frankfurt-Muenster (BFM)-like regimens (MRC/ECOG).** The MRC/ECOG ALL treatment regimen should be considered for patients regardless of age who are thought to be able to withstand the rigors of an intensive program.

   a. **Induction** (consisting of two phases):
      - Phase I, weeks 1 to 4.
         - Vincristine* 1.4 mg/m^2 (maximum 2 mg) IV push on days 1, 8, 15, and 22, *and*
         - Prednisone 60 mg/m^2 by mouth on days 1 to 28 (followed by rapid taper over 7 days), *and*
         - DNR** 60 mg/m^2 IV push on days 1, 8, 15 and 22, *and*
         - L-Asp 10,000 U IV (or intramuscularly) once daily on days 17 to 28.
      - Phase II, weeks 5 to 8, should be postponed until the total WBC exceeds $3 \times 10^3/\mu L$.
         - Cyclophosphamide 650 mg/m^2 IV on days 1, 15 and 29, *and*
         - Cytarabine 75 mg/m^2 IV on days 1 to 4, 8 to 11, 15 to 18, and 22 to 25, *and*
         - 6-Mercaptopurine 60 mg/m^2 by mouth once daily on days 1 to 28.

Direct bilirubin	Dose of vincristine to give	Dose of DNR to give
2–3 mg/dL	100% calculated	50% calculated
>3 mg/dL	50% calculated	25% calculated

   b. **CNS treatment and prophylaxis.** If CNS leukemia is present at diagnosis, MTX IT or via an Ommaya reservoir is given weekly until blasts are cleared form the CNS fluid. Additionally, 24 Gy cranial irradiation and 12 Gy to the spinal cord are administered concurrently with phase II induction. If CNS leukemia is not present at diagnosis, MTX 12.5 mg IT on day 15 in phase I and MTX 12.5 mg IT on days 1, 8, 15, and 22 in phase II are given.

---

* The vincristine dose should be modified to 50% for paresthesia proximal to the distal interphalangeal joints and stopped entirely for major muscle weakness, cranial nerve palsy, or severe ileus.
** DNR and vincristine doses should be modified on a weekly basis according to the serum bilirubin.

c. **Intensification therapy** begins 4 weeks after induction phase II and should be postponed until the WBC is greater than $3 \times 10^3/\mu L$.
   - MTX 3 g/m^2 IV on days 1, 8, and 22
   - Leucovorin rescue starting at 24 hours 10 mg/m^2 by mouth or IV every 6 hours $\times$ 12 or until the serum MTX concentration is less than 5×10^{-8} M, *and*
   - L-Asp 10,000 U on days 2, 9, and 23.

d. **Consolidation therapy** (for patients not proceeding to allo-HSCT). Given after intensification when the WBC is higher than 3000/μL and the platelet count is higher than 100,000/μL.
   - **Cycle I consolidation**
      - Cytarabine 75 mg/m^2 IV on days 1 to 5, *and*
      - Vincristine 2 mg IV on days 1, 8, 15, and 22, *and*
      - Dexamethasone 10 mg/m^2 by mouth on days 1 to 28, *and*
      - Etoposide 100 mg/m^2 IV on days 1 to 5.
   - **Cycle II consolidation** (begins 4 weeks from day 1 of first cycle or when WBC exceeds 3000/μL)
      - Cytarabine 75 mg/m^2 IV on days 1 to 5, *and*
      - Etoposide 100 mg/m^2 IV on days 1 to 5.
   - **Cycle III consolidation** (begins 4 weeks from day 1 of second cycle or when WBC exceeds 3000/μL)
      - DNR 25 mg/m^2 IV on days 1, 8, 15, and 22, *and*
      - Cyclophosphamide 650 mg/m^2 IV on day 29, *and*
      - Cytarabine 75 mg/m^2 IV on days 31 to 34 and 38 to 41, *and*
      - 6-Thioguanine 60 mg/m^2 by mouth on days 29–42.
   - **Cycle IV consolidation** (begins 8 weeks from day 1 of third cycle or when WBC exceeds 3000/μL).
      - Cytarabine 75 mg/m^2 IV on days 1 to 5, *and*
      - Etoposide 100 mg/m^2 IV on days 1 to 5.

e. **Maintenance for adult ALL by MTX- and 6-mercaptopurine-based therapy.** Pulses of vincristine and prednisone are given as "reinforcement" because they have relatively little toxicity. Maintenance therapy should be continued for 2.5 years from start of intensification.
   - 6-Mercaptopurine 75 mg/m^2/day by mouth, *and*
   - Vincristine 2 mg IV every 3 months, *and*
   - Prednisone 60 mg/m^2 by mouth for 5 days every 3 months with vincristine, *and*
   - MTX 20 mg/m^2 by mouth or IV once per week for 2.5 years.

2. **CALGB 881** consists of a five-drug combination devised to achieve more rapid cytoreduction during the induction phase. For B-cell–lineage ALL, it produced an 82% CR rate with 41% DFS at 36 months. Patients in remission receive multiagent consolidation treatment, CNS prophylaxis, late intensification, and maintenance chemotherapy for a total of 24 months. CALGB 8811 should be considered for patients, regardless of age, who are thought to be able to withstand the rigors of an intensive program.

a. **Induction for patients 60 years or younger**
   - Cyclophosphamide 1200 mg/m^2 IV on day 1, *and*
   - DNR 45 mg/m^2 IV on days 1, 2, and 3, *and*
   - Vincristine 2 mg IV on days 1, 8, 15, and 22, *and*
   - Prednisone 60 mg/m^2/day by mouth on days 1 to 21, *and*
   - L-Asp 6000 IU/m^2 SC on days 5, 8, 11, 15, 18, and 22.

b. **Induction for patients older than 60 years**
   - Cyclophosphamide 800 mg/m^2 on day 1, *and*
   - DNR 30 mg/m^2 on days 1, 2, and 3, *and*
   - Prednisone 60 mg/m^2/day on days 1 to 7.

c. **Early intensification (two cycles)**
   - IT MTX 15 mg on day 1, *and*
   - Cyclophosphamide 1000 mg/m^2 IV on day 1, *and*
   - 6-Mercaptopurine 60 mg/m^2/day by mouth on days 1 to 14, *and*
   - Cytarabine 75 mg/m^2/day SC on days 1 to 4 and 8 to 11, *and*
   - Vincristine 2 mg IV on days 15 and 22, *and*
   - L-Asp 6000 U/m^2 SC on days 15, 18, 22, and 25.

d. **CNS prophylaxis and interim maintenance**
   - Cranial irradiation 2400 cGy on days 1 to 12, *and*
   - IT MTX 15 mg on days 1, 8, 15, 22, and 29, *and*
   - 6-Mercaptopurine 60 mg/m^2/day by mouth on days 1 to 70, *and*
   - MTX 20 mg/m^2 by mouth on days 36, 43, 50, 57, and 64.

e. **Late intensification**
   - Doxorubicin 30 mg/m^2 IV on days 1, 8, and 15, *and*
   - Vincristine 2 mg IV on days 1, 8, and 15, *and*
   - Dexamethasone 10 mg/m^2/day by mouth on days 1 to 14, *and*
   - Cyclophosphamide 1000 mg/m^2 IV on day 29, *and*
   - 6-Thioguanine 60 mg/m^2/day by mouth on days 29 to 42, *and*
   - Cytarabine 75 mg/m^2/day SC on days 29 to 32 and 36 to 39.

f. **Prolonged maintenance (monthly until 24 months from diagnosis)**
   - Vincristine 2 mg IV on day 1, *and*
   - Prednisone 60 mg/m^2/day by mouth on days 1 to 5, *and*
   - MTX 20 mg/m^2 by mouth on days 1, 8, 15, and 22, *and*
   - 6-Mercaptopurine 60 mg/m^2/day by mouth on days 1 to 28.

3. **Other vincristine, prednisolone, and daunorubicin (VPD)-based regimens.** A number of variations on the basic VPD program have been described. VPD should be used for patients who are thought not to be able to tolerate a more intensive chemotherapy program. Some options are shown in parentheses.

a. **Induction**
   - Vincristine 2 mg IV on days 1, 8, 15, (22), *and*
   - Prednisone 40 or 60 mg/m^2 by mouth on days 1 to 28 or days 1 to 35, followed by rapid taper over 7 days, *and*
   - DNR 45 mg/m^2 IV on days 1 to 3, *and*
   - L-Asp 500 IU/kg (18,500 IU/m^2) IV on days 22 to 32.

b. **CNS prophylaxis** is given as six doses of IT MTX and whole-brain irradiation starting on approximately day 36.

c. **Maintenance.** Maintenance is usually started once the marrow suppression and the oral toxicity of the CNS prophylaxis have cleared. Maintenance may be given in a pulse or a continuous manner. Although allopurinol is usually not needed after remission is achieved, the dose of 6-mercaptopurine should be decreased by 75% when given concomitantly with allopurinol.

d. **Pulse maintenance** is an 8-week cycle consisting of three courses of MTX and 6-mercaptopurine given every 2 weeks, followed by a 2-week pulse of vincristine and prednisone.

- MTX 7.5 mg/m^2 by mouth on days 1 to 5 during weeks 1, 3, and 5, *and*
- 6-Mercaptopurine 200 mg/m^2 by mouth on days 1 to 5 during weeks 1, 3, and 5, *and*
- Vincristine 2 mg IV on day 1 during weeks 7 and 8, *and*
- Prednisone 40 mg/m^2 by mouth on days 1 to 7 during weeks 7 and 8.

Oral MTX should be taken in a single daily dose because splitting the daily dose significantly increases the mucositis. Approximately three doses of IT MTX are needed once maintenance has started. The schedule should be coordinated so that the IT MTX is given on day 1 of the 5 scheduled days of oral MTX. On those days when IT MTX is given, the oral MTX is not given. Pulse maintenance is given for 3 years.

Dose adjustments for hematologic toxicity from the MTX and 6-mercaptopurine should be made based on blood cell counts obtained before the start of each course.

Dose	ANC (/μL)	Platelets (/μL)
100%	≥2000	≥100,000
75%	1500–1999	75,000–99,999
50%	1000–1499	50,000–74,999
0%	<1000	<50,000

e. **Intensification** with cytarabine and DNR given as "7 + 3" and "5 + 2" does not improve remission duration or OS compared with pulse maintenance in randomized, prospective trials.

4. **Hyper-CVAD**

a. **Odd cycles (1, 3, 5, and 7)**

- Cyclophosphamide 300 mg/m^2 IV every 12 hours on days 1 to 3, *and*
- Mesna 600 mg/m^2/day by continuous infusion on days 1 to 3, *and*
- Vincristine 2 mg IV on days 4 and 11, *and*

- Doxorubicin 50 mg/m^2 IV on day 4, *and*
- Dexamethasone 40 mg/day on days 1 to 4 and days 11 to 14.
- *IT therapy:* MTX 12 mg day 2 each course, *and*
- Cytarabine 100 mg day 7 each course (if CNS leukemia is present, increase therapy to twice weekly until the CSF cell count normalizes).

b. Even cycles (2, 4, 6, and 8).

- MTX 1 g/m^2 IV over 24 hours on day 1, *and*
- Leucovorin 50 mg IV to start 12 hours after MTX, then 15 mg IV every 6 hours until serum MTX less than 1 × 10^{-8} M, *and*
- Cytarabine 3 g/m^2 IV infusion over 1 hour every 12 hours × four doses on days 2 and 3 (reduce cytarabine dose to 1 g/m^2 for patients older than 60 years old), *and*
- *IT therapy:* MTX 12 mg day 2 each cycle, *and*
- Cytarabine 100 mg day 7 each cycle (if CNS leukemia is present, increase therapy to twice weekly until the CSF cell count normalizes).

c. Maintenance therapy for 2 years

- 6-Mercaptopurine 50 mg by mouth twice a day, *and*
- MTX 20 mg/m^2/week by mouth.

5. R-Hyper-CVAD (CD20+ ALL)

- Rituximab 375 mg/m^2 IV over 2 to 6 hours on days 1 and 11 of odd cycles and days 2 and 8 of even cycles; total of eight doses over the first four cycles.

E. Mature (Burkitt) B-cell ALL

Mature B-cell ALL is rare, constituting 2% to 4% of cases of adult ALL and is associated with human immunodeficiency virus (HIV) syndrome. The leukemic cells are characterized by FAB-L3 morphology, expression of monoclonal surface immunoglobulins, and specific nonrandom chromosomal translocations: t(8;14)(q24;q32), t(2;8)(q12;q24), t(8;22)(q24;q11). Characteristic clinical features include frequent CNS involvement, lymphadenopathy, splenomegaly, and high serum LDH level. In the past, the results of the treatment of B-cell ALL in both children and adults had been poor, with a CR rate of about 35% and long-term leukemia-free survival (LFS) of less than 10%. The current pediatric studies designed specifically for B-cell ALL, utilizing shorter-duration, dose-intensive systemic chemotherapy and early CNS prophylaxis/treatment, have substantially improved the CR rate to about 90% and the DFS to 50% to 87%.

With use of these therapeutic strategies in children as a template, clinical trials with young adults have demonstrated long-term survival rates of 70% to 80%. The German BFM group reported the improvement of CR rate from 44% to 74%, the probability of DFS from 0% to 71%, and the OS from 0% to 51% when the intensive treatment was compared with standard ALL regimens.

The hyper-CVAD regimen induced a CR rate of 90% and a cure rate of 70% in patients younger than 60 years of age, and a CR rate of 67% with a cure rate of only 15% in older patients.

Addition of anti-CD20 antibody rituximab to the hyper-CVAD regimen induced CR in 86% of patients, with 3-year OS, EFS, and DFS of 89%, 80%, and 88%, respectively. Nine elderly patients achieved a CR with 3-year OS rate of 89% (1 patient died from infection in CR).

Hyper-CVAD therapy in combination with a highly active antiretroviral therapy (HAART) regimen in HIV-positive patients resulted in a CR rate of 92%, with more than 50% of patients alive at 2 years after the diagnosis. The outcome appeared to be improved in patients taking HAART medications early in the course of the therapy.

For all adult patients with mature B-cell ALL, we recommend HIV testing, CNS prophylaxis, and hyper-CVAD therapy.

F. Minimal residual disease (MRD) in ALL

The aim of induction therapy in ALL is to reduce the leukemia cell population from 10^{12} cells to below the cytologically detectable level of 10^9 cells. At this point, a substantial leukemia cell burden (i.e., MRD) persists and patients relapse within months without subsequent therapy. Various techniques such as flow cytometry and PCR, using either fusion transcript resulting from the chromosomal abnormalities or patient-specific junctional regions of rearranged Ig and TCR genes, can be used to detect approximately one to five blasts/100,000 nucleated cells.

There is a significant correlation between the presence of MRD and early disease recurrence, particularly with greater than 10^{-2} residual blasts per 2×10^5 mononuclear bone marrow cells immediately after the disease remission or greater than 10^{-3} at a later time.

Although adults have higher MRD levels at the completion of induction, and the risk of recurrence is higher with low levels of MRD compared with children, continuous MRD assessment at several points also was predictive in adults. The German Multicenter Study for Adult Acute Lymphoblastic Leukemia prospectively monitored 196 patients with standard-risk ALL at up to nine time points during the first year of therapy with quantitative PCR analysis. Based on the persistence of MRD over time, three risk groups were identified with a 3-year risk of recurrence ranging from 0% (low-risk group) to 94% (high-risk group).

G. CNS disease

Although uncommon at diagnosis (less than 10%), without CNS directed therapy, 50% to 75% of patients will develop CNS disease. Prophylaxis is therefore an essential part of ALL therapy, as it has clearly been shown to reduce the incidence of CNS disease.

1. **Principles of diagnosis, prophylaxis, and management of CNS disease**
   - Obtain the diagnostic lumbar puncture (LP) once the leukemic blasts are cleared from the peripheral blood (to preclude the CNS contamination in the event of traumatic LP). The first dose of IT chemotherapy could be given at the same time.
   - Presence of lymphoblasts in the CSF (5 lymphocytes/μL and blasts on the differential or any lymphoblasts in the CSF) usually signify CNS disease.
   - Patients presenting with clinical symptoms consistent with CNS involvement, such as headache, altered sensorium, and cranial nerve (particularly cranial nerve VI) palsy warrant an *immediate* CNS imaging and LP because neurologic dysfunction is most amenable to therapy within the first 24 hours. Infectious meningitis also must be excluded in the immunocompromised host.
   - Consider Ommaya placement for patients with diagnosed CNS involvement.
   - Isolated CNS relapse usually heralds bone marrow relapse if systemic therapy is not changed. Therefore, isolated CNS relapse is usually treated with systemic reinduction chemotherapy and IT chemotherapy, followed by cranial irradiation.

   Depending on the protocol, CNS prophylaxis includes IT chemotherapy with MTX, Ara-C, and steroids; high-dose systemic chemotherapy with MTX, Ara-C, L-Asp, craniospinal irradiation (XRT); or a combination of the above. None of the combinations have been definitively proven to be superior to the others. The role of XRT has become controversial because of the significant neurologic complications such as seizures, intellectual and cognitive impairment, dementia, and development of secondary CNS malignancy. In addition, most chemotherapy regimens now administer either or both HDAC and high-dose MTX.

   In adults, features that correlate with high-risk of development of CNS disease include mature B-cell ALL, serum LDH higher than 600 u/L, and proliferative index of less than 14% (% S-phase + G_2M-phase).

2. **The commonly used regimens for CNS prophylaxis** include the following:
   - MTX 12 mg/m^2 (maximum 15 mg), diluted in preservative-free saline, given IT once a week for 6 weeks. Some investigators also give 10 mg of hydrocortisone succinate IT to prevent lumbar arachnoiditis. The IT MTX is then given in an "in-and-out" manner. One to two mL of the MTX solution is injected into the spinal canal. Then, 0.5 to 1 mL of spinal fluid is withdrawn back into the syringe. This in-and-out process is repeated until all of the MTX has been given. This method is used to ensure that the MTX is actually given into the subarachnoid space. Leucovorin 5 to 10 mg

may be given orally every 6 hours for four to eight doses to ameliorate the mucositis, although this usually is not needed unless the patient is receiving concurrent systemic MTX. Complications of MTX include chemical arachnoiditis and leukoencephalopathy.

- In the M.D. Anderson hyper-CVAD regimen, IT MTX 12 mg on day 2 and cytarabine 100 mg was administered on day 8 of each of eight cycles to high-risk patients and of each of four cycles in low-risk patients.

- Cranial irradiation with IT MTX is usually initiated within 2 weeks of attaining a CR when classic maintenance is given. Cranial irradiation is usually given to the cranial vault (anteriorly to the posterior pole of the eye and posteriorly to C2) in 0.2-Gy fractions for a total of 18 to 24 Gy. The spine is not irradiated because marrow toxicity significantly limits the ability to give further chemotherapy. Common acute complications of radiation include stomatitis, parotitis, alopecia, marrow suppression, and headaches.

3. **Therapy for overt CNS leukemia** is similar to the CNS prophylaxis.

   - Cranial irradiation is usually given to a total of 30 Gy in 1.5- to 2-Gy fractions.

   - IT chemotherapy is given in the manner described for CNS prophylaxis and is repeated every 3 to 4 days, with appropriate laboratory studies being done with each lumbar puncture. When blast cells are no longer seen on the cytospin preparation, two more doses of IT drug are given, usually followed by a monthly "maintenance" IT injection.

   - Some investigators advocate either a simultaneous or alternating administration of IT Ara-C and MTX.

   - The use of systemic therapy with HDAC 1 to 3 g/m^2 IV infusion over 2 hours every 12 hours is also effective for the treatment of CNS leukemia. A practical approach is to initiate IT chemotherapy until HDAC is started. Further IT therapy can then be given based on the results of subsequent CSF analysis after the HDAC is completed.

   - A slow-release formulation of Ara-C (DepoCyt) that maintains cytotoxic concentrations for approximately 14 days has been demonstrated to be effective for the treatment of lymphomatous meningitis and solid tumors and is under evaluation in acute leukemia.

H. ALL in older adults

The therapeutic advances and improved outcomes in children and young adults with ALL did not occur in older patients with ALL. Likely reasons include fundamental biologic difference in the spectrum of ALL in this patient population, presence of coexisting medical conditions, and decreased ability to tolerate intensive chemotherapy. Additionally, older patients have been frequently excluded from clinical trials. The correlation of age and outcome has been well documented in patients with ALL treated on the five sequential CALGB studies. The CR rates of patients younger than 30 years, between 30 to 59 years, and older than 59 years were 90%, 81%, and 57%, respectively. Based on the data provided by Hoelzer and Pagano et al. for patients older than 60 years treated with intensive chemotherapy from 1990 to 2004, the weighted mean CR rate was 56%; 23% suffered from early mortality and 30% had primary refractory disease.

In a randomized clinical trial evaluating the use of growth factors during chemotherapy for ALL, older patients enjoyed the greatest benefit. Thus, it is recommended to administer growth factors during ALL treatment in older adults.

Full doses of VPD-based induction protocols are used in elderly patients with ALL. Some investigators decrease the dose of vincristine by 50%. The MRC/ECOG and CALGB 8811 regimens should be considered for patients who are thought to be able to tolerate more intensive therapy.

Underlying cardiac disease may preclude the use of an anthracycline for induction therapy. An active program is MTX, vincristine, peg-asp, and dexamethasone (MOAD), developed by the ECOG, which is given in sequential 10-day courses (minimum three, maximum five) until remission is achieved. Once a CR has been attained, two additional courses of MOAD are given.

1. **Induction**
   - MTX 100 mg/m^2 IV on day 1 (increase by 50% on courses 2 and 3 and by 25% each additional course until mild toxicity is achieved), *and*
   - Vincristine 2 mg IV on day 2, *and*
   - L-Asp 500 IU/kg (18,500 IU/m^2) IV infusion on day 2, *and*
   - Dexamethasone 6 mg/m^2/day by mouth on days 1 to 10.
2. **Consolidation** therapy is repeated every 10 days for six courses.
   - MTX (final dose from induction) IV on day 1, *and*
   - L-Asp 500 IU/kg (18,500 IU/m^2) IV infusion on day 2.
3. **Cytoreduction** begins on day 30 of the last consolidation cycle of MTX and L-Asp. Cytoreduction is given monthly for 12 months.
   - Vincristine 2 mg IV on day 1, 30 minutes before MTX, *and*
   - MTX 100 mg/kg (3.7 g/m^2) IV infusion over 6 hours on day 1, *and*
   - Leucovorin 5 mg/kg (185 mg/m^2) divided into 12 doses starting 2 hours after the MTX infusion over days 1 to 3, *and*
   - Dexamethasone 6 mg/m^2/day by mouth on days 2 to 6.
4. **Maintenance** begins on day 30 of the last course of cytoreduction. It is repeated monthly until relapse.
   - Vincristine 2 mg IV on day 1, *and*
   - Dexamethasone 6 mg/m^2/day by mouth on days 1 to 5, *and*
   - MTX 15 mg/m^2 by mouth weekly, *and*
   - 6-Mercaptopurine 100 mg/m^2 by mouth daily.

I. Therapy for Ph1+ ALL

1. **Background**. In the era before tyrosine kinase inhibitors (TKIs), despite only slightly lower rates of CR in Ph1+ ALL patients (60% to 80%) compared to those with Ph1-disease, the long-term DFS was dismal (less than 10%), with allo-HSCT being the only modality offering a meaningful DFS. The MRCUKALLXII/ ECOG2993 international prospective ALL trial compared the outcomes of patients with Ph+ ALL treated with matched-sibling allo-HSCT, matched unrelated allo-HSCT, auto-HSCT, and consolidation/maintenance chemotherapy. The 5-year RR was lower in the allo-HSCT group (29%) than with the auto-HSCT/chemotherapy group (81%), while the 5-year survival rates were 43% and 19%, respectively. The TRM, not surprisingly, was higher in the patients undergoing allo-HSCT: 43% for matched unrelated allo-HSCT, 37% for matched-sibling HSCT, 14% for auto-HSCT, and 8% for chemotherapy.

   However, introduction of TKIs into clinical practice improved the options and outcomes of patients with Ph+ ALL.

   Imatinib mesylate (Gleevec), a potent selective inhibitor of the bcr-abl tyrosine kinase, has been shown in phase I and II clinical trials to have substantial (20% to 58% CR), albeit nonsustained (42 to 123 days) activity in patients with relapsed and refractory Ph+ ALL. Administration of imatinib to 20 patients relapsed after the allo-HSCT induced a CR in 55%. Imatinib monotherapy in previously untreated patients resulted in a CR rate of approximately 95%, without the associated toxicity of chemotherapy. Incorporation of imatinib in the front-line hyper-CVAD chemotherapy is associated with hematologic CR rates consistently higher than 90% and molecular responses higher than 50%. Concurrent administration of imatinib and chemotherapy results in greater antileukemic efficacy than sequential administration.

   Dasatinib (BMS-354825), a second-generation oral kinase inhibitor that targets bcr-abl and SRC kinases, demonstrated significant activity in imatinib-resistant Ph+ ALL. In a recent study, 70% (7 out of 10) of patients with Ph+ ALL and chronic myelogenous leukemia with lymphoid blast crisis achieved a major hematologic response with dasatinib. Early studies of dasatinib and chemotherapy in patients with untreated Ph+ ALL revealed rapid hematologic clearance of bone marrow blasts and residual disease with manageable toxicity profile.

   Nilotinib (AMN107) is a new, orally active, aminopyrimidine-derivative TKI that appears to have some activity in imatinib-resistant Ph+ ALL. One in ten patients with relapsed Ph+ ALL (hematologic relapse) had a partial hematologic response, and one of three patients with molecularly relapsed Ph+ ALL had a complete molecular remission.

Despite high remission rates and favorable DFS, the long-term outcome of TKIs with or without chemotherapy remains to be defined. It has been our practice to proceed with an allo-HSCT for patients achieving adequate responses.

2. Recommendations for Ph+ ALL

- Hyper-CVAD chemotherapy with 600 mg of imatinib, administered daily for 14 days with each cycle; or with induction cycle and then continuously thereafter; if tolerated, dose may be increased to 800 mg for indefinite maintenance therapy if allo-HSCT is not possible.
- Hyper-CVAD chemotherapy with 100 mg of dasatinib, administered for 14 days with each cycle, followed by maintenance 100 mg of dasatinib with vincristine and prednisone for 2 years if allo-HSCT is not an option.
- For eligible patients, allo-HSCT still remains a therapeutic goal.
- The role of TKIs posttransplant remains to be defined.
- TKIs combined with low intensity therapy (vincristine, steroids) is of benefit for older and frail patients who are not candidates for more aggressive therapy and who are at higher risk of induction mortality and death in CR. For example, in GIMEMA LAL201B protocol, 800 mg of imatinib was given with 40 mg/m^2/day of prednisone for 45 days.

J. Salvage therapy for ALL

Although a second remission can usually be achieved in 10% to 50% of adults with ALL, it tends to be short-lived (6 to 7 months). If a second remission can be attained, suitable patients with relapsed ALL should be evaluated for the allo-HSCT. Salvage therapies typically mirror variation of drug combinations used in the front-line protocols, including combinations of vincristine, steroids, and anthracyclines; combinations of MTX and L-Asp; and HDAC-containing regimens. Novel agents are incorporated in to the salvage regimens continuously. None of the programs used for relapse is distinctly superior to the others, and any perceived differences are likely attributable to the usual biases of study selection.

- Vincristine, doxorubicin, and dexamethasone chemotherapy results in CR rates of 39%, median CR duration of 7 months, and median survival of 6 months; 2-year DFS was 20% and OS was 8%.
- "7 + 3" (cytarabine and DNR) as used for the induction of AML is active in ALL. Vincristine and prednisone may be added.
- Etoposide and cytarabine are given every 3 weeks for up to three courses until marrow hypoplasia and remission are achieved. They are then repeated monthly until relapse.
  - Etoposide 60 mg/m^2 IV every 12 hours on days 1 to 5, *and*
  - Cytarabine 100 mg/m^2 IV bolus every 12 hours on days 1 to 5.
- HDAC-based regimens have been reported to induce CR rates in 17% to 70% of patients. HDAC as a single agent has modest

activity in ALL, with a CR rate of about 34% and a median remission duration of 3.6 months. The addition of idarubicin or mitoxantrone increases the response rate to 60%, but the median response time remains 3.4 months.

- Cytarabine and fludarabine comprise an active noncardiotoxic combination. The median response duration is 5.5 months. Neurotoxicity is low. A second course can be given in 3 weeks if needed.
  - Induction
    - Cytarabine 1 g/m^2/day IV over 2 hours on days 1 to 6, *and*
    - Fludarabine 30 mg/m^2/day IV over 30 minutes 4 hours before cytarabine on days 2 to 6.
  - Consolidation is given monthly for two to three courses.
    - Cytarabine 1 g/m^2/day IV over 2 hours on days 1 to 4, *and*
    - Fludarabine 30 mg/m^2/day IV over 30 minutes 4 hours before cytarabine on days 1 to 4.
  - Maintenance
    - 6-Mercaptopurine 50 mg by mouth twice a day, *and*
    - MTX 20 mg/m^2/week by mouth.
- FLAG-IDA induced a 39% CR rate in patients with relapsed/refractory ALL. The responders received the second cycle followed by allo-HSCT and achieved a DFS of 6 months (3 to 38 months) and OS of 9 months (7 to 38 months).
  - Fludarabine 30 mg/m^2/day IV over 30 minutes on days 1 to 5, *and*
  - Cytarabine 2 g/m^2/day IV over 4 hours on days 1 to 5, *and*
  - Idarubicin 10 mg/m^2/day on days 1 to 3, *and*
  - G-CSF 5 μg/kg SC 24 hours after the completion of chemotherapy and until neutrophil regeneration.
- Hyper-CVAD (see Section VIII.H.4) therapy achieves CR rates similar to a combination of HDAC, mitoxantrone, and GM-CSF (44% versus 30%); however, the survival is improved.
- MOAD (see Section VII.H)
- L-Asp has been administered in combination with MTX, anthracyclines, vinca alkaloids, and prednisone with RRs ranging from 33% to 79% and median DFS from 3 to 6 months. Sequential MTX and L-Asp resulted in significant stomatitis (dose-limiting toxicity); 23% of treated patients had allergic reactions to L-Asp.
  - **Induction**
    - MTX 50 to 80 mg/m^2 IV on day 1, *and*
    - L-Asp 20,000 IU/m^2 IV 3 hours after MTX on day 1, *followed by*
    - MTX 120 mg/m^2 IV on day 8, *and*
    - L-Asp 20,000 IU/m^2 IV on day 9.
    - Repeat day 8 and 9 doses for MTX and L-Asp every 7 to 14 days until remission is attained.
  - **Maintenance** is repeated every 2 weeks.
    - MTX 10 to 40 mg/m^2 IV on day 1, *and*
    - L-Asp 10,000 IU/m^2 IV on day 1.

K. Novel and investigational strategies for the therapy of ALL

It is unlikely that altering the sequence of currently available chemotherapeutic agents or increasing their intensity will produce a qualitative improvement in the outcome of adult patients with ALL. A number of experimental approaches are currently being evaluated in clinical trials (Table 18.15). Among those, nelarabine is a soluble prodrug of 9-β-D-arabinofuranosylguanine that has activity in recurrent T-lineage lymphoid malignancies and was approved by the FDA for this indication in 2005. Response rates of 33% and 41% have been achieved in a group of 121 children and 39 adults with T-cell leukemia/lymphoma. The median OS was 20 weeks in adult patients. Neurotoxicity is a major side effect of nelarabine and is both dose- and schedule-dependent; it can be minimized by every other day administration rather than daily. Clofarabine, another nucleoside analogue, has received

TABLE 18.15	Some of the Experimental Agents Being Evaluated for the ALL Therapy

Monoclonal Antibodies
Anti-CD20 (Rituximab)
Anti-CD20 (Ofatumomab)
Anti-CD22 immunotoxin (CAT-3888)
Anti-CD52 (Alemtuzumab)
Anti-CD33 (Gemtuzumab ozogomicin)
Anti-CD7 (+ricin)
Human IgM MoAb (MoAb216)

Farnesyl Transferase Inhibitors
R115777
Sch66336

Tyrosine Kinase Inhibitors
Imatinib mesylate (Gleevec)
Dasatinib (BMS-354825)
Nilotinib (AMN107)
Farnesyl transferase inhibitors

Nucleoside Analogues
Nelarabine (T cell)
Clofarabine
Forodesine

Liposomal and Pegylated Compounds
Liposomal vincristine
Liposomal doxorubicin
Liposomal annamycin
Liposomal cytarabine
Peg-asparaginase

Antifolates
Pemetrexed

DNA Methyltransferase Inhibitors and Histone Deacetylase Inhibitors
LBH589
PDX101
Azacitidine
Decitabine

Mammalian Target of Rapamycin Inhibitors
RAD001

Microtubule-destabilizing Agents
ENMD-1198

FLT-3 Inhibitors
Lestaurtinib
Midostaurin
Tandutinib
Sunitinib

Blinatumomab (recruits T-cells)

FDA approval for pediatric patients with ALL who have failed at least two prior induction regimens. Studies of this drug alone or in combination (with cyclophosphamide, for example) are ongoing.

L. **Hematopoietic stem cell transplantation in ALL**

1. **Auto-HSCT** for patients in first remission appears to offer no advantage over chemotherapy, based on the data for the small prospective trials reported to date and prospective randomized MRCUKALLXII/ECOG2993 ALL data, due to high rates of relapse.

2. **Allo-HSCT**. The optimal patient selection and timing of allo-HSCT remains unresolved. Patients receiving matched-sibling HSCT in first CR reach a survival rate of 50% (20% to 81%). Although allo-HSCT for high-risk patients in first CR has been widely accepted, recent data from the MRCUKALLXII/ECOG2993 International ALL Trial suggest that that advantage may have been overestimated, particularly owing to a high rate of mortality, but the benefit of HSCT may extend to standard-risk patients. This is in contrast to prior studies that have not demonstrated an advantage to allo-HSCT compared to standard chemotherapy for patients with ALL without high-risk features in first CR. However, many of these trials have lacked sufficient numbers of patients, have used varied patient selection criteria, or did not allow for direct, prospective comparisons.

   According to the data collected by the international Bone Marrow Transplant Registry, 9-year DFS was not different for patients treated with chemotherapy and allo-HSCT (32% versus 34%). High TRM in the HSCT group was the main reason for poor outcome, whereas the recurrence rate was twice as high in the chemotherapy group (66% versus 30%)

   The benefit of allo-HSCT in high-risk patients with ALL was shown by a large French multicenter trial (LALA87), which compared the allo-HSCT with chemotherapy or auto-HSCT in first CR. Although 5-year OS for all risk groups combined was not significantly different (48% versus 35%, $p = 0.08$), for patients with high-risk disease, both 5-year OS (44% versus 22%) and DFS (39% versus 14%) were significantly better with allo-HSCT. Similarly, the 10-year OS for the high-risk group was 44% with allo-HSCT and only 11% in the chemotherapy/auto-HSCT arm; in the standard-risk population, the corresponding numbers were 49% and 39% ($p = 0.6$), respectively.

   Prospective data generated from the MRCUKALLXII/ECOG2993 International ALL Trial, which included 1929 patients aged 15 to 59 years, allowed patients with HLA-matched siblings to undergo allo-HSCT; the rest were randomized to receive auto-HSCT or chemotherapy. The results can be summarized as follows: (1) for all patients, CR rate was 90% and 5-year OS was 43%; (2) for Ph1-negative patients treated with matched-sibling allo-HSCT, the 5-year OS was 53% and 45% for the combined cohort of auto-HSCT and consolidation chemotherapy; (3) the 5-year survival for the standard-risk group (defined as Ph1-negative, age under 36 years, time to CR less than 4 weeks, and WBC less than $30,000/\mu L$ for B-cell lineage and less than $100,000/\mu L$ for T-cell lineage) was superior for those who had a donor compared with those who had not (62% versus 52%; $p = 0.02$); (4) the 5-year survival rate for high-risk patients was not significantly different whether patients had a donor or not (41% versus 35%, $p = 0.2$; transplant-related toxicity abrogated the effect of a reduction in the recurrence rate); (5) postremission chemotherapy produced superior EFS and OS compared with auto-HSCT ($p = 0.02$ and $p = 0.03$, respectively).

Despite the high risk of early toxicity, matched-sibling allo-HSCT should be considered for most patients with ALL in first CR, with standard-risk disease.

As less than 30% of suitable patients with ALL have an HLA-matched sibling donor (MSD), extensive work has been aimed at improving the outcome of the transplantations from alternative donor sources, including partially matched related donors, MUDs, and UBC blood. A recently published trial compared the outcomes of auto-HSCT and MUD HSCT in 260 patients with ALL in first and second CR. Although TRM was higher and risk of recurrence was lower in MUD HSCT recipients, the 5-year LFS and OS rates were similar (37% versus 39% and 38% versus 39%, respectively). A similar trend toward comparable outcomes from MUDs and MSDs was observed in other studies. A recently published retrospective analysis of 623 patients with ALL undergoing HSCT from autologous ($n = 209$), MSDs ($n = 245$), unrelated ($n = 100$), and UCB ($n = 69$) sources demonstrated 5-year OS, LFS, and RRs of 29%, 26%, and 43%, respectively. Two-year TRM was 28%. Mismatched unrelated donor transplants yielded higher TRM (relative risk, 2.2; $p < 0.01$) and lower OS (relative risk, 1.5; $p = 0.05$) than MSD and UCB HSCT. Autografting yielded significantly more relapse (68%; $p < 0.01$) and poor LFS (14%; $p = 0.01$). HSCT in first CR yielded much better outcomes than later HSCT. With related donors, MUD, and UCB sources, 5-year LFS was 40%, 42%, and 49%, respectively, while relapse was 31%, 17%, and 27%, respectively. The authors concluded that allo-HSCT, not auto-HSCT, results in durable LFS. Additionally, UCB HSCT led to the outcome similar to that of MSDs or MUDs.

In recent years, the outcomes of allo-HSCT with RIC have been published in small patient series. Low TRM and OS up to 30% at 3 years suggests that RIC HSCT is a viable modality for selected patients who are not candidates for HSCT with standard conditioning.

Based on the available data, we advocate the use of HSCT from MSD and alternative sources for physically fit Ph1+ patients in CR1 as well as patients with relapsed disease in second remission. For Ph1+ patients without a suitable donor, we would continue intensive consolidation chemotherapy accompanied by TKIs followed by maintenance chemotherapy with TKIs.

Selected Readings

Acute Lymphoblastic Leukemia

Annino L, Vegna ML, Camera A, et al. Treatment of adult acute lymphoblastic leukemia (ALL): long-term follow-up of the GIMEMA ALL 0288 randomized study. *Blood.* 2002;99:863–871.

Bachanova V, Verneris MR, DeFor T, Brunstein CG, Weisdorf DJ. Prolonged survival in adults with acute lymphoblastic leukemia after reduced-intensity conditioning with cord blood or sibling donor transplantation. *Blood.* 2009;113(13):2902–2905.

Bassan R, Spinelli O, Oldani E, et al. Improved risk classification for risk-specific therapy based on the molecular study of minimal residual disease (MRD) in adult acute lymphoblastic leukemia (ALL). *Blood.* 2009;113(18):4153–4162.

Brüggemann M, Raff T, Flohr T, et al. Clinical significance of minimal residual disease quantification in adult patients with standard-risk acute lymphoblastic leukemia. *Blood.* 2006;107(3):1116–1123.

Cornelissen JJ, Carston M, Kollman C, et al. Unrelated marrow transplantation for adult patients with poor-risk acute lymphoblastic leukemia: strong graft-versus-leukemia effect and risk factors determining outcome. *Blood.* 2001;97:1572–1577.

Cortes J, Rousselot P, Kim DW, et al. Dasatinib induces complete hematologic and cytogenetic responses in patients with imatinib-resistant or -intolerant chronic myeloid leukemia in blast crisis. *Blood.* 2007;109(8):3207–3213.

Druker BJ, Sawyers CL, Kantarjian H, et al. Activity of a specific inhibitor of the BCR-ABL tyrosine kinase in the blast crisis of chronic myeloid leukemia and acute lymphoblastic leukemia with the Philadelphia chromosome. *N Engl J Med.* 2001;344:1038–1042.

Goldstone AH, Richards SM, Lazarus HM, et al. In adults with standard-risk acute lymphoblastic leukemia, the greatest benefit is achieved from a matched sibling allogeneic transplantation in first complete remission, and an autologous transplantation is less effective than conventional consolidation/maintenance chemotherapy in all patients: final results of the International ALL Trial (MRC UKALL XII/ECOG E2993). *Blood.* 2008;111(4):1827–1833.

Koller CA, Kantarjian HM, Thomas D, et al. The hyper-CVAD regimen improves outcome in relapsed acute lymphoblastic leukemia. *Leukemia.* 1997;11:2039–2044.

Larson RA, Dodge RK, Burns CP, et al. A five-drug remission induction regimen with intensive consolidation for adults with acute lymphoblastic leukemia: cancer and leukemia group B study 8811. *Blood*. 1995;85:2025–2037.

Linker C, Damon L, Ries C, Navarro W. Intensified and shortened cyclical chemotherapy for adult acute lymphoblastic leukemia. *J Clin Oncol*. 2002;20:2464–2471.

Mancini M, Scappaticci D, Cimino G, et al. A comprehensive genetic classification of adult acute lymphoblastic leukemia (ALL): analysis of the GIMEMA 0496 protocol. *Blood*. 2005;105(9):3434–3441.

Moorman AV, Harrison CJ, Buck GA, et al. Karyotype is an independent prognostic factor in adult acute lymphoblastic leukemia (ALL): analysis of cytogenetic data from patients treated on the Medical Research Council (MRC) UKALLXII/ Eastern Cooperative Oncology Group (ECOG) 2993 trial. *Blood*. 2007;109(8): 3189–3197.

Mortuza FY, Papaioannou M, Moreira IM, et al. Minimal residual disease tests provide an independent predictor of clinical outcome in adult acute lymphoblastic leukemia. *J Clin Oncol*. 2002;20:1094–1104.

Secker-Walker LM, Prentice HG, Durrant J, Richards S, Hall R, Harrison G. Cytogenetics adds independent prognostic information in adults with acute lymphoblastic leukaemia on MRC trial UKALL XA. MRC Adult Leukaemia Working Party. *Br J Haematol*. 1997;96:601–610.

Stock W, La M, Sanford B, et al. What determines the outcomes for adolescents and young adults with acute lymphoblastic leukemia treated on cooperative group protocols? A comparison of Children's Cancer Group and Cancer and Leukemia Group B studies. *Blood*. 2008;112(5):1646–1654.

Wetzler M, Dodge RK, Mrózek K, et al. Prospective karyotype analysis in adult acute lymphoblastic leukemia: the Cancer and Leukemia Group B experience. *Blood*. 1999;93:3983–3993.

Acute Myeloid Leukemia

Bloomfield CD, Lawrence D, Byrd JC, et al. Frequency of prolonged remission duration after high-dose cytarabine intensification in acute myeloid leukemia varies by cytogenetic subtype. *Cancer Res*. 1998;58:4173–4179.

Breems DA, Van Putten WL, De Greef GE, et al. Monosomal karyotype in acute myeloid leukemia: a better indicator of poor prognosis than a complex karyotype. *J Clin Oncol*. 2008;26(29):4791–4797.

Büchner T, Berdel WE, Haferlach C, et al. Age-related risk profile and chemotherapy dose response in acute myeloid leukemia: a study by the German Acute Myeloid Leukemia Cooperative Group. *J Clin Oncol*. 2009;27(1):61–69.

Byrd JC, Mrózek K, Dodge RK, et al. Pretreatment cytogenetic abnormalities are predictive of induction success, cumulative incidence of relapse, and overall survival in adult patients with de novo acute myeloid leukemia: results from Cancer and Leukemia Group B (CALGB 8461). *Blood*. 2002;100(13): 4325–4336.

Byrd JC, Dodge RK, Carroll A, et al. Patients with t(8;21)(q22;q22) and acute myeloid leukemia have superior failure-free and overall survival when repetitive cycles of high-dose cytarabine are administered. *J Clin Oncol*. 1999;17: 3767–3675.

Cassileth PA, Harrington DP, Appelbaum FR, et al. Chemotherapy compared with autologous or allogeneic bone marrow transplantation in the management of acute myeloid leukemia in first remission. *N Engl J Med*. 1998;339:1649–1656.

Fenaux P, Mufti GJ, Hellstrom-Lindberg E, et al. Efficacy of azacitidine compared with that of conventional care regimens in the treatment of higher-risk myelo-dysplastic syndromes: a randomised, open-label, phase III study. *Lancet Oncol.* 2009;10(3):223–232.

Fernandez HF, Sun Z, Yao X, et al. Anthracycline dose intensification in acute myeloid leukemia. *N Engl J Med.* 2009;361(13):1249–1259.

Gardin C, Turlure P, Fagot T, et al. Postremission treatment of elderly patients with acute myeloid leukemia in first complete remission after intensive induction che-motherapy: results of the multicenter randomized Acute Leukemia French Asso-ciation (ALFA) 9803 trial. *Blood.* 2007;109(12):5129–5135.

Grimwade D, Walker H, Harrison G, et al. The predictive value of hierarchical cytoge-netic classification in older adults with acute myeloid leukemia (AML): analysis of 1065 patients entered into the United Kingdom Medical Research Council AML11 trial. *Blood.* 2001;98:1312–1320.

Grimwade D, Walker H, Oliver F, et al. The importance of diagnostic cytogenetics on outcome in AML: analysis of 1,612 patients entered into the MRC AML 10 trial. The Medical Research Council Adult and Children's Leukaemia Working Parties. *Blood.* 1998;92:2322–2333.

Löwenberg B, Ossenkoppele GJ, van Putten W, et al. High-dose daunorubicin in older patients with acute myeloid leukemia. *N Engl J Med.* 2009;361(13): 1235–1248.

Mayer RJ, Davis RB, Schiffer CA, et al. Intensive postremission chemotherapy in adults with acute myeloid leukemia. Cancer and Leukemia Group B. *N Engl J Med.* 1994;331:896–903.

Nguyen S, Leblanc T, Fenaux P, et al. A white blood cell index as the main prognostic factor in t(8;21) acute myeloid leukemia (AML): a survey of 161 cases from the French AML Intergroup. *Blood.* 2002;99:3517–3523.

Sievers EL, Larson RA, Stadtmauer EA, et al. Efficacy and safety of gemtuzumab ozo-gamicin in patients with CD33- positive acute myeloid leukemia in first relapse. *J Clin Oncol.* 2001;19:3244–3254.

Slovak ML, Kopecky KJ, Cassileth PA, et al. Karyotypic analysis predicts outcome of preremission and postremission therapy in adult acute myeloid leukemia: a Southwest Oncology Group/Eastern Cooperative Oncology Group Study. *Blood.* 2000;96:4075–4083.

Weick JK, Kopecky KJ, Appelbaum FR, et al. A randomized investigation of high-dose versus standard-dose cytosine arabinoside with daunorubicin in patients with previously untreated acute myeloid leukemia: a Southwest Oncology Group study. *Blood.* 1996;88:2841–2851.

Thomas X, Raffoux E, Botton S, et al. Effect of priming with granulocyte-macrophage colony-stimulating factor in younger adults with newly diagnosed acute myeloid leukemia: a trial by the Acute Leukemia French Association (ALFA) Group. *Leuke-mia.* 2007;21(3):453–461.

Vardiman JW, Thiele J, Arber DA, et al. The 2008 revision of the World Health Organi-zation (WHO) classification of myeloid neoplasms and acute leukemia: rationale and important changes. *Blood.* 2009;114(5):937–951.

Acute Promyelocytic Leukemia

Adès L, Sanz MA, Chevret S, et al. Treatment of newly diagnosed acute promyelocytic leukemia (APL): a comparison of French-Belgian-Swiss and PETHEMA results. *Blood.* 2008;111(3):1078–1084.

Asou N, Kishimoto Y, Kiyoi H, et al. A randomized study with or without intensified maintenance chemotherapy in patients with acute promyelocytic leukemia who have become negative for PML-RARalpha transcript after consolidation therapy: the Japan Adult Leukemia Study Group (JALSG) APL97 study. *Blood.* 2007;110(1):59–66.

Camacho LH, Soignet SL, Chanel S, et al. Leukocytosis and the retinoic acid syndrome in patients with acute promyelocytic leukemia treated with arsenic trioxide. *J Clin Oncol.* 2000;18:2620–2625.

Esteve J, Escoda L, Martín G, et al. Outcome of patients with acute promyelocytic leukemia failing to front-line treatment with all-trans retinoic acid and anthracycline-based chemotherapy (PETHEMA protocols LPA96 and LPA99): benefit of an early intervention. *Leukemia.* 2007;21(3):446–452.

Fenaux P, Chastang C, Chevret S, et al. A randomized comparison of all trans-retinoic acid (ATRA) followed by chemotherapy and ATRA plus chemotherapy and the role of maintenance therapy in newly diagnosed acute promyelocytic leukemia. The European APL Group. *Blood.* 1999;94:1192–1200.

de la Serna J, Montesinos P, Vellenga E, et al. Causes and prognostic factors of remission induction failure in patients with acute promyelocytic leukemia treated with all-trans retinoic acid and idarubicin. *Blood.* 2008;111(7):3395–3402.

Tallman MS, Andersen JW, Schiffer CA, et al. Clinical description of 44 patients with acute promyelocytic leukemia who developed the retinoic acid syndrome. *Blood.* 2000;95:90–95.

Chronic Leukemias

Khaled el-Shami and Bruce D. Cheson

The chronic leukemias have traditionally been grouped together to underscore their differences from the aggressive, acute leukemias. Chronic leukemias can be broadly divided into those arising either from mature lymphocytes or from hematopoietic stem cells or any of their nonlymphoid progenitors. The unifying feature among the chronic leukemias is that, initially, there is relatively normal maturation of the progeny of the neoplastic clone. Malignant hematopoiesis is effective and results initially in increased numbers of mature-appearing cells in the peripheral blood and bone marrow that have few morphologic abnormalities. Functionally, however, both chronic myelogenous leukemia (CML) cells and chronic lymphocytic leukemia (CLL) cells are less functionally competent than their nonleukemic counterparts. The relatively normal morphologic appearance is in marked contrast to the acute leukemias where maturation arrest with consequent bone marrow failure is the hallmark of the disease. Nonetheless, chronic leukemias have heterogeneous biology and natural history and may evolve into aggressive and difficult-to-treat phase(s) with ineffective hematopoiesis resulting in progressive marrow failure and organ infiltration.

I. CHRONIC MYELOGENOUS LEUKEMIA (CML)

CML is a relatively uncommon malignancy, accounting for 15% of adult leukemias in the United States. The annual incidence of CML is 1.5 cases per 100,000 with a slight male predominance. The median age at diagnosis is 53 years. Less than 10% of cases are under 20 years of age. Ionizing radiation is the only known risk factor. There is no known genetic predisposition or sociogeographic preponderance.

CML is a clonal hematopoietic stem cell disorder caused by a balanced translocation between the long arms of chromosomes 9 and 22 [t (9;22)(q34;q11), also known as the Philadelphia (Ph1) chromosome]. The hybrid BCR-ABL gene from the (9;22) translocation has been noted in almost all cases of CML and is considered pathognomonic. This BCL-ABL fusion protein results in constitutive tyrosine kinase signaling activity that mediates the biologic hallmarks of CML through activation of a mitogenic signaling pathways; altered cellular adhesion to the extracellular matrix; inhibition of apoptosis; and downstream activation of a complicated network of signaling pathways including RAS, mitogen-activated protein kinase, Myc, phosphatidylinositol 3 kinase, NF-k-B, and Janus kinase signal transducer and activator of transcription pathways.

The molecular pathogenesis in CML involves three different breakpoint regions in the BCR gene, resulting in distinct disease phenotypes. More than 90% of patients with CML express the 210-kDa oncoprotein, with a minority of patients expressing either a 185-kDa or 230-kDa oncoprotein without significant differences in the natural history of the disease.

CML is a triphasic process consisting of an indolent, chronic phase (CP) that lasts for several years prior to progression to a treatment-resistant accelerated phase, eventually transforming into a blastic phase (BP) similar to an acute leukemia, which is fatal in most cases. The finding in CML that the Ph1 chromosome is present in lymphoid, erythroid, as well as myeloid elements supports the idea that a neoplastic event involves a pluripotent stem cell.

A. Diagnosis

Approximately 90% of patients with CML present in the CP of disease and may be entirely asymptomatic. Symptoms, when present, may include fatigue, bone aches, weight loss, and abdominal discomfort related to splenomegaly. The identification of a marked leukocytosis (usually greater than 25×10^9/L) due to a neutrophilia of all stages of maturation with a myelocyte "bulge" (i.e., myelocytes outnumbering the more mature metamyelocytes), lack of significant circulating blasts, absolute basophilia, frequent thrombocytosis, and mild anemia are key factors in the initial diagnosis. Leukocytes in patients with CML, while morphologically normal, exhibit a cytochemical abnormality with low leukocyte alkaline phosphatase (LAP) or neutrophil alkaline phosphatase when scored. The low LAP score is thought to be a consequence of relatively low levels of granulocyte colony-stimulating factor and is useful in differentiating CML from a reactive leukocytosis or "leukemoid reaction," typically due to infection, in which the score is typically elevated or normal. Other less specific laboratory features include elevated elastase, lactate dehydrogenase, vitamin B_{12} (secondary to production of B_{12}-binding protein haptocorrin by leukocytes), and uric acid levels. A bone marrow aspiration and biopsy is needed in all patients in whom CML is being considered, which will not only confirm the diagnosis, but also provide information necessary to stage and risk-stratify the disease. The bone marrow is invariably hypercellular with a myeloid-to-erythroid ratio in the range of 10 to 30:1. All stages of myeloid maturation are usually seen with myelocyte predominance. Megakaryocytes are increased in number and are characteristically smaller than normal. Up to 40% of patients will display increased reticulin fibrosis, which typically correlates with the degree of megakaryocytosis. Blasts usually account for less than 5% of the marrow cells, and more than 10% indicates transformation to an accelerated phase.

Up to 95% of patients with CML demonstrate the t(9;22) (q32;q11.2) reciprocal translocation that results in the Ph1 chromosome. The rest have either variant translocations, such as complex translocations involving other chromosomes or cryptic translocations of 9q34 and 22q11.2 that cannot be identified by routine cytogenetics. These are referred to as "Ph-negative" and require fluorescence in-situ hybridization (FISH) analysis to identify the BCR-ABL1 fusion gene, or reverse transcription (RT)-polymerase chain reaction (PCR) to identify the BCR-ABL1 fusion mRNA. Therefore, bone marrow samples of patients with suspected CML should be examined both by standard karyotyping (e.g., G-banded metaphase preparation) as well as interphase FISH. Of note, 10% to 15% of patients with CML harbor large deletions flanking the breakpoint on chromosome 9 and/or chromosome 22. Patients with such deletions have a shorter survival and time to progression to accelerated-phase (AP) or BP disease.

While the Ph1 is the initiating event in CML, progression to AP or blast crisis appears to require the acquisition of other nonrandom chromosomal or molecular changes (i.e., clonal evolution, which occurs in 50% to 80% of patients in the accelerated and blast crisis phases and, if noted during the chronic phase, confers a worse prognosis). The most commonly observed karyotypic abnormalities include trisomy 8, trisomy 19, duplication of the Ph1 chromosome, and isochromosome 17q (causing deletion of the P53 gene on 17p). Telomere shortening has also been associated with disease evolution. It is not known how these chromosomal changes contribute to the loss of cell differentiation that characterizes advanced-stage disease.

B. Classification

CML is characterized by three evolutionary phases, each carrying a different clinical and hematologic picture, natural history, and treatment outcome.

1. **Chronic phase (CP)** is the initial presentation of CML in approximately 90% of patients. This phase is marked by immature myeloid cells in the peripheral blood and marked granulocytic hyperplasia in the marrow; however, less than 10% of myeloblasts are present in both peripheral blood and bone marrow. Absolute eosinophilia and basophilia are commonly present (in contrast to reactive leukocytosis). The CP will typically run an indolent course of 3 to 5 years before progressing to the accelerated phase, even without treatment, although the duration can be highly variable.

2. **Accelerated phase (AP)** (Table 19.1) is poorly defined, but is usually marked by a loss of previously controlled white blood cell (WBC) counts and clonal evolution, with the development of new chromosomal abnormalities in addition to the persisting or re-emerged Ph1 chromosome. Peripheral blood counts show one or more of the following: blasts of at least 10%, basophils greater than 20%, or a fall in the platelet count to no more than 100,000/μL, unrelated to ongoing treatment. These laboratory findings are often accompanied by the re-emergence or progression of symptoms such as fever, bone pain, and fatigue, or worsening splenomegaly. The median survival prior to imatinib therapy was only 18 months; however, with imatinib, the estimated 4-year survival rate exceeds 50%.

3. **Blast phase (BP)** (see Table 19.1), also called "blast crisis," is the progressed transformation of CML to acute leukemia. It is defined by the acute leukemia criteria of at least 20% bone marrow blasts.

TABLE 19.1	WHO Criteria for Diagnosis of Accelerated and Blast Phase CML	

Accelerated Phase	**Blast Phase**
Blasts 10%–19% of WBCs in peripheral blood or bone marrow	Blasts ≥20% in peripheral blood or bone marrow
Peripheral blood basophils >20%	Extramedullary blast proliferation
Persistent thrombocytopenia <100 × 10⁹/L unrelated to therapy or persistent thrombocytosis >1000 × 10⁹/L unresponsive to therapy	Large foci or clusters of blasts in the bone marrow biopsy
Increased spleen size or worsening leukocytosis unresponsive to therapy	
Cytogenetic evidence of clonal evolution	

WBC, white blood cell.

However, patients with 20% to 29% blasts seem to carry a better prognosis than those meeting the older criterion of greater than 30% blasts. A majority of cases (50% to 70%) will express a poorly differentiated myeloid phenotype (acute myelogenous leukemia [AML]), while the remainder shows lymphoid (pre-B acute lymphocytic leukemia [ALL]) or an undifferentiated or mixed-lineage phenotype. Recent studies have identified BCR-ABL kinase domain mutations in 30% to 40% of these patients. Persistence of the Ph1 chromosome including additional Ph1 chromosomes and other cytogenetic abnormalities may be present. Extramedullary tumor masses (chloromas) can occur in both the APs and BPs. Durable responses to chemotherapy, using various acute leukemia regimens, are typically uncommon, and median survival in this phase is 3 to 6 months. ALL evolutions in general have a better response and prognosis than AML evolutions. A CP remission can occur with treatment as the blastic progeny clone is eradicated, but the CP Ph1 stem cell typically persists. Transcription factor–induced aberrant lineage priming of leukemic stem cells can bring about variability in subsequent evolution whereby patients achieving remission from a myeloid BP can re-enter a CP then relapse with a lymphoid BP (or vice versa).

C. Prognosis

Separation of these three stages is imprecise, and approximately 25% of patients progress directly from CP to BP. Although the duration of the CP is difficult to predict, a number of factors indicate an increased risk for progression, including greater age, splenomegaly, elevated platelet counts, and higher numbers of peripheral blood myeloblasts, eosinophils, or basophils. The Sokal prognostic system and the Hasford classification utilize a formula factoring in age, spleen size, and the hematologic picture to assign low, intermediate, and high groups differing in prognosis with 5-year survivals of 76%, 55%, and 25%, respectively. Both classifications were developed in patient cohorts receiving interferon, and none have thus far been validated during the imatinib era, limiting their usefulness. Regardless of pretreatment characteristics, the most important and best prognostic predictor of long-term survival is the quality of the response to treatment by minimal residual disease (MRD), which is measured by the degree of cytogenetic and molecular response.

D. Therapy

Hydroxycarbamide (also known as hydroxyurea) is a ribonucleotide reductase inhibitor frequently used to control the high WBC count while confirming the diagnosis of CML. The usual dose of hydroxycarbamide is 40 mg/kg/d. The dose is then adjusted individually to keep the WBC count in a range between 4 and 10×10^9/L.

Hydroxycarbamide does not reduce the percentage of cells bearing the Ph chromosome, and therefore, the risk of transformation to the BP is unchanged. Its use should be limited to temporary control of hematologic manifestations prior to starting definitive therapy. The "imatinib (Gleevec) era" has revolutionized the treatment of CML but also ushered in some questions of treatment uncertainty.

1. **Imatinib (Gleevec)** is a small molecule tyrosine kinase inhibitor (TKI) of the BCR-ABL tyrosine kinase. Targeting and inhibiting the BCR-ABL mitogenic pathway with imatinib has achieved dramatic cytogenetic and molecular levels of responses with prolonged disease control in CML. The most comprehensive source of information about the imatinib therapy for patients with CP disease is the IRIS trial. With a follow-up of 7 years, imatinib was discontinued for adverse events in 5% of patients and for lack of efficacy in 15% of patients. Seventy-five percent of patients with complete cytogenetic response (CCyR) have maintained the response so far. The 6-year event-free survival (EFS), progression-free survival (PFS), and overall survival (OS) rates were 83%, 93%, and 88%, respectively. Based on these results, 400 mg oral daily is deemed the standard initial dosing in CP disease. Maintaining imatinib dosing at greater than 300 mg daily is pharmacologically important to achieve effective inhibitory plasma concentrations. The results of the IRIS trial have been replicated in a prospective, multicenter German CML phase IV study, which reported a 5-year overall survival of 94% and a 2-year EFS of 80%. Studies addressing dose escalation of imatinib in early CP showed that 800 mg of imatinib was well tolerated and is associated with a high rate of cytogenetic and molecular responses, which are also attained more rapidly with the higher dose. However, whether such an approach results in long-term benefit or improvement in survival remains to be seen.

2. **Imatinib can only control, and not completely eradicate, the CML clone**, therefore being unable to cure the disease. Allogeneic stem cell transplantation is the only known curative therapy for CML. The question regarding the timing of transplant during CP CML remains controversial. However, it is clear that imatinib is the initiating therapy in treating CP CML and that close molecular monitoring of the BCR-ABL transcript is important to best manage an individual with CML.

3. **Side effects of imatinib**. Overall, imatinib is well tolerated. Side effects are generally mild and include nausea, peripheral and periorbital edema, muscle cramps, diarrhea, weight gain, and fatigue. Imatinib is metabolized through the CYP450 pathway, causing potential drug interactions. Rare organ damage can occur including liver toxicity, hypophosphatemia, and

potential cardiotoxicity. Myelosuppression is the most common grade 3 to 4 toxicity, with neutropenia and thrombocytopenia during the first few months of treatment. These can be managed with growth factors or dose reductions; however, they may require discontinuation of the drug, which may be temporary or permanent.

4. **Disease monitoring during imatinib therapy** is used to assess for early hematologic treatment toxicity and to evaluate the ongoing and ultimate disease response, with the treatment goal of achieving MRD measured by a CCyR and a 3-log reduction molecular response (Table 19.2). A reasonable approach, modifiable to an individual patient and case, is as follows:
   1. Complete blood count (CBC) weekly until stable, then every 4 to 6 weeks.
   2. Marrow cytogenetics at diagnosis, at 6 and 12 months of initial treatment, and yearly with ongoing treatment.
   3. Peripheral blood quantitative RT-PCR for BCR-ABL mRNA at diagnosis and every 3 months with ongoing treatment.

   The timing and level of response are important management milestones. The earlier a cytogenetic and molecular response is achieved, the longer the ultimate response will last. A partial cytogenetic response (1% to 35% Ph-positive metaphases) by 3 to 6 months predicts an 80% to 95% likelihood of achieving an eventual CCyR. Quantitative PCR on peripheral blood is the monitoring method of choice. There is a significant correlation between the molecular response at 3 months and cytogenetic response at 12 months. At 42 months of follow-up, those patients with a CCyR by 12 months and a major molecular

TABLE 19.2 Response Criteria in CML

Type of Response	Definition
Complete hematologic response	Normalization of complete blood count and differential WBC, resolution of splenomegaly
Minor cytogenetic response	35%–90% Ph+ metaphases
Partial cytogenetic response	1%–34% Ph+ metaphases
Complete cytogenetic response	No Ph+ metaphases
Major cytogenetic response	0%–34% Ph+ metaphases (complete + partial)
Major molecular response	≥3-log reduction of BCR-ABL transcript by qRT-PCR
Complete molecular response	No BCR-ABL transcript by qRT-PCR

PCR, polymerase chain reaction; RT, reverse transcription; WBC, white blood cell.

response (greater than 3-log reduction in BCR-ABL mRNA) had a PFS of 98% compared to 90% if less than 3-log reduction and 75% for patients without a CCyR. There is no absolute latest point in time at which a patient should have a CCyR before considering an altered treatment approach. That must be individualized based on age and other viable treatment options available. In a young patient who is a transplant candidate, if there is not an early optimal response within 6 to 12 months, consideration of this alternative therapy is appropriate.

5. **Imatinib resistance** can either be primary or secondary. Primary resistance without a complete hematologic response (CHR) occurs in approximately 5% of patients. Primary cytogenetic resistance (i.e., failing to achieve a partial cytogenetic response at 6 months or complete at 12 months) occurs in 15% of patients. After 42 months of follow-up, 16% of patients treated in the IRIS study developed secondary resistance or overtly progressed. In patients previously treated with interferon-α, 26% in CP developed resistance or progression. Imatinib resistance is much higher in APs (73%) and BPs (95%). When resistance is observed, a repeat bone marrow with cytogenetics and screening for the new kinase mutations should be performed to identify the T315I mutation, which is a marker of failure for all the currently available TKIs.

   Strategies to overcome imatinib resistance remain challenging. Overt phase progression forces a treatment change, as the current therapy is ineffective. Mutation changes are clearly a harbinger of phase progression, but in a variable time frame. Imatinib dose escalation up to 800 mg can be attempted; however, tolerance and durability remain limiting factors. Switching to second-generation TKIs, either dasatinib or nilotinib (see subsequent discussion) is presently the standard of care for imatinib failure or resistance. The addition of conventional chemotherapy agents, either interferon or cytarabine, may also be considered if unacceptable toxicity to second-generation TKIs develop. An allogeneic stem cell transplant in eligible patients with imatinib resistance may be an additional option.

6. **Alternative treatments**

   a. **Dasatinib (Sprycel)**, a piperazinyl derivative that targets many tyrosine kinases, was selected for its potent inhibitory activity against Src and ABL kinases, including the active conformation of BCR-ABL1 and most mutated forms (except T315I). The drug was shown to be effective for the treatment of Ph+ leukemia and was approved for the treatment of patients with imatinib-intolerant and imatinib-resistant disease who have Ph+ CML in CP, AP, and BP. A prospective, randomized study of four different doses and schedules identified a dose of 100 mg once daily as an efficacious and well-tolerated dose. In patients with imatinib-intolerant disease in CP, the major cytogenetic response (MCyR) and the CCyR rates were 76% and 75%, respectively, with median time to MCyR being 2.8 months. In patients with imatinib-resistant disease in CP, the MCyR and the CCyR rates were 51% and 40%, respectively. The median time to CCyR and major molecular response was 5.5 months. In 80% to 90% of patients in CP, the responses were maintained for 2 years, the PFS was greater than 80%, and the OS was greater than 90%. In 150 patients with imatinib-resistant disease in CP, the results were superior in patients whose therapy was changed to dasatinib 70 mg twice daily compared with those in whom the imatinib dose was increased to 800 mg.

b. **Nilotinib (Tasigna)** Nilotinib is an aminopyrimidine derivative that inhibits the tyrosine kinase activity of the unmutated and several mutated forms of BCR-ABL (except T315I, and to a lesser extent Y253H, E255K, and E255V) with higher in vitro potency and selectivity than imatinib. Similar to dasatinib, nilotinib is effective for the treatment of Ph+ leukemias and was registered for treating imatinib-intolerant and imatinib-resistant patients with Ph+ CML in CP and in AP at a dose of 400 mg twice daily. In 194 patients in imatinib-resistant CP, the MCyR and the CCyR rates were 48% and 30%, respectively, whereas in imatinib-intolerant patients the respective rates were 47% and 35%. For all patients in CP, 1-year OS was 95%, and the proportion of patients remaining in MCyR after 1 year was 96%. Nilotinib was recently tested in a phase II study in upfront therapy of early CP at a dose of 800 mg daily showing a CCyR of 98% and a major molecular response of 70%. In a randomized trial, nilotinib was superior to imatinib as initial therapy and may become the new standard.

c. **Allogeneic stem cell transplant.** As mentioned previously, allogeneic transplantation remains the only known curative treatment for CML. The appropriate patient and the optimal timing of transplantation in CP CML remain controversial. To assist in patient selection, a transplantation risk score has been proposed by the European Blood and Bone Marrow Transplantation Group to assess both transplant-related mortality as well as long-term survival (Table 19.3). In most transplant series, a relationship appears to exist between the interval from diagnosis to transplantation and outcome (i.e., the earlier the disease at the time of transplant, the better the outcome). Five-year survival rates after myeloablative transplantation range from 60% to 80% in CP disease to 25% to 40% in AP and 5% to 10% in BP. It is appropriate to consider

T A B L E 19.3	Allogeneic Stem Cell Transplant and European Group for Blood and Marrow Transplantation Risk Score	

Risk Factor	Score
Disease phase	0 for CP, 1 for AP, and 2 for BP*
Age	0 if <20 years, 1 if 20–40 years, 2 if >40 years
Interval from diagnosis	0 if ≤1 year, 1 if >1 year
Donor type	0 if HLA-matched sibling, 1 for any other alternative donor
Donor-recipient sex match	1 for female donor and male recipient, 0 for any other match

AP, accelerated phase; BP, blastic phase; CP, chronic phase; HLA, human leukocyte antigen.
*The 5-year survival for the cumulative risk score is as follows: 0–1, 70%; 2, 63%; 3, 50%; 4, 32%; >5, 10%.
From Passweg JR, Walker I, Sobocinski KA, Klein JP, Horowitz MM, Giralt SA. Validation and extension of the EBMT Risk Score for patients with chronic myeloid leukaemia (CML) receiving allogeneic haematopoietic stem cell transplants. *Br J Haematol.* 2004;125(5):613–620.

allogeneic transplantation at the first sign of drug therapy failure which, based on the IRIS study, is defined as lack of hematologic response by 3 months to first-line imatinib therapy, no cytogenetic response (Ph+ >95%) by 6 months, less than a partial cytogenetic response by 12 months (Ph+ >35%), and/or lack of CCyR by 18 months. Allogeneic transplant is the appropriate second-line therapy for suitable candidates with an available donor. Patients with advanced phases of the disease should also be considered for transplant as soon as a second CP occurs with either imatinib or a second-generation TKI with or without chemotherapy. Interestingly, prior treatment with TKIs does not negatively impact transplant-related toxicity or the outcome with allogeneic stem cell transplant. For patients without a human leukocyte antigen (HLA)-matched sibling, transplantation with a matched unrelated donor is an acceptable alternative. An important advance has been the development of techniques that permit molecular typing, which have demonstrated that only about 55% of individuals who are serologically identical are highly matched by molecular typing. Patients who receive transplants from molecularly matched donors have better outcomes. Fortunately, because of the relatively indolent nature of CML, adequate time is usually available to search for a matched unrelated donor through the National Marrow Donor Program and other donor registries. Age, disease stage at time of transplant, and degree of HLA matching all have been strongly correlated with outcome of transplant. For good-risk patients (age less than 40 years, first CP, and an HLA-matched sibling donor; see Table 19.3), leukemia-free survival of approximately 60% can be achieved. Reduced-intensity transplants have improved the outlook for older patients, particularly those older than 50 years of age or those with comorbid medical conditions.

Relapse following allografting can be managed with donor lymphocyte infusion (DLI), which results in molecular remissions within 3 to 12 months in as many as 60% to 80% of patients relapsing in CP and in up to 90% in those with molecular relapse. While the toxicity of DLI, including graft-versus-host disease (GVHD) and/or marrow aplasia, can be substantial, it continues to be the most effective therapy for relapse following stem cell transplant.

d. **Interferon-α and cytarabine** no longer have a role as primary therapy in CML given the results of the IRIS trial and availability of imatinib and second-generation TKIs. However, interferon-α, often in conjunction with low-dose cytarabine, has been shown in randomized clinical trials to result in improved 5-year survival ranging from 50% to 60% compared with busulphan and hydroxycarbamide. The combination of interferon-α and cytarabine achieve a 55% CHR and 15% complete clinical response. Importantly, half of the patients achieving a CCyR maintained it even after stopping interferon-α and may in fact be cured. As such, this combination can be used in patients who are resistant to all available TKIs (e.g., T315I mutation) either as the sole therapeutic modality or as a bridge to allogeneic stem cell transplantation.

7. **Advanced-phase CML**. It is conventional now to start treating patients who present in advanced phases (a term including APs and BPs) with a starting dose of imatinib at 600 to 800 mg daily; however, the response is more robust in CP of CML than in patients with advanced CML. Patients with "early" AP may obtain long-term responses to imatinib as a single agent, while those in blastic transformation (BT; BP) may have extremely short responses requiring a more aggressive initial strategy. Thus, they may be considered for treatment with dasatinib with its wider spectrum of activity against Src and Src family kinases. For patients in lymphoid BT, extrapolation from results obtained with treatment of Ph-positive ALL suggest that combining imatinib with standard ALL treatment may be the best initial approach. Once remission is achieved, maintenance treatment with cytotoxic drugs together with a TKI can then be continued. Neuroprophylaxis is also advisable. For patients presenting in myeloid BT, the combined use of a TKI with therapy appropriate to the AML induction regimen may be an optimal approach.

Recently, dasatinib at 140 mg daily combined with daunorubicin and cytarabine has been shown to be well tolerated with induction of remission in half the patients and a median survival of 12 months. Unfortunately, even with aggressive treatment options, the probability of relapse in both lymphoid and myeloid BT remains high, and may be reduced by considering allogeneic stem cell transplantation while the patient is in remission. Transplantation during BP CML is associated with an approximately 80% risk of relapse with a 5-year survival of only about 5%. Thus, BT CML remains an extremely high-risk disease with a dismal prognosis, unlike CP CML; diligent molecular monitoring at more frequent intervals in these patients may help detect this disease phase earlier without delaying treatment.

E. Conclusion

In conclusion, for patients with CP CML, targeted therapies such as imatinib have changed the treatment paradigm. While transplantation remains the only curative approach for CML, the high response rates and tolerability of imatinib at 400 mg daily render it the standard treatment for patients with newly diagnosed CML. Other TKIs such as dasatinib or nilotinib are second-line agents. However, recent data suggest that even nilotinib may be more effective for the initial treatment of this disease. Allogeneic stem cell transplantation should be strongly considered in instances of drug therapy failure and for patients in AP or BP (typically following downstaging with drug therapy to a second chronic phase). While new treatment options for this disease continue to emerge, several unanswered questions remain: What is the optimal therapy for imatinib failure? What are the indications for allografting in the presence of second-generation TKIs? Should the second-generation TKIs be used in upfront therapy of early chronic phase? Should the mutational analysis guide the choice of TKI? Answers to these and other questions will be forthcoming as the algorithm for treatment of CML continues to evolve.

II. CHRONIC LYMPHOCYTIC LEUKEMIA (CLL)

CLL is the most common leukemia in Western countries with over 15,000 new cases projected in the United States in 2009. There are no evident etiologic factors, although there is a clear familial incidence with 10% to 15% of patients having a family history of a hematologic malignancy. Whereas more than half of patients are diagnosed over 70 years of age, about 10% to 15% of patients with CLL are younger than 50 years of age and 20% are younger than 55 years. Younger patients are more likely to die from CLL-related events, whereas older patients more often die from secondary malignancies and non-CLL causes.

A. Diagnosis and staging

In the World Health Organization classification, CLL and small lymphocytic lymphoma (SLL) are considered together as CLL/SLL, the distinction being the number of circulating B-cells with a threshold of 5000/μL. About half of the cases of CLL are asymptomatic at presentation and diagnosed incidentally.

1. **Examination of a peripheral blood smear in CLL** reveals a relatively homogeneous population of mature-appearing lymphocytes, with occasional smudge cells, occasionally with prolymphocytes that are larger with prominent nucleoli. The diagnosis of prolymphocytic leukemia (PLL) requires that greater than 55% of circulating lymphocytes are prolymphocytes. Other lymphoid malignancies that can be confused with CLL include hairy cell leukemia (HCL), marginal zone or follicular lymphoma, and T-cell leukemias.

2. **The characteristic immunophenotype of CLL B-cells** distinguishes this disease from these other entities: CLL cells are positive for CD19 and CD20 (generally dim), as well as CD23 and CD5, and are monoclonal with respect to expression of kappa or lambda light chains. Of note is that CD5/CD20+ B-cells can be detected in the peripheral blood of up to 5% of the normal population; this occurrence has been referred to as monoclonal lymphocytosis of undetermined significance, which, without other evidence of the disease, rarely evolves into CLL.

3. **Staging of the patient with CLL** includes assessment of renal and hepatic function, uric acid and lactate dehydrogenase, quantitative immunoglobulins, and a direct antiglobulin test (DAT). A bone marrow aspiration or biopsy is not needed to make the diagnosis; however, it is strongly recommended prior to therapy as it provides a baseline against which to compare the results of treatment and provides an assessment of the normal blood elements. A lymph node biopsy is rarely indicated in CLL unless there is a concern of Richter transformation. Whether computed tomography (CT) scans should be incorporated into routine practice is controversial. Patients with stage 0 CLL who have lymphadenopathy on CT have a greater likelihood of progressive disease.

   a. **Staging systems.** For more than 30 years, CLL has been staged according to the classifications published by Rai, used in the United States, and Binet, applied in much of Europe, which use physical examination and peripheral blood counts to separate patients into clinically meaningful risk groups (Table 19.4). The two systems have similar prognostic value.

   Considerable heterogeneity in patient outcome within stages suggests the importance of other prognostic factors (Table 19.5). Over the past decade, there have been new important and clinically relevant insights into the genetics, biology, and immunology of CLL, which may predict the time to disease progression, requirement for therapy, and survival.

TABLE 19.4 CLL Staging Systems

Rai	Findings	Survival (Months)
0	Lymphocytosis only	>120
I	Lymphocytosis plus lymphadenopathy	95
II	Lymphocytosis plus splenomegaly or hepatomegaly	72
III	Lymphocytosis plus anemia (Hgb <11 g/dL)	30
IV	Lymphocytosis plus thrombocytopenia (platelets <100,000/μL)	30

Binet	Findings	Survival (Months)
A	Hgb ≥10 g/dL, platelets ≥100,000/μL, <3 involved areas*	>120
B	Hgb ≥10 g/dL, platelets ≥100,000/μL, ≥3 involved areas*	84
C	Hgb <10 g/dL or platelets <100,000/μL	24

Hgb, hemoglobin.
*Involved areas include cervical, axillary, or inguinal nodes; spleen or liver.
Data from Passweg JR, Walker I, Sobocinski KA, Klein JP, Horowitz MM, Giralt SA. Validation and extension of the EBMT Risk Score for patients with chronic myeloid leukaemia (CML) receiving allogeneic haematopoietic stem cell transplants. *Br J Haematol.* 2004;125(5):613–620; Rai KR, Sawitsky A, Cronkite EP, Chanana AD, Levy RN, Pasternack BS. Clinical staging of chronic lymphocytic leukemia. *Blood.* 1975;46(2):219–234; Binet JL, Auquier A, Dighiero G, Chastang C, Piguet H, Goasguen J, Vaugier G, Potron G, Colona P, Oberling F, Thomas M, Tchernia G, Jacquillat C, Boivin P, Lesty C, Duault MT, Monconduit M, Belabbes S, Gremy F. A new prognostic classification of chronic lymphocytic leukemia derived from a multivariate survival analysis. *Cancer.* 1981;48(1):198–206.

   b. Cytogenetic abnormalities. FISH studies identify nonrandom chromosomal abnormalities in 80% of cases that are almost exclusively deletions or trisomy, without translocations. The most common abnormality is a 13q deletion, which occurs in about half of cases either alone or in combination with another abnormality. Normal karyotypes and trisomy 12 are the

TABLE 19.5 Factors Associated With Poor Prognosis in CLL

Older age
Advanced stage
Male sex
Diffuse pattern of bone marrow involvement
Short (<6 months) lymphocyte doubling time
High β2-microglobulin
Poor risk cytogenetics (17p-, 11q-, or complex abnormalities)
Unmutated IgVH status
High CD38 expression
High ZAP-70 expression
Poor or brief response to therapy

IgVH, immunoglobulin variable region gene; ZAP, zeta-associated protein.

next in frequency followed by del(11q) and del(17p) (p53 mutation). There is a strong correlation between these findings and outcome; del(13q) confers a favorable prognosis, while normal cytogenetics and trisomy 12 have an intermediate outcome. The prognosis of patients with a del(11q) (mutation of ATM gene) is poorer. Those with a del(17p) (deletions or mutations in p53) and those with complex cytogenetic abnormalities generally exhibit a reduced likelihood of response to treatment and a poor survival. Cytogenetic abnormalities are not stable over time, and FISH might be repeated when there is a change in the clinical picture.

c. **A number of other biomarkers have clinical implications.** CLL can be distinguished into two groups based on the level of cellular differentiation as characterized by whether they exhibit an unmutated (or pregerminal center) or mutated (or memory B-cell) immunoglobulin heavy chain gene mutation (immunoglobulin variable region genes). The former is associated with a significantly worse outcome. Other potential surrogates for mutational status have been investigated. When the two cell populations were subjected to DNA microarray analysis, zeta-associated protein (ZAP)-70 is differentially expressed in the unmutated cells. Some studies suggest that ZAP-70 may even be a better predictor of outcome than mutational status. CD38 expression on CLL cells is also an independent, negative prognostic factor. There currently is no defined role for these new prognostic factors in the clinical management of patients with CLL. Moreover, some patients have a mix of high- and low-risk features. These biomarkers should be reserved for clinical trials to stratify patients among various therapies to better characterize their role in directing therapy.

B. **Complications of CLL**
1. **Other malignancies.** Long-term complications related to the disease or its treatment include an increased risk for common solid tumors including skin cancers and those of the gastrointestinal tract. Thus, patients should be encouraged to undergo routine screening for appropriate tumor types. In addition, about 15% of patients with CLL may transform to a more aggressive lymphoid malignancy including PLL and Richter syndrome, a diffuse large B-cell lymphoma that is particularly resistant to standard chemotherapy. Patients with CLL may also develop or even have coexisting AML, CML, ALL, and multiple myeloma.
2. **Autoimmunity.** At least 25% of patients will develop a positive DAT, but fewer than 5% develop autoimmune hemolytic anemia. Other patients may develop pure red cell aplasia. Immune thrombocytopenia is also a common consequence of the disease and its treatment. These consequences can often be successfully

treated with corticosteroids or rituximab. Other immune complications are uncommon.

3. **Recurrent infections.** Patients with CLL are at an increased risk for infections as a consequence of hypogammaglobulinemia and abnormal activation of the complement system. Historically, the most common pathogens were those that require opsonization for bacterial killing, such as *Streptococcus pneumoniae, Staphylococcus aureus*, and *Haemophilus influenzae*. The increased use of immunosuppressive agents such as fludarabine and alemtuzumab has markedly increased the risk for infections with opportunistic organisms such as *Candida, Listeria, Pneumocystis*, cytomegalovirus, aspergillus, herpes infections, and others that were rarely encountered before the widespread use of these agents. Nevertheless, the use of prophylactic intravenous immunoglobulins is discouraged, as they are expensive, in short supply, have associated adverse reactions, and appear to protect patients from bacterial infections that are only mild to moderate in severity, not severe, and not viral or fungal infections. Thus, the administration of prophylactic intravenous immunoglobulins should be reserved for patients with recurrent bacterial infections.

C. Therapy of CLL

Most patients with CLL are asymptomatic at presentation. Randomized trials have failed to demonstrate an advantage to early intervention in such patients. Thus, watchful waiting is an acceptable approach, checking counts and performing a physical examination every 3 to 6 months. Indications for initiating therapy have been published by the National Cancer Institute (NCI)-sponsored Working Group, more recently reinforced by the International Workshop on CLL (IWCLL) recommendations, and include disease-related symptoms, massive and/or progressive lymphadenopathy or hepatosplenomegaly, recurrent infections, thrombocytopenia, or anemia. The decision to treat may be supported by a doubling of the lymphocyte count in a period of 6 months or less.

1. **Initial therapy.** Major changes have taken place in the initial therapy of CLL in recent years. Fludarabine-based therapy has replaced alkylating agent regimens, such as chlorambucil, as the standard initial treatment of CLL. Randomized trials have shown higher complete response (CR) and overall response rates with fludarabine compared to chlorambucil, with a longer time to progression, and even a survival advantage without an increase in secondary malignancies. The addition of cyclophosphamide to fludarabine improves the response rate and PFS compared with fludarabine alone, but without a survival benefit and with an increase in toxicities. Acceptable regimens include the following:

   ▪ Fludarabine 25 mg/m^2 intravenously (IV) over 10 to 30 minutes on days 1 to 5 every 28 days.

- Fludarabine 30 mg/m^2/day IV on days 1 to 3 and cyclophosphamide 250 mg/m^2 IV on days 1 to 3, each given as separate 30-minute infusions; cycle is repeated every 28 days.
- Chlorambucil may be used in the frail elderly, being well tolerated with minimal nausea and no alopecia. Various schedules are used, including daily oral doses of 2 to 6 mg by mouth with adjustments according to biweekly CBC.

2. **Monoclonal antibody-based therapy of CLL.** The availability of active and safe monoclonal antibodies has dramatically altered the treatment of CLL.

   a. **Rituximab.** The first major advance in the treatment of CLL in many years was afforded by the availability of rituximab, a chimeric anti-CD20 monoclonal antibody that, as a single agent in patients with relapse or refractory disease, has limited activity, inducing about 15% partial remissions of brief duration, but with a 50% to 70% single-agent response rate in previously untreated patients. The potential role for this agent was first realized by Byrd and coworkers from the Cancer and Leukemia Group B who conducted a randomized phase II trial of concurrent versus sequential fludarabine and rituximab demonstrating an overall response rate of 90% with 47% complete remissions. Keating and coworkers developed the fludarabine, cyclophosphamide, and rituximab (FCR) regimen with a response rate of 95% including 72% complete remissions. In both studies, a survival benefit was suggested using historical controls. The German CLL study group (GCLLSG) recently provided data from the CLL-8 trial, a randomized phase III comparison of fludarabine and cyclophosphamide versus FCR for the initial treatment of 817 patients with CLL. They were able to demonstrate not only a significant prolongation of PFS (51.8 months versus 32.8 months), but also an apparent survival advantage for FCR as well (87.2% versus 82.5% at 3 years, $p = 0.012$). This study, and a second one in relapsed/refractory disease, confirms the role of rituximab in the treatment of this disease and led to the recent approval of this combination by the U.S. Food and Drug Administration (FDA) as initial treatment or for relapse. Whether FCR is indeed superior to fludarabine and rituximab (FR) is controversial. A phase III trial is currently comparing FR with FCR. The FR regimen is as follows:

      - Rituximab is given over three infusions during cycle 1, then once per cycle thereafter. Day 1 of cycle 1, 50 mg/m^2 IV over 4 hours; day 3 of cycle 1, 325 mg/m^2 IV, initially at 50 mg/hr, but escalating the rate as tolerated; day 5 of cycle 1, 375 mg/m^2 IV over 1 to 2 hours. On days 1 of subsequent cycles (every 4 weeks), 375 mg/m^2 IV over 1 to 2 hours for a total of six cycles.

- Fludarabine 25 mg/m^2/day IV over 30 minutes on days 1 through 5 of each treatment cycle, given after the rituximab on days it is given.

The FCR regimen is as follows. Note dose reductions for those 70 and older.

- Rituximab is given over two infusions during cycle 1, then once per cycle thereafter. Day 1 of cycle 1, 50 mg/m^2 IV over 4 hours; day 3 of cycle 1, 325 mg/m^2 IV, initially at 50 mg/hr, but escalating the rate as tolerated. On days 1 of subsequent cycles (every 4 weeks), 375 to 500 mg/m^2 IV over 1 to 2 hours for a total of six cycles. (Nonstandard dose may require longer infusion.)

- In patients younger than 70 years of age, fludarabine 25 mg/m^2/day IV over 30 minutes on days 1 through 3 of each treatment cycle, given after the rituximab on days it is given. In patients 70 years of age and older, fludarabine 20 mg/m^2/day IV over 30 minutes on days 1 through 3 of each treatment cycle, given after the rituximab on days it is given.

- In patients younger than 70 years of age, cyclophosphamide 250 mg/m^2/day IV over 30 minutes days 1 through 3 of each treatment cycle, given after the rituximab on days it is given. In patients 70 years of age or older, cyclophosphamide 150 mg/m^2/day IV over 30 minutes days 1 through 3 of each treatment cycle, given after the rituximab on days it is given.

b. **Alemtuzumab.** The first antibody approved by the FDA for CLL was alemtuzumab, a humanized anti-CD52 monoclonal antibody. Alemtuzumab induces responses in 30% to 40% of patients with CLL failing after alkylating agents and fludarabine. The currently recommended schedule of administration for alemtuzumab is to escalate the dose from 3 mg as a 2-hour IV infusion on day 1 and, if tolerated, 10 mg as a 2-hour IV infusion on day 2, then 30 mg as a 2-hour IV infusion three times weekly as tolerated for up to 12 weeks. Because of an increased occurrence of *Pneumocystis jiroveci (carinii)* and herpesvirus infections, antimicrobial prophylaxis is essential, with weekly PCR for cytomegalovirus. The subcutaneous mode of administration appears to preserve activity with reduced fevers, rigors, and other toxicities. In a randomized comparison of alemtuzumab with chlorambucil in previously untreated patients with CLL, the antibody induced an overall response rate of 83.2% with 24.2% CRs, 7.4% of which were negative for MRD, compared with 55.4%, 2%, and 0%, respectively for chlorambucil. PFS also favored the alemtuzumab arm at 14.6 months versus 11.7 months. Toxicity was not substantially different between the arms.

c. **Ofatumumab.** Ofatumumab is a human anti-CD20 antibody that binds to a different epitope than rituximab. Ofatumumab has activity in patients with CLL who are refractory to fludarabine and alemtuzumab (FA-ref) or with bulky disease refractory to fludarabine (BF-ref), as the latter are not considered suitable candidates for alemtuzumab. In a study of 138 patients (59 FA-ref, 79 BF-ref), 63% of which had Rai stage III/IV disease and had received a median of five prior regimens, 59% of FA-ref and 54% of BF-ref patients had received prior rituximab. Ofatumumab was dosed at 300 mg IV at an initial rate of 3.6 mg/hour on day 1 followed 1 week later by 2000 mg for weekly doses 2 to 12 (see Chapter 33 for details). The overall response rate was 58% for the FA-ref group with a median PFS of 5.7 months, and 47% with 5.9 months in the BF-ref group. The median OS was 13.7 months and 15.4 months, respectively. Results were reported to be independent of prior rituximab therapy.

3. **Bendamustine.** One of the most active drugs in CLL is bendamustine, a bifunctional alkylating agent developed in East Germany in the 1960s. Following numerous reports of its activity in pretreated CLL, it was approved by the FDA for CLL based largely on a randomized trial demonstrating superiority over chlorambucil with respect to overall response rate (68% versus 31%), CRs (31% versus 2%), and median PFS (21.6 months versus 8.3 months), without a major difference in adverse effects. Because of its efficacy and tolerability, bendamustine is well suited for older patients. Moreover, it can be safely administered to patients with mild to moderate renal impairment without dose reduction.

Based on its impressive single agent activity (100 mg/m^2 IV over 30 minutes on days 1 and 2 of a 28-day cycle, up to six cycles), the GCLLSG combined it with rituximab in 48 patients with relapsed and refractory disease and achieved an overall response rate of 77% with 15% CRs, and, notably, 78% of fludarabine-refractory patients responded. Based on these important results, they conducted the CLL-8 trial in 177 previously untreated patients. The 91% response rate with 33% CRs led to a randomized comparison in previously untreated patients against FCR in CLL-10, which could redefine the treatment for this disease.

4. **Other new agents.** New drugs with promise in CLL include lenalidomide (Revlimid), a second-generation immunomodulatory agent, which has been approved for patients with myelodysplastic syndrome and the 5q-chromosome abnormality, and for those with relapsed/refractory multiple myeloma. In two studies in patients with relapsed and refractory CLL, the response rate to lenalidomide was about 30% to 50%, with activity even in patients

with unfavorable cytogenetics. Major side effects include tumor lysis syndrome and a flare reaction. Combinations with other agents such as rituximab or bendamustine are in development.

Flavopiridol is a cyclin-dependent kinase inhibitor. In early studies, a lack of activity was observed in CLL. Byrd and coworkers treated 42 high-risk patients with a pharmacologically derived regimen of administration and achieved a 45% partial response rate lasting a median of greater than a year. Further development of this agent is under way.

5. **Other agents.** A number of small molecules that target the apoptotic pathways in clinical development include ABT-263 and obatoclax. Fostamatinib disodium inhibits the downstream effects of activation of the B-cell receptor and induces responses in half of patients with CLL/SLL.

6. **Stem cell transplantation.** Autologous stem cell transplantation has a limited role in CLL. The data on allogeneic BMT are primarily limited to younger patients with CLL and are associated with considerable morbidity and mortality. Submyeloablative preparative regimens may achieve successful engraftment without substantial acute GVHD; however, chronic GVHD has been a serious problem. Nevertheless, long-term disease-free survival

TABLE 19.6 Response Criteria for CLL

CR
- Absence of disease-related symptoms
- Absence of peripheral blood clonal lymphocytosis (bone marrow only in clinical trials)
- Absence of lymphadenopathy and hepatosplenomegaly
- Neutrophils ≥1500/μL
- Platelets >100,000/μL
- Hemoglobin >11 g/dL (untransfused)

CRi
- Same as CR, but with persistent anemia, neutropenia, or thrombocytopenia (for clinical trials, not yet validated)

PR
- Decrease by ≥50% in peripheral blood lymphocytes
- Decrease by ≥50% in the sum of the products of diameters of up to six nodes; no new nodes; no increase in any nodes
- Decrease by ≥50% in hepatosplenomegaly
- Plus one of the following
    - Neutrophils ≥1500/μL or ≥50% from baseline
    - Platelets >100,000/μL or ≥50% from baseline
    - Hemoglobin >11g/dL or ≥50% from baseline

CR, complete remission; CRi, incomplete CR; PR, partial response.

can be achieved, and this option is promising, especially for younger patients who are refractory to their initial therapy or who have only a transient response to treatment.

7. **Response Assessment in CLL.** With the availability of effective treatments for CLL, standardized response criteria are essential. In 1988, the NCI-sponsored Working Group published the first widely accepted response criteria that were updated in 1996, and reinforced by the IWCLL in 2008 (Table 19.6). MRD eradication appears to be associated with prolongation of survival. Consolidation of response with agents such as alemtuzumab has been successful in eradicating MRD but with prohibitive toxicity.

III. RELATED B-CELL LEUKEMIAS

A. Prolymphocytic leukemia (PLL)

PLL may be of either B-cell or T-cell lineage. What was formerly called T-CLL or chronic T-cell lymphocytosis was renamed in the World Health Organization classification as T-PLL. Patients with B-PLL tend to be older than those with CLL, with a median age of 70 years at presentation. The main complaints include abdominal discomfort, fevers, and weight loss. Virtually all have advanced-stage disease at presentation, with a larger spleen and a higher WBC count, but less lymphadenopathy than CLL. PLL cells are large, with a round nucleus and a prominent nucleolus. In de novo PLL, most of the peripheral blood mononuclear cells tend to be prolymphocytes; in the setting of an aggressive transformation from CLL, there is a dimorphic population in the peripheral blood. The immunophenotype is different from CLL; the cells are positive for CD19, CD20, and CD24, and strongly express CD22, surface immunoglobulins, and FMC7. Fewer than a third express CD5 or CD23.

Patients with PLL tend to respond poorly to either single-agent or combination chemotherapy, with overall response rates of less than 25% and rare CRs. The median survival for de novo PLL is 3 years, and it is less than a year for T-PLL. Small series and anecdotal cases suggest activity for nucleoside analogs and alemtuzumab in PLL. Allogeneic stem cell transplantation should be considered for younger patients whose disease is responsive to induction therapy.

B. Hairy cell leukemia (HCL)

HCL is diagnosed in about 500 new patients each year in the United States, generally in older persons, with a strong male predominance. Patients generally present with symptoms referable to cytopenias. The most common signs include palpable splenomegaly (72% to 86%), hepatomegaly (13% to 20%), hairy cells in the peripheral blood (85% to 89%), thrombocytopenia (less than 100,000/µL: 53%), anemia (hemoglobin less than 12/dL: 71% to 77%), and neutropenia (absolute neutrophil count less than 500/µL: 32% to 39%). The lymphocytes in the peripheral blood generally have an eccentric, spongiform, kidney-shaped nucleus, with characteristic filamentous cytoplasmic projections. The malignant cells express the B-cell antigens CD19, CD20, as well as the monocyte antigen CD11c, and specifically CD103. Bone marrow biopsy is generally required to confirm the diagnosis, as the aspirate is often not obtainable.

Treatment is indicated in the setting of massive or progressive splenomegaly, worsening blood counts, recurrent infections, greater than 20,000 hairy cells/μL of peripheral blood, or bulky lymphadenopathy. Until the early 1980s, splenectomy was the standard treatment for HCL. Splenectomy is now reserved for the rare patient who is refractory to treatment and has splenomegaly that is either symptomatic or is resulting in cytopenias.

1. **The purine analogs** revolutionized the treatment of patients with HCL. Pentostatin (2^1-deoxycoformycin, DCF) at doses of 4 mg/m^2 IV every other week for 4 to 6 months achieves CR in 60% to 89% of previously treated or untreated patients, including those who have failed interferon, with overall response rates of 80% to 90%. About 25% of patients have relapsed with more than 5 years of follow-up.

2. **Cladribine**. Using a 7-day continuous infusion or a 2-hour infusion for 5 to 7 days, cladribine (CdA) at 3.3 to 5.2 mg/m^2 (see Chapter 33) achieves responses in 80% to more than 90% of patients, including 65% to 80% complete remissions. These responses tend to be durable, with 20% to 30% of patients relapsing with prolonged follow-up. In many cases, relapse is characterized only by an increase in bone marrow hairy cells, with no indication for treatment. Most patients who require retreatment achieve a second durable response.

    The results with DCF are equivalent to those with CdA. The shorter duration of treatment makes CdA somewhat more attractive, although it may be associated with greater neurotoxicity and myelosuppression.

3. **Rituximab** has also shown promise for patients with HCL who fail purine analog therapy as it has an anti-CD22 pseudomonas exotoxin immunoconjugate.

Selected Readings

Chronic Myelogenous Leukemia

Apperley JF. Part II: management of resistance to imatinib in chronic myeloid leukaemia. *Lancet Oncol.* 2007;8:1116–1128.

Baccarani M, Cortes J, Pane F, et al. Chronic myeloid leukemia: an update of concepts and management recommendations of European LeukemiaNet. *J Clin Oncol.* 2009;27:6041–6051.

Barrett J. Allogeneic stem cell transplantation for chronic myeloid leukemia. *Semin Hematol.* 2003;40:59–71.

Cortes J, Jabbour E, Kantarjian H, et al. Dynamics of BCR-ABL kinase domain mutations in chronic myeloid leukemia after sequential treatment with multiple tyrosine kinase inhibitors. *Blood.* 2007;110:4005–4011.

Cortes J, Kantarjian H, Goldberg S, et al. High-dose imatinib in newly diagnosed chronic-phase chronic myeloid leukemia: high rates of rapid cytogenetic and molecular responses. *J Clin Oncol.* 2009;27:4754–4759.

Cortes J, O'Brian S, Kantarjian H. Discontinuation of imatinib therapy after achieving a molecular response. *Blood.* 2004;104:2204–2205.

Cortes J, Rousselot P, Kim DW, et al. Dasatinib induces complete hematologic and cytogenetic responses in patients with imatinib-resistant or -intolerant chronic myeloid leukemia in blast crisis. *Blood.* 2007;109:3207–3212.

Cortes J, Talpaz M, O'Brien S, et al. Molecular responses in patients with chronic myelogenous leukemia in chronic phase treated with imatinib mesylate. *Clin Cancer Res.* 2005;11:3425–3432.

Druker BJ, Guilhot F, O'Brien SG, et al. Five-year follow-up of patients receiving imatinib for chronic myeloid leukemia. *N Engl J Med.* 2006;355:2408–2417.

Gratwohl A, Hermans J, Goldman JM, et al. Risk assessment for patients with chronic myeloid leukaemia before allogeneic bone marrow transplantation. *Lancet.* 1998;352:1087–1092.

Guilhot F, Apperley J, Kim DW, et al. Dasatinib induces significant hematologic and cytogenetic responses in patients with imatinib-resistant or -intolerant chronic myeloid leukemia in accelerated phase. *Blood.* 2007;109:4143–4150.

Jones D, Kamel-Reid S, Bahler D, et al. Laboratory practice guidelines for detecting and reporting BCR-ABL drug resistance mutations in chronic myelogenous leukemia and acute lymphoblastic leukemia. *J Mol Diagn.* 2009;11:4–11.

Kantarjian H, Pasquini R, Hamerschlak N, et al. Dasatinib or high-dose imatinib for chronic-phase chronic myeloid leukemia after failure of first-line imatinib: a randomized phase 2 trial. *Blood.* 2007;109:5143–5150.

Kantarjian H, Schiffer C, Jones D, Cortes J. Monitoring the response and course of chronic myeloid leukemia in the modern era of BCR-ABL tyrosine kinase inhibitors: practical advice on the use and interpretation of monitoring methods. *Blood.* 2008;111:1774–1780.

Kantarjian HM, Giles F, Gattermann N, et al. Nilotinib (formerly AMN107), a highly selective BCR-ABL tyrosine kinase inhibitor, is effective in patients with Philadelphia chromosome-positive chronic myelogenous leukemia in chronic phase following imatinib resistance and intolerance. *Blood.* 2007;110:3540–3546.

le Coutre P, Ottmann OG, Giles F, et al. Nilotinib (formerly AMN107), a highly selective BCR-ABL tyrosine kinase inhibitor, is active in patients with imatinib-resistant or -intolerant accelerated-phase chronic myelogenous leukemia. *Blood.* 2008;111:1834–1839.

Quintas-Cardama A, Kantarjian H, Cortes J. Flying under the radar: the new wave of BCR-ABL inhibitors. *Nat Rev Drug Discov.* 2007;6:834–848.

Saglio G, Kim D-K, Issaragrisil S, et al. Nilotinib demonstrates superior efficacy compared with imatinib in patients with newly diagnosed chronic myeloid leukemia in chronic phase: results from the international randomized phase III ENESTnd trial. *Blood.* 2009;114(22):abstract LBA-1.

Chronic Lymphocytic Leukemia

Binet JL, Auquier A, Digheiro G, et al. A new prognostic classification of chronic lymphocytic leukemia derived from a multivariate survival analysis. *Cancer.* 1981;48: 198–206.

Binet JL, Caligaris-Capio F, Catovsky D, et al. Perspectives on the use of new diagnostic tools in the treatment of chronic lymphocytic leukemia. *Blood.* 2006;107:859–861.

Byrd JC, Rai K, Peterson BL, Appelbaum FR, et al. Addition of rituximab to fludarabine may prolong progression-free survival and overall survival in patients with previously untreated chronic lymphocytic leukemia: an updated retrospective comparative analysis of CALGB 9712 and CALGB 9011. *Blood.* 2005;105(1):49–53.

Chanan-Khan A, Miller KC, Musialo L, et al. Clinical efficacy of lenalidomide in patients with relapsed or refractory chronic lymphocytic leukemia: results of a phase II study. *J Clin Oncol.* 2006;24:5343–5349.

Cheson BD, Bennett JM, Grever M, et al. National Cancer Institute-Sponsored Working Group guidelines for chronic lymphocytic leukemia: revised guidelines for diagnosis and treatment. *Blood.* 1996;87:4990–4997.

Cheson BD, Rummel MJ. Bendamustine: rebirth of an old drug. *J Clin Oncol.* 2009;27:1492–1501.

Ferragoli A, Lee BN, Schlette EJ, et al. Lenalidomide induces complete and partial remissions in patients with relapsed and refractory chronic lymphocytic leukemia. *Blood.* 2008;111:5291–5297.

Fischer K, Cramer P, Stilgenbauer S, et al. Bendamustine combined with rituximab (BR) in first-line therapy of advanced CLL: a multicenter phase II trial of the German CLL Study Group (GCLLSG). *Blood.* 2009;114:89(abstract #205).

Hallek M, Cheson BD, Catovsky D, et al. Guidelines for the diagnosis and treatment of chronic lymphocytic leukemia: a report from the International Workshop on Chronic Lymphocytic Leukemia updating the National Cancer Institute-Working Group Guidelines. *Blood.* 2008;111:5446–5456.

Hallek M, FIngerle-Rowson G, Fink AM, et al. First-line treatment with fludarabine (F), cyclophosphamide (C), and rituximab (R)(FCR) improves overall survival (OS) in previously untreated patients (pts) with advanced chronic lymphocytic leukemia (CLL): results of a randomized phase III trial on behalf of an international group of investigators and the German CLL Study Group. *Blood.* 2009;114(22):223–224 (abstract 535).

Hillmen P, Skotnicki AB, Robak T, et al. Alemtuzumab compared with chlorambucil as first-line therapy for chronic lymphocytic leukemia. *J Clin Oncol.* 2007;25:5616–5623.

Keating MJ, O'Brien S, Albitar M, et al. Early results of a chemoimmunotherapy regimen of fludarabine, cyclophosphamide, and rituximab as initial therapy for chronic lymphocytic leukemia. *J Clin Oncol.* 2005;23(18):4079–4088.

Knauf WU, Lissichkov T, Aldaoud A, et al. Phase III randomized study of bendamustine compared with chlorambucil in previously untreated patients with chronic lymphocytic leukemia. *J Clin Oncol.* 2009;27:4378–4384.

Moreton P, Kennedy B, Lucas G, et al. Eradication of minimal residual disease in B-cell chronic lymphocytic leukemia after alemtuzumab therapy is associated with prolonged survival. *J Clin Oncol.* 2005;23:2971–2979.

Rai KR, Sawitsky A, Conkite EP, Chanana AD, Levy RN, Pasternack BS. Clinical staging of chronic lymphocytic leukemia. *Blood.* 1975;46:219–234.

Wierda W, Kipps T, Mayer J, et al. High activity of single-agent ofatumumab, a novel CD20 monoclonal antibody, in fludarabine- and alemtuzumab-refractory or bulky fludarabine-refractory chronic lymphocytic leukemia, regardless of prior rituximab exposure. *Haematologica.* 2009;94:369 (abstract 0919).

Wierda WG, Kipps TJ, Dürig J, et al. Ofatumumab combined with fludarabine and cyclophosphamide (O-FC) shows high activity in patients with previously untreated chronic lymphocytic leukemia (CLL): results from a randomized, multicenter, international, two-dose, parallel group, phase II trial. *Blood.* 2009;114:abstract #207.

20 Myeloproliferative Neoplasms and Myelodysplastic Syndromes

Elias Jabbour and Hagop Kantarjian

I. MYELOPROLIFERATIVE NEOPLASMS (MPNs)

The MPNs are clonal disorders of pluripotent hematopoietic stem cells or of lineage-committed progenitor cells. MPNs are characterized by autonomous and sustained overproduction of morphologically and functionally mature granulocytes, erythrocytes, or platelets. Although one cellular element is most strikingly increased, it is not uncommon to have modest or even major elevations in other myeloid elements (e.g., thrombocytosis and leukocytosis in patients with polycythemia vera [PV]). Bone marrow aspirates and biopsy specimens typically show hyperplasia of all myeloid lineages (panmyelosis). Morphologic maturation and cellular function are essentially normal, although platelet dysfunction occasionally contributes to bleeding. The overproduction of blood elements in MPNs now appears related to "switched-on" tyrosine kinase signaling pathways. For chronic myelogenous leukemia (see Chapter 19), this arises from the t(9;22) translocation and the BCR-ABL gene product. For the MPNs discussed in this chapter, a single nucleotide mutation in the gene for JAK2, a tyrosine kinase normally activated by erythropoietin and other cytokines, plays an analogous role. JAK2 V617F is present in 74% to 97% of patients with PV, and in 30% to 50% of patients with essential thrombocythemia (ET) and primary myelofibrosis (PMF). Positivity for JAK2 V617F gives important diagnostic confirmation for MPN, though negative results do not exclude MPN.

A. Polycythemia vera (PV)

1. **Diagnosis.** PV must be distinguished from relative or spurious polycythemia (normal red blood cell [RBC] mass, decreased plasma volume) and from secondary erythrocytosis (increased RBC mass due to hypoxia, carboxyhemoglobinemia, inappropriate erythropoietin syndromes with tumors or renal disease, etc.). PV is suspected in patients with hemoglobin levels greater than 18.5 g/dL in men or 16.5 g/dL in women or hemoglobin levels greater than 17 g/dL in men or 15 g/dL in women if associated with a documented and sustained increase of at least 2 g/dL from an individual's baseline value. Diagnostic evaluation begins with peripheral JAK2 V617F mutation screen and measurement of serum erythropoietin

levels. This is because JAK2 is present in 97% of patients with PV and is not associated with other causes of increased hemoglobin/hematocrit levels; similarly, a subnormal serum erythropoietin level is expected and encountered in more than 90% of patients with PV but not in secondary or apparent polycythemia. However, neither the absence of JAK2 nor the presence of a normal erythropoietin level rules out the diagnosis of PV.

The presence of a JAK2 V617F in suspected PV is highly supportive of the diagnosis, regardless of the serum erythropoietin level. In the absence of a JAK2 V617F mutation, the serum erythropoietin level is useful to guide further evaluation. If the serum erythropoietin level is subnormal, a JAK2 exon 12 mutation screen should be performed. In the setting of a negative JAK2 mutation and a normal erythropoietin level, the diagnosis of PV is unlikely and evaluation should focus on secondary causes of erythrocytosis.

The diagnosis of PV requires meeting either both major criteria and one minor criterion or the first major criterion and two minor criteria:

- Major criteria
  - Hemoglobin greater than 18.5 g/dL in men, 16.5 g/dL in women, or other evidence of increased red cell volume
  - Presence of JAK2 V617F or other functionally similar mutation such as JAK2 exon 12 mutation.
- Minor criteria
  - Bone marrow biopsy showing hypercellularity for age with trilineage myeloproliferation
  - Serum erythropoietin level below the normal reference range
  - Endogenous erythroid colony formation in vitro.

2. **Aims of therapy.** PV is generally an indolent disorder with the decision to treat based on risk stratification. Low-risk patients (i.e., those with no history of thrombosis, age less than 60 years, or platelets below $1 \times 10^6/\mu L$) are usually treated with phlebotomy and/or aspirin (ASA). The goal of phlebotomy is to keep the hematocrit level below 45% in men and below 42% in women. Initially, phlebotomy is used to reduce hyperviscosity by decreasing the red cell mass, and subsequent phlebotomies help maintain the red cell mass in a normal range. For patients with high-risk features (i.e., history of thrombosis, or an age greater than 60 years), treatment consists of phlebotomy, ASA, and/or cytoreductive therapy with hydroxyurea. Control of hypertension and diabetes and avoidance of smoking are also important.

3. **Treatment regimens**
   a. **Phlebotomy.** Removal of 350 to 500 mL of blood every 2 to 4 days (less often in the elderly or in patients with cardiac disease) is the standard initial approach; the goal is getting the

hematocrit to 40% to 45%. The blood count is then checked monthly, and phlebotomy is repeated as needed to maintain the hematocrit at no more than 45%. Rapid lowering of the hematocrit may also be achieved in emergency situations by erythropheresis. Elective surgery should be deferred until the hematocrit has been stable at no more than 45% for 2 to 4 months. Platelet function should be evaluated before surgery or invasive procedures.

b. **Antithrombotic therapy.** Concomitantly with phlebotomy, use of low-dose ASA is now widely regarded as standard therapy, following a large European study (ECLAP) utilizing 100 mg ASA daily that showed an approximately 60% reduction in thrombotic events. Higher doses of ASA (325 mg daily) carry risk of bleeding, especially in patients with platelet counts greater than $1.5 \times 10^6/\mu L$, in whom acquired von Willebrand disease may be seen. The exact thrombogenic role of platelets in MPNs is not clear, but hydroxyurea and anagrelide have been shown to lower platelet counts and reduce the risk of thrombosis.

c. **Myelosuppressive agents.** Myelosuppressive agents are indicated in conjunction with phlebotomy for persistent thrombocytosis, recurrent thrombosis, enlarging spleen, or similar problems. They may also reduce the risk of progression to myelofibrosis compared with phlebotomy alone. Most alkylating agents carry a high risk of inducing a secondary myelodysplastic syndrome (MDS) or leukemia and should no longer be used. Currently recommended choices are as follows:

(1) **Hydroxyurea** 10 to 30 mg/kg by mouth daily. Weekly blood cell counts are required initially, with dose adjustments to maintain the hematocrit at no more than 45%, the platelet count at 100,000 to 500,000/μL, and the white blood cell (WBC) count at greater than 3000/μL. Side effects are usually minimal, but long-term use may cause painful leg ulcers and aphthous stomatitis. For younger patients and cases difficult to control with hydroxyurea, acceptable alternatives include the following.

(2) **Interferon-α** is usually effective in controlling hematocrit, platelet count, and splenomegaly and in relieving pruritus. The starting dose is 1 to 3×10^6 U/m^2 three times weekly (pegylated interferon once weekly may also be an option—see Section I.B.2.c.). Common side effects include myalgia, fever, and asthenia, usually controlled with acetaminophen. Leukemogenic effects are presumably absent, but high cost is a deterrent to long-term use.

(3) **Radioactive phosphorus** (^{32}P) 2.3 mCi/m^2 intravenously (IV) (5 mCi maximum single dose). Repeat in 12 weeks if the response is inadequate (25% dose escalation optional).

Lack of response after three doses mandates a switch to other forms of therapy. Use of ^{32}P entails an approximately 10% risk of leukemia by 10 years, and it is best reserved for the elderly and patients refractory to other modalities. Supplemental phlebotomies may be required for patients with satisfactory platelet and WBC counts but with rising hematocrit levels.

(4) **Busulfan** appears to have less leukemogenic potential than other alkylating agents and is appropriate in patients whose disease is not controlled by other treatments or in the elderly. It is best given in short courses over several weeks (to avoid prolonged marrow suppression) at 2 to 4 mg/day.

(5) **Anagrelide** selectively inhibits platelet production, and platelets start to fall in 7 to 14 days. The WBC count is unaffected; hemoglobin may fall slightly. Responses to anagrelide have been reported in more than 80% of patients with MPNs, and thrombotic risk is reduced. Recommended starting dose is 0.5 mg by mouth once a day. Average dose for control is 2.4 mg daily. Side effects include headache (44%), palpitations, diarrhea, asthenia, and fluid retention. It should be used with caution in cardiac patients and is contraindicated in pregnancy.

d. **Ancillary treatments.** To control hyperuricemia, allopurinol 300 mg/day is usually effective. Pruritus is a frequent problem, but usually abates with myelosuppressive therapy. Cyproheptadine 5 to 20 mg/day or paroxetine 20 mg/day may be helpful; interferon-α is also frequently effective. ASA is often helpful for erythromelalgia (hot, red, painful digits) and is commonly used to prevent thrombosis.

4. **Evolution and outcome.** The median survival in patients with PV exceeds 15 years and the 10-year risk of developing either myelofibrosis (MF; <4% and 10%, respectively) or acute myeloid leukemia (AML; <2% and 6%, respectively) is relatively low. To date, drug therapy has not been shown to favorably affect these figures. Therefore, at present, drugs should not be used with the intent to either prolong survival or prevent disease transformation into AML or MF.

B. **Essential thrombocythemia (ET)**

1. **Diagnosis.** Diagnosis of ET requires a persistent elevation of the platelet count above $450 \times 10^3/\mu L$ plus the absence of known causes of reactive or secondary thrombocytosis (e.g., iron deficiency, malignancy, chronic inflammatory disease). After excluding obvious causes of reactive thrombocytosis (iron deficiency, trauma, infection, etc.), peripheral blood testing for the JAK2 V617F mutation is helpful. The presence of JAK2 V617F confirms

clonal thrombocytosis but careful review of the peripheral blood smear and bone marrow histology with cytogenetics must also be performed to confirm the diagnosis of ET. Chronic myeloid leukemia (CML) can often present with thrombocytosis, therefore the presence of BCR–ABL must be excluded. As stated previously, the absence of JAK2 does not rule out the possibility of ET given that a large proportion of patients do not carry the mutation. Only 4% of patients with ET without a JAK2 V617F mutation will have a mutation in the MPL gene; however, if present, it does suggest clonal thrombocytosis. Moderate leukocytosis is common. Palpable splenomegaly is present in less than 50% of patients. Platelet function studies may show either spontaneous aggregation or impaired response to agonists. Microvascular occlusion may cause digital gangrene, transient ischemic attacks, visual complaints, and paresthesias. Large-artery thrombotic episodes are also common. Deep venous thrombosis is uncommon. The risk of hemorrhagic problems is significant, particularly with a platelet count greater than $1500 \times 10^3/\mu L$. The diagnosis of ET requires meeting four criteria, as follows:

- Sustained platelet count of at least $450 \times 10^3/\mu L$
- Bone marrow biopsy specimen showing proliferation mainly of the megakaryocytic lineage with increased numbers of enlarged, mature megakaryocytes. No significant increase or left-shift of neutrophil granulopoiesis or erythropoiesis.
- Not meeting World Health Organization (WHO) criteria for PV or primary myelofibrosis, BCR–ABL-positive CML, or MDS or other myeloid neoplasm
- Demonstration of JAK2 V617F or other clonal marker or, in the absence of JAK2 V617F, no evidence of reactive thrombocytosis

2. **Treatment regimens.** Given its typically indolent course, the primary goal of treatment in patients with ET is the prevention of complications from thrombocytosis, such as microvascular disturbances or hemorrhagic events caused by acquired von Willebrand disease. ASA therapy is often used to reduce microvascular symptoms for patients with all risk categories. Hydroxyurea, to reduce platelet counts, in combination with low-dose ASA, has been shown to decrease the risk of arterial thrombosis in patients with high-risk ET, such as those older than 60 years with platelets greater than $1000 \times 10^3/\mu L$ or a history of hypertension, diabetes requiring treatment, or ischemia, thrombosis, embolism, or hemorrhage related to ET. For patients with ET whose platelet counts are refractory to therapy with ASA or other salicylates, therapy with interferon-α (including in pegylated preparations), anagrelide, or hydroxyurea can be used. Anagrelide was developed to prevent platelet aggregation

but was subsequently found to reduce platelet counts in ET and PMF when used at low dose.

a. Hydroxyurea 10 to 30 mg/kg by mouth daily, with dosage adjustments on the basis of weekly blood counts, should give satisfactory response in 2 to 6 weeks. Its use in combination with low-dose ASA may give optimal protection against arterial thrombosis and evolution to myelofibrosis.

b. Anagrelide can be a reasonable alternative to hydroxyurea and perhaps is preferable in younger patients. Anagrelide plus ASA was inferior to hydroxyurea plus ASA in a large recent trial, however. This agent should not be used in pregnancy.

c. Interferon-α. Most patients with ET respond to this agent, at an initial dose of 3×10^6 U/day subcutaneously (SC). Maintenance doses of 3×10^6 U three times weekly usually suffice. Pegylated interferon at an initial dose of 1.5 to 4.5 μg/kg/wk SC seems comparable in efficacy and side effects. Use of interferon in pregnancy is considered safe.

d. ^{32}P and alkylating agents. These agents are effective but carry increased risk of secondary leukemia. Nitrogen mustard (mechlorethamine 0.15 to 0.3 mg/kg [6 to 12 mg/m^2] IV) can be helpful when rapid reduction in platelet count is needed. Busulfan 2 to 4 mg/day initial dose is appropriate in selected elderly patients resistant to other agents.

e. ASA 81 to 325 mg/day may control erythromelalgia and similar vaso-occlusive problems but is contraindicated in patients with a history of hemorrhagic symptoms. ASA may be useful in pregnant patients, in whom the preceding agents are contraindicated.

3. Evolution and outcome. The course of ET is often indolent, particularly in young patients. The median survival exceeds 15 years, and some patients appear to have normal life expectancy. Transformation to PMF, MDS, or acute leukemia occurs in 5% to 10%. Thrombosis is the major cause of ET-related death.

C. Primary myelofibrosis (PMF)

1. Diagnosis. This is a clonal disorder of the hematopoietic stem cell, marked by an intense reactive (nonclonal) fibrosis of the marrow; splenomegaly (frequently massive), reflecting ectopic hematopoiesis in the spleen and portal hypertension; and the presence of immature granulocytes and nucleated RBCs in the peripheral blood (leukoerythroblastic blood picture) plus teardrop RBCs and giant platelets. Mild to moderate elevations of WBC and platelet counts are common initially; cytopenias dominate later on.

JAK2 V617F mutation is present in approximately 50% of patients with PMF. An abnormal karyotype is also demonstrable in approximately 50% and connotes shortened survival time. Other adverse prognostic factors include advanced age, anemia, WBC count of less than 4000/µL or greater than 30,000/µL, thrombocytopenia, blasts in peripheral blood, and hypercatabolic symptoms (weight loss, night sweats, fever). Diseases causing secondary marrow fibrosis, such as metastatic carcinoma, hairy-cell leukemia, and granulomatous infections, must be excluded. Similar to ET, the presence of a JAK2 V617F or an MPL mutation can be helpful to rule out reactive marrow fibrosis. However, the absence of both of these molecular markers does not exclude the presence of an MPN. Therefore, causes of reactive marrow fibrosis must be excluded in cases where no clonal marker is found. Again, bone marrow histology in combination with other clinical and laboratory features helps to establish the diagnosis of PMF. BCR–ABL should be performed to rule out the presence of CML and criteria for another myeloid neoplasm should not be met. The minor criteria, which help to establish a diagnosis of PMF, include leukoerythroblastosis, increased serum lactate dehydrogenase, anemia, and palpable splenomegaly. Major causes of death in PMF include marrow failure, infection, portal hypertension, and leukemic transformation. Cases of MDS with marrow fibrosis are easily confused with PMF. Postpolycythemic myelofibrosis is clinically indistinguishable but carries a poor prognosis, evolving to acute leukemia in 25% to 50% of patients (compared to 5% to 20% for de novo PMF). Acute megakaryoblastic leukemia (M7) may also present with a myelofibrotic picture and be confused with PMF.

The diagnosis of PMF requires meeting all three major criteria and two minor criteria:

- Major criteria
  - Presence of megakaryocyte proliferation and atypia, accompanied by either reticulin or collagen fibrosis; or, in the absence of significant reticulin fibrosis, the megakaryocyte changes must be accompanied by an increased marrow cellularity characterized by granulocytic proliferation and often decreased erythropoiesis (i.e., prefibrotic cellular-phase disease)
  - Not meeting WHO criteria for PV, CML, MDS, or other myeloid disorders
  - Demonstration of JAK2 V617F or other clonal marker (e.g., MPL W515K/L); or, in the absence of the above clonal markers no evidence of secondary bone marrow fibrosis.
- Minor criteria
  - Leukoerythroblastosis
  - Increased serum lactate dehydrogenase level
  - Anemia
  - Palpable splenomegaly.

2. **Treatment regimens.** PMF has a much more aggressive course than ET and PV, and treatments include androgen preparations (e.g., fluoxymesterone or danazol), corticosteroids, erythropoietin, and lenalidomide. Splenectomy should be considered for patients with portal hypertension, to improve anemia (due to sequestration) or for symptomatic relief of abdominal pain or problems with alimentation. Radiation therapy may be beneficial for palliative relief; however, a significant increase in the risk of neutropenia and infection is seen.

Allogeneic hematopoietic stem cell transplantation (allo-HSCT) is considered the only curable treatment option for patients with PMF. This option should be considered in young patients with intermediate-/high-risk PMF. For patients older than 60 years of age, a reasonable option would be a reduced-intensity conditioning regimen. Studies assessing the efficacy of JAK kinase inhibitors are ongoing and, in the setting of clinical benefit, may eventually change the course of the disease. Intervention is indicated in the following situations.

a. **Anemia.** Androgens (e.g., testosterone enanthate 600 mg intramuscularly weekly or fluoxymesterone 10 mg by mouth two or three times a day for men; danazol 400 to 600 mg by mouth daily for women) are recommended and reduce transfusion requirements in 30% to 50% of patients. Corticosteroids (e.g., prednisone 40 mg/m^2 by mouth daily) should be tried if overt hemolysis is present. Erythropoietin is helpful in a small percent of patients but requires large doses; response is unlikely if serum erythropoietin level is greater than 200 mU/mL. In limited studies, improvement in cytopenias or transfusion requirements has been reported in 20% to 50% of patients with PMF receiving low-dose thalidomide (50 mg/day) or lenalidomide (5 to 10 mg/day).

PMF patients routinely become transfusion-dependent; early institution of iron-chelating agents is advisable.

b. **Splenomegaly.** Massive splenomegaly may lead to cytopenias, portal hypertension, variceal bleeding, abdominal pain, or compression of adjacent organs. Anorexia, fatigue, and hypercatabolic complaints may be prominent. The first option for control by myelosuppressive therapy is hydroxyurea, given as for PV. Melphalan (2.5 mg by mouth three times weekly, with escalations up to 2.5 mg daily as tolerated), and busulfan (2 mg/day in older patients) can also be considered. Interferon-α produces responses in some cases as well.

Radiation 50 to 200 cGy is effective in improving splenomegaly but causes cytopenias in 40% of patients. Radiation occasionally is indicated for extramedullary hematopoietic tumors causing compression syndromes or for bone pain.

Splenectomy is indicated in carefully selected cases but carries significant perioperative mortality and morbidity from bleeding, sepsis, and postoperative thrombocytosis.

c. **Curative intent.** Allo-HSCT from appropriately matched donors appears to be potentially curative, but transplant-related mortality is high in patients with PMF who are older than 45 years. Younger patients with expected survival of no more than 5 years may be reasonable candidates. Engraftment rates are equal to those in other hematologic disorders, and a "graft versus myelofibrosis" effect has been demonstrated. Encouraging early results with nonmyeloablative allo-HSCT suggest that this modality may be the most appropriate option and is feasible in older patients with PMF.

3. **Novel therapies**

a. **JAK2 inhibitors.** The discovery of the JAK pathways in patients with PMF led to the conduct of several clinical studies with JAK2 inhibitors. INCB018424 is a JAK2 inhibitor in advanced clinical trials. It is a potent selective inhibitor of JAK1 and JAK2, has demonstrated encouraging clinical activity in a phase I/II study in over 100 patients with PMF and MF post PV/ET. INCB018424 was associated with 50% or greater reduction in splenomegaly in 35% of patients treated with 10 mg twice a day or 50 mg once a day, and in 59% of patients dosed with 25 mg twice a day. Patients experienced rapid improvement of well-being, and weight gain was most pronounced in patients with the lowest body mass index values at baseline. This may be due to the associated profound reductions in inflammatory cytokines in virtually all patients. The treatment was well tolerated, the primary toxicity being grade 3 or 4 reversible thrombocytopenia.

b. **Immunomodulatory agents (IMiDs).** These agents have engendered an interesting clinical activity in a subset of patients with PMF, including improvements in anemia, thrombocytopenia, and splenomegaly, thought to be due to their effect on bone marrow environment. Thalidomide and lenalidomide induced responses in 16% to 34% of patients. The combination of lenalidomide and prednisone may be more effective and safer than single-agent IMiD therapy. New agents like pomalidomide are under study.

c. **Hypomethylating agents.** Azacitidine and decitabine are being assessed in ongoing clinical trials.

II. MYELODYSPLASTIC SYNDROMES (MDSs)

This is a diverse group of hematopoietic stem cell clonal neoplasms characterized by ineffective hematopoiesis and dysplastic morphologic changes in one or more lineages. The disease has a median age of 65 to 70 years, is the most frequent hematologic malignancy in the over-65 age group, and affects 20,000 to 30,000 cases annually in the United States. For the population over 60 years of age, the incidence is 1 in 500. Eighty percent of cases occur de novo and have no specific etiology or known cause. In the remaining 20% of cases, an association with prior chemotherapy use can be identified, most frequently high-dose alkylator or topoisomerase-II inhibitor-based regimens, or exposure to radiation. Whether a specific inciting cause can be identified or not, the pathophysiologic process of MDS is DNA damage in a pluripotential bone marrow stem cell with a dynamic balance of secondary and associated changes in proliferation, differentiation, and apoptosis intrinsic cellular pathways along with extrinsic marrow microenviroment, angiogenic, cytokine, and immune effects. Clonal cytogenetic abnormalities can be identified in 40% to 50% of de novo cases, most typically a loss of chromosome material involving chromosomes 5, 7, 11, 20, or Y, or trisomy of chromosome 8. Cytogenetic abnormalities in chromosomes 5 or 7 will be identifiable in 95% of therapy-related cases, with half of cases also having complex cytogenetic changes involving three or more chromosomes.

A. Diagnosis

The typical clinical picture is an elderly patient with macrocytic anemia, with or without thrombopenia and neutropenia. Initial diagnostic studies needed are complete blood count with differential and peripheral smear review, bone marrow aspirate and biopsy with cytogenetics, reticulocyte count, serum erythropoietin level prior to transfusion, serum iron-total iron binding capacity-ferritin, B_{12} and folate levels, along with human immunodeficiency virus status if a clinical concern, and human leukocyte antigen (HLA) typing in young patients if a candidate for transplant or aggressive immunosuppressive therapy. There is no single diagnostic test, however. A confirmed diagnosis is made from the hematologic picture of cytopenias and dysplastic lineage morphology supported by associated marrow cytogenetic findings, if abnormal. The typical dysplastic features seen in the marrow and peripheral blood include megaloblastoid precursors, budding and irregular nuclear outline of normoblasts, hypochromia and basophilic stippling of red blood cells, iron-laden sideroblasts, hyposegmentation (bilobed Pelger-Huet-like forms are characteristic) and hypogranularity of neutrophils, hypolobar and/or micromegakaryocytes, and hypogranular platelets. Platelet and neutrophil functional abnormalities exist, further contributing to the symptomatic cytopenias. The bone marrow is most often hypercellular (but 10% to 20% will be hypocellular) with a low reticulocyte count. Abnormal localization of immature precursors is often seen on the marrow core biopsy. A variable number of myeloblasts will be seen from less than 5% up to 20%. Differential diagnosis includes B_{12} and folate deficiency, lead poisoning and alcohol abuse in patients with sideroblastic anemia, aplastic anemia in patients with hypoplastic marrows, PMF if marrow fibrosis is present, and paroxysmal nocturnal hemoglobinuria.

B. Classification

The French-American-British (FAB) classification for MDS put forth in 1982 continues to be useful (Table 20.1). More recently, WHO modified this classification to better correlate with more homogeneous subsets and natural histories (Table 20.2). The major changes (1) lowered the percentage of marrow blasts to define full blown acute myelogenous leukemia at greater than or equal to 20%, removing refractory anemia with excess blasts (RAEB) in transformation as a category; (2) separated out the 5q- syndrome, given its different clinical picture and treatment; and (3) moved chronic myelomonocytic leukemia to a separate category of myelodysplastic/myeloproliferative disease.

C. Prognosis

Acute leukemia transformation potential and survival correlate to some degree with both the FAB and WHO classifications, but even more so with the International Prognostic Scoring System (IPSS). The IPSS (Table 20.3) assigns a score based on the percent of marrow blasts, initial marrow cytogenetics, and the number of peripheral cytopenias to provide a better prognostic risk stratification for an individual; the IPSS can be very helpful in guiding management decisions. However, recent studies have highlighted issues with the IPSS model in relation to the exclusion of many subgroups that now represent a large proportion of patients with MDS (e.g., secondary MDS, chronic myelomonocytic leukemia with leukocytosis, prior therapy) and its lack of applicability to most patients on investigational programs, because many would have received prior therapies and would have had MDS for a significant length of time. A multivariate analysis of

TABLE 20.1 MDS Subtypes: FAB Classification

FAB Subtype	Marrow Blasts (%)	Peripheral Blood Blasts (%)	Other Findings	Median Survival (months)
RA	<5	≤1	—	43
RARS	<5	≤1	≥15% ring sideroblasts	73
RAEB	5–20	<5	—	12
RAEBt*	20–30 *or*	≥5 *or*	Presence of Auer rods	5
CMML	≤20	<5	Monocytes >1000/μL	20

CMML, chronic myelomonocytic leukemia; RA, refractory anemia; RAEB, refractory anemia with excess blasts; RAEBt, refractory anemia with excess blasts in transformation; RARS, refractory anemia with ringed sideroblasts.
*In a subsequent revised scheme, RAEBt cases are reclassified as acute leukemia.

	WHO Classification of MDS and Pertinent Features	
Subtype	**Blood Findings**	**Bone Marrow Findings**
RA	Anemia; no blasts	Erythroid dysplasia only; <5% blasts
RARS	Anemia; no blasts	RA + 15% or greater ringed sideroblasts
RCMD	Bi- or pancytopenia; no blasts	Dysplasia in >10% cells in two or more lineages
RCMD-RS	RCMD	RCMD + 15% or greater ringed sideroblasts
RAEB		
RAEB-1	No Auer rods and ,5% blasts;	Uni- or multilineage dysplasia plus no Auer rods and 5%–9% blasts;
RAEB-2	Auer rods or 5%–19% blasts	Auer rods or 10%–19% blasts
MDS-U	Cytopenias; no blasts	Unilineage dysplasia in granulocytes or megakaryocytes; <5% blasts
MDS with isolated del(5q-)	Anemia; <5% blasts	Normal to increased megakaryocytes

MDS-U, myelodysplastic syndrome, unclassified; RA, refractory anemia; RAEB, refractory anemia with excess blasts; RARS, refractory anemia with ringed sideroblasts; RCMD, refractory cytopenia with multilineage dysplasia; RCMD-RS, refractory cytopenia with multilineage dysplasia and increased ringed sideroblasts.

prognostic factors in 1915 patients with MDS identified the following adverse, independent factors as continuous and categoric values (p <0.001): poor performance status, older age, thrombocytopenia, anemia, increased bone marrow blasts, leukocytosis, chromosome 7 or complex (≥3) abnormalities, and prior transfusions. The new MDS prognostic model divides patients into four prognostic groups with significantly different outcomes (Table 20.4). The new model accounts for duration of MDS and prior therapy. It is applicable to any patient with MDS at any time during the course of MDS.

D. Therapy

The management of MDS is guided by the scoring systems previously elucidated including patient's age, IPSS category, serum erythropoietin level, cytogenetics if 5q- present, and by assessing HLA status in a candidate for allo-HSCT or immunosuppressive therapy. All patients should receive appropriate blood product transfusion support.

1. General approach

a. Low-risk patients (IPSS low and intermediate-1):

- If serum erythropoietin level is less than 500 mU/mL, treat with growth factors (erythropoietin analog, adding granulocyte colony-stimulating factor [G-CSF] if no hematocrit response).

- Azacitidine, decitabine, or lenalidomide if no clinical response to growth factors.

TABLE 20.3 IPSS for MDS

Prognostic Factor	Score value				
	0	0.5	1.0	1.5	2.0
Marrow blasts (%)	<5	5–10	—	11–20	21–30
Karyotype*	Good	Intermediate	Poor	—	—
Cytopenias†	0–1	2–3	—	—	—

Risk category	Total Score	Median Survival (yr)
Low	0	5.7
Intermediate-1	0.5–1.0	3.5
Intermediate-2	1.5–2.0	1.2
High	2.5	0.4

*Good, normal karyotype, −Y, 5q⁻, or 20q⁻. Poor, chromosome 7 abnormal (monosomy, 7q⁻, etc.); or complex (three separate abnormalities). Intermediate, all other abnormal karyotypes.
†Cytopenias defined by hemoglobin <10 g/dL, neutrophils <1500/μL, and platelets <100,000/μL. (Note that the IPSS conforms to the FAB classification, and includes patients with refractory anemia with excess blasts in transformation who would be classified as AML under the WHO system.)

    b. High-risk patients (IPSS intermediate-2 and high):
- If young and a donor available, allo-HSCT.
- If not a transplant candidate, azacitidine, decitabine, or lenalidomide.

    c. 5q- cytogenetics: lenalidomide.

    d. MDS with hypoplastic features:
- Antithymocyte globulin (ATG)
- Cyclosporine A
- Alemtuzumab.

2. Growth factors. Erythropoietin analogs, either epoetin or darbepoetin, can effectively achieve a meaningful hemoglobin improvement in 15% to 25% of patients. In patients with a serum erythropoietin level less than 500 mU/mL, a trial of an erythropoietin analog is indicated. Low-risk patients do respond better than high-risk patients. Usually, higher dosing than used in chemotherapy-associated anemias is needed. An adequate therapeutic trial of 8 to 12 weeks is appropriate. G-CSF can be synergistic with erythropoietin therapy, enhancing the erythroid response rate potential up to 40%. This synergism is particularly effective in patients with greater than 15% ringed sideroblasts. These growth factors need to be continued to maintain the achieved benefit.

    a. Recombinant human erythropoietin 40,000 to 60,000 units SC 2 to 3 times weekly; taper to smallest effective dosing schedule if response, and continue.

TABLE 20.4	The M.D. Anderson Scoring System for MDS	
Prognostic Factor		**Points**
Performance status ≥2		2
Age, years		
60–64		1
≥65		2
Platelets, × 10³/μL		
<30		3
30–49		2
50–199		1
Hemoglobin <12 g/dL		2
Bone marrow blasts, %		
5–10		1
11–29		2
WBC >20 × 10³/μL		2
Karyotype: Chromosome 7 abnormality or complex (≥3) abnormalities		3
Prior transfusion, yes		1

WBC, white blood cell.
Low risk (score 0–4): the median survival is 54 months and the 3-year survival rate is 63%; intermediate-1 risk (score 5–6): the median survival is 25 months and the 3-year survival rate is 34%; intermediate-2 risk (score 7–8): the median survival is 14 months and the 3-year survival rate is 16%; high risk (score ≥9): the median survival is 6 months and the 3-year survival rate is 4%.

   b. Darbepoetin 150 to 300 μg SC weekly. If an inadequate or no response to the erythropoietin analog alone and clinically still indicated, add G-CSF.

   c. G-CSF (filgrastim) 1 to 2 μg/kg SC two to three times weekly, with the erythropoietin analog.

3. **Specific agents**

   a. Azacitidine is a hypomethylating agent inhibiting DNA methyltransferase, reversing the epigenetic silencing of gene transcription. The exact mechanism of action in MDS is most likely multifactorial. In a landmark phase III trial compared to conventional care, azacitidine showed a survival improvement (24 months versus 15 months) and improved quality-of-life parameters. It is now approved by the U.S. Food and Drug Administration (FDA) in all types of MDS at the dose of 75 mg/m^2 SC or IV daily for 7 days every 28 days with a possibility of continuing treatment as long as there is a favorable benefit/tolerance balance. The most common toxicity is myelosuppression with a 20% treatment-related infection rate. It is generally very well tolerated and can be administered in the outpatient setting.

b. **Decitabine (Dacogen)** is another hypomethylating agent DNA methyltransferase inhibitor that has shown significant activity in MDS. Initial European phase II studies showed 50% hematologic response rates, notably even higher in IPSS high-risk patients. A landmark phase III trial compared to supportive care confirmed significant response rates (17% complete or partial response by International Working Group criteria, plus an additional 13% with hematologic improvement) and a longer time to acute leukemia transformation or death, in particular among those patients with an IPSS intermediate-2/high-risk score, or not previously treated. Overall survival was prolonged in patients responding to decitabine compared to nonresponders (23.5 months versus 13.7 months). It is now approved by the FDA for use in MDS. Decitabine was originally approved at the dose of 15 mg/m^2 as a 3-hour infusion IV every 8 hours for 3 consecutive days (9 total doses) every 6 weeks $\times$ four cycles continuously, as long as it is effective. Myelosuppression with cytopenic complications is an expected and frequent toxicity of decitabine, especially in the already-cytopenic MDS patient. Other side effects include nausea, diarrhea or constipation, and cough. More convenient dosing schedules were evaluated. The M.D. Anderson experience has reported overall clinical benefit in 76% of patients treated with a modified schedule of 20 mg/m^2 IV over 1 hour daily for 5 consecutive days every 4 weeks. The efficacy of this regimen was confirmed in the ADOPT trial. Decitabine is currently approved in the United States at the dose of 20 mg/m^2 IV over 1 hour daily for 5 consecutive days every 4 weeks.

c. **Lenalidomide** is a thalidomide-related immunomodulator with greater potency. It has with a wide range of biologic effects including suppression of angiogenesis, inhibition of inflammatory cytokines, potentiation of immune pathways, and other cellular ligand-induced responses. A landmark phase II study showed dramatic erythroid responses in erythropoietin-resistant patients. Major erythroid responses and cytogenetic responses occurred in 83% of patients with a 5q- deletion, but were not limited to this 5q- subset. Overall, 68% of patients with a low IPSS score, 50% with intermediate-1 IPSS, and over half of patients with normal cytogenetics had erythroid responses. High-risk MDS patients had a much less frequent hematologic response (20%) but those patients with RAEB responding also demonstrated decreased blast counts. It is approved by the FDA in patients with 5q- MDS. Lenalidomide 10 mg orally daily is given continuously so long as this dose is tolerated; the dose can be reduced to a 21 out of 28 day schedule or 5-mg dosing if persistent or severe hematologic toxicity occurs. Marrow suppression with neutropenia and thrombocytopenia, the most frequent toxicity, is dose dependent and requires dose interruption in over half of patients. Other systemic side effects include low-grade pruritus, diarrhea, rash, and fatigue.

4. **Allogeneic hemapoietic stem cell transplant (allo-HSCT).** This remains the only curative therapy but is limited to younger patients and preferably with a matched related donor. Treatment-related mortality and chronic morbidity remain very high. Given the older age group with MDS, less than 10% of patients are considered transplant candidates. It should always be considered in younger patients in IPSS high-risk or intermediate-2-risk category with suitable sibling donors. Transplant studies show disease-free survival ranges from 29% to 40%, nonrelapse mortality of 37% to 50%, and relapse even with a sibling donor of 23% to 48%. Reduced-intensity conditioning transplants appear to carry promise for use in an older population but are still fraught with significantly high mortalities.

5. **Intensive chemotherapy.** There is no clear consensus regarding the role of intensive chemotherapy in MDS. Its use is typically restricted to patients in IPSS intermediate- and high-risk groups. Induction chemotherapy utilizing acute leukemia-type regimens (e.g., anthracycline/cytosine arabinoside) can induce complete responses in 50% to 60% of patients with MDS, but remissions tend to be brief and outcomes correlate strongly with karyotype-associated chemoresistance mechanisms. Topotecan, a topoisomerase I inhibitor, has been postulated to have selectively favorable effectiveness in MDS, but its role is not well established as responses are brief and myelotoxicity is very high. The role of intensive chemotherapy in treating MDS is limited to young patients with high-risk disease serving as a bridge to an allo-HSCT. In hopes of minimizing toxicity, low-dose chemotherapy has been utilized, most notably with cytarabine at doses of 5 to 20 mg/m^2 daily, as an every 12-hour SC injection, continued for 10 to 20 days. Hematologic responses are seen in 20% to 30% of patients, but without any significant survival benefit, and serious marrow suppression may result. The effectiveness, tolerability, and availability of azacitidine and decitabine have now largely supplanted the use of low-dose chemotherapies in MDS.

6. **Immunotherapy.** The immunosuppressive effects of ATG can be quite effective achieving transfusion independence along with other cytopenia responses in one-third of a select subset of patients with MDS, namely those who are younger, with hypocellular marrow, normal cytogenetics, shorter duration of transfusion dependency, and those who are HLA DR15 positive.

   ■ **ATG** 40 mg/kg per day × 4 days (common toxicities include infusion reactions, serum sickness [coadministration of prednisone may alleviate this] and immunosuppression).

Other immunosuppressive agents have been tried with mixed success. Prednisone is occasionally helpful in improving cytopenias (approximately 10% response rate overall), particularly in those patients with evidence of hemolysis. Cyclosporine has shown high response rates in limited studies, utilizing 5 to 6 mg/kg/day initially, then monitored with dose adjustments to maintain serum levels of 100 to 300 ng/mL.

- **Alemtuzumab** given at the dose of 10 mg IV daily was recently used in 21 patients with MDS. Responses were reported in 74%: five out of seven patients with abnormal cytogenetics achieved a complete cytogenetic response. The estimated 3-year relapse-free survival is 50%.

7. **Other agents** have shown some limited hematologic benefit in MDS. However, with the availability of azacitidine, decitabine, and lenalidomide, and with a very narrow therapeutic index for either amifostine or arsenic trioxide, their use should be rare except in a clinical trial.

Pyridoxine 100 to 200 mg daily is a reasonable trial in patients with increased ringed sideroblasts; however, benefit is infrequent. Developmental therapies targeting angiogenesis, apoptosis, cytokine, farnesyl transferase, tyrosine kinase, and histone deacetylase or other DNA methyltransferase epigenetic pathways alone and in combination are being evaluated in clinical trials.

8. **Supportive care**
   a. **Anemia**. RBC transfusions will become needed in most patients with MDS to maintain quality of life. A hemoglobin goal (usually above 9 g/dL) must be individualized based on symptom need and improvement. Leukocyte-depleted packed RBC should be used in all patients, with cytomegalovirus (CMV)-negative (if the patient is CMV negative) and irradiated blood products in potential allo-HSCT candidates.
   b. **Iron overload and chelation therapy.** Secondary hemochromatosis with cardiac, hepatic, endocrine, and hematopoietic dysfunction can develop after 20 to 30 units of red cell transfusion. Chelation therapy can improve visceral and marrow function, and should be a strong consideration in patients with an ongoing transfusion need who are expected to survive several years, as well as in patients with overt iron overload-related visceral dysfunction. Monitoring of ferritin levels should begin at a 20 to 30 unit transfusion threshold, with institution of a chelating agent when the ferritin is greater than 2500 µg/L. The treatment goal is to lower ferritin to less than 1000 µg/L.
      - Deferoxamine (Desferal) 1 to 2 g by overnight (8 to 12 hrs) infusion SC 5 to 7 nights per week; *or*

◾ Deferasirox (Exjade) 20 mg/kg oral daily dispersed in water or orange/apple juice taken on an empty stomach. Toxicities are similar to deferoxamine with nausea and vomiting, diarrhea, pyrexia, and abdominal pain but also potential increased serum creatinine. The availability of this more convenient oral chelator will likely greatly improve this aspect of supportive care in MDS.

c. Infections. Neutropenia and neutrophil dysfunction contribute to a high risk of bacterial infections in MDS. Antibiotics remain the mainstay of management, but prophylactic antibiotics are of unknown benefit. G-CSF can raise the neutrophil count in 90% of patients with MDS, and its short-term use may be appropriate in infected, severely neutropenic patients; indications for long-term use of G-CSF are limited.

d. Bleeding. Symptomatic thrombocytopenia requires platelet transfusion support. Single-donor platelets delay alloimmunization, but this will eventually develop in the majority (30% to 70%) of patients, limiting subsequent platelet transfusion increments. There is not an absolute thrombocytopenia transfusion threshold, but platelet counts below 10,000/µL carry a spontaneous central nervous system hemorrhage risk. Two additional adjuncts to thrombocytopenic bleeding control are as follows:

◾ Aminocaproic acid 4 g IV over 1 hour, followed by 1 gram/hour continuous infusion; or orally in a similar dosing schedule, or by a more convenient 2 to 4 g schedule orally every 4 to 6 hours. Tachyphylaxis and loss of antifibrinolytic stabilization will often occur after 48 consecutive hours of therapy.

◾ Interleukin-11/oprelvekin is a thrombopoietic cytokine that has increased platelet counts after chemotherapy. A low-dose regimen of 10 µg/kg/day can raise platelet counts in selected patients with bone marrow failure.

Acknowledgments

The authors are indebted to Drs. Peter White and Paul R. Walker, who contributed to previous editions of this chapter. Several sections in this revision of the handbook represent their work.

Selected Readings

Myeloproliferative Diseases

Barosi G, Hoffman R. Idiopathic myelofibrosis. *Sem Hematol.* 2005;42:248–258.

Harrison CN, Campbell PJ, Buck G, et al. Hydroxyurea compared with anagrelide in high-risk essential thrombocythemia. *N Engl J Med.* 2005;353:33–45.

Harrison CN. Platelets and thrombosis in myeloproliferative diseases. In: *American Society of Hematology education program book*. Washington, DC: American Society of Hematology; 2005:409–415.

Kralovics R, Passamonti F, Buser AS, et al. A gain of function mutation of *JAK 2* in myeloproliferative disorders. *New Engl J Med*. 2005;352:1779–1790.

Landolfi R, Marchioli R, Kutti J, et al. Efficacy and safety of low-dose aspirin in polycythemia vera. *New Engl J Med*. 2004;350:114–124.

Marchioli R, Finazzi G, Landolfi R, et al. Vascular and neoplastic risk in a large cohort of patients with polycythemia vera. *J Clin Oncol*. 2005;23:2224–2232.

Wadleigh M, Tefferi A. Classification and diagnosis of myeloproliferative neoplasms according to the 2008 World Health Organization criteria. *Int J Hematol*. 2010;91:174–179.

Myelodysplastic Syndromes

Greenberg PL, Baer MR, Bennett JM, et al. Myelodysplastic syndromes: clinical practice guidelines in oncology. *J Natl Compr Canc Netw*. 2006;4:58–77.

Greenberg P, Cox C, Le Beau NM, et al. International scoring system for evaluating prognosis in myelodysplastic syndromes. *Blood*. 1997;89:2079–2088.

Greenberg PL. Myelodysplastic syndromes: iron overload consequences and current chelating therapies. *J Natl Compr Canc Netw*. 2006;4:91–96.

Jadersten M, Montgomery SM, Dybedal I, et al. Long-term outcome of treatment of anemia in MDS with erythropoietin and G-CSF. *Blood*. 2005;106:803–811.

Kantarjian H, Issa J-P, Rosenfield C, et al. Decitabine improves patient outcomes in myelodysplastic syndromes. *Cancer*. 2006;106:1794–1803.

Kantarjian H, O'Brien S, Giles, F, et al. Decitabine low-dose schedule (100 mg/m^2/ course) in myelodysplastic syndrome (MDS): comparison of 3 different dose schedules. *Blood*. 2005;106:2522a.

Kurzrock R, Cortes J, Thomas DA, et al. Pilot study of low-dose interleukin-11 in patients with bone marrow failure. *J Clin Oncol*. 2001;19:4165–4172.

List A, Kurtin S, Roe DJ, et al. Efficacy of lenalidomide in myelodysplastic syndromes. *N Engl J Med*. 2005;352:549–557.

Silverman LR, Demakos EP, Peterson BL, et al. Randomized controlled trial of azacytidine in patients with the myelodysplastic syndrome: a study of the Cancer and Leukemia Group B. *J Clin Oncol*. 2002;20:2429–2440.

Vardiman JW, Harris NL, Brunning RD. The World Health Organization (WHO) classification of the myeloid neoplasms. *Blood*. 2002;100:2292–2302.

Hodgkin Lymphoma

Richard S. Stein and David S. Morgan

Hodgkin lymphoma (HL) is a lymphoproliferative malignancy that accounts for approximately 1% of cancers in the United States. Most patients present with disease limited to lymph nodes or to lymph nodes and the spleen. The bone marrow is involved in approximately 5% of cases. HL generally spreads in a contiguous fashion, making the use of radiation therapy (RT) feasible for many patients. The average age at presentation is 32 years with a bimodal incidence curve; one peak occurs before age 25 years and the other at age 55 years.

Most patients with HL are cured with primary therapy. Patients with advanced disease can be cured with combination chemotherapy, while those with limited disease can be cured either with limited combination chemotherapy and limited RT, or with more extensive RT alone. A major focus of HL therapy in the last 40 years has been the recognition of and the attempt to limit long-term side effects of therapy. Thus, the recent trend has been away from extensive RT alone for limited-stage disease.

While HL is highly curable at presentation, a significant minority will not respond or will relapse after initial treatment. Many of these patients can be cured by salvage therapy. Salvage chemotherapy may produce cures in patients initially treated with RT. Readministration of standard-dose chemotherapy or, more commonly, the administration of high-dose chemotherapy in conjunction with autologous stem cell transplantation may produce cures in patients initially treated with combination chemotherapy. Nevertheless, the potential for cure should not lead clinicians and patients to lose sight of the fact that approximately 20% to 25% of patients with HL eventually die of the disease.

For most cancers, disease-free survival (DFS) is a valuable surrogate marker for overall survival and thus evaluating DFS is a useful method for choosing optimal initial therapy. However, for HL, the success of salvage therapy means that the treatment options that are associated with superior DFS may not necessarily produce superior overall survival when the results of salvage therapy are considered, and this makes the selection of initial therapy somewhat subtler. In fact, because radiation and chemotherapy have significant long-term consequences such as secondary malignancies (associated with larger RT fields) or acute leukemia (associated with combined-modality therapy), DFS may overestimate the value of a specific therapy. Therefore, for each stage of HL, more than one rational therapeutic option may exist.

I. DIAGNOSIS AND PATHOLOGY

The diagnosis of HL requires excisional biopsy of an involved node and review of the material by a hematopathologist. Lymph node biopsy is recommended for any patient with lymphadenopathy greater than 1 cm in diameter and persisting for more than 4 weeks. Lymphoma, including HL, may be suspected when the nodes are freely movable and rubbery rather than stony hard. However, these clinical features are not specific for HL or for lymphoma in general. Key features of the histopathology of HL include the presence of Reed-Sternberg (RS) cells (or variants) in a mixed inflammatory background. The RS cells of classical HL (see subsequent discussion) are of B-cell origin, stain for CD15 and CD30, and are negative for CD45 and CD20. Whenever the diagnosis of HL is made in a patient presenting at an extranodal site or at a nodal site below the diaphragm, the diagnosis should be subjected to greater than usual scrutiny.

The current World Health Organization classification divides HL into two major groups: classical HL and nodular lymphocyte predominant HL (NLPHL). Classical HL includes the four subtypes: nodular sclerosis HL (approximately 70% of cases), mixed cellularity HL (approximately 20%), lymphocyte-rich HL (less than 5%), and lymphocyte depletion HL (less than 5%). NLPHL (5% of all HL) is a B-cell neoplasm characterized by variant RS cells ("L and H cells" or "popcorn cells") that are positive for CD20 and negative for CD30 and CD15. In immunophenotype and behavior, NLPHL bears similarities to low-grade non-HL.

In the past, much was made of the prognostic significance of the subtypes of classical HL. Most of the difference is explained by the fact that stage covaries with histology. For instance, the average patient with mixed cellularity HL presents at a more advanced stage than the average patient with the nodular sclerosis HL. Thus it is generally true that patients with nodular sclerosis HL do better than patients with mixed cellularity HL. However, when one stratifies patients by stage, the impact of histopathology on prognosis is minimal.

II. STAGING

Accurate staging is critical to determining the optimal therapy for the patient with HL. It also provides a baseline so that the completeness of a response can be determined when therapy has been completed.

A. Cotswold staging system

The Cotswold modification of the Ann Arbor Staging System (Table 21.1) is used for patients with HL. Clinically, patients are placed in one of four stages based on anatomic extent of disease and are further classified as to the absence, "A," or presence, "B," of systemic symptoms (see subsequent discussion). In addition, the subscript E (e.g., II_E) may be used to denote involvement of an

TABLE 21.1	Cotswold Modification of the Ann Arbor Staging System for HL
Stage I	Involvement of a single lymph node region
Stage II	Involvement of two or more lymph nodes regions on the same side of the diaphragm
Stage III$_1$	Involvement of lymph node regions on both sides of the diaphragm. Abdominal disease is limited to the upper abdomen (i.e., spleen, splenic hilar, celiac, and/or porta hepatis nodes).
Stage III$_2$	Involvement of lymph node regions on both sides of the diaphragm. Abdominal disease includes para-aortic, mesenteric, iliac, or inguinal nodes, with or without disease in the upper abdomen.
Stage IV	Diffuse or disseminated involvement of one or more extralymphatic tissues or organs, with or without associated lymph node involvement
A	No symptoms
B	Fever, drenching sweats, weight loss
X	Bulky disease greater than one-third widening of the mediastinum
E	Involvement of a single extranodal site contiguous to a nodal site

extralymphatic site primarily or, more commonly, to denote direct extension into an organ, such as a large mediastinal mass extending into the lung. Stage III HL is subdivided into two substages, stages III$_1$ and III$_2$, based on the extent of intra-abdominal disease. However, as current treatment recommendations are the same for both substages, this distinction is of little clinical relevance.

B. Prognostic score for advanced HL (International Prognostic Score [IPS])

In 1998, Hasenclever and Diehl created a prognostic model for advanced HL based on a multivariate analysis of patients. Seven factors were identified as having prognostic value: serum albumin <4 gm/dL, hemoglobin <10.5 gm/dL, male sex, stage IV disease, age ≥45 years, white cell count ≥15,000/μL, and lymphocyte count either <600/μL or <8% of the white cell count. In the paper presenting the model, the prognostic score correlated with both freedom from progression and overall survival rate. However, the utility of the IPS is limited by the fact that most patients had a score of 0 to 3, with only 12% of patients having a score of 4 and only 7% of patients having a score of 5 to 7.

C. Staging tests

Before the advent of modern radiographic and nuclear medicine techniques, clinicians made use of the knowledge that HL tends to spread in a contiguous manner, and elegant and detailed descriptions of patterns of disease were made. For instance, it was recognized that because the thoracic duct makes the left supraclavicular area and the abdomen contiguous sites, abdominal disease is found in 40% of patients with left supraclavicular presentations and in only 8% of patients with right supraclavicular presentations. While such fascinating associations were useful before modern imaging was available, today they are largely superseded by computed tomography (CT) and positron emission tomography (PET) scans. Procedures used in the staging of HL are as follows.

1. **History taking.** As with any patient, the staging of the patient with HL begins with a history and a physical exam. Special attention should be given to symptoms such as bone pain that might signal a specific extranodal site of disease. The symptoms that are considered "B symptoms" are fever, night sweats, and weight loss greater than 10% of body weight. Fever in HL can have any pattern. The pattern of days of high fever separated by days without fever, so-called Pel-Ebstein fever, has been associated with HL for over a century but is quite rare in modern times when the diagnosis of HL is usually made early in the course of disease and effective therapy is initiated. Pain at the site of HL in association with alcohol ingestion is a rare finding but may give hints as to visceral sites of involvement.

2. **Complete physical examination.** Attention must be paid to all lymph node regions and the spleen. Splenomegaly is seen at presentation in approximately 10% of patients with HL and does not necessarily indicate splenic involvement by HL.

3. **Laboratory tests.** Complete blood counts, erythrocyte sedimentation rate (ESR), serum alkaline phosphatase, and tests of liver and kidney function should be obtained. Hepatic enzymes may be elevated "nonspecifically" in patients with HL and do not necessarily indicate hepatic involvement by HL.

4. **Chest radiographs and CT scans** of the neck, chest, abdomen, and pelvis are routinely obtained in patients with HL.

5. **PET scans,** especially PET/CT fusion scans, have been shown to be highly sensitive in HL and may "upstage" patients in comparison to CT scans alone. The PET scan is also useful for detecting relapse and persistent disease and therefore should be obtained at baseline for comparison with later scans. The PET scan is especially helpful when the posttreatment CT scan shows a residual mass, which could be either an inactive residual mass or persistent HL. The value of PET has been shown in many studies and was most clearly shown in a study by Gallamini and associates in which the PET scan was repeated after two cycles of doxorubicin, bleomycin, vinblastine, and dacarbazine (ABVD) chemotherapy. Therapy was not changed based on the PET findings (i.e., ABVD was continued). Two-year progression-free survival was 13% for patients who were PET-positive as compared to 95% in patients who had become PET-negative ($p < 0.0001$). Whether or not changing the chemotherapy in patients with a positive PET can alter the poor prognosis of those patients is the subject of ongoing clinical trials.

6. **Bone marrow biopsy**. The test is rarely positive except in patients who are found to have at least stage III disease by other tests. However, because of the potential use of autologous bone marrow transplantation (ABMT) or stem cell transplantation as salvage therapy, a bone marrow biopsy is a reasonable baseline study in all patients with HL. Alternatively, if chemotherapy is planned and if blood counts are normal, the test may be omitted until the time that stem cell transplantation is considered.

7. **Staging laparotomy**. With the widespread availability of PET scans, and the tendency to treat even limited disease with chemotherapy, staging laparotomy is of historical interest only.

III. THERAPY OF HODGKIN LYMPHOMA

A. General considerations

Therapy of HL must be considered on a stage-by-stage basis. The incidence of various stages of HL is presented in Table 21.2, which also presents an estimated cure rate for each stage. Historically, potentially curative RT was available before curative chemotherapy was defined, and therefore there has been a traditional bias to use radiation as the sole modality of therapy or as part of combination therapy whenever possible. Thus, RT has been used for limited-stage HL, and even stage IIIa HL in the recent past, even after more effective, and safer, chemotherapy had been advocated for use in HL. Indeed, there are only limited data for the use of chemotherapy alone in stage I and II HL.

Late complications of RT for HL include breast cancer, lung cancer, hypothyroidism, thyroid cancer, musculoskeletal atrophy or growth deficit, coronary artery disease, cardiomyopathy, and valvular heart disease. While the incidence of each of these complications is fairly low, the cumulative risk of death from all of these complications may be as much as 15% at 15 years following treatment. It is therefore reasonable to consider decreasing

TABLE 21.2	HL: Incidence of Stages and Results of Therapy	
Stage	**Relative Incidence (%)**	**Potential Cure Rate (%)**
IA	10	95
IIA	35	85
IB, IIB	13	70
III$_1$A	12	85
III$_2$A	8	65
IIIB	12	60
IVA, IVB	10	60

the field and dose of RT or eliminating it entirely as an approach to limited-stage disease. We now have numerous reports of combined modality therapy for limited-stage HL showing excellent DFS; however, there are no data showing that the overall survival of patients with limited-stage HL can be improved with this alteration of therapy. Studies designed to illustrate the superiority of combined modality therapy with respect to the incidence of late side effects may require 15 to 20 years of follow-up. Thus, after decades of general agreement that RT was the optimal approach to limited-stage HL, there has been a shift to incorporating chemotherapy in the treatment of limited-stage HL.

Chemotherapy has been established as the optimal therapy for advanced-stage disease. A series of U.S. cooperative group studies in the 1980s and 1990s established ABVD as the most effective and least toxic of the candidate regimens, and most authorities, at least in North America, would agree that this regimen is the standard for use alone in advanced disease and for sequencing with RT in limited-disease stages. Two multidrug regimens, Stanford V from the Stanford group and BEACOPP (Table 21.3) and its variation from the German Hodgkin Study Group, have been proposed as alternatives, but have not been widely adopted in North America. The standard regimens should not be altered arbitrarily as dose reductions may decrease the possibility of cure. Although most patients receive six cycles of chemotherapy (e.g., ABVD) for advanced-stage disease, the data actually support administering a minimum of six cycles, with therapy being given until a complete remission (CR) has been achieved and then administered for an additional two cycles.

B. Radiotherapy (RT)

Studies conducted in the 1960s established that the optimal dose for local control if RT used as a single modality was 36 to 40 Gy given over 3.5 to 4 weeks.

With modern equipment, adequate radiation can be administered to involved areas while shielding adjacent tissues. As a result, radiation pneumonitis and radiation pericarditis occur only rarely. Because of the common occurrence of hypothyroidism and the less common occurrence of thyroid cancer in patients who receive radiation to the thyroid gland, thyroid-stimulating hormone (TSH) levels should be monitored yearly in these patients starting at 8 to 10 years following administration of RT. Patients with elevated levels of TSH, even if clinically euthyroid, should be placed on thyroid hormone replacement to limit stimulation of the radiated thyroid gland by elevated levels of TSH. While RT alone has not been associated with an increased risk of acute leukemia, the use of RT in conjunction with combination chemotherapy (especially alkylator therapy as in the outdated mechlorethamine, Oncovin

TABLE 21.3	Chemotherapy Regimens Used in the Treatment of HL
Regimen	**Drugs and Dosages**
MOPP	Mechlorethamine 6 mg/m² IV on days 1 and 8
	Vincristine (Oncovin) 1.4 mg/m² IV on days 1 and 8 (not to exceed 2.5 mg)
	Procarbazine 100 mg/m² PO on days 1–14
	Prednisone 40 mg/m² PO on days 1–14, cycles 1 and 4 only
	Repeat cycle every 28 days.
ABVD	Doxorubicin (Adriamycin) 25 mg/m² IV on days 1 and 15
	Vinblastine 6 mg/m² IV on days 1 and 15
	Bleomycin 10 U/m² IV on days 1 and 15
	Dacarbazine 375 mg/m² IV on days 1 and 15
	Repeat cycle every 28 days.
Stanford V	Vinblastine 6 mg/m² IV weeks 1, 3, 5, 7, 9, and 11
	Doxorubicin 25 mg/m² IV weeks 1, 3, 5, 7, 9, and 11
	Vincristine 1.4 mg/m² IV (not to exceed 2 mg) weeks 2, 4, 6, 8, 10, and 12
	Bleomycin 5 U/m² IV weeks 2, 4, 6, 8, 10, and 12
	Mechlorethamine 6 mg/m² IV weeks 1, 5, and 9
	Etoposide 60 mg/m² IV daily × 2 weeks 3, 7, and 11
	Prednisone 40 mg/m² PO every other day on weeks 1–10, with tapering weeks 11 and 12
	No repeat.
BEACOPP*	Bleomycin 10 U/m² IV on day 8
	Etoposide 100 mg/m² IV om days 1, 2, and 3
	Doxorubicin 25 mg/m² IV on day 1
	Cyclophosphamide 650 mg/m² IV on day 1
	Vincristine 1.4 mg/m² IV (not to exceed 2 mg)
	Procarbazine 100 mg/m² PO on days 1–7
	Prednisone 40 mg/m² PO on days 1–14
	Repeat every 3 weeks.

IV, intravenously; PO, by mouth.
*Escalated BEACOPP increases the etoposide dose to 200 mg/m² daily × 3, increases doxorubicin to 35 mg/m² day × 1, and increases cyclophosphamide to 1200 mg/m² on day 1. Other drugs and doses remain the same.

[vincristine], procarbazine, and prednisone [MOPP] regimen) has been associated with a risk of acute nonlymphocytic leukemia as high as 7% to 10% in the decade following therapy.

Women receiving RT for HL are at higher risk of developing breast cancer, and the risk is higher the younger the woman is at the time RT is administered. Women who receive RT for HL should receive yearly mammograms starting 8 years following the completion of therapy.

C. Treatment by stage of disease

1. **Stages IA and IIA.** Patients with stage IA disease were traditionally treated with mantle irradiation when the disease occurred above the diaphragm (as it does in 90% of cases) or with pelvic

RT when the disease presented in an inguinal node. Patients with stage IIA disease presenting above the diaphragm were previously treated with mantle plus para-aortic–splenic RT. In the last decade, however, evidence has accumulated that RT, as traditionally used in Hodgkin disease, is associated with an increase in late malignancies to the point that second malignancies, rather than Hodgkin disease, are the major cause of death in stage IA and IIA patients treated with extended-field RT alone. While certain patients who are not candidates for chemotherapy might still be treated with RT alone, the current standard of care for stage IA and IIA, based on excellent DFS, is an abbreviated course of chemotherapy such as four cycles of ABVD followed by involved-field-only, limited-dose RT.

2. **Stage II$_X$ disease with bulky mediastinal mass.** Patients with bulky mediastinal masses (disease diameter greater than 10 cm or greater than one-third of the chest diameter) present a special problem. When these patients, who are generally at stage II$_X$, are treated with RT alone, the risk of relapse approaches 50%. "Full course" combination chemotherapy with RT is most commonly employed in these patients.

   However, the value of a combined modality approach for all stage II$_X$ patients is not obvious. As the majority of stage II$_x$ patients have residual disease when evaluated by CT scans following completion of chemotherapy, treating patents with chemotherapy alone was not feasible when CT scans were the best method of evaluating residual disease.

   The introduction of PET scans and the documentation that relapse rates are markedly increased in PET-positive patients as compared to patients who are PET-negative following the completion of chemotherapy has simplified this issue. One logical approach is to treat stage II$_X$ patients with combination chemotherapy and to give low-dose RT (20 Gy) only to patients who have residual disease on the basis of the PET scan obtained on completion of chemotherapy. When this is done, radiation is administered only to the area of residual disease. Long-term follow-up will be necessary to determine the ultimate value of using the PET scan to select patients who will not receive RT in this clinical situation.

3. **Stages IB and IIB and stages I or II with other unfavorable characteristics.** Several cooperative groups have identified unfavorable features in limited-stage patients, including elevated ESR, mixed cellularity subtype, and B symptoms. In the RT-only era, these patients were often treated with extended-field RT, presumably with the thought that these features were associated with more extensive, occult disease. While the available data do not allow firm treatment recommendations to be made,

unfavorable stage I and II patients are most often treated as if they had more advanced-stage disease (i.e., with "full-course chemotherapy").

4. **Stages III and IV.** Combination chemotherapy is the standard approach for these stages of HL, and the standard chemotherapy regimen in North America is ABVD. The data support the use of six to eight cycles, using the rule of "two cycles past the best response." This approach does not incorporate PET scanning. A common, though technically unproven, approach is to stop the therapy if the PET is negative after six cycles.

D. **Chemotherapy**

In 1970, the demonstration by investigators at the National Cancer Institute that MOPP chemotherapy could cure advanced HL was one of the major milestones of the modern chemotherapy era as it was the first demonstration that a previously incurable advanced adult cancer could be cured by combination chemotherapy. This has provided the rationale for the use of combination chemotherapy in medical oncology. However, more recent studies have indicated that the classic MOPP regimen is not the optimal regimen for patients with advanced HL.

1. **Dose and duration of therapy.** Arguments regarding selection of the "best" regimen should not obscure the following principles:

   ▨ Drugs should be administered in accordance with prescribed doses and schedules and not modified for toxicities such as nausea and vomiting (which should be controlled with antiemetics).

   ▨ Full doses should be given when cytopenias are due to bone marrow involvement with HL.

   ▨ Vinca alkaloids should be decreased only in the presence of ileus, motor weakness, or numbness involving the whole fingers, not just the fingertips.

   ▨ Patients should be treated for a minimum of six cycles, but also until a CR is documented, and then for another two cycles. If tests are equivocal, it is better to treat with additional cycles rather than to prematurely discontinue therapy. However, many clinicians would stop therapy if a PET scan were negative after the sixth cycle.

2. **Classical MOPP therapy.** When MOPP was initially administered in the late 1960s, 81% of patients achieved a CR. Of these patients, 66% (representing 53% of the total series) remained in CR for 5 years, and an identical percentage remained in CR for 10 years. Thus, while late relapses have been seen on occasion, 5-year DFS represents cure for most patients. Because salvage therapy can cure patients who are not cured by initial chemotherapy, the figure of 53% represents a minimal estimate for the cure of advanced HL.

3. **ABVD** was developed by Bonadonna and colleagues in Milan as a nonleukemogenic, nonsterilizing regimen that was not cross-resistant to MOPP. In a large randomized trial, ABVD was shown to be superior to MOPP with respect to remission rates and survival. In a randomized cooperative group clinical trial, reported in 1992, Canellos and associates reported a freedom from progression rate of 61% in patients receiving ABVD; however, more recent studies have shown failure-free survival rates of 75% to 88% using ABVD.

Chemotherapy regimens that alternate cycles of MOPP with cycles of ABVD or which administer the regimens sequentially have been studied in clinical trials. None was superior in efficacy or in toxicity profile to ABVD.

Although some investigators have combined chemotherapy with RT as treatment of advanced disease, there is no evidence that the routine addition of RT to combination chemotherapy can improve results enough to compensate for the leukemogenic risk of that practice. Additionally, while one might consider supplementing combination chemotherapy with local RT to sites of previously bulky disease, if the area in question has become negative by repeat PET scan following the completion of chemotherapy, the logic of that approach is minimal.

Also, as high-intensity therapy in conjunction with stem cell transplantation has been shown to be effective salvage therapy of HL, more intense induction regimens have been studied in HL. Favorable results have been reported by German investigators using BEACOPP (and escalated BEACOPP) and by investigators at Stanford using Stanford V. Doses of these regimens are included in Table 21.3. A recently reported randomized trial demonstrated that Stanford V was equivalent to but not superior to ABVD with respect to DFS and overall survival. The incidence of serious toxicities of the two regimens was similar, though more pulmonary toxicity was seen in patients receiving ABVD and more nonpulmonary toxicity was observed in patients receiving Stanford V. The results of a U.S. cooperative group trial (Eastern Cooperative Oncology Group 2496) comparing Stanford V and ABVD are still pending.

BEACOPP has never been compared directly with ABVD, although it has been shown to be superior to an alternating regimen of cyclophosphamide, prednisone, procarbazine, and vincristine, and ABVD. However, because ABVD is generally regarded as superior to MOPP alternating with ABVD, it is not clear that the excess toxicity of BEACOPP, including sterility, justifies its use as standard chemotherapy in all patients receiving chemotherapy.

In the absence of definitive data that BEACOPP represents a superior therapeutic choice, it has been suggested that chemotherapy for Hodgkin disease should be stratified based on the basis of either risk (baseline prognostic status) or on the early response to therapy. For example, Dann and associates[5] have demonstrated the feasibility of using standard BEACOPP for patients with an IPS of less than 2 and escalated BEACOPP for patients with an IPS of at least 3. Of course this begs the question of whether either BEACOPP regimen is necessary.

A further option is to alter therapy based on the early response to therapy. For example, in the aforementioned BEACOPP/escalated BEACOPP study, patients receiving escalated BEACOPP who became PET-negative after two cycles were switched to standard BEACOPP; patients receiving standard BEACOPP and remaining PET-positive after two cycles were switched to escalated BEACOPP. As yet, there are no data showing the superiority of this approach, but the results of the trial are awaited.

4. **Salvage therapy**. Salvage therapy may produce cures in patients with HL who relapse following initial therapy. However, the chance of curing a patient with relapsed HL is greater if the relapse is nodal than if the relapse is visceral. Additionally, the chance of cure is greater when the initial stage of disease was limited than when the initial stage was advanced.

For the rare patient treated with RT alone who experiences a limited nodal relapse, additional RT may be considered. If the recurrence represents a marginal miss at the edge of a radiation field, this may be feasible. However, if the recurrence is within a treatment field, further irradiation of the area is usually contraindicated and chemotherapy is needed. Furthermore, as fewer patients are treated with RT alone, this option is rarely clinically relevant.

For patients who relapse following chemotherapy, the variable that best predicts the chance of cure is the disease-free interval. The data is clearest for patients treated with MOPP. Among patients initially treated with MOPP therapy, patients whose first CR lasted less than 1 year had a second CR rate of 29%, and only 14% of these second remissions lasted more than 4 years. Among patients whose first CR lasted more than 1 year, 93% achieved a second CR, and 45% of second CRs were projected to last more than 20 years. While the drugs used to obtain the first CR may be successful as salvage therapy, the general trend is to use drugs to which the patient has not been exposed. Thus, for patients treated with MOPP, the ABVD combination is the most commonly used salvage therapy. As ABVD has become the standard therapy, the regimens generally considered as salvage are ifosfamide, carboplatin, and etoposide (known as ICE); etoposide, methylprednisone, cytarabine, and cisplatin (known as ESHAP); and gemcitabine, vinorelbine, and doxorubicin (known as GND; Table 21.4).

However, rather than rely on salvage chemotherapy alone, the more common approach to salvage therapy is to follow a few cycles of salvage chemotherapy with high-dose chemotherapy in conjunction with ABMT or peripheral blood stem cell transplantation (PBSCT).

High-dose therapy in conjunction with ABMT or PBSCT is based on the rationale that bone marrow toxicity limits the dosages of the drugs that are most effective in HL. When autologous marrow or stem cells are stored and reinfused following chemotherapy, drug doses can be escalated to levels that would ordinarily be fatal in the absence of stem cell reinfusion. A number of standard preparative regimens exist for use in conjunction with ABMT and PBSCT, and some of these regimens are presented in Table 21.5.

Controlled trials comparing preparative regimens for autologous transplantation have not been conducted, and in view of the heterogeneity of relapsed patients with respect to prior therapy, sensitivity to therapy, site of relapse, and disease-free interval, it is impossible to compare regimens across studies. Nevertheless, as improvements in supportive

TABLE 21.4 Salvage Regimens in the Treatment of HL

Regimen	Drugs and Dosages
ICE pre–stem cell transplant	Ifosfamide 5000 mg/m^2 IV on day 2 over 24 hours
	Mesna same dose as ifosfamide, continuously with ifosfamide, with an additional dose after ifosfamide
	VP-16 100 mg/m^2 IV on days 1, 2, and 3
	Carboplatin AUC = 5, maximum 800 mg on day 2
ICE in heavily pretreated patients	Ifosfamide 1000 mg/m^2 IV on days 1 and 2 (t = 0 to t = 1 hr)
	Mesna 333 mg/m^2 IV 30 minutes prior to ifosfamide and 4 and 8 hrs after each dose of ifosfamide
	VP-16 150 mg/m^2 IV BID on days 1 and 2
	Carboplatin 200 mg/m^2 IV on days 1 and 2
ESHAP	VP-16 60 mg/m^2 IV daily on days 1–4
	Methylprednisolone 500 mg IV daily on days 1–4
	Cisplatin 25 mg/m^2 IV daily by continuous infusion over 24 hours on days 1–4
	Cytabarine 2000 mg/m^2 IV on day 5

AUC, area under the curve; BID, twice a day; IV, intravenously.

Regimen	Drugs and Dosages

TABLE 21.5 Regimens Used as Preparative Regimens for Autologous Transplantation in HL

Regimen	Drugs and Dosages
CBV	Cyclophosphamide 1800 mg/m^2 IV on days –7, –6, –5, and –4
	Carmustine 600 mg/m^2 IV on day –3
	Etoposide (VP-16) 800 mg/m^2 IV on days –7, –6, and –5
CBV	Cyclophosphamide 1500 mg/m^2 IV on days –5, –4, –3, and –2
	Carmustine 300 mg/m^2 IV on day –5
	Etoposide (VP-16) 300 mg/m^2 IV on days –5, –4, and –3
BEAM	Carmustine 300 mg/m^2 IV on day –6
	Etoposide (VP-16) 100–200 mg/m^2 IV on days –5, –4, –3, and –2
	Cytosine arabinoside 200–400 mg/m^2 IV on days –5, –4, –3, and –2
	Melphalan 140 mg/m^2 IV on day –1

IV, intravenously.
Day 0 is the day of reinfusion of progenitor cells. Therefore, day –5 would be 5 days before reinfusion.

care, such as the use of granulocyte colony-stimulating factor (filgrastim) or granulocyte–macrophage colony-stimulating factor (sargramostim), have lowered treatment-related mortality to approximately 5%, it appears that long-term DFS may occur in approximately 50% of patients treated with ABMT or PBSCT. Patients who achieved long disease-free intervals with standard treatment seem to have the best chance for long-term DFS, and some studies have suggested that good performance status and persistent sensitivity to standard chemotherapy may predict an excellent response to autologous transplantation.

E. **Treatment of symptoms**

Fever, and occasionally pruritis, may be disabling for some patients with HL. The basic approach to these problems is to treat the disease. However, if disease is drug resistant, that approach may be an oversimplification. Indomethacin 25 to 50 mg by mouth twice a day may be helpful in these patients. Anecdotal experience also supports the use of other nonsteroidal anti-inflammatory agents in these patients.

IV. **FOLLOW-UP**

Patients with HL who achieve a CR and who later relapse usually do so at a site of previous disease. Our policy for follow-up is to see the patient every 2 months for the first year, every 3 months for the second year, every 4 months during the third year, every 6 months during the fourth year, and every year thereafter. There is no standard panel of tests for routine follow-up, but our practice is to obtain CT scans or a whole body PET/CT every 6 months for 1 to 2 years, then every year for the next 3 to 4 years. If such tests suggest that disease has recurred, it is advisable to obtain pathologic confirmation before initiating salvage therapy.

Because of the risk of acute leukemia following therapy, we obtain complete blood counts at the time of each visit in patients who have received combination chemotherapy during the previous 8 years. Monitoring for hypothyroidism was discussed in the section on RT. While elevated sedimentation rates and lactic dehydrogenase levels may provide hints of relapse, we have not routinely used these tests for follow-up monitoring in our practice. Because women who receive RT above the diaphragm are at increased risk of breast cancer, we recommend yearly mammograms in these patients starting at age 40 or at 8 years following the completion of RT.

Selected Readings

Andrieu JM, Ifrah N, Payen C, Fermanian J, Coscas Y, Flandrin G. Increased risk of secondary leukemia after extended field radiation combined with MOPP chemotherapy for Hodgkin's disease. *J Clin Oncol.* 1990;8:1148–1154.

Bonadonna G, Zucali R, Monfardini S, et al. Combination chemotherapy of Hodgkin's disease with adriamycin, bleomycin, vinblastine, and imidazole carboxamide versus MOPP. *Cancer.* 1975;36:252–259.

Canellos GP, Anderson JR, Propert KJ, et al. Chemotherapy of advanced Hodgkin's disease with MOPP, ABVD, or MOPP alternating with ABVD. *N Engl J Med.* 1992;327:1478–1484.

Dann EJ, Bar-Shalom R, Tamir A, et al. Risk-adapted BEACOPP regimen can reduce the cumulative dose of chemotherapy for standard and high-risk Hodgkin lymphoma with no impairment of outcome. *Blood.* 2007;109:905–909.

DeVita VT Jr, Serpick AA, Carbone PP. Combination chemotherapy in the treatment of advanced Hodgkin's disease. *Ann Intern Med.* 1970;73:881–895.

Diehl V, Franklin J, Hasenclever D, et al. BEACOPP, a new dose-escalated and accelerated regimen, is at least as effective as COPP/ABVD in patients with advanced stage Hodgkin's lymphoma: interim report from a trial of the German Hodgkin's Lymphoma Study Group. *J Clin Oncol.* 1998;16:3810–3821.

Diehl V, Franklin J, Pfreundschuh M, et al. Standard and increased dose BEACOPP chemotherapy compared with COPP-ABVD for advanced Hodgkin's disease. *N Engl J Med.* 2003;348:2386–2395.

Gallamini A, Hutchings M, Rigacci L, et al. Early interim 2-[^{18}F]Fluoro-2-deoxy-D-glucose positron emission tomography is prognostically superior to International Prognostic Score in advanced stage Hodgkin's lymphoma: a report from a joint Italian-Danish Study. *J Clin Oncol.* 2007;25:3746–3752.

Glick JH, Young ML, Harrington D, et al. MOPP/ABV hybrid chemotherapy for advanced Hodgkin's disease significantly improves failure-free and overall survival: the 8-year results of the intergroup trial. *J Clin Oncol.* 1998;16:19–26.

Hancock SL, Cox RS, McDougall IR. Thyroid diseases after treatment of Hodgkin's disease. *N Engl J Med.* 1991;325:599–605.

Hasenclever D, Diehl V. A prognostic score for advanced Hodgkin's disease. *N Engl J Med.* 1998;339:1506–1514.

Horning SJ, Williams J, Bartlett NL, et al. Assessment of the Stanford V regimen and consolidative radiotherapy for bulky and advanced Hodgkin's disease: Eastern Cooperative Oncology Group pilot study E1492. *J Clin Oncol.* 2000;18:972–980.

Hoskin PJ, Lowry L, Horwich A, et al. Randomized comparison of the Stanford V regimen and ABVD in the treatment of advanced Hodkin's lymphoma: United Kingdom National Cancer Research Institute Lymphoma Group Study ISRCTN 64141244. *J Clin Oncol.* 2009;27:5390–5396.

Klimo P, Connors JM. An update on the Vancouver experience in the management of advanced Hodgkin's disease treated with MOPP/ABV hybrid regimen. *Semin Hematol.* 1988;25(suppl 2):34–40.

Lister TA, Crowther D. Staging for Hodgkin's disease. *Semin Oncol.* 1990;17:696.

Longo DL, Duffey PL, Young RC, et al. Conventional-dose salvage combination chemotherapy in patients relapsing with Hodgkin's disease after combination chemotherapy: the low probability of cure. *J Clin Oncol.* 1992;10:210–218.

Salzman JR, Kaplan HS. Effect of prior splenectomy on hematologic tolerance during total lymphoid radiotherapy of patients with Hodgkin's disease. *Cancer.* 1972;27:472.

Specht L, Gray RG, Clarke MJ, et al. Influence of more extensive radiotherapy and adjuvant chemotherapy on long-term outcome of early stage Hodgkin's disease: a meta-analysis of 23 randomized trials involving 3,888 patients. International Hodgkin's Disease Collaborative Group. *J Clin Oncol.* 1998;16:830–848.

Stein S, Golomb HM, Wiernik PH, et al. Anatomic substages of stage IIIA Hodgkin's disease. *Cancer Treat Rep.* 1982;66:733–741.

Vose JM, Bierman PJ, Armitage JO. Hodgkin's disease: the role of bone marrow transplantation. *Semin Oncol.* 1990;17:749–757.

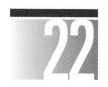

Non-Hodgkin Lymphoma
Mark Roschewski and Wyndham H. Wilson

I. INTRODUCTION

Non-Hodgkin lymphomas (NHLs) are a heterogeneous group of malignant neoplasms in which lymphocytes—either of B-cell, T-cell, or natural killer (NK)–cell origin—have arrested at various stages of differentiation, have acquired the ability to clonally proliferate, and do not undergo apoptosis in a typical fashion. Tremendous variation exists in their molecular profiles, mode of presentation, natural history, and response to therapy. Tumor clonality is established by demonstrating immunoglobulin (Ig) gene rearrangement in B-cells, T-cell receptor rearrangement in T-cells, or more sophisticated methods such as the finding of a reciprocal cytogenetic translocation or molecular rearrangements by fluorescent in situ hybridization or polymerase chain reaction (PCR). The malignant clone most commonly proliferates within the lymphatic system, spleen, and bone marrow, but it can also occur in almost any extranodal site such as the bones, central nervous system (CNS), gastrointestinal tract, and the skin. The inciting events in NHL are multifactorial and result from a combination of alterations in antitumor immunity, changes in the local microenvironment of the tumor, and occasionally antigen selection with certain lymphomas now having established relationships with both viral and bacterial pathogens. Still, although advances in molecular medicine have provided exciting insights into the biology of NHL, the full characterization of lymphomagenesis is not complete, and the precise etiology of most cases of NHL is considered unknown.

II. EPIDEMIOLOGY AND RISK FACTORS OF NHL

A. Epidemiology

NHL is the most common hematologic malignancy in the United States, with an estimated 65,540 cases of NHL in the United States in 2010 (35,380 male and 30,160 female) and approximately 20,210 people dying of the disease. It accounts for 4% to 5% of new cases of cancer as well as 3% to 4% of cancer-related deaths. NHL is the sixth most common cause of cancer in both men and women but shows a male predominance in almost all subtypes. From the early 1970s to the 1990s, the incidence of NHL in the United States had been increasing steadily at a compound rate of about 4% in a fashion that prompted some to describe it as an epidemic, but the incidence since 1991 has been stable for men and slowed to an annual rise of 1.1% for women. Death rates from NHL no longer continue to rise and have actually been decreasing by 3.0% in men and 3.7% in women. The 1-year survival rates for all subtypes of NHL are 80%, but drop to 56% at 10 years. B-cell lymphomas represent about 80% to 85% of all cases, with T-cell lymphomas being represented in the other 15% to 20% of cases and NK-cell lymphomas extremely rare. Even though NHL can affect persons of any age, including children, the incidence of NHL clearly increases steadily from childhood through the age of 80 years. Much of the increase in incidence has been in patients in their sixth and seventh decade of life, and the median age of individuals with NHL has correspondingly risen with the incidence; the median age of patients at the time of diagnosis of NHL is currently between 60 and 65 years of age, which has implications regarding therapeutic decisions.

NHL is also increasing in incidence worldwide, and some geographical distribution exists in certain subtypes of NHL (Table 22.1). Overall, the highest reported incidence rates are in the United States, Europe, and Australia, with the lowest rates reported

TABLE 22.1 Geographical Distribution of Certain NHLs	
Lymphoma	**Distribution**
Adult T-cell lymphocytic leukemia	Caribbean, Southern Japan, Africa
Angioimmunoblastic T-cell lymphoma	Europe > North America
Burkitt lymphoma (endemic form)	Children in equatorial Africa
Gastric lymphoma	Northern Italy
T-/NK cell lymphomas, nasal-type	China, Native Americans
Small intestinal lymphomas	Middle East

NHL, non-Hodgkin lymphoma; NK, natural killer.

in Asia. Ethnicity does not seem to directly correlate with risks of developing NHL, but there does seem to be some disparity in outcomes after treatment that is related to a patient's socioeconomic status. For example, shorter survival has been associated with low socioeconomic status among elderly patients with follicular lymphoma, but this relationship has yet to be demonstrated in younger patients with NHL. Whether this disparity in outcome represents poorer access to care, true ethnic differences to therapy, or differences in tumor biology are not yet defined.

B. Risk factors

The increase in diagnoses of NHL in the 1970s to 1990s was due, in part, to the improvement in diagnostic techniques, but another reason was the increase in cases of HIV and AIDS over the same period of time. Many additional factors have also contributed to the incidence in NHL and are listed in Table 22.2. The mode of

TABLE 22.2 Factors Associated With an Increased Risk of NHL
Immunosuppression
Congenital immunodeficiency syndromes
Male gender
Increasing age
Family history of NHL
Drugs
Immunosuppressive agents
Phenytoin
Methotrexate
Tumor necrosis factor inhibitors
Occupational exposures
Exposure to herbicides, pesticides, wood dust, epoxy glue, solvents
Farming, forestry, painting, carpentry, tanning

NHL, non-Hodgkin lymphoma.

presentation of NHL may differ based on geography, with extra-nodal presentations occurring in only 15% to 25% of adult cases in the United States but in higher percentages in Europe and the Far East. Familial aggregation of NHL plays only a small role in the rise with a two- to fourfold increased risk for NHL in close relatives of patients with lymphoma or other hematopoietic neoplasms. Lymphomagenesis and the study of its inciting events has best been studied in patients with underlying immunodeficiency states. These conditions can be divided into congenital (or primary) immunodeficiencies and acquired (or secondary) immunodeficiencies (Table 22.3). Common components to all of these disorders are defects in immunoregulation, particularly in T-cell immunity, resulting in unregulated B-cell proliferation in lymphoid tissue, often in association with chronic exposures to antigens such as the Epstein-Barr virus (EBV) genome. Chronic inflammation, immune hyperactivity, and immune dysregulation are all elements of autoimmune disorders that predispose patients to lymphoma. Most NHLs that occur in association with immune suppression are B-cell lymphomas, with the exception of the increased risk of T-cell lymphoma seen in ataxia telangiectasia and a small percentage of posttransplant lymphoproliferative disorders (PTLDs), which are of T-cell origin. Rare, extranodal T-cell lymphomas, such as enteropathy-associated T-cell lymphoma (EATCL), will occur in the setting of celiac sprue, and hepatosplenic T-cell lymphoma (HSTCL) typically occurs in patients with a history of solid organ transplantation, inflammatory bowel disease, systemic lupus, Hodgkin lymphoma, and malarial infection.

TABLE 22.3   Conditions That Predispose to NHL

Congenital	Acquired
Ataxia telangiectasia	Solid organ transplantation
Wiskott-Aldrich syndrome	Stem cell transplantation (higher if T-cell depleted)
	Acquired immunodeficiency syndrome
Severe combined immunodeficiency	Sjögren syndrome
Common variable immunodeficiency	Rheumatoid arthritis
Hyper immunoglobulin M (Job syndrome)	Hashimoto thyroiditis
X-linked hypogammaglobulinemia	Inflammatory bowel disease
X-linked lymphoproliferative syndrome	Celiac sprue
Autoimmune lymphoproliferative syndrome	Malarial infection
	Hodgkin lymphoma

In addition to HIV, other viruses have specific clinical associations with subtypes of NHL (Table 22.4). Chronic hepatitis C infection is often associated with an underlying indolent B-cell lymphoma, and *Helicobacter pylori* infection can be demonstrated in over 90% of cases of low grade B-cell lymphoma of mucosa-associated lymphoid tissue (MALT) of the stomach. In some cases of antigen-associated lymphomas, eradication of the infectious agent has resulted in partial or complete remission (CR) of the lymphoma.

III. PATHOLOGIC CLASSIFICATION OF NHL

The classification systems for lymphomas have changed dramatically and frequently since they were first introduced in the 1950s and have been a source of tremendous confusion to clinicians and controversy among hematopathologists. Even the distinction between "lymphoma" and "leukemia" has been a source of potential confusion as many entities cannot be exclusively categorized. In general, if the site of origin is the bone marrow, the disorder may be classified as a form of lymphocytic leukemia, but when disease is present in both nodes and marrow, the distinction between leukemia and lymphoma is somewhat arbitrary. In view of its clinical diversity, accurate classification of NHL is essential for scientific and clinical purposes.

TABLE 22.4 Infectious Agents Associated With NHL

Infectious Agent	Lymphoma
EBV	Burkitt lymphoma, EBV$^+$ DLBCL of the elderly, extranodal NK/T-cell lymphoma, lymphomatoid granulomatosis, PTLD, systemic EBV$^+$ T-cell lymphoproliferative disorder of childhood, hydroa vacciniforme-like T-cell lymphoma
Human T-cell lymphotropic virus type I	ATLL
Helicobacter pylori	Gastric MALT
Hepatitis C	Splenic marginal zone lymphoma; lymphoplasmacytic lymphoma, nodal marginal zone lymphoma, DLBCL
Human herpesvirus 8	Primary effusion lymphoma, plasmablastic lymphoma
Human immunodeficiency virus	DLBCL, Burkitt lymphoma, PCNSL, primary effusion lymphoma, plasmablastic lymphoma
Borrelia burgdorferi	Cutaneous B-cell lymphoma
Chlamydia psittaci	Ocular adnexal MALT
Chlamydia trachomatis	
Chlamydia pneumoniae	
Campylobacter jejuni	Small intestine MALT

ATLL, adult T-cell leukemia/lymphoma; DLBCL, diffuse large B-cell lymphoma; EBV, Epstein-Barr virus; MALT, mucosa-associated lymphoid tissue; NK, natural killer; PCNSL, primary central nervous system lymphoma; PTLD, posttransplant lymphoproliferative disorder.

Ideally, a classification system should identify types of NHL that are scientifically and clinically meaningful as well as those that are relatively homogeneous from a clinical, morphologic, immunologic, and genetic point of view. The systems have evolved along with available technology and scientific discovery from ones that rely heavily on morphologic descriptions to the current working system that incorporates morphology, immunophenotypic characteristics based on both immunohistochemistry and flow cytometry (Tables 22.5 and 22.6), cytogenetic and molecular abnormalities (Tables 22.7 and 22.8), and even clinical variables.

In 1956, Henry Rappaport of the U.S. Armed Forces Institute of Pathology proposed a very simple and reproducible classification system based on the growth pattern of the disease (nodular versus diffuse) as well as the appearance of the predominant cell as well-differentiated, poorly differentiated, undifferentiated, or histiocytic. This was followed in the 1970s by the Lukes-Colins-Lennert classification system that related morphology to lymphocyte lineage by dividing entities into B-cell and T-cell disorders based on their cell surface markers; however, they still did not address clinical concerns and were not uniformly utilized internationally.

In the 1980s, the New Working Formulation defined broad categories of lymphoma based on general clinical prognosis of either low-grade, intermediate-grade, or high-grade in order to assist the clinician in treating the lymphoma. The system, however, did not include information regarding immunophenotype, and therefore was difficult to reproduce and did not foster recognition of new entities.

In 1994, the International Lymphoma Study Group developed a consensus list of diseases that could be recognized by pathologists and that appeared to be distinct clinical entities called the Revised European–American Classification of Lymphoid Neoplasms classification system, which ultimately became the World Health Organization (WHO) classification system: the first international consensus on the classification of hematologic malignancies. The original classification system, published in 2001, defined diseases by four features: morphology, immunophenotype, genetics, and clinical information. The updated 2008 version (Table 22.9) increases the use of both molecular profiles and clinical presentations to define separate clinicopathologic entities.

Gene expression profiling (GEP) is a powerful new technique that allows assessment of the expression of thousands of genes simultaneously on a solid platform. Once this ability to measure gene expression patterns in lymphomas became available, it has become increasingly apparent that the clinical behavior of lymphoid neoplasms is driven by their molecular makeup. The importance of underlying molecular definitions of entities is apparent in the updated

TABLE 22.5 Immunophenotype of Common Mature B-Cell Neoplasms (All CD20+)*

Histology	SIg	CIg	CD 5	CD 10	CD 23	CD 43	CD 103	BCL6	MUM1	Cyclin D1
CLL/SLL	+	-/+	+	-	+	+	-	-	+ (PC)	-
LPL	+/-	+	-	-	-	-/+	-	-	+	-
Splenic marginal zone	+	-/+	-	-	-	-	-	-	-	-
Hairy cell leukemia	+	-	-	-	-	-	+	-	-	+/-
MALT lymphoma	+	+/-	-	-	-/+	-/+	-	-	+	-
Follicular lymphoma	+	-	-	+/-	-/+	-	-	+	-/+	-
Mantle cell lymphoma	+	-	+	-	NA	+	-	-	-	+
DLBCL	+/-	-/+	-	-/+	NA	-/+	NA	+/-	+/-	-
Burkitt lymphoma	+	-	-	+	-	+/-	NA	+	-/+	-

CLL, chronic lymphocytic leukemia; DLBCL, diffuse large B-cell lymphoma; LPL, lymphoplasmacytoid lymphoma; MALT, mucosa-associated lymphoid tissue; NA, not applicable; SLL, small lymphocytic lymphoma.
*These are not absolute, and individual cases can vary slightly.

TABLE 22.6 Immunophenotypic Features of Common Mature T-Cell and NK-Cell Neoplasms*

Histology	CD 3	4	8	7	5	2	30	25	56	EBV
T-cell PLL	+	+	+/−	+	+	+	−	−	−	−
T-cell LGL	+	−	+	−/+	−/+	+	−/+	++	−	−
ATLL	+	+	−	−	+	+	−/+	++	−	+
Aggressive NK-cell	+C	−	−/+	−	−	+	−	−	+	+
Extranodal NK-/T-cell	+C	−	−/+	−	−	+	−	−	+	+
Enteropathy-associated T-cell	+	−	−/+	+	−	+	−/+	−/+	−/+	−
Hepatosplenic T-cell	+	−	+/−	+	−	+	−	−	+	−
SPTCL	+	−	+	+	−/+	+	−	−	+	−
MF/SS	+	+	−/+	−/+	+/−	+	−	−	−	−
Primary cutaneous γδ	+	−	−/+	−/+	−	+	−	+	+	−
Primary cutaneous CD30+	+	+	−/+	−	+/−	+	+	+	−	−
AITL	+	+	−	+	+	+	−	−	−	−
PTCL-NOS	−/+	+/−	−/+	−/+	−/+	+	−/+	−	−	−
ALCL, ALK+	−/+	+/−	−/+	−/+	+/−	+/−	++	++	+/−	−
ALCL, ALK−	+/−	+/−	−/+	−/+	+/−	+/−	++	++	+/−	−

AITL, angioimmunoblastic T-cell lymphoma; ALCL, anaplastic large cell lymphoma; ATLL, adult T-cell leukemia/lymphoma; C, cytoplasmic only; EBV, Epstein-Barr virus; LGL, large granular lymphocytic; MF/SS, mycosis fungoides/Sézary syndrome; NK, natural killer; NOS, not otherwise specified; PLL, prolymphocytic leukemia; PTCL, peripheral T-cell lymphoma; SPTCL, subcutaneous panniculitis-like T-cell lymphoma.
*These are not absolute and individual cases can vary slightly.

Histology	Cytogenetics	Oncogene/ Protein	Immunoglobulin Gene Rearrangements	
			Heavy	κ λ
SLL*	t(14; 19) Trisomy 12, 13q	Bcl-3	+	+
Lymphoplasmacytoid lymphoma			+	+
Follicular center cell grade I and II	t(14; 18)	Bcl-2	+	
Marginal zone†	Trisomy 3 t(11; 18)		+	
Mantle cell lymphoma	t(11; 14)	Cyclin-D1	+	
Follicular center cell grade III‡	t(14; 18)	Bcl-2	+	
Large B-cell**	t(3;14)(q27;q32)	Bcl-6 Bcl-2		+
Primary mediastinal (thymic) large B-cell			+	+
Lymphoblastic lymphoma/ leukemia			+	+/−
Burkitt lymphoma	t(8; 14)(q24;q32)	c-myc	+	
	t(2; 8)(11p; q24)			λ +
	t(8; 22)(q24;q11)			κ +

DLBCL, diffuse large B-cell lymphoma; NHL, non-Hodgkin lymphoma; SLL, small lymphocytic lymphoma.
*Trisomy 12 is seen in 30% of cases and abnormalities in 13q are present in 25% of patients.
†Cytogenetic abnormalities have been seen in extranodal marginal zone NHL.
‡t(14; 18) is present in 75% to 95% of follicular center cell NHL.
**Bcl-2 rearrangements occur in up to 30% and Bcl-6 in up to 45% of cases of DLBCL.

WHO 2008 classification system. Newly recognized entities in the WHO 2008 classification system include "grey-zone" lymphomas, which are intermediate between two types of lymphomas. The inclusion of these entities demonstrates that, in some cases, the ability to distinguish between lymphomas requires an understanding of their complete genetic makeup and cannot easily be separated based on clinical data, morphology, immunophenotypic profile, or even cytogenetics alone.

IV. STAGING AND PROGNOSIS OF NHL

A. Making the diagnosis

One of the most critical, yet often overlooked, aspects surrounding prediction of the prognosis in NHLs is ensuring the accuracy of

22.8 Molecular Characteristics of T-Cell Lymphomas

Histology	Cytogenetics	Oncogene	TCR Gene Rearrangements
T-CLL/T-PLL	Inv14(q11; q32), Trisomy 8q	Bcl-3	+
Mycosis fungoides			+
Peripheral T-cell lymphoma			+/−
Angioimmunoblastic	Trisomy 3, 5 EBV+		+
ATLL	HTLV I integration+		+
Enteropathy T-cell	EBV−		β +
Hepatosplenic γ/δ			δγ+
ALCL	t(2;5)	Alk+	+
Precursor T-cell lymphoblastic lymphoma/leukemia	Variable T(7;9)	Tcl-4	Variable

ALCL, anaplastic large cell lymphoma; ATLL, adult T-cell leukemia/lymphoma; CLL, chronic lymphocytic leukemia; EBV, Epstein-Barr virus; HTLV, human T-lymphotropic virus; PLL, prolymphocytic leukemia.

the pathologic diagnosis. This starts with the appropriateness of the original biopsy procurement procedure, adequacy of the tissue specimen, and the selection of a representative site. In general, fine needle aspiration is not sufficient to accurately classify NHLs given the multiple tests required to accurately classify them. Great preference is placed on excisional lymph node biopsies in order to preserve nodal architecture, while multiple core needle biopsies will suffice in situations where involved nodes are not easily accessible. One should have a low threshold for considering rebiopsy in circumstances where the original biopsy is nondiagnostic or any level of uncertainty remains. Diagnoses made from referring centers are concordant with academic medical centers in almost 95% of cases, but when T-cell lymphomas are suspected, expertise is essential as the discordant rate can be as high as 15%.

B. Ann Arbor staging

1. **Recommended workup and imaging.** Determining the true extent of disease prior to initiating therapy is important both for determining the treatment plan as well as predicting the likelihood of achieving a complete response to therapy. The staging evaluation of the patient with NHL begins with a history focused on the pace of the disease at presentation, the presence or absence of B symptoms (fevers, chills, drenching night sweats), possible sites of nodal and extranodal involvement, and signs suggestive of a possible underlying immunodeficiency. When performing the physical examination, special care must be

TABLE 22.9 WHO 2008 Classification of Lymphoid Neoplasms

Precursor Lymphoid Neoplasms
B lymphoblastic leukemia/lymphoma NOS
B lymphoblastic leukemia/lymphoma with recurrent genetic abnormalities
- t(9:22)(q34;q11.2); BCR-ABL1
- t(v;11q23); MLL rearranged
- t(12:21)(p13;q22); TEL-AML1 (ETV6-RUNX1)
- With hyperdiploidy
- With hypodiploidy
- t(5:14)(q31;q32); IL3-IGH
- t(1:19)(q23;p13.3); E2A-PBX1(TCF3-PBX1)
T lymphoblastic leukemia/lymphoma

Mature B-Cell Neoplasms
Small lymphocytic lymphoma/chronic lymphocytic leukemia
B-cell prolymphocytic leukemia
Splenic B-cell marginal zone lymphoma
Hairy cell leukemia
Splenic B-cell lymphoma/leukemia, unclassifiable
- Splenic diffuse red pulp small B-cell lymphoma
- Hairy cell leukemia-variant
Lymphoplasmacytic lymphoma
Heavy chain diseases
- Gamma heavy chain disease
- Mu heavy chain disease
- Alpha heavy chain disease
Plasma cell neoplasms
- Monoclonal gammopathy of undetermined significance
- Plasma cell myeloma
- Solitary plasmacytoma of bone
- Extraosseous plasmacytoma
- Monoclonal immunoglobulin deposition diseases
Extranodal marginal zone B-cell lymphoma of mucosa-associated lymphoid tissue
Nodal marginal zone B-cell lymphoma
Follicular lymphoma
Primary cutaneous follicle center lymphoma
Mantle cell lymphoma
DLBCL, NOS
- T-cell/histiocyte-rich large B-cell lymphoma
- Primary DLBCL of the CNS
- Primary cutaneous DLBCL, leg type
- EBV-positive DLBCL of the elderly
DLBCL associated with chronic inflammation
Lymphomatoid granulomatosis
Primary mediastinal (thymic) large B-cell lymphoma
Intravascular large B-cell lymphoma
ALK+ large B-cell lymphoma

(continued)

Plasmablastic lymphoma
Large B-cell lymphoma arising in HHV8-associated multicentric Castleman disease
Primary effusion lymphoma
Burkitt lymphoma
B-cell lymphoma, unclassifiable, with features intermediate between DLBCL and Burkitt lymphoma
B-cell lymphoma, unclassifiable, with features intermediate between DLBCL and classical Hodgkin lymphoma

Mature T- and NK-Cell Neoplasms
T-cell prolymphocytic leukemia
T-cell large granular lymphocyte leukemia
Chronic lymphoproliferative disorder of NK cells
Aggressive NK-cell leukemia
EBV-positive T-cell lymphoproliferative diseases of childhood
■ Systemic EBV+ T-cell lymphoproliferative disease of childhood
■ Hydroa vacciniforme-like lymphoma
Adult T-cell lymphoma/leukemia
Extranodal NK-/T-cell lymphoma nasal type
Enteropathy-associated T-cell lymphoma
Hepatosplenic T-cell lymphoma
Subcutaneous panniculitis-like T-cell lymphoma
Mycosis fungoides (cutaneous T-cell lymphoma)
Sézary syndrome
Primary cutaneous CD30-positive T-cell lymphoproliferative disorders
Primary cutaneous peripheral T-cell lymphomas, rare subtypes
■ Primary cutaneous gamma-delta T-cell lymphoma
■ Primary cutaneous CD8-positive aggressive epidermotropic cytotoxic T-cell lymphoma
■ Primary cutaneous CD4-positive small/medium T-cell lymphoma
Peripheral T-cell lymphoma, NOS
Angioimmunoblastic T-cell lymphoma
Anaplastic large-cell lymphoma, ALK+
Anaplastic large-cell lymphoma, ALK−

Immunodeficiency-Associated Lymphoproliferative Disorders
Lymphoproliferative diseases associated with primary immune disorders
Lymphomas associated with HIV infection
PTLD
■ Plasmacytic hyperplasia and infectious-mononucleosis–like PTLD
■ Polymorphic PTLD
■ Monomorphic PTLD
■ Classical Hodgkin lymphoma–type PTLD
Other iatrogenic immunodeficiency-associated lymphoproliferative disorders

CNS, central nervous system; DLBCL, diffuse large B-cell lymphoma; EBV, Epstein-Barr virus; HHV8, human herpesvirus 8; HIV, human immunodeficiency virus; NK, natural killer; NOS, not otherwise specified; PTLD, posttransplant lymphoproliferative disorder; WHO, World Health Organization.

given to examining the Waldeyer ring, epitrochlear nodes, and popliteal nodes, which may be difficult to measure on radiographic imaging, as well as examining for sites of extranodal involvement such as the skin and abdomen for signs of hepatosplenomegaly. Recommended tests that supplement the history and physical examination at the time of diagnosis are listed in Table 22.10.

The Cotswold modification of the Ann Arbor classification is generally used to stage patients with newly diagnosed NHL and is shown in Table 22.11. Anatomic-based imaging such as contrast-enhanced computed tomography (CT) scans (or magnetic resonance imaging for patients with contrast allergies) are the gold standard for determining which nodal chains are involved with lymphoma. Lymph nodes are considered involved if the long axis is $\geq$1.5 cm (regardless of short axis) or if the long axis is $\geq$1.1 cm and the short axis is >1.0 cm. Lymph nodes that are $\leq$1.0 cm in both axes are considered uninvolved. Determining the stage of lymphomatous involvement based on anatomic imaging alone misses nodes that are involved but not enlarged and can easily miss extranodal sites of disease such as bony involvement which may affect treatment recommendations. Accurate assessment of disease involvement is not only essential at baseline but also when evaluating the response at the end of treatment; functional imaging such as positron emission tomography (PET) scans can greatly aid in this matter.

TABLE 22.10	Recommended Workup of Newly Diagnosed NHL

- Adequate biopsy specimen with tissue sent for flow cytometry and molecular studies
- Complete blood count
- Lactate dehydrogenase
- Comprehensive metabolic panel
- Uric acid
- Beta-2 microglobulin
- Human immunodeficiency virus
- Hepatitis B surface antigen
- Chest-abdominal-pelvic CT with contrast
- ^{18}Fluoro-2-deoxy-D-glucose PET/CT scan
- Lumbar puncture with flow cytometry of cerebrospinal fluid
- Unilateral (or bilateral) bone marrow biopsy with aspirate
- Assessment of ejection fraction with multigated acquisition scan or echocardiogram
- Pregnancy testing in women
- Discussion of fertility issues

CT, computed tomography; NHL, non-Hodgkin lymphoma; PET, positron emission tomography.

TABLE 22.11	Staging System for NHL

Ann Arbor Staging Classification for NHLs

Stage	Description
I	Involvement of a single lymph node region (I) or involvement of a single extralymphatic organ or site (IE)
II	Involvement of two or more lymph node regions or lymphatic structures on the same side of the diaphragm alone (II) or with involvement of limited, contiguous extralymphatic organ or tissue (IIE)
III	Involvement of lymph node regions on both sides of the diaphragm (III) which may include the spleen (IIIS) or limited, contiguous extralymphatic organ or site (IIIE) or both (IIIES)
IV	Diffuse or disseminated foci of involvement of one or more extralymphatic organs or tissues, with or without associated lymphatic involvement
A	Asymptomatic
B	Unexplained persistent or recurrent fever with temperature higher than 38°C or recurrent drenching night sweats within 1 month or unexplained loss of more than 10% body weight within 6 months
E	Limited direct extension into extralymphatic organ from adjacent lymph node
X	Bulky disease (mediastinal tumor width greater than one-third transthoracic diameter at T5-T6 or tumor diameter larger than 10 cm)

NHL, non-Hodgkin lymphoma.

2. PET/CT imaging. [18]Fluorodeoxyglucose (FDG)-PET scans and PET/CT scans exploit the enhanced rate of glucose utilization (both uptake and phosphorylation) seen in many tumor cells as compared to normal surrounding cells (the Warburg effect). Thus, [18]FDG-PET scans can provide a semiquantitative measurement of tumor involvement in NHLs, which has proven to have superior sensitivity compared to anatomic imaging alone.

PET/CT scans are not without drawbacks, however, as [18]FDG uptake in tumor cells and the subsequent appearance on PET scan is dependent on a number of variables related to the tumor such as blood flow, glucose transporters, tumor cell number, and tumor proliferation, but also related to nontumor variables such as the fat content of the patient, technicalities regarding the procurement of the images, resolution of the scanner, and clinician interpretation. Nonetheless, PET scans and PET/CT scans have essentially become the standard of care in the United States for aiding in the initial evaluation and staging of patients with newly diagnosed aggressive lymphomas. It is estimated that using PET/CT at diagnosis will "upstage" about 15% to 20% of patients with NHL, but the impact of this on treatment options or ultimate outcomes has not yet been elucidated.

C. International Prognostic Index (IPI)

The prognosis of patients with newly diagnosed NHL is clearly related to more than just Ann Arbor staging, and it is standard practice to determine the IPI at diagnosis in patients with intermediate-grade lymphoma such as diffuse large B-cell lymphoma (DLBCL). The IPI score accurately stratifies patients into quartiles with differing probabilities of both complete response as well as 5-year disease-free survival (DFS) in DLBCL based on the age, stage, performance status, number of extranodal sites of disease, and lactate dehydrogenase (LDH) level. For all patients, 5-year survival was 73% for low-risk patients, 51% for low/intermediate-risk patients, 43% for high/intermediate-risk patients, and 26% for high-risk patients (Table 22.12). For patients under the age of 60 years, a slightly modified age-adjusted prognostic system was developed in which the 5-year survival was 83% for low-risk patients, 69% for low/intermediate-risk patients, 46% for high/intermediate-risk patients, and 32% for high-risk patients (Table 22.13).

D. Gene expression profiling (GEP) as prognostic marker

As opposed to clinical variables that may be dominated by extent of disease burden, there has been great interest in attempting to define and predict the clinical behavior of lymphomas based on the expression of genes on tissue microarray. With the advent of GEP,

TABLE 22.12 International Prognostic Index for NHL

Risk Factors	Definition		Risk Category	Number of Risk Factors
Age	>60 years		Low	0–1
LDH	>1 X normal	Predictive Model	Low Intermediate	2
ECOG Performance Status	>1	Aggressive NHL	High Intermediate	3
Stage	III/IV		High	4–5
Extranodal sites	>1			

Risk Category	% Cases	CR	Five-year DFS of CR	Overall Survival*
Low	35	87%	70%	73%
Low/intermediate	27	67%	51%	51%
High/intermediate	22	55%	49%	43%
High	16	44%	42%	26%

CR, complete remission; DFS, disease-free survival; ECOG, Eastern Cooperative Oncology Group; NHL, non-Hodgkin lymphoma.
*Histologies: Diffuse mixed, diffuse large, and immunoblastic.

	TABLE 22.13	Age-Adjusted International Prognostic Index for DLBCL*

Patients aged <60 years	0 points	1 point
Stage	I or II	III or IV
Performance status	0 or 1	≥2
Lactate dehydrogenase	Normal	Elevated

DLBCL, diffuse large B-cell lymphoma.
*Risk category: Low risk, 0 points; low/intermediate risk, 1 point; high/intermediate risk, 2 points; high risk, 3 points.

which can simultaneously analyze the overexpression or underexpression of thousands of genes at one time on an individual's tissue sample, it has become possible to predict outcomes based on the molecular profile of the tissue. The best example of this exists in DLBCL, which can be subdivided into three categorical subtypes: germinal center B-cell (GCB) subtype, activated B-cell (ABC) subtype, and primary mediastinal B-cell lymphoma (PMBL). All three of these subtypes have a widely different prognosis (independent of IPI score), with the GCB subtype responding more favorably to standard chemotherapy regimens than the ABC subtype and the mediastinal B subtype with the best overall prognosis (59%, 30%, and 64% 5-year survivals, respectively).

E. Functional biomarkers

In addition to providing a tool for staging patients, [18]FDG-PET scanning also has the potential to serve as an interim functional biomarker during therapy for aggressive lymphomas to predict which patients are responding to therapy and which ones are likely to be refractory. A risk-adapted approach such as that based on interim PET scanning is based on the principle that even though many patients are cured of their lymphoma, a significant minority will be resistant to chemotherapy. Early identification of the patients who will ultimately be failed by their chemotherapy may allow for a change in treatment. Changes suggestive of treatment response occur much earlier in functional imaging than anatomic imaging and this strategy has prompted research into its use. Unfortunately, the promise of this risk-adapted approach is still a research question as the current positive predictive value of [18]FDG-PET scanning is suboptimal. Patients who have a negative PET, however, after only one or two cycles of chemotherapy have a much more favorable prognosis than their counterparts.

V. MANAGEMENT OF INDOLENT NHL

Indolent lymphoma is a term used to describe the natural history of NHLs that frequently are managed with low-intensity strategies at the time of diagnosis as they may not cause direct symptoms to patients for months or even years. They should not be considered "good lymphomas," however, because the majority of patients ultimately die of their cancer. Indolent NHLs are generally considered incurable with conventional chemoimmunotherapy strategies. Of particular concern is the fact that indolent lymphomas maintain a perpetual risk of transformation into a more aggressive lymphoma; no reliable predictive variables exist to identify the patients at risk for such transformation. The second most frequent subtype of NHL overall (~20%) and prototypical indolent lymphoma specifically is follicular lymphoma (FL). The principles applied to the diagnosis and management of FL can be applied to most other indolent NHLs. Small lymphocytic lymphoma (SLL) is now known to be biologically identical to chronic lymphocytic leukemia (CLL) and is defined by the lack of a leukemic component. CLL/SLL has unique properties which necessitate that it be considered separately from NHL.

A. **Follicular lymphoma (FL) pathology**

FL is characterized by the translocation t(14;18), which places the BCL2 oncogene under the control of the Ig H enhancer, leading to dysregulated and impaired apoptosis. Histologically, two principal cells exist in the normal follicle center (germinal center): the centrocyte (small cleaved cell) and the centroblast (large noncleaved cells). In the 2008 WHO classification of FL, a grading system exists by which one can categorize FL into grades I to IIIa-b based on the ratio of centroblasts/centrocytes. Grade 3b FL (sheets of centroblasts) is clinically indistinguishable from DLBCL and is commonly treated with algorithms appropriate for intermediate-grade NHLs whereas grades 1 to 3a are considered truly indolent NHLs.

B. **Prognostic scoring systems for FL**

FL is typically a widespread disease at presentation that frequently involves multiple nodal chains and the bone marrow, even in cases in which the natural history of the tumor growth will be slow. Also, it is common for patients to experience no symptoms attributable to the disease despite the widespread amount of tumor burden. Thus, prognostic scoring models have been developed to help predict the course of disease.

On the basis of multivariate analysis collected on over 4000 patients and ultimately validated on almost 1000 patients, a five-variable prognostic index was constructed: the Follicular Lymphoma International Prognostic Index (FLIPI; Table 22.14). The scoring system was found to discriminate outcomes better than the IPI, and it does separate patients into three risk groups with variable 5-year overall survival (OS) rates, but it is based on a cumbersome method of determining the number of nodal sites involved (Groupe d'Etude des Lymphomes Folliculaires criteria) and predated the use of the monoclonal anti-CD20 therapy rituximab,

Follicular Lymphoma International Prognostic Index (FLIPI)

Score one point for each factor:
Age ≥60 years
Ann Arbor stage III–IV
Hemoglobin level <12 g/dL
Serum lactate dehydrogenase level > upper limit of normal
Number of nodal sites ≥5

Score	Risk Group	Five-year OS
0 to 1	Low	90.6%
2	Intermediate	77.6%
≥3	High	52.5%

OS, overall survival.

which may render its use obsolete. Despite its widespread use, however, the FLIPI does not define for clinicians which patients should be treated at time of diagnosis.

In an attempt to improve on the FLIPI, an international project was conducted on over 1000 patients with newly diagnosed FL; all were treated with rituximab-based regimens. A prognostic score was also determined from this data set of five variables that could also separate patients into three separate risk groups, termed the F2 (Table 22.15). Even though the F2 model has been available for only a short period of time, it has the strengths of using easily obtainable clinical variables and was derived from patients treated with rituximab. Validation of its prognostic value with current treatment strategies will be required.

 F2 Prognostic Model

Score one point for each factor:
Age >60 years
Hemoglobin level <12 g/dL
Serum B2 microglobulin > upper limit of normal
Longest diameter of the largest involved lymph node longer than 6 cm
Bone marrow involvement

Score	Risk Group	Three-year PFS	Five-year PFS
0	Low	90.9%	79.5%
1–2	Intermediate	69.3%	51.2%
3–5	High	51.3%	18.8%

PFS, progression-free survival.

C. Front-line treatment principles of indolent NHL

Myriad treatment options exist for patients with newly diagnosed untreated FL, but no curative standard therapy has been identified. The life expectancy of FL patients has been prolonged with the use of rituximab, but it is still characterized by being highly responsive to initial therapies with relapse of disease inevitable. Patients typically undergo many different therapies in their lifetimes. The only potentially curative therapy is allogeneic stem cell transplantation, which is only an option for highly selected patients and carries an unacceptably high risk of treatment-related mortality (TRM) in most patients.

"Watchful waiting" or "dynamic observation" is an appropriate strategy in many patients until the disease progression causes undesired symptoms, progressive cytopenias, or threatens the function of an organ. Discussing this strategy with patients who are otherwise fit for therapy is challenging given the fact that many of them have advanced-stage disease and feel uncomfortable with delaying therapy. All available data, however, suggests that early administration of therapy does not ultimately improve outcomes and certainly carries inherent risks that observation does not. If this strategy is employed, then careful attention should be placed on the pace of the disease as well as the identification of signs of histologic transformation, and PET/CT scanning may add supplemental information in this regard.

Rituximab is a chimeric monoclonal antibody against CD20 that has revolutionized the treatment of all B-cell NHLs since its introduction in the early 2000s. The use of rituximab as a single agent in indolent NHLs is an attractive treatment option for infirm patients because it has relatively few toxicities other than infusional ones and can be given to patients with underlying organ dysfunction. The use of rituximab as a single agent at 375 mg/m^2 for four or eight doses, most often weekly but at various intervals, in FL yields response rates as high as 73% with progression-free survival (PFS) up to 3 years in duration. Extended duration therapy up to 2 years or longer may be an even more effective strategy for some patients and appears to be safe. In general, however, single-agent rituximab is not terribly effective for patients with bulky nodes that are greater than 10 cm and should be reserved for patients who are not candidates for combination chemotherapy.

Most patients with FL are initially treated with one of a handful of standard combination chemotherapy regimens with the addition of rituximab (Table 22.16). All of these regimens produce overall response rates in excess of 90% with approximately 50% complete responses, but can vary in the duration of maintaining that response and have varying toxicities. The use of anthracyclines

TABLE 22.16	Indolent Lymphoma Initial Treatment
Chemoimmunotherapy	**Treatment Description**
R-CVP	Rituximab 375 mg/m^2 IV on day 1 only
	Cyclophosphamide 750 mg/m^2 IV on day 1 only
	Vincristine 1.4 mg/m^2 IV push on day 1 only (maximum 2 mg)
	Prednisone 100 mg/m^2 PO on days 1–5
	Each cycle is 21 days
R-FND	Rituximab 375 mg/m^2 IV on day 1 only
	Fludarabine 25 mg/m^2 IV on days 1–3
	Mitoxantrone 10 mg/m^2 IV on day 1
	Dexamethasone 20 mg/m^2 PO on days 1–5
	Each cycle is 21 days
BR	Rituximab 375 mg/m^2 IV on day 1 only
	*Bendamustine 90 mg/m^2 IV on days 1 and 2
	Each cycle is 28 days

FDA, U.S. Food and Drug Administration; IV, intravenously; PO, by mouth.
*This dose of bendamustine is less than the FDA-approved dose of 120 mg/m^2 given every 21 days.

is not mandatory in patients with untreated FL, but according to the National LymphoCare study, which examined practice patterns in both community- and academic-based institutions, rituximab plus cyclophosphamide, doxorubicin, vincristine, and prednisolone (R-CHOP) remains the most commonly prescribed regimen in the United States with some geographical variation. Other strategies would be to save anthracycline-based therapies for signs of transformation, but no consensus exists. Bendamustine-rituximab is a newly available regimen based on an old chemotherapeutic developed in East Germany in the 1940s that has shown surprisingly high response rates and PFS but with less toxicity in a recent randomized study compared to R-CHOP. Given the fact that this regimen is easily tolerated by patients, it may eventually replace R-CHOP as the preferred regimen in the United States for untreated patients with FL and other indolent lymphomas.

One treatment strategy that has impressive results in phase II studies but remains largely underutilized is the use of the anti-CD20 radioimmunoconjugates such as iodine[131]-tositumomab (Bexxar) and ibritumomab tiuxetan (Zevalin). These agents, collectively known as radioimmunotherapy, are U.S. Food and Drug Administration (FDA)-approved for use as both the initial therapy of indolent NHL as well as in a consolidative strategy after initial combination chemotherapy. Barriers to its widespread use, however, include cost and reimbursement issues, unfamiliarity with the conjugates, and the fact that other services (such as nuclear medicine or radiation-oncology) are required to use these agents. Additionally, concerns linger regarding the long-term risks of treatment-related complications such as myelodysplasia or acute myelogenous leukemia, and long-term safety data are currently lacking.

Because none of the above strategies can claim superiority to other strategies based on controlled data, the list of potential options is long in patients with untreated indolent lymphomas. Many different strategies are employed with different types of patients and there is not currently one standard approach. However, it is probably important to avoid bone marrow toxic agents (fludarabine) in patients who may be candidates for autologous transplantation in the future.

D. Maintenance therapy in indolent NHL

Given that relapse is considered definite after initial therapy for indolent lymphoma, great emphasis has been placed on finding effective strategies at maintenance therapy. Interferon-α was the first agent tried in this setting, but it did not produce significant results in all patients and was difficult to tolerate in many. There have been several attempts at using cancer vaccines in consolidation after chemotherapy with mixed results. Because rituximab has limited long-term toxicities, it has been an attractive agent for this purpose. Its use after initial chemotherapy and now chemoimmunotherapy with the recently reported results of the PRIMA trial has demonstrated a benefit in PFS, but there has been no OS benefit yet. No consensus currently exists on the appropriate duration or schedule of maintenance therapy, however, and toxicities such as hypogammaglobulinemia and reversible neutropenia have been observed. Until long-term data exists demonstrating a clear OS benefit without unexpected toxicities, this cannot be recommended to all patients, but it appears to be a promising method of prolonging response duration and treatment-free intervals in many patients with indolent lymphomas.

E. Other indolent lymphomas

1. MALT lymphoma. The treatment principles applied to FL do not apply to all indolent lymphomas, and some lymphomas such as extranodal MALT lymphomas (MALTomas) may respond to treatment of underlying associated pathogens. MALTomas can occur at a number of sites including conjunctiva, thyroid, salivary gland, and gastrointestinal tract and are frequently antigen-driven. MALTomas that arise in immunocompetent patients tend to be localized and are associated with a better survival than other low-grade lymphomas. Of particular importance is the fact that many gastric MALTomas associated with *H. pylori* will respond to antibiotic therapy directed at the bacteria alone and will not require either radiation or chemotherapy.

TABLE 22.17	Staging System for Cutaneous T-Cell Lymphoma

Stage I: Limited or generalized plaques without adenopathy or histologic involvement of lymph nodes

Stage II: Limited or generalized plaques with adenopathy, or cutaneous tumors without adenopathy; without histologic involvement of lymph nodes or viscera

Stage III: Generalized erythroderma, with or without adenopathy; without histologic involvement of lymph nodes or viscera

Stage IV: Histologic involvement of lymph nodes or viscera with any skin lesions; with or without adenopathy

2. **Cutaneous T-cell lymphomas (CTCL; mycosis fungoides).** Another subset of indolent NHLs that deserves special attention are the cutaneous lymphomas. Cutaneous lymphomas include a wide variety of diseases of both B-cell and T-cell origin which present primarily involving the skin and are predominantly indolent. These NHLs are frequently misdiagnosed as other skin disorders such as eczema, and it is not uncommon for patients to be followed for many years before an accurate diagnosis is made. The most common cutaneous lymphoma is CTCL, also known as mycosis fungoides. When there is generalized erythroderma and involvement of the peripheral blood, the syndrome is known as Sézary syndrome. Prognosis in CTCL depends on stage of disease, and special staging systems for CTCL exist (Table 22.17). Clinical stage IA disease is so indolent that it does not impact on normal life expectancy, while prognosis worsens with more advanced stage of disease. The disease may exist as plaques in the skin for many years before progressing to involve skin tumors, lymphadenopathy, or visceral disease. Often, this clinical progression occurs in association with a pathologic transformation to a more aggressive lymphoma. If disease is limited to the skin, topical therapy such as topical nitrogen mustard, electron beam radiotherapy, or psoralen (often in conjunction with ultraviolet radiation) may be employed. Combination chemotherapy regimens such as those used for intermediate-grade lymphoma may be used for disease involving nodes or viscera. Other approaches to this disease include the use of denileukin diftitox, an antibody to CD25, and bexarotene, a novel retinoid X receptor–selective retinoid (see Chapter 14).

VI. MANAGEMENT OF INTERMEDIATE-GRADE NHL

A. Diffuse large B-cell lymphoma (DLBCL)

DLBCL is the most common lymphoid neoplasm in adults, representing about 30% of cases diagnosed in the United State annually. In most cases, it is very responsive to combination chemoimmunotherapy regimens, and an approach with curative intent is appropriate in most cases of newly diagnosed DLBCL. Still, a significant minority of patients will relapse after initial response to chemotherapy or be primarily refractory. The molecular mechanisms underlying DLBCL have been elegantly defined recently, and we now know that tremendous genetic heterogeneity exists and that the different subsets are accompanied accordingly with a different prognosis. Molecular profiling and DNA microarray studies have demonstrated that the relationship with the stroma (microenvironment) as well as disease subtype as defined by GEP are important in determining the behavior of DLBCLs. Novel agents with rational targets are beginning to enter the clinical arena in the treatment of DLBCL, and exciting treatment breakthroughs are likely to follow.

As previously mentioned, the Lymphoma/Leukemia Molecular Profiling Project has essentially established three subtypes of DLBCL with very different molecular profiles: the GCB subtype, the ABC subtype, and PMBL subtype. Forthcoming from the elucidation that different subtypes of DLBCL exist has been the realization that they are addicted to different signal transduction pathways for their survival. Upfront treatment decisions are not yet routinely altered based on the underlying tissue subtype, but a potentially attainable goal in the future is to define a more "personalized" treatment approach based on the expression of genes unique to individual patients' tumors.

Another emerging concept related to the biology of DLBCL is the fact that certain subsets of DLBCL contain molecular mutations that portend a particularly grave prognosis. It is now recognized that 5% to 10% of DLBCL cases actually possess a rearrangement in the c-myc oncogene, which makes them highly proliferative and less responsive to standard regimens. Two different groups have retrospectively reported their experience with c-myc$^+$ DLBCLs and both found distinctly poor OS in this subset of patients. The 2008 edition of the WHO classification scheme recognizes that some cases of c-myc$^+$ DLBCL may be very difficult to distinguish from Burkitt lymphoma (BL), and a landmark study was able to demonstrate that based on GEP, some cases of DLBCL may actually have a BL-like molecular signature.

In addition to c-myc$^+$ DLBCLs, another subset of DLBCLs with a poor prognosis are those that have a "double-hit" with the BCL2 translocation t(14;18) (as seen in FL) in addition to the c-myc translocation. These tumors are particularly troublesome because they have developed mutations in both proliferation and impaired apoptosis. No consensus exists on the correct approach to patients in these poor-risk subgroups, but it is becoming increasingly important to identify these patients prior to treating them with standard regimens as they all do uniformly poorly.

B. Initial treatment of advanced-stage intermediate-grade NHL

Treatment principles of combining chemotherapeutic agents without overlapping toxicities and giving the maximally tolerated dose have defined the approach to DLBCL since the advent of chemotherapy in the 1960s. Anthracyclines as a class of agents established themselves many years ago as the single most important drug in the treatment of aggressive lymphomas. In the 1980s, single institution phase II studies of dose-intensive regimens such as cyclophosphamide, doxorubicin, etoposide, bleomycin, vincristine, methotrexate, and prednisone (known as Pro-MACE-CytaBOM); methotrexate, bleomycin, doxorubicin, cyclophosphamide, vincristine, and dexamethasone (known as m-BACOD); and methotrexate plus leucovorin rescue, doxorubicin, cyclophosphamide, vincristine, prednisone, and bleomycin (known as MACOP-B) began to report what appeared to be markedly improved response rates compared to conventional response rates seen with cyclophosphamide, doxorubicin, vincristine, and prednisolone (CHOP) therapy. However, a landmark study in 1993 re-established CHOP therapy as the backbone by which all challengers are to be compared based on OS.

Prior to rituximab, only about 30% to 40% of patients were cured of their DLBCL if found in advanced stages. Almost immediately on its availability, rituximab overcame some of the chemoresistance of DLBCL (possibly via overcoming BCL2 overexpression) and has become standardly incorporated into every regimen used in this disease with essentially the same result of improving outcomes. Every time chemotherapy with rituximab has been compared to chemotherapy without rituximab, it has been demonstrated superior. Thus, the current standard of care is to administer R-CHOP for six to eight cycles every 3 weeks for patients without contraindication for advanced-stage DLBCL (Table 22.18). Efforts to give the regimen in a "dose-dense" fashion every 14 days with support with growth factors has been advocated by some and show feasibility, but formal comparisons of R-CHOP-14 to R-CHOP-21 disappointingly demonstrated no clear superiority.

In comparison to the bolus administration of chemotherapy in the R-CHOP regimen, the dose-adjusted etoposide, doxorubicin, vincristine, cyclophosphamide, prednisone, and rituximab (EPOCH-R) regimen utilizes infusional administration of agents over 96 hours in an effort to affect cells that are not dividing on the first day of administration. Also, the regimen adjusts the dose of the doxorubicin, etoposide, and cyclophosphamide with subsequent cycles using the absolute neutrophil count as a biomarker. The dose-adjusted EPOCH-R regimen is designed to be effective in more proliferative tumors, and response rates in single institution studies and a multi-institutional phase II trial demonstrate

	Chemotherapy Regimens for Intermediately Aggressive B-NHL

Combination Chemotherapy	Treatment Description
R-CHOP	Rituximab 375 mg/m^2 IV on day 1
	Cyclophosphamide 750 mg/m^2 IV on day 1
	Doxorubicin 50 mg/m^2 IV on day 1
	Vincristine 1.4 mg/m^2 IV push on day 1 (maximum 2 mg)
	Prednisone 50 mg/m^2 per day PO on days 1–5
	Each cycle is 21 days
R-EPOCH (dose adjusted)*	Rituximab 375 mg/m^2 IV on day 1
	Etoposide 50 mg/m^2 per day by continuous IV infusion for 96 hours
	Doxorubicin 10 mg/m^2 per day by continuous IV infusion for 96 hours
	Vincristine 0.4 mg/m^2 per day by continuous IV infusion for 96 hours (no cap)
	Prednisone 60 mg/m^2 per dose PO every 12 hours for 5 days
	Cyclophosphamide 750 mg/m^2 IV on day 5 only
	Filgrastim 5 μg/kg per day SC starting day 6
	Treatment is repeated every 21 days

IV, intravenously; NHL, non-Hodgkin lymphoma; PO, by mouth; SC, subcutaneously.
*EPOCH is adjusted with each cycle based on the absolute neutrophil count nadir and platelet count.

response rates that are higher than those seen in R-CHOP; results of a formal phase III comparison between EPOCH-R and CHOP-R are anxiously awaited. Until a regimen such as EPOCH-R demonstrates superiority either in all patients with DLBCL or certain subgroups, R-CHOP will remain the most widely used regimen in DLBCL.

C. Initial treatment of localized intermediate-grade NHL

The contemporary treatment options for patients with early-stage (stage I or II) DLBCL usually employ R-CHOP therapy but utilize fewer cycles and often include consolidative radiation therapy to sites of involvement. Unlike Hodgkin lymphoma, there is almost no role for radiation therapy alone in early-stage DLBCL because the disease does not spread to contiguous nodes as predictably as HL and commonly has disseminated tumor cells that escape detection at diagnosis. Combined modality therapy with brief duration chemotherapy followed by radiation became the standard approach based on a Southwest Oncology Group trial in the late 1990s that demonstrated an OS benefit to this approach, but whether or not rituximab has obviated the need for radiation therapy has not yet been determined. Thus, most patients will be offered a combination of R-CHOP for two to three cycles followed by consolidative radiation to sites of involvement. Reported 5-year OS rates with this approach are in excess of 90%. In patients in whom the risk of radiation may outweigh its benefit in the long term (young women with nonbulky mediastinal masses), it may be reasonable to use R-CHOP for six cycles in lieu of consolidative radiotherapy. The standard therapy for patients with bulky disease (>10 cm), however, remains consolidative radiation therapy.

D. CNS prophylaxis

Involvement of the CNS at the time of diagnosis of DLBCL is uncommon with incidence rates of only 5%, but at the time of relapse, uncontrolled disease in the CNS is a very poor prognostic sign. Thus, efforts to predict who is at risk to develop CNS disease have focused on patients with an extranodal disease presentation and/or an elevated LDH at diagnosis. By convention, patients with at least two sites of extranodal involvement (including bone marrow) and an elevated LDH as well as those with "sanctuary sites" involved at presentation (testis, nasopharynx, orbit) are offered CNS prophylaxis with intrathecal therapy: usually methotrexate with or without cytarabine. The administration of CNS prophylaxis, however, is very much understudied and no consensus exists. Therefore, significant variation exists in the patients selected as well as the number and total doses of prophylaxis given.

E. Primary mediastinal B-cell lymphoma (PMBL)

As previously mentioned, PMBL has been identified on the basis of DNA microarray profiles to have a unique molecular profile that carries a relatively good prognosis with current treatment strategies. Clinically, it has some unique features, including the fact that it commonly affects persons of young age (classically women) and at the time of initial presentation usually stays within the mediastinum. Bone marrow involvement and nodal chains below the diaphragm are very uncommon, making the Ann Arbor staging system unhelpful in this disease. Thus, all patients with PMBL are treated with advanced-stage disease principles of six to eight cycles of R-CHOP usually followed by mediastinal radiation irrespective of stage. Recently reported data suggests that with the use of dose-adjusted EPOCH-R, mediastinal radiation may be safely omitted, but this finding requires further validation.

F. Response assessment of DLBCL

Of equal importance to finding an effective treatment regimen is the ability to determine its effect at the end of the therapy. An International Working Group has published guidelines that determine the response to therapy based on the bidimensional measurements of involved nodal groups at the time of diagnosis and again at the end of therapy. If all nodes have regressed to no more than 1 cm in size and symptoms of disease have disappeared, the patient is considered in CR. If the sum of the product of diameters has reduced by 50% but not all nodes are no more than 1 cm, then it is considered a partial response. As residual necrotic tissue and inflammatory cells often prevent bulky nodal groups from ever getting to no more than 1 cm, the use of PET/CT scanning at the end of therapy is highly useful. In patients who present with bulky mediastinal nodes (such as patients with PMBL), the use of PET/CT scans to confirm a complete response is almost mandatory to differentiate between residual tumor cells and dead cells.

G. Mantle cell lymphoma (MCL)

MCL is an uncommon NHL derived from naïve small B lymphocytes. These lymphomas have a diffuse pattern; are generally CD5 positive, CD23 negative, positive for cyclin D-1; and are associated with a t(11;14) chromosomal translocation. MCL essentially shares the worst features of both indolent NHLs and aggressive NHLs in that it is practically incurable but usually requires therapy at diagnosis to prevent a rapid downhill course. Current therapies have slightly improved the median survival of MCL from 3 to 4 years to closer to 7 years, but it is still one of the NHLs with the worst prognosis.

The proliferation signature of MCL as defined by GEP has proven to be highly predictive of outcome in that patients with more proliferative variants of MCL have a much worse prognosis than patients with low proliferative variants. In fact, a subset of patients with MCL can often go several years without therapy while enjoying a lack of progression of disease. Clinical, pathologic, and radiographic variables have all been used to attempt to identify which patients can be observed and which need immediate therapy, but it is currently difficult to accurately identify these subsets prospectively. A prognostic score similar to the IPI, termed the MIPI (Table 22.19) has been developed and is currently undergoing validation in numerous prospective studies.

Despite the poor prognosis, MCL is very sensitive to both chemotherapy and radiation with the overall response rate being in excess of 90% with R-CHOP therapy. These responses, however, are usually of brief duration, and relapsed MCL is often unresponsive to conventional chemotherapy. Thus, the most common strategy for otherwise fit individuals with MCL is to undergo treatment with intense regimens with cytarabine-based combinations and to consolidate with high-dose therapy with stem cell rescue in first CR (Table 22.20). It is likely that this approach is not curative, but long-term data are not yet available and it is the current standard approach for fit patients with newly diagnosed MCL.

H. Peripheral T-cell lymphomas (PTCLs)

It has become apparent that PTCLs have a worse prognosis than that of their B-cell intermediate-grade lymphoma counterparts,

TABLE 22.19	Mantle Cell Lymphoma International Prognostic Index			
Points	**Age, years**	**ECOG PS**	**LDH (ULN)**	**WBC 10^9/L**
0	<50	0–1	<0.67	<6.7
1	50–59	—	0.67–0.99	6.70–9.99
2	60–69	3–4	1.00–1.49	10.00–14.99
3	≥70	—	≥1.50	≥15.00

0–3 points = low risk
4–5 points = intermediate risk
6–11 points = high risk

Risk Category	**Median OS**
Low risk	Not yet reached
Intermediate risk	51 months
High risk	29 months

ECOG, Eastern Cooperative Oncology Group; LDH, lactate dehydrogenase; OS, overall survival; PS, performance status; ULN, upper limit of normal; WBC, white blood count.

and as a result, have a relatively poor prognosis except for the ALK+ anaplastic large cell lymphomas (ALCLs). PTCLs are a heterogeneous group of lymphomas that constitute only 5% to 7% of adult NHLs diagnosed in the United States. The International T-cell/NK Lymphoma Project demonstrated that the use of an anthracycline in PTCLs does not correlate to improved outcomes compared to nonanthracycline–based therapies, bringing into question the conventional approach of using CHOP as initial therapy in most cases of PTCL.

Unfortunately, with the exception of CHOP for ALK$^+$ ALCL, an optimal therapy for PTCLs has not yet been defined, and practice patterns vary markedly between institutions. Agents that seem to have activity and are being explored include gemcitabine, alemtuzumab (a monoclonal antibody that targets CD52), pentostatin, histone deacetylase inhibitors, and the immunomodulatory drug lenalidomide. Patients with PTCL should be encouraged to participate in well-designed clinical trials whenever possible in order to help determine optimal first-line treatment algorithms.

In September 2009, the FDA approved the first agent specifically for the treatment of relapsed/refractory PTCL in the form of the novel antifolate drug pralatrexate. The approval was based on a multicenter phase II trial that demonstrated significant activity of pralatrexate in patients who had been refractory to many previous therapeutic regimens.

TABLE 22.20	Chemotherapy Regimens for Mantle Cell Lymphoma

Combination Chemotherapy	Treatment Description
R-HyperCVAD/ MA *Cycles 1, 3, 5, and 7*	Rituximab 375 mg/m^2 IV infusional protocol on day 1 only Cyclophosphamide 300 mg/m^2 IV every 12 hours for six doses on days 2–4 Vincristine 1.4 mg (maximum 2 mg) IV push on days 5 and 12 Doxorubicin 50 mg/m^2 via CIVI over 72 hours on days 5–7 Dexamethasone 40 mg/day IV or PO on days 2–5 and 12–15 Mesna 600 mg/m^2 IV daily starting 1 hour before cyclophosphamide and completed 12 hours after the last cyclophosphamide dose
R-HyperCVAD/ MA *Cycles 2, 4, 6, and 8*	Rituximab 375 mg/m^2 IV infusional protocol on day 1 only Cytarabine 3000 mg/m^2 per dose IV over 1 hour every 12 hours $\times$ 4 doses on days 3 and 4 (reduce cytarabine dose to 1 g/m^2 for patients over 60 years old or creatinine >1.5) Methotrexate 1 g/m^2 IV over 24 hours on day 1 Leucovorin 50 mg IV to start 12 hours after methotrexate, then 15 mg IV every 6 hours until serum methotrexate <1 $\times$ 10^{-8} M Filgrastim (G-CSF) should be administered starting on day 4 until granulocyte recovery occurs Treatment cycles started based on blood counts ($\sim$ every 21 days)
MCL 2 regimen	*Cycles 1, 3, and 5* (MAXI CHOP) Rituximab 375 mg/m^2 IV on day 1 Cyclophosphamide 1200 mg/m^2 IV on day 1 Doxorubicin 75 mg/m^2 IV on day 1 Vincristine 2 mg IV push on day 1 Prednisone 100 mg per day PO on days 1–5 *Cycles 2, 4, and 6* Rituximab 375 mg/m^2 IV on days 1 and 9 Cytarabine 3000 mg/m^2 per dose IV over 3 hours every 12 hours $\times$ 4 doses (reduce cytarabine dose to 2 g/m^2 for patients over 60 years old) Filgrastim (G-CSF) should be administered starting on day 4 until granulocyte recovery occurs

CIVI, continuous intravenous infusion; G-CSF, granulocyte colony-stimulating factor; IV, intravenously; PO, by mouth.

I. **Rare, extranodal T-cell lymphomas**

HSTCL, subcutaneous panniculitis-like T-cell lymphoma, and EATCL are rare subtypes of PTCLs that often present with primarily extranodal disease. Despite the fact that these tumors have distinct clinical and pathologic features, they are often diagnosed after significant delay. Also, the use of anthracycline-based combination chemotherapy that is highly effective in B-cell counterparts is not effective in these disorders. The combination of delay in diagnosis, aggressive natural history of these tumors, and ineffective therapies has resulted in a poor prognosis in most cases. In patients who do achieve remissions with initial therapy, consideration should be given to consolidation with allogeneic stem cell transplantation given the dismal prognosis, especially for HSTCL, cutaneous γδ T-cell lymphoma, and the anaplastic variant of EATCL.

VII. MANAGEMENT OF HIGHLY AGGRESSIVE NHL

A. Lymphoblastic lymphoma (LBL)

LBL is a highly aggressive lymphoma regarded as a variant of acute lymphoblastic leukemia (ALL) that is rapidly fatal without prompt initiation of combination chemotherapy. In adults, it is most commonly of T-cell lineage (85% to 90% of cases), but can also be of B-cell lineage, and demonstrates a male predominance. Tissue specimens are often composed of small- or medium-sized blast cells with scant cytoplasm that are positive for immature markers such as CD99 and TdT. LBL commonly presents with a mediastinal mass (60% to 70% of patients), elevated LDH levels, and B symptoms; bone marrow involvement is present in about 20% of cases. Although all patients with LBL should receive intrathecal therapy as part of their regimen, actual CNS involvement at the time of diagnosis is less than 10%. R-CHOP and other regimens used for intermediate-grade NHLs are not effective in LBL. ALL-like regimens with CNS prophylaxis are required to effectively treat LBL and typically are administered in three phases (induction, consolidation, and maintenance) with prolonged administration lasting up to 24 to 36 months (cases of B-cell lineage do not typically require prolonged maintenance therapy). A major determining factor in treatment outcomes is the underlying cytogenetic and molecular profile of the tumor. Patients with the t(9;22) translocation have a poor prognosis whereas those with t(12;21) and HOX mutations have a better prognosis. Outcomes in adults treated for LBL are inferior to pediatric outcomes, which may reflect disease biology or adherence to treatment protocols.

B. Burkitt lymphoma (BL)

BL is composed of post–germinal center mature B-cells with a highly aggressive presentation and natural history. Morphologically, Burkitt tumor cells are small noncleaved cells arranged in a monotonous pattern and may have a "starry sky" appearance. It is often subdivided into cases that are endemic, sporadic, and associated with underlying HIV. All cases of BL are associated with a c-MYC translocation and most commonly arise from the reciprocal t(8;14) translocation although variant translocations of t(2;8) and t(8;22) exist.

In the United States, BL tends to occur in younger patients and is associated with a higher incidence of gastrointestinal disease. R-CHOP is substandard therapy for BL, and high-intensity brief-duration regimens such as the R-Hyper-CVAD regimen (rituximab plus hyper-cyclophosphamide, vincristine, doxorubicin, and dexamethasone), or the cyclophosphamide, vincristine, doxorubicin, high-dose methotrexate/ifosfamide, etoposide, high-dose cytarabine (known as CODOX-M/IVAC) regimen (Table 22.21) have been associated with long-term DFS in almost 50% of patients. Patients with disease involving the CNS or bone marrow have a worse prognosis than those patients with limited-stage disease. The role of stem cell transplantation as routine consolidation following initial high-dose therapy or in relapsed disease has not been established by clinical trials.

C. Tumor lysis prophylaxis

Highly aggressive lymphomas such as LBL and BL are composed of rapidly proliferative tumor cells that have the potential to cause spontaneous lysis of tumor cells even before the administration of combination chemotherapy. When tumor cells lyse, they release intracellular cations such as potassium, uric acid, and phosphorus, which can be toxic to renal tubules. This potentially fatal clinical scenario is termed the tumor lysis syndrome and is becoming increasingly common as regimens become more effective (see Chapter 29).

TABLE 22.21 CODOX-M/IVAC for Burkitt Lymphoma

Cycles 1 and 3
Cyclophosphamide 800 mg/m^2 IV on day 1
Vincristine 1.5 mg/m^2 (maximum 2 mg) IV on days 1 and 8
Doxorubicin 40 mg/m^2 IV on day 1
Cytarabine 70 mg intrathecal on days 1 and 3
Cyclophosphamide 200 mg/m^2 IV on days 2, 3, 4, and 5
Methotrexate 1200 mg/m^2 IV over 1 hour starting on day 10, followed immediately by 240 mg/m^2 hourly for 23 hours
Leucovorin 192 mg/ m^2 IV at hour 36 of methotrexate therapy
Leucovorin 12 mg/m^2 IV every 6 hours until methotrexate level is $<5 \times 10^{-8}$ M
G-CSF 5 mg/kg SC daily starting day 13
Methotrexate 12 mg intrathecal on day 15
Leucovorin 15 mg PO 24 hours after intrathecal methotrexate

Cycles 2 and 4
Etoposide 60 mg/m^2 IV over 1 hour daily on days 1–5
Ifosfamide 1500 mg/m^2 IV over 1 hour daily on days 1–5
Mesna 360 mg/m^2 IV with ifosfamide, then every 3 hours for seven additional doses each 24 hours
Cytarabine 2 gm/m^2 IV over 3 hours every 12 hours for four total doses on days 1 and 2
Methotrexate 12 mg intrathecal on day 5
Leucovorin 15 mg PO 24 hours after methotrexate
G-CSF 5 mcg/kg SC daily starting day 7

G-CSF, granulocyte colony-stimulating factor; IV, intravenously; SC, subcutaneously.

VIII. THERAPY OF RELAPSED NHL

A. Salvage chemotherapy

Up to 50% of patients with DLBCL will ultimately relapse after initial chemoimmunotherapy; the number is higher with MCL and PTCL, meaning that large numbers of patients will ultimately need second-line or "salvage" chemotherapy. Aggressive NHLs such as DLBCL that have relapsed after response to initial chemotherapy are still curable in a significant minority of cases and the duration of response (DOR) can sometimes be used as a surrogate for chemotherapy sensitivity. One of the most important prognostic markers of relapsed NHL is whether it remains chemosensitive or has become resistant to chemotherapy. Tumors that have become chemoresistant or are primarily refractory to initial chemotherapy (defined as never achieving CR or a DOR <6 months) uniformly have a dismal prognosis and are likely incurable.

Despite the importance of salvage chemotherapy, the optimal regimen remains a research question as comparative data is lacking. Typically, a platinum-based regimen (Table 22.22) is administered for two to three cycles (usually with rituximab) and patients are then taken to high-dose therapy with stem cell rescue (autologous transplant) if they demonstrate chemosensitivity. The standard practice of taking every patient to

TABLE 22.22	Salvage Chemotherapy Regimens in Aggressive NHL
Regimen	**Treatment Description**
DHAP	Cisplatin 100 mg/m^2 by continuous IV infusion for 24 hours on day 1
	Cytarabine 2000 mg/m^2 per dose IV over 3 hours every 12 hours for two doses on day 2
	Dexamethasone 40 mg per day PO or IV for 4 days on days 1–4
	Treatment is repeated every 21 days
ESHAP	Etoposide 40 mg/m^2 per day over 1 hour IV for 4 days, days 1–4
	Methylprednisolone 250–500 mg per day IV on days 1–5
	Cytarabine 2000 mg/m^2 IV over 2 hours on day 5
	Cisplatin 25 mg/m^2 per day by continuous IV infusion on days 1–4
	Treatment is repeated every 21 days
ICE	Ifosfamide 5000 mg/m^2 over 24 hours by continuous IV infusion starting on day 2, mixed with equal amounts of mesna
	Etoposide 100 mg/m^2 IV twice a day on days 1–3
	Carboplatin AUC = 5 (maximum dose of 800 mg) IV on day 2
	G-CSF administered a 5 μg/kg SC on days 7–14
	Treatment is repeated every 14 days but if ANC <1000 or platelets <50,000, then administer at 21-day intervals

ANC, absolute neutrophil count; AUC, area under the curve; IV, intravenously; NHL, non-Hodgkin lymphoma; PO, by mouth; SC, subcutaneously.

autologous transplant in first relapse is based on the PARMA study published in the pre-rituximab era that demonstrated an OS advantage to this approach versus chemotherapy alone, with up to 30% of patients enjoying long-term DFS. In the current era of rituximab being given with initial therapy in almost all cases, however, less is known about the biology of disease relapse and its response to salvage chemotherapy. The recently presented results of the international, multicenter CORAL study suggest that fewer patients (approximately 15%) will be salvaged with autologous transplantation done in second CR, suggesting the need for an alternative approach that utilizes novel agents. In the era of PET/CT scanning, an emerging concept is that patients with residual ^{18}FDG-PET positivity prior to transplant may not benefit from high-dose therapy and should not be offered this approach.

High-dose chemotherapy with stem cell transplantation can also be offered to patients with relapsed low-grade NHL, but since this is not a curative procedure, enthusiasm for this approach is not high. Additionally, the use of high doses of chemotherapy carry a risk of treatment-related myelodysplasia and acute myeloid leukemia, and patients with indolent NHL often get multiple therapies in their lifetime which increases that risk. However, younger patients with indolent NHLs such as FL have been salvaged with autologous transplantation in first CR with an improvement in PFS but not OS being demonstrated.

B. Allogeneic transplantation in relapsed NHL

Myeloablative allogeneic transplantation has traditionally been reserved as a "last ditch" option for select patients with relapsed both indolent and aggressive NHLs that have failed all other therapies. Even though the graft-versus-leukemia effect can be very potent in NHL, the TRM and incidence of at least grade III graft-versus-host disease has been a significant barrier to widespread use of this approach. Nevertheless, it appears that allogeneic transplantation is a potentially curative approach in carefully selected patients with relapsed NHL; with the use of reduced-intensity preparative regimens, more patients are becoming eligible for this high-risk/high-reward therapy.

C. Novel/targeted agents

Numerous agents with novel mechanisms are being tested in relapsed/refractory NHLs in an effort to address this unmet clinical need. Many of these agents are considered "targeted" agents that attempt to selectively inhibit tumor cells in a more selective manner than conventional DNA-damaging agents. Molecular biology has uncovered many pathways important for proliferation and impaired apoptosis, which are the targets of many of these agents. In addition, some novel agents are thought to work by affecting the tumor cell's interactions with the local microenvironment, which may be providing protection from the effects of chemotherapy. Agents that are currently being studied include immunomodulating agents (such as lenalidomide), proteasome inhibitors (such as bortezomib), BCL2 inhibitors, histone deacetylase inhibitors, mammalian target of rapamycin inhibitors, PI3k/AkT inhibitors, MEK inhibitors, PARP inhibitors, cyclin-dependent kinase inhibitors, Bruton tyrosine kinase inhibitors, and novel monoclonal antibodies targeting both CD20 and CD19. Many of these agents are likely to be important in the management of NHL moving forward.

IX. RADIATION THERAPY IN NHL

NHL is very sensitive to the tumoricidal effects of radiation therapy, and it remains an essential treatment modality to improve local control in the contemporary management of patients with NHL. Enthusiasm for widespread use of radiation therapy has been somewhat tempered, however, by concerns about its inherent risks of localized tissue destruction; premature risks of coronary artery and valvular heart disease; secondary malignancies such as carcinomas of the breast, lung, and thyroid; and sarcomas that frequently present 15 to 25 years after patients are cured of their NHL. Additionally, as chemotherapeutic strategies improve and functional imaging modalities such as PET/CT can better define tumor responses in residual nodal masses, questions arise regarding the need for consolidative radiation.

Current indications for radiation therapy include a potential curative approach in limited-stage indolent NHL such as FL or gastric MALT as well as consolidative therapy to sites of tumor bulk in patients with mediastinal lymphomas and primary CNS lymphoma (PCNSL). Another potential method by which to take advantage of the effects of radiation is to employ the use of "targeted radiation" in the form of anti-CD20 radioimmunoconjugates such as iodine[131]- tositumomab (Bexxar) or ibritumomab tiuxetan (Zevalin), which are particularly attractive in low-volume disease in patients with indolent lymphomas, either in the relapsed setting or as a consolidative approach after initial chemotherapy. It is important to use caution in patients with significant bone marrow involvement, however.

Currently used modalities for employing radiation therapy may eventually be replaced with advanced modes of high-precision radiotherapy that utilize computer-controlled linear accelerators to deliver precise radiation doses to a malignant tumor or specific areas within the tumor such as intensity modulated radiotherapy and three-dimensional proton beam therapy (PBT). These advancements in the field purport to deliver higher doses and more precise therapy to tumor cells while at the same time minimizing the dose to surrounding normal critical structures. Another potential advantage of using PBT is that clinical data from cancer survivors thus far has not demonstrated an increased risk of secondary malignancies.

X. SUBGROUPS AND SPECIAL CONSIDERATIONS IN NHL

A. AIDS-related lymphomas

Among patients with HIV infection, 3% to 6% will develop NHL, and this is considered an AIDS-defining illness. The lymphoid neoplasms that are associated with HIV include DLBCL, PCNSL, primary effusion lymphoma, plasmablastic lymphoma of the oral cavity, and BL (see Table 22.4) and concomitant infection with human herpesvirus 8 and EBV also appear to play a role in pathogenesis. NHL is typically a late manifestation of HIV, with most cases occurring when the cluster of differentiation 4 (CD4) cell count is less than 200 mm^3 except for BL which can occur with any CD4 count (see Chapter 25 for further discussion of the HIV- and AIDS-related lymphomas).

B. Post-transplant lymphoproliferative disorders (PTLDs)

Abnormal expansions of lymphoid cells (either B-cell or T-cell) in patients who have undergone either solid organ or hematopoietic stem cell transplantation are defined as PTLDs. Given the broad definition, PTLDs are a clinically heterogeneous group of disorders with marked variation in clinical behavior ranging from benign expansions to aggressive and fatal NHL.

Risk factors for the development of PTLD are listed in Table 22.23. EBV plays a pivotal role in the development the majority of PTLDs. In fact, many transplant centers now routinely

TABLE 22.23	Risk Factors for PTLDs

Seronegative for EBV pretransplantation (HSCT recipients)
Age >50 years at time of transplantation
Use of a second transplantation
Less than 1 year since transplantation
ATG or OKT3 (antiCD3 monoclonal antibody) as prophylaxis
Unrelated or mismatched HLA grafts
Use of a T-cell depleted graft
Acute or chronic GVHD
Cardiac transplant > renal transplant

ATG, antithymocyte globulin; EBV, Epstein-Barr virus; GVHD, graft-verus-host disease; HLA, human leucocyte antigen; HSCT, hematopoietic stem cell transplantation; PTLD, posttransplant lymphoproliferative disorder.

monitor periodic PCR for EBV and will preemptively treat cases of a rapidly rising viral load of EBV with rituximab.

If the PTLD is limited in extent, one can employ therapy designed at increasing the host response to EBV, such as withdrawing or decreasing immunosuppression, administering interferon, or giving lymphocytes from individuals who have had EBV infection. Such therapy is most effective in limited disease and in patients in whom the lymphocytes are polyclonal.

Radiotherapy or surgery can be effective in localized and accessible disease, but for more advanced disease and for disease in which the lymphocytes are monoclonal, combination chemotherapy with or without rituximab or donor lymphocyte infusions for stem cell transplant patients is often necessary. Unfortunately, response rates are lower for transplant-associated lymphomas than for de novo lymphomas, and long-term survival has been disappointing.

C. Primary central nervous system lymphoma (PCNSL)

PCNSL is defined as a NHL that is confined to the CNS and has no systemic involvement. PCNSL has risen more rapidly than other extranodal sites in part due to the association with HIV, but it has risen in immunocompetent hosts as well. It is of a B-cell origin in almost all cases in the United States and typically of an intermediate-grade histology, such as in DLBCL. For reasons that are not entirely clear, it very infrequently metastasizes outside of the CNS even though very sensitive techniques such as PCR can detect tumor cells in the peripheral blood of a significant minority of patients with PCNSL. The diagnosis can be made with direct tissue biopsy or demonstration of lymphoma cells on examination of the cerebrospinal fluid (CSF). Of note, the presence of a positive PCR for EBV DNA found in CSF is virtually diagnostic of PCNSL. If PCNSL is considered in the differential diagnosis of patients who present with isolated brain lesions, it is important to attempt diagnostic studies prior to the administration of steroids as tumor cells are very sensitive to steroids and the opportunity to accurately characterize the lymphoma may be lost.

Treatment with radiation therapy alone is generally associated with poor OS, and radiotherapy alone is no longer recommended for patients with PCNSL who are able to undergo more intensive therapies. The current standard is a multimodality approach that utilizes combination chemotherapy with agents that cross the blood–brain barrier such as high-dose methotrexate and cytarabine (with the addition of rituximab if of B-cell lineage) followed by consolidative whole-brain radiotherapy (WBRT). Such approaches can achieve overall response rates greater than 90%, but 2-year PFS rates are approximately 50% to 55% and relapse is a common clinical problem. Due to concerns of both acute and long-term toxicities on both central and peripheral neurologic function associated with WBRT, some regimens attempt to use chemotherapy alone, but response rates tend to be lower. The overall effect on OS with the omission of WBRT, however, is not yet clear.

D. Testicular lymphomas

Testicular lymphomas represent the most common testicular tumor seen in men over the age of 60 years, with DLBCL being the most common histologic type. Primary testicular lymphoma (PTL) is a rare entity with a distinct natural history compared to nodal DLBCL that frequently affects the contralateral testis, lung pleura, and soft tissues. Recent reports suggest that the majority of these tumors are of the ABC subtype of DLBCL with marked proliferative activity. Therapy consists of a multimodality approach of surgical removal of the primary tumor, systemic chemoimmunotherapy, and radiation of the contralateral testis. Additionally, as PTL originates in an immunoprivileged site, prophylactic treatment of the CNS is uniformly administered. Despite this approach, PTL has an inferior outcome compared to nodal DLBCL and can be associated with late relapses.

E. NHL in the elderly

NHL in patients over the age of 60 years deserves special mention because the median age at diagnosis of NHL is between 60 and 65 years, the U.S. population is aging, and age consistently is determined to be a prognostic marker in outcomes in NHL despite no known biologic differences in the disease associated with age. Thus, a common clinical problem involves the selection of appropriate therapy for a patient with intermediate-grade NHL over the age of 70 years or older than 60 years with significant comorbid disease. Patients in this category have been underrepresented in the prospective clinical trials that have defined our standard treatment approaches, with data regarding patients over the age of 80 years being virtually nonexistent. Concerns about the potential toxicities for these patients frequently leads to empiric dose reductions or dose delays that likely compromise the potential for cure. Available data, however, suggest that when CHOP is used in lower doses, remission rates decline and survival is shortened. In the Group d'Etude des Lymphome d'Adulte LN 98-5 trial, 399 patients with DLBCL aged 60 to 80 years were treated with R-CHOP versus CHOP. The addition of rituximab was associated with a 15% improvement in CR rate with associated improvements in DFS and OS. In this trial, the most common $\geq$G3 toxicity was infection, cardiac toxicities $\geq$G3 were seen in only 8% of patients, and other toxicities were consistent with those expected with the use of CHOP in younger populations. It is likely that, with the use of supportive medications such as granulocyte colony-stimulating factor, many patients over the age of 60 years can be offered standard treatments at standard doses and experience similar toxicities as younger patients with NHL, but identifying patients over the age of 60 years (and especially 80 years) who are at risk for excessive toxicities remains a significant clinical challenge.

Selected Readings

Alizadeh AA, Eisen MB, Davis RE, et al. Distinct types of diffuse large B-cell lymphoma identified by gene expression profiling. *Nature.* 2000;403:503–511.

American Cancer Society. *Cancer facts & figures, 2010.* Atlanta, GA: American Cancer Society; 2010.

Anderson JR, Armitage JO, Weisenburger DD. Epidemiology of the non-Hodgkin's lymphomas: distributions of the major subtypes differ by geographic locations. Non-Hodgkin's Lymphoma Classification Project. *Ann Oncol.* 1998;9:717.

Armitage JO. How I treat patients with diffuse large B-cell lymphoma. *Blood.* 2007; 110:29–36.

Barrans S, Crouch S, Smith A, et al. Rearrangement of *MYC* is associated with poor prognosis in patients with diffuse large B-cell lymphoma treated in the era of rituximab. *J Clin Oncol.* 2010;26:1–6.

Cairo MS, Coiffier B, Reiter A, et al. Recommendations for the evaluation of risk and prophylaxis of tumour lysis syndrome (TLS) in adults and children with malignant diseases: an expert TLS panel consensus. *Br J Haematol.* 2010;149:578–586.

Cheson BD, Pfistner B, Juweid ME, et al. Revised response criteria for malignant lymphoma. *J Clin Oncol.* 2007;25:579–586.

Coiffier B, Lepage E, Briere J, et al. CHOP chemotherapy plus rituximab compared with CHOP alone in elderly patients with diffuse large-B-cell lymphoma. *N Engl J Med.* 2002;346:235–242.

Czuczman MS, Grillo-Lopez AJ, White CA, et al. Treatment of patients with low grade B-cell lymphoma with the combination of chimeric anti CD20 monoclonal antibody and CHOP. *J Clin Oncol.* 1999;17:268–276.

Dave SS, Fu H, Wright GW, et al. Molecular diagnosis of Burkitt's lymphoma. *N Engl J Med.* 2006;354(23):2431–2442.

Dunleavy K, Little RF, Pittaluga S, et al. The role of tumor histogenesis, FDG-PET, and short-course EPOCH with dose-dense rituximab (SC-EPOCH-RR) in HIV-associated diffuse large B-cell lymphoma. *Blood.* 2010;115:3017–3024.

Federico M, Bellei M, Marcheselli L, et al. Follicular lymphoma International Prognostic Index 2: a new prognostic index for follicular lymphoma developed by the International Follicular Lymphoma Prognostic Factor Project. *J Clin Oncol.* 2009;27:4555–4562.

Feugier P, Van Hoof A, Sebban C, et al. Long-term results of the R-CHOP study in the treatment of elderly patients with diffuse large B-cell lymphoma: a study by the Groupe d'Etude des Lymphomes de l'Adulte. *J Clin Oncol.* 2005;23(18):4117–4126.

Fisher RI, Gaynor ER, Dahlberg S, et al. Comparison of a standard regimen (CHOP) with three intensive chemotherapy regimens for advanced non-Hodgkin's lymphoma. *N Engl J Med.* 1993;328:1002–1006.

Friedberg JW, Taylor MD, Cerhan JR, et al. Follicular lymphoma in the United States: first report of the National LymphoCare Study. *J Clin Oncol.* 2009;27:1202–1208.

Geisler CH, Kolstad A, Laurell A, et al. Long-term progression-free survival of mantle cell lymphoma after intensive front-line immunochemotherapy with in vivo-purged stem cell rescue: a nonrandomized phase 2 multicenter study by the Nordic Lymphoma Group. *Blood.* 2008;112(7):2687–2693.

Gisselbrecht C, Glass B, Mounier N, et al. Salvage regimens with autologous transplantation for relapsed large B-cell lymphoma in the rituximab era. *J Clin Oncol.* 2010;28:4184–4190.

Hainsworth JD, Litchy S, Burris HA, et al. Rituximab as first-line and maintenance therapy for patients with indolent non-Hodgkin's lymphoma. *J Clin Oncol.* 2002;20:4261–4267.

Hans CP, Weisenburger DD, Greiner TC, et al. Confirmation of the molecular classification of diffuse large B-cell lymphoma by immunohistochemistry using a tissue microarray. *Blood.* 2004;103:275–282.

Hoster E, Dreyling M, Klapper W, et al. A new prognostic index (MIPI) for patients with advanced-stage mantle cell lymphoma. *Blood.* 2008;111:558–565.

Hummel M, Bentink S, Berger H, et al. A biologic definition of Burkitt's lymphoma from transcriptional and genomic profiling. *N Engl J Med.* 2006;354(23):2419–2430.

International Non-Hodgkin's Lymphoma Prognostic Factors Project. A predictive model for aggressive non-Hodgkin's lymphoma. *N Engl J Med.* 1993;329: 987–994.

Kaminski MS, Tuck M, Estes J, et al. 131-I-tositmomab therapy as initial treatment for follicular lymphoma. *N Engl J Med.* 2005;352:441–449.

Keegan T, McClure L, Foran J, et al. Improvements in survival after follicular lymphoma by race/ethnicity and socioeconomic status: a population-based study. *J Clin Oncol.* 2009;27:3044–3051.

Kwee TC, Kwee RM, Nievelstein RA. Imaging in staging of malignant lymphoma: a systematic review. *Blood.* 2008;111:504–516.

Lacasce A, Howard O, Lib S, et al. Modified magrath regimens for adults with Burkitt and Burkitt-like lymphomas: preserved efficacy with decreased toxicity. *Leuk Lymphoma.* 2004;45(4):761–767.

LaCasce AS, Kho ME, Friedberg JW, et al. Comparison of referring and final pathology for patients with non-Hodgkin's lymphoma in the National Comprehensive Cancer Network. *J Clin Oncol.* 2008;26:1–6.

Lenz G, Wright G, Dave SS, et al. Stromal gene signatures in large-B-cell lymphomas. *N Engl J Med.* 2008;359:2313–2323.

Levine AM, Seneviratne L, Espina BM, et al. Evolving characteristics of AIDS related lymphoma. *Blood.* 2000;96:4084–4090.

Link BK, Martin P, Kaminski MS, et al. Cyclophosphamide, vincristine, and prednisone followed by tositumomab and iodine-131–tositumomab in patients with untreated low-grade follicular lymphoma: eight-year follow-up of a multicenter phase II study. *J Clin Oncol.* 2010;28:3035–3041.

Marcus R, Imrie K, Belch A, et al. CVP chemotherapy plus rituximab compared with CVP as first-line treatment for advanced follicular lymphoma. *Blood.* 2005;105:1417–1423.

McMaster ML, Greer, JP, Greco FA, et al. Effective treatment of small non-cleaved cell lymphoma with high intensity, brief duration chemotherapy. *J Clin Oncol.* 1991;9:941–946.

Miller TP, Dahlberg S, Cassady JR, et al. Chemotherapy alone compared with chemotherapy plus radiotherapy for localized intermediate and high-grade non-Hodgkin's lymphoma. *N Engl J Med.* 1998;339:21–26.

Pfreundschuh M, Trümper L, Österborg A, et al. CHOP-like chemotherapy plus rituximab versus CHOP-like chemotherapy alone in young patients with good-prognosis diffuse large-B-cell lymphoma: a randomised controlled trial by the MabThera International Trial (MInT) Group. *Lancet Oncol.* 2006;7:379–391.

Prince HM, Whittaker S, Hoppe RT. How I treat mycosis fungoides and Sézary syndrome. *Blood.* 2009;114:4337–4353.

Robinson KS, Williams ME, van der Jagt RH, et al. Phase II multicenter study of bendamustine plus rituximab in patients with relapsed indolent B-cell and mantle cell non-Hodgkin's lymphoma. *J Clin Oncol.* 2008;26:4473–4479.

Romaguera JE, Fayad LE, Feng L, et al. Ten-year follow-up after intense chemoimmunotherapy with Rituximab-HyperCVAD alternating with Rituximab-high dose methotrexate/cytarabine (R-MA) and without stem cell transplantation in patients with untreated aggressive mantle cell lymphoma. *Br J Haematol.* 2010;150(2):200–208.

Roschewski M, Wilson WH. Biology and management of rare primary extranodal T-cell lymphomas. *Oncology (Williston Park).* 2010;24(1):94–100.

Rosenwald A, Wright G, Chan WC, et al. The use of molecular profiling to predict survival after chemotherapy for diffuse large B-cell lymphoma. *N Engl J Med.* 2002;346:1937–1947.

Rummel MJ, Niederle N, Maschmeyer G, et al. Bendamustine plus rituximab is superior in respect of progression free survival and CR rate when compared to CHOP plus rituximab as first-line treatment of patients with advanced follicular, indolent, and mantle cell lymphomas: final results of a randomized phase III study of the StiL (Study Group Indolent Lymphomas, Germany). *Blood.* 2009;114:405.

Savage KJ, Johnson NA, Ben-Neriah S, et al. *MYC* gene rearrangements are associated with a poor prognosis in diffuse large B-cell lymphoma patients treated with R-CHOP chemotherapy. *Blood.* 2009;114:3533–3537.

Seam P, Juweid ME, Cheson BD. The Role of FDG-PET scans in patients with lymphoma. *Blood.* 2007;110:3507–3516.

Sebban C, Brice P, Delarue R, et al. Impact of rituximab and/or high-dose therapy with autotransplant at time of relapse in patients with follicular lymphoma: a GELA study. *J Clin Oncol.* 2008;26(21):3614–3620.

Sehn LH, Donaldson J, Chhanabhai M, et al. Introduction of combined CHOP plus rituximab therapy dramatically improved outcome of diffuse large B-cell lymphoma in British Columbia. *J Clin Oncol.* 2005;23:5027–5033.

Solal-Ce'ligny P, Roy P, Colombat P, et al. Follicular lymphoma International Prognostic Index. *Blood.* 2004;104:1258–1265.

Swerdlow S, Campo E, Harris N, et al. (eds). *WHO Classification of tumours of haematopoeitic and lymphoid tissues.* 4th ed. Geneva, Switzerland: WHO Press; 2008.

Thomas DA, Cortes J, O'Brien S, et al. Hyper-CVAD program in Burkitt's type adult acute lymphoblastic lymphoma. *J Clin Oncol.* 1999;17:2461–2470.

Valasquez W, Cabanillas F, Salvador P, et al. Effective salvage therapy for lymphoma with cisplatin in combination with high-dose Ara-C and dexamethasone (DHAP). *Blood.* 1988;71:117–122.

Valasquez WS, McLaughlin P, Tucker S, et al. ESHAP—an effective chemotherapy regiment in refractory and relapsing lymphoma: a 4-year follow up study. *J Clin Oncol.* 1994;12:1169–1176.

van Oers MHJ, Van Glabbeke M, Giurgea L, et al. Rituximab maintenance treatment of relapsed/resistant follicular non-Hodgkin's lymphoma: long-term outcome of the EORTC 20981 phase III randomized Intergroup study. *J Clin Oncol.* 2010;28:1–7.

Wang M, Burau K, Fang S, et al. Ethnic variations in diagnosis, treatment, socioeconomic status, and survival in a large population-based cohort of elderly patients with non-Hodgkin lymphoma. *Cancer.* 2008;113:3231–3241.

Zinzani PL, Fanti S, Battista G, et al. Predictive role of positron emission tomography (PET) in the outcome of lymphoma patients. *Br J Cancer.* 2004;91:850–854.

Zinzani PL, Pulsoni A, Perrotti A, et al. Fludarabine plus mitoxantrone with and without rituximab versus CHOP with and without rituximab as frontline treatment for patients with follicular lymphoma. *J Clin Oncol.* 2004;22:2654–2661.

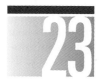

Multiple Myeloma, Other Plasma Cell Disorders, and Primary Amyloidosis

Rachid Baz and Mohamad A. Hussein

I. INTRODUCTION

A. Types of plasma cell dyscrasias

Plasma cell dyscrasias represent a heterogeneous group of conditions characterized by an increased number of plasma cells or by the productions of a monoclonal protein. The following plasma cell dyscrasias will be discussed in this chapter: monoclonal gammopathy of undetermined significance (MGUS), multiple myeloma (MM), Waldenström macroglobulinemia (WM), amyloidosis, and solitary plasmacytomas. Light chain deposition disease, heavy chain diseases, immunoglobulin D MM, nonsecretory MM, osteosclerotic myeloma or POEMS (*p*olyneuropathy, *o*rganomegaly, *e*ndocrinopathy, *m*onoclonal gammopathy, and *s*kin changes) syndrome and primary plasma cell leukemia are beyond the scope of this text.

B. Monoclonal protein (M-protein)

An M-protein is detected in the serum, urine, or both of most patients with plasma cell dyscrasias. The so-called M-protein is thought to be a measure of plasma cell burden, although a correlation is not always evident. A notable discordance between the M-protein and disease burden could be noted in heavily pretreated patients where the malignant cells might have dedifferentiated and have become less secretory or nonsecretory. This is often accompanied by an increase in the serum lactate dehydrogenase. Exceptions aside, most plasma cell dyscrasias are best followed by serial measurements of the M-protein and parameters of end organ dysfunction. Current standard criteria rely on changes in the M-protein for determining response and progression after treatment. The basic immunoglobulin (Ig) unit comprises two identical heavy chains (G, A, M, D or E) and two identical light chains (kappa or lambda). The serum protein electrophoresis is used to quantify the monoclonal component of the globulin; it fails to do so, however, when the concentration of the latter is low because of lack of secretion or if the M-protein is excreted in the urine. If there is a high clinical suspicion for the presence of an M-protein despite a negative serum protein electrophoresis, an immunoelectrophoresis should be performed on both the serum and the urine, as up to 15% of patients may have a negative serum immunofixation with positive urine immunofixation. The urinary light-chain excretion (expressed in grams per 24 hours) is used to follow the urinary M-protein. This is calculated from the 24-hour urine protein and the percent contribution of light chain to proteinuria on the urine protein electrophoresis. It is critical to assess the percent contribution of the light chain to the proteinuria especially in patients with other comorbidities such as hypertension and diabetes mellitus, where the patient could present with an M-protein with the proteinuria consisting mainly of albumin secondary to the other medical processes. Newer assays for serum free light chain are becoming increasingly available and often result in the detection of increased free light chains in the serum of many patients with nonsecretory MM (negative immune fixation of the serum and urine) and amyloid light-chain (AL) amyloidosis. The latter assay does not demonstrate monoclonality of the light chain but relies on the ratio of kappa to lambda light chain to infer an excess of one of the light chains. While some investigators have correlated changes in the free light chain induced by therapy with outcomes and the use of the serum, and the free light-chain test has been incorporated in the International Myeloma Working Group response criteria, the precise role of these markers beyond their contribution to the diagnosis has not been thoroughly validated. Infections, autoimmune disorders, and poor renal function make interpretation of the free light-chain assay difficult.

II. MONOCLONAL GAMMOPATHY OF UNCERTAIN SIGNIFICANCE (MGUS)

MGUS is usually characterized by a low M-protein (less than 3 g/dL), the absence of bone lesions, less than 10% plasma cells on the bone marrow biopsy, and the absence of attributable end organ damage such as anemia, hypercalcemia, and renal dysfunction. The prevalence of MGUS increases with age and has been described in as many as 3% of all individuals over 70 years of age. The rate of progression from MGUS to MM or other lymphoproliferative disorders varies based on several factors, the most notable of which is the level of the serum M-protein. A high serum M-protein ($\geq$1.5 g/dL), a higher bone marrow plasma cell burden, and possibly an abnormal kappa to lambda ratio on free light-chain testing puts select patients at higher risk of progression to MM. While patients with lower risk MGUS may be followed on a yearly or biannual basis, patients with higher risk of progression probably benefit from closer follow-up and may be eligible for enrollment in prevention clinical trials. In a small number of patients, MGUS could be associated with peripheral neuropathy. The majority of patients with MGUS and peripheral neuropathy in association with an Ig M-protein have anti-myelin-associated glycoprotein antibodies. This group of patients responds favorably to therapy with single-agent rituximab.

III. MULTIPLE MYELOMA (MM)
A. General considerations and aims of therapy
1. **Diagnosis.** MM is a clonal B-cell tumor of slowly proliferating plasma cells within the bone marrow. Table 23.1 illustrates diagnostic criteria required for a diagnosis of MM. The Durie and Salmon staging system was initially used for the staging of patients with MM (Table 23.2). Its use has fallen out of favor due to difficulties inherent to its use. A staging system is the International Staging System, which is illustrated in Table 23.3. It relies on the serum β2-microglobulin and on serum albumin. It was found to accurately prognosticate patient outcomes.

With the increased awareness, an increasing number of patients are being diagnosed with monoclonal gammopathy

TABLE 23.1	Diagnostic Criteria of MGUS and Multiple Myeloma	
MGUS	**Asymptomatic MM**	**Symptomatic MM**
Serum M-protein <30 g/L and clonal bone marrow plasmacytosis <10%	Serum M-protein ≥30 g/L or clonal bone marrow plasmacytosis ≥10%	M protein in the serum or urine and clonal bone marrow plasmacytosis or plasmacytoma
No other B-cell lymphoproliferative disorder	No related organ and tissue impairment	Related organ and tissue impairment*
No related organ and tissue impairment		

M-protein, monoclonal protein; MGUS, monoclonal gammopathy of undetermined significance; MM, multiple myeloma.
*Related organ tissue impairment includes the following:
- Hypercalcemia
- Renal dysfunction
- Anemia: hemoglobin 2 g/dL below the lower limit of normal
- Lytic bone lesions (solitary plasmacytoma requires >30% plasma cells)
- Symptomatic hyperviscosity
- Amyloidosis (requires >30% plasma cells)
- Recurrent bacterial infections (>2/year).

TABLE 23.2 Durie-Salmon Staging System

Stage*	Criteria

I	All of the following:
	1. Hemoglobin >10 g/dL
	2. Serum calcium value normal (≤12 mg/dL)
	3. On radiograph, normal bone structure or solitary bone plasmacytoma only
	4. Low M-component production rates
	   a. IgG value <5 g/dL
	   b. IgA value <3 g/dL
	   c. Urine light-chain M component on electrophoresis <4 g/24 hours

II	Fitting neither stage I nor stage III

III	One or more of the following:
	1. Hemoglobin <8.5 g/dL
	2. Serum calcium value >12 mg/dL
	3. Advanced lytic bone lesions
	4. High monoclonal component production rates
	   a. IgG value >7 g/dL
	   b. IgA value >5 g/dL
	   c. Urine light-chain M component on electrophoresis >12 g/24 hours

IG, immunglobulin.
*Stages I, II, and III are further designated A for serum creatinine <2 and B for serum creatinine ≥2.
From Durie BG, Salmon SE. A clinical staging system for multiple myeloma. Correlation of measured myeloma cell mass with presenting clinical features, response to treatment, and survival. *Cancer.* 1975;36:842.

TABLE 23.3 ISS Staging System for Multiple Myeloma

Better response to therapy	**Stage I Factors:** beta-2 microglobulin <3.5 mg/dL Albumin ≥3.5 g/dL	Most favorable prognosis

↕	**Stage II Factors:**
	beta-2 microglobulin
	  <3.5 mg/dL
	Albumin <3.5 g/dL *or*
	  beta-2 microglobulin
	  ≥3.5–<5.5 mg/dL
		↕

Lesser response to therapy	**Stage III Factors:** beta-2 microglobulin ≥5.5 mg/dL	Less favorable prognosis

ISS, International Staging System.

incidentally, and the decision to monitor or actively treat has become difficult with the old nomenclature.

a. **End organ damage.** The International Myeloma Working Group has presented the concept of MM with active or inactive disease based on the presence or absence of end organ damage, respectively.

b. **Criteria defining end organ damage** are anemia, renal failure, hypercalcemia, severe osteoporosis or lytic bony disease, or other organ abnormality that is attributable to the plasma cell dyscrasia.

c. **Patients without end organ damage** (MGUS or inactive myeloma) should be monitored carefully as early intervention does not affect the outcome of the disease. Patients with inactive MM should be considered for enrollment clinical trials aimed at preventing or retarding the progression to active disease.

d. **Alternatively,** patients who meet the criteria for MGUS but demonstrate end organ damage related to the plasma cell dyscrasia must be classified as active MM and should receive active therapy.

2. **Epidemiology.** The annual incidence of MM is 4 per 100,000 population, with a peak incidence between the sixth and seventh decade of life. Patients of African-American descent have an incidence of MGUS and MM approaching twice the incidence for Caucasians in the United States. Several agents have been strongly associated with the development of MM, ionizing radiation being the most commonly described risk factor. Nickel, agricultural chemicals, petroleum products, and other aromatic hydrocarbons, benzene, and silicon have been considered potential risk factors as well. One particular note is made for Agent Orange exposure by Vietnam veterans imparting an increased incidence of MM.

3. **Goals of therapy.** Despite recent advances in the treatment of MM, the disease remains incurable. Accordingly, therapy is aimed at improving symptoms and preventing complications of the disease, thus improving quality of life and survival. These goals could be achieved with different approaches: one aim is to transform the disease into a chronic process by using frequent low morbidity therapies, while the other approach attempts to eradicate the disease with intensive therapy. The cure versus control paradigm remains a subject of considerable debate, and it remains unclear which treatment methodology is superior. However, there is evidence that certain subgroups of patients might benefit from one or the other approach, and therapy aimed at control of the myeloma may be inappropriate for patients with more aggressive risk features. Because of these uncertainties and because standard first-line therapy is not well defined, patients with MM,

regardless of age, stage of disease, or number of previous therapies, must be considered for clinical trials enrollment.

In addition to the management of the malignant plasma cell clone, particular attention must be made to end organ dysfunction including skeletal health, prevention of infections, and thrombotic, neuronal, and renal complications. Accordingly, response to therapy is based on changes to the M-protein concentration, the percentage of plasma cells in the bone marrow, as well as monitoring end organs for improvement in function. The cooperative oncology groups in the United States and Europe have adopted different cutoffs to define response. Table 23.4 illustrates the uniform response criteria as defined by the International Myeloma Working Group.

4. **Prognostic factors.** Severe anemia, hypercalcemia, advanced lytic lesions, and very high M-protein are all associated with a high tumor burden and a poor survival and are the basis of the Durie and Salmon staging system. Renal failure, although not clearly correlated with disease burden, is associated with worse outcomes. Other established clinical poor prognostic factors include the following: advanced age, poor performance status at presentation, high serum lactate dehydrogenase level, lower platelet counts, bone marrow with greater than 50% plasma cells, greater than 2% bone marrow plasmablasts, high plasma cell labeling index, elevated serum β_2-microglobulin, and low serum albumin. The latter two are the basis for the Southwest Oncology Group (SWOG) and International Myeloma Working Group staging systems. The identification of cytogenetic prognostic factors using metaphase karyotyping relies on cellular growth, which is difficult as the MM plasma cells have a low in vitro proliferative rate and thus such information is available only in 20% to 40% of the patients. The presence of abnormalities with this method, however, is meaningful. Genomic prognostic factors include the deletion of chromosome 13, translocation of the immunoglobulin heavy chain [t(4;14), t(14;16)], and loss of 17p13. The t(11;14), on the other hand, is not thought to portend a worse outcome. Recently, interphase fluorescence in situ hybridization (FISH) has been used to detect specific cytogenetic abnormalities. Even though FISH analysis is more sensitive at detecting certain abnormalities such as chromosome 13, this might not be clinically meaningful without other additional poor prognosticators. Nonhyperdiploid karyotypes are frequently associated with immunoglobulin heavy chain rearrangements and worse clinical outcomes.

B. **Initial treatment**
1. **General measures.** Patients with a new diagnosis of MM occasionally have associated complications that require immediate attention, such as hypercalcemia, renal failure, severe cytopenias,

	Uniform Response Criteria as Defined by the International Myeloma Working Group
CR	■ Negative immunofixation on the serum and urine, *and* ■ Disappearance of any soft-tissue plasmacytomas, *and* ■ No more than 5% plasma cells in the bone marrow (confirmation with repeat bone marrow is not needed)
Stringent CR	■ CR as defined above, *and* ■ Normal serum FLC ratio, *and* ■ Absence of clonal cells in the bone marrow by immunohistochemistry or immunofluorescence, based on a κ/λ ratio of >4:1 or <1:2 performed on a minimum of 100 plasma cells (confirmation with repeat bone marrow is not needed)
Very good partial remission	■ Serum and urine M-protein detectable by immunofixation but not on electrophoresis, *or* ■ At least 90% reduction in serum M-protein plus urine M-protein level of <100 mg per 24 hours
Partial remission	■ At least 50% reduction of serum M-protein and reduction in 24-hour urinary M-protein by ≥90%, or to <200 mg per 24 hours ■ If the serum and urine M-protein are unmeasurable,* a ≥50% decrease in the difference between involved and uninvolved FLC levels is required in place of the M-protein criteria ■ In addition to the above listed criteria, if present at baseline, a ≥50% reduction in the size of soft-tissue plasmacytomas is also required
Stable disease	■ Not meeting criteria for CR, very good partial remission, partial remission, or progressive disease
Progressive disease	■ Increase of ≥25% from baseline in serum monoclonal component, and the absolute increase must be ≥0.5 g/dL. If the starting monoclonal component is ≥5 g/dL, increases ≥1 g/dL are sufficient to define relapse. ■ Increase of ≥25% from baseline in urine monoclonal component, and the absolute increase must be ≥200 mg/24 hours ■ Only in patients without measurable serum and urine M-protein levels: increase of ≥25% from baseline in the difference between involved and uninvolved FLC levels, and the absolute difference must be >10 mg/dL ■ Increase of ≥25% from baseline in bone marrow plasma cell percentage, and the absolute % must be ≥10% (relapse from CR has the 5% cutoff versus 10% for other categories of relapse) ■ Definite development of new bone lesions or soft-tissue plasmacytomas or definite increase in the size of existing bone lesions or soft-tissue plasmacytomas ■ Development of hypercalcemia (corrected serum calcium >11.5 mg/dL or >2.65 mmol/L) that can be attributed solely to the plasma cell proliferative disorder

CR, complete remission; FLC, free light-chain; M-protein, monoclonal protein.
*All relapse categories require two consecutive assessments made at any time before classification as relapse or disease progression and/or the institution of any new therapy.
Measurable disease is defined as:
■ Serum M-protein ≥1 g/dL (≥10 g/L)
■ Urine M-protein ≥200 mg/24 hours
■ Serum FLC assay: involved FLC level ≥10 mg/dL (≥100 mg/L) provided serum FLC ratio is abnormal.

and spinal cord compression. These complications should be promptly identified and managed either simultaneously or before the start of therapy. Alternatively, asymptomatic patients and those with smoldering MM may be followed without specific therapy until clear evidence of progression. Ambulation and hydration should be maintained throughout the initial therapy. Avoidance of nonsteroidal anti-inflammatory drugs (NSAIDs), aminoglycosides, and intravenous contrast agents is important for renal health. If radiologic procedures involving the use of intravenous contrast agents are to be considered, appropriate hydration and the use of *N*-acetyl-cysteine should be considered. The use of bisphosphonates (either pamidronate or zoledronic acid) is recommended for nearly every patient with myeloma with normal renal function, in particularly those with bony disease (see Section III.C.5). The authors recommend holding the initiation of the bisphosphonates in the first cycle of therapy to help decrease renal complications from the use of these agents. In addition, because of the increased awareness for osteonecrosis of the jaw, a rare complication of bisphosphonate therapy, a dental evaluation prior to starting therapy should be considered.

2. **Systemic therapy for the newly diagnosed patient** (see Section IV.B.3 for specific regimens). While a plethora of therapeutic options for the treatment of patients with newly diagnosed MM are available, there is no standard first-line therapy. In this text, we will define non–high-dose therapy as *traditional* therapy and high-dose therapy with stem cell rescue as *intensive* therapy. The precise role of novel therapeutic agents (such as bortezomib, lenalidomide, and thalidomide) in the management of newly diagnosed MM remains unclear and is the subject of ongoing clinical trials. As therapy for MM does not result in cures, treatment recommendations are often individualized and based on a patient's comorbidities, performance status, and preference, as well as disease characteristics. For example, if high-dose therapy is considered during the course of therapy, avoidance of agents that impair stem cell collection is important (e.g., melphalan and other alkylating agents). In the patient with significant symptoms from the disease, the choice of highly active first-line therapy that results in rapid responses is reasonable. Similarly, in patients with renal dysfunction at presentation, the choice of agents with a safe renal profile is recommended (e.g., bortezomib-based therapy).

Patients with poor prognostic factors at presentation [chromosome 13 deletion by metaphase cytogenetics or t(4;14), high β2 microglobulin, or increased plasma cell labeling index] fare poorly with all traditional therapies. Accordingly, these patients are best managed by enrollment in clinical trials. Alternatively, it is intuitive, though unproven, that intensive therapy (combination novel agent induction therapy followed by consideration of high-dose therapy) would result in improved outcomes. While some reports suggest that bortezomib-based therapy overcomes the negative implications of high-risk disease, these observations are based on small numbers and relatively short follow-up, and other investigations did not confirm these findings.

For patients eligible for intensive therapy, the use of dexamethasone in combination with an immunomodulator (lenalidomide) or a proteasome inhibitor is reasonable. At the time of best response, collection of stem cells is recommended. Lenalidomide-based therapy is usually continued until progression or until high-dose therapy, while bortezomib-based therapy is usually planned for six to eight cycles (or until high-dose therapy).

While many patients over the age of 65 years remain excellent candidates for intensive therapy, high-dose therapy may not be appropriate for some; therapy with melphalan, prednisone, and either thalidomide or bortezomib has been demonstrated to be superior to melphalan and prednisone. In addition, therapy with low-dose dexamethasone and lenalidomide may also be reasonable. In addition, for the much older patient with significant comorbidities, less intensive therapy may be appropriate (e.g., melphalan or cyclophosphamide in combination with prednisone). Chemotherapeutic regimens are described below.

3. **Traditional chemotherapy recommendations.** While numerous additional chemotherapeutic regimens have been described, only commonly used agents in the treatment of MM are reviewed below.

   a. **Dexamethasone** is considered the standard corticosteroid for many induction regimens for MM. Recently, the Eastern Cooperative Oncology Group study comparing lenalidomide and low-dose dexamethasone to lenalidomide and high-dose dexamethasone demonstrated a survival benefit in the lower dose of dexamethasone. This was more pronounced in patients older than 65 years but was noted in all age groups. High-dose dexamethasone, for a few cycles, in combination with lenalidomide remains reasonable in younger patients with high disease burden.

   High-dose dexamethasone is given at a dose of 40 mg by mouth on days 1 to 4, 9 to 12, and 17 to 20. Cycles are repeated every 28 days. Low-dose dexamethasone consists of 40 mg by mouth weekly or on days 1 to 4 of a 28-day cycle. Significant early toxicities include hyperglycemia, dyspepsia, fatigue, and muscle weakness. Additionally, patients often report agitation and insomnia with the use of this schedule of dexamethasone.

Longer term toxicities include increased infections, cataract, osteoporosis, and avascular necrosis of femoral heads. As a single agent in patients with newly diagnosed myeloma, responses are observed in about 50% of patients, and the median time to response is approximately 1 month. However, the median duration of response is only 6 months. As such, single-agent dexamethasone is generally not the treatment of choice.

b. **Thalidomide and dexamethasone.** The addition of thalidomide to the above schedule of dexamethasone results in an increased response rate (about 70%) at the cost of additional toxicity (in the form of thromboembolic events, rash, sedation, peripheral neuropathy, and constipation). While thalidomide was started at 200 mg daily at bedtime on the pivotal clinical trial, our experience suggests improved patient tolerance with a more gradual start of thalidomide.

We recommend initiating thalidomide at 50 mg daily at bedtime and increasing the daily dose by 50 mg increments every week to a desired target dose not exceeding 200 mg daily or as dictated by patient tolerance. It should be noted, however, that there is no known minimal dose required for response: some (though rare) patients respond to dosages as low as 50 mg three times a week.

In addition, in responding patients receiving high-dose dexamethasone, reduction of dexamethasone to 40 mg on days 1 to 4 monthly (or low-dose dexamethasone) results in improved patient tolerance.

With the increased risks of thromboembolic events (about 17% of patients receiving this combination), we recommend the use of prophylactic low dose aspirin (81 mg). Other investigators have used different prophylactic strategies, which include low-molecular-weight heparin and therapeutic anticoagulation with warfarin. A recent randomized trial of these thromboprophylactic strategies did not demonstrate the superiority of any one of the above regimens. Given that thalidomide use has been associated with the development of neuropathy with long-term use, this agent has largely been replaced with lenalidomide in this setting. This regimen may be considered in patients with significant cytopenias or renal insufficiency with disease refractory to bortezomib.

c. **Lenalidomide and dexamethasone.** Lenalidomide is an immunomodulatory drug with more potent tumor necrosis factor-α inhibition than thalidomide. In addition, lenalidomide has a different adverse event profile than thalidomide and does not usually cause significant sedation or neuropathy; it does result in myelosuppression. In patients with relapsed or refractory MM, the combination of lenalidomide and dexamethasone resulted in responses in approximately 60% of patients with a progression-free survival of approximately 12 months.

Lenalidomide is usually started at 25 mg by mouth daily for 21 of 28 days. Lower starting doses are recommended in patients with renal dysfunction as lenalidomide is renally cleared. Lenalidomide toxicities include thromboembolic events, myelosuppression, rash, and diarrhea. Myelosuppression is often noted early during the course of therapy, and febrile neutropenia is rare. Lenalidomide with low-dose dexamethasone results in a response in 75% to 90% of patients. The optimal duration of therapy with lenalidomide is unclear. Because in clinical trials this agent was used until progression, we recommend a similar approach in patients tolerating this agent well and not proceeding with immediate high-dose therapy. After two cycles of therapy, consideration for decreasing the frequency of dexamethasone to 4 days must be given. In addition, in responding patients after 1 year of therapy, omitting dexamethasone and continuing with single-agent lenalidomide is reasonable. Long-term lenalidomide therapy may make stem cell collection difficult, and the use of chemotherapy in combination with granulocyte colony-stimulating factor (G-CSF) may be needed for stem cell collection.

d. **Melphalan and prednisone (MP)** has fallen out of favor with the availability of novel agents, and combinations of thalidomide or bortezomib with MP have resulted in superior survival than MP alone. Nonetheless, MP remains a reasonable option for very elderly patients with many comorbidities. MP results in about a 50% overall response rate in patients with newly diagnosed myeloma and a median time to progression of about 15 months. While a number of different dosages and schedules for MP exists, we recommend the following:

- Melphalan 9 mg/m^2 by mouth on days 1 to 4, *and*
- Prednisone 100 mg by mouth on days 1 to 4.

For reliable absorption, melphalan should be taken on an empty stomach. Repeat the cycle every 4 to 6 weeks depending on recovery of counts. MP is usually given for six to nine cycles, and treatment beyond 1 year does increase risks of myelodysplasia. Responses to MP tend to occur slower on average, making this a less attractive regimen in patients with significant symptoms. On the other hand, MP is well tolerated in patients with myeloma, with myelosuppression being the most significant adverse event. MP should not be used in patients who are candidates for intensive therapy as it may impair stem cell collection.

e. **Melphalan, prednisone, and thalidomide (MPT).** Thalidomide has been added to MP in the MPT regimen. Similar recommendations to Section IV.B.3.b pertaining to the use of thalidomide can be made. In addition, thalidomide up to 100 mg at bedtime is usually recommended. In some studies involving MPT, thalidomide was continued for 1 year after MP therapy was discontinued, while in other MPT studies thalidomide was discontinued at the time of stopping MP. In patients with a good tolerance to thalidomide, continuing such therapy would be reasonable.

f. **Bortezomib** is a proteasome inhibitor approved for relapsed or refractory MM and more recently for newly diagnosed disease in combination with MP. In addition, combination therapy with dexamethasone or pegylated liposomal doxorubicin or with thalidomide or lenalidomide has shown promising results. As a single agent in relapsed and refractory patients, it was shown to result in a response rate of about 30% to 40% and a median time to progression of 6 to 7 months. This was found to be superior to high-dose dexamethasone.

   ▪ Bortezomib is given at 1.3 mg/m^2 intravenously over 3 to 5 seconds on days 1, 4, 8, and 11 on a 21-day cycle.

   ▪ Dexamethasone 20 mg on the day of and the day after bortezomib is often added after two cycles in patients with suboptimal responses. The addition of steroids, however, results in only a modest improvement in the response and/or the quality of the response.

   Treatment is continued for a maximum of eight cycles. Grade 3 and 4 adverse events of bortezomib include the following: thrombocytopenia (30%), neutropenia (14%), anemia (10%), and neuropathy (8%). Neuropathy should be monitored carefully with special attention to autonomic neuropathy in the form of paralytic ileus and delayed peripheral neuropathy after the discontinuation of therapy. Neuropathy is often painful in nature but is also reversible in about two-thirds of patients after 3 to 6 months of discontinuation of therapy. Bortezomib-based therapy is often the treatment of choice in patients with significant renal impairment.

g. **Melphalan, prednisone, and bortezomib (VMP).** Two 3-week bortezomib cycles are added to a 6-week MP cycle in standard VMP. In addition, "lite" and "superlite" VMP regimens, in which bortezomib is given on a standard schedule for the first cycle and subsequently weekly or bortezomib is given weekly instead of twice weekly, respectively, have been described. These reduced intensity regimens result in less grade 3 neuropathy and gastrointestinal toxicity than standard VMP. While VMP "lite" and "superlite" have comparable response rates to VMP, efficacy was not compared in a randomized study, and these reduced intensity regimens did not demonstrate a survival advantage to MP as standard VMP has. The risk of varicella zoster reactivation can be effectively reduced/eliminated with the use of acyclovir prophylaxis, which is recommended for all bortezomib-containing regimens.

■ Standard VMP
  ■ Bortezomib 1.3 mg/m^2 on days 1, 4, 8, 11, 22, 25, 29, and 32 for four cycles followed by bortezomib 1.3 mg/m^2 on days 1, 8, 22, and 29 for five cycles
  ■ Melphalan 9 mg/m^2 on days 1 to 4
  ■ Prednisone 60 mg/m^2 on days 1 to 4
  ■ Cycles are repeated every 6 weeks.
■ VMP lite
  ■ Similar MP dosing with bortezomib given on days 1, 4, 8, 11, 22, 25, 29, and 32 for one cycle and on days 1, 8, 22, and 29 for eight cycles.
■ VMP superlite
  ■ Similar MP dosing with bortezomib given on days 1, 8, 22, and 29 for all nine cycles.

h. **Cyclophosphamide and prednisone (CP)** is a forgotten alternative to MP. Cyclophosphamide does not need dose adjustments for renal failure, making it a useful agent in patients with a decreased performance status and/or comorbidities. It results in a response rate of about 50% and a progression-free survival of 12 to 15 months in treatment naïve patients. CP is given as follows:
  ■ Cyclophosphamide 1000 mg/m^2 intravenously (IV) on day 1, *and*
  ■ Prednisone 100 mg by mouth on days 1 to 5
  ■ Cycles are repeated every 21 days.

   CP is well tolerated and, in distinction to MP, does not result in significant compromise to stem cell reserve. Furthermore, thalidomide and bortezomib have been added to this backbone with demonstrated efficacy.

i. **Bortezomib, lenalidomide, and dexamethasone (RVD).** The combination of lenalidomide, bortezomib, and dexamethasone was evaluated in patients with newly diagnosed as well as previously treated MM. In newly diagnosed myeloma, the combination has a demonstrated high response rate and appears to be well tolerated. An ongoing intergroup trial will be comparing this combination to lenalidomide and dexamethasone in newly diagnosed patients. However, it remains unclear if the high response rate for this triplet will translate into improved patient outcomes. For newly diagnosed patients, RVD is administered as follows:
  ■ Lenalidomide 25 mg by mouth on days 1 to 14
  ■ Bortezomib 1.3 mg/m^2 IV on days 1, 4, 8, and 11
  ■ Dexamethasone 20 mg by mouth on days 1, 2, 4, 5, 8, 9, 11, and 12
  ■ Cycles are repeated every 21 days.

Supportive therapy includes acyclovir and aspirin prophylaxis for varicella zoster virus reactivation and thromboembolic disease, respectively.

In relapsed and refractory myeloma, the RVD regimen has demonstrated the ability to induce responses in patients refractory to both lenalidomide and bortezomib. Due to the marrow compromise often present in patients with relapsed and refractory myeloma, the lenalidomide starting dose is 15 mg orally on days 1 to 14 of a standard bortezomib cycle.

j. **Bortezomib and pegylated liposomal doxorubicin.** Bortezomib has been combined with pegylated liposomal doxorubicin. A pivotal phase III trial, which led to the approval of pegylated liposomal doxorubicin, compared this combination to single-agent bortezomib in patients with relapsed and refractory myeloma. The combination results in a similar overall response rate to single-agent bortezomib, but the quality responses (very good partial responses and better) were increased with combination therapy. This translated to improved progression-free and overall survival. Pegylated liposomal doxorubicin (30 mg/m^2) was given on day 4 of a standard bortezomib cycle in this combination, but in our experience, it can also be safely given on day 1 of the cycle. Notable toxicities of pegylated liposomal doxorubicin include palmar plantar erythrodysesthesia syndrome (hand-foot syndrome), myelosuppression, and cardiotoxicity. In addition, dexamethasone can be added to this regimen, and intriguing early results with this combination have been reported but have not been replicated.

4. **Treatment of patients with relapsed or refractory MM.** Despite original responses to therapy, virtually all patients develop recurrent or refractory MM. In patients who experience a relapse more than 1 year after receiving chemotherapy, remission can frequently be obtained using the same regimen. Patients relapsing earlier will likely require an alternate treatment regimen. Patients with refractory myeloma have evidence of progressive disease while receiving active therapy or within 60 days from last therapy despite possible original responses. This patient population has a worse outcome than relapsed patients do. Enrollment of patients with relapsed or refractory myeloma into clinical trials should be a first consideration in the choice of antineoplastic therapy. A number of novel therapeutic tools are emerging in the treatment of MM. These include novel immunomodulatory drugs (pomalidomide), novel proteasome inhibitors (carfilzomib), histone deacetylase inhibitors (LBH589, vorinostat), mammalian target of rapamycin inhibitors (temsirolimus), and RANK-L antibodies (denosumab). Many of these

will likely be approved first for the treatment of relapsed or refractory patients prior to gaining indication in newly diagnosed patients.

5. **High-dose therapy with bone marrow or peripheral blood stem cell transplantation.** The role of high-dose therapy and autologous stem cell transplantation for MM in the era of novel agents remains poorly defined. Initial reports of high-dose therapy generated significant enthusiasm for this approach, as it was associated with a survival advantage over standard therapy using alkylating agents. Contemporary clinical trials comparing high-dose therapy to conventional therapy have failed to consistently confirm the results of initial trials, likely because of the improvement in standard therapies and the availability of novel active salvage therapies. Despite the lack of consistent overall survival advantage, early high-dose therapy does offer a prolongation in the Time Without Symptoms of Disease or Toxicity of Treatment, a quality-of-life measure surrogate. With the advent of novel agents, the role of high-dose therapy and its timing in MM therapeutic armamentarium will require revalidation.

For patients electing to proceed to high-dose therapy, available induction therapies include the use of lenalidomide or thalidomide-dexamethasone or bortezomib-dexamethasone. Three-agent induction has been shown to result in a higher rate of quality responses prior to high-dose therapy compared to two-agent induction. While this may translate in improved posttransplant quality responses, it remains unclear whether three-agent induction will improve survival. As such, the use of three-agent induction therapy should be considered only in the context of clinical trials.

Stem cells can be derived from the peripheral blood or the bone marrow. The former can be done with the use of G-CSF with or without chemotherapy. Novel agents to facilitate stem cell collection (plerixafor) have entered the clinical arena. Peripheral stem cell rescue results in faster engraftment as compared to bone marrow stem cell rescue and has accordingly supplanted the former in clinical use. High-dose therapy is usually in the form of melphalan given at 200 mg/m^2 for younger patients with intact renal function. Total-body radiation has mostly been abandoned in this setting in view of inferior results associated with its use. While purging the graft of malignant cells seems intuitively useful, it has not been shown to improve outcomes, and in vivo purging (with systemic therapy) remains the preferred modality. High-dose therapy with peripheral stem cell rescue has been carried out in an outpatient setting at some transplant centers but remains an inpatient therapy for 2 to 3 weeks at most other centers.

Advances in high-dose therapy will likely involve defining the role of vaccination and immunomodulatory drugs post autologous stem cell transplantation and supportive care improvement needed to further increase the safety of this approach.

6. **Duration of therapy and role of maintenance therapy.** Patients with stable M-protein for greater than 6 months (the so-called plateau phase) appear to have a favorable prognosis and should be monitored carefully at least every 3 months. No study has conclusively demonstrated benefit by continuing chemotherapy beyond 1 year in responding patients (except with treatment with immunomodulators, in which therapy is usually continued until progressive disease or significant toxicity). Several investigators have noted earlier re-emergence of active myeloma after complete cessation of therapy, hence suggesting a benefit for maintenance therapy. A study by SWOG has shown that maintenance therapy with prednisone given at 50 mg every other day improves overall and progression-free survival when compared to maintenance therapy with 10 mg of prednisone every other day. While interferon maintenance resulted in a prolonged progression-free survival, overall survival was not increased and toxicity from interferon was notable. The use of thalidomide to maintain responses observed after intensive therapy has been associated with a survival benefit in patients, not in a very good partial response or better after high-dose therapy. On the other hand, patients receiving continued thalidomide should be closely monitored for peripheral neuropathy, and doses as low as 50 mg every other day are often all that patients are able to tolerate. Thalidomide maintenance is currently not routinely recommended for all patients post intensive therapy. Emerging data from the Cancer and Leukemia Group B and the Institute for Functional Medicine have evaluated maintenance with lenalidomide. Both studies reported a significant benefit to lenalidomide maintenance on progression-free survival, while overall survival remains not statistically different with maintenance lenalidomide. The consideration of lenalidomide maintenance should be individualized with discussion of risks and benefits with the patient.

7. **Role of radiotherapy.** While radiotherapy is sometimes curative in patients with solitary plasmacytomas, its use in patients with MM is palliative and adjunctive to the use of systemic therapy. Patients with symptomatic extraskeletal plasmacytomas, large lytic lesions threatening fracture of long bones, spinal cord or root compression by plasma cells, and certain pathologic fractures are good candidates for radiotherapy. Conservative use of radiotherapy is wise as radiation of bone marrow can impair marrow reserves and render the patient less able to tolerate subsequent therapy.

C. Complications of disease or therapy

Notable toxicity of each chemotherapeutic agent is described in Chapter 33. In addition, complications characteristic of MM are described here.

1. **Hypercalcemia.** Once a very frequent complication of MM, hypercalcemia is less often noted, likely as a result of more widespread use of bisphosphonate therapy for bone health. The pathophysiology of hypercalcemia in patients with MM is related to increased osteoclast activation as a result of binding of the latter to malignant plasma cells. Receptor activator of nuclear factor-κB (RANK)-ligand produced by bone marrow stromal cells is the best-described cytokine mediating this effect. Antibodies to RANK-ligand are entering the clinical arena and are currently being tested in clinical trials in patients with MM. Symptoms of hypercalcemia are often protean, often overlap with adverse events of thalidomide, and require a strong index of suspicion. Symptoms include anorexia, constipation, polyuria, and lethargy. Coma and death can be the result of untreated hypercalcemia. Dehydration and potentially reversible renal dysfunction are frequently associated with hypercalcemia. Treatment of hypercalcemia involves aggressive saline hydration, use of loop diuretics once fluid overload occurs, use of corticosteroids (such as prednisone 60 mg for 7 days), and bisphosphonate therapy. Calcitonin is sometimes used, and hemodialysis is reserved for refractory cases. When hypercalcemia occurs in previously untreated patients, prompt initiation of therapy for the MM in addition to the above usually results in effective, durable control.

   a. **Bisphosphonates**
      - Pamidronate 90 mg given as a 2-hour IV infusion that can be repeated every 30 days *or*
      - Zoledronic acid 4 mg IV over 15 to 30 minutes in the absence of renal dysfunction.

   b. **Calcitonin** 100 to 300 U subcutaneously every 8 to 12 hours for up to 2 to 3 days. Calcitonin is usually given with prednisone 60 mg by mouth daily to prolong its effectiveness.

   c. **Hemodialysis** is very effective but rarely needed.

2. **Infections** (see Chapter 27). Patients with MM are at increased risks for infectious complications usually related to capsulated microorganisms. Deficiency of normal immunoglobulins, diminished bone marrow reserves, therapies for MM, and immobilization due to skeletal disease are important predisposing factors. Prompt evaluation of fever or other manifestations of infection and institution of empiric antimicrobial therapy is essential. The prophylactic and therapeutic use of growth factors (such as G-CSF) is often given consideration. Intravenous Ig is administered to patients with recurrent significant infectious complications.

3. **Hyperviscosity.** This is a rare manifestation of MM and is more commonly observed in patients with WM. It may present as central nervous system impairment (which is often subtle and noted as difficulty concentrating, visual changes, and headaches) and occasionally congestive heart failure. Plasmapheresis is used for the treatment of symptomatic hyperviscosity; however, therapy should be combined with systemic therapy directed at the plasma cell clone, as benefits of plasmapheresis are short lived.

4. **Renal dysfunction.** The possible causes of renal dysfunction in patients with MM include the following: myeloma kidney or cast nephropathy, drugs (such as NSAIDs, bisphosphonates, and intravenous contrast agents), hypercalcemia, hyperuricemia and urate nephropathy, amyloid deposition, pyelonephritis and other infections, hyperviscosity syndrome, plasma cell infiltration of both kidneys (rare), and renal tubular acidosis. In addition, patients with MM are particularly susceptible to intravascular volume depletion and prerenal azotemia. Adequate hydration, avoidance of possible culprit drugs when possible, high index of suspicion, and early identification of etiology will result in improved renal outcomes, as most of the causes of renal dysfunction are reversible. Patients with MM with severe renal dysfunction, in whom readily identifiable causes of renal dysfunction have been ruled out, may be assumed to have cast nephropathy without the need for a biopsy. Plasmapheresis in addition to institution of chemotherapy should be considered in such selected cases. While plasmapheresis does not impact overall survival, it may result in improved dialysis-free survival. In patients with severe renal failure that have not improved with the previously discussed interventions, hemodialysis should be considered if chemotherapy offers the potential for a prolonged remission.

5. **Skeletal destruction.** This remains a major cause of disability, pain, and immobilization for patients with MM. Adopting a multidisciplinary approach to the patient with bone disease cannot be overemphasized. Bisphosphonates are best given monthly in the first 1 to 2 years and less frequently thereafter. They have been shown to reduce the incidence of skeletal-related events. Pamidronate and zoledronic acid have both been associated with the development of osteonecrosis of the jaw. A dentist experienced in management of this complication should promptly evaluate patients with symptoms referable to the jaw or teeth. In addition, bisphosphonates should be held for 1 month prior and 2 months after any elective dental procedure or after confirmation of the total healing after the procedure. Radiation therapy is often used to palliate painful lytic lesions. Surgical intervention is used for prevention of impending fractures of

weight-bearing bones and the treatment of compression fractures causing pain and loss of height (kyphoplasty).

6. **Anemia**. Anemia is frequently observed in patients with MM. MM and its treatment are etiologic in most patients. In addition, a subset of patients was found to have vitamin B_{12} and folate deficiency and treatment with erythropoietic agents is thought to result in decreases in iron stores. Thus, monitoring vitamin B_{12}, folate, and iron levels is recommended. The use of recombinant human erythropoietin results in responses of the anemia in about 80% of patients.

7. **Leukemia**. Acute myeloid leukemia develops in up to 4% of patients with myeloma who have received alkylator-based chemotherapy (melphalan). Myelodysplasia is present at diagnosis in a subset of patients as it, like myeloma, occurs in older age groups. Leukemia in this setting appears to be caused by the interaction of a carcinogenic drug with a predisposed host. With the avoidance of long-term therapy with alkylating agents, the incidence of this complication is declining. In addition, myelodysplastic syndrome post high-dose therapy and autologous stem cell transplant is increasingly recognized in patients with myeloma who currently enjoy longer survival than with previous therapies.

IV. WM (LYMPHOPLASMACYTIC LYMPHOMA)
A. Diagnosis and presentation

WM is a B-cell lymphoproliferative disorder characterized by the production of a monoclonal Ig of the IgM subtype and by intertrabecular bone marrow infiltration with a lymphoplasmacytic infiltrate. The second international workshop on WM has proposed the following diagnostic criteria: an IgM M-protein of any concentration, bone marrow infiltration with small lymphocytes exhibiting plasmacytoid differentiation, and with a suggestive immunophenotype (expression of surface IgM, CD19, CD20, CD25, CD27, FMC7, and CD138 without the expression of CD5, CD10, CD23, and CD103).

Symptoms attributable to WM are related to tumor infiltration or to the M-protein. The former results in constitutional symptoms (fevers, sweats, and weight loss), cytopenias (secondary to bone marrow involvement), lymphadenopathy, and hepatosplenomegaly. Symptoms related to the M-protein include hyperviscosity, cryoglobulinemia, cold agglutinin, neuropathy, and amyloidosis.

B. General considerations and aims of therapy

There is no cure for WM. Treatment is palliative and aimed at reduction of symptoms and prevention of complications of the disease. Increasing numbers of patients without signs or symptoms are being diagnosed with WM. Expectant observation is the recommended approach for patients with asymptomatic WM. The level of the M-protein should not be used as an indication for treatment. The choice of the therapeutic option in a symptomatic individual is guided by disease characteristics as well as patient characteristics. The available therapies include the following: oral alkylating agents, nucleoside analogs, rituximab monotherapy, and a combination of chemotherapy, rituximab, and autologous stem cell transplantation. Novel therapies include thalidomide, alemtuzumab, and bortezomib. Limited randomized clinical trials have been conducted for WM, and treatment recommendations rely mostly on phase II studies. Patients with WM are monitored by repeated measurements of one or more of the following: the serum M-protein, the serum viscosity when that is elevated, and by serial computed tomography scan. A complete response is defined as the disappearance of the M-protein and by resolution of infiltration of lymph node and visceral organs confirmed on two separate evaluations 6 weeks apart. A partial response is defined as a greater than 50% reduction in the M-protein and a greater than 50% reduction in lymphadenopathy with the resolutions of symptoms related to WM. Progressive disease is defined as a greater than 25% increase in the M-protein, worsening of cytopenias, organ infiltration, or disease-related symptoms. After the documentation of the best response, continued therapy is not clearly beneficial. The median survival of patients with WM has historically been 5 to 10 years, likely as a consequence of the older patient population and comorbidities.

B. **Treatment**

1. **Cytopenias** in patients with WM are related to bone marrow involvement and occasionally to hypersplenism. Anemia in patients with WM is common and often responds to erythropoietic agents. While transfusions are generally safe, it is generally done with caution in patients with hyperviscosity as red blood cells contribute to whole blood viscosity. Thrombocytopenia and anemia usually are indications to initiate treatment, and improvement in these cytopenias is often regarded as evidence of response to therapy. Platelet transfusions are occasionally needed, especially after chemotherapy is given to the patient with baseline thrombocytopenia.

2. **Hyperviscosity.** Hyperviscosity syndrome readily responds to plasmapheresis. Plasmapheresis should not be regarded as a long-term treatment, and consolidation of that response with chemotherapy is ultimately needed to render patients independent of that procedure.

3. **Chemotherapy**

   a. **Oral alkylating agents**
      - Chlorambucil 2 to 6 mg by mouth daily, *or*
      - Cyclophosphamide 50 to 100 mg by mouth daily.
      - Prednisone 40 to 60 mg by mouth on days 1 to 4 every 4 weeks is often added.

While complete responses are rare with the use of alkylating agents, partial responses approach 50% in some series. The time to response has been slow with alkylating agents. The use of alkylating agents should be considered in older patients in whom rapid control of the disease is not necessary.

b. **Nucleoside analog**
  - Fludarabine 25 mg/m^2 IV on days 1 to 5
  - Cycles are repeated every 28 days.

  While many patients are able to tolerate this regimen, older individuals and patients with significant cytopenias at baseline are best treated with a reduced dose. Two to three days of fludarabine 25 mg/m^2 in the first two cycles are recommended; consider dose increases if the patient is able to tolerate therapy well and responses are suboptimal. Nucleoside analogs have been shown to result in a higher response rate than oral alkylators, but a survival benefit has not been demonstrated. The time to response is shortened by the use of nucleoside analogs. We recommend the use of these agents in younger patients in whom autologous stem cell transplantation is not considered and who require a fast tumor control.

c. **Rituximab**
  - Rituximab 375 mg/m^2 IV weekly for four doses (consider repeating for another four doses).

  Rituximab is a monoclonal antibody targeting CD20 on B-lymphocytes. Response rates range from 20% to 70% in newly diagnosed patients and around 30% in relapsed patients. Time to response to rituximab is in the order of 3 months. A flare reaction has been described in patients treated with rituximab and is characterized by a transient increase in the serum IgM of patients. A serum IgM lower than 5 grams is predictive of response to this agent. We recommend the use of this agent in younger patients with minimal symptoms of their disease and with a lower serum IgM level.

d. **High-dose therapy and autologous stem cell transplantation.** Autologous stem cell transplantation has resulted in high rates of responses (approaching 90%) and lasting responses (progression-free survival approaching 70 months) in a small series of patients. The small number of patients, the nonrandomized nature of the studies, and potential for treatment-related morbidity makes it difficult to routinely recommend this approach for most patients. It should, however, be considered in younger patients after cytoreductive treatment with rituximab. Treatment with alkylating agents and nucleoside analogs may impair the ability to collect stem cells and should be judiciously used in younger patients.

V. AMYLOIDOSIS

Only AL (primary) amyloidosis, with or without associated plasma cell neoplasms, is considered in this section. In these disorders, fragments of Ig light chain accumulate and deposit in the affected tissues. These deposits are characterized by a pathognomonic apple green birefringence on polarized microscopy. These deposits lead to organ dysfunction. AL amyloidosis characteristically infiltrates the tongue, heart, skin, ligaments, and muscle and occasionally the kidney, liver, and spleen. The diagnosis requires biopsy of the affected organ; although occasionally, a fat pat biopsy may obviate that need. In patients with documented lymphomas or plasma cell neoplasms, treatment is directed at the underlying neoplasm, but the decline in the amount of amyloid deposits is often minimal. With primary amyloidosis without a demonstrable underlying neoplasm, treatment with alkylator-based therapy such as MP has been used historically and is of moderate benefits. The use of high-dose dexamethasone is often prescribed as well. High-dose therapy with stem cell rescue is considered in only a minority of patients as most patients are not eligible and the procedure-related mortality remains high in this patient group. Patients with cardiac amyloidosis have dismal outcomes often measured in months if they have concomitant heart failure. Recently, bortezomib-based therapy has been shown to result in high hematologic responses, but long-term follow-up and organ responses have not been clearly defined with this therapy. Novel effective therapies are needed and enrollment of patients onto clinical trials should be considered early.

Selected Readings

Attal M, Harousseau JL, Stoppa AM, et al. A prospective, randomized trial of autologous bone marrow transplantation and chemotherapy in multiple myeloma. Intergroupe Francais du Myelome. *N Engl J Med.* 1996;335:91–97.

Barlogie B, Kyle RA, Anderson KC, et al. Standard chemotherapy compared with high-dose chemoradiotherapy for multiple myeloma: final results of phase III US Intergroup Trial S9321. *J Clin Oncol.* 2006;24:929–936.

Baz R, Li L, Kottke-Marchant K, et al. The role of aspirin in the prevention of thrombotic complications of thalidomide and anthracycline-based chemotherapy for multiple myeloma. *Mayo Clin Proc.* 2005;80:1568–1574.

Bergsagel PL, Kuehl WM. Molecular pathogenesis and a consequent classification of multiple myeloma. *J Clin Oncol.* 2005;23:6333–6338.

Bladé J, Kyle RA. Nonsecretory myeloma, immunoglobulin D myeloma, and plasma cell leukemia. *Hematol Oncol Clin North Am.* 1999;13:1259–1272.

Dhodapkar MV, Hussein MA, Rasmussen E, et al. Clinical efficacy of high-dose dexamethasone with maintenance dexamethasone/alpha interferon in patients with primary systemic amyloidosis: results of United States Intergroup Trial Southwest Oncology Group (SWOG) S9628. *Blood.* 2004;104:3520–3526.

Dimopoulos MA, Kyle RA, Anagnostopoulos A, Treon SP. Diagnosis and management of Waldenstrom's macroglobulinemia. *J Clin Oncol.* 2005;23:1564–1577.

Durie BG, Salmon SE. A clinical staging system for multiple myeloma. Correlation of measured myeloma cell mass with presenting clinical features, response to treatment, and survival. *Cancer.* 1975;36:842–854.

Durie BG, Harousseau JL, San Miguel JF, et al. International uniform response criteria for multiple myeloma. *Leukemia.* 2006;20:1467–1473.

Fonseca R, Barlogie B, Bataille R, et al. Genetics and cytogenetics of multiple myeloma: a workshop report. *Cancer Res.* 2004;64:1546–1558.

Frassica DA, Frassica FJ, Schray MF, Sim FH, Kyle RA. Solitary plasmacytoma of bone: Mayo Clinic experience. *Int J Radiat Oncol Biol Phys.* 1989;16:43–48.

Greipp PR, San Miguel J, Durie BG, et al. International staging system for multiple myeloma. *J Clin Oncol.* 2005;23:3412–3420.

Jacobson JL, Hussein MA, Barlogie B, et al. A new staging system for multiple myeloma patients based on the Southwest Oncology Group (SWOG) experience. *Br J Haematol.* 2003;122:441–450.

Owen RG, Treon SP, Al-Katib A, et al. Clinicopathological definition of Waldenstrom's macroglobulinemia: consensus panel recommendations from the Second International Workshop on Waldenstrom's Macroglobulinemia. *Semin Oncol.* 2003; 30:110–115.

Rajkumar SV, Blood E, Vesole D, et al. Phase III clinical trial of thalidomide plus dexamethasone compared with dexamethasone alone in newly diagnosed multiple myeloma: a clinical trial coordinated by the Eastern Cooperative Oncology Group. *J Clin Oncol.* 2006;24:431–436.

Rajkumar SV, Hayman SR, Lacy MQ, et al. Combination therapy with lenalidomide plus dexamethasone (Rev/Dex) for newly diagnosed myeloma. *Blood.* 2005;106: 4050–4053.

Richardson PG, Sonneveld P, Schuster MW, et al. Bortezomib or high-dose dexamethasone for relapsed multiple myeloma. *N Engl J Med.* 2005;352:2487–2498.

Rifkin RM, Gregory SA, Mohrbacher A, Hussein MA. Pegylated liposomal doxorubicin, vincristine, and dexamethasone provide significant reduction in toxicity compared with doxorubicin, vincristine, and dexamethasone in patients with newly diagnosed multiple myeloma: a Phase III multicenter randomized trial. *Cancer.* 2006;106:848–858.

San Miguel JF, Schlag R, Khuageva NK, et al. Bortezomib plus melphalan and prednisone for initial treatment of multiple myeloma. *N Engl J Med.* 2008;359:906–917.

Segeren CM, Sonneveld P, van der Holt B, et al. Overall and event-free survival are not improved by the use of myeloablative therapy following intensified chemotherapy in previously untreated patients with multiple myeloma: a prospective randomized phase 3 study. *Blood.* 2000;101:2144–2151.

Srkalovic G, Elson P, Trebisky B, Karam MA, Hussein MA. Use of melphalan, thalidomide, and dexamethasone in treatment of refractory and relapsed multiple myeloma. *Med Oncol.* 2002;19:219–226.

Stewart AK, Fonseca R. Prognostic and therapeutic significance of myeloma genetics and gene expression profiling. *J Clin Oncol.* 2005;23:6339–6344.

Treon SP, Gertz MA, Dimopoulos M, et al. Update on treatment recommendations from the Third International Workshop on Waldenstrom's macroglobulinemia. *Blood.* 2006;107:3443–3446.

Weber DM, Chen C, Niesvizky R, et al. Lenalidomide plus dexamethasone for relapsed multiple myeloma in North America. *N Engl J Med.* 2007;357:2133–2142.

24 Metastatic Cancer of Unknown Origin

James M. Leonardo

The primary site remains unknown in about 5% to 10% of patients with newly diagnosed cancer (excluding nonmelanoma skin cancer), despite a detailed pretreatment evaluation. Even after extensive evaluation and postmortem examination, a primary tumor is not found in up to 30% of these patients. However, the frequency of cancers with truly occult primary sites is decreasing, in part because of advances in technology to detect the primary site(s). The problem of metastatic cancer of unknown origin raises difficult questions for both diagnosis and treatment. Although the median survival time of patients with cancer of unknown origin has been reported to be 6 to 9 months, subgroups of patients have been defined who have a more favorable outlook with aggressive management. With current therapy modalities, the overall survival of these patients appears to be improving. A major responsibility of the clinician is to identify those patients with a characteristic presentation who might benefit from a specific strategy and to identify the increasingly large group of patients who might benefit from a trial of chemotherapy.

Tumors thought to be more amenable to treatment, and thus have a more favorable prognosis, include poorly differentiated cancers with midline distribution, squamous cell carcinoma (SCC) involving cervical lymph nodes, papillary adenocarcinoma of the peritoneal cavity in women, and adenocarcinoma involving only axillary lymph nodes in women. Conversely, adverse prognostic findings include adenocarcinoma metastatic to the liver or other organs, nonpapillary malignant ascites, and multiple metastases to brain, bones, or lungs.

I. GENERAL CONSIDERATIONS AND AIMS OF THERAPY

A. Histology and presenting clinical manifestations

Moderately differentiated adenocarcinoma and poorly differentiated carcinoma or adenocarcinoma respectively comprise up to 60% and 30% of all cancers of unknown origin. SCC and poorly differentiated cancers other than adenocarcinoma each account for about 5% of unknown primary tumors. Other histologies that may present as cancer of unknown origin include lymphomas, germ cell tumors, and neuroendocrine carcinomas. These histologies are particularly important to identify because they represent tumors that may be effectively managed with systemic chemotherapy. Nearly half of all patients with unknown primaries and well over half of those with adenocarcinoma present with hepatomegaly, abdominal mass, or other abdominal symptoms. Lymphadenopathy is the presenting clinical manifestation in 15% to 25% of patients. Lower cervical or supraclavicular lymph nodes usually contain adenocarcinoma or undifferentiated carcinoma, and middle to high cervical adenopathy generally represents SCC. Between 10% and 20% of patients present with manifestations of bone, lung, or pleural involvement, whereas fewer than 10% present with evidence of central nervous system disease. Most of the latter group is eventually found to have either lung or gastrointestinal tract primaries.

A few presentations of advanced carcinoma of unknown primary site have been recognized as being more treatable and thus having a more favorable prognosis than others. Poorly differentiated carcinoma or adenocarcinoma, especially with predominant sites of involvement in the mediastinum, retroperitoneum, lymph nodes, or lungs, and adenocarcinoma in women predominantly involving the peritoneal surfaces may respond to platinum-based chemotherapy regimens designed for germ cell or ovarian cancers and result in occasional long-term disease-free survival. Women with axillary adenopathy and adenocarcinoma or undifferentiated carcinoma may occasionally enjoy sustained responses to therapy directed against breast cancer.

B. Sites of origin

It is sometimes possible to predict the most likely primary sites from the histology and location of the metastatic lesion of unknown origin. Pancreas and lung are the most common ultimately determined sites of origin. Together, they represent more than 40% of the adenocarcinomas of unknown origin in which the site can be ultimately determined. Colorectal, gastric, and hepatobiliary carcinoma each represent about another 10%.

In general, adenocarcinomas or undifferentiated carcinomas presenting with hepatic metastases or left supraclavicular adenopathy are eventually demonstrated to be of gastrointestinal origin. SCCs that present in the supraclavicular or low cervical lymph nodes are usually from lung primaries, whereas similar lesions of higher cervical nodes are more likely to have originated from occult primary lesions in the head and neck region.

The pattern of metastatic involvement associated with occult primary tumors may differ from that associated with overt primaries. For example, occult lung cancer rarely involves bone, a common site of metastasis from overt lung cancer; however, bone metastases appear to be more common in patients with gastrointestinal cancer who have occult primaries than in those who have overt primaries. Nonetheless, occult primaries can metastasize to any site and, in general, one should not rely on the pattern of metastatic spread to predict the site of origin.

C. Aims of diagnostic evaluation

The first objective in the management of a patient newly diagnosed with cancer of unknown origin is to plan the appropriate diagnostic evaluation. There are three chief aims of this evaluation:

1. Identify a tumor in which cure or effective disease control is possible.
2. Determine if the tumor is regionally confined or widely metastatic.
3. Identify any complication for which immediate local therapy is indicated.

D. Goals of treatment

In patients with tumors for which effective systemic therapy is available and in patients with disease regionally confined to peripheral lymph nodes alone, the primary goal of treatment is prolongation of life through extended disease control; in some cases, cure should be considered. These patients represent approximately 25% of patients with occult primaries. For the remaining patients, the chance of prolonging life has been less likely, but with the advent of new cytotoxic agents and targeted drugs, prospects for this group are improving. Treatment should also address palliation of symptoms and preservation of the best possible quality of life.

II. DIAGNOSTIC EVALUATION

A. Initial workup

The initial evaluation of a patient presenting with a metastatic tumor should include a complete history and physical examination including a breast, pelvic, and rectal examination in women and prostate and testicular examination in men. Routine laboratory studies (complete blood count, electrolytes, creatinine, blood urea nitrogen, and calcium, as well as liver function testing) should also be done early on in the evaluation. The clinical scenario should determine whether more specialized laboratory testing is appropriate. It is wholly reasonable to measure cancer antigen (CA)-125 in the setting of a woman with ascites, for example. Imaging studies should include a chest radiograph at minimum; additional studies such as mammography may be useful depending on the location of the metastases and symptoms. Computed tomography (CT) scanning is now being routinely used to evaluate patients with occult primary tumors and may be responsible for the decreased frequency of cancers that remain of truly unknown origin. The role of [^{18}F]fluorodeoxyglucose positron emission tomography (PET)-CT scanning is not clear, but some series have reported a usefulness of this modality for identifying the primary site, particularly when the presentation is in cervical lymph nodes. Although not recommended as part of the routine evaluation of all patients with occult primary cancers, PET-CT scans may be particularly useful with occult primary tumors with a single site of metastasis when therapy with a curative intent is planned. More invasive testing, such as bronchoscopy, endoscopy, or colonoscopy, should be guided by the patient's symptoms.

B. Analysis of the biopsy specimen

If possible, the pathologist should receive fresh, unfixed material to allow electron microscopy, histochemistry, immunohistology, and hormone receptor studies to be done, if needed, after routine examination. Careful review of the biopsy material should be undertaken to attempt to classify the tumor conclusively as SCC, adenocarcinoma, or other identifiable histology. Up to 40% of cancers of unknown origin are undifferentiated or poorly differentiated tumors based on evaluation of hematoxylin and eosin–stained material. Electron microscopy, when available, may be useful for the further classification of these tumors through the identification of desmosomes and intercellular bridges (SCC); tight junctions, microvilli, and acinar spaces (adenocarcinoma); premelanosomes (amelanotic melanoma); neurosecretory granules (small-cell or neuroendocrine carcinoma); and absence of junctions (lymphoma). Immunohistochemistry is an indispensable part of the evaluation of carcinoma of unknown primary site. The expression of cytokeratins, particularly CK7 and CK20, may be useful in narrowing down the origin of a tumor. Immunohistochemical studies on the tumor may be used to demonstrate the presence of prostatic acid phosphatase or prostate-specific antigen (PSA; prostate carcinoma), human chorionic gonadotropin (β-hCG; germ cell tumors), α-fetoprotein (germ cell tumors or hepatocellular carcinoma), or monoclonal immunoglobulin (lymphoma, plasmacytoma). Immunoglobulin or T-cell receptor gene rearrangements may be helpful in identifying tumors of lymphoid origin. Undifferentiated carcinomas or adenocarcinomas in women should be evaluated for estrogen and progesterone receptors. Mucin positivity is helpful in eliminating the possibility of renal cell carcinoma.

Molecular profiling of tumors has emerged as a powerful new tool to aid in determining the site of origin. This methodology relies on the observation that different tumor types exhibit unique qualitative and quantitative patterns of expression of genes, which can be measured using DNA microarray analysis. These analyses can be done on formalin-fixed, paraffin-embedded tissue or fresh frozen specimens. In one large, retrospective study with 547 specimens, the tissue of origin was correctly identified in 88% of the specimens. Although this promising technology is now widely available, prospective trials are needed to determine if these data can determine optimum treatment for cancers with occult primaries and prolong survival.

Clearly, the use of many of these specialized studies must be balanced against their expense. If judiciously applied, they can aid in the identification of some of the undifferentiated or poorly differentiated tumors of unknown origin and help to focus their subsequent diagnostic evaluation and management.

C. Squamous cell carcinoma (SCC)

One exception to the policy of seeking a definitive histologic diagnosis as the first step in evaluating a tumor of unknown origin is when the patient presents with a potentially resectable neck mass (other than supraclavicular adenopathy) and no other apparent lesion. In these patients, a head and neck primary should be sought by detailed head and neck examination, radiographs of the sinuses, and, if necessary, panendoscopy under general anesthesia, including laryngoscopy, bronchoscopy, esophagoscopy, and nasopharyngoscopy with blind biopsy of the base of the tongue, piriform sinuses, nasopharynx, and tonsillar fossae if no gross primary is found. A CT scan of the head and neck may also be of value. PET-CT scanning has also been utilized in this setting. If this workup is not diagnostic, biopsy of the neck mass is undertaken. This order of evaluation is chosen so that if a resectable SCC of the head and neck is found, the neck mass can be removed as part of the curative procedure.

For SCCs with apparent involvement of only one lymph node group, the possibility of long-term survival exists if proper treatment is carried out. The diagnostic evaluation depends on the lymph node region involved. The most common lymph node presentation for SCCs of unknown origin is in the cervical or supraclavicular region. Cervical lymph node metastases above the supraclavicular region usually originate from head and neck primary lesions. The diagnostic approach to these lesions is discussed in the preceding paragraph. Because surgery, irradiation, or both, with curative intent, are employed if disease is localized to this region, distant metastases should be excluded with a bone scan, a chest radiograph, and, in some instances, a chest CT scan. SCC of supraclavicular lymph nodes is usually of lung or esophageal origin and seldom represents regionally confined disease. Evaluation is the same as that for disease that extends beyond regional lymph nodes.

SCC in axillary or inguinal lymph nodes is rarely associated with an occult primary. Regional skin and lung should be examined as possible primary sites with axillary disease, whereas the skin, anus, and genitalia should be carefully examined when the presentation is SCC in the inguinal nodes.

SCC with generalized lymphadenopathy or, more commonly, with disease that extends beyond the lymph nodes, represents disease that cannot be satisfactorily controlled by present day techniques. The search for the primary lesions should be done mainly by a chest radiograph and careful physical examination of the appropriate organs. Serum chemistries, including the calcium level, should be determined. Further diagnostic studies are needed only if indicated by signs, symptoms, or abnormalities on the initial studies.

D. Adenocarcinoma and poorly differentiated carcinoma

Women with adenocarcinoma or poorly differentiated carcinoma of unknown origin should undergo mammography, careful pelvic examination, and hormone receptor evaluation of the tumor. In men, serum acid phosphatase, PSA, β-hCG, and α-fetoprotein should be determined to help exclude prostate and germ cell tumors, respectively. An elevated CA-27-29 or CA-15-3 level would point toward a breast primary. All patients should have stools and urine examined for occult blood, and the serum should be tested for abnormalities in the liver chemistries, creatinine, and electrolytes. With disease apparently confined to axillary lymph nodes, mammography is particularly important in women and should be considered in men as well. If there is a strong suspicion of breast cancer and the mammogram is negative, magnetic resonance imaging should be considered. Undifferentiated carcinoma found only in middle to high cervical lymph nodes should be evaluated in the same manner as described in Section II.C for cervical node SCC.

Traditional contrast studies such as intravenous pyelogram, barium enema, and upper gastrointestinal series are not indicated unless specifically suggested by signs or symptoms (e.g., occult blood in the stool). Abdominal CT scan with intravenous contrast medium is a reasonable option in view of the frequency with which it detects carcinoma of the pancreas or hepatobiliary cancer in this setting.

E. Malignant melanoma

The finding of malignant melanoma confined to a single lymph node group and without a detectable primary lesion represents stage II disease and is associated with a 30% 5-year survival rate after lymphadenectomy. Evaluation to exclude more extensive disease should include a history, physical examination (emphasizing skin and ophthalmoscopic examination), chest radiograph, liver chemistries, liver scan, and brain CT scan.

III. TREATMENT

A. General strategy

The importance of identifying tumors that may be treated effectively, such as lymphomas, germ cell tumors, trophoblastic tumors, and breast, prostate, ovarian, and neuroendocrine carcinomas, is readily apparent. Once identified, these lesions should be treated as described in their respective chapters. In patients whose primary lesion remains obscure, a therapeutic distinction must be made between those with disease confined to one lymph node region and those with more widespread disease or involvement of visceral organs. In the former, some may be treated with curative intent, whereas in the latter, the aims of treatment are palliative.

B. Squamous cell carcinoma (SCC)

Patients with SCC confined to the cervical lymph nodes above the supraclavicular region should receive full-course radiotherapy to a field extending from the base of the skull to the clavicles. Alternatively, they may be treated with radical lymph node dissection followed by radiation therapy. In either case, the irradiation is designed to include any possible head and neck primary carcinoma. Survival of patients so treated is at least as good as that for patients with known head and neck primaries. More limited lymph node dissection or regional irradiation may also be indicated for SCC confined to unilateral involvement of the axillary or inguinal nodes.

More widespread SCCs of unknown origin are treated with a palliative intent. No treatment except for local radiotherapy to symptomatic lesions is the standard approach. In patients with symptomatic or progressive disease who desire chemotherapy, regimens designed mainly for head and neck (see Chapter 5) or non–small-cell lung cancer (see Chapter 6) should be considered.

C. Adenocarcinoma and poorly differentiated carcinoma

In women, if these carcinomas are confined to the unilateral axillary lymph nodes, they should be considered possible breast cancer and treated accordingly as stage II disease (see Chapter 9). A woman with adenocarcinoma or poorly differentiated carcinoma predominantly confined to the peritoneal surface should be considered for a platinum-based ovarian cancer regimen. Undifferentiated carcinoma confined to the middle or high cervical lymph nodes should be treated actively as SCC (see Section II.C). Men with adenocarcinoma of unknown primary and a positive tumor or serum PSA should have a trial of hormonal therapy.

Patients with more advanced adenocarcinoma or poorly differentiated carcinoma in which the evaluation previously described in Section II does not suggest breast, prostate, or other highly treatable primary or a primary site should be managed according to the histology. Platinum-based combination chemotherapy may be valuable in the treatment of poorly differentiated carcinoma and poorly differentiated adenocarcinoma. Newer regimens containing paclitaxel, docetaxel, or gemcitabine have shown efficacy in phase II studies of patients with occult primary tumors. In patients with mediastinal or retroperitoneal tumors, the germ cell regimen of bleomycin, etoposide, and cisplatin (BEP) or etoposide and cisplatin (EP) has been studied in a series of 220 patients. This combination may produce more than a 60% objective response rate and more than a 20% complete response rate with up to a 13% long-term survival rate.

▪ BEP

  ▪ Cisplatin 20 mg/m^2 intravenously (IV) over 30 minutes on days 1 to 5, *and*

  ▪ Etoposide 100 mg/m^2 IV on days 1 to 5, *and*

- Bleomycin 30 U IV push weekly on days 1, 8, and 15
- Repeat cycle every 21 days regardless of blood cell counts for two (adjuvant therapy), three (good-risk patients), or four (intermediate or poor risk) cycles.

Patients with widespread adenocarcinoma that is well or moderately well differentiated may be responsive to systemic therapy. Combinations such as paclitaxel, carboplatin, and oral etoposide (PCE) or gemcitabine and carboplatin followed by paclitaxel yield objective responses in 25% to 45% of patients.

- PCE
  - Paclitaxel 200 mg/m^2 as a 1-hour IV infusion on day 1, *and*
  - Carboplatin area under the curve (AUC) 6 IV over 30 to 60 minutes on day 1, *and*
  - Etoposide 50 to 100 mg by mouth on alternate days between days 1 and 10.
- Gemcitabine and carboplatin
  - Carboplatin AUC of 5 on day 1
  - Gemcitabine 1000 mg/m^2 IV on days 1 and 8.
- Repeat each cycle every 3 weeks.

Both regimens are worthy of consideration in patients with good performance status because occasional durable responses have occurred. Reports on both of these regimens are based on limited accrual phase II studies. Responding patients show improvement within two cycles, and chemotherapy should be stopped after two cycles if no improvement is seen. PCE is also effective in patients with poorly differentiated adenocarcinoma and poorly differentiated carcinoma and may be considered as an alternative to BEP.

D. Malignant melanoma

For disease confined to a single lymph node group, radical lymph node dissection yields long-term survival in 30% of treated patients. Treatment of disseminated melanoma is discussed in Chapter 14.

E. Neuroendocrine carcinoma

Poorly differentiated neuroendocrine carcinoma may represent up to 13% of cases of poorly differentiated carcinoma or adenocarcinoma. The diagnosis is secured by recognition of neurosecretory granules on electron microscopy. Localized lesions are uncommon and should be treated with surgery or radiation therapy. Metastatic disease frequently responds to platinum-based chemotherapy such as EP or newer regimens, such as irinotecan and cisplatin.

- EP
  - Etoposide 120 mg/m^2 IV on days 1 to 3 *or* 120 mg/m^2 by mouth twice a day on days 1 to 3, *and*
  - Cisplatin 60 mg/m^2 IV on day 1.

IV. FUTURE DIRECTIONS

Advances in our understanding of the molecular events leading to carcinogenesis and metastasis have led to the development of gene profiling for specific types of cancer. Retrospective studies of archival breast tumor specimens, for example, in which genetic profiles are identified and compared to the known treatment outcomes, have led to prospective studies in which gene profiles are being used to guide specific therapy. Similar retrospective analyses have also been done with many other tumor types and have led to the development of DNA microarray assays which are now widely available. It is likely that genetic profiling will be used routinely as an essential step in the characterization of most tumors. This approach should identify the tissue of origin of most tumors, leading to a further decline in the apparent incidence of true occult primary tumors. More importantly, cost-effective, targeted therapies that act at defined points in the cancer cell could then be chosen based on the molecular characteristics of the tumor rather than the purported tissue or organ of origin.

Acknowledgments

The author is indebted to Dr. Martin Oken who contributed to this chapter in previous editions and whose work has been included in this revision of the handbook.

Selected Readings

Abbruzzese JL, Abbruzzese MC, Hess KR, et al. Unknown primary carcinoma: natural history and prognostic factors in 657 consecutive patients. *J Clin Oncol.* 1994;12:1272–1284.

Altman E, Cadman E. An analysis of 1539 patients with cancer of unknown primary site. *Cancer.* 1986;57:120–124.

Ettinger DS, Aguinik M, Cates JMM, et al. Occult primary (cancer of unknown primary [CUP]). *NCCN Practice Guidelines in Oncology* Version 2.2011; NCCN.org.

Greco FA, Burris HA III, Litchy S, et al. Gemcitabine, carboplatin, and paclitaxel for patients with carcinoma of unknown primary site: a Minnie Pearl Cancer Center Research Network Study. *J Clin Oncol.* 2002;20:1651–1656.

Greco FA, Vaughn WK, Hainsworth JD. Advanced poorly differentiated carcinoma of unknown primary site: recognition of a treatable syndrome. *Ann Intern Med.* 1986;104:547–556.

Hainsworth JD, Erland JB, Kalman LA, et al. Carcinoma of unknown primary site: treatment with one-hour paclitaxel, carboplatin, and extended schedule etoposide. *J Clin Oncol.* 1997;15:2385–2393.

Hainsworth JD, Greco FA. Treatment of patients with cancer of an unknown primary site. *N Engl J Med.* 1993;329:257–263.

Hainsworth JD, Johnson DH, Greco FA. Cisplatin-based combination chemotherapy in the treatment of poorly differentiated carcinoma and poorly differentiated adenocarcinoma of unknown primary site: results of a 12-year experience. *J Clin Oncol.* 1992;10:912–922.

Hainsworth JD, Johnson DH, Greco FA. Poorly differentiated neuroendocrine carcinoma of unknown primary site: a newly recognized clinicopathologic entity. *Ann Intern Med.* 1988;109:364–371.

Hainsworth JD, Spigel DR, Raefsky EL, et al. Combination chemotherapy with gemcitabine and irinotecan in patients with previously treated carcinoma of an unknown primary site: a Minnie Pearl Cancer Research Network Phase II trial. *Cancer.* 2005;104(9):1992–1997.

Kolesnikov-Gauthier H, Levy E, Merlet P, et al. FDG PET in patients with cancer of an unknown primary. *Nucl Med Commun.* 2005;26(12):1059–1066.

Lenzi R, Hess KR, Abbruzzese MC. Poorly differentiated carcinoma and poorly differentiated adenocarcinoma of unknown origin: favorable subsets of patients with unknown-primary carcinoma. *J Clin Oncol.* 1997;15:2056–2066.

Moertel CG. Adenocarcinoma of unknown origin. *Ann Intern Med.* 1979;91:646–647.

Monzon, FA, Lyons-Weiler M, Buturovic LJ, et al. Multicenter validation of a 1,550-gene expression profile for identification of tumor tissue of origin. *J Clin Oncol.* 2009;27:2503–2508.

Stokkel MP, Terhoard CH, Hordij KFJ, et al. The detection of unknown primary tumors in patients with cervical metastases by dual-head positron emission tomography. *Oral Oncol.* 1999;35:390–394.

Strnad CM, Grosh WW, Baxter J, et al. Peritoneal carcinomatosis of unknown primary site in women: a distinctive subset of adenocarcinoma. *Ann Intern Med.* 1989;11:213–217.

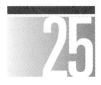

HIV-Associated Malignancies

Thomas S. Uldrick, Mark N. Polizzotto, and Robert Yarchoan

Patients with HIV infection have an increased susceptibility to several cancers. Three malignancies confer a diagnosis of AIDS when they arise in an HIV-infected patient: Kaposi sarcoma (KS), aggressive B-cell non-Hodgkin lymphoma (NHL), and cervical cancer. The incidence of some non-AIDS–defining malignancies (NADM) is also increased in people with HIV/AIDS.

With the availability of potent combination antiretroviral therapy (cART), the epidemiology of cancer in patients with HIV has changed. While AIDS-defining tumors are still the most common cancers in people with HIV, the incidence of KS and some NHL subtypes has decreased. However, as HIV-infected patients are living longer, as the number of people living with HIV/AIDS is increasing, and as the HIV-infected population is aging in the developed world, NADM are becoming an increasing public health concern. Cancers with increased incidence in HIV-infected patients include lung cancer, anal cancer, Hodgkin lymphoma (HL), certain head and neck cancers, and Merkel cell carcinoma. Liver cancer is also increased in people with HIV due to frequent coinfection with hepatitis B virus (HBV) and/or hepatitis C virus (HCV) and alcohol use. Many of these tumors have established viral associations. While certain common cancers such as breast or colon cancer are not more common in HIV-infected individuals, the burden of these NADM is also increasing as the population infected with HIV ages. Information on optimal treatment approaches to these cancers in the setting of HIV infection is needed.

The outlook for patients with AIDS-defining tumors has improved markedly in the last 15 years as a result of both the introduction of cART and improved specific therapy for several of these malignancies. However, given the recent epidemiologic trends in HIV-associated malignancies and the dramatic decline in infectious complications of AIDS, malignancies are now a leading, if not the foremost, cause of mortality in the HIV-infected population where cART is available, with about half the deaths from AIDS-defining malignancies and half from NADM. This is a rapidly evolving field, and several lines of research are contributing to improved therapies. Patients should therefore be considered for clinical trials when possible.

I. KAPOSI SARCOMA (KS)-ASSOCIATED HERPESVIRUS AND ASSOCIATED TUMORS

A. **KS-associated herpesvirus (KSHV),** also called human herpesvirus-8, is a gammaherpesvirus related to Epstein-Barr virus (EBV). KSHV is the causal agent of three tumors: KS, multicentric Castleman disease (MCD), and primary effusion lymphoma (PEL). KS derives from endothelial cells, and MCD and PEL from B-lymphocytes. KSHV infection occurs endemically in certain regions, such as sub-Saharan Africa and parts of the Mediterranean basin, and at lower levels worldwide. In the United States, KSHV seroprevalence is generally low, but the rate is more than 15% in men who have sex with men (MSM). In the immunocompetent host, clinical manifestations of KSHV infection are uncommon. However, HIV infection and other forms of immunodeficiency substantially increase the risk of KSHV-associated malignancies.

B. **KS**

1. **Epidemiology.** KS is a multifocal angioproliferative tumor. The tumor is comprised of spindle cells and infiltrating mononuclear cells around leaky vascular slits; blood in these slits gives KS its characteristic coloration. Clonality studies in KS are conflicting. Generally, it is thought to be oligoclonal or polyclonal, but it may have a monoclonal component, especially in advanced disease. Four epidemiologic categories of KS are described, each caused by KSHV. Classical KS is an uncommon, generally indolent tumor predominantly seen in older men in the Mediterranean basin. Endemic KS occurs in Africa and more often develops in women and younger patients. Iatrogenic KS occurs in solid organ transplant patients and other patients on chronic

immunosuppressive agents. AIDS-associated KS is also called epidemic KS. After peaking in the early-1990s, epidemic KS incidence declined rapidly in developed countries, likely due to the use of nucleoside anti-HIV therapy and then cART. It is the second most common tumor in people with HIV/AIDS in the United States. In sub-Saharan Africa, where prevalence of both HIV and KSHV is high and access to cART remains limited, KS remains one of the most common tumors.

2. **Presentation and patient evaluation.** Early KS usually manifests as red, purple, or brown papules or plaques on the skin or mucous membranes. Lesions may occur at any site but there is a predilection for the extremities, ears, nose, and palate. Advanced lesions are often nodular and may become confluent or ulcerate. Involvement of lymph nodes and dermal lymphatics leading to edema is seen in advanced cases and may result in permanent impairment. KS involvement of visceral organs such as the lungs or gastrointestinal tract and effusions in serous body cavities are other manifestations of advanced disease. Gastrointestinal KS may present as occult blood loss or with other gastrointestinal symptoms. Pulmonary disease may manifest with cough, dyspnea, or hemoptysis, and may be life threatening. Radiographic findings in the chest include reticulonodular or nodular infiltrates, with or without effusions, and may be difficult to differentiate from infection. Endoscopy and bronchoscopy are useful in visually demonstrating luminal lesions. Given the risk of bleeding, endobronchial biopsy is rarely performed. The natural history of KS is variable, and even in the absence of treatment, KS commonly waxes and wanes.

Evaluation of a patient with KS should focus on the extent of disease, KS-associated symptoms (pain, edema, disfigurement, secondary infections), rate of progression, association with cART, and the use of immunosuppressive agents including glucocorticoids. Other important factors include the history of HIV treatment, opportunistic infections, nadir and current cluster of differentiation 4 (CD4) lymphocyte counts, and HIV viral load. Physical exam should include documentation of the extent of cutaneous and mucosal involvement, evaluation of lymph nodes and spleen, fecal occult blood test for occult gastrointestinal blood loss, and baseline chest radiography for asymptomatic pulmonary involvement. A biopsy should be performed when possible to exclude other cutaneous processes. Computed tomography (CT) scans and endoscopy are not indicated unless the initial evaluation suggests visceral disease. Pathologic evaluation of pleural effusions or lymphadenopathy should be performed when feasible, if present. Patients with KS are at elevated risk of PEL and MCD, and physicians should be alert for these tumors (see subsequent discussion).

	AIDS Clinical Trials Group Staging for Epidemic KS*	

	Relative Risk	
	Good Risk (0)[†]	**Poor Risk (1)**[‡]
Disease status		
Tumor (T)	Confined to skin, minimal oral disease, or both	Edema; extensive oral ulcers; visceral and gastrointestinal disease
Immune status (I)[a]	CD4 count ≥150/μL	CD4 count <150/μL
Systemic illness (S)	No prior opportunistic infection or thrush; no B symptoms	Prior opportunistic infection or thrush; B symptoms; performance status <70%; other HIV-related illness

KS, Kaposi sarcoma.
*Modified by validation study.
[†] Requires all in this column.
[‡] If any in this column.

3. **Staging.** KS is a multicentric tumor that does not fit TNM categorization. Prior to the availability of cART, the AIDS Clinical Trials Group developed and validated a staging system that reflects various prognostic factors (Table 25.1). Patients are defined as good (designated with subscript 0) or poor (designated with subscript 1) risk on the basis of tumor burden (T), immune function assessed by CD4 count (I), and systemic illness (S) assessed by history of opportunistic infections, systemic symptoms, and performance status. Before the availability of cART, patients who were poor risk in any category were considered as being at poor risk overall. In the post-cART era, CD4 count is a less important prognosticator, and two overall risk categories are utilized: patients with a heavy burden of disease and systemic illness (T_1S_1) are poor risk compared to all other patients (T_1S_0, T_0S_1, or T_0S_0). Patients with pulmonary involvement have the highest risk of death and may require urgent evaluation and therapy.

4. **Treatment.** All patients with HIV-associated KS should receive cART. The Department of Health and Human Services (DHHS) guidelines for treatment of HIV provide current information on topics including optimal drug therapy and interactions at http://www.aidsinfo.nih.gov/guidelines/. Effective HIV suppression and immune reconstitution can lead to sufficient tumor regression, especially in patients with limited (T_0) disease, and it can improve response durability and overall survival in patients with any stage disease. However, some patients have initial worsening of KS on starting cART, believed to be due to immune reactivation syndrome.

A number of other therapies are effective in KS and should be considered in light of the risks, potential benefits, and needs of each individual patient. KS is not curable, and the goal of therapy is to induce durable responses or minimize the extent of disease while minimizing toxicity. Some patients, especially those with severe KS and low CD4 counts, may require intermittent therapy for years. Most patients with HIV-associated KS will either respond to cART or require systemic therapy, and local therapy is now rarely used. Systemic therapy is generally indicated for bulky, rapidly progressing, symptomatic, or life-threatening disease. In addition, it is worth considering for patients with disfiguring or other psychological distressing disease manifestations. Except for diagnostic biopsy, surgery is rarely indicated in settings where cytotoxic chemotherapeutic drugs are available.

a. **Local therapy.** Radiotherapy including electron beam therapy, topical therapy, cryotherapy, or intralesional injection of vinblastine or other cytotoxics can be used for localized KS. Topical alitretinoin 0.1% gel is specifically approved for this indication. The overall response rate with 12 weeks of therapy is 35% to 37%. Radiation therapy is also highly effective for local control; it is generally reserved for disease that is limited but causing severe pain or distress. Short-term local toxicities are usually manageable, but radiation can lead to "woody" skin and other long-term ill effects. Doses range from an 8 Gy single dose to fractionated therapy to a total of 16 to 30 Gy and are individualized for a given patient.

b. **Systemic therapy**

(1) **Chemotherapy.** Several cytotoxic chemotherapy agents are effective, providing rapid improvement in KS-related symptoms in the majority of patients (Table 25.2). Liposomal doxorubicin (20 mg/m^2 every 3 weeks) is generally the agent of choice. It is equivalent or superior in activity to older regimens containing bleomycin and vincristine, with or without doxorubicin, and less toxic. An absolute neutrophil count of 750 cells/μL is adequate to deliver therapy, although granulocyte colony-stimulating factor (G-CSF) support

TABLE 25.2   Selected Systemic Treatment Regimens for KS

Regimens

Chemotherapy	Commonly used dosing regimen
Liposomal doxorubicin (Doxil)	20 mg/m^2 IV every 3 weeks
Paclitaxel	100 mg/m^2 IV every 2 weeks, *or* 135 mg/m^2 IV every 3 weeks

Biologic response modifier	
Interferon-α2b	$1–10 \times 10^6$ IU/d SC

IV, intravenously; KS, Kaposi sarcoma; SC, subcutaneously.

between cycles may be necessary. Treatment should generally be continued until maximal response is obtained. Treatment duration is variable. If possible, patients should not receive a cumulative lifetime anthracycline dose of over 550 mg/m^2 because of the risk of severe, irreversible cardiotoxicity. The sense of some practitioners is that the risk is less with a liposomal formulation; however, this dose should not be exceeded without careful cardiac monitoring and an awareness of the risks involved.

For second-line therapy, paclitaxel 100 mg/m^2 every 2 weeks or 135 mg/m^2 every 3 weeks has produced response rates of 50% to 70% when used without cART. Paclitaxel is substantially more toxic than liposomal doxorubicin, especially in patients with HIV-associated immunosuppression, and careful monitoring of blood counts is required. Caution should be used with medications that inhibit CYP3A4, such as protease inhibitors, or CYP2C8 (including trimethoprim), as these may increase the toxicity, and paclitaxel dose reduction may be necessary.

Lastly, oral etoposide 50 mg/day for days 1 to 7 of a 14-day cycle is active, with an overall response rate of 36% in previously treated patients, the majority of whom were not receiving cART. This may be particularly useful in resource-limited settings. Monitoring of complete blood counts is required.

(2) Immune modulators. Interferon-α (IFN-α) is the best-studied immunotherapy in KS. Responses have been reported with doses ranging from 1×10^6 IU/day to 36×10^6 IU three times per week (see Table 25.2). Common side effects include cytopenias and elevated transaminases. Fatigue, fevers, and flulike symptoms are common but decline with continued therapy and can be managed with acetaminophen or nonsteroidal anti-inflammatory drugs. Patients should be monitored for depression and hypothyroidism. Most practitioners begin with low-dose IFN-α, 1 to 5×10^6 IU subcutaneous injection daily, and gradually increase the dose as tolerated.

C. KSHV-associated MCD (KSHV-MCD)

1. Epidemiology. There are several forms of Castleman disease, including a unicentric hyaline-vascular form, a multicentric plasma cell form, and a multicentric form associated with KSHV. Nearly all Castleman disease arising in the setting of HIV infection is KSHV-MCD. This polyclonal hyperproliferative B-cell disorder is considered to be rare, although its incidence is not well defined. In contrast with KS, there is evidence that MCD has become more common since the advent of cART. While most commonly seen in the setting of HIV, KSHV-MCD may occur in elderly or immunocompromised patients.

2. **Presentation.** KSHV-MCD is characterized by intermittent flares of inflammatory symptoms, including fevers, fatigue, cachexia, and edema, together with lymphadenopathy and/or splenomegaly. Gastrointestinal symptoms and cough are also common. Flares are often severe and can be fatal. Many symptoms are attributable to a KSHV-encoded viral interleukin-6. There is no validated staging or prognostic system. KSHV-MCD should be considered in the differential diagnosis of patients with HIV and unexplained inflammatory symptoms or autoimmune phenomena, particularly anemia or thrombocytopenia. The clinical course waxes and wanes, but untreated, it is frequently fatal within 2 years of diagnosis, with patients succumbing to the severe inflammatory syndrome or progressing to lymphoma.

3. **Evaluation.** Diagnosis of KSHV-MCD generally involves an excisional lymph node biopsy, including demonstration of characteristic pathologic changes and KSHV-infected cells by immunohistochemistry. Physical exam should focus on adenopathy, splenomegaly, edema, and evaluation for concurrent KS. Common laboratory abnormalities include anemia, thrombocytopenia, hypoalbuminemia, hyponatremia, and elevated inflammatory markers such as C-reactive protein. Lactate dehydrogenase (LDH) is generally not elevated. Patients with MCD should undergo CT of neck, chest, abdomen and pelvis.

4. **Treatment.** There is no standard therapy for KSHV-MCD. HIV-infected patients should receive cART. Several agents have reported activity in case series or small studies. Perhaps best studied is the anti-CD20 monoclonal antibody rituximab. Most patients respond initially to rituximab-containing regimens, although relapses are common. Rituximab monotherapy may be insufficient in advanced disease, and it has been associated with exacerbation of intercurrent KS. Other potentially active agents include ganciclovir, IFN-α, and NHL chemotherapy regimens. Survival of over 2 years is now relatively common. However, given the many uncertainties in managing patients with KSHV-MCD, consideration should be given to referral to a clinical trial.

D. **Primary effusion lymphoma (PEL)**

1. **Epidemiology.** PEL is a rare variant of B-cell NHL notable for its unusual presentation and aggressive clinical course. The great majority of reported cases occur in people with HIV, where it represents less than 4% of all lymphomas.

2. **Presentation.** PEL usually presents as a lymphomatous effusions in serous body cavities, frequently in patients with other KSHV-associated malignancies. Many cases are pleural, but peritoneal, pericardial, and leptomeningeal presentations are seen. Extracavitary PEL may rarely present in other locations, including lymph nodes and the gastrointestinal tract.

3. **Evaluation.** Diagnosis of PEL depends on the demonstration of KSHV infection of tumor cells. In more than 70% of cases, tumor cells are coinfected with EBV. Common B-cell surface markers (CD19, CD20, CD79a) are absent, while activation markers (CD30, CD38, CD71, CD138) are often present; presence of immunoglobulin gene rearrangements confirms B-cell monoclonality. Evaluation of disease extent should be performed as for NHL (see Section II).

4. **Treatment.** There are few data to guide the choice of therapy in PEL. Case series using doxorubicin-based regimens report initial complete response (CR) rates as high as 40%, but rapid relapse is common. Median survival is less than 6 months, although a few long-term remissions have been described. The potential role of novel therapies is being explored, and patients should be treated within clinical studies if possible.

II. NON-HODGKIN LYMPHOMA (NHL)

A. Background

NHL is now the most common cancer in HIV-infected patients in the United States. Histologies associated with HIV include both germinal center (GC) and non-GC subtypes of diffuse large B-cell lymphoma (DLBCL), Burkitt lymphoma (BL), plasmablastic lymphoma, primary central nervous system lymphoma (PCNSL), and PEL.

B. Presentation and patient evaluation

HIV-associated NHL often presents with constitutional symptoms (fevers, night sweats, and weight loss) and enlarging lymph nodes. Extranodal presentations occur more commonly than in HIV-uninfected patients, at sites including the gastrointestinal tract, bone marrow, liver, and central nervous system (CNS). Diagnosis depends on excisional lymph node biopsy or biopsy of an involved extranodal site, and review by pathologists with expertise in lymphoma is advised.

C. Staging

Staging should include CT of the head, neck, chest, abdomen and pelvis, [18]fluorodeoxyglucose (FDG)-positron emission tomography (PET), LDH, complete blood count with differential, bone marrow biopsy, and lumbar puncture with evaluation of cerebral spinal fluid by cytology and flow cytometry. Evaluation of cardiac function using echocardiography or multigated acquisition scan is recommended. Magnetic resonance imaging (MRI) of the brain with gadolinium should be strongly considered to evaluate for CNS involvement, or other CNS complications of AIDS in patients with low CD4 counts. HIV viral load, CD4 count, and HBV core antibody and surface antigen, as well as HCV serology, should be evaluated. Patients with detectable HBV core antibody or surface antigen should be screened for a quantitative HBV viral load.

Ann Arbor staging classification is used in HIV-related NHL; however, assessment of prognosis in HIV-associated lymphoma also depends largely on tumor biology. The International Prognostic Index, when applied to patients with DLBCL receiving rituximab plus cyclophosphamide, doxorubicin, vincristine, and prednisolone (R-CHOP), is valid in patients with HIV. For patients with DLBCL, immunohistochemical analysis to determine GC versus non-GC subtypes using Hans criteria provides prognostic information. When treated with short-course dose-adjusted etoposide, prednisone, doxorubicin, cyclophosphamide, vincristine, and rituximab (SC-EPOCH-RR), patients with non-GC have a worse outcome than patients with GC (5-year progression-free survival 44% for non-GC versus 95% for GC). Patients with low CD4 counts have a worse prognosis, reflecting both a propensity to develop more aggressive NHL subtypes and increased risk for death from AIDS-related infections during and after chemotherapy.

D. Treatment

1. **General approach.** Patients with HIV-associated NHL should be treated with curative intent whenever possible. Prior to cART, modified regimens using lower doses of drugs to reduce toxicity were often used, and the median survival was approximately 2 years. However, studies in the cART era have shown that prognosis improves with therapies that mirror those used in HIV-negative patients, albeit with particular attention to the prevention of infection. CR and prolonged progression-free survival are now achievable in a high percentage of patients.

   Decisions regarding use of cART during lymphoma therapy are based on expert opinion. Its use is not essential; studies of dose-adjusted EPOCH (DA-EPOCH) in HIV-associated lymphoma have achieved excellent results withholding cART during lymphoma treatment. However, other studies have maintained patients on cART during therapy, and most specialists will continue well-tolerated cART regimens. In patients who have not yet started on cART, opinions vary. Optimized cART should not interfere with delivery of full-dose chemotherapy. Caution regarding possible drug–drug interactions is required. Ritonavir should generally be avoided due to strong inhibition of CYP3A4. Other protease inhibitors also inhibit CYP3A4 to varying degrees; nonprotease inhibitor cART regimens are preferred. Zidovudine should be avoided due to its additive hematotoxicity. If withheld, cART should be introduced immediately after completion of therapy.

   Patients should receive prophylaxis against *Pneumocystis* pneumonia regardless of the CD4 count, preferably with trimethoprim/sulfamethoxazole (one double-strength tablet three times weekly throughout therapy, continued thereafter until CD4 >200 cells/μL). Patients with fewer than 50 to 100 CD4 cells/μL require azithromycin 1200 mg weekly as prophylaxis against *Mycobacterium avium* complex infection. Those with detectable hepatitis B viremia require HBV antiviral therapy. Care is required to ensure therapy of intercurrent HBV is tailored to avoid compromising HIV control. Single-agent therapy for HBV will increase the likelihood of a specific HIV-mutation, M184V, which renders patients resistant to several important antiretroviral agents. Patients with mucosal candidal infections should not receive azoles concurrently with chemotherapy.

2. **Systemic therapy.** The tolerability and efficacy of several rituximab-containing combination chemotherapy regimens have been evaluated in HIV-associated lymphoma. DA-EPOCH-R, SC-EPOCH-RR, R-CHOP, and rituximab plus cyclophosphamide, doxorubicin, and etoposide (R-CDE) have all been evaluated prospectively, although they have not been directly compared (Table 25.3).

TABLE 25.3 Initial Chemotherapy Regimens for HIV-associated NHL

Regimen	
DA-EPOCH-R/ SC-EPOCH-RR **(every 21 days)**	
Etoposide	50 mg/m²/d CIV × 4 days
Vincristine	0.4 mg/m²/d CIV × 4 days (no cap)
Doxorubicin	10 mg/m²/d CIV × 4 days
Cyclophosphamide*	*AIDS Malignancy Consortium*
	375 mg/m² IV on day 5 if CD4 ≥100 cells/mL
	187 mg/m² IV on day 5 if CD 4 <100 cells/mL
	National Cancer Institute
	750 mg/m² IV on day 5
Prednisone	60 mg/m² PO on days 1–5
Rituximab†	375 mg/m² on day 1 (+/− 375 mg/m² day 6)
G-CSF	Starting on day 6, continue until ANC >5000 after nadir
R-CHOP (every 21 days)	
Cyclophosphamide	750 mg/m² IV on day 1
Doxorubicin	50 mg/m² IV on day 1
Vincristine	1.4 mg/m² IV on day 1, not to exceed 2 mg total
Prednisone	100 mg/m² PO on days 1–5
Rituximab	375 mg/m² on day 1
R-CDE (every 28 days)	
Cyclophosphamide	200 mg/m²/24 hours CIV on days 1–4
Doxorubicin	12.5 mg/m²/24 hours CIV on days 1–4
Etoposide	60 mg/m²/24 hours CIV on days 1–4
Rituximab	375 mg/m² on day 1
G-CSF	Starting on day 6, continue until ANC recovery after nadir

ANC, absolute neutrophil count; CIV, continuous intravenous; G-CSF, granulocyte colony-stimulating factor; NHL, non-Hodgkin lymphoma; PO, by mouth.
*The AMC study by Sparano et al. employed a stratified cyclophosphamide dosing scheme of 375 mg/m² IV on day 5 if CD4 ≥100 cells/mm³ and 187 mg/m² IV if CD4 <100/mm³. The National Cancer Institute study by Dunleavy et al. employed 750 mg/m² during the first cycle, which is the dose used in HIV-uninfected patients.
†Dose-dense rituximab as evaluated by Dunleavy et al. includes a day 6 dose of rituximab.

Rituximab improves CR rates and overall survival in a range of lymphomas in HIV-negative patients, and there is an emerging consensus that it should also be incorporated in the setting of HIV, although in patients with poor immune function ($<$50 CD4 cells/μL), rituximab may confer enhanced risk of infection.

Three studies have used EPOCH as a platform for the treatment of HIV-associated NHL. Infusional DA-EPOCH, which used a stratified dose of cyclophosphamide based on initial CD4 count and withheld cART until completion of chemotherapy, led to a 77% CR rate with 30 months median follow-up; overall survival was 74%. Subsequently, four to six cycles of DA-EPOCH with concurrent or sequential rituximab was evaluated. Patients with BL and Burkitt-like lymphoma were included. This protocol maintained a dose stratification of cyclophosphamide based on CD4 count (see Table 25.3), and 76% of patients received concurrent cART. In patients receiving concurrent rituximab, the CR

TABLE 25.4	Dosage Modifications used in DA-EPOCH in AIDS-NHL, based on Previous Cycle
Toxicity	**Dose Adjustment**
Hematologic toxicities	
ANC nadir $\geq$500/μL and Platelet nadir $\geq$25,000/μL	Escalate cyclophosphamide in increments of 187 mg/m^2 to maximum of 750 mg/m^2
ANC nadir $<$500/μL on one occasion Platelet nadir $<$25,000/μL on one occasion or less	Maintain current dose
ANC nadir $<$500/μL for two to four occasions and/or Platelet nadir $<$25,000/μL for two to four occasions	Decrease cyclophosphamide by increments of 187 mg/m^2 If no cyclophosphamide was given in previous cycle, decrease etoposide, doxorubicin, and vincristine by 25%
ANC nadir $<$500/μL for at least five occasions and/or Platelet nadir $<$25,000/μL for at least five occasions	Decrease cyclophosphamide by increments of 375 mg/m^2
Neurologic toxicity	
Constipation $>$ grade 3 Sensory neuropathy $>$ grade 3 Motor neuropathy $>$ grade 1	Decrease vincristine by 0.3 mg/m^2/day
Motor neuropathy $>$ grade 2	Discontinue vincristine

ANC, absolute neutrophil count; NHL, non-Hodgkin lymphoma.
Complete blood counts (CBC) should be checked twice weekly for patients on DA-EPOCH. Decisions for dose adjustments are based on this CBC monitoring schedule. Reductions for thrombocytopenia are not required if attributed to immune thrombocytopenia.

rate was 73%, with a 2-year overall survival of 63%. DA-EPOCH followed by rituximab yielded inferior CR rates with no decrease in infective toxicity. A further development of DA-EPOCH incorporated standard doses of cyclophosphamide and dose-dense rituximab. The number of courses administered was based on assessment of response by interim FDG-PET and CT, delivering a minimum of three (80% of patients) and maximum of six cycles with one cycle beyond stable imaging (SC-EPOCH-RR). The observed CR rate was 91% in DLBCL. With 48 months median follow-up, progression-free survival and overall survival were 84% and 64%, respectively. Notably, the estimated 5-year progression-free survival was 95% for those with GC DLBCL. However, validation of the approach—particularly the generalizability of the use of interim FDG-PET—is required before its adoption outside of clinical trials.

Another infusional regimen, R-CDE, has been evaluated in three separate phase II studies, presented together in a pooled analysis. These studies included patients with BL. R-CDE was administered with G-CSF support every 4 weeks, with a planned six cycles. In these studies, 76% of patients received concurrent cART. The CR rate was 70%, and the estimated 2-year overall survival rate was 64%. This regimen was associated with a high rate of both opportunistic and neutropenia-related infections.

Although the survival of patients with HIV-associated NHL has improved considerably, additional studies are needed to optimize treatment, and patients with HIV-associated NHL should continue to be enrolled in clinical studies when possible. For patients not referred for clinical studies, one of the three discussed regimens (DA-EPOCH-R, R-CHOP, or R-CDE; see Table 25.3) is recommended. The consensus now is that patients, even those with poor immune function, should be offered established regimens at standard doses whenever possible, as delivery of less intensive therapy may compromise outcomes.

3. **CNS prophylaxis and treatment.** CNS involvement at presentation occurs in less than 10% of patients with HIV-associated lymphoma and is particularly common in patients with EBV-associated disease, BL, or extranodal involvement. In those patients where staging, including lumbar puncture, shows no evidence of CNS disease at presentation, CNS prophylaxis should be instituted. The prophylaxis utilized varies between studies, but most investigators employ intrathecal methotrexate (12 mg) or cytosine arabinoside (50 mg) for a total of four to eight doses. A single dose of leucovorin 25 mg, given orally 24 hours after methotrexate, is advisable. Patients with documented leptomeningeal disease generally have a poor prognosis. Several intensive intraventricular and intrathecal methotrexate schedules

have shown activity. Most commonly, therapy is administered using an Ommaya reservoir twice weekly until 2 weeks after negative flow cytometry is documented (for a minimum of eight doses), and then continued weekly for 6 to 8 weeks, then monthly for 6 months.

4. **Burkitt lymphoma (BL)** is characterized by a very high rate of cell cycling (the proliferative index may approach 100%), an aggressive clinical course, and propensity to acquire chemotherapy resistance rapidly if treated improperly. Until recently, clinical trials of AIDS-related NHL included both DLBCL and BL. However, it is now appreciated that there are substantial differences in response of these diseases to therapy, and they must be considered separately. Combination dose intensive and infusional regimens are the standard of care for HIV-negative BL, and similar approaches are now being employed for AIDS-related BL.

    DA-EPOCH-R with a risk-adapted approach (employing cyclophosphamide 750 mg/m^2), and cyclophosphamide, vincristine, doxorubicin, and methotrexate plus ifosfamide, etoposide, and cytarabine (CODOX-M/IVAC) with rituximab each deliver high CR rates and are being evaluated in studies that include patients with HIV. There is evidence that patients with BL have a relatively poorer outcome with R-CDE or R-CHOP, and there is an expert consensus that these regimens should not be used. Particular attention to the risk of tumor lysis with induction is needed in BL. Intravenous hydration; monitoring of uric acid, calcium, potassium, and phosphate; and allopurinol prophylaxis should be employed during the first cycle of chemotherapy.

5. **Plasmablastic lymphoma (PBL)** is a rare EBV-associated B-cell NHL. While most commonly reported in the setting of HIV, PBL also occurs in organ transplantation patients and elderly individuals. It most commonly presents with extranodal disease within the oral cavity but may occur at other extranodal or nodal sites. Ann Arbor staging is not prognostic, and patients with stage I disease should be treated the same as those with systemic disease. PBL is characterized by a high proliferative index and aggressive clinical course. Historically, the prognosis has been poor, with median survival less than 2 years. CHOP has often been used with poor outcomes. Nonetheless, intensive regimens such as DA-EPOCH and CODOX-M/IVAC are recommended.

6. **Use of high-dose therapy (HDT) and stem cell transplantation.** Increasingly, data support the feasibility and effectiveness of HDT with autologous peripheral blood stem cell transplantation (PBSCT) in patients with relapsed HIV-NHL and HIV-associated HL. In the largest study of HDT-PBSCT, the Italian Cooperative

Group on AIDS and Tumors evaluated 50 patients: 31 with NHL and 19 with HL; 27 patients actually received transplantation. By intent-to-treat analysis with median follow-up of 44 months, overall and progression-free survival were each approximately 50%. Limiting analysis to those who received transplant, overall and progression-free survival were 75%. These results are comparable to results in HIV-negative patients. The role of this approach is still unclear. Nonetheless, if an HIV-infected patient requires second-line therapy for NHL or HL, early consideration of the role of transplantation is critical, as disease progression and consequent compromised performance status impact transplant feasibility.

III. PRIMARY CENTRAL NERVOUS SYSTEM LYMPHOMA (PCNSL)
A. Background

PCNSL typically occurs in patients with fewer than 50 CD4 cells/μL. Most are high-grade DLBCLs. The EBV genome is identified in nearly all investigated cases of HIV-associated PCNSL, and patients with AIDS-associated PCNSL have defects in EBV-specific CD4 activity, supporting the role of dysregulated lymphoproliferation of EBV-infected B-cells in its pathogenesis. The incidence of PCNSL has declined sharply since the introduction of cART, largely because the number of patients with under 50 CD4 cells/μL has decreased.

B. Presentation and diagnosis

Patients with AIDS-PCNSL may present with a headache, focal neurologic deficits, ataxia, or altered mental status. CT or MRI of the head typically shows single or multiple, periventricular, contrast-enhancing masses with surrounding edema. Lesions may be difficult to distinguish from those of toxoplasmosis. Given the changing epidemiology of HIV and HIV-associated malignancies, the differential diagnosis should also include other infections, such as tuberculosis. EBV-negative PCNSL, other CNS tumors, or metastatic cancer should also be considered, especially in patients with a CD4 count of more than 50 cells/μL. PCNSL is a curable malignancy with an extremely poor outcome if not treated. Expedited evaluation of patients with intracranial masses is therefore required.

Historically, AIDS patients with intracranial masses were often given an empiric trial of antitoxoplasmosis therapy. However, this approach is no longer considered acceptable except under unusual circumstances. Imaging should include MRI with gadolinium. Evaluation of CSF should include cytology, flow cytometry, and EBV polymerase chain reaction (PCR) in addition to evaluation of infectious etiologies. The presence of EBV by PCR in the cerebrospinal fluid is a sensitive marker for PCNSL, but EBV may be detectable in the cerebrospinal fluid in other settings. Patients with

HIV-PCNSL should undergo ophthalmologic evaluation for ocular involvement. In the context of a patient with 50 CD4 cells/μL or less, the combination of a high titer EBV viral load in the cerebrospinal fluid, a ring-enhancing brain mass on MRI, and a positive thallium scan or CNS FDG-PET may be considered highly suggestive of PCNSL, even without a tissue diagnosis. Whenever possible, patients in whom PCNSL is suspected should undergo stereotactic biopsy of the brain lesion. In patients who meet the criteria above, and who are too unstable for brain biopsy, empiric treatment for PCNSL may be warranted after careful consideration of the diagnostic possibilities, risks, and benefits. As 95% of HIV-positive patients with toxoplasmosis have serologic evidence of *Toxoplasma* sp. infection, the *Toxoplasma* titer can be a useful adjunct to determine a course of action. However, concurrent PCNSL and toxoplasmosis has been described.

C. Treatment

There is no standard therapy for HIV-associated PCNSL, and patients should be considered for referral to a clinical trial when possible. Therapy should include cART, which has been shown in retrospective studies to improve overall survival. After a pathologic diagnosis is made, a short course of dexamethasone may help control the mass effect of the tumor. Prior to cART, whole-brain radiation therapy (WBRT) was considered the standard of care. WBRT can be associated with severe late toxicity, but this was not a major concern in an era when the median survival in AIDS-associated PCNSL was 2 to 5 months. With the availability of cART, radiation-sparing approaches with curative intent that reduce the likelihood of late CNS toxicities are warranted. High dose methotrexate, 8 mg/m² every 2 weeks with leucovorin rescue, crosses the blood-brain barrier, is minimally hematotoxic, and is the backbone of PCNSL regimens in non-immunosuppressed patients. PCNSL is strongly CD20 positive, and inclusion of rituximab may also be beneficial. HIV-infected patients with EBV-negative PCNSL should be considered for radiation-sparing combination regimens used in HIV-uninfected patients, especially if they have CD4 greater than 100 cells/μL. If chemotherapeutic approaches fail, WBRT salvage therapy can be considered.

IV. HUMAN PAPILLOMAVIRUS (HPV)–ASSOCIATED CANCERS

A. Background

HIV-infected patients have an increased incidence of several cancers caused by HPV, including cancer of the cervix, anus, penis, vulva, oral pharynx, and tonsil. This increase is related to an increased exposure to oncogenic strains of HPV and an impaired ability to clear these strains because of HIV-associated immunodeficiency.

HIV-infected women have about a fivefold increased incidence of cervical cancer as compared to HIV-uninfected women, and cervical cancer became an AIDS-defining cancer in 1993. Virtually all cervical cancer is caused by oncogenic strains of HPV. HIV-infected women also have a four- to fivefold increased risk of cervical intraepithelial neoplasia (CIN), and cervical cancer screening is an integral component of health care for HIV-infected women. HIV-infected individuals, and especially MSM, have a high incidence of anal intraepithelial neoplasia (AIN) and persistence of HPV infection in the anus. People with HIV are at a 100-fold increased risk of anal cancer, and its incidence is increasing. In addition, there is evidence that other HPV-associated cancers, especially cancers of the oral pharynx and tonsil, are increasing in the last decade.

B. **Cervical cancer**
  1. **Screening and treatment of premalignant lesions.** The U.S. Preventative Services Task Force guidelines recommend that women with HIV should have evaluation of cervical cytology twice in the first year after diagnosis and then annually if the results are normal. Additional evaluation of HPV DNA during the first year, with a subsequent screening frequency of 6 months in women with detectable high-risk subtypes of HPV and yearly in those without high-risk HPV, has also been proposed as a more individualized screening algorithm. The management of premalignant cervical lesions in women with HIV is more complicated than that in HIV-negative women due to higher rates of positive margins and recurrent CIN, especially in women with low CD4 counts. Low-grade lesions (CIN1) are generally observed closely, while higher grade lesions (CIN2 or higher) are generally treated. Initiation of cART and associated immune reconstitution has been associated with regression of lesions over time in certain cases, and may decrease the risk of recurrence. Treatment options for CIN include ablative therapy, loop excision of the transformation zone, or conization procedures, and should be individualized based on the size and location of the lesion.
  2. **Staging and treatment.** The International Federation of Gynecology and Obstetrics staging system, used for non–HIV-infected patients, is used in this population as well. More recently, FDG-PET has been incorporated in the initial assessment of women with cervical cancer, largely due to the prognostic value of FDG-avid para-aortic lymph nodes. However, this modality has not been evaluated in women with HIV and cervical cancer, and results should be interpreted with the understanding that uncontrolled HIV viremia alone

is associated with lymph node FDG-avidity. Treatment is based on clinical stage. There are no clinical trials specific to HIV-infected women with cervical cancer. In the absence of information to the contrary, HIV-positive women with invasive cervical cancer should be treated in the same manner as those without HIV infection.

C. Anal cancer

1. **Screening and treatment of premalignant lesions.** The annual incidence of anal cancer in patients with HIV in the United States, estimated at 80 per 100,000 individuals, is much higher than that of the general population. Given the biologic similarities to cervical cancer and the effectiveness of cervical cancer screening, programs to screen HIV-infected men and women for AIN and treat high-grade lesions are being developed. This approach has the potential to prevent anal cancer by detecting and treating premalignant lesions. However, it has not yet been tested in prospective studies. A major difference between anal and cervical cancer is the greater difficulty in doing preventive surgery on precancerous lesions of the anus. The primary tool to screen for anal cancer is cytology of the anal epithelium. Abnormal cytology should be followed up with anoscopy if possible. Treatment decisions are based on the grade of the lesion. Current options for high-grade AIN include local treatment with topical immune modulator or antiviral agents, electrocautery, laser or infrared coagulation, and surgery.

2. **Treatment.** The standard of care for stages I to III anal cancer is concurrent chemoradiation, and patients with HIV should receive standard regimens. Given the concern of hematologic toxicity associated with mitomycin-C–based chemoradiation in patients with HIV, cisplatin-based regimens have been advocated by some. However, with the availability of cART, outcomes in patients with HIV receiving concurrent chemoradiation, including mitomycin-C–based therapy, appear to be comparable to that of the general population. The alternative to chemoradiation is surgical abdominoperineal resection (APR), which leaves patients with a permanent colostomy. APR is an option for patients with poor performance status or who do not wish to undergo concurrent chemoradiation, but should generally be employed only for the management of locoregional recurrence. Patients with HIV and anal cancer should be treated within clinical studies where possible.

V. NON-AIDS–DEFINING MALIGNANCIES (NADMs)

NADMs are an increasing public health concern, yet much remains to be learned about their epidemiology, pathogenesis, and optimal treatment. For some cancers, there are known biologic differences between those that arise in HIV-infected and uninfected patients (i.e., HIV-infected patients are more likely than the general population to present with mixed cellularity and lymphocyte-depleted HL subtypes). For other cancers, such biologic differences have not been established. Until recently, HIV-infected patients have generally been excluded from most cancer clinical trials of NADM, leading to a lack of specific data to guide therapy. A recent National Cancer Institute initiative encourages enrollment of HIV-infected patients in clinical trials where possible. In the absence of specific evidence, standard therapeutic approaches should generally be considered, especially in patients with good performance status.

Special considerations in the setting of HIV include the role of cART and of prophylaxis for opportunistic infections. For surgically managed tumors, cART should be prescribed based on DHHS guidelines. In patients for whom chemotherapy or radiation is required, most specialists recommend the use of cART in the absence of a clear contraindication. Potential drug–drug interactions between antiretroviral agents and chemotherapeutic agents should be considered, as outlined previously. Protease inhibitors, especially nelfinavir, may also have radiosensitizing effects. Generally, trimethoprim/sulfamethoxazole is recommended for patients with under 200 CD4 cells/μL, but more liberal use may be warranted in this setting, especially in patients receiving lymphotoxic regimens.

Selected Readings

Background

Biggar RJ, Engels EA, Ly S, et al. Survival after cancer diagnosis in persons with AIDS. *J Acquir Immune Defic Syndr*. 2005;39:293–299.

Bonnet F, Burty C, Lewden C, et al. Changes in cancer mortality among HIV-infected patients: the Mortalite 2005 Survey. *Clin Infect Dis*. 2009;48:633–639.

Engels EA, Biggar RJ, Hall HI, et al. Cancer risk in people infected with human immunodeficiency virus in the United States. *Int J Cancer*. 2008;123:187–194.

Yarchoan R, Tosato G, Little RF. Therapy insight: AIDS-related malignancies—the influence of antiviral therapy on pathogenesis and management. *Nature Clin Prac Oncology*. 2005;2:406–415.

Kaposi Sarcoma

Bower M, Weir J, Francis N, et al. The effect of HAART in 254 consecutive patients with AIDS related Kaposi's sarcoma. *AIDS*. 2009;23:1701–1706.

Krown SE, Testa MA, Huang J. AIDS-related Kaposi's sarcoma: prospective validation of the AIDS Clinical Trials Group staging classification. AIDS Clinical Trials Group Oncology Committee. *J Clin Oncol*. 1997;15:3085–3092.

Krown SE, Lee KY, Lin L, Fischl MA, Ambinder R, Von Roenn JH. Interferon-alpha 2b with protease inhibitor-based antiretroviral therapy in patients with AIDS-associated Kaposi sarcoma—An AIDS malignancy consortium phase I trial. *J Acquir Immune Defic Syndr.* 2006;41:149–153.

Martin-Carbonero L, Palacios R, Valencia E, et al. Long-term prognosis of HIV-infected patients with Kaposi sarcoma treated with pegylated liposomal doxorubicin. *Clin Infect Dis.* 2008;47:410–417.

Nasti G, Talamini R, Antinori A, et al. AIDS-related Kaposi's sarcoma: evaluation of potential new prognostic factors and assessment of the AIDS Clinical Trial Group Staging System in the Haart Era—the Italian Cooperative Group on AIDS and Tumors and the Italian Cohort of Patients Naive From Antiretrovirals. *J Clin Oncol.* 2003;21:2876–2882.

Northfelt DW, Dezube BJ, Thommes JA, et al. Pegylated-liposomal doxorubicin versus doxorubicin, bleomycin, and vincristine in the treatment of AIDS-related Kaposi's sarcoma: results of a randomized phase III clinical trial. *J Clin Oncol.* 1998;16: 2445–2451.

Saville MW, Lietzau J, Pluda JM, et al. Treatment of HIV-associated Kaposi's sarcoma with paclitaxel. *Lancet.* 1995;346:26–28.

Multicentric Castleman Disease

Bower M, Powles T, Williams S, et al. Brief communication: rituximab in HIV-associated multicentric Castleman disease. *Ann Intern Med.* 2007;147:836–839.

Casper C, Nichols WG, Huang ML, Corey L, Wald A. Remission of HHV-8 and HIV-associated multicentric Castleman disease with ganciclovir treatment. *Blood.* 2004;103:1632–1634.

Oksenhendler E, Duarte M, Soulier J, et al. Multicentric Castleman's disease in HIV infection: a clinical and pathological study of 20 patients. *AIDS.* 1996;10:61–67.

Primary Effusion Lymphoma

Boulanger E, Gérard L, Gabarre J, et al. Prognostic factors and outcome of human herpesvirus 8-associated primary effusion lymphoma in patients with AIDS. *J Clin Oncol.* 2005;23:4372–4380.

Zelenetz AD, the NCCN Non-Hodgkin's Lymphoma Panel. Non-Hodgkin's lymphoma. In: *NCCN Practice Guidelines in Oncology.* 1st ed. Fort Washington, PA: National Comprehensive Cancer Network; 2010.

Non-Hodgkin Lymphoma

Dunleavy K, Little RF, Pittaluga S, et al. The role of tumor histogenesis, FDG-PET, and short course EPOCH with dose-dense rituximab (SC-EPOCH-RR) in HIV-associated diffuse large B-cell lymphoma. *Blood.* 2010;114:3017–3024.

Kaplan LD, Lee JY, Ambinder RF, et al. Rituximab does not improve clinical outcome in a randomized phase 3 trial of CHOP with or without rituximab in patients with HIV-associated non-Hodgkin's lymphoma: AIDS-malignancies consortium trial 010. *Blood.* 2005;106:1538–1543.

Lim ST, Karim R, Nathwani BN, Tulpule A, Espina B, Levine AM. AIDS-related Burkitt's lymphoma versus diffuse large-cell lymphoma in the pre-highly active antiretroviral therapy (HAART) and HAART eras: significant differences in survival with standard chemotherapy. *J Clin Oncol.* 2005;23:4430–4438.

Little RF, Pittaluga S, Grant N, et al. Highly effective treatment of acquired immunodeficiency syndrome-related lymphoma with dose-adjusted EPOCH: impact of antiretroviral therapy suspension and tumor biology. *Blood.* 2003;101:4653–4659.

Miralles P, Berenguer J, Ribera JM, et al. Prognosis of AIDS-related systemic non-Hodgkin lymphoma treated with chemotherapy and highly active antiretroviral therapy depends exclusively on tumor-related factors. *J Acquir Immune Defic Syndr.* 2007;44:167–173.

Re A, Michieli M, Casari S et al. High-dose therapy and autologous peripheral blood stem cell transplantation as salvage treatment for AIDS-related lymphoma: long-term results of the Italian Cooperative Group on AIDS and Tumors (GICAT) study with analysis of prognostic factors. *Blood.* 2009;114:1306–1313.

Ribera JM, Oriol A, Morgades M, et al. Safety and efficacy of cyclophosphamide, adriamycin, vincristine, prednisone and rituximab in patients with human immunodeficiency virus-associated diffuse large B-cell lymphoma: results of a phase II trial. *Br J Haematol.* 2008;140:411–419.

Sparano JA, Lee JY, Kaplan LD, et al. Rituximab plus concurrent infusional EPOCH chemotherapy is highly effective in HIV-associated, B-cell non-Hodgkin's lymphoma. *Blood* 2010;115:3008–3016.

Spina M, Jaeger U, Sparano JA, et al. Rituximab plus infusional cyclophosphamide, doxorubicin, and etoposide in HIV-associated non-Hodgkin lymphoma: pooled results from 3 phase 2 trials. *Blood.* 2005;105:1891–1897.

Wang ES, Straus DJ, Teruya-Feldstein J, et al. Intensive chemotherapy with cyclophosphamide, doxorubicin, high-dose methotrexate/ifosfamide, etoposide and high-dose cytarabine (CODOX-M/IVAC) for human immunodeficiency virus-associated Burkitt lymphoma. *Cancer.* 2003;6:1196–1205.

Primary Central Nervous System Lymphoma

Antinori A, De Rossi G, Ammassari A, et al. Value of combined approach with thallium-201 single-photon emission computed tomography and Epstein-Barr virus DNA polymerase chain reaction in CSF for the diagnosis of AIDS-related primary CNS lymphoma. *J Clin Oncol.* 1999;17:554–560.

Corcoran C, Rebe K, van der Plas H, Myer L, Hardie DR. The predictive value of cerebrospinal fluid Epstein-Barr viral load as a marker of primary central nervous system lymphoma in HIV-infected persons. *J Clin Virol.* 2008;42:433–436.

Hoffmann C, Tabrizian S, Wolf E, et al. Survival of AIDS patients with primary central nervous system lymphoma is dramatically improved by HAART-induced immune recovery. *AIDS.* 2001;15:2119–2127.

Human Papillomavirus–Associated Cancers

Abramowitz L, Mathieu N, Roudot-Thoraval F, et al. Epidermoid anal cancer prognosis comparison among HIV+ and HIV- patients. *Aliment Pharmacol Ther.* 2009;30:414–421.

Frisch M, Biggar RJ, Goedert JJ. Human papillomavirus-associated cancers in patients with human immunodeficiency virus infection and acquired immunodeficiency syndrome. *J Natl Cancer Inst.* 2000;92:1500–1510.

Minkoff H, Zhong Y, Burk RD, et al. Influence of adherent and effective antiretroviral therapy use on human papillomavirus infection and squamous intraepithelial lesions in human immunodeficiency virus-positive women. *J Infect Dis.* 2010;201:681–690.

Palefsky JM. Anal cancer prevention in HIV-positive men and women. *Curr Opin Oncol.* 2009;21:433–438.

Wexler A, Berson AM, Goldstone SE, et al. Invasive anal squamous-cell carcinoma in the HIV-positive patient: outcome in the era of highly active antiretroviral therapy. *Dis Colon Rectum.* 2008;51:73–81.

Wright TC Jr, Ellerbrock TV, Chiasson MA, Van Devanter N, Sun XW. Cervical intraepithelial neoplasia in women infected with human immunodeficiency virus: prevalence, risk factors, and validity of Papanicolaou smears. New York Cervical Disease Study. *Obstet Gynecol.* 1994;84:591–597.

Non-AIDS–Defining Malignancies

Deeken JF, Pantanowitz L, Dezube BJ. Targeted therapies to treat non-AIDS-defining cancers in patients with HIV on HAART therapy: treatment considerations and research outlook. *Curr Opin Oncol.* 2009;21:445–454.

Persad GC, Little RF, Grady C. Including persons with HIV infection in cancer clinical trials. *J Clin Oncol.* 2008;26:1027–1032.

SECTION III: SUPPORTIVE CARE OF PATIENTS WITH CANCER

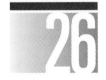

Side Effects of Chemotherapy and Molecular Targeted Therapy

Janelle M. Tipton

The supportive care of patients receiving cancer chemotherapy and molecular targeted therapy has improved considerably over the last two decades. Contributions to the substantial improvements include better understanding of the pathophysiology of specific side effects, increased knowledge and attention to risk factors, and availability of newer agents for prevention and management of side effects. The side effects of systemic cancer treatment may be acute, self-limited, and mild, or can be chronic, permanent, and potentially life threatening in nature. Although much progress has been made, the management of side effects continues to be of utmost importance for the tolerability of therapy and effect on overall quality of life. In addition, inadequately controlled side effects may lead to increased use of healthcare resources and costs, and may occasionally impact adherence to therapy. The implementation of evidence-based interventions has received recent emphasis and is critical in making appropriate clinical decisions for patient safety and the management of side effects.

I. ACUTE REACTIONS

A. Extravasation

Extravasation is defined as the leakage or infiltration of drug into the subcutaneous tissues. Vesicant drugs that extravasate are capable of causing tissue necrosis or sloughing. Irritant drugs cause inflammation or pain at the site of extravasation. Common vesicant and irritant agents and potential antidotes are listed in Table 26.1.

1. **Risk factors for peripheral extravasation** include small, fragile veins; venipuncture technique; site of venipuncture; drug administration technique; presence of superior vena cava syndrome; peripheral neuropathy; limited vein selection due to lymph node dissection; and concurrent use of medications that may cause somnolence, altered mental status, excessive movements, vomiting, and coughing.

2. **The incidence of extravasation** for vesicant chemotherapy is recorded as 0.01% to 6.5% in the literature. Extravasation may also occur with central venous catheters. Potential causes for central venous catheter extravasation include backflow secondary to fibrin sheath or thrombosis in the central venous catheter; needle dislodgement from a venous access port; central venous catheter damage, breakage, or separation; and displacement or migration of the catheter from the vein.

3. **Common signs and symptoms of extravasation** are pain or burning at the intravenous (IV) site, redness, swelling, inability to obtain a blood return, and change in the quality of the infusion. Any of these complaints or observations should be considered a symptom of extravasation until proven otherwise.

4. **Procedures to manage peripheral extravasation** are imperative to have in place, including guidelines or orders for extravasation management of vesicant and irritant agents before administration. If an extravasation is suspected, the following actions should be taken:

   1. Stop administration of the chemotherapy agent.
   2. Leave the needle/catheter in place and immobilize the extremity.
   3. Attempt to aspirate any residual drug in the tubing, needle, or suspected extravasation site.
   4. Notify the physician.
   5. Administer the appropriate antidote, as shown in Table 26.1. This may include instillation of a drug antidote or application of heat or cold to the site. Consideration for antidote order sets and verification of antidote accessibility is recommended prior to administration.
   6. Provide the patient and/or caregiver with instructions, including the need to elevate the site for 48 hours and the continuation of antidote measures as appropriate.
   7. Discuss the need for further intervention with the physician and photograph if indicated.

| TABLE 26.1 | Common Vesicant and Irritant Drugs and Potential Antidotes |

Chemotherapy Agent	Pharmacologic Antidote	Nonpharmacologic Antidote	Method of Administration
Mechlorethamine HCl	Sodium thiosulfate	Apply ice for 6–12 hours following sodium thiosulfate antidote injection	Prepare one-sixth M solution: If 10% sodium thiosulfate solution, mix 4 mL with 6 mL sterile water for injection. Through existing IV line, inject 2 mL for every 1 mL extravasated. Inject SC if needle is removed.
Mitomycin Dactinomycin	No known drug antidote	Topical cooling	Apply ice pack for 15–20 minutes at least four times a day for the first 24 hours.
Doxorubicin Daunorubicin Epirubicin Idarubicin	Dexrazoxane (Totect)	Topical cooling	Dexrazoxane should be used as soon as possible and within 6 hours of the anthracycline extravasation. Administration of dexrazoxane is IV for 3 consecutive days (Day 1: 1000 mg/m^2; Day 2: 1000 mg/m^2; Day 3: 500 mg/m^2) into a large vein in an area other than the extravasation area (i.e., preferably the opposite arm) over 1–2 hours. Apply cold pad with circulating ice water, ice pack, or Cryo-Gel (Cryopak, Edison, NJ) pack for 15–20 minutes at least four times a day for first 24–48 hours. Topical cooling should be removed 15 minutes before, and during, dexrazoxane administration.
Vinblastine Vincristine Vindesine Vinorelbine	Hyaluronidase (Amphadase; 150 units/1 mL; Hydase 150 units/1 mL; Vitrase: 150 units/mL)	Warm compresses	Apply heat for 15–20 minutes at least four times a day for first 24–48 hours. Hyaluronidase is instilled as five 0.2 mL injections SC into extravasated area, using a small-gauge needle (25 g). Change needle with each injection. Hyaluronidase is stored in refrigerator.
Oxaliplatin	Case reports that use of high-dose dexamethasone (8 mg twice daily for up to 14 days) has reduced inflammation.	Warm compresses	A warm compress applied to extravasation site is preferable.
Docetaxel Paclitaxel	None	Topical cooling	Apply ice pack for 15–20 minutes at least four times a day for first 24 hours.

IV, intravenous; SC, subcutaneously.

   8. Document extravasation occurrence according to institutional guidelines.
   9. Continued monitoring of extravasation site at 24 hours, 1 week, 2 weeks, and additionally as guideline recommends. Secondary complications such as infection and pain may occur. Follow-up photographs at these time periods, if possible, are helpful in monitoring extent of injury and progress in healing.

5. Procedures for central extravasation are also critically important to follow, as extravasation of chemotherapy agents in the upper torso or neck area is difficult to manage and may result in extensive defects, requiring reconstructive surgery. Extreme caution should be taken by nurses administering chemotherapy by this route. Procedures followed in central extravasation are similar to peripheral extravasation. Assessment of lack of blood return, patient reports in changes of sensation, pain, burning, or swelling at the central venous catheter site or chest warrant immediate discontinuation of chemotherapy. Prompt administration of the appropriate antidote is recommended, but if the extravasation has been extensive, these actions may not prevent damage. Collaboration with the physician regarding the need for further studies to identify the cause of the extravasation will be necessary as well as decisions for future plans for venous access.

B. Infusion reactions: hypersensitivity, anaphylaxis, and cytokine-release syndrome

Specific drugs with the potential for hypersensitivity with or without an anaphylactic response should be administered under constant supervision of a competent and experienced nurse and with a physician readily available, preferably during the daytime hours. Important preassessment data to be documented include the patient's allergy history, though this information may not predict an allergic reaction to chemotherapy. Other risk factors include previous exposure to the agent and failure to administer effective prophylactic medications. Drugs with the highest risk of immediate hypersensitivity reactions are asparaginase, murine monoclonal antibodies (e.g., ibritumomab tiuxetan), the taxanes (e.g., paclitaxel and docetaxel), and platinum compounds (e.g., cisplatin, carboplatin, and oxaliplatin). Drugs with a low to moderate risk include the anthracyclines, bleomycin, IV melphalan, etoposide, and humanized (e.g., trastuzumab) or chimeric (e.g., rituximab) monoclonal antibodies. Test doses or skin tests may be performed if there is an increased suspicion for hypersensitivity. This is most commonly done for carboplatin, bleomycin, and asparaginase. A skin testing protocol for carboplatin skin testing is shown in Table 26.2.

   1. Type I hypersensitivity reactions (which may or may not be immune-mediated) are the most common chemotherapy-induced type of reactions. These reactions characteristically occur within

▬▬TABLE▬▬ 26.2	Sample Carboplatin Skin Testing Protocol

1. All patients receiving their sixth and subsequent doses of carboplatin will have skin test dosing.
2. The planned carboplatin dose is diluted in 50 mL of 0.9% sodium chloride. A 0.02 mL aliquot is withdrawn and administered intradermally.
3. Following the intradermal injection, the injection site is examined at 5, 15, and 30 minutes.
4. A positive skin test is a wheal of ≥5 mm in diameter, with surrounding redness. A strongly positive skin test was one with ≥1 cm in diameter. If a patient develops a positive skin test, the physician is notified.
5. If the skin test is negative, the patient is then pretreated for the carboplatin with antiemetics, dexamethasone, diphenhydramine, and famotidine. Thirty minutes after the premedications are given, the carboplatin is given.

1 hour of receiving the drug; however, with paclitaxel, the hypersensitivity reactions often occur within the first 10 minutes of the start of the infusion. Common manifestations of a grade 1 or 2 type I reaction include flushing, urticaria, fever, chills, rigors, dyspnea, and mild hypotension. Grade 3 and 4 reactions may involve bronchospasm, hypotension requiring treatment, and angioedema. Less common signs and symptoms of infusion reactions include back or abdominal pain, nausea, vomiting, and diarrhea, incontinence, and anxiety. With appropriate premedication, the incidence of the hypersensitivity reactions has markedly decreased. Commonly used premedications include dexamethasone, diphenhydramine, and an H_2-histamine antagonist such as cimetidine, ranitidine, or famotidine. Emergency equipment should be immediately accessible, including oxygen, an Ambu respiratory assist bag (Ambu, Inc., Glen Burnie, MD), and suction equipment. The following parenteral drugs should also be stocked in the treatment area: epinephrine 1:1000 or 1:10,000 solution, diphenhydramine 25 to 50 mg, methylprednisolone 125 mg, and dexamethasone 20 mg. The development of a clinical guideline for hypersensitivity reactions, with or without true anaphylaxis, may be helpful in preparing for a potential reaction, reducing delays in response time to a reaction, and standardizing the management of a reaction with standing orders. Table 26.3 provides a sample preprinted standing order for the management of hypersensitivity and anaphylactic reactions.

2. **Cytokine-release syndrome,** which is commonly referred to as infusion reaction, is a symptom complex that occurs most frequently when monoclonal antibodies are administered. This reaction is believed to be primarily related to the release of cytokines from targeted cells and other immune cells. Most

TABLE 26.3	Sample Standing Orders for Hypersensitivity Reactions to Chemotherapy Agents

1. Have the following medications available:
   a. Diphenhydramine 50 IV
   b. Methylprednisolone 125 mg IV or equivalent hydrocortisone
   c. Epinephrine (1:10,000) 10-mL single-dose vial (or 1 mL of 1:1000, 1-mg vial).
2. If signs/symptoms of hypersensitivity occur (such as urticaria [hives], respiratory distress, bronchospasm, hypotension, angioedema, flushing, chest/back pain, anxiety), stop infusion of chemotherapy/biotherapy agent.
3. Maintain IV access with IV normal saline at 200 mL/hr until blood pressure stabilizes.
4. Administer oxygen at 2–4 L/min and measure pulse oximetry.
5. Administer methylprednisolone 125 mg IV push.
6. Administer diphenhydramine (Benadryl) 50 mg IV push.
7. Continuously monitor blood pressure, pulse, and oxygen saturation.
8. Notify physician immediately for further orders.
9. If symptoms do not resolve or worsen, administer epinephrine as directed by physician.
10. Initiate a code if airway patency is not maintained or cardiopulmonary arrest occurs.

IV, intravenous.

monoclonal antibodies have the potential to cause this syndrome, and the appearance may be similar to the type I hypersensitivity reaction. In contrast, however, the cytokine-release reactions may be managed by short-term cessation of the infusion, administration of histamine blockers, and restarting the infusion at a slower rate. Table 26.4 compares the differences between chemotherapy and biotherapy infusion reactions.

3. **Retreatment and rechallenge** of patients who have experienced paclitaxel-associated and platinum hypersensitivity reactions are supported in the literature. If a rechallenge is considered, the drug should be administered in the appropriate setting where immediate emergency situations may be handled. The decision to reinstitute the agent should be based on the clinical importance of using the drug in the particular disease setting. Patients have been successfully retreated within hours to days of the initial paclitaxel reactions at full doses; however, rechallenge with platinum compounds are generally less successful.

   a. **Reinstitution of paclitaxel.** Patient management after experiencing a hypersensitivity reaction includes immediate discontinuation of the paclitaxel infusion at the onset of symptoms and rapid administration of additional diphenhydramine and methylprednisolone. Following stabilization of the patient and waiting approximately 30 minutes, the paclitaxel infusion is reinitiated, with initial infusion rates at 10% to 25% of the total infusion rate. If tolerated, the rate can be gradually increased over the next several hours. Nursing care

TABLE 26.4	Infusion Reactions: The Comparison of Chemotherapy and Biotherapy Agents	
Characteristic	**Chemotherapy**	**Biotherapy**
Reaction type	Type I hypersensitivity	Cytokine release
Timing of reaction	Platinum: after multiple cycles	Most MoAbs: first infusion
	Taxanes: first or second infusion	Rituximab: any infusion
Prevention	Premedication	Premedication
Management/ Rechallenge	Grade 1 or 2: premedication— reinitiate infusion at slower rate	Dependent on grade Interruption Premedication
	Grade 3 or 4: not likely to rechallenge	Reinitiate at slower rate
Grading	1: Transient flushing/rash/ fever >38°C	1: Mild reaction: No infusion interruption
	2: Rash; flushing; urticaria, dyspnea, fever >38°C	2: Infusion interruption; responds promptly to symptomatic treatment (drugs, fluids); prophylactic medications indicated for ≤24 hours
	3: Symptomatic bronchospasm, with/without urticaria; parenteral medications indicated; allergy-related angioedema; hypotension	3: Prolonged/recurrences of symptoms after initial improvement; hospitalization indicated
	4: Anaphylaxis	4: Life-threatening; pressors or ventilator needed
	5: Death	5: Death

MoAb, monoclonal antibody.

would also include vital signs every 5 minutes or continuous observation for the first 15 minutes, then every 15 minutes through the first hour, then hourly until completed. An alternative is to pretreat the patient for 24 hours with dexamethasone 10 mg × 3 orally and to restart the infusion at the rate indicated above on the second day.

b. **Desensitization approaches.** Rechallenge after a severe hypersensitivity reaction of the second episode of hypersensitivity reaction to paclitaxel and platinum agents (cisplatin, carboplatin, oxaliplatin) are documented in the literature; however, planning for the desensitization is necessary. Regimens including dexamethasone 20 mg orally at 36 and 12 hours before chemotherapy and the morning of chemotherapy have been studied. A full 30 minutes before the chemotherapy, other IV premedications such as dexamethasone 20 mg, diphenhydramine 50 mg, and a H_2-histamine antagonist are given. For paclitaxel, the desensitization procedure continues with administration of a test dose of 2 mg in 100 mL of normal saline over 30 minutes. If there is no reaction, 10 mg in 100 mL of normal saline is given over 30 minutes, followed by the remaining full dose in 500 mL of normal saline over 3 hours if there is still no reaction. If a reaction is experienced, the usual diphenhydramine and methylprednisolone medications are given.

II. NAUSEA AND VOMITING

Patients who are about to begin chemotherapy are often concerned and apprehensive about nausea and vomiting. Nausea and vomiting can be distressing enough to the patient to cause extreme physiologic and psychological discomfort, culminating in withdrawal from therapy. With the advent of more effective antiemetic regimens in the last 20 years, many improvements in the prevention and control of nausea and vomiting have led to a better quality of life for patients receiving chemotherapy. The goal of therapy is to prevent the three phases of nausea and vomiting: that which occurs before the treatment is administered (anticipatory), that which follows within the first 24 hours after the treatment (acute), and that which occurs more than 24 hours after the treatment (delayed). It is also important to assess nausea and vomiting separately because they are different events and may have different causes. Factors related to the chemotherapy that can affect the likelihood and severity of symptoms include the specific agents used, the doses of the drugs, and the schedule and route of administration. Other patient characteristics that may affect emesis include history of poor emetic control, history of alcoholism, age, gender, anxiety level, and history of motion sickness.

A. Emetic potential of the drug

To plan an effective approach to control nausea and vomiting, the chemotherapeutic agents are grouped according to their emetic potential (Table 26.5). This type of categorization is helpful in making decisions regarding possible antiemetics to be used and how aggressive the antiemetic regimen should be for patients receiving chemotherapy for the first time or in subsequent treatments. It is important to select appropriate antiemetics from the various antiemetic classes and to not undertreat the patient for nausea and vomiting in the initial chemotherapy cycle. Failure to control nausea and/or vomiting may result in a conditioned response and subsequent anticipatory nausea and vomiting.

B. Antiemetic drugs

Agents that have been effective in preventing and treating nausea and vomiting (Table 26.6) come from various pharmacologic classes. They work by different mechanisms that may relate to the pathophysiologic processes causing nausea and vomiting. Within the last 20 years, it was discovered that agents that block predominately the serotonin 5-hydroxytryptamine subtype 3 ($5\text{-}HT_3$) receptors, rather than the dopamine receptors, have greater efficacy in the prevention of nausea and vomiting. More recent research indicates that the tachykinins, including a peptide called substance P, play an important role in emesis. Substance P binds to the neurokinin

	Emetogenic Potential for Commonly Used Chemotherapeutic Agents*	
TABLE 26.5		

Highly Emetogenic Agents ($\geq$75% potential for nausea, vomiting, or both)	Moderately Emetogenic Agents (50%–75% potential for nausea, vomiting, or both)	Mildly Emetogenic gents (25%–50% potential for nausea, vomiting, or both)
Carmustine	Arsenic trioxide	Asparaginase
Cisplatin ($>$40 mg/m^2)	Azacitidine	Bevacizumab
Cyclophosphamide ($>$1 g/m^2)	Bendamustine	Bleomycin
Cytarabine ($>$1 g/m^2)	Carboplatin	Busulfan
Dacarbazine (days 1 and 2)	Cisplatin ($<$40 mg/m^2)	Capecitabine
Dactinomycin	Clofarabine	Cetuximab
Doxorubicin ($>$60 mg/m^2)	Cyclophosphamide	Cladribine
Epirubicin	(200 mg/m^2 to 1 g/m^2)	Cyclophosphamide ($<$200 mg/m^2)
Ifosfamide ($>$1.2 g/m^2)	Cytarabine	Cytarabine ($<$200 mg/m^2)
Mechlorethamine	(200 mg/m^2 to 1 g/m^2)	Decitabine
Methotrexate ($>$1 g/m^2)	Daunorubicin	Docetaxel
Mitomycin ($>$15 mg/m^2)	Doxorubicin ($<$60 mg/m^2)	Fludarabine
Oxaliplatin	Etoposide	Fluorouracil
Streptozocin	Idarubicin	Gemcitabine
	Ifosfamide ($<$1.2 g/m^2)	Gemtuzumab
	Irinotecan	Hydroxyurea
	Methotrexate	Imatinib
	(50 mg/m^2 to 1 g/m^2)	Ixabepilone
	Mitomycin ($<$15 mg/m^2)	Liposomal doxorubicin
	Mitoxantrone	Melphalan
	Procarbazine	Mercaptopurine
	Temozolomide	Methotrexate ($<$50 mg/m^2)
	Topotecan	Paclitaxel
		Pemetrexed
		Rituximab
		Thioguanine
		Thiotepa
		Trastuzumab
		Vinblastine
		Vincristine
		Vinorelbine

*High-dose therapy requiring progenitor cell support is not included in this table.

type 1 (NK-1) receptor. Thus, the NK-1-receptor antagonists are now validated in their role in inhibiting nausea and vomiting with moderately and highly emetogenic chemotherapy. NK-1-receptor antagonists are thought to improve acute nausea and vomiting associated with chemotherapy when combined with standard regimens (i.e., dexamethasone and 5-HT$_3$ receptor antagonists) and to have additional effect during the period of delayed nausea and vomiting, alone or in combination with dexamethasone.

TABLE 26.6 Agents Used for Chemotherapy-Induced Nausea and Vomiting

Agent	Route of Administration	Dose	Comments
Phenothiazines			
Prochlorperazine (Compazine)	PO	10 mg every 4–6 hours	Some EPS; potential for postural hypotension when given IV
	IM or IV	2–10 mg every 4–6 hours	
	PR	25 mg every 12 hours	
Thiethylperazine (Torecan)	PO; IM; PR	10 mg every 6–8 hours	Some EPS
Trimethobenzamide (Tigan)	PO	250 mg every 4–6 hours	Some EPS
	IM or PR	200 mg every 4–6 hours	
Butyrophenones			
Haloperidol (Haldol)	IM; PO; IV	2–5 mg every 2–4 hours	Some EPS
Droperidol (Inapsine)	IV; IM	0.5–2.5 mg every 4 hours	Causes sedation, cardiac arrhythmias, EPS, hypotension. Not recommended.
Substituted benzamide			
Metoclopramide (Reglan)	PO; IV	10–40 mg once a day to 1- to 2-mg/kg dose at 2-hour intervals	EPS common in higher doses, which should be given with diphenhydramine; EPS worse with younger patients; may have diarrhea in higher doses
Benzodiazepines			
Lorazepam (Ativan)	PO or SL	1–2 mg every 4–6 hours	Causes sedation, amnesia, and confusion
	IV	0.5–2 mg every 4–6 hours	
Corticosteroids			
Dexamethasone (Decadron)	IV	4–20 mg (10–20 mg × 1), otherwise every 4–6 hours	Potential for agitation, delirium
	PO	4–8 mg every 4 hours	
Serotonin (5-HT₃) antagonists			
Ondansetron (Zofran)	IV	8–32 mg × 1	For highly emetogenic chemotherapy; lower doses effective for less emetogenic regimens
		0.15 mg/kg, every 4 hours × 3	
	PO	8 mg twice a day	
Granisetron (Kytril)	IV	1 mg × 1	Similar to ondansetron
	PO	1–2 mg × 1	
Dolasetron (Anzemet)	PO	100 mg before chemotherapy (once daily)	Similar to above. Oral form only recommended due to potential life-threatening cardiac arrythmias.
Palonosetron	IV	0.25 mg IV	

(continued)

TABLE 26.6	**Agents Used for Chemotherapy-Induced Nausea and Vomiting** *(continued)*		
Agent	**Route of Administration**	**Dose**	**Comments**
Cannabinoids			
Dronabinol (Marinol)	PO	2.5–10 mg every 4–6 hours	Causes sedation, may be habit forming, a controlled substance
NK-1 Receptor Antagonists			
Aprepitant (Emend)	PO	Tri-pack: 125 mg 30 minutes prior to chemotherapy on day 1, then 80 mg daily on days 2 and 3	

EPS, extrapyramidal symptoms; IM, intramuscularly; IV, intravenous; PO, by mouth; PR, per rectum; SL, sublingual.

C. Combination antiemetic therapy

Several antiemetic regimens are effective, but their design should be based on two general principles:

■ Combinations of antiemetics are more effective than single agents.

■ Preemptive treatment and scheduled administration are more effective than reactive therapy to prevent nausea and vomiting early in therapy and to manage potential delayed nausea and vomiting in the days following treatment.

Table 26.7 shows examples of antiemetic regimens that may be used when the chemotherapy has a high, moderate, and low emetic potential.

D. Nonpharmacologic interventions

Patients who are likely to experience or who have experienced anticipatory nausea and vomiting related to chemotherapy may benefit from the use of nonpharmacologic interventions in addition to the pharmacologic agents taken. The use of acupuncture, acupressure, guided imagery, music therapy, and progressive muscle relaxation are often effective in preventing nausea and vomiting. Many of these are forms of distraction that assist patients in maintaining a feeling of control over their treatment effects. Massage therapy, hypnosis, exercise, and acustimulation with wristband devices have insufficient data, and further studies are needed to support their use as interventions. With increasing attention to complementary therapies, it is hoped that more clinical studies will determine their value in patient care. Patients who are able to have little or no nausea and vomiting with their first chemotherapy treatment often assert that positive thinking is helpful as well. Patients may also prepare for their

TABLE 26.7   Examples of Regimens for Antiemetic Prevention and Management of Chemotherapy-Induced Nausea and Vomiting

Level I: patients receiving a mildly emetogenic agent
Dexamethasone 8–10 mg PO/IV before chemotherapy
with or without
Prochlorperazine 10 mg PO before chemotherapy, then 10 mg PO every 4–6 hours when necessary, *or*
Lorazepam 1 mg PO every 4–6 hours when necessary, *or both*

Level II: patients receiving a moderately emetogenic agent or patients receiving a mildly emetogenic agent who have failed to respond to or are intolerant of at least two level I regimens
Aprepitant* 125 mg PO before chemotherapy on day 1, then 80 mg PO daily on days 2 and 3, *and*
Palonosetron† 0.25 mg IV before chemotherapy, *and*
Dexamethasone 10–12 mg IV/PO before chemotherapy, then 8 mg PO daily on days 2–4
with or without
Lorazepam 1 mg PO or IV before chemotherapy every 4–6 hours when necessary, *or*
Prochlorperazine 10 mg PO every 4–6 hours when necessary, *or both*

Level III: patients receiving a highly emetogenic agent or patients receiving two or more moderately emetogenic agents or patients who have failed a level II regimen
Aprepitant* 125 mg PO before chemotherapy on day 1, then 80 mg PO daily on days 2 and 3, *and*
Palonosetron‡ 0.25 mg IV before chemotherapy, *and*
Dexamethasone 10–12 mg PO/IV before chemotherapy, then 8 mg PO on days 2–4, *and*
Lorazepam 1 mg PO or IV before chemotherapy, then every 4–6 hours when necessary
In addition, for delayed nausea and vomiting:
Metoclopramide 40 mg PO every 6 hours × 4 days, *with*
Dexamethasone 4 mg PO every 6 hours × 3 days, then 4 mg PO every 12 hours × 1 day
   (if not given already with aprepitant)
Give antiemetics 20–30 minutes prior to chemotherapy when using the IV route and 1 hour prior to chemotherapy when using the PO route. Given in this fashion, oral medication is usually as effective as the same medication IV, and the cost is considerably less.

IV, intravenous; PO, by mouth.
*Alternatively, could administer fosaprepitant 115 mg IV on day 1, followed by aprepitant 80 mg PO on days 2 and 3.
†Alternatives (5-HT$_3$): ondansetron 16–24 mg IV × 1 before chemotherapy, *or* dolasetron 100 mg PO, or granisetron 1 mg PO or IV before chemotherapy.
‡Alternatives (5-HT$_3$ antagonists): ondansetron 32 mg IV before chemotherapy; dolasetron 100 mg PO, or granisetron 1 mg PO or IV before chemotherapy.

chemotherapy treatments by eating foods that do not have offensive odors or spicy tastes. Clear liquids, foods served at room temperature, soda crackers, and carbonated beverages are sometimes good suggestions. Following chemotherapy, smaller, more frequent meals are less likely to promote the development of nausea and vomiting.

E. **Herbal remedies: ginger**

There have long been anecdotally based recommendations for the use of ginger to help prevent and minimize chemotherapy-induced nausea and vomiting. Few randomized controlled trials have been done to evaluate ginger as an intervention in this patient population. Early studies show safety and little toxicity; therefore, its use may be considered, but the actual benefit has not been established, and difficulty remains with respect to dosages and schedules.

III. OTHER SHORT-TERM COMPLICATIONS RELATED TO CANCER CHEMOTHERAPY

A. Stomatitis and other oral complications

The oral mucosa is vulnerable to the effects of chemotherapy and radiotherapy because of its rapid growth and cell turnover rate. Radiotherapy also interferes with the production of saliva and may increase oral complications because of a consequent reduction in the protective effect of the saliva. It is crucial to manage oral complications effectively because patients may experience considerable discomfort or develop secondary infections from the disruption of the oral mucosa. The likelihood of the development of stomatitis from a drug is dependent on the agent, the dose, and the schedule of administration. Continuous rather than intermittent administration is more likely to cause stomatitis with the antimetabolites.

1. **Specific chemotherapy agents that may cause stomatitis** include the following:
   - Antimetabolites: methotrexate, fluorouracil (particularly continuous infusion), capecitabine, cytarabine, irinotecan
   - Antitumor antibiotics: doxorubicin, idarubicin, dactinomycin, mitomycin, bleomycin
   - Plant alkaloids: vincristine, vinblastine, vinorelbine
   - Taxanes: docetaxel, paclitaxel
   - Alkylating agents: high doses of busulfan, cyclophosphamide
   - Biologic agents: interleukins, lymphokine-activated killer cell therapy

2. **Prevention and early detection.** If oral complications are anticipated, it is important to implement a good oral hygiene program before the initiation of therapy. Dental consultation is recommended for those at risk, and particularly in specific groups of patients, including those with bone marrow transplant, leukemia, or head and neck malignancies. Maintaining good nutrition and dental hygiene are also primary preventive measures. Normal saline is the preferred mouth rinse. Alternative rinsing agents such as sodium bicarbonate or nonalcoholic mouthwashes, if preferred by patients, may be used. Chlorhexidine and hydrogen peroxide mouth rinses should *not* be used. For patients receiving bolus fluorouracil, it is recommended that patients perform oral cryotherapy. This involves holding ice chips in the mouth starting 5 minutes prior to the bolus of fluorouracil and for 30 minutes after the administration of the drug.

This intervention is effective for bolus administration only and should not be done when oxaliplatin is also given, due to the potential for increase in acute neurotoxicity. Systematic oral assessments should be integrated into the physical examination at regular intervals. Special attention should be given to the tongue, the gingiva, the buccal mucosa, the soft palate, and the lips. It is also important to assess the patient for soreness, functional ability to swallow, and any effects on eating.

3. **Management of oral complications.** Although the primary goal is prevention, once oral complications develop, the focus of care should shift to the continuation of good oral hygiene and treatment of symptoms. Agents used for oral care are categorized according to function: cleansing agents, lubricating agents, analgesic agents, and preventive agents. Commercial mouthwashes and lemon glycerin swabs are not recommended for use because of their irritating and drying effects. If painful ulcerations do develop, topical relief may be best obtained by using single agent topical analgesics such as Ulcerease (Med-Derm Pharmaceuticals, Johnson City, TN) or lidocaine. Compounded analgesic mouth rinses such as "magic mouthwash" consisting of various components such as lidocaine, diphenhydramine, antacids, and/or sodium bicarbonate may be helpful, but do not have clear evidence of benefit. Systemic pain control measures such as oral or parenteral narcotics should be implemented if topical analgesics are ineffective.

4. **Xerostomia** that follows radiation therapy to the mouth area may require treatment with artificial saliva. It may also be benefited by the administration of pilocarpine 5 to 10 mg by mouth twice a day before meals. Before the initiation of radiation therapy to the head and neck area, dental consultation is necessary to evaluate oral hygiene, the state of repair of the teeth, and the health of the gums. Amifostine is a protective agent for xerostomia and is sometimes used concurrently with radiation to the head and neck.

5. **Secondary oral infections** should be treated promptly and as accurately as possible. Fungal infections may be treated with nystatin suspension, clotrimazole troches, or oral fluconazole. Viral infections may be reactivated after chemotherapy and are commonly treated with oral or IV acyclovir. The benefit of prophylactic use of antiviral agents or antifungal agents is not well established. However, in patients with a known history of cold sores or positive herpes simplex virus titers, it may be advantageous to administer prophylactic acyclovir.

Patients with dentures should be encouraged to remove them during the period after chemotherapy when they are at risk for infection, except at mealtime. In addition, the dentures should be cleansed before use. Although removal of the dentures may be detrimental to the patient's self-esteem, irritation of the dentures can lead to inflammation, ulceration, and secondary infection.

B. Fatigue

Cancer treatment–related fatigue has become an increasingly reported side effect of cancer therapy, and it can be the most distressing. An estimated 80% to 100% of patients experience fatigue. Cancer treatment–related fatigue is a subjective feeling of tiredness that is disproportionate to the level of exertion. This symptom often interferes with activities of daily living and can be part of a symptom cluster, which can be debilitating if left untreated. Any chemotherapy or biotherapy agent may cause fatigue and all patients should be screened for potential etiologic factors and appropriate management.

1. **Interventions** recommended for fatigue include exercise, education, energy conservation and activity management, measures to optimize sleep quality, massage, and behavioral therapies such as relaxation and healing touch. Exercise has the strongest and most cumulative evidence in support as an intervention for fatigue. Exercise interventions should be individualized and based on the patient's specific disease and treatment. Medical management may have some benefit, particularly psychostimulants such as methylphenidate and modafinil, and antidepressants if depression is a causal factor. While erythropoiesis-stimulating agents should be used with caution, they may have some benefit in correcting fatigue associated with anemia.

C. Diarrhea

Among the many causes of diarrhea in patients with cancer are chemotherapy, radiotherapy, the cancer itself, medications, supplemental feedings, and anxiety. Chemotherapy may result in osmotic diarrhea or secretory diarrhea, and often is associated with destruction of actively dividing epithelial cells of the gastrointestinal tract. Secretory diarrhea also may result from infectious causes (e.g., *Clostridium difficile* or other enterocolitis-causing bacteria), with or without concurrent neutropenia. Prolonged diarrhea can lead to discomfort, severe electrolyte imbalances and dehydration, altered social life, and poor quality of life. In the past, little attention has been paid to the prompt evaluation and management of diarrhea, but with increasing use of agents such as irinotecan, the observation of severe and potentially life-threatening problems has heightened awareness of this side effect. The elderly, in particular, may be at increased risk for treatment-related diarrhea and may require close monitoring.

1. **Chemotherapy and biologic agents** may contribute to the development of diarrhea and most commonly include the antimetabolites such as fluorouracil, capecitabine, methotrexate, cytarabine, and

irinotecan. In addition, agents such as dactinomycin, hydroxyurea, idarubicin, the nitrosoureas, and paclitaxel may cause diarrhea. When diarrhea from fluorouracil or irinotecan is present while on therapy, it is a sign of toxicity that must be monitored closely because it can escalate rapidly to severe levels at which the drug must be held or discontinued. Diarrhea also has been noted with interferon-α and interleukin-2 and with oral small molecule targeted therapies, such as lapatinib, erlotinib, sorafenib, and sunitinib; diarrhea can be a problem but is manageable with proper education and reporting. High-dose chemotherapy regimens used in stem cell transplantation may also be associated with severe diarrhea and may be caused by acute graft-versus-host disease.

2. **Assessment** of a patient experiencing diarrhea should begin with a baseline history of usual elimination patterns, pattern of symptoms, and concurrent medications. The duration of the diarrhea and frequency of stool passage should be noted with reference to a stool diary if indicated. The physical examination may disclose abdominal tenderness, signs of dehydration, and disruption in perianal or peristomal skin integrity. Laboratory data may be obtained to assess serum chemistries, complete blood count, and stool samples for *C. difficile* toxin and other enteropathic bacteria.

3. **Management** of treatment-related diarrhea is often symptomatic and requires little or no alteration in cancer therapy. Agents that decrease bowel motility should not be used for longer than 24 hours unless significant infections have been excluded. In the absence of obvious inflammation and infection, it is appropriate to treat most patients with nonspecific treatment for diarrhea, including opioids (loperamide, diphenoxylate, and codeine), anticholinergics (atropine and scopolamine), or both. Octreotide is often effective in controlling chemotherapy-related diarrhea as well as diarrhea associated with the carcinoid syndrome. Table 26.8 lists common agents used to treat diarrhea. Nonpharmacologic measures that may also assist in the prevention and management of diarrhea are a low-residue diet and increased fluids. If the diarrhea is severe, IV hydration is necessary to prevent serious hypovolemia, electrolyte disturbances, and shock. In patients who experience severe irinotecan-associated diarrhea, antibiotic therapy such as ciprofloxacin is recommended because of a high incidence of an infectious contribution to gastrointestinal problems, which may include a functional ileus.

D. **Constipation**

In patients whose cancer has resulted in debility or immobility or in those who require narcotic analgesics, constipation can be a particular problem. Constipation may also develop in patients who have received neurotoxic chemotherapy agents including the vinca alkaloids, etoposide, and cisplatin, each of which may cause autonomic

TABLE 26.8	Pharmacologic Management Strategies for Diarrhea
Agent	**Comments**
Kaolin pectin (Kaopectate)	30–60 mL PO after each loose stool
Loperamide (Imodium)	Two capsules (4 mg) PO 4 hours initially, then add 1 capsule (2 mg) after each loose stool; should not exceed 16 capsules daily
Diphenoxylate hydrochloride, with atropine sulfate (Lomotil)	1–2 tablets PO 4 hours; should not exceed eight tablets daily; there may be anticholinergic effects due to atropine
Atropine	Used with early-onset cholinergic diarrhea (i.e., irinotecan) 0.25–1 mg PO or SC
Octreotide	May be useful for fluorouracil-induced diarrhea; starting dose: 0.05–0.1 mg SC twice a day; may be increased to 1.8 mg/d in refractory diarrhea Sandostatin LAR® Depot is indicated for carcinoid and VIPomas. It is a slow-release drug that is dosed at 20–30 mg every 4 weeks.

PO, by mouth; SC, subcutaneously; VIPoma, vasoactive intestinal peptide tumor.

dysfunction. Decreased bowel motility due to intra-abdominal disease, hypercalcemia, dehydration, and antiemetic use can also contribute to constipation. Chronic constipation in patients with cancer is a problem that is more easily prevented than treated. A diet high in bulk fiber, fresh fruits, and vegetables, as well as adequate fluid intake, may help to minimize constipation. Patients started on narcotic analgesics should also begin a bowel regimen, first with mild stool softeners and bulk laxatives and then proceeding to stimulants or osmotic laxatives if the milder regimen is not effective. Methyl-naltrexone is a new agent now approved for use with opioid-induced constipation and has clear evidence-based benefit. A bowel regimen example for a patient at risk for constipation is as follows:

1. Docusate sodium 100 mg twice a day alone or with casanthranol one capsule twice a day
2. If no bowel movement, add:
   a. Senna at bedtime (dose varies with the preparation), *or*
   b. Milk of magnesia 30 mL at bedtime.
3. If no bowel movement with the above, may add:
   a. Bisacodyl one to three tablets or one 10-mg suppository at bedtime, *or*
   b. Lactulose one to four tablespoons daily *or*
   c. Polyethylene glycol 17 g daily.
4. Other more aggressive alternatives, if there is no impaction, include:
   a. Fleet enema
   b. Magnesium citrate 1 bottle
   c. Tap-water enema.

E. Altered nutritional status

Patients with cancer often experience progressive loss of appetite and sometimes severe malnutrition during the course of the disease and treatment. Malnutrition may result from a side effect of the therapy or a direct effect of the cancer (e.g., gut obstruction or hepatic or brain metastases). The resulting effects of malnutrition are a poorer response to therapy, increased incidence of infections, and an overall worsening of patient well-being. Many times, one of the presenting signs that leads to the diagnosis of cancer is weight loss; therefore, the patient is most likely already experiencing some alteration in nutritional status. Malnutrition is reported to occur in 50% to 80% of patients with advanced disease. Nutritional management of the patient with cancer involves early intervention using a supportive healthcare team.

1. **Effects of chemotherapy and radiation therapy on nutrition.** Chemotherapy has a major effect on nutritional status because of the direct insult on the gastrointestinal tract. Among the gastrointestinal effects are anorexia, nausea, vomiting, taste alterations, stomatitis, esophagitis, colitis, constipation, and diarrhea. Not only are the effects physiologic in nature, but the added psychologic impact of the disease and therapy can also result in anxiety and depression, which can contribute to the lack of interest in food. Any patient receiving concurrent therapy with chemotherapy and radiation therapy to the head/neck or aerodigestive tract will likely experience difficulty in swallowing, appetite, and inadequate nutritional intake. Such high-risk patients need early assessment by a clinical dietician and proactive interventions, including consideration of a feeding tube.

2. **Nutritional assessment.** Early in the patient's treatment, a thorough nutritional assessment should be completed by the healthcare team. The assessment should include diet history; nutrient intake; anthropometric measurements (height, weight, and skin-fold thickness and midarm circumference, if possible); laboratory tests for anemia, serum albumin, and prealbumin; and an evaluation of activity and functional status. A good nutritional assessment may help to identify patients who are already at risk of malnutrition or those who may be prone to develop problems during the course of the illness and treatment.

3. **Nutritional intervention.** Nutritional intervention should be considered during the initial and ongoing assessments. Situations that warrant nutritional intervention include involuntary weight loss (more than 10% within the last 6 months, especially when combined with weakness and fatigue), history of recent physiologic stress, serum albumin below 3.2 g/dL, or severe immunocompromise. Nurses, dietitians, and even family members can identify problems and may be the first to act to promote weight

gain. Various approaches to help increase weight are changes in diet; symptomatic treatment of nausea and vomiting, stomatitis, and other gastrointestinal effects of chemotherapy; and supplemental nutrition. Individual dietary counseling is recommended in the literature to be an effective intervention.

    a. Nutritional supplements. Several nutritional supplements are commercially available for oral use. One benefit of nutritional supplements is that they are a concentrated form of nutrition for protein and calories. Some of the disadvantages are the unappealing taste and the high cost to the consumer. Some patients and their families are able to develop some creative high-protein and -calorie supplements using household items with some suggestions from the healthcare team.

    b. Tube feedings. Enteral nutrition through a nasogastric, gastrostomy, or jejunostomy tube may be an alternative if oral intake is not possible. Enteral feedings are the recommended route if the gastrointestinal tract is functional. Advantages of enteral feeding include lower cost and fewer complications than with parenteral feedings and maintenance of normal gastrointestinal function. Some care and maintenance are involved with feeding tubes, and patients and their families need to be given information regarding available options for feeding.

    c. Total parenteral nutrition (TPN). Parenteral nutrition should be considered in patients who do not have a functioning gastrointestinal tract or in those for whom supplemental nutrition is anticipated for a short period of time. Patients who receive TPN usually require the insertion of a central venous catheter, which may result in other iatrogenic complications such as pneumothorax, vein thrombosis, and catheter-related infections. In many situations, TPN used in the patient with cancer increases morbidity, especially from infection, without improving survival. Thus, TPN has considerable economic, ethical, and medical consequences that must be evaluated in conjunction with the patient's overall prognosis.

    4. Pharmacologic interventions. A recent area of interest is pharmacologic appetite stimulation. Current evidence supports the use of corticosteroids and progestins, one of which is megestrol acetate oral suspension 800 mg/day (20 mL/day).

F. Neurotoxicity

The incidence of neurotoxicity associated with chemotherapy is increasing, potentially because of the greater use of high-dose chemotherapy and newer drugs causing neurotoxicity used in combination. In many cases, early detection and treatment of neurotoxicity (i.e., reduction of drug dose or discontinuation) allow for the reversal of symptoms. The neurotoxic symptoms may manifest as altered level of consciousness or coma, cerebellar dysfunction, ototoxicity, or peripheral neuropathy, which may be temporary but can cause significant changes in functional ability that persist as a long-term effect. It is also important to assess renal function because poor renal function may reduce clearance of the chemotherapy agent, leading to increased neurotoxicity.

1. **Chemotherapy and biologic agents** with known potential for neurotoxicity include high-dose cytarabine, high-dose methotrexate, vincristine, vinblastine, vinorelbine, ifosfamide, cisplatin, carboplatin, oxaliplatin, paclitaxel, docetaxel, ixabepilone, procarbazine, bortezomib, thalidomide, interleukin-2, and the interferons.

2. **Prevention and early detection** of neurotoxicity is key to the prevention of permanent neurologic damage. Assessment of symptoms of neurotoxicity should be documented on a routine basis. In certain treatment regimens, altering the drug sequence can markedly decrease the symptoms.

3. **Management** of peripheral neurotoxicity is being studied, with the goal of slowing, halting, and reversing the neuropathy. Dose reduction of the suspect agent, particularly with the microtubule inhibitors and epothilones, may be warranted, depending on the grade and duration of neuropathy. There is very little evidence to support specific interventions for peripheral neuropathy. Anecdotally, B complex vitamins such as pyroxidine or vitamin B_6 may be used, 100 mg twice a day in attempt to minimize the peripheral neuropathy. Glutamine, anticonvulsants (gabapentin, pregabalin, or carbamazepine), or tricyclic antidepressants (amitriptyline) have been studied in phase II trials and may be considered. Topical analgesics and opioids may also be effective. Conventional nondrug interventions with some report of effectiveness include exercise, physical therapy, massage, and transcutaneous electrical nerve stimulation. Patient safety is critical and patient education on self-care measures is recommended.

G. **Palmar–plantar erythrodysesthesia (PPE) or hand–foot syndrome**
PPE is dose-limiting and the most common cumulative toxicity associated with continuous-infusion fluorouracil in the past but has captured recent attention with newer chemotherapy drugs such as capecitabine and liposomal doxorubicin with high incidence. PPE is a toxic drug reaction that begins as a cutaneous eruption of the integument on the palms of the hands and plantar surfaces of the feet. It has been postulated that PPE occurs because of drug extravasation in the microcapillaries of the hands and feet due to local everyday trauma or by drug concentration and accumulation in sweat glands found in the palms and soles with resultant tissue damage. PPE is time exposure–dependent and occurs with protracted, chronic exposure over long periods (i.e., more than 3 to 4 weeks).

Prevention or minimization of PPE has been observed through regional cooling during the infusion of pegylated liposomal doxorubicin by having patients keep ice packs around the wrists and ankles, and consume iced liquids. These interventions were continued for 24 hours after completion of the chemotherapy. A second retrospective study also showed benefit of regional cooling during the chemotherapy infusion. While regional cooling decreased the frequency and severity of PPE in patients in the intervention group, data are not sufficient to support routine use in clinical practice. Conversely, this intervention appears promising, and the minimal cost, relatively simple procedure, and well-tolerated intervention may be helpful. Other preventive interventions that have few studies or case report support include pyroxidine, oral corticosteroids, supportive care with topical wound care, and patient education.

1. **Chemotherapy agents** with a known potential for the development for PPE include fluorouracil (primarily with continuous infusions), capecitabine, doxorubicin, and liposome-encapsulated doxorubicin.

2. **Clinical findings** of PPE include tingling, numbness, pain, dryness, erythema, swelling, rash, blister formation, and pruritus of the hands and feet. Clinical knowledge of the potential for PPE and early assessment is imperative for adjustments of dose or withholding of therapy.

3. **Management of PPE** and symptomatic treatment result from prompt identification of symptoms. The grading scale for PPE is shown in Table 26.9. At the first sign of PPE, the drug should be stopped, the interval between doses should be increased, or the drug dose should be reduced. If identified at grade 2 toxicity, symptoms typically improve within a few days of stopping the drug. If untreated, grade 2 side effects may quickly progress to grade 3 or 4, requiring more intense medical concern and intervention. Depending on the drug used, recommendations

TABLE 26.9 Hand–Foot Syndrome (Palmar–Plantar Erythrodysesthesia) Grading Scale

Grade 1	Grade 2	Grade 3	Grade 4
Painless erythema, or swelling, numbness, dysesthesia/paresthesia, and tingling that do not disrupt activities of daily living	Painful erythema with swelling that affects activities of daily living, blisters or ulcerations less than 2 cm	Moist desquamation, ulceration, blistering, and severe pain, interference with normal daily activities, cannot wear regular clothing	Diffuse or local process causing infectious complications, a bedridden state, or hospitalization

Based on National Cancer Institute of Canada CTG Expanded Common Toxicity Criteria.

are available for dose modifications. In situations where PPE is likely, education on preventative measures should be given to patients before beginning the drug. Patients should be counseled to avoid tight-fitting shoes and rings or repetitive rubbing pressure to the hands or feet. Other precautionary measures include avoiding excessive pressure and heat on the skin for 3 to 5 days after treatment, avoidance of hot baths, showers, or hot tubs (hot water for 24 hours prior to and 72 hours after treatment), and friction-causing activities such as exercise for 3 to 5 days after treatment. Patients should also be advised to use emollients such as Bag Balm (Dairy Association Co., Lyndonville, VT), Udderly Smooth (Redex Industries, Salem, OH), or other petroleum- or lanolin-containing creams liberally and frequently. Patients should also be instructed to notify their healthcare providers at the first signs or symptoms of PPE. If the grade of toxicity worsens, supportive care related to analgesia and prevention of infection is important. Further studies need to be done to evaluate which interventions are helpful for PPE and do not exacerbate the skin toxicity.

H. Skin reactions

With the advent of epidermal growth factor receptor (EGFR) antagonist drugs and small molecule targeted therapies, dermatologic toxicities have become relevant to patients and oncology healthcare providers. The dermatologic toxicities can vary in their type, time of onset, severity, duration, and response to therapeutic interventions. Reactions can include dry skin, rashes, pruritus, blistering, and desquamation. While such reactions do not often lead to alteration in therapy, they do pose a new challenge for symptomatic treatment.

1. **Common EGFR inhibitors and small molecule targeted therapies** known to cause skin reactions include cetuximab, panitumumab, erlotinib, lapatinib, sunitinib, and sorafenib.

2. **Clinical findings** for EGFR skin reactions are primarily a pustulopapular rash that is often mild to moderate in severity. The rash can cause pruritus and some discomfort, and patients may have difficulty coping with the appearance and body image changes. While often not severe in nature, the rash may contribute to the development of secondary infections.

3. **Management of skin reactions** from consensus guidelines emphasizes the importance of utilizing an interdisciplinary approach to management, involving specialists in oncology and dermatology. Important to any skin reaction is the understanding of the etiology and aggravating factors. As more data becomes available, particular agents to avoid as well as therapeutic options are critical in supportive care. For example, traditional acne medications and retinoids may actually enhance inflammation

and exacerbate the rash, and alcohol-based gels and lotions may irritate the skin and exacerbate xerosis. A proactive, stepwise intervention strategy based on rash severity may be helpful. For a localized and minimally symptomatic rash, no intervention or topical hydrocortisone 1% or 2.5% cream and/or clindamycin 1% gel may be used. Reassessment within a few weeks is recommended by a healthcare professional or patient self-report if the reaction worsens or does not improve. For a moderate reaction, where there is a more generalized rash with some mild symptoms such as pruritus, options may include hydrocortisone cream 2.5%, clindamycin 1% gel, or pimecrolimus 1% cream in addition to doxycycline 100 mg by mouth twice a day or minocycline 100 mg by mouth twice a day. If the rash continues to worsen, symptoms are severe and impact functional status, and the potential for superinfection is present, a corticoid dose pack may need to be added to the moderate reaction interventions.

Selected Readings

Eaton LH, Tipton JM. *Putting Evidence into Practice: Improving Oncology Patient Outcomes.* Pittsburgh: Oncology Nursing Society; 2009.

Grunberg S, Clark-Snow RA, Koeller, J. Chemotherapy-induced nausea and vomiting: contemporary approaches to optimal management. *Support Care Cancer.* 2010 Jan 19 [Epub ahead of print].

Hesketh PJ. Chemotherapy-induced nausea and vomiting. *New Engl J Med.* 2007; 358:2482–2494.

Jacobson JO, Polovich M, McNiff KK, et al. American Society of Clinical Oncology/Oncology Nursing Society chemotherapy administration safety standards. *J Clin Oncol.* 2009;25:1–7.

Lenz HJ. Management and preparedness for infusion and hypersensitivity reactions. *Oncologist.* 2007;12:601–609.

Lorusso P. Toward evidence-based management of dermatologic effects of EGFR inhibitors. *Oncology.* 2009;28:2.

Lynch TJ, Kim ES, Eaby B, Garey J, West DP, Lacouture ME. Epidermal growth factor receptor inhibitor-associated cutaneous toxicities: an evolving paradigm in clinical management. *The Oncologist.* 2007;12:610–621.

Mouridsen HT, Langer SW, Buter J, et al. Treatment of anthracycline extravasation with Savene (dexrazoxane): results from two prospective clinical multicentre studies. *Ann Oncol.* 2007;18:546–550.

National Comprehensive Cancer Network. Antiemesis practice guidelines in oncology, Version 1.2010. Retrieved from www.nccn.org

Polovich M, Whitford JM, Olsen, M (Eds). *Chemotherapy and Biotherapy Guidelines and Recommendations for Practice.* 3rd ed. Pittsburgh: Oncology Nursing Society; 2009.

Schulmeister L. Managing extravasations. *Clin J Oncol Nurs.* 2005;9:472–475.

Richardson G, Dobish R. Chemotherapy induced diarrhea. *J Oncol Pharm Pract.* 2007;13:181–198.

Schulmeister L. Totect™: a new agent for treating anthracycline extravasation. *Clin J Oncol Nurs.* 2007;11:387–395.

Spence RR, Heesch KC, Brown WJ. Exercise and cancer rehabilitation: a systematic review. *Cancer Treat Rev.* 2010;36:185–194.

Swain SM, Arezzo JC. Neuropathy associated with microtubule inhibitors: diagnosis, incidence, & management. *Clin Adv Hemat Oncol.* 2008;6:455–467.

Tariman JD, Love G, McCullagh E, Sandifer S, IMF Nurse Leadership Board. Peripheral neuropathy associated with novel therapies in patients with multiple myeloma: consensus statement of the IMF Nurse Leadership Board. *Clin J Oncol Nurs.* 2008;12(suppl):29–35.

Van Gerpen R. Chemotherapy and biotherapy-induced hypersensitivity reactions. *J Infus Nurs.* 2009;32:157–165.

Vogel WH. Infusion reactions: diagnosis, assessment, and management. *Clin J Oncol Nurs.* 2010;14:E10–21.

Von Moos R, Thuerlimann BJ, Aspro M, et al. Pegylated liposomal doxorubicin-associated hand-foot syndrome: Recommendations of an international panel of experts. *Eur J Cancer.* 2008;44:781–790.

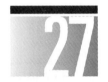

Infections: Etiology, Treatment, and Prevention

Thomas J. Walsh and Joan M. Duggan

Infectious diseases are an important cause of morbidity and mortality in immunocompromised patients with cancer. Advances in the diagnosis, treatment, and prevention of these infections have been critical in improving outcome of oncology patients, particularly those with hematologic malignancies. The critical components of infectious disease supportive care include the following: recognition of risk factors that impair host defenses, understanding of the likely pathogens and their resistance patterns within one's own institution, meticulous diagnostic evaluation of symptomatic or febrile patients, and prompt initiation of a rationally based antimicrobial regimen that is active against the most likely microorganisms.

I. ETIOLOGY OF INFECTIONS IN PATIENTS WITH CANCER

A. General considerations

Infections develop in patients with cancer as the result of quantitative or qualitative defects in their innate or adaptive host defense systems. Among these components are circulating phagocytic cells, cell-mediated immunity (CMI), circulating immunoglobulins, the reticuloendothelial system (RES), endogenous cytokines, intact mucocutaneous barriers, and patency of hollow visci. Defects commonly occur in more than one system of innate and adaptive host defenses due to a multitude of etiologies, including the underlying malignancy and its treatment. Alterations of these host defense systems increase the risk for development of specific infections. The relationship between altered host defenses and infections caused by specific pathogens is delineated in Table 27.1.

B. Circulating phagocytic cells

Neutrophils (PMNs) and monocytes are key effector cells of the innate host defense system against most bacterial and fungal pathogens encountered in patients with cancer. Neutropenia (defined as an absolute neutrophil count [ANC] of <500 PMNs/µL) increases the risk of infection in direct relation to its duration and depth. Patients with persistent neutropenia (defined as >10 days) or those with profound neutropenia (<100 PMNs/µL) have a markedly increased risk of developing serious bacterial and fungal infections. Neutropenia may develop as the direct result of a leukemic process infiltrating normal bone marrow with suppression of myelopoiesis or following cytotoxic chemotherapy. Development of mucositis in association with chemotherapy-induced neutropenia further increases the risk of infection. Neutropenia is associated with an increased risk of development of life-threatening infections caused by the endogenous mucocutaneous bacterial flora, as well as *Candida* spp. from the alimentary tract and *Aspergillus* spp. and other filamentous fungi from the external environment.

C. Cell-mediated immunity (CMI)

Altered CMI may result from the primary neoplastic process, such as Hodgkin lymphoma or hairy cell leukemia, or from therapeutic interventions, such as corticosteroids and fludarabine. Although fludarabine may induce a profound depletion of CD4 lymphocytes (T-helper cells), corticosteroids have less of an effect on the absolute number while still profoundly compromising their function. Altered CMI is associated with an increased risk of infections caused by intracellular bacterial pathogens (e.g., *Listeria monocytogenes*, *Mycobacterium* spp., and *Salmonella* spp.), many fungal organisms (e.g., *Pneumocystis*, *Cryptococcus neoformans*, *Histoplasma capsulatum*), and DNA viruses (e.g., varicella zoster virus [VZV], cytomegalovirus [CMV], Epstein-Barr virus [EBV]). As corticosteroids also affect PMN, monocyte, and macrophage function, invasive aspergillosis may also develop in patients receiving sustained and elevated dosages.

D. Circulating immunoglobulins

Hypogammaglobulinemia or dysimmunoglobulinemia may develop in patients with multiple myeloma or chronic lymphocytic leukemia. These defects in adaptive immunity are strongly associated with infections caused by encapsulated bacteria, particularly *Streptococcus pneumoniae*, *Haemophilus influenzae*, and *Neisseria meningitidis*.

TABLE 27.1	Relationship Between Altered Host Defenses and Organisms Causing Infection in Patients with Cancer				
Altered Host Defense	Gram-Positive Bacteria	Gram-Negative Bacteria	Fungi	Viruses	Other Pathogens
Neutropenia	*Staphylococcus* species (e.g., *S. aureus*, coagulase-negative staphylococci) α-hemolytic streptococci (e.g., *Streptococcus mitis*) *Enterococcus faecalis* and *E. faecium*	Enterobacteriaceae (e.g., *Escherichia coli, Klebsiella* spp., *Enterobacter* spp.) *Pseudomonas aeruginosa*	*Candida* species (e.g., *C. albicans, C. tropicalis,* and *C. glabrata*) *Aspergillus,* spp. Mucorales *Fusarium* spp., *Scedosporium* spp. *Trichosporon* spp.	HSV (associated with chemotherapy-induced mucositis)	
Decreased cell-mediated immunity	*Nocardia* spp.	*Listeria monocytogenes* *Salmonella* spp. *Legionella* spp.	*Pneumocystis, Cryptococcus neoformans* *Histoplasma capsulatum* *Coccidioides* spp.	HSV VZV CMV EBV	*Mycobacterium* spp. (e.g., *M. tuberculosis, M. avium* complex) *Toxoplasma gondii* *Strongyloides stercoralis*
Hypogammaglobulinemia, dysimmunoglobulinemia, or asplenia	*Streptococcus pneumoniae*	*Haemophilus influenzae* *Neisseria meningitidis* *Capnocytophaga canimorsus*	—	—	*Plasmodium falciparum* *Ehrlichia chaffeensis* *Anaplasma phagocytophilum* *Babesia microti*

Disruption of mucocutaneous barriers					
Vascular catheters	Coagulase-negative staphylococci S. aureus	P. aeruginosa Acinetobacter bau-mannii Stenotrophomonas maltophilia	Candida species*	—	—
Mucositis of the alimentary tract	α-hemolytic strepto-cocci (e.g., S. mitis) Enterococcus spp. Clostridium septicum	E. coli Klebsiella spp. Enterobacter spp., P. aeruginosa	Candida species	—	—
Postoperative wounds	Coagulase-negative staphylococci S. aureus Group A streptococci Enterococcus spp.	Enterobacteriaceae	—	—	—
Urinary tract catheters	Enterococcus spp.	Enterobacteriaciae, P. aeruginosa	—	—	—
Obstruction of hollow visci	Aerobic and an-aerobic respiratory, gastrointestinal, and genitourinary bacterial flora	Aerobic and anaer-obic respiratory, gastrointestinal, and genitourinary bacterial flora	—	—	—

CMV, cytomegalovirus; EBV, Epstein-Barr virus; HSV, herpes simplex virus; VZV, varicella zoster virus.

*The portal of entry of Candida spp. in most neutropenic patients is thought to be the gastrointestinal tract.

E. Reticuloendothelial system (RES)

Alterations of the RES most commonly develop as the result of splenectomy. Among its important functions, the spleen serves as a mechanical filter for removing opsonized or nonopsonized bacterial pathogens, as well as a setting for IVIG production. There is an increased risk in splenectomized patients for development of fulminant infections caused by *S. pneumoniae, H. influenzae, Capnocytophaga canimorsus, Babesia microti, Ehrlichia chaffeensis, Anaplasma phagocytophilum,* and *Plasmodium falciparum.*

F. Endogenous cytokines and chemokines

An elaborate network of immunoregulatory cytokines and chemokines regulates the effector cells of the innate host defense systems. These molecules mediate their effect through an intricate system of cell surface receptors. The expanding use of monoclonal antibodies to inhibit immunoregulatory molecules and their receptors has resulted in new forms of immunosuppression. For example, infliximab, which binds to tumor necrosis factor (TNF)-α, is associated with an increased risk of tuberculosis and histoplasmosis.

G. Intact mucocutaneous barriers

Cytotoxic chemotherapy, particularly regimens containing cytarabine, high-dose methotrexate, and etoposide, may cause severe mucosal disruption, which may result in the translocation of pathogenic endogenous bacterial and fungal pathogens, such as *Escherichia coli, Klebsiella pneumoniae,* and *Candida* spp., from the intestinal tract or *Streptococcus mitis* from the oral cavity. Vascular catheters disrupt the normal cutaneous barriers and provide a conduit for staphylococci to enter the bloodstream.

Normal bacterial flora further contribute to mucosal host defense by suppressing the growth of more pathogenic organisms. Use of broad-spectrum antibacterial agents may reduce the normal bacterial flora and allows more resistant organisms to fill the void on mucosal surfaces. Normal gastrointestinal flora also protect against the emergence of *Clostridium difficile* colitis. Prior use of broad-spectrum antibiotics is the strongest predictive variable for the development of *C. difficile* colitis in numerous studies.

H. Obstruction of hollow visci

Solid tumors or lymphoid malignancies that obstruct the upper and lower respiratory tract, biliary tree, intestines, and urinary tract result in accumulation of bacteria that are normally cleared by these structures. Obstructions in the upper respiratory tract may result in sinusitis and in the lower respiratory tract as postobstructive pneumonia caused by respiratory flora, including anaerobes. Obstructions of the gastrointestinal and biliary tract may result in polymicrobial bacteremia and ascending cholangitis. By comparison, obstruction of the urinary tract is more often associated with aerobic gram-negative bacteremia.

II. DIAGNOSIS OF INFECTIONS IN PATIENTS WITH CANCER

A. General overview

The initial assessment of possible infection in a patient with cancer includes a careful history assessing risks and symptoms, physical examination assessing for hemodynamic stability and localizing signs, and prompt completion of a laboratory diagnostic evaluation. As early symptoms and signs of infection are attenuated in immunocompromised patients, attention to subtle details in history and physical exam are important. Any clinical features suggesting infection in an immunocompromised patient with cancer should prompt initiation of broad-spectrum antibiotics. For example, the presence of localizing abdominal pain in a neutropenic patient in the absence of fever should prompt the initiation of empirical antibacterial therapy. The clinical assessment of immunocompromised febrile patients with cancer should attempt to localize the possible source of infection. Clinical localization helps to guide therapy for likely pathogens.

B. Clinical history

The clinical history is directed toward elucidating risk factors for infection and localizing symptoms. Immunocompromised patients may have minimal symptomatic findings. Deep-seated infection may present as simply fever and malaise. Pneumonia in a neutropenic patient may present initially with only mild dyspnea or cough. Patients should be queried for any history of localizing pain.

Suspected infection in neutropenic patients constitutes a medical emergency. Understanding the patient's current immune deficits is important and can guide therapy.

1. **Cancer treatment.** Understanding the current underlying neoplastic process and current therapy will help to assess a patient's immune status.

   a. **Chemotherapeutic and biologic agents.** Many commonly used chemotherapeutic drugs are cytotoxic, resulting in significant lymphopenia and/or neutropenia. The duration, severity, and type of myelosuppression can be related to the type of chemotherapeutic agent, the amount of drug exposure, and the underlying degree of myelosuppression.

      (1) **Neutropenia.** Alkylating agents, anthracyclines, cytarabine, methotrexate, carboplatin, busulfan, 5-fluorouracil, and nitrosoureas are examples of drugs that commonly cause dose-dependent neutropenia, depending on the protocol.

      (2) **Cluster of differentiation 4 (CD4) and 8 cell suppression (cellular immune system suppression).** The following chemotherapeutic agents may result in prolonged suppression of the T-helper/suppressor arm of the immune system:

      ■ Alemtuzumab: median duration of lymphopenia is 28 days

- Corticosteroids: severe T-cell function suppression can be seen with a dose equal to or more than 15 mg prednisone/day for a month or more.
- Purine analogs (cladribine, fludarabine, and pentostatin) may result in CD4 cell count suppression to 200 or less for several years after therapy.

(3) Suppressed B-cell function (altered humoral immunity). The following chemotherapeutic and biologic agents may cause suppression of antibody production by B cells:

- Alkylating agents (cyclophosphamide, chlorambucil, melphalan)
- Corticosteroids: use of greater than 40 mg/day of prednisone equivalent may decrease antibody production
- Methotrexate
- Rituximab

(4) Cytokine suppression. Infliximab, adalimumab, and etanercept may be used in autoimmune diseases or for graft-versus-host disease in recipients of hematopoietic stem cell transplantation (HSCT). Such agents result in altered TNF-α response with an increased risk of infections with conditions such as tuberculosis, histoplasmosis, and aspergillosis.

2. Type of malignancy

  a. Solid tumors. These malignancies can cause significant obstruction in affected tissues, leading to infection behind the obstruction. For example, postobstructive pneumonias are common in patients with bronchogenic carcinomas. Colonic carcinomas may cause obstruction or perforation and may simulate diverticular abscesses. Tissue necrosis secondary to malignancy may also create an area of potential sequestrum, which can become infected during an episode of bacteremia or from translocation of bacteria from a normally nonsterile area to a sterile area. For example, hepatic metastases may serve as a nidus for recurrent bacteremias of enteric gram-negative bacteria. Some solid tumors may mimic an infectious etiology without any microbial involvement, such as the presence of fever and malaise in a patient with renal cell carcinoma.

  b. Hematologic malignancies. Leukemias and lymphomas may cause severe immunodysregulation. Lymphoblastic leukemias and lymphomas also may cause B symptoms, including fever. In contrast, fever associated with nonlymphocytic leukemias is usually caused by an infection complicating neutropenia rather than B symptoms.

C. Clinical evaluation

The physical examination should be thorough with special emphasis on areas of symptomatology and likely mucocutaneous portals of entry. Like the clinical history, the review of systems and clinical examination can present with subtle or atypical findings in the presence of severe infection. Special attention should be directed to the following areas and potential infectious etiologies.

1. **Review of systems/symptoms of infection**
    - Head, eyes, ears, nose, and throat (HEENT): changes in vision, ear or sinus discomfort, oral lesions, changes in dentition
    - Lungs: cough, hemoptysis, shortness of breath, pleuritic chest pain
    - Abdomen: dysphagia, odynophagia, abdominal pain, perianal pain or pruritus, bleeding, diarrhea, nausea or vomiting
    - Skin: any new skin lesions or skin changes
    - Genitourinary (GU) system: urinary frequency, dysuria, urinary urgency, hematuria, GU discharge, flank tenderness, decreased urination
    - Central nervous system (CNS): altered mental status, new onset focal deficits, seizures
    - Catheter sites: redness, tenderness at the insertion site including along the subcutaneous tract of the catheter.

2. **Signs of infection** in immunocompromised patients with malignancy may be subtle or atypical, so a thorough physical examination focusing on changes or alteration in function is essential. Special attention should be directed to the areas listed in Table 27.2 and the associated potential etiologic agents.
    a. **HEENT**
        (1) **Ophthalmic assessment.** Hemorrhages; necrosis of the retina; yellow lesions adjacent to scarred retina ("headlight in fog"); white, infiltrative lesions on the retina; chorioretinitis with retinal detachment; or fulminant endophthalmitis are all signs of serious infection. New anisocoria or extraocular muscle palsy suggests a space-occupying lesion, cavernous sinus infection, or orbital infiltrative process.
        (2) **Paranasal sinuses.** Sinus tenderness, orbital cellulitis, or edema can indicate bacterial or fungal infection of the sinuses. Black material along the nasal turbinate mucosa may indicate mucormycosis.
        (3) **Oropharynx and dentition.** Bacterial infections, especially anaerobic infections, may present with marginal gingivitis, loosened teeth, pain or discomfort in the teeth or gums, or referred pain to the sinus area in addition to frank abscess formation. The presence of a draining sinus tract may be significant for Actinomycosis. Hemipalatal erythema suggests ipsilateral maxillary sinus infection involving the palatine blood vessels. Ulcerations can be caused by a variety of infectious agents, including viruses, fungi, and *Mycobacterium tuberculosis*. Viral ulcerations

TABLE 27.2 Potential Etiologic Agents of Infection and Associated Signs and Symptoms in Immunocompromised Oncology Patients

Clinical Change	Potential Etiologic Agent
HEENT	
Changes in vision	
Retinal hemorrhage	*Staphylococcus aureus* (endocarditis), CMV, and in neutropenic hosts *Candida* spp. or *Aspergillus* spp.
Retinal necrosis	HSV, VZV
Retinal exudate with scarring	Toxoplasmosis
Vitreal opacities (non-neutropenic patients), chorioretinitis, or endophthalmitis	*Candida* spp., *Trichosporon* spp., *Histoplasma capsulatum*
Sinus tenderness	
Black discharge or orbital cellulitis/edema	Mucormycosis (zygomycosis)
Oropharynx	
Painful, bleeding gums, marginal gingivitis	Oral anaerobes
Ulcerations	
Shallow, painful	HSV, coxsackievirus
Deep, painful	*Histoplasmosis*
Erythema or white plaques	*Candida*
Cardiovascular	
Murmur or line infection	*Staphylococcus epidermidis*, *S. aureus*
Chest pain, dyspnea, pleural rub, pericarditis	*Aspergillus* spp., *Streptococcus pneumoniae*, *S. aureus*, coxsackievirus
Pulmonary	
Consolidation	*S. pneumoniae*, *Legionella* spp., *Haemophilus influenzae*, *Pseudomonas aeruginosa*, *Aspergillus* spp., or other angioinvasive mold
Diffuse interstitial pattern/patchy alveolar infiltrate	CMV, PCP, *Mycoplasma*, other viruses (e.g., influenza, adenovirus)
Nodule, halo sign, wedge-shaped infiltrate, crescent sign	*Aspergillus* spp, Mucorales, *Fusarium* spp., *Scedosporium* spp., other angioinvasive mold, *P. aeruginosa*
Postobstructive	Anaerobes + gram-negative bacilli *S. aureus*, *P. aeruginosa*
Abdomen	
Pain, nausea/vomiting—suspect typhlitis	Polymicrobial: gram-positive cocci, gram-negative bacilli, anaerobes
Perianal or rectal discomfort—suspect anorectal infection	Polymicrobic; gram-positive cocci, gram-negative rods, anaerobes
Diarrhea	*Clostridium difficile*

(continued)

TABLE 27.2	Potential Etiologic Agents of Infection and Associated Signs and Symptoms in Immunocompromised Oncology Patients *(continued)*
Clinical Change	**Potential Etiologic Agent**
Skin	
Petechiae/purpura	Coxsackievirus, echovirus, CMV, *Neisseria meningitidis*, *Haemophilus* spp., *Rickettsia* spp., *S. aureus*, *S. pneumoniae*, *Capnocytophaga canimorsus*, *Listeria monocytogenes*
Macules/papules	*Pseudomonas* and other gram-negative rods, *S. aureus*, *Rickettsia* spp., *Candida*, *Aspergillus*, endemic mycosis, viral infections (multiple), mycobacterium
Vesicles/bullae	VZV, HSV
Ecthyma gangrenosum	*Pseudomonas* spp., *Aspergillus* spp., Mucorales, *Fusarium* spp., *Scedosporium* spp., *Vibrio vulnificus* and other gram-negative bacilli, *S. aureus*
Lines	
Pain, swelling, erythema	*S. aureus*, *Candida*, Gram-negative bacilli (e.g., *Pseudomonas*), coagulase-negative *Staphylococcus* spp.

CMV, cytomegalovirus; HEENT, head, eyes, ears, nose, and throat; HSV, herpes simplex virus; PCP, *Pneumocystis* pneumonia; VZV, varicella zoster virus.

are generally shallow and painful, and may have extensive oropharyngeal involvement in the patient with cancer. The viruses that usually cause ulcerations are the herpes viruses and coxsackie viruses (herpangina). Fungal infections such as histoplasmosis may present with painful, deep ulcers with heaped up edges. *Candida* can present with characteristic white plaques on the buccal mucosa (thrush) or, less commonly, erythema of the mucosal surfaces or angular cheilitis.

b. **Cardiovascular system.** The presence of new murmurs or suspected line infections should prompt an evaluation for endocarditis. The most common cause of endocarditis in this population is *Staphylococcus aureus*. Pericarditis and pericardial tamponade are uncommon, but should be suspected in patients with chest pain, shortness of breath, fever, and/or pericardial rub. A variety of infectious agents can cause pericarditis, including common agents such as *S. aureus*, *S. pneumoniae*, and coxsackie viruses and less common agents such as *Candida* spp. and *Aspergillus* spp., and the Mucorales in patients with cancer with prolonged neutropenia or corticosteroids.

   c. Lungs. Signs of consolidation and/or pleural effusion may indicate the presence of pneumonia (including postobstructive pneumonia). In neutropenic hosts, pneumonia may present with minimal changes on examination. Also, atypical pulmonary infections such as *Pneumocystis* pneumonia (PCP) can present initially with minimal or no changes on pulmonary examination.

   d. Abdomen. Peritonitis may present with minimal findings of pain, rebound, or rigidity and can be somewhat benign initially, especially in neutropenic hosts with neutropenic enterocolitis (typhlitis) or patients receiving narcotics or corticosteroids. Perianal infections can present with minimal discomfort or pruritus and, on physical examination, may reveal only minimal erythema, tenderness, or swelling.

   e. Skin. All areas of the skin including perineal area, soles, and palms should be thoroughly examined for new lesions. The pattern of skin involvement and type of lesions are important. Some of the following skin changes can signal disseminated infection with the following microbes.

      (1) Petechiae and purpura. Both viral and bacterial infections may present with scattered petechiae or purpura. *N. meningitidis* is the most common bacterial agent causing petechiae, especially in asplenic patients.

      (2) Macules and papules. A wide variety of gram-negative bacteria (including *Pseudomonas* and *Enterobacteriaceae*) may present with papules or macules, as can *S. aureus* and atypical bacteria such as rickettsial species. Disseminated fungal infections (including *Candida*, *Cryptococcus*, *Histoplasma*, *Coccidioides*, *Fusarium*, *Scedosporium*, and *Aspergillus*) may present with maculopapular, umbilicated, or nodular skin lesions. Common viral illnesses (and childhood viral illnesses such as adenovirus, rubella, or rubeola) may present with maculopapular eruptions as well. Mycobacterial infections such as *Mycobacterium haemophilum* may present with nodules.

      (3) Vesicles and bullae. Classic herpes virus infections, such as varicella or herpes simplex virus (HSV), may have vesicles in localized areas (dermatomal or mucocutaneous) or extensive cutaneous dissemination with other organ system involvement such as lungs or CNS. Several bacterial infections may present with rapidly evolving vesicles or bullae (ecthyma gangrenosum) in immunocompromised hosts such as *Vibrio vulnificus* and *Pseudomonas* spp. Lesions with these infections can initially present as macules with or without vesicles but quickly evolve into hemorrhagic bullae. These bullae later slough, revealing a deep underlying ulceration with surrounding erythema. Other infectious causes of ecthyma gangrenosum include fungal infections, such as mucormycosis and aspergillosis, *S. aureus*, and a variety of gram-negative bacilli.

   f. Vascular catheters. Infections in vascular catheters may present with minimal erythema, tenderness, and swelling along the exit and entrance sites, as well as along the tunnel (for chronic indwelling catheters)

D. Microbiologic evaluation

Any patient with cancer with suspected infection should have a complete microbiologic evaluation of blood, urine, and, when available, sputum. Immunocompromised patients with radiographically evident pneumonia should be evaluated for bronchoalveolar lavage. Other specimens should be obtained depending on the patient's presentation (e.g., stool, skin biopsy, cerebrospinal fluid). Diagnostic studies such as blood cultures may need to be repeated periodically to document adequate response to therapy or to identify the etiology of infection.

   1. Blood cultures. Blood cultures are the single most important microbiologic test to be ordered and should be obtained in all patients with fever or suspected infection. In patients with multilumen catheters, each lumen should be separately sampled. Peripheral blood cultures should be drawn in patients without catheters. Initially, two to three sets of blood cultures are drawn and may be repeated in 48 to 72 hours, or sooner if the patient is clinically unstable. Ideally, 10 mL of blood should be drawn in each bottle in adults up to a total of 30 mL. Most commercially available blood culture systems are able to detect *Candida* species in the blood. While antimicrobial therapy should not be delayed pending results of blood cultures, antibiotics should be initiated after the blood cultures are obtained, provided the cultures are obtained promptly.

   ■ Vascular catheter-related infections. In patients with longer-term percutaneous indwelling central catheters (PICCs), subcutaneously implanted catheters, and other central catheters, blood cultures should be drawn through all lumens. The presence of organisms in blood cultures in immunocompromised patients is usually considered significant.

   2. Sputum. Expectorated sputum in non-neutropenic patients with suspected respiratory tract infection should be obtained for Gram stain, culture, and susceptibility. If patients cannot produce a sputum sample and a pulmonary source of infection is suspected, bronchoscopy is indicated, where feasible. When bronchoscopy is performed on an immunocompromised host, the following studies should be obtained on lavage specimens: routine Gram stain, culture, fungal stains and culture, acid-fast bacillus stains and cultures, culture for *Legionella* spp., modified acid-fast stains (for *Nocardia*), viral cultures, immunoassays or polymerase chain reaction (PCR), and immunoassay or silver stain for *Pneumocystis*.

3. **Urine.** Urine should be sent for Gram stain, culture, and urinalysis. Leukocytes are typically absent in urinalysis in a neutropenic host with urinary tract infections (UTIs).

4. **Stool.** If patients have loose stools, initial specimens at the time of admission should be sent for routine culture (often this includes *Salmonella*, *Shigella*, *Campylobacter*, *Yersinia*, and *E. coli* 0157.H7), *C. difficile* toxin, ova and parasites, *Giardia* antigen, and cryptosporidium antigen. Except for *C. difficile* toxin, these tests have a low yield in patients who have been hospitalized for more than 3 days and then develop diarrhea. The exception to this is reactivation of a parasitic cause of diarrhea (such as *Strongyloides stercoralis*).

5. **Cerebrospinal fluid.** Lumbar punctures are not indicated in the routine evaluation of patients with fever unless a meningeal source is suspected (e.g., significant headache, focal deficits, altered mental status, or nuchal rigidity). A relative contraindication to lumbar puncture is thrombocytopenia ($<$50,000) or coagulopathy. When cerebrospinal fluid is obtained, it should be sent at a minimum for cell count with differential, glucose, protein, routine culture and Gram stain, and cryptococcal antigen. Other tests such as acid-fast bacillus smear and cultures and fungal smear and cultures should be ordered if clinically warranted.

6. **Other microbiologic tests.** Other microbiologic tests that can be clinically useful in the appropriate clinical context include the following:

   ■ Serum and bronchoalveolar lavage galactomannan for detection of invasive aspergillosis
   ■ Serum $(1 \rightarrow 3)$-β-D-glucan for detection of invasive fungal infections, particularly disseminated candidiasis and invasive pulmonary aspergillosis
   ■ CMV PCR of blood.
   ■ Legionella urine antigen ($>$93% sensitive in detecting *Legionella pneumophila* serogroup)
   ■ Histoplasmosis urinary antigen
   ■ HSV PCR of cerebrospinal fluid.

E. **Diagnostic imaging**

   1. **Chest radiographs (CXRs).** All patients with malignancy and suspected infection should have a baseline CXR, including a lateral view if possible.

2. **Computed tomography (CT)** scans should be ordered on an individualized basis. Patients with pulmonary complaints should undergo a CT scan of the chest if the CXR is noncontributory. Patients with abdominal complaints should have a CT of the abdomen and pelvis.

3. **Magnetic resonance imaging** scans are especially useful in evaluating the brain and spine, hepatobiliary system and pancreas, soft tissue, and bone.

4. **Ultrasound.** Ultrasounds are noninvasive or minimally invasive tests without the need for intravenous (IV) contrast. Patients with suspected endocarditis should receive a transesophageal echocardiogram (TEE) unless contraindicated. Ultrasonography is especially useful in imaging the liver, biliary tree and gallbladder, pancreas, and kidneys.

5. **Other imaging tests.** Positron emission tomography (PET) scans detect differential glucose metabolism of normal and abnormal tissues. While PET scans cannot definitively differentiate between infection and underlying malignancy, they have been used increasingly in detecting unsuspected infectious foci when the location of the malignancy is known to be elsewhere. Other imaging studies such as gallium scans or tagged white blood cell (WBC) scans are relatively nonspecific.

F. **Other tests**

All patients with cancer with suspected infection should have a complete blood count with differential and basic chemistry profile including electrolytes, blood urea nitrogen, creatinine, and liver function tests in order to assess possible multiple organ system dysfunction and presence of neutropenia.

G. **Invasive diagnostic procedures**

Bronchoscopy should be performed when feasible in patients with pneumonia without etiology, pneumonia with failure to improve with empirical therapy, or suspected pulmonary site of infection with a negative CXR or CT scan (especially in neutropenic patients). In addition to routine Gram stains and cultures, bone marrow aspirates and liver biopsies are often sent for acid-fast bacillus smears and cultures, fungal smears and cultures, viral cultures, and histopathology for stains such as Warthin-Starry. Consultation with the clinical microbiology laboratory and pathology laboratory is important before obtaining these specimens.

III. TREATMENT
A. **General overview**

Fever or suspected infection in a patient with cancer requires urgent evaluation and initiation of treatment. In certain populations (patients with neutropenia, asplenia), it constitutes a medical emergency. Antibiotic therapy should not be withheld while the workup for a fever source is in progress, but empirical therapy against the most likely pathogens should be promptly instituted. If possible, however, blood cultures should be drawn before antibiotics are initiated if this does not result in a treatment delay. Empiric therapy in febrile neutropenic and non-neutropenic hosts with suspected infection is reviewed as well as directed therapy against specific pathogens. Commonly used dosages of antimicrobials are listed in Table 27.3.

B. **Fever and neutropenia**

An excellent guideline for the management of febrile neutropenic patients has been recently updated by the Infectious Diseases Society of America (IDSA, 2011).

1. **Fever in neutropenic patients** is usually defined as two episodes of temperatures greater than 100.4°F or one episode of temperature greater than 101°F in a patient with a neutrophil count of less than 500 cells/μL or WBC count less than 1000 cells/μL with neutrophils predicted to be less than 500 cells/μL. Most fevers in neutropenic patients stem from bacteria and fungi that are normal colonizers of the skin and alimentary canal. Mucosal damage with secondary bacterial and fungal translocation is thought to be an important initial step in the pathogenesis of febrile neutropenia.

2. **Microbiology.** The most common organisms causing fever in neutropenic hosts are gram-positive cocci, such as *Staphylococcus* species (*S. epidermidis* and, occasionally, *S. aureus*), *Streptococcus*, *Enterococcus*, and *Pseudomonas*, and other gram-negative bacilli (such as *Enterobacter* and *Proteus* spp.) and anaerobes (such as *Bacteroides* and *Clostridium* spp.). Fungi such as *Candida* species occasionally can cause primary infections, but usually occur as secondary infections.

3. **Empirical antibiotic therapy.** All neutropenic patients with fever without localizing source or suspected infection in the absence of fever should receive urgent empirical antibiotic therapy to cover aerobic gram-negative bacilli, including *Pseudomonas aeruginosa*. The extent of coverage of gram-positive organisms such as *Staphylococcus* species and *Streptococcus* species depends on the risk for skin and soft-tissue infections and of mucositis, respectively. Antifungal agents are not usually included in the initial empirical antibiotic regimen unless a fungal infection is suspected (i.e., use of hyperalimentation).

a. **Monotherapy.** Use of a single broad-spectrum antimicrobial such as a third- or fourth-generation cephalosporin or a carbapenem has been shown in randomized clinic trials to be as effective as multidrug treatment regimens for febrile neutropenia. Treatment options for empirical therapy include the following:

▪ Ceftazidime

▪ Cefepime

TABLE 27.3 Dosages of Commonly Used Antibiotics in Adult Oncology Patients

Antibacterials	Renal Adjustment Required for Cr Cl <50	Comments
Vancomycin 1 g IV every 12 hours	Yes	Monitor peak and trough
		Nephrotoxicity increased with aminoglycosides
Piperacillin-tazobactam 3.375 g IV every 6 hours	Yes	Piperacillin needs aminoglycosides for synergy with *Pseudomonas* infections
Amoxicillin-clavulanate 875 mg PO every 12 hours	Yes	Diarrhea common
Imipenem-cilastatin 0.5 g IV every 6 hours	Yes	Seizures can occur if dose not reduced for renal insufficiency
Meropenem 1 g IV every 8 hours	Yes	Approved for meningitis in patients ≥3 months of age
Aztreonam 2 g IV every 8 hours	Yes	Can use in patients with β-lactam allergy
Ciprofloxacin 400 mg IV every 12 hours	Yes	
Ceftriaxone 2 g IV every 2 hours	No	High doses can result in sludge in gallbladder—no *Pseudomonas* or enterococcal coverage
Cefepime 2 g IV every 8 hours	Yes	Covers *Pseudomonas*, not *Enterococcus*
Ceftazidime 2 g IV every 8 h	Yes	Covers *Pseudomonas*, not *Enterococcus*
Trimethoprim-sulfamethoxazole 1 double-strength tablet PO every 12 hours	Yes	Can increase creatinine/PCP doses—5 mg/kg every 8 hours IV based on a trimethoprim component
Metronidazole 500 mg PO every 6 hours	No	Dose adjustment with dialysis—avoid alcohol
Linezolid 600 mg PO or IV every 12 hours	No	Anemia, thrombocytopenia, leukopenia common—monitor CBC weekly if treatment >2 weeks.
Daptomycin 4 mg/kg IV every day	Yes	Not effective in pneumonia
Quinupristin/dalfopristin 7.5 mg/kg IV every 8 h	Yes	Infuse through central line
Gentamicin—dosing varies based on clinical scenarios; once-daily dosing is preferred for reduced toxicity	Yes	Nephrotoxicity/ototoxicity common—monitor peak and trough Use ideal body weight or adjusted body weight with obesity

(continued)

TABLE 27.3 Dosages of Commonly Used Antibiotics in Adult Oncology Patients *(continued)*

Antibacterials	Renal Adjustment Required for Cr Cl <50	Comments
Antifungal agents		
Amphotericin B up to 1.0 mg/kg/day	No, unless due to drug itself	Nephrotoxicity (increased with radiographic contrast, cisplatin, other nephrotoxic agents)
Fluconazole 200–400 mg IV every day	Yes	Drug–drug interactions common
Voriconazole 6 mg/kg × 2 loading doses followed by 4 mg/kg IV every 12 hours maintenance dose 400 mg PO every 12 hours on day 1, then 200 mg PO every 12 hours if >40 kg	No	Assess risk-benefit in patients with Cr Cl <50
Caspofungin 70 mg IV on day 1, then 50 mg IV every day	No	Decrease dose with liver dysfunction
Antiviral agents		
Ganciclovir 5 mg/kg IV every 12 hours	Yes	Neutropenia, thrombocytopenia
Valganciclovir 900 mg PO every 12 hours	Yes	Prodrug of ganciclovir—oral form only
Foscarnet 60 mg/kg IV every 8 hours	Yes	Significant renal toxicity
Acyclovir 10–12 mg/kg IV every 8 hours	Yes	Not active against CMV. Seizures can occur if dose is not adjusted for renal insufficiency.

CBC, complete blood count; CMV, cytomegalovirus; Cr Cl, creatinine clearance; IV, intravenous; PCP, *Pneumocystis* pneumonia; PO, by mouth.

- ■ Carbapenems (imipenem-cilastatin or meropenem)
- ■ Piperacillin–tazobactam
- ■ For patients with severe penicillin allergies, aztreonam plus vancomycin is appropriate. Linezolid may be an appropriate substitute for vancomycin.

b. Two-drug therapy. Multidrug therapy does not offer any specific clinical advantages over monotherapy against aerobic gram-negative bacilli in clinical trials using carbapenems or antipseudomonal cephalosporins.

c. Severe penicillin allergy. Aztreonam and vancomycin should provide effective coverage against the most likely pathogens.

    d. Vancomycin. Vancomycin should be included in the initial antibiotic regimen of febrile neutropenic patients if any of the following additional clinical situations are noted:
- Suspected catheter infection
- Cellulitis or mucositis
- Known colonization or previous infection with methicillin-resistant *S. aureus* (MRSA)
- Blood cultures with gram-positive organisms
- Sepsis, hypotension, or signs of cardiovascular or endovascular infection (e.g., new murmur, petechiae)
- Significant institutional presence of β-lactam–resistant gram-positive organisms
- Use of quinolones as antibiotic prophylaxis before the onset of fever.

4. Duration of antimicrobial therapy

    a. In patients in whom a source of infection is found, standard therapy should be continued for the standard duration (i.e., treat Group A streptococcal pharyngitis with penicillin for 10 days).

    b. In patients in whom no specific infection is found, antimicrobial therapy can be discontinued when the neutrophil count is more than 500 cells/μL and the patient is afebrile for more than 48 hours and without signs of infection.

    c. In patients who become afebrile within 3 to 5 days but remain neutropenic, no specific treatment strategy is well defined. Options include the following:
- Continue empirical antimicrobial therapy for 5 to 7 afebrile days.
- Continue empirical antimicrobial therapy during the period of neutropenia.

5. Continued fever in neutropenic patients on empirical therapy without a source. Patients with febrile neutropenia should undergo a thorough history and physical examination daily to evaluate for a source of infection, including a review of all laboratory tests, microbiology data, and radiologic studies. If a source of fever is found, antimicrobial therapy should be adjusted accordingly for most likely etiologic organisms.

    a. If no source of fever is found after 5 days and a change of antibiotic therapy is not indicated on the basis of the results of the workup, an empirical antifungal agent should be added.

    b. Options include amphotericin B compounds, voriconazole, or caspofungin. Both caspofungin and voriconazole have been shown to be as effective as liposomal amphotericin B. Fluconazole is generally not recommended for empirical antifungal therapy, as it does not cover *Aspergillus* or *Candida* species such as *Candida krusei* or *Candida glabrata*.

C. Empirical therapy in non-neutropenic patients

Patients with infection and neutrophil count greater than 1000 cells/μL may present with fever or infection from a known or unknown source. Urgent evaluation and initiation of prompt empirical therapy is indicated.

1. Patients with altered CMI. Patients with altered cellular immunity due to treatment or underlying diseases (such as non-Hodgkin lymphoma in a patient with acquired immune deficiency syndrome) may present with fever without a known source.

   a. Microbiology. In addition to common bacterial pathogens such as *S. pneumoniae* or *S. aureus*, patients with altered CMI are at risk for infection with atypical organisms such as PCP, *Mycobacterium*, *Nocardia*, *Listeria*, viral infections such as CMV, and fungal infections such as *Cryptococcus*.

   b. Treatment. In patients with altered CMI, diagnostic evaluation of fever before initiating treatment is important if the patient is clinically stable. Workup before antimicrobial therapy should include at a minimum blood cultures, acid-fast bacillus blood cultures, viral cultures, urinalysis and culture, and CXR or CT scan of chest and abdomen. Urgent infectious disease consultation is recommended for the clinically unstable patient with suspected infection and altered CMI.

2. Patients with altered humoral immunity and/or splenectomy. Patients with hypogammaglobulinemia or agammaglobulinemia may lack opsonizing antibodies to encapsulated bacteria.

   a. Microbiology. Encapsulated bacteria such as *S. pneumoniae*, *H. influenzae*, *N. meningitidis*, *C. canimorsus*, and encapsulated strains of other bacteria such as *S. aureus* and *E. coli* are potential pathogens.

   b. Treatment. Antibiotic therapy in patients with asplenia and/or altered humoral immunity must be instituted immediately as a delay in treatment may lead to death. Treatment is aimed at covering the major pathogens. An appropriate empirical antibiotic regimen would be vancomycin and a third-generation cephalosporin such as ceftriaxone. In patients with severe penicillin allergy, a fluoroquinolone such as levofloxacin could be substituted for ceftriaxone. In patients with documented or suspected bacteremia, the duration of therapy is at least 14 days.

3. Nosocomial infections are generally defined as infections occurring in a healthcare setting 48 hours after admission. These infections are often multidrug resistant, resulting in severely limited treatment options. They can be associated with high morbidity and mortality.

   a. Lungs. Hospital-acquired pneumonia is commonly polymicrobic with resistant gram-negative bacilli (such as *Pseudomonas*, *Klebsiella*, and *Acinetobacter* species) and gram-positive

cocci (such as MRSA). In hospitalized patients, the oropharynx becomes colonized with microbes from the hospital
environment within 48 hours. Microaspiration of oropharyngeal bacteria is the main cause of pneumonia. Empirical
antimicrobial therapy should be directed against common
multidrug resistant organisms such as *Pseudomonas* species
or MRSA. Examples of an initial empirical regimen for nosocomial pneumonia would be as follows:

- Antipseudomonal β-lactam (cefepime or ceftazidime) *or*
- Carbapenem (imipenem-cilastatin, meropenem) *or*
- Piperacillin-tazobactam + antipseudomonal fluoroquinolone (levofloxacin or ciprofloxacin) + vancomycin or
  linezolid.

Duration of therapy is approximately 3 weeks in immunocompromised hosts.

b. Vascular catheters. Intravascular catheter-related infections
are common nosocomial infections and can occur in central
venous catheters (CVCs) (tunneled and nontunneled), arterial catheters, and implantable devices. They are a major
cause of morbidity and mortality, and may result in significant complications such as endocarditis or distant metastasis or infection. The most common organisms involved in
line infections are *Staphylococcus* species (*S. epidermidis*,
S. aureus), gram-negative rods, and *Candida* species. Treatment of catheter-related infections usually requires removal
of the catheter if possible, in addition to systemic antibiotics.
In recent retrospective studies, however, catheter retention
in CVC infections with coagulase negative staphylococci, the
most commonly recovered organism, did not impact infection resolution but did increase recurrence.

**(1) Empirical antibiotic therapy in patients with a nontunneled
CVC.** In patients with a suspected indwelling line infection with an easily removable venous access catheter
(i.e., PICC line and severe infection), the line should be
removed and inserted at a new site if possible. Semiquantitative cultures of the catheter tip should be performed.
Empirical antibiotic therapy with vancomycin and an
antipseudomonal penicillin or cephalosporin is indicated. If the patient has been receiving hyperalimentation through the line, empirical therapy against *Candida*
species with amphotericin B or caspofungin may be also
needed. Owing to the increasing incidence of resistant
Candida species, fluconazole should not be used empiri-
cally for suspected fungemia. If associated septic thrombophlebitis is present, surgical excision or drainage of the
vein is generally required.

If *S. aureus* is present on blood cultures, a TEE should be performed to rule out infective endocarditis in non-neutropenic patients. If there is no evidence of endocarditis, 2 weeks of antistaphylococcal therapy guided by susceptibility data can be used. Otherwise, 4 to 6 weeks is indicated. Infection with distant colonization (such as osteomyelitis) may require more than 6 weeks. In patients with positive fungal blood cultures, an ophthalmologic examination to rule out endophthalmitis is indicated. Blood cultures need to be repeated until they are negative, and antifungal therapy is continued for 2 weeks after documented clearance of the fungemia. Infection with gram-negative bacilli is generally treated for 2 weeks as well. In patients with coagulase-negative staphylococcus (*S. epidermidis*), treatment may be indicated for 5 to 7 days after catheter removal.

If the catheter is not removed in nonvirulent infections such as *S. epidermidis* line infections, an attempt can be made to clear the catheter infection using intraluminal ("antibiotic lock therapy") IV antibiotics. A common antibiotic regimen for antibiotic lock therapy for *S. epidermidis* is vancomycin at 1 to 5 mg/mL instilled into the catheter lumen(s) to fill all lumens completely for more than 12 hours/day for 2 weeks in combination with IV antibiotics. A wide range of study results using antibiotic lock therapy to clear *S. epidermidis* line infections have been published with success rates of 18% to 100%, but in general successful clearance of infection is usually less than 50%.

(2) Empirical antibiotic therapy in patients with a tunneled CVC. In patients in whom the CVC cannot be easily removed, it is important (if possible) to determine if the catheter is the actual source of infection. Insertion site infections, tunnel infections, clinically unstable patients with possible vascular catheter infection, evidence of metastatic disease or infection with *Candida* species, atypical mycobacteria, *Bacillus* spp., or *S. aureus* require catheter removal and treatment. Salvage therapy of the line with systemic antibiotic therapy and antibiotic lock therapy can be attempted in selected stable patients with nonvirulent pathogens such as *S. epidermidis*, but clinical deterioration, continued bacteremia, or failure to improve requires catheter removal.

c. Foley catheter/UTIs. Complicated UTIs in hospitalized patients with or without Foley catheters are commonly caused by *E. coli* and *Enterococcus* species. Other microbes that can cause nosocomial infection of the urinary tract include *Pseudomonas* species, and other *Enterobacteriaceae* bacteria/gram-negative rods (*Proteus*, *Klebsiella*, *Providencia*). *S. epidermidis* may cause catheter-associated UTIs. The presence of *S. aureus* in the urine should prompt a search for bacteremia and metastatic staphylococcal infection. Treatment involves removal of the Foley catheter and correction of any associated obstructions or renal-related problems (e.g., azotemia), if possible. Empirical therapy for complicated UTIs could include quinolones with good urinary concentration such as ciprofloxacin or levofloxacin, extended spectrum β-lactams such as ticarcillin-clavulanate or piperacillin-tazobactam, or carbapenems such as imipenem-cilastatin or meropenem. Antibiotic resistance in commonly occurring gram-negative rods (such as *E. coli*) to trimethoprim-sulfamethoxazole (TMP-SMZ) is equal to or more than 20% in most areas, making this a poor choice for empirical therapy in immunocompromised hosts.

Duration of therapy is usually 2 weeks but patients should be improving and afebrile within 72 hours. Patients who remain febrile or who are initially clinically unstable should undergo ultrasound or CT to rule out perinephric abscess or obstruction.

d. Diarrhea

(1) The major nosocomial pathogen causing diarrhea is *C. difficile*. Recently, an epidemic strain of binary toxin producing *C. difficile* associated with an aggressive form of colitis has been described. In addition, hospitalized patients with neutropenia and diarrhea may also develop neutropenic enterocolitis (typhlitis). Typhlitis is probably caused by mucosal disruption and enteric bacterial invasion of the mucosa during neutropenia. Clostridial organisms (e.g., as *Clostridium septicum*), *Pseudomonas*, anaerobes, and occasionally *Candida* are commonly occurring pathogens. Fungemia and/or bacteremia also can be associated with typhlitis. Evaluation of a hospitalized patient with diarrhea and/or neutropenia should include *C. difficile* toxin assay and CT of the abdomen. For diarrhea developing in the hospital, unless reactivation of a parasitic illness is suspected (e.g., *Strongyloides*), ova and parasite examination of stool has a relatively low yield.

(2) Empirical therapy of suspected *C. difficile* colitis is metronidazole 500 mg orally three times a day or 250 mg orally four times a day. Metronidazole is preferred initially over vancomycin. Both are equally effective but use of vancomycin may lead to vancomycin-resistant enterococcus (VRE).

(3) **In patients with suspected typhlitis,** broad-spectrum antibiotic therapy with good anaerobic coverage is indicated, such as ceftazidime plus metronidazole or imipenem-cilastatin, meropenem, or piperacillin-tazobactam. If *C. difficile* colitis has not been excluded, oral metronidazole should be added as well. In patients with continued fever or clinical deterioration, an antifungal agent such as caspofungin should be added. Initial surgical consultation is recommended for patients with suspected typhlitis because perforation or clinical deterioration may require urgent laparotomy and resection of the involved bowel.

D. **Directed therapy against specific pathogens**
Before the results of susceptibility testing, empirical therapy against specific or suspected pathogens needs to be chosen on the basis of the most likely patterns of resistance. Microbial susceptibility profiles are influenced by a number of factors, including earlier antibiotic exposure, clinical scenario of infection, and institutional and community resistance patterns (Table 27.4).

1. *S. aureus.* As previously mentioned, risk factors for MRSA infection include catheter infections, cellulitis, mucositis, previous colonization with resistant organisms, sepsis or possible endovascular

TABLE 27.4   Directed Therapy Against Specific Pathogens

Organism	Antibiotics
Staphylococcus aureus	
Methicillin-sensitive	Nafcillin, cefazolin, ceftriaxone
Methicillin-resistant	Vancomycin, linezolid, daptomycin, quinupristin-dalfopristin
Staphylococcus epidermidis	Vancomycin, linezolid, daptomycin, quinupristin-dalfopristin
Enterococcus	Vancomycin, linezolid, daptomycin, quinupristin-dalfopristin, penicillin/amoxicillin + aminoglycoside
Pseudomonas	Cefepime, piperacillin, imipenem or meropenem, ciprofloxacin, aztreonam + aminoglycoside
Candida	
C. albicans	Fluconazole, amphotericin B, voriconazole, caspofungin
C. glabrata	Amphotericin B, caspofungin, voriconazole
C. krusei	Amphotericin B, caspofungin, voriconazole
Aspergillus	Voriconazole, amphotericin B, caspofungin
Pneumocystis jiroveci (formerly *carinii*)	Trimethoprim-sulfamethoxazole, pentamidine, atovaquone
Cytomegalovirus	Ganciclovir, valganciclovir, foscarnet, cidofovir

infections, earlier use of quinolones, or significant institutional presence of MRSA. Good treatment options for MRSA include vancomycin, linezolid, daptomycin, and quinupristin-dalfopristin. For methicillin-susceptible *S. aureus*, good treatment options include β-lactam antibiotics such as nafcillin, cefazolin or ceftriaxone, and β-lactam/β-lactamase inhibitor combinations such as piperacillin-tazobactam or vancomycin, if allergic to β-lactams. Bacteriostatic antibiotics such as TMP–SMZ, clindamycin, or doxycycline should generally not be used as first-line therapy in patients with severe *S. aureus* infections.

2. *S. epidermidis.* Coagulase-negative staphylococci are often resistant to β-lactams (>80%). When these infections are suspected (often line-associated), good initial antibiotic choices include vancomycin, linezolid, daptomycin, or quinupristin-dalfopristin.

3. *Enterococcus.* Treatment of enterococcal endocarditis or other severe enterococcal infection generally requires synergy with a β-lactam (penicillin or amoxicillin) or glycopeptide (such as vancomycin) in combination with an aminoglycoside at synergistic doses. Cephalosporins have no activity against *Enterococcus*. Linezolid is bacteriostatic against VRE, but has been used successfully in cases of severe enterococcal infection as monotherapy. Other antibiotics with activity against enterococcus include daptomycin and quinupristin-dalfopristin (active against *Enterococcus faecium*, but not *Enterococcus faecalis*). Nitrofurantoins, quinolones such as ciprofloxacin, and doxycycline also have some enterococcal activity, but should be used only for UTIs after data are available on susceptibility.

4. *P. aeruginosa.* Serious *Pseudomonas* infections (e.g., bacteremia, ecthyma gangrenosum) may require synergistic combinations of antipseudomonal β-lactams (such as piperacillin or cefepime) and an aminoglycoside. Other treatment options include monotherapy with an antipseudomonal β-lactam, imipenem or meropenem, ciprofloxacin, or aztreonam. Resistance can occur with treatment, resulting in treatment failure.

5. *Candida* **species.** *Candida albicans* is usually susceptible to fluconazole, amphotericin B, caspofungin, micafungin, anidulafungin, and voriconazole. *C. glabrata* and *C. krusei* have decreased susceptibility to fluconazole (85% and 5% sensitive, respectively) but are usually susceptible to amphotericin B, caspofungin, and voriconazole. Two other commonly seen *Candida* species (*Candida parapsilosis* and *Candida tropicalis*) are usually susceptible to fluconazole, amphotericin B, voriconazole, and echinocandins, but have decreased sensitivity to itraconazole. Newer agents such as posaconazole are generally not used as first-line *Candida* agents.

6. ***Aspergillus.*** *Aspergillus* species (*Aspergillus fumigatus*, *Aspergillus flavus*, *Aspergillus terreus*, and *Aspergillus niger*) are resistant to fluconazole. Voriconazole was more effective than amphotericin B in one large study of invasive aspergillosis in immunocompromised hosts. In addition to amphotericin B and voriconazole, echinocandins have activity in invasive aspergillosis. Combination therapy with echinocandins and voriconazole has been successfully used in patients with invasive aspergillosis, but large-scale randomized studies are lacking.

7. **PCP.** TMP-SMZ at high doses (5 mg/kg IV every 8 hours) is the primary treatment for PCP. If the PaO_2 is less than 70 mm Hg, prednisone 40 mg orally every 12 hours is added for 5 days, then 20 mg daily for 11 days. Other commonly used treatment choices for PCP include pentamidine (IV) or atovaquone (oral).

8. **CMV** can cause a variety of end-organ diseases. CMV pneumonia is generally treated with high-dose ganciclovir (2.5 mg/kg IV every 8 hours) with IV IVIG. CMV retinitis can be treated with oral valganciclovir or IV ganciclovir. Other antivirals with CMV activity include foscarnet and cidofovir.

IV. INFECTIONS IN RECIPIENTS OF HEMATOPOIETIC STEM CELL TRANSPLANT (HSCT)

The management of recipients of HSCT with infection is extremely complex and depends on a number of variables: type of transplantation, latent infections in the recipient, timing of humoral and cellular reconstitution, development of graft-versus-host disease, conditioning regimen, and time after transplantation. Several excellent reviews of infection in recipients of HSCT are available and are listed in "Selected Readings."

A. **Evaluation of infection based on temporal approach**

One classic approach to the evaluation of infection in patients with bone marrow transplant is to divide the transplant immunodeficiencies and pathogen susceptibilities into three separate periods: pre-engraftment, early postengraftment, and late postengraftment. Engraftment is defined as the time when a patient can sustain an ANC greater than 500 cells/µL and platelet count of more than 20,000 µL for three or more consecutive days without transfusion.

1. **Pre-engraftment (phase I: generally first month after transplant).** Pathogens likely to cause infection in the pre-engraftment period include the following:

   - Viral: HSV, seasonal respiratory and enteric viruses
   - Bacteria: *S. epidermidis*, *S. aureus*, viridans streptococcus, *Pseudomonas* species, Enterobacteriaceae, and other gram-negative rods
   - Fungus: *Candida* species, *Aspergillus*.

2. **Early postengraftment (phase II: generally first 30 to 100 days after transplant).** Pathogens likely to cause infection in this phase include the following:
   - Other human herpesviruses such as EBV, seasonal respiratory viruses, and enteric viruses
   - Bacterial: *L. monocytogenes*, *Legionella* species, *S. epidermidis*, *Streptococcus* species, and *S. aureus*
   - Fungus: *Aspergillus* and other molds (e.g., *Zygomycetes*, *Pseudallescheria boydii*), and *Pneumocystis*
   - Parasites: *Toxoplasma gondii* and *S. stercoralis*.

3. **Late postengraftment (phase III: generally more than 100 days after transplant).** Pathogens likely to cause infection in this phase include the following:
   - Viral: VZV, EBV, and other human herpesviruses (e.g., CMV, human herpesvirus-8), hepatitis B, hepatitis C, seasonal respiratory viruses, and enteric viruses
   - Bacteria: encapsulated bacteria such as *S. pneumonia*, *H. influenza*, and *N. meningitidis*
   - Fungi: *Pneumocystis*, *Aspergillus*, and other molds
   - Parasitic: *T. gondii*.

V. PROPHYLAXIS OF INFECTION IN PATIENTS WITH CANCER

Given the high rate of infection in oncology patients and the associated morbidity and mortality, multiple studies have evaluated preventive strategies for fungal, bacterial, and viral infections in different oncology populations.

A. **Prophylaxis of infection in patients not treated with HSCT**

1. **Antibacterial prophylaxis.** Multiple randomized placebo controlled studies of antibiotic prophylaxis in afebrile neutropenic patients have been performed over the last 30 years with differing results. Many studies have shown reductions in febrile illnesses using antibiotic prophylaxis during afebrile neutropenia, but significant side effects have been noted. These include fungal superinfection and development of resistant organisms. The most widely studied prophylactic antibiotics have been oral nonabsorbable antibiotics for selective gastrointestinal decontamination (e.g., aminoglycosides, oral vancomycin) and systemically absorbed antibiotics such as TMP-SMZ and fluoroquinolones. Oral nonabsorbable antibiotics for prophylaxis in afebrile neutropenic patients with cancer are not recommended on the basis of previous studies, but controversy exists regarding the use of TMP-SMZ and quinolones.

   a. **TMP-SMZ.** Studies on use of TMP-SMZ for the most part have shown some decrease in infection rates in afebrile neutropenia with little effect on overall mortality. The development of resistant organisms and potential bone marrow suppression are important disadvantages in the routine prophylactic use of TMP-SMZ. The current 2011 IDSA guidelines for use of antimicrobial agents in neutropenic patients with cancer recommend prophylactic use of TMP-SMZ only for PCP in patients at risk.

   b. **Fluoroquinolones.** Oral quinolones have been studied extensively for prophylaxis in afebrile neutropenic patients with mixed results. Use of agents such as ciprofloxacin in randomized trials has shown a decrease in gram-negative bacillary infections, but an increase in infections with resistant organisms and gram-positive cocci. More recent studies of levofloxacin demonstrate improved outcome. The current 2011 IDSA guidelines for use of antimicrobial agents in neutropenic patients with cancer recommend consideration of prophylactic use of quinolones in neutropenic patients. However, a recent meta-analysis of antibiotic prophylaxis in neutropenia patients showed potential reduction in mortality with fluoroquinolone use.

2. **Antifungal prophylaxis.** The 2011 IDSA guidelines for antimicrobial prophylaxis in neutropenic patients recommends against use of fluconazole for antifungal prophylaxis and consideration of use of posaconazole. Several studies have shown a decrease in fungal infections and associated mortalities in patients receiving fluconazole and posaconazole prophylaxis. Additional studies are in progress for specific oncologic populations, such as those with acute myeloid leukemia. Use of newer agents such as posaconazole has resulted in decreased fungal infections and improved overall survival, but with increased side effects in patients with neutropenia.

3. **Antiviral prophylaxis** with oral acyclovir in HSV-Ab–positive patients reduces the frequency of mucocutaneous HSV infection.

B. **Prophylaxis of infection in HSCT**

The American Society for Blood and Marrow Transplantation and the IDSA recommend prophylaxis for encapsulated bacteria, *Pneumocystis*, HSV, and VZV (with prophylactic or pre-emptive therapy for CMV) and antifungal prophylaxis for patients receiving chronic corticosteroids and until engraftment. In addition, they recommend antibiotic prophylaxis for patients undergoing dental procedures as per the current American Heart Association guidelines for endocarditis prophylaxis.

1. **Bacterial prophylaxis.** There are no recommendations for use of specific antibiotics for bacterial prophylaxis in patients with HSCT. Physicians who use single antibiotics for prophylaxis of encapsulated organisms after transplant should choose agents on the basis of factors such as local antimicrobial resistance

patterns. IVIG can be used in patients with severe hypogamma-globinemia during the early postengraftment phase.

2. **Fungal prophylaxis.** Fluconazole 400 mg orally per day until engraftment is currently recommended.

3. **PCP and toxoplasmosis prophylaxis.** One TMP-SMZ double-strength tablet daily or three times per week. Prophylaxis for PCP should begin before transplantation.

4. **Viral prophylaxis.** Multiple strategies (prophylaxis or pre-emptive) exist to decrease the incidence of CMV infection and reactivation in patients with HSCT. One strategy is the use of IV ganciclovir 5 g/kg IV every 12 hours for 1 week, then 5 days/week until day 100 posttransplant in seropositive patients at risk. Prophylaxis against HSV reactivation is recommended for HSV seropositive transplant recipients. Acyclovir (200 mg orally three times per day) can be given at the start of conditioning until engraftment or resolution of mucositis.

5. **Other prophylactic strategies**

a. **Vaccination.** The following vaccines are commonly given 12 to 24 months after HSCT transplantation in adults: tetanus-diphtheria toxoid vaccine, hepatitis B series, 23-valent pneumococcal polysaccharide vaccine, influenza vaccine, and inactivated polio vaccine. Measles, mumps, and rubella (MMR) vaccine and varicella vaccine are contraindicated. No recommendation has yet been made on the use of meningococcal vaccine or the newly developed tetanus-diphtheria-acellular pertussis vaccine for adults due to limited data.

b. **Infection control measures.** Strict attention to infection control measures should be practiced by recipients of HSCT, caregivers, and healthcare workers, especially strict attention to hand washing. Some unique aspects of infection control include the following;

- While in the hospital, strict attention should be paid to air flow and air filtration, possible exposure to construction in the hospital environment, and exposure to healthcare workers with seemingly minor infections such as adenovirus conjunctivitis.
- Recipients of HSCT should avoid exposure to respiratory and enteric viruses (i.e., wear surgical mask during close contact with people with respiratory illness).
- Contact with sick pets should be minimized and excellent pet health should be maintained.
- Patients should avoid reptiles, chicks, ducklings, and exotic pets.
- Patients should avoid well water.
- Strict attention to food safety practices (e.g., use of separate cutting boards for raw chicken, cleaning of surfaces

and knives after each use, and washing all produce) should be practiced by everyone involved in meal preparation for recipients of HSCT.

▧ Use of a low microbial diet is recommended (cooked foods are preferred; avoid sushi and salad dressings made with raw eggs).

▧ Vaccination of family members and household contacts should be done as per current Advisory Committee on Immunization Practices guidelines. Currently, family members and household contacts should receive all age-appropriate vaccinations and influenza, hepatitis A, MMR, and varicella vaccinations, if indicated. Oral polio vaccine should be avoided. Updated information about vaccines can be accessed at www.cdc.gov/vaccines.

Selected Readings

Bucaneve G, Micozzi A, Menichetti F, et al. Levofloxacin to prevent bacterial infection in patients with cancer and neutropenia. *N Engl J Med.* 2005;353:977–987.

Centers for Disease Control and Prevention. Guidelines for preventing opportunistic infections among hematopoietic stem cell transplant recipients: recommendations of CDC, the Infectious Disease Society of America, and the American Society of Blood and Marrow Transplantation. *MMWR Morb Mortal Wkly Rep.* 2000;49(RR-10):1–128.

Centers for Disease Control and Prevention. Recommended adult immunization schedule–United States, October 2005-September 2006. *MMWR.* 2005; 54(48):Q1–Q4.

Cornely OA, Maertens J, Winston DJ, et al. Posaconazole vs. fluconazole or itraconazole prophylaxis in patients with neutropenia. *N Engl J Med.* 2007;356:348–359.

Cullen M, Steven N, Billingham L, et al. Antibacterial prophylaxis after chemotherapy for solid tumors and lymphomas. *N Engl J Med.* 2005;353:988–998.

Freifeld AG, Bow EJ, Sepkowitz KA, et al. Clinical practice guideline for the use of antimicrobial agents in neutropenic patients with cancer: 2010 update by the Infectious Diseases Society of America. *Clin Infect Dis.* 2011;52:427–431.

Gafter-Gvili A, Fraser A, Paul M, Leibovici L. Meta-analysis: antibiotic prophylaxis reduces mortality in neutropenic patients. *Ann Intern Med.* 2005;142(12 Pt 1):979–995.

Garey KVV, Rege M, Pai MP, et al. Time to initiation of fluconazole therapy impacts mortality in patients with candidemia: a multi-institutional study. *Clin Infec Dis.* 2006;43:25–31.

Hall K, Farr B. Diagnosis and management of long-term central venous catheter infections. *J Vasc Interv Radiol.* 2004;15:327–334.

Helbig JH, Uldum SA, Bernander S, et al. Clinical utility of urinary antigen detection for diagnosis of community-acquired, travel-associated and nosocomial legionnaires' disease. *J Clin Microbiol.* 2003;41:838–840.

Jaksic B, Martinelli G, Perez-Oteyza J, Hartman CS, Leonard LB, Tack KJ. Efficacy and safety of linezolid compared with vancomycin in a randomized, double-blind study of febrile neutropenic patients with cancer. *Clin Infec Dis.* 2006; 42:1813–1814.

McDonald LC, Killgore GE, Thompson A, et al. An epidemic, toxin gene-variant strain of Clostridium difficile. *N Engl J Med*. 2005;353:2442–2449.

Mermel L, Farr B, Sherertz RJ, et al. Guidelines for the management of intravascular catheter-related infections. *Clin Infect Dis*. 2001;32:1249–1272.

Pappas PG, Rex JH, Sobel JD, et al. Guidelines for treatment of candidiasis. *Clin Infect Dis*. 2004;38:161–189.

Raad I, Kassar R, Ghannam D, Chaftari AM, Hachem R, Jiang Y. Management of the catheter in documented catheter-related coagulase-negative staphyloccal bacteremia: remove or retain? *Clin Infect Dis*. 2009;49:1187–1194.

Rizzo JD, Wingard JR, Tichelli A, et al. Recommended screen and preventive practices for long-term survivors after hematopoietic cell transplantation: joint recommendations of the European Group for Blood and Marrow Transplantation, the Center for International Blood and Marrow Transplant Research, and the American Society of Blood and Marrow Transplantation (EBMT/CIBMTRA/ASBMT). *Bone Marrow Transplant*. 2006;37:249–261.

Rubin RH, Young LS. *Clinical Approach to Infections in the Compromised Host*. New York: Kluwer Academic Klenum Publishers; 2002.

Sable CA, Donowitz GR, Infections in bone marrow transplant recipients. *Clin Infect Dis*. 1994;18:223.

Safdar N, Fine JP, Maki DG. Meta-analysis: methods for diagnosing intravascular device-related bloodstream infection. *Ann Intern Med*. 2005;142(6):451–466.

Sung L, Nathan P, Shabbir MH, Tomlinson GA, Beyene J. Meta-analysis: effect of prophylactic hematopoietic colony-stimulating factors on mortality and outcomes of infection. *Ann Intern Med*. 2007;147:400–411.

Van Burik J, Weisdoft D. Infections in recipients of hematopoietic stem cell transplantation. In: Mandel GL, Bennett JE, Dolin R, eds. *Principles and Practices of Infectious Diseases*. Philadelphia: Elsevier Churchill Livingstone; 2005.

Vetter E, Torgerson C, Feuker A, et al. Comparison of the BACTEC MYCO/F lytic bottle to the isolator tube, BACTEC Plus Aerobic F/bottle, and BACTEC Anaerobic Lytic/10 bottle and comparison of the BACTEC Plus Aerobic F/bottle to the isolator tube for recovery of bacteria, mycobacteria and fungi from blood. *J Clin Microbiol*. 2001;39(12):4380–4386.

Walsh TJ, Pappas P, Winston DJ, et al. Voriconazole compared with liposomal amphotericin B for empirical antifungal therapy in patients with neutropenia and persistent fever. *N Engl J Med*. 2002;346(4):225–234.

Walsh TJ, Teppler H, Donowitz GR, et al. Caspofungin versus liposomal amphotericin B for empirical antifungal therapy in patients with persistent fever and neutropenia. *N Engl J Med*. 2004;351:1391–1402.

Transfusion Therapy, Bleeding, and Clotting

Mary R. Smith and NurJehan Quraishy

Disorders of the hemostatic mechanisms are common in patients with malignancy. Active cancer accounts for 20% of new venous thromboembolism (VTE) events. Patients who present with unprovoked VTE have a 10% risk of developing cancer within the next 2 years. Abnormalities associated with thromboembolic events cause significantly more morbidity and mortality than disorders leading to hemorrhage.

I. THROMBOEMBOLISM IN CANCER

A. Pathophysiology

The thromboembolic risk associated with neoplasia reflects an imbalance between platelet number, platelet function, levels of coagulation factors, and generation of thromboplastins compared with the levels of inhibitors of hemostasis and fibrinolytic activity. Thrombosis may be minor and localized or widespread and associated with multiple-organ damage. There may also be hemorrhage of varying degrees of severity in association with the thromboembolic events.

1. **Factors that may affect the risk of thromboembolism** vary widely from patient to patient and include the following:
   - Specific type of tumor: adenocarcinomas (ovary, pancreas, colon, stomach, lung, and kidney)
   - Nutritional status of the patient
   - Type of chemotherapy
   - Response to chemotherapy (e.g., tumor lysis syndrome)
   - Liver and renal function
   - Patient immobility and venous stasis
     - Surgery (twice the risk for VTE and three times the risk for pulmonary embolism [PE] compared to patients without cancer)
     - Arterial and venous catheters.
2. **Factors that can initiate thrombus formation** are common to many cancers:
   - Circulating tumor cells adhere to the vascular endothelium and form a nidus for clot formation.
   - Tumors may penetrate the vessel, destroying the endothelium and promoting clot formation.
   - Neovascularization associated with many tumors may stimulate clotting.

- ■ Arterial thrombosis associated with tumors may result from vasospasm.
- ■ A systemic hypercoagulable state develops (e.g., decreased protein C).
- ■ External compression of vessels by tumor masses impedes blood flow and leads to stasis and clot development.

   3. Platelet abnormalities associated with an increased risk of thromboembolism include thrombocytosis and increased platelet adhesion and aggregation. Tumors may produce substances that cause increased platelet aggregation with subsequent release of platelet factor 3 and ensuing acceleration of coagulation.

B. Clinical syndromes

A variety of noteworthy clinical syndromes are associated with the "hypercoagulable state" of malignancy and of its treatment.

   1. Disseminated intravascular coagulation (DIC) is a syndrome with many signs, symptoms, and laboratory abnormalities (Table 28.1). As many as 90% of patients with metastatic neoplasms have some laboratory manifestation of DIC, but only a small fraction of these patients suffer morbidity from the coagulation process or subsequent depletion of coagulation factors and consequent bleeding due to DIC. The initiating factor for DIC is apparent in some situations but unknown in others.

TABLE 28.1	Laboratory Diagnosis of DIC	
Laboratory Tests	**Acute DIC**	**Chronic DIC**
Screening		
PT, aPTT	Usually prolonged	Normal
Platelets	Usually decreased	Normal or slightly decreased
Fibrinogen	Usually decreased but may be normal*	Usually normal*
Confirmatory†		
Fibrin monomer	Positive	Positive
FDP	Strongly positive	Positive
D-Dimer	Positive	Positive
Thrombin time	Normal or abnormal	Usually normal
Factor assays	Decreased factors V and VIII	Normal factors V and VIII
Antithrombin III	May be reduced	Usually normal

aPTT, activated partial thromboplastin time; DIC, disseminated intravascular coagulation; FDP, fibrinogen degradation products; PT, prothrombin time.

*Fibrinogen is usually elevated in advanced malignancy or acute leukemia that is not complicated by DIC. Thus, a normal fibrinogen level may actually be decreased for the physiologic state of the patient.

†Changes indicated are confirmatory if present; the absence of the indicated findings in some of the confirmatory tests does not exclude the diagnosis.

Among the common initiators of DIC are the following:

■ Thromboplastic substances in granules from promyelocytes of acute promyelocytic leukemia (DIC may worsen with therapy). There is a significant concomitant fibrinolysis in many patients.

■ Sialic acid from mucin produced by adenocarcinomas of the lung or gastrointestinal tract

■ Trypsin released from pancreatic cancer

■ Impaired fibrinolysis associated with hepatocellular carcinoma

■ DIC in any patient may be fostered by sepsis or other causes of the systemic inflammatory response syndrome (SIRS).

2. **Lupus anticoagulant in neoplastic disease.** The lupus anticoagulant is an antiphospholipid antibody (immunoglobulin G or M). Antiphospholipid antibodies are reported to be associated with a number of malignant disorders including hairy cell leukemia, lymphoma, Waldenström macroglobulinemia, and epithelial neoplasms. The lupus anticoagulant leads to a prolonged activated partial thromboplastin time (aPTT) but is paradoxically associated with an increased risk of thrombosis.

3. **Trousseau syndrome (tumor-associated thrombophlebitis).** Suspect the possibility of neoplasia in the following circumstances:

■ An unexplained thromboembolic event occurs after the age of 40 years.

■ Thromboses occur in unusual sites.

■ The thromboses affect superficial as well as deep veins.

■ The thromboses are migratory.

■ The thromboses tend not to respond to the "usual" anticoagulant therapies.

■ An unexplained thrombosis occurs more than once.

4. **Thrombotic events that occur after surgery** for tumors of the lung, ovary, pancreas, or stomach.

5. **Nonbacterial thrombotic endocarditis** may be found in association with carcinoma of the lung. These thrombi are formed from accumulations of platelets and fibrin. The mitral valve is the most frequent site of origin of these thrombi, which frequently embolize.

6. **Thrombotic thrombocytopenic purpura (TTP)** is a poorly understood syndrome characterized by thrombocytopenia, microangiopathic hemolytic anemia, fever, fluctuating neurologic signs and symptoms, and acute renal failure. TTP and the hemolytic-uremic syndrome (thrombocytopenia, hemolysis, and acute renal failure) have been associated with untreated malignancies as well as with a number of drugs used for treating malignant disease. The agent most often reported is mitomycin, but other drugs including bleomycin, cisplatin, cyclophosphamide, gemcitabine, and vinca alkaloids may also be associated with these syndromes. TTP may be difficult to diagnose in this setting because the

chemotherapy suppresses platelet production, some agents may impair renal function, and many of the features of DIC are similar to those of TTP. Careful review of the peripheral blood smear is required to identify the changes in red blood cells (RBCs) that are associated with a microangiopathic hemolytic process.

There is growing evidence that damage to the endothelium is seen in association with TTP. For many patients with TTP, von Willebrand-cleaving protease (ADAMTS13) levels are very low or absent, leading to the accumulation of unusual large multimers of von Willebrand factor (vWF) and subsequent platelet clumping. The von Willebrand-cleaving proteolytic activity is thought to be inhibited by an anti-vWF–cleaving protease immunoglobulin G antibodies.

The prognosis of patients with TTP is poor, and its therapy has been varied. Plasmapheresis and transfusion with fresh frozen plasma (FFP) appear to be the best modalities of therapy. Plasmapheresis is most frequently used as it not only replaces the von Willebrand-cleaving protease missing or decreased in patients with TTP but also removes the anti-vWF–cleaving protease antibody.

Complications from platelet transfusions are not as common in TTP associated with malignancy and bone marrow transplantation as in other cases of TTP; thus, platelet transfusion can be used especially if there is a threat of bleeding.

7. **Thromboembolism associated with chemotherapy**
   a. **The use of central arterial or venous catheters** has markedly facilitated the delivery of chemotherapy, but all such catheters are associated with a 5% increase in the risk of vascular thrombosis. This risk level is lower than was previously suspected. The empiric use of low doses of warfarin (1 mg/day) or low-dose low-molecular-weight heparin (LMWH) has been evaluated in recent randomized trials, and both drugs failed to show any reduction in symptomatic catheter-associated thrombosis. The risk of catheter-associated thrombosis appears to be higher in children. In a recent large randomized trial, there was an increased risk of bleeding in patients treated with low-dose warfarin.
   b. **Many chemotherapy agents** cause significant chemical phlebitis. The most common offending agents are mechlorethamine (nitrogen mustard), anthracyclines, nitrosoureas, mitomycin, fluorouracil, dacarbazine, and epipodophyllotoxins.
   c. **L-asparaginase** inhibits the synthesis of proteins, including coagulation factors. This inhibition may cause either hemorrhage or thrombosis. Patients with pre-existing hemostatic disorders are at particular risk for complications when using L-asparaginase. L-asparaginase also decreases antithrombin-III (AT-III) activity.

d. **Tamoxifen**, when used as an adjuvant, has been associated with a two- to sixfold increased risk of thromboembolic events. This effect may be magnified when tamoxifen is combined with chemotherapeutic agents. When tamoxifen is used for primary prevention, the risk of deep vein thrombosis and PE is 1.6% and 3.0%, respectively. Other selective estrogen receptor modulators, like raloxifene, are also associated with an increase in the risk of thromboembolic events. Aromatase inhibitors have a lower risk of thromboembolism than tamoxifen and are preferred for postmenopausal women, particularly if there are additional risk factors for thrombosis.

e. **Estrogens** may increase the risk of thromboembolism. This is likely due, at least in part, to a decrease in protein S and an increase in coagulation factors.

f. **Superior vena cava syndrome** is nearly always associated with thrombosis in the thoracic venous system cephalad to the site of obstruction and may lead to upper-extremity thrombosis.

g. **Antiangiogenic or targeted therapy** may be associated with a significant increase in the risk of VTE events. Thalidomide and lenalidomide in combination with corticosteroids or chemotherapy increases the risk of symptomatic VTE in patients with multiple myeloma. Prophylaxis with low doses of anticoagulation therapy has not been formally evaluated in this group of patients.

C. **Principles of therapy for thrombosis associated with neoplasia**

1. **Discrete vascular thrombosis**

a. **General guidelines.** Therapy should be directed at controlling the neoplasm. As an anticoagulant, heparin is superior to warfarin in these patients. Warfarin and antiplatelet drugs have been used with varying degrees of success in some patients with thromboembolism associated with tumors. The use of heparin, warfarin, and antiplatelet agents alone or in combination may be associated with normalization of hemostatic parameters. Despite this, patients with malignant disease are often resistant to anticoagulant therapy and may continue to have thrombotic events even while receiving what appears to be adequate treatment. Great care must be exercised in the use of both heparin and warfarin in patients with malignant disease because hemorrhage into areas of necrotic tumor can be hazardous. The use of anticoagulant therapy is generally contraindicated in patients with central nervous system metastases. Bulky disease is a relative contraindication, especially if central necrosis of the tumor is suspected and particularly if the lesion is in the mediastinum or pleural spaces.

The decision to treat thromboembolism occurring in a patient with malignancy may be difficult. One must carefully weigh the risks of therapy against expected benefits. The patient's life expectancy, concurrent therapy, and type of malignancy also influence the decision.

b. Heparin. Low doses of heparin (5000 U given via the subcutaneous [SC] route every 12 hours) can be used to protect patients with malignant disease from thromboembolism during perioperative periods.

Heparin may be used as the initial or long-term therapy for thromboembolic events in patients with malignant disease. Heparin may be administered either by the intravenous (IV) or SC routes. Generally, the IV route is preferred for initial therapy so that the anticoagulant effect begins at once and adjustment of doses can be easily achieved. An initial dose of 5000 U (70 U/kg) of heparin is given as an IV bolus followed by 1000 to 1200 U (15 U/kg)/h as a continuous infusion. One should check the aPTT 1 hour after the heparin bolus to ensure that the patient is heparinizable (i.e., not AT-III deficient), 6 hours after beginning therapy, and 6 hours after any change in the dose of heparin. Some patients with malignant disease may appear to be refractory to heparin; in all likelihood, this reflects low levels of AT-III, owing to poor production or increased consumption, both of which may occur in patients with malignant disease. (Infusion therapy with L-asparaginase has been associated with reduced levels of AT-III.) As long as the AT-III activity is above 50% of normal, it is usually possible to achieve the desired anticoagulant effect if adequate doses of heparin are given. If AT-III activity is less than 50% of normal, AT-III may be replaced using AT-III concentrates or FFP.

Heparin may be administered by the SC route for both the acute and the chronic management of thromboembolism associated with malignancy. Using the SC route may be less desirable when treating acute events because the onset of anticoagulant effect is somewhat slower (2 to 3 hours), and adjusting the therapeutic effect may be more difficult. SC heparin can be considered for chronic therapy provided that the patient can manage the twice-daily injection and weekly monitoring of the aPTT. In a patient who has been receiving IV heparin, half the total dose of IV heparin received in the previous 24 hours should be given SC twice a day (e.g., 1000 U/h by IV infusion equals 12,000 U SC twice a day). For the patient being started on SC heparin, the initial dose is 7500 to 10,000 U SC twice a day. The aPTT should be checked 6 hours after the third dose of heparin. Otherwise, the aPTT should be checked 6 hours after a SC dose of heparin. The goal for the aPTT should be similar to that of IV heparin, namely, 1.5 to 2 times the patient's baseline aPTT.

LMWHs should now be considered as the first line of therapy or prevention of VTE in patients with malignant disease. LMWH is preferred to unfractionated heparin as it can be given as an outpatient more easily and has a lower risk of heparin-associated thrombocytopenia. LMWH may have specific antineoplastic effects separate from its effect to reduce VTE. There are a number of ongoing trials designed to evaluate this antineoplastic effect. Monitoring of LMWH is indicated if the patient suffers from liver or kidney dysfunction or if the patient is significantly malnourished or debilitated. One must use anti-Xa levels as the aPTT is not indicative of the anticoagulant effect of LMWH.

c. **Warfarin.** In the past, warfarin was the therapy of choice for the chronic management of thromboembolic events associated with malignant disease. The use of warfarin in this setting is of concern because patients with malignant disease are frequently taking multiple medications that can alter the patient's response to warfarin. An additional concern about the use of warfarin in patients with malignancy is the development of purpura fulminans. This complication may be due to lower-than-normal protein C levels in patients who had DIC before initiation of warfarin therapy. Warfarin should not be used as the primary drug to manage VTE events or future prevention of events in patients with malignant disease.

d. **The use of platelet-inhibiting drugs** such as aspirin, other non-steroidal anti-inflammatory agents, and dipyridamole has met with varying degrees of success in the prevention of repeated thromboembolic events in patients with malignant disease. Care must be taken with the use of such drugs, especially in thrombocytopenic patients, because the risk of bleeding associated with thrombocytopenia is increased.

e. **Fibrinolytic therapy.** Systemic malignancy is a relative contraindication to fibrinolytic therapy.

f. **Vascular interruption devices** such as inferior vena cava filters should only be used in patients who cannot tolerate anticoagulant therapy or who develop emboli while on adequate anticoagulant therapy.

g. **Anticoagulation therapy** should be continued as long as the patient is receiving anticancer therapy or has evidence of active cancer.

2. **Disseminated intravascular coagulation.** Therapy for DIC includes the following:
   ■ Urgently correct shock (if present).
   ■ Treat the underlying disease process. When it is not possible to treat the underlying disease process, it is unlikely that the complicating DIC can be successfully managed.

▩ Replace depleted blood components (e.g., platelets, cryoprecipitated antihemophilic factor [AHF] for fibrinogen and factor VIII, FFP for other factors) if clinically significant bleeding is present.

▩ Consider the use of heparin only in the following situations:

   ▩ In patients with acute promyelocytic leukemia (see Chapter 18).

   ▩ When there is clear evidence of ongoing end-organ damage due to microvascular thrombosis.

   ▩ If venous thrombosis occurs.

These latter two complications of DIC are most likely to occur as a component of SIRS, and the treatment of the underlying cause of SIRS is necessary in addition to treatment with heparin. There is no evidence that chronic warfarin therapy is of value for treating the chronic DIC seen in some patients with neoplasia if thromboses are absent. Warfarin may predispose to the development of purpura fulminans in the presence of chronic DIC due to acquired protein C deficiency.

II. BLEEDING IN PATIENTS WITH CANCER

A. Tumor invasion

It is well recognized that bleeding may be a warning sign of cancer. Bloody sputum may indicate carcinoma of the lung, blood in the urine may be a sign of carcinoma of the bladder or kidney, blood in the stool may be due to carcinoma of the alimentary tract, and postmenopausal vaginal bleeding may be caused by endometrial carcinoma. In each of these instances, bleeding can be directly related to the invasive properties of cancer and disruption of normal tissue integrity.

B. Hemostatic abnormalities

Often, bleeding in patients with cancer is not due to the direct effects of the neoplasm but rather to indirect effects of the cancer or its therapy on one of the components of the hemostatic system. Because of the frequency and the special management problems caused by abnormalities in the hemostatic system in patients with cancer, it is important to consider the possible causes and corrective measures in detail.

1. **Increased vascular fragility** may be due to chronic corticosteroid therapy, chronic malnutrition, or "senile purpura." Bleeding is usually not severe, but bruising, particularly around IV sites, is common. Hemostatic therapy is not necessary.

2. **Thrombocytopenia** may occur for a variety of reasons. Some of the more common causes are as follows.

   a. **Chemotherapy and radiotherapy** regularly cause depression of platelet production. Serial blood cell counts must be monitored while patients are being treated.

b. **Bone marrow invasion or replacement** causing thrombocytopenia is commonly seen only with leukemias or lymphomas but may occur in other cancers that invade the bone marrow.

c. **Splenomegaly with splenic sequestration** is most common with leukemia or lymphoma.

d. **Folate deficiency** with decreased platelet production is common in patients with cancer because of poor nutrition. Dietary history should provide the clues to the diagnosis.

e. **Neoplasm-induced immune thrombocytopenic purpura.** Patients with lymphoproliferative malignancies (e.g., chronic lymphocytic leukemia, Hodgkin disease) often develop immune thrombocytopenic purpura (ITP). ITP may also be the presenting symptom of a nonhematologic malignancy. Usually, the ITP improves with prednisone 1 mg/kg/day followed by treatment of the malignancy.

f. **Drug-induced immune thrombocytopenia.** Many nonchemotherapy medications used to treat patients with malignancy can cause immune thrombocytopenia. Offending agents to consider are heparin, vancomycin, H_2-receptor antagonists, penicillins, cephalosporins, interferon, sulfa-containing antibiotics, diuretics, and hypoglycemic agents.

g. **Graft-versus-host disease** developed after bone marrow transplantation may produce a chronic (often isolated) immune-mediated thrombocytopenia. The platelet count may respond to increased immunosuppression.

3. **Abnormalities of platelet function** must be suspected in patients who have a normal or near-normal platelet count and signs or symptoms of bleeding and a documented prolonged bleeding time. Most cases are secondary to drug effects including aspirin and other nonsteroidal anti-inflammatory agents, antibiotics (e.g., ticarcillin), antidepressants (e.g., tricyclic drugs), tranquilizers, and alcohol. Consider any drug that the patient is taking as a possible offender until proved otherwise. The presence of fibrin degradation products is a common cause of platelet dysfunction in patients with malignancy who also have DIC. Platelet dysfunction may occur in patients with malignant paraproteinemias as a result of the coating of the platelet surfaces by the immunoglobulin. When renal failure develops or is present in such patients, the platelet dysfunction is magnified.

4. **Coagulation factor deficiencies** may develop in patients with malignancy for several reasons:
   - Acute (decompensated) DIC depletes most clotting factors but to variable degrees.

- Liver failure causes deficiency of all clotting factors except factor VIII.
- Malnutrition leads to deficiency of factors II, VII, IX, and X (the vitamin K–dependent factors).
- Fibrinolysis may be due to the release of urokinase in prostate cancer or secondary to DIC. This may produce hypofibrinogenemia as well as fibrin split products, which act as circulating anticoagulants.
- Functionally abnormal clotting factors are occasionally seen. The most commonly diagnosed abnormality is dysfibrinogenemia.

5. **Acquired circulating anticoagulants** may develop in patients with a number of different tumors. Many of these anticoagulants are heparinoid in nature. The most common associations are with carcinoma of the lung and myeloma. Other anticoagulants act as antithrombins; in this case, the most common association is with carcinoma of the breast.

6. **Chemotherapy and other drug-induced bleeding**
   a. **Mithramycin,** although rarely used now, may lead to platelet dysfunction and a reduction in multiple coagulation factors. Hemorrhage due to these effects may occur in up to half of patients treated with mithramycin.
   b. **Anthracyclines** may be associated with primary fibrinolysis or fibrinogenolysis and hemorrhage.
   c. **Dactinomycin** is a powerful vitamin K antagonist that causes defective synthesis of all vitamin K–dependent proteins (factors II, VII, IX, and X, protein C, and protein S).
   d. **Melphalan, cytarabine, doxorubicin, vincristine, and vinblastine** are all associated with platelet dysfunction.
   e. **Mitomycin, daunorubicin, cytarabine, bleomycin, cisplatin, tamoxifen, pentostatin, gemcitabine, atorvastatin, clopidogrel, ticlopidine, cyclosporine, sulfonamides, tacrolimus, sirolimus, "crack" cocaine, penicillin, rifampin, penicillamine, oral contraceptives, arsenic, quinine, and iodine** are all associated with TTP.

III. LABORATORY EVALUATION OF HEMOSTASIS IN PATIENTS WITH MALIGNANCY

About half of all patients with cancer and about 90% of those with metastases manifest abnormalities of one or more routine coagulation parameters (Table 28.2). These abnormalities may be minor early in the patient's disease, but as the disease progresses, the hemostatic abnormalities become more pronounced. Serial coagulation tests may offer the clinician a clue to response to therapy or recurrence of malignant disease and are more valuable than a single determination in patients with no symptoms of hemostatic disruption.

TABLE 28.2	Coagulation Tests That May Show an Abnormality in Patients With Cancer Without Clinical Bleeding or Thrombosis	
Test	**Common Results in Patients With Malignancy**
Antithrombin III	Decreased
β-Thromboglobulin	Increased
Cryofibrinogen	Present
D-Dimer	Increased
Factor VIII	Increased
Fibronectin	Decreased
Fibrin monomer (soluble)	Present
Fibrinogen	Increased
Fibrin(ogen) degradation products	Present
Fibrinopeptide A	Increased
Fibrinopeptide B	Increased
Plasmin	Increased
Plasminogen	Decreased
Platelet count	Increased or decreased
Platelet factor 4	Increased
Protein C	Decreased

A. Screening tests for bleeding

The following tests provide an adequate screening battery: platelet count, bleeding time or whole blood platelet function screening testing, aPTT, prothrombin time (PT), thrombin time, and fibrinogen level.

B. Interpretation of screening laboratory studies

Abnormal results of the screening tests reflect hematologic problems caused by blood vessels, platelets, or coagulation factors. The following list provides clues to the interpretation of the screening test results that help determine the most likely cause or causes of the patient's bleeding.

1. Platelet count. A normal platelet count it 150,000 to 450,000/μL. If thrombocytopenia is less than 100,000/μL, consider the following:

- Bone marrow failure
- Increased consumption of platelets
- Splenic pooling of platelets.

    Thrombocytosis with a platelet count of more than 500,000/μL has the following characteristics:

- It is common in patients with neoplasms.
- It may be seen in association with iron deficiency (e.g., secondary to gut neoplasm).
- It usually poses no risk of arterial thrombosis unless the patient has a myeloproliferative disorder.

2. **Bleeding time.** This is a useful screening test if the platelet count is normal and platelet dysfunction is suspected.
   - A normal bleeding time requires normal platelet number, normal platelet function, and normal function of the blood vessels and connective tissues.
   - A prolonged bleeding time may be due to thrombocytopenia, abnormal platelet function, and, rarely, inadequate vessel functions. The bleeding time may be spuriously prolonged in elderly people with "tissue-paper" skin.
   - The following formula is a rough rule of thumb to be used to estimate what the bleeding time should be in patients who have platelet counts between 10,000 and 100,000/μL. Although it was derived using the Mielke template, the principle should still hold for contemporary bleeding time devices: bleeding time (min) = 30 − ([platelet count/μL]/4000). (Whole blood platelet function screening testing is replacing the bleeding time in many laboratories. This method of screening for platelet function abnormalities appears to be a better predictor for the risk of bleeding due to platelet function abnormalities than the bleeding time.)
3. **Prolonged PT.** This is seen in the presence of the following:
   - Deficiency of one or more of the following clotting factors: VII, X, V, II (prothrombin), or I (fibrinogen); oral anticoagulant therapy leads to a deficiency of factors II, VII, IX, and X
   - Circulating anticoagulants against factor VII, X, V, or II
   - Dysfibrinogenemia.
4. **Prolonged aPTT.** This is seen in the presence of the following:
   - Deficiency of any of the following clotting factors: XII, XI, IX, VIII, X, V, II, or I. Factor XII deficiency is not associated with bleeding. Fletcher and Fitzgerald factor deficiencies (both rare) may also prolong the aPTT.
   - Circulating anticoagulants directed against the factors mentioned above or the lupus inhibitor.
   - Anticoagulant therapy with heparin or oral anticoagulants.
5. **Prolonged thrombin time.** Prolongation of the thrombin time may be due to the following:
   - Hypofibrinogenemia (fibrinogen less than 100 mg/dL)
   - Some forms of dysfibrinogenemia
   - Fibrin-fibrinogen split products
   - Heparin therapy
   - Paraproteins.

   If the thrombin time is prolonged, further studies to clarify the cause may be required.
6. **Low fibrinogen level.** When evaluating the results of a fibrinogen assay, one must be familiar with the assay method used. Many laboratories use immunologic assays, which measure both functionally normal and abnormal fibrinogens. If such an assay is in use,

the thrombin time can be used to evaluate the functional integrity of the fibrinogen. A low functional fibrinogen level means that production is decreased, consumption is increased, or a dysfibrinogen is present. Fibrinogen is an acute-phase reactant and is often elevated with advanced malignancy. A fibrinogen level in the normal range may actually be relatively low for the patient's physiologic state and thus may be a sign of DIC (see Table 28.1).

C. **Laboratory findings in patients with DIC**
Acute DIC is often associated with significant hemorrhage, whereas chronic DIC may be asymptomatic or associated with thromboses. Screening and confirmatory laboratory tests are shown in Table 28.1.

D. **Review of peripheral smear**
Review of peripheral smear for schistocytes and decreased numbers of platelets is needed if TTP is suspected.

IV. TREATMENT OF HEMORRHAGIC SYNDROMES IN PATIENTS WITH MALIGNANT DISEASE

A. **Transfusion therapy**
1. **General guidelines**
   a. **Regard elective transfusion with allogeneic blood as an outcome to be avoided.** Blood is not risk-free. Consider the factors that will influence the use of blood products, including the following:
      - Alternative forms of therapy that could control bleeding (e.g., topical measures or desmopressin).
      - How symptomatic is the patient? Do not treat an abnormal laboratory test in a symptom-free patient. For example, patients with chronic DIC may demonstrate prolongation of both the PT and the aPTT and mild to moderate thrombocytopenia. If there is no demonstrable bleeding, transfusion therapy is not necessary.
   b. **Use the specific blood component needed by the patient.**
   c. **Minimize complications** of transfusion by using the following:
      - Only the amount and type of blood product indicated for the patient in the specific clinical setting.
      - Leukocyte-reduced blood products, irradiated blood, or both, when indicated.
   d. **Obtain a class I human leukocyte antigen (HLA) type** on the patient at diagnosis to allow for better support of platelet transfusions.
2. **Blood component therapy**
   a. **RBC transfusions**
      (1) **Available forms of RBCs for transfusion.** The primary component available for red cell transfusion is RBCs.
      (2) **Criteria for transfusing RBCs.** Chemotherapy-induced anemia is common in patients with cancer and should preferably be managed by erythropoiesis-stimulating agents, such as recombinant erythropoietin and/or hematinics such as iron,

folic acid, and vitamin B_{12}, as applicable. RBCs are indicated for the treatment of symptomatic anemia to increase the oxygen-carrying capacity by increasing red cell mass. RBCs should not be used to increase well-being, promote wound healing, increase oncotic pressure, or as a source of blood volume.

Transfusion should be based on clinical assessment and not a laboratory value. In general, RBC transfusion may be indicated in the following circumstances:

- Hemoglobin less than 7 g/dL if clinically indicated. Acceptable transfusion goal is to maintain hemoglobin at 7 to 9 g/dL.
- Any hemoglobin level in the presence of acute life-threatening hemorrhage with evidence of hemodynamic instability or inadequate oxygen delivery.
- Hemodynamically stable anemia with hemoglobin less than 10 g/dL with acute coronary syndrome (either angina or acute myocardial infarction).
- Hemoglobin less than 10 g/dL causing or contributing to symptomatic anemia (not explained by other causes), with excessive fatigue, dyspnea on exertion, syncope, or with signs such as tachycardia, tachypnea, and postural hypotension.

(3) **Expected response.** One unit of RBCs will increase the hemoglobin by approximately 1.0 g/dL (hematocrit by 3%) in a stable nonbleeding patient. However, the response may vary depending on the hemoglobin content of the unit and the patient's blood volume.

(4) **Check hemoglobin.** Hemoglobin equilibrates in 15 minutes in a stable nonbleeding patient. Use the posttransfusion hemoglobin along with the patient's clinical status to determine if additional RBCs transfusion is needed.

b. **Platelet transfusions**

(1) **Available forms of platelets for transfusion.** Platelets may be ordered and transfused in various ways. Because most patients with an underlying malignancy have the potential for needing long-term platelet support, platelet products should be leukocyte reduced from the initiation of transfusion (see Section IV.A.3). In general, patients who need platelet support can be started with platelets (whole-blood–derived platelet concentrates) or apheresis platelets (single-donor platelets). Many blood centers have geared up production of apheresis platelets, and this product may be more readily available in some places than in others. There are no solid data to suggest that starting with apheresis platelets decreases the incidence of alloimmunization. In fact, the Trial to Reduce Alloimmunization to Platelets

Study Group (1997) did not show any benefit in the use of platelet apheresis products over whole-blood–derived platelets. HLA-compatible platelets or crossmatched platelets should be reserved for patients who have become refractory to whole-blood–derived platelets or apheresis platelets and are alloimmunized [see Section IV.A.2.b.(4)]. Patients who are candidates for bone marrow transplantation should receive single-donor platelets (if available) from the initiation of platelet therapy. Patients who are candidates for transplantation with bone marrow from an HLA-matched sibling should not receive apheresis products from the potential donor before the transplantation.

(a) **Platelets (whole-blood–derived platelet concentrates, random-donor platelets, or platelet concentrates).** Four to six U (usually pooled in one bag) are considered an adequate dose for a 70-kg adult.

(b) **Apheresis platelets obtained by apheresis (single-donor platelets).** These come as a single pack and represent the platelets obtained by apheresis from a single donor. One unit of platelets obtained by apheresis is equivalent to 6 to 8 U of platelet concentrates.

(2) **Check platelet count** 10 minutes to 1 hour, and then 24 hours, after platelet transfusion to estimate recovery and survival of platelets in the patient. Each unit of platelet concentrate should increase the platelet count by about 7000/μL. The expected 1-hour posttransfusion rise in platelets is 15,000 platelets/μL divided by the patient's body surface area in square meters for each unit of platelet concentrate (thus, for a person of 2 m^2, 6 U should produce a rise of 45,000/μL [6 $\times$ 15,000/2]). The corrected count increment (CCI) may also be used to determine the response. The CCI is determined by the platelet count increment (posttransfusion – pretransfusion count) multiplied by the body surface area in m^2 and divided by the platelet count in the product. A CCI of greater than 7500 between 10 minutes to 1 hour posttransfusion is considered an adequate response and represents 20% to 30% platelet recovery. At 24 hours, a CCI of greater than 4500 is adequate. A reduced CCI at 18 to 24 hours after a normal CCI at 10 minutes to 1 hour is believed to represent increased consumption of platelets due to nonimmune clinical events [see Section IV.A.2.b(4)]; in some patients, it may represent immune destruction.

(3) **Criteria for transfusing platelets**

(a) **For patients with reduced platelet production,** criteria for transfusion are shown in Table 28.3.

Guidelines for Platelet Transfusion in Patients With Reduced Platelet Production

Platelet Count	Recommendation
0–5000/μL	Transfuse with platelets even if there is no evidence of bleeding
6000–10,000/μL	Transfuse with platelets if there is: ■ Fresh minor hemorrhage ■ Temperature of 38°C or active infection ■ Rapid decline in platelet count (>50%/d) ■ Headache ■ Significant gastrointestinal blood loss ■ Recent chemotherapy that may be expected to cause severe stomatitis or gastrointestinal ulceration ■ Presence of confluent petechiae (as opposed to scattered petechiae) ■ Continuous bleeding from a wound or other sites ■ Planned minor procedure such as a bone marrow biopsy
11,000–20,000/μL	Transfuse with platelets if there is more rapid bleeding or if more complicated procedures are anticipated
>20,000/μL	If major surgery is planned or when life-threatening bleeding occurs, the platelet count should be increased to at least 50,000/μL. For intracranial surgery or ophthalmic surgery, transfuse to a platelet count of at least 100,000/μL (bleeding time must be checked before surgery and must be normal). In fully anticoagulated patients, it is advisable to keep the platelet count to at least 50,000/μL.

(b) Increased platelet destruction. Platelet transfusions are of limited benefit in patients with thrombocytopenia due to increased destruction as a result of either antibodies or consumption. If potentially life-threatening bleeding complicates thrombocytopenia due to increased destruction, platelet transfusions may be given; however, only small increments in the platelet count usually occur. IV γ-globulin 1 g/kg IV daily × 2 days given before the platelet transfusions might improve the response.

(c) Dysfunctional platelets. One must stop any drugs known to cause platelet dysfunction. Although the use of platelet transfusions should be considered, pharmacologic methods of enhancing platelet function, such as desmopressin, should be used if possible (see Section IV.B.1).

(4) Refractoriness to platelet transfusions is defined as a CCI of less than 7500 at 10 minutes to 1 hour or less than 4500 at 18 to 24 hours after transfusion of 5 to 6 U of platelet concentrates or 1 U of apheresis platelets after two or more transfusions. Refractoriness may be the result of alloimmunization (i.e., formation of alloantibodies to HLA or rarely platelet-specific antigens) or to other immune or nonimmune causes such as fever, septicemia, DIC, splenomegaly, drugs, infections, or bleeding. Alloimmunization is the most difficult form to treat and therefore is best prevented (see Section IV.A.3).

(a) **Evaluation.** Patients who become refractory to platelet transfusions should have a laboratory evaluation for alloimmunization. They should also be evaluated for infection and DIC. Further, all potentially offending medications should be stopped.

(b) **Therapy.** The therapeutic modalities for ITP (corticosteroids, IV globulin, danazol) are generally ineffective for platelet refractoriness due to alloimmunization. Two therapeutic options exist, as follows.

(i) **HLA-compatible platelets.** These platelets may be provided using two approaches: the donor platelets have HLA class I antigens similar to the patient: HLA antigen matching; an alternative approach is to provide platelets that lack HLA class I antigens to which the patient has made antibodies: the antibody specificity prediction method. A combination of the two may provide the best match.

(ii) **Crossmatched platelets.** Because platelets are available at most blood centers, if a blood center performs crossmatching, it is often easier to obtain crossmatched platelets as no specific donor qualification is required. This product is as effective as HLA-compatible platelets in producing a platelet response in the alloimmunized patient. Either platelet concentrates or apheresed platelets can be crossmatched with the recipient. Nonreactive or, in extenuating circumstances, the least reactive platelets can then be selected for transfusion.

c. **Coagulation factor support**

(1) **FFP** contains all clotting factors (but not platelets) and should be used for multiple coagulation factor deficiencies. FFP requires 20 to 30 minutes to thaw and must be thawed at 37°C. Once thawed, FFP (thawed plasma) must be transfused within 5 days of thawing as long as it is maintained at 1 to 6°C.

(2) **Plasma frozen within 24 hours of phlebotomy is often used interchangeably with FFP.**

(3) **Cryoprecipitated antihemophilic factor** is a source of factor VIII-vWF complex, fibrinogen, and factor XIII. Each bag of cryoprecipitated AHF contains about 50% of the factor VIII-vWF complex (minimum of 80 U) and 20% to 40% of the fibrinogen (minimum of 150 mg) harvested from 1 U of blood. Cryoprecipitated AHF is stored in a frozen state and has the advantage of concentrating the clotting factors in a small volume (10 to 15 mL/bag). It is used primarily in deficiencies of fibrinogen. The goal is to keep the fibrinogen level higher than 100 mg/dL. The usual dosage of cryoprecipitated AHF to correct hypofibrinogenemia is one bag of cryoprecipitated AHF for every 10 kg of body weight. Because 50% is recovered after transfusion, this may raise the fibrinogen level only by about 50 mg/dL. Larger doses may be needed for severe hypofibrinogenemia or "flaming" DIC. The dose of cryoprecipitated AHF may be calculated using the following formula: number of bags = desired increase in fibrinogen level in mg/dL × plasma volume/average fibrinogen per bag (average fibrinogen content may be obtained from the blood supplier). The patient is evaluated to determine if the laboratory values have been corrected.

(4) **Factor IX concentrates** are available as factor IX complex concentrates, which contain factors II, VII, IX, and X, or as coagulation factor IX concentrates. The latter are highly purified factor IX concentrates with few or no other coagulation factors. Several precautions are worth noting regarding the factor IX concentrates:

- This concentrate is made from pooled plasma but is treated with viral attenuation processes such as dry or vapor heat in the case of factor IX complex concentrates (therefore, the risk of hepatitis is significant) and solvent-detergent or monoclonal antibody in the case of coagulation factor IX concentrates. The dose depends on the preparation to be used. The goal is to bring the factor concentration to no more than 50% of normal.

- There is a small risk of DIC resulting from the use of factor IX complex concentrates. Newborns and patients with liver dysfunction are at increased risk. The coagulation factor concentrates are far less thrombogenic and should be used in cases at increased risk for venous thrombosis or DIC.

- Factor IX concentrates are stored in the lyophilized state. Do not shake when reconstituting.

3. **Leukocyte reduction.** Patients who have not previously received transfusions and who will need long-term blood product support should receive leukocyte-reduced ($<5 \times 10^6$ leukocytes/bag)

blood products. Leukocyte reduction may prevent febrile trans-fusion reactions, prevent cytomegalovirus (CMV) infections, and delay or prevent alloimmunization. Controversy still exists as to whether tumor recurrence and infections are a result of immu-nomodulatory effects of blood transfusion and if they can be re-duced by leukoreduction. There is also ongoing controversy as to whether leukocyte-reduced blood products should be provided to all patients, not just patients at risk. Leukocyte reduction does not prevent graft-versus-host disease, but irradiation does (see Section IV.A.5).

Two methods of leukocyte reduction by filtration are cur-rently available: bedside and prestorage.

a. **Bedside filtration** involves leukocyte reduction at the time of transfusion. Disadvantages include plugging of the filter, the presence of leukocyte breakdown products, bag breakage, and lack of consistency of products. Filters are available for RBCs and platelets.

b. **Prestorage leukocyte-reduced RBCs** are RBCs that have been leukocyte-reduced generally within 8 to 24 hours of collec-tion. Advantages are fewer leukocyte breakdown products, ease of administration, and consistent quality (95% of prod-ucts with less than 5×10^6 leukocytes/bag). Cost may be perceived as a disadvantage. However, this is offset by the ex-pense of stocking filters, training of staff in the use of filters, and breakage. Likewise, whole-blood–derived platelets may be prestorage leukocyte reduced by filtration. Some aphere-sis machines leukocyte reduce apheresis platelets during collection.

4. **CMV-seronegative cellular blood products.** Only patients known to be anti-CMV negative with impaired immunity should be considered for the use of CMV-negative screened blood. This group includes children, for the most part. Some insti-tutions also consider provision of CMV-seronegative units for bone marrow transplant candidates. The use of CMV-seronegative blood seriously restricts the potential donor pool for these patients. Leukocyte-reduced blood products ($<5.0 \times 10^6$/bag) are considered CMV-"safe" products and may be used as an alternative to CMV-seronegative products based on institutional policy. Only cellular blood products transmit CMV.

White blood cell (WBC) depletion filters also remove CMV because CMV resides in the WBCs. Irradiation of blood prod-ucts does not render them CMV-free. Frozen deglycerolized blood is considered free of CMV contamination.

5. **Irradiated blood products.** These prevent the development of graft-versus-host disease. Irradiated blood products, in the case

of patients with cancer or hematologic malignancies, are indicated in the following situations:

- Congenital immunodeficiency
- Bone marrow, peripheral blood stem cell, or umbilical cord stem cell transplantation
- Directed blood donations to blood relatives
- HLA-compatible or crossmatched platelets
- Granulocyte transfusions
- High-dose chemotherapy with growth factor or stem cell rescue
- Hodgkin lymphoma
- Leukemia and non-Hodgkin lymphoma (relative indications)
- Purine analogues, such as, fludarabine treatment
- Significant lymphocytopenia with alemtuzumab treatment.

B. Other forms of therapy

1. **Desmopressin** 0.3 μg/kg IV over 30 minutes every 12 to 24 hours for 2 to 4 days may be used to elevate factor VIII and vWF levels as well as improve platelet function. Tachyphylaxis may occur if therapy is continued for longer periods. Intranasal desmopressin 0.25 mL twice a day using a solution containing 1.3 mg/mL has been given for minor bleeding episodes.

2. **Fibrin glue.** This is a topical biologic adhesive. Its effects imitate the final stages of coagulation. The glue consists of a solution of concentrated human fibrinogen, which is activated by the addition of bovine thrombin and calcium chloride. The resulting clot promotes hemostasis and tissue sealing. The clot is completely absorbed during the healing process. The best adhesive and hemostatic effect is obtained by applying the two solutions simultaneously to the open wound surface. Fibrin glue has been used primarily in surgical settings. It has been most effective when used for surface, low-pressure bleeding. There is a small risk of anaphylactic reaction because of the bovine origin of the thrombin.

3. **Antifibrinolytic agents.** ε-Aminocaproic acid (EACA) and tranexamic acid have been used to control bleeding associated with primary fibrinolysis as seen in patients with prostatic carcinoma and in a small number of patients with refractory thrombocytopenia. Great care must be taken in the use of these agents because of a possible increased risk of thrombosis. EACA may be used topically to control small-area, small-volume bleeding.

4. **Oprelvekin (interleukin-11)** may be used for the treatment and prevention of chemotherapy-related thrombocytopenia. Oprelvekin is a thrombopoietic growth factor that directly stimulates the proliferation of hematopoietic stem cells and megakaryocyte progenitor cells as well as megakaryocyte maturation, resulting in increased platelet production. It may cause substantial fluid retention and should be used with caution in patients who have

congestive heart failure (CHF), those with a history of CHF, and those being treated for CHF. One must also be cautious using this agent in patients who are receiving diuretic therapy or ifosfamide because sudden deaths have been reported as a result of severe hypokalemia. Oprelvekin should be used to prevent thrombocytopenia, which would be severe enough to require platelet transfusions. Therapy usually begins 6 to 24 hours after the completion of chemotherapy, and patients should be monitored for any signs or symptoms of allergic reactions or cardiac dysfunction.

Selected Readings

Anand SS, Wells PS, Hunt D, et al. Does this patient have deep vein thrombosis? *JAMA*. 1998;279:1094–1099.

Ansell J, Hirsh J, Hylek E, et al. Pharmacology and management of the vitamin K antagonists. *Chest*. 2008;133:160S–198S.

Baker WF Jr. Thrombosis and hemostasis in cardiology: review of pathophysiology and clinical practice. II. Recommendations for anti-thrombotic therapy. *Clin Appl Thromb Hemost*. 1998;4:143–147.

Blajchman MA, Goldman M, Freedman JJ, Sher GD. Proceedings of a consensus conference: prevention of post-transfusion CMV in the era of universal reduction. *Transfus Med Rev*. 2001;15:1–20.

Callum JL, Karkouti K, Lin Y. Cryoprecipitate: the current state of knowledge. *Transfus Med Rev*. 2009;23:177–188.

AABB, American Red Cross, America's Blood Centers, Armed Services Blood Program. *Circular of Information for the Use of Human Blood and Blood Components*. Bethesda, MD: AABB; 2009.

Dwyre DM, Holland PV. Transfusion-associated graft-versus-host disease. *Vox Sang*. 2008;95:85–93.

Hillyer CD, Emmens RK, Zago-Novaretti M, et al. Methods for the reduction of transfusion transmitted cytomegalovirus infection: filtration versus the use of seronegative donor units. *Transfusion*. 1994;34:929–934.

Hull RD, Pineo GF. Prophylaxis of deep vein thrombosis and pulmonary embolism: current recommendations. *Clin Appl Thromb Hemost*. 1998;4:96–104.

Humphries JE. Transfusion therapy in acquired coagulopathies. *Hematol Oncol Clin North Am*. 1994;8:1181–1201.

Klein HG, Spahn DR, Corson JL. Red blood cell transfusion in clinical practice. *Lancet*. 2007;370:415–426.

Lee AY. Thrombosis and cancer: the role of screening for occult cancer and recognizing the underlying biological mechanisms. *Hematology Am Soc Hematol Educ Program*. 2006;438–443.

Legler TJ, Fischer I, Dittman J, et al. Frequency and course of refractoriness in multiply transfused patients. *Ann Hematol*. 1997;74:185–189.

Napolitano LM, Kurek S, Luchette FA, et al. Clinical practice guideline: red blood cell transfusion in adult trauma and critical care. *Crit Care Med*. 2009;37: 3124–3157.

National Comprehensive Cancer Network (NCCN). NCCN Clinical Practice Guidelines in Oncology. Cancer- and chemotherapy-induced anemia. www.nccn.org.

Preiksaitis JK. The cytomegalovirus-"safe" blood product: is leukoreduction equivalent to antibody screening? *Transfus Med Rev.* 2000;14:112–136.

Rizzo DJ, Somerfield MR, Hagerty KL, et al. Use of epoetin and darbepoetin in patients with cancer: 2007 American society of clinical oncology/American society of hematology clinical practice guideline update. *J Clin Oncol.* 2008;26:132–149.

Schiffer CA, Anderson KC, Bennett CL, et al. Platelet transfusion for patients with cancer: clinical practice guidelines of the American Society of Clinical Oncology. *J Clin Oncol.* 2001;19:1519–1538.

Shlicter SJ. Platelet transfusion therapy. *Hematol Oncol Clin N Am.* 2007;21:697–729.

Shlicter SJ, Kaufman RM, Assmann SF, et al. Dose of prophylactic platelet transfusions and prevention of hemorrhage. *N Engl J Med.* 2010;362:600–613.

The Thrombosis Interest Group of Canada: http://www.tigc.org/eguidelines/cancer06.htm.

Vassallo RR. New paradigms in the management of alloimmune refractoriness to platelet transfusions. *Curr Opin Hematol.* 2007;14:655–663.

Wiesen AR, Hospenthal DR, Byrd JC, et al. Equilibration of hemoglobin concentration after transfusion in medical inpatients not actively bleeding. *Ann Intern Med.* 1994;121:278–280.

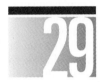

Oncology Emergencies and Critical Care Issues: Spinal Cord Compression, Cerebral Edema, Superior Vena Cava Syndrome, Anaphylaxis, Respiratory Failure, Tumor Lysis Syndrome, Hypercalcemia, and Bone Metastasis

Roland T. Skeel

Spinal cord compression, cerebral edema, superior vena cava syndrome (SVCS), anaphylaxis, respiratory failure, tumor lysis syndrome, hypercalcemia, and bone metastasis can be major causes of morbidity and, in some cases, potential mortality in patients with cancer. Because of the critical nature of these complications of cancer and its treatment, oncologists, oncology nurses, and other oncology health professionals must be prepared to recognize the signs and symptoms of these disorders promptly so that appropriate therapy can be instituted without delay.

I. SPINAL CORD COMPRESSION

A. Tumors

The most common tumors resulting in spinal cord compression are breast cancer, lung cancer, prostate cancer, and renal cancer, although it may also occur with sarcoma, multiple myeloma, and lymphoma. Purely intradural or epidural lesions are uncommon because more than three-fourths of cases arise from metastasis to either a vertebral body or other bony parts of the vertebra or, less commonly, by direct extension from a paravertebral soft-tissue mass. Seventy percent of the bone lesions are osteolytic, 10% are osteoblastic, and 20% are mixed. More than 85% of patients with metastases to the vertebra have lesions that involve more than one vertebral body.

B. Symptoms and signs

The most common early symptoms seen in patients with spinal cord compression are localized vertebral or radicular pain. These are not from the cord compression per se but rather from involvement of the vertebral structures and nerve roots at the level of the compression. Localized tenderness to pressure or percussion over the involved vertebrae is often found on physical examination. Because pain is seen initially in up to 90% of patients, localized back pain, radicular pain, or spinal tenderness in a patient with cancer should evoke clinical suspicion and prompt further evaluation to determine whether the patient has potential or early cord compression. Muscle weakness, evidenced by subjective symptoms or objective physical findings, is present in 75% of patients by the time of diagnosis. The clinician must be aware that progression of this symptom can vary from a gradual increase in weakness over several days to a precipitous loss of function over several hours that may worsen rapidly to the point of paraplegia. If muscle weakness is present, it is incumbent on the physician to act urgently to obtain consultation with the neurosurgeon and the radiation oncologist. It is not appropriate to wait until the next morning! By the time there is muscle weakness, most patients also have sensory deficits below the level of the compression and often have changes in bladder and bowel sphincter function. When compression is diagnosed late or if treatment is not started emergently, only 25% of patients who are unable to walk when treatment is started regain full ambulation.

C. Diagnosis

Magnetic resonance imaging (MRI) is the diagnostic modality of choice, although high-resolution computed tomography (CT) with myelography is an alternative. Plain radiographs and bone scans give evidence of metastases to vertebrae, but in and of themselves are not diagnostic of spinal cord involvement.

When there is evidence of bony involvement of the spine on a plain radiograph, CT scan, or bone scan, the approach is to obtain an MRI for those patients who have subjective or objective evidence of weakness, radicular pain, paresthesia, or sphincter dysfunction, because these patients are at highest risk of spinal cord compression. Routine MRIs in patients who have completely asymptomatic bony spine metastases (without pain, tenderness, or neurologic findings on a comprehensive clinical examination) are not cost-effective. In patients with only localized pain or tenderness to correspond with the bone scan or radiographic findings, the yield of additional tests is also low. Thus, the clinical determination of whether to obtain additional invasive or costly diagnostic tests is more difficult and requires a careful assessment of all clinical features of the patient. All patients with metastasis to the spine require close follow-up, and they and their families must be urged to report relevant symptoms immediately.

D. Treatment

As noted above, immediate consultation with radiation oncology and neurosurgery is imperative. Because of potentially precipitous deterioration when neurologic deficits have developed, treatment should be started immediately.

1. **Corticosteroids.** When a radiologic study identifies the level of cord compression or a neurologic deficit is detected on physical examination, dexamethasone should be started immediately to reduce spinal cord edema. A recommended dose is 10 to 20 mg intravenously (IV) as a loading dose and then 4 to 6 mg by mouth or IV four times daily to be continued through the initial weeks of radiation therapy. Higher doses up to 96 mg daily have marginal benefit and toxicity is clearly greater. At the completion of the radiotherapy, the dexamethasone therapy may be tapered.

2. **Initial interventional therapy**

   a. **Although the preferences of individual physicians and centers vary,** the immediate initiation of radiotherapy once cord compression is diagnosed and corticosteroids have been started, providing the spine is stable and the tumor is likely to be sensitive to radiotherapy, is generally recommended. This is based on several studies that showed no significant improvement in outcome for patients treated with surgery plus radiation versus those treated with radiation alone. However, when there is spine instability, a tumor that is not likely to be sensitive to radiotherapy, or rapid progression of weakness, the surgical option may be preferable. One recent randomized study found that initial surgery was better for preserving the patient's ability to walk, perhaps owing to improved surgical techniques.

   b. **Dose and schedule of radiotherapy.** Radiation therapy is most frequently given at a total dose of 30 to 45 Gy with daily dose fractions of 200 to 250 cGy. Alternatively, 400 cGy daily may be given initially for the first 3 days of therapy and then subsequently decreased to standard-dose levels for the completion of the radiation course. Short-course therapies with higher dose fractions have also been used. These appear to have similar functional outcome in patients with a short prognosis, but local control is maintained for a longer time when long-course (standard) therapy is used. The longer course is thus recommended for patients with better prognosis from their overall disease.

c. **The clinical response to radiation** is dependent not only on the degree of cord involvement and the duration of symptoms but also on the underlying cell type. In general, patients with severe deficits such as complete paraplegia or a long duration of neurologic deficit are unlikely to have return to normal function. This underscores the need to diagnose and treat these patients rapidly. Lymphoma, myeloma, and other hematologic malignancies, along with breast, prostate, and small cell lung carcinoma, tend to be more responsive than adenocarcinomas of the gastrointestinal tract, non-small–cell lung cancer, renal cancer, and others.

3. **Surgery** plays a crucial role for some patients. Traditional approaches include decompressive laminectomy for posterior lesions or anterior approaches for other lesions. Newer treatment options include minimally invasive vertebroplasty and kyphoplasty, which may effectively maintain function, reduce pain in appropriately selected patients, and have a shorter recovery time than other procedures. Clear indications for surgery include worsening of neurologic signs or symptoms or the appearance of new neurologic findings during the course of radiation treatment, vertebral collapse at presentation, a question of spinal stability, tumor type expected to be refractory to radiotherapy, and disease recurrence within a prior radiation port. In selected patients, the use of surgery to remove disease in the vertebral bodies followed by stabilization can result in dramatic improvement in pain and function.

II. CEREBRAL EDEMA
A. Clinical evaluation
1. **Neurologic signs and symptoms.** Intracranial metastases are commonly manifested by a variety of neurologic symptoms and signs, including headache, change in mentation, visual disturbances, cranial nerve deficits, focal motor or sensory abnormalities, difficulty with coordination, and seizures. In the more critical condition of brainstem herniation, there may be gradual to rapid loss of consciousness, neck stiffness, unilateral or bilateral pupillary abnormalities, ipsilateral hemiparesis, or respiratory

dysfunction; the specific findings depend on whether there is uncal, central, or tonsillar herniation. Any new neurologic complaint from a patient with cancer should be viewed with a high index of suspicion that it represents metastasis, especially if metastasis to the brain is commonly associated with the patient's tumor type.

The history and physical examination provide the first clue to the presence of a metastatic lesion or associated cerebral edema. In general, a history of gradual progression of neurologic symptoms before the development of a significant deficit is more consistent with a metastatic lesion, whereas the absence of symptoms followed by the abrupt onset of a severe deficit is suggestive of a cerebrovascular event.

2. **Radiologic studies.** MRI is the imaging modality of choice because it has greater sensitivity than CT in detecting the presence of metastatic lesions, evaluating the posterior fossa, and determining the extent of cerebral edema. While CT is sufficient to detect the presence of cerebral edema in a majority of patients, it is necessary to realize that CT fails to diagnose some lesions and may underestimate cerebral edema. If CT of the brain with and without contrast reveals no definite abnormality in the presence of persistent neurologic findings, MRI is the recommended next step. Delay of appropriate imaging studies (either CT or MRI) to examine plain skull radiographs or to obtain radionuclide studies in patients experiencing neurologic difficulties is not warranted.

Warning: In a patient with cancer who has focal neurologic signs or symptoms, headache, or alteration in consciousness, a lumbar puncture to evaluate for possible neoplastic meningeal spread should not be done until a CT scan or MRI shows no evidence of mass, midline shift, or increased intracranial pressure. To do the lumbar puncture without this assurance could precipitate brainstem herniation, which is often rapidly fatal.

B. **Treatment**

1. **Symptomatic therapy.** Once the presence of cerebral edema is established, dexamethasone 10 to 20 mg IV to load followed by 4 to 6 mg IV or by mouth four times daily should be started. The rationale for the use of steroids centers around the etiology of cerebral edema. It appears that the invasion of malignant cells releases leukotrienes and other soluble mediators responsible for vasodilation, increased capillary permeability, and subsequent edema. Dexamethasone inhibits the conversion of arachidonic acid to leukotrienes, thereby decreasing vascular permeability. Additionally, steroids appear to have a direct stabilizing effect on brain capillaries. There is some evidence to suggest that patients who do not have lessening of cerebral

edema with the dexamethasone dose just described may respond to higher doses (50 to 100 mg/day). Because of the risk of gastrointestinal bleeding and other side effects of doses higher than 32 mg/day, higher doses are usually not given for more than 48 to 72 hours.

Patients with severe cerebral edema leading to a life-threatening rise in intracranial pressure or brainstem herniation should also receive mannitol 50 to 100 g (in a 20% to 25% solution) infused IV over approximately 30 minutes. This may be repeated every 6 hours if needed, although serum electrolytes and urine output must be monitored closely. Patients with severe cerebral edema should be intubated to allow for mechanical hyperventilation to reduce the carbon dioxide pressure to 25 to 30 mm Hg in order to decrease intracranial pressure.

2. **Therapy of the intracerebral tumor.** Once the patient has been stabilized, appropriate therapy for the cause underlying the cerebral edema should be implemented. Radiation is the usual modality for most metastases, but surgery may be considered in addition for suitable candidates with easily accessible lesions; combined surgery and radiotherapy may result in a longer disease-free and total survival if there are only one or two metastatic lesions and the systemic disease is controlled. Stereotactic radiosurgery combined with whole brain radiation is an effective and equivalent alternative to surgery plus whole brain radiation, providing the lesions are not too large and limited in number.

3. **Nonmalignant causes of cerebral edema,** such as subdural hematoma in thrombocytopenic patients and brain abscess, toxoplasmosis, or other infections in immunocompromised patients, must always be considered.

III. SUPERIOR VENA CAVA SYNDROME (SVCS)

The superior vena cava is a thin-walled vessel located to the right of the midline just anterior to the right mainstem bronchus. It is ultimately responsible for the venous drainage of the head, neck, and arms. Its location places it near lymph nodes that are commonly involved by malignant cells from primary lung tumors and from lymphomas. Lymph node distention or the presence of a mediastinal tumor mass may compress the adjacent superior vena cava, leading to SVCS. Similarly, the presence of a thrombus due to a hypercoagulable state secondary to underlying malignancy or a thrombus developing around an indwelling central venous catheter may also lead to the development of this syndrome.

A. Symptoms and signs

Patients who develop SVCS commonly complain of dyspnea, orthopnea, paroxysmal nocturnal dyspnea, and facial, neck, and upper-extremity swelling. Associated symptoms may include cough, hoarseness, and chest or neck pain. Headache and mental status changes also may be seen. A patient's symptoms may be gradual and progressive, with only mild facial swelling being present early in the course of this disorder. These early changes may be so subtle that the patient is unaware of them. Alternatively, if a clot develops in the superior vena cava in association with narrowing of the vessel, as often happens when the caval compression is severe, the signs and symptoms may appear suddenly. Physical examination may reveal a spectrum of findings from facial edema to marked respiratory distress. Neck vein distention, facial edema or cyanosis, and tachypnea are commonly seen. Other potential physical findings include the presence of prominent collateral vessels on the thorax, upper-extremity edema, paralysis of the vocal cords, and mental status changes.

B. Radiologic evaluation

Patients may often be diagnosed by physical findings plus the presence of a mediastinal mass on chest radiographs. CT scan with contrast will confirm the diagnosis and delineate the extent of obstruction. It permits a detailed examination of surrounding anatomy, including adjacent lymphadenopathy, may differentiate between extrinsic compression and an intrinsic lesion (primary thrombus), and aids in treatment planning for radiation therapy.

SVCS may also occur in patients with subclavian or internal jugular IV catheters. The injection of contrast material into these catheters is useful to determine the origin and extent of the thrombus. Determination of the cause and the appropriate treatment depends on both the clinical situation and the radiologic findings.

C. Tissue diagnosis

Although some patients present with such severe respiratory compromise as to require emergent treatment, most patients are clinically stable and may undergo biopsy for a tissue diagnosis if they are not previously known to have cancer. Tissue may be acquired through multiple methods including bronchoscopy, CT-guided biopsy, mediastinoscopy, mediastinotomy, and thoracoscopy. Thoracotomy is the most invasive option and is rarely needed. Because of increased venous pressure and dilated veins distal to the obstruction, extreme care must be taken to ensure adequate hemostasis after any biopsy procedure.

D. Treatment

Initially, patients with SVCS may be treated with oxygen for dyspnea, furosemide 20 to 40 mg IV to reduce edema, and dexamethasone 16 mg IV or by mouth daily in divided doses. The benefit of dexamethasone is not clear. In patients with lymphoma, there is probably a lympholytic effect with resultant decrease in tumor mass; in patients with most other tumors, the effect is probably limited to decreasing any local inflammatory reaction from the tumor and from subsequent initial radiotherapy.

1. **Neoplasms.** Therapy for SVCS ultimately involves radiation therapy for most tumors but possibly chemotherapy as a single modality for particularly sensitive tumor types such as small-cell lung cancer, lymphomas, and germ cell cancers. Radiation therapy may be given in relatively high-dose fractions (e.g., 4 Gy) for several days, followed by a reversion to "standard doses" thereafter. Dexamethasone is continued for about 1 week after the start of radiation treatment.

2. **Thrombi.** All patients require anticoagulation, initially with a heparin to limit propagation of the clot. A newer highly effective treatment for the relief of signs and symptoms is percutaneous stent placement in the superior vena cava. Anticoagulation with heparin after stent placement is recommended because clot formation is common, even when external pressure was the primary cause of the obstruction. Depending on the situation, therapeutic doses of warfarin may be used after initial heparin to prevent return of the clot, though it is generally less effective than heparin or enoxaparin (see Chapter 28).

IV. ANAPHYLAXIS AND OTHER ACUTE INFUSION REACTIONS (SEE CHAPTER 26, SECTION I.B)

A. Causes

Anaphylaxis, although infrequent, is one of the most catastrophic potential side effects of biologic agents and chemotherapy. Anaphylaxis is a hyperimmune reaction mediated by the release of immunoglobulin E. This emergency situation may arise in oncology patients who are exposed to serum products, bacterial products such as L-asparaginase, certain cytotoxic agents (such as paclitaxel [Taxol] or the Cremophor component of paclitaxel), monoclonal antibodies, antibiotics such as penicillin, and iodine-based contrast material. However, virtually any drug can lead to a hyperimmune response resulting in anaphylaxis. Some acute hypersensitivity infusion reactions have similar manifestations, but occur predominantly during initial treatments (e.g., monoclonal antibodies) or late in the course of treatment (e.g., carboplatin), and may have alternate mechanisms of action. An example is the acute infusion reaction that may also occur with the use of rituximab or other agents in patients with chronic lymphocytic leukemia (CLL) or lymphomas, particularly when they have a high tumor burden. In this circumstance, the manifestations of the hypersensitivity reactions are not from a classical immunologic response, but more likely the result of a sudden release of cytokines causing hypotension or hypertension, dyspnea, and other manifestations.

B. Clinical manifestations

Patients may display anxiety, dyspnea, urge to defecate, and presyncopal symptoms. Urticaria, generalized itching, and evidence of bronchospasm and upper-airway angioedema may occur. Peripheral vasodilation may be manifest by facial flushing or pallor, can result in significant hypotension, and may lead to syncope. With carboplatin, the reaction may be immediate during the infusion or not start until hours later.

C. Management

Prompt recognition and treatment can be invaluable in blunting an adverse response and may prevent a reaction from becoming life-threatening. Patients must be assessed rapidly to ensure that an open airway is present and maintained. Supplemental oxygen should be given for respiratory symptoms. Endotracheal intubation may be necessary. If severe laryngeal edema rather than bronchospasm is the cause of respiratory distress, tracheostomy or cricothyrotomy is necessary.

1. Epinephrine 0.3 to 0.5 mg (0.3 to 0.5 mL of 1:1000 epinephrine or 3 to 5 mL of a 1:10,000 solution) IV is given every 10 minutes for severe reactions with laryngeal stridor, major bronchospasm, or severe hypotension, for a maximum of three doses (1 mg) or until the episode resolves, whichever occurs first. For milder reactions, a dose of 0.2 to 0.3 mL of 1:1000 epinephrine may be given subcutaneously (SC) and repeated every 15 minutes twice. In the event of life-threatening anaphylaxis, 0.5 mg (5 mL of a 1:10,000 solution) should be given IV; this dose may be repeated once in 10 minutes if needed. Because of the cardiovascular stress associated with epinephrine, its use in relatively minor allergic reactions, such as pruritus alone, should be avoided. Alternatively, epinephrine may be administered through the endotracheal tube if IV access is unavailable.

2. IV fluids (either normal saline or lactated Ringer solution) may be given for hypotension. Hypotension unresponsive to these measures requires the use of vasopressors such as dopamine.

3. Albuterol or metaproterenol aerosol treatments can be used to treat bronchospasm.

4. Diphenhydramine 25 mg IV may be followed by a second dose, if necessary. Blood pressure must be monitored because hypotension can result.

5. Corticosteroids have a slow onset of action measured in hours. Although their administration may be reasonable for their later effects, they do not have a primary role in the acute management of this emergent condition. Hydrocortisone 100 to 500 mg IV or methylprednisolone 125 mg IV may be given for their later effects.

6. Cimetidine 300 mg IV or other H_2-blockers may be given for urticaria; it has no significant role in acute, severe episodes, although it has a preventive role in averting reactions from paclitaxel along with dexamethasone and diphenhydramine.

V. RESPIRATORY FAILURE

A. Causes

Respiratory failure in patients with cancer may have many potential causes:

- Bacterial or other pneumonias, especially in patients who are neutropenic due to therapy
- Sepsis (and other causes of the systemic inflammatory response syndrome)
- Interstitial pulmonary spread of cancer
- Overwhelming parenchymal pulmonary metastases
- Radiation injury
- Lung damage from chemotherapy agents (such as bleomycin, mitomycin, high-dose cyclophosphamide, or methotrexate)
- Pulmonary edema secondary to cardiac damage from cytotoxic agents (like doxorubicin) or capillary leak syndrome from biologic agents (such as interleukin [IL]-2)
- Retinoic acid syndrome from tretinoin (all-*trans*-retinoic acid) therapy of acute promyelocytic leukemia
- Pulmonary emboli, either multiple small or single large
- Adult respiratory distress syndrome.

B. Management

The management of severe respiratory failure requires intubation and mechanical ventilation, which is usually managed by pulmonologists or critical care specialists. However, because the prognosis of most patients with advanced solid tumors who develop respiratory failure is poor, careful consideration of a patient's entire medical situation must be made. Relevant factors include the patient's underlying medical illnesses, such as concurrent cardiopulmonary disease, and their particular tumor type and potential for response to antineoplastic therapy. It is prudent—some would say imperative—to ascertain well in advance of the emergency the goals of the patient and the wishes of patients and their families regarding intensive care unit support and full resuscitative measures.

C. Prevention

If possible, progressive steps to prevent or lessen the possibility of the development of respiratory failure should be undertaken. These include the following.

1. **Careful monitoring of granulocyte counts** to be aware of patients at risk for bacterial infection.

2. **Routine lung auscultation of patients receiving agents with potential pulmonary toxicity** followed by appropriate action in the event of pulmonary findings. This may include giving furosemide if indicated and discontinuing offending agents (like bleomycin) before the development of serious symptoms. Reasons for discontinuing bleomycin therapy include unexplained exertional

dyspnea, fine bibasilar rales, fine bibasilar reticular shadows on chest radiograph, and significant fall in pulmonary function tests from pretreatment levels.

3. **Ensuring that patients are ambulatory or that antithrombotic precautions are taken for hospitalized patients who are bedridden.**
4. **Consideration of underlying cardiopulmonary disease, prior chest irradiation, and so forth** before patients are considered to be candidates for systemic therapy is most important. Concurrent illnesses may proscribe the selection of or modify the dosing of cytotoxic agents (such as cisplatin, which requires substantial IV hydration) and biologic agents (like IL-2, before which patients' cardiac and pulmonary function should be tested).

VI. TUMOR LYSIS SYNDROME

This syndrome may be seen with any tumor that is undergoing rapid cell turnover as a result of high growth fraction or high cell death due to therapy. In general, acute leukemia, high and intermediate grade lymphoma, and, less commonly, solid tumors such as small-cell lung cancer and germ cell cancers undergoing therapy are the most commonly associated tumor types. Tumor lysis syndrome is usually distinguished from the acute infusion reactions such as those seen with the use of rituximab or other agents (see Section IV.A) in patients with CLL or low-grade lymphoma. Tumor lysis syndrome is characterized by the metabolic abnormalities of hyperuricemia, hyperkalemia, and hyperphosphatemia leading to hypocalcemia. Patients with underlying chronic renal insufficiency are more susceptible to develop tumor lysis syndrome because of their limited capacity to excrete the products of rapid tumor cell destruction. Severe clinical situations, including acute renal failure, and serious cardiac dysrhythmia, including ventricular tachycardia and ventricular fibrillation, may develop. It is therefore important for physicians to be aware of which patients might be at risk for this syndrome, attempt to prevent its onset, monitor patients' blood chemistry values carefully, and initiate treatment promptly.

A. Prevention

It is useful to start all patients who have tumor types or therapy that predispose to this complication on allopurinol 600 to 1200 mg/day by mouth in divided doses for 1 or 2 days at least 24 hours before initiating chemotherapy, and continuing with 300 mg by mouth twice a day for 2 to 3 days after the start of therapy. Thereafter, patients may receive allopurinol 300 mg/day by mouth.

For patients who must be treated immediately, allopurinol is started at the same dose just described, urine should be alkalinized (pH 7), and IV fluid hydration with a "brisk diuresis" to maintain 100 to 150 mL/h output of urine provided. This can be achieved through the use of IV crystalloid, with 1 ampule (44.6 mEq) of sodium bicarbonate in each liter of IV solution. If the desired urine output is not reached after adequate hydration, furosemide 20 mg IV may be given to facilitate diuresis. If routine monitoring of urine shows pH less than 7, an additional ampule of sodium bicarbonate may be added to each liter of infused fluid. Acetazolamide 250 mg by mouth once a day may also be added to keep urine alkaline.

The recombinant urate oxidase, rasburicase, is generally a safe and effective alternative to allopurinol, though it may cause anaphylaxis, hemolysis in patients with G6PD deficiency, or methemoglobinemia. The recommended dose of rasburicase is 0.15 mg/kg/day for 5 days, but excellent control of hyperuricemia may be achieved with a lower dose of 3 to 7.5 mg/day. It is preferable in some situations, such as with the use of bendamustine where the concurrent use of allopurinol has been associated with severe cutaneous reactions (Stevens-Johnson syndrome and toxic epidermal necrolysis).

B. Monitoring

During the course of chemotherapy for patients at risk of tumor lysis syndrome, serum electrolytes, phosphate, calcium, uric acid, and creatinine levels should be checked before therapy and at least daily thereafter. Patients at high risk (e.g., high-grade lymphoma with large bulk) should have these parameters checked every 6 hours for the first 24 to 48 hours. In addition, patients who show any initial or subsequent abnormality in any of these parameters should have appropriate therapy initiated and have measurements of abnormal parameters repeated every 6 to 12 hours until completion of chemotherapy and normalization of laboratory values.

C. Treatment

Patients who have evidence of tumor lysis syndrome must have adequate hydration with half-normal saline solution. Oral aluminum hydroxide can be used to treat hyperphosphatemia.

Hyperkalemia may be treated in multiple ways. However, the clinician must differentiate between methods that reduce serum potassium by driving this ion intracellularly (as is done with dextrose and insulin or sodium bicarbonate) and methods that lead to actual potassium loss out of the body (as with furosemide [urine] and with sodium polystyrene sulfonate resin [Kayexalate; gut]). If hyperkalemia or hypocalcemia occurs, an electrocardiogram should be obtained, with continuous monitoring of the cardiac rhythm until these abnormalities are corrected. In addition, because of the potential cardiac arrhythmias secondary to hyperkalemia with hypocalcemia, cardioprotection could be achieved through the use of IV calcium.

We recommend the following.

1. **For patients with mild elevation of potassium (serum potassium no higher than 5.5 mEq/L),** increasing IV hydration using normal saline solution with a single dose (20 mg) of IV furosemide is often

sufficient. An alternative to normal saline is the use of two ampules of sodium bicarbonate (89 mEq) in 1 L of 5% dextrose/water, although alkalinization per se is probably not beneficial.

2. **For patients with serum potassium levels between 5.5 and 6.0 mEq/L,** increased IV fluids, furosemide, and oral sodium polystyrene sulfonate resin 30 g with sorbitol may be used.

3. **For patients with serum potassium levels of more than 6.0 mEq/L or evidence of cardiac arrhythmia,** several options may be combined. IV calcium gluconate, 10 mL of a 10% solution, or one ampule, is given first, followed by increased IV fluids, furosemide, plus one ampule of 50% dextrose and 10 U of regular insulin IV. Albuterol may be used to augment the effect of the insulin. Oral sodium polystyrene sulfonate resin with sorbitol also may be used except in patients with a history of congestive heart failure or reduced left ventricular function. Dialysis may be necessary for refractory hyperkalemia.

VII. HYPERCALCEMIA

A. Causes of tumor hypercalcemia

1. **Associated tumors.** Hypercalcemia is relatively common in patients with malignancy. In one study, it was shown that the most common cause of hypercalcemia in hospitalized patients is malignancy. Hypercalcemia of malignancy can be associated with bone metastasis, or it may occur in the absence of any direct bone involvement by the tumor. Based on the findings of a study of 433 patients with hypercalcemia of cancer, 86% of the patients had identifiable bone metastasis. More than half ($n = 225$) of the cases were accounted for by patients with breast carcinoma, and cancer of the lung and kidneys accounted for a smaller proportion. Patients with hematologic malignancies accounted for approximately 15% of the cases. These patients usually had hypercalcemia in the presence of diffuse tumor involvement of bone, although in a small percentage there was no evidence of bone involvement.

2. **Humoral mediators.** In approximately 10% of the cases of malignancy, hypercalcemia develops in the absence of radiographic or scintigraphic evidence of bone involvement. In this group of patients, the pathogenesis of hypercalcemia appears to be secondary to humoral mediators, including parathyroid hormone–related protein, other osteoclast-activating factors, and a number of cytokines, with potential bone-resorbing activities, including IL-6, receptor activator for nuclear factor κ B ligand (RANKL), macrophage inflammatory protein-1α, and tumor necrosis factor-α.

B. Symptoms, signs, and laboratory findings

Hypercalcemia often produces symptoms in patients with cancer and, in fact, may be the patients' major problem. Polyuria and nocturia, resulting from the impaired ability of the kidneys to concentrate the urine, occur early. Anorexia, nausea, constipation, muscle weakness, and fatigue are common. As the hypercalcemia progresses, severe dehydration, azotemia, mental obtundation, coma, and cardiovascular collapse may appear. In addition to hypercalcemia, the laboratory studies may reveal hypokalemia and increased blood urea nitrogen and creatinine levels. Patients with hypercalcemia of malignancy frequently have hypochloremic metabolic alkalosis. Bone involvement is best evaluated by a bone scan, which is often positive in the absence of radiographic evidence of bone involvement.

C. Treatment

The management of hypercalcemia of malignancy has two objectives: reducing elevated levels of serum calcium and treating the underlying cause. When hypercalcemia is mild to moderate (corrected [for albumin concentration] serum calcium less than 12 mg/dL) and the patient is not symptomatic, adequate hydration and measures directed against the tumor (e.g., surgery, chemotherapy, or radiation therapy) may suffice. Severe hypercalcemia, on the other hand, may be a life-threatening condition requiring emergency treatment. Therefore, for more severe degrees of hypercalcemia, other measures must be taken, including enhancement of calcium excretion by the kidney in patients with adequate renal function and the use of agents that decrease bone resorption.

The agents used for treatment of hypercalcemia have differences in the time of onset and duration of action as well as in their potency. Therefore, effective treatment of severe hypercalcemia requires the use of more than one modality of therapy.

A suggested approach to the treatment of severe hypercalcemia is as follows:

- Rehydration with 0.9% sodium chloride
- Bisphosphonate therapy—either pamidronate or zoledronic acid
- Continuing saline diuresis (0.9% sodium chloride + furosemide).

1. Rehydration. Rehydration and restoration of intravascular volume comprise the most important initial step in the therapy of hypercalcemia. Rehydration should be accomplished using 0.9% sodium chloride (normal saline) and often requires the administration of 4 to 6 L over the first 24 hours. Rehydration alone causes only a mild decrease of the serum calcium levels (about 10%). However, rehydration improves renal function, facilitating urinary calcium excretion.

2. Saline diuresis. After adequate restoration of intravascular volume, forced saline diuresis may be used. Sodium competitively inhibits the tubular resorption of calcium. Therefore, the IV infusion of saline causes a significant increase in calcium clearance. The infusion of normal saline (0.9% sodium chloride) at a rate of 250 to 500 mL/h, accompanied by the IV administration of 20 to 80 mg of furosemide every 2 to 4 hours, results in significant calcium diuresis and mild lowering of the serum calcium in the majority of patients. This type of therapy requires strict monitoring of cardiopulmonary status to avoid fluid overload. Also, it requires ready access to the laboratory to prevent electrolyte imbalance, as the urinary losses of sodium, potassium, magnesium, and water must be replaced to maintain metabolic balance. The infusion of saline at lower rates of 125 to 150 mL/h plus the addition of furosemide 40 to 80 mg IV once or twice a day may reduce the serum calcium until other measures aimed at inhibiting bone resorption take effect.

3. **Bisphosphonates**
   a. **Mechanism of action.** The bisphosphonates are potent inhibitors of normal and abnormal osteoclastic bone resorption. They bind to the surface of calcium phosphate crystals and inhibit crystal growth and dissolution. In addition, they may directly inhibit osteoclast resorptive activity.
   b. **Pamidronate and zoledronic acid** are very potent inhibitors of bone resorption and highly effective agents for the treatment of hypercalcemia of malignancy. Pamidronate was the treatment of choice for hypercalcemia of malignancy for several years, but has largely been replaced by zoledronic acid, which is at least as effective in the treatment of hypercalcemia and can be given over a shorter period of time.
      (1) **Dosage and administration.** For symptomatic, moderate hypercalcemia (corrected serum calcium 12 to 13.5 mg/dL), the recommended dose of pamidronate is 60 to 90 mg given IV as a single dose over 4 to 24 hours. The maximum recommended dose of zoledronic acid in hypercalcemia of malignancy is 4 mg, given as a single-dose IV infusion over no less than 15 minutes. Doses are often adjusted according to renal function. Repeat doses may be given in 3 to 4 days if inadequate response has been seen.
      (2) **Side effects.** Pamidronate and zoledronic acid are usually well tolerated. Mild fever with temperature elevations of 1°C have been noted occasionally in patients after drug administration. The transient fever is presumed to be due to release of cytokines from osteoclasts. Pain, redness, swelling, and induration at the site of infusion occur in approximately 20% of patients. Hypocalcemia, hypophosphatemia, or hypomagnesemia may be seen in 15% of patients. Both should be used with caution in patients with decreased renal function. Osteonecrosis of the jaw in association with dental procedures and conditions can be

a debilitating side effect of the bisphosphonates and requires the skill of an experienced dentist or oral surgeon.

4. **Glucocorticoids.** Large initial doses of hydrocortisone 250 to 500 mg IV every 8 hours (or its equivalent) can be effective in the treatment of hypercalcemia associated with lymphoproliferative diseases such as non-Hodgkin lymphoma and multiple myeloma and in patients with breast cancer metastatic to bone. However, it may take several days for glucocorticoids to lower the serum calcium level. Maintenance therapy should be started with prednisone 10 to 30 mg/day by mouth. The mechanisms by which glucocorticoids lower the serum calcium are multiple and involved.

5. **Oral phosphate supplements.** Oral phosphate therapy at dosages of 1.5 to 3.0 g/day of elemental phosphorus as an adjunct for the chronic treatment of hypercalcemia of malignancy is no longer commonly used. Phosphate supplements should never be given to patients with renal failure or when hyperphosphatemia is present, as soft-tissue calcification may occur. Monitoring of the level of calcium and phosphorus as well as the calcium times phosphorus ion product is important to prevent metastatic calcifications.

6. **Other agents.** Salmon calcitonin use is uncommon because of the requirement for frequent administration and the rapid development of therapeutic refractoriness. However, it does have a rapid duration of action and may be administered to patients with congestive heart failure and hypercalcemia. Calcitonin salmon is given at 4 IU/kg every 12 hours SC or intramuscularly. The dose may be increased to 8 IU/kg every 12 hours after 24 to 48 hours if response is unsatisfactory.

VIII. BONE METASTASIS

Metastases to bone occur frequently from many types of tumors and have great potential for morbidity. Bone involvement can be a source of constant pain, limiting a patient's activity and quality of life. The consequences of spinal involvement have been discussed previously. The occurrence of a pathologic fracture in a weight-bearing bone has catastrophic implications: Patients who are consequently immobilized or bedridden are predisposed to a variety of complications including deep venous thrombi, pulmonary emboli, aspiration pneumonia, and decubitus ulcers as well as psychosocial consequences, including depression.

A. Clinical findings

Bone involvement with metastatic disease can be manifested by a spectrum of clinical presentations. This can vary from constant aching pain through nocturnal exacerbations of pain to sharp pains brought on by pressure, weight bearing, other use, or range of motion of the affected site. Tenderness of an affected bone area may or may not be present. Tenderness or sharp pain with weight bearing often implies a greater degree of disruption of the bony architecture and thus a greater potential for fracture, particularly in a weight-bearing area.

B. Radiologic findings

Radiologic findings often depend on the type of malignancy involved as well as the extent of the metastases. For example, multiple myeloma commonly has pure osteolytic lesions. Consequently, radionuclide bone scans are rarely useful in the evaluation of patients with this disease and a metastatic skeletal survey (plain radiographs) is preferable. In contrast, prostate cancer most commonly has purely osteoblastic lesions. Therefore, a radionuclide bone scan would be the diagnostic test of choice. In general, most tumor types have the potential to yield either type of bone lesion or both, and a radionuclide bone scan may be done to permit a "global view" in these patients. Although a fluorodeoxyglucose positron emission tomography scan can also pick up bone metastasis, unless there is a reason to look at nonbony areas for other sites of disease, it is not necessary to use and is considerably more expensive.

The presence of "hot spots" in the spine, in weight-bearing bones such as the femur, or in other major long bones such as the humerus should lead the clinician to assess the patient further with plain radiographs of these bones. Patients who display significant cortical thinning of long bones or large lytic bone metastases are at high risk of developing pathologic fractures with great morbidity. These patients should be evaluated by orthopedic surgery for consideration of prophylactic surgery to stabilize the affected bone and by radiation oncology for treatment of the tumor to permit regeneration of normal bone.

C. Treatment

1. Surgery. Because rapid return of the patient to as normal a life as possible is an overriding concern when treating patients with metastatic disease, surgical stabilization is most often the initial step in treating pathologic fractures of long bones. If the fracture is the initial manifestation of tumor relapse, biopsy confirmation can also be obtained. Whereas fractures at sites of significant residual bony architecture can be satisfactorily stabilized with an intramedullary rod or pin, marked lytic destruction may necessitate additional structural support such as methylmethacrylate cement to fill the intramedullary canal and cortical defects. Pathologic fractures of non–weight-bearing bones can be managed by splinting (ribs) or sling immobilization (humerus or clavicle) while delivering radiotherapy to promote healing. Fixation may also be used in the upper extremities to speed recovery of function, particularly of the humerus. Surgical stabilization of the spine may also be used in selected circumstances (provided the patient has an anticipated survival time of more than 3 months) with open or minimally invasive procedures such as kyphoplasty and vertebroplasty, and can result in significant pain relief and reduction in risk of cord and nerve root compression.

2. **External-beam therapy.** Radiation doses of 15 to 20 Gy in three to five fractions lead to complete relief of pain in about 50% of patients, with an additional 30% of patients having some decrease in pain; 80% to 90% show significant improvement with 30 to 40 Gy. The alleviation of symptoms can be expected within 2 to 3 weeks. For patients who may be expected to have more prolonged survival, higher doses over a larger number of fractions may be used. Most patients receive optimal results from courses of 30 Gy in 10 fractions (2 weeks) or 40 Gy in 15 fractions (3 weeks).

   Radiotherapy fields should include the area of evident bone involvement, as shown on radiograph and bone scan, with a sufficient extension to prevent relapse at the portal margin. It is seldom necessary to treat an entire long bone unless the entire bone is involved because encroachment on marrow reserve may compromise any systemic chemotherapy that might also be indicated.

3. **Strontium-89 therapy.** A different approach to the therapy of symptomatic bone metastases is through the use of radioisotopes, such as strontium-89, which is given by IV injection. This isotope is highly selective for bone, is an emitter of beta radiation, and has low penetration into surrounding tissue. The affinity of strontium to metastatic bone disease is reported to be 2 to 25 times greater than its affinity to normal bone. This therapy is especially useful in patients with breast or prostate cancer who have many metastatic bone sites or who have received maximal external-beam irradiation to a specific site. Pain relief may occur as early as 1 to 2 weeks after the first injection. Ten percent to twenty percent of patients experience complete pain relief. Another 50% to 60% have at least a moderate reduction in symptoms. Responses last 3 to 6 months. Patients who experience some relief of symptoms may receive multiple doses at 3-month intervals if there has been adequate hematologic recovery.

   The toxicity of strontium-89 is primarily hematologic, involving both leukocytes and platelets. About 10% of patients may experience a transient "flare" of their bone pain. This flare reaction often foreshadows a response to treatment. Other radioisotopes for the palliation of painful bone metastases include samarium-153 and rhenium-186.

4. **Bisphosphonates.** Pamidronate and zoledronic acid are specific inhibitors of osteoclastic activity. They not only are effective for the treatment of hypercalcemia associated with malignancy but can reduce bone pain and reduce fractures, especially in multiple myeloma, breast cancer, and prostate cancer. Zoledronic acid appears to be more effective than pamidronate in reducing the risk of skeletal-related events.

Selected Readings

Allon M, Shanklin N. Effect of bicarbonate administration on plasma potassium in dialysis patients: interactions with insulin and albuterol. *Am J Kidney Dis.* 1996;28:508–514.

Arrambide K, Toto RD. Tumor lysis syndrome. *Semin Nephrol.* 1993;13:273–280.

Brown JE, Neville-Webbe H, Coleman RE. The role of bisphosphonates in breast and prostate cancers. *Endocr Relat Cancer.* 2004;11:207–224.

Ciesielski-Carlucci C, Leong P, Jacobs C. Case report of anaphylaxis from cisplatin/paclitaxel and a review of their hypersensitivity reaction profiles. *Am J Clin Oncol.* 1997;20:373–375.

Cooper PR, Errico TJ, Martin R, et al. A systematic approach to spinal reconstruction after anterior decompression for neoplastic disease of the thoracic and lumbar spine. *Neurosurgery.* 1993;32:1–8.

Courtheoux P, Alkofer B, Al Refai M, Gervais R, Le Rochais JP, Icard P. Stent placement in superior vena cava syndrome. *Ann Thorac Surg.* 2003;75:158–161.

Escalante CP. Causes and management of superior vena cava syndrome. *Oncology.* 1993;7:61.

Garmatis CJ, Chu FC. The effectiveness of radiation therapy in the treatment of bone metastases from breast cancer. *Radiology.* 1978;126:235.

George R, Jeba J, Ramkumar G, et al. Interventions for the treatment of metastatic extradural spinal cord compression in adults. *Cochrane Database Syst Rev.* 2008;(4):CD006716.

Gray BH, Olin JW, Graor RA, et al. Safety and efficacy of thrombolytic therapy for superior vena cava syndrome. *Chest.* 1991;99:54–59.

Greenberg A. Hyperkalemia: treatment options. *Semin Nephrol.* 1998;18:46–57.

Kademani D, Koka S, Lacy MQ, Rajkumar SV. Primary surgical therapy for osteonecrosis of the jaw secondary to bisphosphonate therapy. *Mayo Clin Proc.* 2006;81:1100–1103.

Major P, Lortholary A, Hon J, et al. Zoledronic acid is superior to pamidronate in the treatment of hypercalcemia of malignancy: a pooled analysis of two randomized, controlled clinical trials. *J Clin Oncol.* 2001;19:558–567.

Man Z, Otero AB, Rendo P, et al. Use of pamidronate for multiple myeloma osteolytic lesions. *Lancet.* 1990;335:663.

Noel G, Bollet MA, Noel S, et al. Linac stereotactic radiosurgery: an effective and safe treatment for elderly patients with brain metastases. *Int J Radiat Oncol Biol Phys.* 2005;63:1555–1561.

Patchell RA, Tibbs PA, Regine WF, et al. Direct decompressive surgical resection in the treatment of spinal cord compression caused by metastatic cancer: a randomised trial. *Lancet.* 2005;366:643–648.

Porter AT, Davis LP. Systemic radionuclide therapy of bone metastases with strontium-89. *Oncology.* 1994;8:93.

Rades D, Fehlauer F, Schulte R, et al. Prognostic factors for local control and survival after radiotherapy of metastatic spinal cord compression. *J Clin Oncol.* 2006;24:3388–3393.

Rades D, Stalpers LJ, Schulte R, et al. Defining the appropriate radiotherapy regimen for metastatic spinal cord compression in non-small cell lung cancer patients. *Eur J Cancer.* 2006;42:1052–1056.

Seifert V, Zimmerman M, Stolke D, et al. Spondylectomy, microsurgical decompression and osteosynthesis in the treatment of complex disorders of the cervical spine. *Acta Neurochir (Wien).* 1993;124:104–113.

Stafinski T, Jhangri GS, Yan E, Menon D. Effectiveness of stereotactic radiosurgery alone or in combination with whole brain radiotherapy compared to conventional surgery and/or whole brain radiotherapy for the treatment of one or more brain metastases: a systematic review and meta-analysis. *Cancer Treat Rev.* 2006; 32:203–213.

Thiebaud D, Leyvraz S, von Fliedner V, et al. Treatment of bone metastases from breast cancer and myeloma with pamidronate. *Eur J Cancer.* 1991;27:37–41.

Weissman DE. Steroid treatment of CNS metastases. *J Clin Oncol.* 1988;6:543–551.

Witham TF, Khavkin YA, Gallia GL, Wolinsky JP, Gokaslan ZL. Surgery insight: current management of epidural spinal cord compression from metastatic spine disease. *Nat Clin Pract Neurol.* 2006;2:87–94.

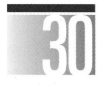

Malignant Pleural, Peritoneal, and Pericardial Effusions and Meningeal Infiltrates

Rekha T. Chaudhary

Malignant pleural, peritoneal, and pericardial effusions and malignant meningeal infiltrates are uncommon early in the course of the malignancy. They occur more frequently with disseminated disease and often herald a poor prognosis. Although pleural and peritoneal effusions may initially have little adverse effect on quality of life, when progressive, they can result in incapacitating disability and death. Effusions can denote a poor prognosis; for example, the median survival after a diagnosis of a malignant pleural effusion is 4 months. It is therefore necessary for the clinician to have a high index of suspicion for these problems and to be prepared to take appropriate action and deliver palliative treatment promptly.

I. PLEURAL EFFUSIONS

A. Causes

Malignant pleural effusions arise in association with malignant cells lining the pleura, exuded into the pleural space, or blocking veins or lymphatics. The most common malignancy associated with pleural effusions in women is carcinoma of the breast; in men, it is carcinoma of the lung. Other causes of malignant pleural effusions include lymphoma, mesothelioma, and carcinomas of the ovary, gastrointestinal tract, urinary tract, and uterus. Malignancy is not the only cause of effusions, even in patients with known neoplastic disease; therefore, it is important to attempt to exclude other possible causes such as congestive heart failure, infection, and pulmonary infarction.

B. **Diagnosis**

1. **Clinical diagnosis.** Effusions may be asymptomatic or may be suspected because of respiratory symptoms such as shortness of breath with exertion or at rest, orthopnea, paroxysmal nocturnal dyspnea, or occasionally chest pressure or cough. The patient may feel more comfortable when lying on one side when the effusion is unilateral. On physical examination, dullness to percussion, decreased tactile fremitus, diminished breath sounds, and egophony are typical signs over the area of the effusion.

2. **A chest radiograph** should be obtained to confirm the clinical impression. If fluid appears to be present, a lateral decubitus film must be obtained to help estimate the volume of the effusion and how free it is within the pleural space.

3. **Diagnostic thoracentesis** should be performed. Ultrasonographic guidance is helpful if loculation is present. Fluid should be obtained for bacterial, acid-fast, and fungal cultures, for cytologic examination, and for determining protein concentration (greater than 3 g/dL in most exudates), lactate dehydrogenase (LDH) level, specific gravity, and cell count. The cytologic examination is important, because if the results are positive, as in 50% to 70% of patients with malignant effusion, the diagnosis is established. Other parameters of the pleural fluid that may be helpful in establishing that the fluid is an exudate and not a transudate include a specific gravity of more than 1.015, protein concentration that is more than 0.5 times the serum protein concentration, LDH level more than 0.6 times the serum LDH level, and low glucose level. A cytologic examination of fluid from a newly discovered pleural effusion is wise, regardless of whether the patient is known to have malignancy, because for nearly half of all malignant effusions, this finding is the first sign of malignancy. Analyzing pleural fluid for carcinoembryonic antigen (CEA) may be helpful in some patients. Levels higher than 20 ng/mL are suggestive of adenocarcinoma, although they do not substitute for a tissue diagnosis in patients who have no history of malignancy. CEA elevations may be seen in adenocarcinomas from various primary sites including the breast, lung, and gastrointestinal tract. Elevated levels between 10 and 20 ng/mL

may reflect malignancy or benign disorders such as pulmonary infection. The role of assessing other tumor markers on a routine basis has not been established. Likewise, the utility of monoclonal antibodies and gene rearrangement studies in patients with lymphomas to distinguish reactive mesothelial or lymphocytic cells from malignant cells has yet to be determined. The routine use of a "panel of tumor markers" is costly, time-consuming, and not recommended.

4. **Pleural biopsy** may be helpful in establishing the diagnosis in up to 20% of patients for whom the pleural fluid cytology results are negative.

5. **Thoracotomy or pleuroscopy** with direct biopsy may be done in patients who have negative cytology and pleural biopsy results but in whom there is still high suspicion of malignancy.

C. Treatment

As malignant pleural effusions are generally a sign of systemic rather than localized disease, the best therapy is treatment that effectively treats the malignancy systemically. Unfortunately, effective systemic treatment is often not possible, particularly when the malignancy is commonly refractory to systemic treatment (e.g., in non–small-cell carcinoma of the lung) or in patients who have previously been heavily treated and in whom systemic therapy is no longer effective. In these circumstances, locoregional therapy is required for palliation of the patient's symptoms.

1. **Drainage.** Many malignant pleural effusions recur within 1 to 3 days after simple thoracentesis; about 97% recur within 1 month. Chest tube drainage (closed tube thoracotomy) allows the pleural surfaces to oppose each other and, if maintained for several days, may result in obliteration of the space and improvement in the effusion for several weeks to months. It does not appear to be as effective when used alone as when a cytotoxic or sclerosing agent is added, and therefore, one of these agents is commonly instilled into the space while the chest tube is in place. Repeated thoracentesis is an option in patients who reaccumulate slowly (greater than 1 month).

2. **Cytotoxic and sclerosing agents or pleurodesis.** The most widely used agents for intrapleural administration are bleomycin, doxycycline, and talc. Other agents, including fluorouracil, interferon-α, and methylprednisolone acetate, have been less commonly used. Randomized studies have suggested that bleomycin may be more effective than doxycycline (in part because doxycycline sometimes requires multiple dose administrations) and that talc is either equal to or slightly better than bleomycin in terms of recurrence. The agents vary in toxicity, ease of administration, and cost. Additionally, institutional experience often determines the agent utilized. Nevertheless, for optimal

effectiveness, drainage of pleural fluid as completely as possible is required before instillation.

a. **Method of administration.** The drug to be used is diluted in 50 to 100 mL of saline and instilled through the thoracostomy tube into the chest cavity after the effusion has been drained for at least 24 hours and the rate of collection is less than 100 mL/24 h. Throughout the procedure, care must be taken to avoid any air leak. The thoracostomy tube is clamped, and the patient is successively repositioned on his or her front, back, and sides for 15-minute periods during the next 2 to 6 hours. The tube is then reconnected to gravity drainage or suction for at least 18 hours to ensure that the pleural surfaces remain opposed and to prevent the rapid accumulation of any fluid in reaction to the instillation. Some clinicians repeat the instillation daily for a total of 2 to 3 days. For most of the agents, this has no proven benefit. Exceptions include methylprednisolone acetate and doxycycline, which appear to be more effective with additional doses. If the drainage is less than 40 to 50 mL over the previous 12 hours, the tube may be removed and a chest radiograph obtained to be certain that pneumothorax has not occurred during removal of the tube. If the thoracostomy tube continues to drain more than 100 mL/24 h after the last instillation, it may be necessary to leave it in place for an additional 48 to 72 hours to ensure that a maximum amount of adhesion between the pleural surfaces has taken place. Because the use of sclerotic agents can be painful, it is prudent for the clinician to consider the use of scheduled narcotic analgesia, particularly during the initial 24 hours.

b. **Recommended agents.** Efficacy, side effects, cost, and institutional (operator) experience must be considered when choosing a sclerosing agent. Bleomycin, in one prospective study, was shown to be more effective than tetracycline. It is also more expensive per dose than the other agents. Talc is the least expensive, but this must be balanced against the costs of related procedures, including thoracoscopy and anesthesia. Talc is probably superior to bleomycin in terms of recurrence rate of effusions at 90 days and later.

(1) **Bleomycin** 1 mg/kg or 40 mg/m^2 has relatively little myelosuppressive effect and is highly effective.

(2) **Talc** 5 g is given typically as a powder (poudrage). It is highly effective but requires thoracoscopy and general anesthesia. Rarely, adult respiratory distress syndrome has been reported, primarily with doses greater than 10 g. If the patient is a high risk for general anesthesia, talc slurry may be administered at the bedside, though it is probably less effective than the thoracoscopic poudrage.

    (3) Doxycycline 500 mg may cause pleuritic chest pain. An injection of 10 mL of 1% lidocaine (100 mg) through the chest tube may reduce this symptom.

  c. Alternative agents

    (1) Fluorouracil 2 to 3 g (total dose) may have a theoretical advantage in sensitive carcinomas, but whether that advantage has practical significance is not established. Pain is generally minimal. Occasional patients may experience a depressed white blood cell count, especially at the higher dose.

    (2) Interferon-α 50×10^6 U typically causes influenza-like symptoms. Lower doses appear to be ineffective. Patients should be premedicated with acetaminophen 650 mg before and then 6 hours after interferon administration. Meperidine 25 mg intravenously by slow push may be given for rigors from interferon.

    (3) Methylprednisolone acetate 80 to 160 mg appears to be well tolerated.

  d. Responses. Chest tube drainage together with instillation of one of the agents discussed in Section I.C.2.b or c controls pleural effusions more than 75% of the time. The durations of response are often short, with a median between 3 and 6 months unless the patient's systemic disease comes under adequate control. In that circumstance, the effusion may not recur for years or at least until the systemic disease once more emerges.

  e. Side effects common to most agents include chest pain, fever, and occasional hypotension. These effects are usually not severe and may be controlled by standard symptomatic management. Fever after pleurodesis is usually not due to infection.

3. Indwelling pleural catheter placement is another option for patients who have recurrent pleural effusions. It involves placement of a soft, flexible, valved catheter connected to a drainage kit into the pleural space. Patients must be willing to care for the catheter on an outpatient basis but in contrast to a standard chest tube and pleurodesis, it allows the patient to be treated as an outpatient. It has similar efficacy to pleurodesis, but carries an added risk of infection owing to the indwelling catheter. Spontaneous pleurodesis may occur after 1 month or more of pleural catheter placement.

4. Thoracotomy and pleural stripping may be tried subsequently for effusions refractory to other medical treatment, when the prognosis is otherwise good.

II. PERITONEAL EFFUSIONS

A. Causes

Malignant peritoneal effusions usually occur in association with diffuse seeding of the peritoneal surface with small malignant deposits.

The impairment of subphrenic lymphatic or portal venous flow may result in peritoneal effusions. Alternatively, it has been postulated that a "capillary leak" phenomenon mediated by tumor cells or immune effector cells could be a contributing factor. Carcinoma of the ovary is the most commonly associated malignancy in women, whereas in men, gastrointestinal carcinomas are most common. Other neoplasms that may cause peritoneal effusions include carcinoma of unknown primary, lymphoma, mesothelioma, and carcinomas of the uterus and breast. Liver metastasis by itself, unless it is far advanced, is not usually associated with symptomatic peritoneal effusions.

B. **Diagnosis**

1. **Symptoms and signs.** Patients may be completely symptom-free or have so much fluid that they have severe abdominal distention, abdominal pain, and respiratory distress. In the presence of peritoneal metastases, there may be abnormal bowel motility that at times resembles a paralytic ileus and may result in loss of appetite, early satiety, nausea, and vomiting. On examination, the lower abdomen and flanks bulge when the patient is supine. Confirmatory signs include shifting dullness, a fluid wave, diminished bowel sounds, or the "puddle sign" (periumbilical dullness when the patient rests on knees and elbows).

2. **Radiographic studies.** Ascites may be suggested on a recumbent film of the abdomen, although radiographs are less sensitive than computed tomography (CT) or ultrasound in detecting fluid. CT is also helpful in defining whether there are enlarged retroperitoneal nodes, tumor masses in the abdomen or pelvis, or liver metastases in association with the ascites.

3. **Paracentesis** is used to distinguish malignancy from other causes of peritoneal effusions, including congestive heart failure, hepatic cirrhosis, and peritonitis. Malignant cells are found in about half of patients in whom the effusion is due to malignancy. Other tests are less reliable, and treatment decisions must often be based on incomplete data. Elevated LDH and protein levels, along with a negative Gram stain and cultures, are supportive but nonspecific for malignancy. The use of monoclonal antibodies to identify tumor cells is still experimental. The serum-ascites albumin gradient (SAAG) is also useful. The SAAG is simply calculated by subtracting the ascitic fluid albumin from the serum albumin. If the gradient is at least 1.1 g/dL, the ascites is most likely from portal hypertension, congestive heart failure, or from massive hepatic metastases in a patient with cancer. If the gradient is less than 1.1 g/dL in a patient with cancer, the more likely cause is peritoneal metastasis or another inflammatory condition.

C. Therapy

As with malignant pleural effusions, malignant peritoneal effusions as a rule are optimally treated with effective systemic therapy. (The possible exception to this is peritoneal effusions from carcinoma of the ovary. In this circumstance, there may be an advantage to intraperitoneal therapy, at least as one component of therapy, because most systemic disease is on the peritoneal surface.) If the patient is resistant to all further systemic treatment, regional treatment should be tried, but the likelihood of success is less and the complications greater with peritoneal effusions than with pleural effusions. Success probably is less because of the greater likelihood of loculations to areas inaccessible to therapy and the impossibility of obliterating the peritoneal space in the same way that the pleural space can be obliterated. Complications are greater because of the increase in adhesions caused by instillation therapy and the resultant increase in obstructive bowel problems.

1. **Paracentesis** may be helpful in acutely relieving intra-abdominal pressure. If the ascites has caused impairment of respiration, paracentesis may give temporary relief. Rapid withdrawal of large volumes of fluid (more than 1 L) can result in hypotension and shock, however, and if frequent paracenteses are performed, severe hypoalbuminemia and electrolyte imbalance may result. Repeated procedures could also subject the patient to increased risk of peritonitis or bowel injury. This procedure thus results in only temporary benefit.

2. **Bed rest and dietary salt restriction,** although helpful in the treatment of various nonmalignant causes of ascites, are of less benefit in malignant ascites.

3. **Diuretics** may be helpful in reducing ascites, but care must be taken not to be too vigorous in attempts at diuresis because of the possibility of dehydration and hypotension. A reasonable choice of diuretic is a combination of either furosemide 40 mg or hydrochlorothiazide 50 to 100 mg/day and spironolactone 50 to 100 mg/day.

4. **Intracavitary therapy.** Radioisotopes, cytotoxic drugs, and sclerosing agents have been used with some benefit for treating malignant ascites, but overall probably fewer than half of patients have a satisfactory response. The utility of these agents has less to do with direct tumor cytotoxicity and more with the induction of a local inflammatory response with subsequent sclerosis. The radioactive isotopes gold-198 and phosphorus-32 should be used only by those with experience and appropriate certification. Cytotoxic agents such as fluorouracil are associated with less risk to the person administering the therapy.

   a. **Method.** The peritoneal fluid should be drained slowly through a Tenckhoff catheter over a 24- to 36-hour period.

The potential distribution of the therapeutic agent can be determined by instilling technetium-99m–glucoheptonate macroaggregated albumin in 50 mL of saline and obtaining an abdominal scintigram. Two liters of warmed 1.5% peritoneal dialysate solution is instilled, allowed to remain for 2 hours, and then drained. The chemotherapeutic agent is next mixed with 2 L of fresh 1.5% dialysate solution containing 1000 U of heparin/L. After warming, this solution is instilled through the Tenckhoff catheter. For some agents, draining after 4 hours is recommended.

  b. Agents
    (1) Cisplatin 50 to 100 mg/m^2 (especially for carcinoma of the ovary). Drainage is optional. Saline diuresis is recommended. Dosages higher than 100 mg/m^2 should not be used without protection by intravenous sodium thiosulfate. Cisplatin is repeated every 3 weeks.
    (2) Fluorouracil 1000 mg (total dose) in normal saline with 25 mEq of sodium bicarbonate/L. Drainage is optional. Treatment is given on days 1 to 4 monthly.
    (3) Mitoxantrone 10 mg/m^2. Drainage is optional. This dose has been administered on a weekly basis, although white blood cell counts must be monitored.
    (4) Interferon-α 50 × 10^6 U (for ovarian cancer). Drainage is optional. This dose has been administered weekly for 4 weeks or longer. Patients should be premedicated with acetaminophen before and every 4 hours on the day of therapy.
    (5) Floxuridine 3 g in 1.5 to 2 L of normal saline given daily for 3 days every 3 to 4 weeks has been used in colon, gastric, and ovarian cancer.
    (6) Other agents that have been used intraperitoneally include carboplatin, paclitaxel, methotrexate, cytosine arabinoside, etoposide, bleomycin, thiotepa, and doxorubicin. High-dose interleukin (IL)-2 with lymphokine-activated killer cells has shown activity in ovarian and colorectal cancer but at the cost of significant toxicity, including peritoneal fibrosis, which in general has prevented the administration of more than one or two cycles. Lower-dose IL-2, 6 × 10^6 IU, on days 1 and 7 has been used successfully.
  5. Peritoneal-venous shunts (Denver shunt, LeVeen shunt) may offer palliative relief for refractory ascites because recurrent paracentesis leads to infection and leakage of peritoneal fluid through the paracentesis sites. Potential disadvantages are shunt occlusion, the systemic dissemination of cancer, and disseminated intravascular coagulation.

III. PERICARDIAL EFFUSIONS

Although 5% to 10% of patients dying with disseminated malignancy have cardiac or pericardial metastases, far fewer have symptomatic pericardial effusion. However, although malignant pericardial effusions are not particularly common, they are of great importance because of their potential to cause acute cardiac tamponade and death.

A. Causes

The most common neoplasms causing pericardial effusions are carcinomas of the lung and breast, lymphomas, and melanoma.

B. Diagnosis

1. **Clinical diagnosis.** Patients with developing cardiac tamponade may exhibit a variety of grave symptoms including extreme anxiety, dyspnea, orthopnea, precordial chest pain, cough, and hoarseness. On examination, they are likely to have engorged neck veins, generalized edema, tachycardia, distant heart tones, lateral displacement of the cardiac apex, a low systolic blood pressure and low pulse pressure, and a paradoxical pulse. They may also have tachypnea and a pericardial friction rub.

2. **Electrocardiogram** (ECG) may show nonspecific low-voltage, T-wave abnormalities, elevation of ST segments, and ventricular alternans or the more specific total electrical alternans. Premature beats and atrial fibrillation also occur.

3. **Chest radiograph** typically shows an enlarged cardiac silhouette, often with a bulging appearance suggestive of an effusion ("water-bottle heart"). There is frequently an associated pleural effusion.

4. **Echocardiography** can confirm the diagnosis and provide important information on the location of the effusion within the pericardium.

5. **Pericardiocentesis** reveals neoplastic cells on cytologic examination in more than 75% of patients.

C. Treatment

1. **Volume expansion and vasopressor support** are applied (if necessary) to maintain blood pressure. Adequate oxygenation must be maintained. Diuretics are contraindicated.

2. **Pericardiocentesis** under ECG and blood pressure monitoring should be done in emergent circumstances. If the patient can be stabilized or in cases of pericardial effusion without tamponade, pericardiocentesis under two-dimensional ECG is preferable because it significantly reduces the incidence of cardiac laceration, arrhythmia, and tension pneumothorax as a complication of the procedure.

3. **Instillation of chemotherapeutic or sclerosing agents.** Because pain may be associated with the intrapericardial therapy, lidocaine (Xylocaine) 100 mg may be administered intrapericardially as a local anesthetic. (Check with the cardiologist on the safety for each patient.) After the cytotoxic or sclerosing agent is instilled,

the pericardial catheter is clamped for 1 to 2 hours and then allowed to drain. One of the following agents may be used.

a. **Fluorouracil** 500 to 1000 mg in aqueous solution as supplied commercially. This dose is generally not repeated.

b. **Thiotepa** 25 mg/m^2 in 10 mL of normal saline may be preferred in tumors deemed sensitive to alkylating agents. Myelosuppression may occur. The dose is usually not repeated.

Complications of intrapericardial therapy include arrhythmias, pain, and fever.

4. **Radiotherapy** with radioisotopes or 2000 to 4000 cGy of external-beam therapy may help control effusions.

5. **Systemic chemotherapy** (with standard regimens) after pericardiocentesis is a possible alternative for newly diagnosed, potentially responsive malignancies such as lymphomas. Chemotherapy, intrapericardial or systemic, or radiotherapy controls the effusion for at least 30 days in 60% to 70% of patients.

6. **Surgery** to create a pericardial window may be necessary and can be effective for several months. It is not recommended, however, unless simpler measures fail.

IV. MALIGNANT SUBARACHNOID INFILTRATES

A. Causes

Leptomeningeal involvement with non–central nervous system cancer is an uncommon complication of most neoplasms, although in children with acute lymphocytic leukemia who have not received prophylactic treatment, the incidence approaches 50%. Of the nonleukemic diseases, breast carcinoma and lymphomas (primarily Burkitt and T-cell lymphoblastic) account for about 30% each in cases of malignant subarachnoid infiltrates. Carcinoma of the lung and melanoma account for 10% to 12% each.

B. Diagnosis

1. **Clinical diagnosis.** Patients commonly present with headache, change in mental status, cranial nerve dysfunction, or spinal root–derived pain, paresthesia, or weakness. Any onset of change in neurologic status, particularly of cerebral, cranial nerve, or spinal root origin, should alert the clinician to the possibility of subarachnoid infiltrates.

2. **Diagnostic studies**

   a. **CT or magnetic resonance imaging (MRI) of the head** should be done to look for any intracranial mass. If none is present, a lumbar puncture should be done.

   b. **A lumbar puncture** is done to obtain 8 to 12 mL of cerebrospinal fluid (CSF) fluid; 4 mL may be frozen to use for subsequent studies when initial evaluation is inconclusive. The following are evaluated or performed:

   ▪ Opening pressure

   ▪ Cytology of centrifugal specimen for malignant cells

- Total cell count and differential
- CSF chemistry, including glucose and protein
- Microbiologic studies as indicated by the clinical situation: India ink or cryptococcal antigen determination, Gram stain, cultures (routine, acid-fast, fungi), serum toxoplasma titer, CSF viral (e.g., Epstein-Barr virus, cytomegalovirus, HIV, and herpes simplex virus) polymerase chain reaction, and other special studies.

  c. **MRI of the spine** (or less commonly, myelography with CT follow-up) is performed if signs or symptoms of cord compression are present.

C. Treatment

Malignant subarachnoid infiltrates may be treated with radiotherapy, intrathecal chemotherapy, or a combination of the two.

1. **Radiotherapy.** The radiation field is usually limited to the most involved field (frequently the brain), and intrathecal chemotherapy is used to control the infiltrates elsewhere. This technique is used even though the entire neuraxis is usually involved because total craniospinal irradiation causes severe myelosuppression, which limits the patient's tolerance to concurrent or subsequent cytotoxic chemotherapy.

2. **Chemotherapy** may be administered by lumbar puncture or preferably into a surgically implanted (Ommaya) reservoir that communicates with the lateral ventricle. The latter has the advantages of being easily accessible in patients who require repeated treatments and of giving a better distribution of drug than can be obtained through lumbar puncture. When the Ommaya reservoir is used, a volume of CSF equal to that to be injected (6 to 10 mL) should be removed through the reservoir with a small-caliber needle. The chemotherapy should then be given as a slow injection. When the chemotherapy is given through lumbar puncture, the volume of injection (usually 7 to 10 mL) should be greater than that of the CSF withdrawn, so as to have a higher closing than opening pressure. This method facilitates distribution of the drug and minimizes postlumbar puncture headache. The most commonly used drugs for intrathecal therapy are the following.

   a. **Methotrexate** 12 mg/m^2 (maximum 15 mg) twice weekly until the CSF clears of malignant cells, then monthly.

   b. **Cytarabine** 30 mg/m^2 (maximum 50 mg) twice weekly until the CSF clears of malignant cells, then monthly.

   c. **Liposomal cytarabine** 50 mg (total dose) is given every 14 days for two doses. If the CSF clears, give 50 mg every 14 days for two additional doses. Then give 50 mg every 4 weeks for two additional doses (total of six doses).

    d. Thiotepa 2 to 10 mg/m^2 twice weekly until the CSF clears of malignant cells, then monthly.

        Each of the agents is given in preservative-free saline or, if available, buffered preservative-free diluent similar to Elliot B solution. Any subsequent flush solution should be of similar composition. Other drugs used to treat effusions (e.g., fluorouracil, mechlorethamine, or radioisotopes) must *not* be used to treat meningeal disease.

D. Response to treatment

Most patients with meningeal leukemia or lymphoma respond to a combination of radiotherapy and intrathecal chemotherapy. Carcinomas are less likely to improve, but mild to moderate improvement may be seen in up to 50% of patients.

E. Complications

Aseptic meningitis or arachnoiditis, seizures, acute encephalopathy, myelopathy, leukoencephalopathy, and radicular neuropathy may result from intrathecal chemotherapy with or without radiotherapy. Bone marrow suppression is not usually severe unless the patient undergoes spinal irradiation or systemic chemotherapy as well. Oral leucovorin can be given after the intrathecal methotrexate (10 mg leucovorin by mouth every 6 hours for six to eight doses, starting either at the same time or 24 hours after the methotrexate) to prevent marrow toxicity. Serious complications are infrequent, however, and in patients with advanced metastatic disease, they usually are not a major problem.

Selected Readings

Pleural Effusions

Andrews CO, Gora W. Pleural effusions: pathophysiology and management. *Ann Pharmacother.* 1994;28:894–903.

de Campos JR, Vargas FS, de Campos Werebe E, et al. Thoracoscopy talc poudrage: a 15-year experience. *Chest.* 2001;119:801–806.

Diacon AH, Wyser C, Bollinger CT, et al. Prospective randomized comparison of thoracoscopic talc poudrage under local anesthesia versus bleomycin instillation for pleurodesis in malignant pleural effusions. *Am J Respir Crit Care Med.* 2000;162:1445–1449.

Fuller DK. Bleomycin versus doxycyclines: a patient-oriented approach to pleurodesis. *Ann Pharmacother.* 1993;27:794.

Herrington JD. Chemical pleurodesis, with doxycycline 1 g. *Pharmacotherapy.* 1996;16:290–295.

Johnson WW. The malignant pleural effusion: a review of cytopathologic diagnoses of 584 specimens from 472 consecutive patients. *Cancer.* 1985;56:905.

Kessinger A, Wigton RS. Intracavitary bleomycin and tetracycline in the management of malignant pleural effusions: a randomized study. *J Surg Oncol.* 1997;36:81–83.

Patz EF Jr, McAdams HP, Erasmus JJ, et al. Sclerotherapy for malignant pleural effusions: a prospective randomized trial of bleomycin vs. doxycyline with small-bore catheter drainage. *Chest.* 1998;113:1305–1311.

Putnam JB Jr, Walsh GL, Swisher SG, et al. Outpatient management of malignant pleural effusion by a chronic indwelling catheter. *Ann Thorac Surg.* 2000;69:369–375.

Stefani A, Natali P, Casali C, Morandi U. Talc poudrage versus talc slurry in the treatment of malignant pleural effusion. A prospective comparative study. *Eur J Cardiothorac Surg.* 2006;30:827–832.

Tremblay A, Mason C, Michaud G. Use of tunnelled catheters for malignant pleural effusions in patients fit for pleurodesis. *Eur Respir J.* 2007;30(4):759–762.

Van Hoff DD, LiVolsi V. Diagnostic reliability of needle biopsy of the parietal pleura: a review of 272 biopsies. *Am J Clin Pathol.* 1975;64:200.

Walker-Renard PB, Vaughan LM, Sahn SA. Chemical pleurodesis for malignant pleural effusions. *Ann Intern Med.* 1994;120:56–64.

Peritoneal Effusions

Lacy JH, Wieman TJ, Shivley EH. Management of malignant ascites. *Surg Gynecol Obstet.* 1984;159:397.

Muggia FM, Liu PY, Alberts DS, et al. Intraperitoneal mitoxantrone or floxuridine: effects on time-to-failure and survival in patients with minimal residual ovarian cancer after second-look laparotomy: a randomized phase II study by the Southwest Oncology Group. *Gynecol Oncol.* 1996;61:395–402.

Speyer JL, Beller U, Colombo N, et al. Intraperitoneal carboplatin: favorable results in women with minimal residual ovarian cancer after cisplatin therapy. *J Clin Oncol.* 1990;8:1335–1341.

Sugarbaker PH, Gianola FJ, Speyer JC, et al. Prospective, randomized trial of intravenous versus intraperitoneal 5-fluorouracil in patients with advanced primary colon or rectal cancer. *Surgery.* 1985;95:414.

Pericardial Effusions

Buzaid AC, Garewal HS, Greenberg BR. Managing malignant pericardial effusion. *West J Med.* 1989;150:174–179.

Callahan JA, Seward JB, Nishimura RA, et al. Two-dimensional echocardiographically guided pericardiocentesis: experience in 117 consecutive patients. *Am J Cardiol.* 1985;55:476–479.

Helms SR, Carlson MD. Cardiovascular emergencies. *Semin Oncol.* 1989;16:463.

Liu G, Crump M, Gross PE, et al. Prospective comparison of the sclerosing agents doxycycline and bleomycin for the primary management of malignant pericardial effusion and cardiac tamponade. *J Clin Oncol.* 1996;14:3141–3147.

Maher ER, Buckman R. Intrapericardial installation of bleomycin in malignant pericardial effusion. *Am Heart J.* 1986;111:613–614.

Runyon BA, Montano AA, Akriviadis EA, Antillon MR, Irving MA, McHutchison JG. The serum-ascites albumin gradient is superior to the exudate-transudate concept in the differential diagnosis of ascites. *Ann Intern Med.* 1992;117(3):215–220.

Shepherd FA, Ginsberg JS, Evans WK, et al. Tetracycline sclerosis in the management of pericardial effusion. *J Clin Oncol.* 1985;3:1678–1682.

Malignant Subarachnoid Infiltrates

Glantz MJ, Jaeckle KA, Chamberlain MC, et al. A randomized controlled trial comparing intrathecal sustained-release cytarabine (Depocyt) to intrathecal methotrexate in patients with neoplastic meningitis from solid tumors. *Clin Cancer Res.* 1999;5:3394–3402.

Grossman SA, Krabak MJ. Leptomeningeal carcinomatosis. *Cancer Treat Rev.* 1999;25: 103–119.

Grossman SA. Advances in the treatment of central nervous system metastases: treatment of leptomeningeal metastasis. In: *American Society of Clinical Oncology, Educational Book.* Alexandria, VA: American Society of Clinical Oncology; 2001: 598–604.

Gutin PH, Levi JA, Wiernik PH, et al. Treatment of malignant meningeal disease with intrathecal thiotepa: a phase II study. *Cancer Treat Rep.* 1977;61:885–887.

Jaeckle KA, Phuphanich S, van den Bent MJ, et al. Intrathecal treatment of neoplastic meningitis due to breast cancer with a slow-release formulation of cytarabine. *Br J Cancer.* 2001;84:157–163.

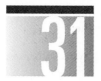

Cancer Pain

Richard T. Lee and Michael J. Fisch

It is likely that 85% of patients with cancer could be free of significant pain with the techniques we have available today. Most pain from cancer can be adequately controlled with analgesics given by mouth. When this is not possible, various more sophisticated pain management techniques can provide good pain control. Unfortunately, poorly controlled pain and/or analgesic side effects have significant effects on the quality of life of patients and their families. For example, symptoms such as depressed mood, fatigue, anorexia, and sleep disturbance are associated with poor pain control. Likewise, opioid side effects may cause chronic nausea, anorexia, constipation, dehydration, sedation, and confusion. Consequently, overall performance status and adherence to anticancer treatment regimens may deteriorate in the presence of poor pain management. Desperate patients and families may seek relief through unproven therapies or even from physician-assisted suicide. Improving the practice of anticipating, evaluating, and treating pain will benefit most patients.

I. PREVALENCE, SEVERITY, AND RISK FOR PAIN

Most cancer patients with terminal disease need expert pain management. Between 60% and 80% of such patients have significant pain at some point in their trajectory of illness, and nearly 20% of oncology outpatients have moderate to severe pain at any given outpatient visit. Sometimes, chronic pain will be expressed by the patient in confusing terms ("stiffness," "nagging") or masquerade as other symptoms (fatigue, apathy, anxiety, anorexia). For this reason, the estimates of the prevalence and impact of chronic pain in this population are probably conservative. Nevertheless, in the United States, 60% of all outpatients with metastatic disease have cancer-related pain, and one-third report pain so severe that it significantly impairs their quality of life. Multicenter studies indicate that about 40% of outpatients with cancer pain do not receive analgesics potent enough to manage their pain, especially among minority patients, female patients, and older patients.

II. ETIOLOGY OF CANCER PAIN

A. Direct tumor involvement

This is the most common cause of pain and is present in about two-thirds of those with pain from metastatic cancer. Tumor invasion of bone is the physical cause of pain in about 50% of these patients. The remaining 50% of patients experience tumor-related pain that is due to nerve compression, tumor infiltration, or involvement of the gastrointestinal tract or soft tissue.

B. Persistent pain after treatment

Persistent pain from long-term effects of surgery, radiotherapy, and chemotherapy accounts for an additional 20% of all who report pain with cancer, with a small residual group experiencing pain from non–cancer-related conditions. Chronic pain is a common problem for cancer survivors with some studies indicating nearly a third reporting active pain symptoms.

C. Complex, chronic pain

Most patients with advanced cancer have pain at multiple sites caused by multiple mechanisms. Pain production occurs either by stimulation of peripheral pain receptors or by damage to afferent nerve fibers. Peripheral pain receptors can be stimulated by pressure, compression, and traction as well as by disease-related chemical changes. Pain due to stimulation of pain receptors is called *nociceptive pain*. Damage to visceral, somatic, or autonomic nerve trunks produces *neurogenic* or *neuropathic pain*. Neuropathic pain is thought to be caused by spontaneous activity in nerves damaged by disease or treatment. Patients with cancer often simultaneously experience nociceptive and neuropathic pain. In addition to evaluating the broad possible causes of pain production, the evaluating clinician should also consider the relevant mechanisms of pain *perception* and *expression*. Pain perception refers to the transmission of the nociception to the central nervous system (CNS). Peripheral nerve fibers include myelinated $A\delta$ fibers that are responsible for the transmission of sharp pain and unmyelinated C fibers that carry dull and burning pain. These primary sensory afferents have their cell bodies in the dorsal horn, where the pathways decussate and ascend along the spinothalamic tracts to the thalamus and cortex. Repetitive or continuous stimulation of the peripheral nerves can increase the excitability of the secondary neurons and spread the neurologic region of pain perception and transmission. The N-methyl-D-aspartate (NMDA) receptor is involved in the neurobiology of this "wind-up" phenomenon as well as in the development of tolerance to opioid analgesics. Understanding this biology of pain perception helps account for the observation that some patients experience pain that endures even after the tumor or injury has resolved, and sometimes the pain is more severe than one might expect from the nerve or tissue insult itself. Of course, the clinician can directly observe only pain expression; the production and perception of the pain can be inferred only from indirect clues. Pain expression, that is, how patients report or show their pain, can be influenced by multiple factors (mood, cultural beliefs, etc.). For this reason, effective pain assessment and management necessitates a comprehensive understanding of the patient as a person.

III. ASSESSMENT OF PAIN

Proper pain management requires a clear understanding of the characteristics of pain production, perception, and expression, as described previously. The changing expression of cancer pain demands repeated assessment because new causes of pain can emerge rapidly and pain severity can increase quickly. In patients with advanced disease, pain from multiple causes is the rule and not the exception. A careful history includes asking questions concerning the location, severity, and quality of the pain as well as the aspects of the patient's daily routine that may be adversely affected by the pain experience.

Health professionals should also consider a comprehensive evaluation of pain that incorporates several dimensions of health including physical, psychospiritual, and sociocultural. Just as pain may affect patients' moods, anxiety or depression also has been shown to alter patients' perception of pain. Additionally, sociocultural differences in the meaning of pain will alter how patients experience and express their pain symptoms. Identifying these key factors will assist with successful pain management.

A. Pain severity

Inadequate pain assessment and poor physician–patient communication about pain are major barriers to good pain care. Physicians and nurses tend to underestimate pain intensity, especially when it is severe. Patients whose physicians underestimate their pain are at high risk for poor pain management and compromised function. A small minority of patients with cancer may complain of pain in a dramatic fashion, but many more patients underreport the severity of their pain and the lack of adequate pain relief.

Several studies have confirmed that there are multiple reasons for this hesitancy to report pain, including the following:

- Reluctance to acknowledge that the disease is progressing
- Reluctance to divert the physician's attention from treating the disease
- Reluctance to tell the physician that pain treatments are not working.

Patients may not want to be put on opioid analgesics because of the following reasons:

- Fear of addiction
- Concern about possible neurotoxic side effects of opioids (sedation, confusion)
- Frustration over gastrointestinal side effects of opioids (nausea, constipation, anorexia)
- Fear that using opioids "too early" will endanger pain relief when they have more pain
- Fear that opioid use means that death is near
- Having accepted religious or societal norms or teachings that pain should be endured.

Presenting information that addresses these concerns in a straightforward manner will allay most of these fears and should be considered as an essential step in providing pain control. It is important that patients understand that they will function better if their pain is controlled and their opioid side effects are prevented or managed effectively. Patient education materials available from state cancer pain initiatives and from the National Cancer Institute (www.cancer.gov), the American Cancer Society (www.cancer.org), the National Comprehensive Cancer Network (NCCN; www.nccn.org), and the American Society of Clinical Oncology (www.cancer.net) can be very useful for both patients and families and should be given to patients when they develop pain.

Communication about pain is greatly aided by having patients use a scale to rate the severity of their pain. A simple rating scale ranges from 0 to 10, with 0 being "no pain" and 10 being pain "as bad as you can imagine." Used properly, pain severity scales can be invaluable for titrating analgesics and monitoring increases in pain with progressive disease. Mild pain is often well tolerated with minimal impact on a patient's activities. However, there is a threshold beyond which pain is especially disruptive. This threshold has been reached when patients rate the severity of their pain at 5 or greater on a 0 to 10 scale. When pain is too great (7 or greater on this scale), it becomes the primary focus of attention and compromises most activities that are not directly related to pain. Although it may not be possible to eliminate pain totally, reducing its severity to 4 or less should be a minimum standard of pain therapy.

Often, patients may have difficultly relating to a scale of 0 to 10 or communication may be limited due to neurologic deficits. When initially assessing pain, asking what pain level is tolerable to them may assist with a goal pain score. Other times, patients may indicate only minimal changes in their pain score while showing signs of significant improvement. Rather than using the 0 to 10 scale, others may respond better to mild, moderate, or severe while others may be better able to describe differences in pain by stating by what percentage the pain has changed. When communication is limited, questions may focus on behaviors such as sleep, the provider may ask family members about changes in behavior or irritability, or the provider may consider nonverbal cues such as wrinkling of the forehead. Providing patients with different ways in which to express their pain score as well as the provider's ability to collect information will assist with assessing treatment interventions.

In some instances, patients may develop chronically high levels of pain expression that do not respond to appropriate initial analgesic dosing and coprescribing of medications to prevent nausea and constipation. The proper care of this subset of patients often requires a multidisciplinary approach; it includes regular administration of pain medication plus counseling and sometimes use of antidepressants or anxiolytic agents. Skillful switching of opioid medications (often called "opioid rotation" or "opioid switching") can produce a more favorable ratio of analgesia to opioid side effects. Interventional pain procedures may be appropriate in selected cases as well. Such procedures may include nerve blocks (such as a celiac plexus block) or neuraxial delivery of opioids and other adjuvant medications (such as epidural or intrathecal therapies).

B. Diagnostic steps

Those who treat patients with cancer should be familiar with the common pain syndromes associated with the disease:

1. Having the patient show the area of pain on a drawing of a human figure aids identification of the syndrome. This can be particularly helpful in indicating areas of referred pain that commonly coincide with nerve compression.

2. Careful questioning concerning the characteristics of the pain is a key component of diagnosis. For example, pain characterized as "burning" or "shooting" may indicate neuropathic pain.

3. In addition to severity, these characteristics include the temporal pattern of the pain (constant or episodic) and its quality. Episodic or "incident" pain (such as severe pain when standing) requires a different strategy for management than chronic pain.

4. Other important characteristics of pain are its relationship to physical activity and what seems to alleviate the pain.

5. The physical examination includes examination of the painful area as well as neurologic and orthopedic assessment. A brief assessment of mood and cognition is also appropriate. Impaired cognition can confound symptom assessment dramatically.

6. Because bone metastases are a common cause of pain and pain can occur with changes in bone density that is not detectable on radiographs, bone scans can be helpful. Magnetic resonance imaging (MRI) is useful in the evaluation of retroperitoneal, paravertebral, and pelvic areas as well as the base of the skull.

C. The impact of pain on the patient

When pain is of moderate or greater severity, one can assume that it has a negative impact on the patient's quality of life. That impact, including problems with sleep and depression, must be evaluated and treated when appropriate. A reduced number of hours of sleep compared with the last pain-free interval, difficulties with sleep onset, frequent interruptions of sleep, and early morning awakening suggest the need for appropriate pharmacologic intervention. Just as patients hesitate to report severe pain, they may hesitate to report depression. Family caregivers can often provide important clues regarding the presence or absence of a mood disturbance. Significant depression should be treated. Treatment approaches may include use of antidepressants, counseling, and/ or referral to a behavioral health specialist. Sometimes a patient will accept only one of the suggested options, thus requiring some degree of flexibility on the part of the clinician in order to achieve the best results.

It is important to make an attempt to differentiate between physical pain and psychological distress. Accurate pain assessment in patients who are cognitively impaired, particularly those with agitation, may be extremely difficult. A small number of patients in severe psychosocial distress express their concerns as a report of physical pain. These patients present with symptoms that may be attributable to either agitated delirium or pain. Although it is important to recognize severe somatization and to provide psychiatric referral or counseling to these patients, it is equally important to recognize true physical pain. Because of the possible misinterpretation by patients that the medical establishment is atrributing their pain as entirely psychological in nature, a frank discussion with patients regarding the difficulty many patients have distinguishing between physical and emotional pain, which often occur together, may help patients understand your approach and often provide an opportunity to acknowledge different sources of pain they may not have considered. Ultimately, the treatment approach for this difficult situation includes concomitant provision of pain treatment(s) and management of the patient's underlying psychological distress.

D. Addiction/aberrant drug-taking behaviors

Some patients with alcohol or drug addiction may request analgesics for their psychological effects or may have aberrant drug-taking behaviors. Aberrant drug-taking behaviors may include requests for frequent, early renewals; unauthorized dose escalations; reports of lost or stolen prescriptions; adamant requests for specific medications; and acquisition of similar drugs from other medical sources. Patients with past or current substance use disorders may also be difficult to treat because of fear of exposure to opioid analgesics and their potential vulnerability to addiction. In any case, these behaviors or fears should be discussed openly and in nonjudgmental terms with the patient. Ultimately, an agreement should be reached about the use of opioids for the management of pain (as opposed to mood alterations), and some details about the expectations and responsibilities of both the physician and the patient should be delineated. With this group of patients, long-acting opioids or continuous infusion is often preferable to short-acting opioids or patient-controlled analgesia. Although their care is more complex, patients with drug or alcohol addiction should not be denied appropriate pain medications.

IV. TREATMENT

A. General aspects

All healthcare professionals who see patients with cancer should be familiar with standard guidelines for management of cancer pain such as those published by the NCCN or the Agency for Healthcare Research and Quality. An example of a cancer pain practice guideline is shown in Table 31.1. This guideline incorporates basic principles of cancer pain assessment, initial treatment, and routine management of opioid side effects.

The prompt relief of pain from cancer frequently involves the use of simultaneously rather than serially administered combinations of drug and other adjunctive therapies. Identification of a treatable neoplasm as a factor in pain production calls for appropriate radiotherapy (e.g., to bone metastases), chemotherapy, or, in some instances, surgical debulking. Until such treatment can be effective (this may take days to weeks), the patient's pain must be managed with analgesics with or without other specific interventional pain procedures. In some instances, analgesics are the only effective palliative treatment available because of the patient's condition, the physical basis of the pain, or limited treatment options. The principles of pharmacologic management of pain are evolving through studies of analgesic effectiveness and research on the use of combinations of palliative medications.

There is a growing consensus concerning the types of drugs to use, their routes of administration, and how best to schedule them. The first step is to assess the severity of the pain. Simple

31.1   An Example of a Pain Practice Guideline

A. Comprehensive pain assessment
  1. Evaluation of pain. Determine level using 0–10 intensity scale, location, onset, duration, frequency, quality (somatic, visceral, neuropathic), history, etiology, associated symptoms, what modifies the pain, side effects associated with treatment of pain, and response to other pain medications.
    No pain (0) Mild (1–3) Moderate (4–6) Severe (7–10)
  2. Evaluation of past medical history (oncologic or other significant medical illnesses) including medication history
  3. Physical examination
  4. Evaluation of relevant laboratory and imaging studies
  5. Evaluation of risk factors for undertreatment of pain, including underreporting, extremes of age, gender, cultural barriers, communication barriers, and a history of substance abuse
  6. Evaluation of psychosocial issues (patient distress, family support, psychiatric history, special issues relating to pain [meaning of pain for patient/family, patient/family knowledge of and beliefs surrounding pain])
B. Overall management plans
  1. If pain = 0, reassess at each subsequent visit or interaction
  2. Manage pain related to oncologic emergencies, if any
    a. Such pain requires assessment and treatment (e.g., surgery, steroids, radiotherapy, antibiotics) along with an emergent consultation
    b. Oncologic emergencies include:
      ■ Bowel obstruction/perforation
      ■ Brain metastasis
      ■ Leptomeningeal metastasis
      ■ Fracture or impending fracture of weight-bearing bone
      ■ Epidural metastasis/spinal cord compression
      ■ Pain related to infection.
  3. Manage non–emergency-related pain
C. Management of non–emergency-related pain
  1. If pain = 1–3
    ■ NSAIDs (including COX-2 agents) and acetaminophen. If ineffective: opioids (hydrocodone scheduled or as needed)
    ■ Overall reassessment at each subsequent visit or interaction.
  2. If pain = 4–6
    ■ Oral opioids
    ■ Morphine 15 mg orally every 4 hours as needed or scheduled
    ■ Oxycodone 5 mg orally every 4 hours as needed or scheduled
    ■ Hydromorphone 2 mg orally every 4 hours as needed or scheduled
    ■ Adjuvants: NSAIDs, antidepressants, antiepileptics, etc.
    ■ Overall reassessment in 24–48 hours.
  3. If pain = 7–10 (possible pain crisis)
    ■ Oral opioids: morphine 20 mg orally every 4 hours as needed (opioid-naive)
    ■ Thirty percent increase in current opioid regimen (sustained- and immediate-release [rescue] opioids)
    ■ Morphine, hydromorphone, or oxycodone for rescue dosing

(continued)

An Example of a Pain Practice Guideline *(continued)*

- Consider intravenous opioid titration (PCA pump may be used to titrate)
- Reassess frequently, based on clinical situation.

D. Additional steps for pain that was rated 4–10
1. Re-evaluate opioid titration
2. Re-evaluate pain diagnosis
3. Consider consults from specialty services*
4. All patients receiving opioids should begin:
   - Bowel regimen (such as oral senna 1 tablet twice daily)
   - Antiemetics as needed (such as metoclopramide 10 mg 30 minutes before meals and at bedtime)
   - Educational activities regarding pain management
   - Psychosocial support as needed.

E. At the time of re-evaluation for patients whose pain was 4–10
1. If pain now = 1–3
   - Consider conversion to a sustained-release agent with rescue medications
   - Continue adjuvants or add them as needed
   - Reassess and modify side effects of pain treatment
   - Provide psychosocial support
   - Provide educational activities
   - Reassess pain every week until comfortable, then every visit.
2. If pain now = 4–6
   - Continue opioid titration
   - Consider specific pain problems
   - Consider consults from specialty services*
   - Continue psychosocial support
   - Continue educational activities.
3. If pain now = 7–10[†] (possible pain crisis)
   - Continue opioid titration
   - Re-evaluate working diagnosis
   - Consider specific pain problems
   - Obtain consults from specialty services*
   - Continue psychosocial support.

COX, cyclooxygenase; NSAID, nonsteroidal anti-inflammatory drug; PCA, patient-controlled analgesia.
*Postoperative pain service, cancer pain section, department of symptom control and palliative care, or other specialties as needed (i.e., radiotherapy).
[†]Some patients with chronic pain syndromes will report high pain scores on an ongoing basis. Generally, this situation is not a crisis. This practice guideline was created by the National Comprehensive Cancer Network and modified by the University of Texas M.D. Anderson Cancer Center under the supervision of Allen Burton, MD, and Charles Cleeland, PhD.

categories such as mild, moderate, and severe are often sufficient. Second is the choice of analgesic drug to be used (nonopioid, opioid, or a combination of both), which is commonly based on the severity level. The next step is the choice of adjuvant drugs, which can increase analgesic effectiveness and can produce other palliative effects to counter the disruptive consequences of pain. Finally, some consideration should be made on follow-up assessment of the interventions to ensure adequate relief is achieved.

B. Nonsteroidal anti-inflammatory drugs (NSAIDs)

1. Mechanism of action and selection of agents. NSAIDs constitute the majority of nonopioid analgesics. Their effect on the inflammatory process is a key to their analgesic property. Tumor growth produces inflammatory and mechanical effects in adjacent tissues that can trigger the release of prostaglandins, bradykinin, and serotonin, which in turn may precipitate or exacerbate pain in the surrounding tissues. Prostaglandins are frequently associated with painful bone metastases because of their involvement in bone reabsorption. NSAIDs appear to exert their analgesic, antipyretic, and anti-inflammatory actions by blocking the synthesis of prostaglandins. Table 31.2 gives the usual starting doses and dose ranges for several commonly used NSAIDs. The concern about NSAIDs are due to reports of cardiac toxicity associated with celecoxib as well as most other agents in this class. It is appropriate to discuss the cardiac toxicity of these agents in the context of the risk/benefit ratio relative to the condition(s) for which they are being prescribed.

By virtue of their different mechanisms of action and toxicity profiles, NSAIDs and opioids are often administered together. Enteric-coated aspirin is one of the first-choice drugs for mild to moderate cancer pain. Other NSAIDs such as ibuprofen, diflunisal, naproxen, and choline magnesium trisalicylate have established value in the management of clinical pain. These drugs are better tolerated than aspirin but are usually significantly more expensive. Individual differences in analgesic response to the various NSAIDs clearly occur but are not yet well understood.

Cyclooxygenase (COX)-2 NSAIDs are inhibitors of COX-2, the enzyme expressed in inflamed tissues, and have minimal

TABLE 31.2	Starting Doses and Dose Ranges of Some Nonsteroidal Analgesic Agents		
Drug	**Starting Dose (mg)**	**Frequency**	**Dose Range**
Aspirin	650	Every 4–6 hours	Up to 1300 mg every 6 hours
Choline magnesium trisalicylate	500	Every 6 hours	Up to 1000 mg every 6 hours
Ibuprofen	400	Every 4–6 hours	Up to 2400 mg daily
Naproxen	250	Every 8–12 hours	Up to 1250 mg daily
Diclofenac	25	Every 6 hours	Up to 150 mg daily
Piroxicam	10	Every 12–24 hours	Up to 20 mg daily
Celecoxib	100	Every 24 hours	Up to 400 mg daily

or no effects on COX-1, the enzyme expressed normally in the stomach and kidney. These NSAIDs are widely used because of their once- or twice-daily dosing schedule and the roughly 50% relative reduction in significant gastrointestinal adverse events compared with those induced by other NSAIDs.

2. **Side effects.** NSAIDs have a number of potentially serious side effects, including gastritis and gastrointestinal hemorrhage, bleeding due to platelet inhibition, renal failure, and cardiac toxicity. Most of these side effects are related to the prostaglandin inhibitory effect of NSAIDs and are therefore common to all of these drugs. Renal failure due to the inhibition of renal medullary prostaglandins can be of particular concern for patients who are also receiving opioids. Decreased renal elimination of active opioid metabolites can result in somnolence, confusion, hallucinations, or generalized myoclonus. Therefore, kidney function should be monitored in patients receiving a combination of NSAIDs and opioids.

Gastrointestinal complications include gastric pain, nausea, vomiting, hemorrhage, and, in extreme cases, perforation. Gastrointestinal damage is mediated by prostaglandin inhibition. The most common form of nephrotoxicity associated with NSAIDs is renal failure related to prostaglandin inhibition and consequent vasodilation. Hepatic injury has been reported with the use of aspirin, benoxaprofen, and phenylbutazone and, less commonly, with diclofenac, ibuprofen, indomethacin, naproxen, pirprofen, and sulindac. Sulindac, however, appears to be associated with a higher incidence of cholestasis.

NSAID use is also associated with various hypersensitivity reactions involving the skin (rash, eruption, itching), blood vessels (angioneurotic edema, vasomotor disorders), and respiratory system (rhinitis, asthma). In particular, aspirin may cause anaphylactic crisis, a syndrome characterized by dyspnea, sudden weakness, sweating, and collapse. Undesirable hematologic effects of NSAIDs include platelet dysfunction, aplastic anemia, and agranulocytosis. Factors often considered in the empiric selection of an NSAID for a given patient include its relative toxicity, cost, and dosage schedule and the patient's prior experience. The use of certain aspirin analogs (choline magnesium trisalicylate) has been associated with a low incidence of gastropathy and platelet dysfunction. The effects of NSAIDs used as single agents in the management of cancer pain are characterized by a ceiling effect, beyond which further increases in dose do not enhance analgesia.

C. **Opioid analgesics**

1. **When to start therapy.** The choice of using an opioid analgesic as opposed to a nonopioid analgesic follows from an assessment

of the severity of pain. The decision is relatively easy when pain is mild (choose nonopioid) or severe (choose opioid, usually in combination with a nonopioid). The choice is more difficult when the patient reports moderate pain, especially when there is reason to suspect that the patient may be underreporting pain severity. Several studies have documented that the pain of many patients with cancer are inadequately managed because of the physician's reluctance to use opioids in dosages and with schedules known to be sufficient to relieve moderate pain.

Opioid analgesics should be prescribed promptly as soon as there is evidence that pain is not well controlled with non-opioid analgesics. When pain is moderate to severe, it is also appropriate to use a strong opioid as a first-line treatment for cancer pain.

2. **Schedule of treatment and selection of dose.** Except for a minority of patients whose pain is clearly episodic (often called "incidental pain"), analgesics should be given on an around-the-clock basis, with the time interval based on the duration of effectiveness of the drug and the patient's report of the duration of effectiveness. There is evidence that the total opioid requirement is lower when opioids are given on a scheduled basis, thereby preventing peaks of pain. Putting patients in the position of having to ask for medication or continually making a judgment about whether their pain is severe enough to take analgesics focuses their attention on pain, reminds them of their need for drugs, and allows pain to reach a severity not readily controlled by the same doses that would be effective with scheduled administration. When writing a scheduled dose of opioids, adding notation that patients may refuse doses will allow the patient to remain in control of pain medication dosing and often avoid unnecessary anxiety and conflict between nursing staff and patients. Nevertheless, there may be large individual differences in the required dose of opioid, depending on such factors as the patient's opioid use history, activity level, and metabolism. The patient's report of pain severity and pain relief is the best guideline for opioid titration.

3. **The so-called weak opioids,** including codeine and hydrocodone, usually formulated in combination with acetaminophen or aspirin, can provide patients with good pain relief for long periods of time. As disease advances, oral administration of the more potent opioids provides most patients with pain relief. There is considerable agreement that propoxyphene is not ideal for chronic use because of its low efficacy at commercially available doses; because of the presence of a toxic metabolite, which is a CNS stimulant, at higher doses; because it has a long serum half-life; and because it has no analgesic properties. Oral

administration is preferred, but the physician must remain flexible to changes that are dictated by the patient's ability to use orally administered drugs. This may include the use of opioid and nonopioid suppositories and other alternative routes of administration (transdermal, sublingual, rectal, subcutaneous).

4. **Oral morphine,** either in an immediate- or sustained-release preparation, is the analgesic of choice for moderate to severe cancer pain. Long-acting formulations of morphine and other strong opioids may be convenient for both the patient and the healthcare staff, but they are usually most expensive. Immediate-release morphine is much cheaper, however, and is as effective for chronic pain relief when administered on a regular schedule. A typical starting dose for immediate-release oral morphine is 15 to 30 mg every 4 hours in patients who are not currently receiving opioids. When a patient is switching from another opioid (usually codeine or oxycodone) to morphine, it is important to calculate the equianalgesic morphine dose as a basis for determining what morphine-equivalent doses are the threshold for pain control (Table 31.3). The starting dose may not be sufficient and relatively rapid upward titration may be needed, especially if pain is severe.

The upward titration of morphine and other oral opioid analgesics can be done by giving a supplemental "boost" using 25% to 50% of the scheduled dose 2 hours after the scheduled dose if there is still mild to moderate pain and the patient is

---

TABLE 31.3   Dose Equivalence of Selected Opioids

Drug	Approximate Equianalgesic Dose	
	Oral	**Parenteral**
Morphine	30 mg every 3–4 hours*	10 mg every 3–4 hours
Hydromorphone	4–8 mg every 3–4 hours	1.5 mg every 3–4 hours
Codeine[†]	130 mg every 3–4 hours	
Hydrocodone[†]	30 mg every 3–4 hours	
Oxycodone[†]	20 mg every 3–4 hours	
Transdermal fentanyl	25-μg/h patch = 8–22 mg/24 hours IV or IM morphine sulfate = roughly 50 mg/d of oral morphine sulfate; 50-μg/h patch = roughly 60 mg MS-Contin every 12 hours	

IM, intramuscularly; IV, intravenously.
*Slow-release formulations of oral morphine that are available have 8- to 12-hour durations of analgesic action.
[†]Codeine, hydrocodone, and oxycodone are often given as combination products with aspirin, acetaminophen, or both.
Adapted from Weissman DE, Dahl JL, Dinndorf PA. *Handbook of cancer pain management* (4th ed.). Madison: Wisconsin Cancer Pain Initiative; 1993.

not overly sedated or lethargic. However if severe pain remains, a supplemental dose of 50% to 100% would be indicated. The scheduled dose is then set at 125% to 200% of the initial scheduled dose. Because of the time it takes to achieve a steady state, there may need to be some readjustment downward if the patient is unduly sleepy or is lethargic at the time of the scheduled dose. The supplemental dose may be given after any scheduled dose (even if there was an increase in the scheduled dose) as long as a sufficient time has passed for the drug to be absorbed from the stomach. An alternative way to titrate is simply to add 50% to the next scheduled dose, but staying with the previously determined schedule (usually every 4 hours). When the doses of opioid are higher (e.g., morphine 100 mg every 4 hours), some clinicians use less, for example, 20% to 30% (20 to 30 mg) as the boost, but incrementally add to the dose with each scheduled treatment until adequate pain relief has been achieved. It is often best to have the patient check in with a physician or nurse 1 to 3 days after a significant dose or medication adjustment to be sure the treatment plan is understood, safe, and effective.

5. **Long-acting preparations.** When an effective dose of short-acting morphine has been established, the required 24-hour dose for a long-acting preparation can be calculated. An additional supply of short-acting morphine, given when necessary, will help the patient manage "breakthrough" pain. Consistent need for this additional short-acting morphine (e.g., three or four doses daily) dictates an upward adjustment of the dose of sustained-release drug. Orders for immediate-release morphine should allow for some upward titration of dose by the patient or by the nurse. Each dose of short-acting morphine for breakthrough pain is usually 5% to 15% of the 24-hour dose of long-acting morphine. If more than this is required, it is usually an indication for increasing the dose of the long-acting preparation or considering some other adjuvant or interventional approaches.

6. **Although the opioid agonist–antagonist analgesics** have established effectiveness in the control of acute (especially procedurally related) pain, their use in chronic cancer pain is limited by the possibility of precipitous withdrawal in the patient who has been taking morphine-type drugs, by their analgesic ceiling effect (when the drug does not provide more pain relief), and by the lack of an oral form of administration.

7. **Methadone** is an agonist opioid analgesic that has the advantages of extremely low cost (often 10- to 30-fold less expensive than other strong opioids), efficacy in neuropathic pain, slow development of tolerance, and lack of known active metabolites. Because of its long and unpredictable half-life and

relatively unknown equianalgesic dose compared with other opioids, methadone has generally been used by pain specialists with experience in its use. The methadone preparation widely utilized in the United States is a racemic mix of the D-isomer and L-isomer of methadone. The D-isomer has antagonist activity at the NMDA receptor, and this produces clinically relevant benefits in the control of neuropathic pain.

The relative potency of methadone increases with higher morphine-equivalent doses. Thus, when converting from another opioid to methadone, the calculated equianalgesic dose of methadone should be decreased by 75% to 90%. A guideline for choosing an appropriate initial dose of methadone based on the oral morphine-equivalent daily dose of the previous opioid is shown in Table 31.4. For example, a patient who has been using sustained-release morphine at 80 mg every 8 hours (240 mg/day) would be appropriately switched to methadone at a dose of 10 mg every 8 hours (30 mg/day, an 8:1 conversion ratio). In contrast, a patient who is taking sustained-release morphine at a total daily dose of 60 mg/day might be switched to an oral methadone dose of 5 mg every 8 hours (15 mg/day, a 4:1 conversion ratio).

Methadone is available as a pill, an elixir, and for parenteral use. The oral bioavailability of the drug is excellent (50% to 80%). Methadone is roughly twice as potent via intravenous (IV) or intramuscular routes compared with oral administration. Thus, a patient with well-controlled pain on a stable oral methadone dose of 10 mg every 8 hours would be switched to IV methadone at 5 mg every 8 hours if necessary. Subcutaneous (SC) use of methadone may cause skin irritation in some patients.

Methadone is metabolized primarily by the hepatic cytochrome-P450-system isoenzyme CYP3A4, and to a lesser extent by isoenzyme CYP2D6. Drugs that inhibit CYP3A4 cause

TABLE 31.4	Suggested Dosing of Oral Methadone Based on Morphine-Equivalent Daily Dose*
Oral MEDD (mg/d)	**Initial Dose Ratio (Oral Morphine/Oral Methadone)**
<30	2:1
30–99	4:1
100–299	8:1
300–499	12:1

MEDD, morphone-equivalent daily dose.
*Great caution must be used when converting to methadone when very high opioid doses have been used. Often, only a portion of the total opioid dose is converted initially, with further conversions taking place over several days to weeks.

Drugs Causing Methadone Levels to Drift Upward (higher effects)	Drugs Causing Methadone Levels to Drift Downward (lower effects)
Ciprofloxacin	Rifampin
Ketoconazole, itraconazole, fluconazole	Phenytoin
Erythromycin, clarithromycin	Corticosteroids
Grapefruit juice	Carbamazepine
HIV protease inhibitors (indinavir, nelfinavir, ritonavir, saquinavir)	St. John's wort
Verapamil, diltiazem	Modafinil
Aprepitant	Efavirenz
Nefazodone	Nevirapine

For a more complete listing of CYP3A4 interactions, see http://medicine.iupui.edu/clinpharm/ddis/table.asp.

the methadone levels to drift upward, and drugs that induce the metabolism of CYP3A4 will cause the methadone levels to drift downward. Important drugs to consider when prescribing methadone are summarized in Table 31.5.

Methadone is one of a long list of medications that can cause prolongation of the QT interval and torsades de pointes ventricular tachycardia. This is caused by inhibition of the rapid component of the delayed rectifier potassium ion current. Other common drugs that share this attribute include haloperidol, chlorpromazine, clarithromycin, pentamidine, and others. The level of risk associated with these drugs is low and depends on the dose and the population being treated. Oral methadone can be safely administered in the low doses (<100 mg/day) that are generally prescribed for the treatment of cancer pain, and routine electrocardiograms are not performed at our institution when prescribing oral methadone. Caution should be taken when prescribing methadone to certain patients who may be at higher risk of QT prolongation.

8. **Alternative potent opioids** include levorphanol, which has a longer half-life than morphine, and single-entity oxycodone and hydromorphone, which have half-lives similar to morphine. Equivalent starting doses can be selected from Table 31.3, but if the patient has been on high doses of morphine, care must be taken to reduce the dose by 25% to 50% of the calculated equianalgesic dose to account for incomplete cross-tolerance that may increase the relative potency of the newly prescribed agent.

9. **Alternative routes.** About 70% of patients benefit from the use of an alternative route for opioid administration sometime before death. The duration for which patients need these routes varies between hours and months. Although intermittent injections

can be effective for a brief period of time, this method is painful for the patient, time-consuming for the nursing staff, and difficult to manage at home.

a. **IV infusions** of opioids produce stable blood levels of drug that are safe and effective for treating both postoperative and cancer pain. IV infusion using a patient-controlled analgesia pump may be very effective in gaining rapid control over pain that has gotten out of hand. It may also be of value when the patient cannot take medications orally and does not wish to take suppositories. The main problem associated with continuous IV infusions is the prolonged maintenance of an IV line. Patients may need to be subjected to numerous venipunctures when peripheral IV lines are used. Totally implantable IV catheters represent a major improvement, permitting long-term IV access. However, these catheters are expensive and need to be surgically implanted, and their maintenance requires considerable nursing expertise and patient teaching. If such a catheter is already available in a patient with advanced cancer who has pain, it certainly could be used for the administration of opioids. Starting doses of morphine for severe pain are 2 to 3 mg hourly as a continuous infusion, with patient-controlled boosts of 1 mg every 6 to 15 minutes. At the end of 24 hours, 50% of the patient boosts can be added to the total 24-hour dose of the continuous infusion until the patient is requiring less than one boost hourly. At that time, a shift to oral analgesics can be started, if the patient is able to take oral medications. If the doses of IV morphine are high, shifting to appropriate oral doses may take several days. It is usually safe and effective to give a 24-hour dose of long-acting morphine orally that is equal in milligrams (not equianalgesic) to the 24-hour IV requirement and simultaneously to reduce the IV dose (continuous infusion rate) by half. Boosts can be given by mouth, but the patient should have the IV boost option as reassurance. The next day, the 24-hour IV dose required (continuous plus boosts) can be added orally to the previous day's oral dose (long-acting plus short-acting) and the infusion further reduced. The same process is repeated until the patient is getting adequate pain relief with the oral morphine. The infusion can usually be stopped and needed boosts given orally by the third or fourth day.

b. **SC route.** This route has been found to be safe and effective for the administration of morphine and hydromorphone. SC opioids can be administered as a continuous infusion using a pump (use as small a volume as possible, e.g., less than 5 mL/h) or as an intermittent injection. A butterfly needle can be left under the skin for about 7 days, making both intermittent injections and continuous infusion painless. The needles are frequently inserted in the subclavicular region, anterior chest, or abdominal wall. This allows patients to have free limbs.

c. **Rectal route.** Most of the experience reported in the literature is with the short-term use of rectal opioids for the management of acute pain. Both solid and liquid solutions have been used. Although there is considerable interindividual variation in the bioavailability of rectally administered morphine, there is general consensus that this drug is well absorbed after rectal administration. A number of authors have treated terminally ill cancer patients with rectal morphine, with good pain control until death. Advantages of the rectal route include the absence of the need for the insertion of needles and the use of portable pumps. However, rectal administration can be uncomfortable or psychologically distressing for some patients; absorption may be decreased by the presence of stool in the rectum, by diarrhea, or simply by normal bowel movements; and progressive titration may be difficult because of the limited availability of different commercial preparations.

d. **Transdermal route.** Pharmacokinetic data suggest that transdermal fentanyl is well absorbed, although there is considerable delay in reaching steady-state blood levels and a slowly declining plasma concentration after removal of the skin patch. The 72-hour dosing of the patch makes it convenient to use, and treatment appears to be well tolerated. The transdermal route is generally worth avoiding if the enteral route is readily available. Transdermal preparations are usually more expensive and more difficult to titrate compared with oral opioids. However, this route is quite useful for patients with chronic malignant bowel obstruction or similar chronic problems with the oral route. These skin patches range in doses from 12 mcg/hour to 100 mcg/hour.

e. **Transmucosal route.** Fentanyl citrate can also be formulated in a candied matrix to allow it to be administered orally as a lozenge on a stick. Oral transmucosal fentanyl citrate (OTFC) appears to be rapidly effective for breakthrough pain or for procedures. Dose-equivalency studies have suggested that OTFC is about 10 times more potent than parenteral morphine. Starting doses for the lozenges are usually 200 μg, with dosing intervals of 4 to 6 hours. Drug dose requires titrating up as with other agents with single doses of up to 600 μg. This transmucosal route has been used sparingly because the lozenges are expensive and require the patient to rub the lozenge against the buccal mucosa to enhance absorption. Another formulation that is available is a transmucosal buccal tablet;

it has been developed and approved for breakthrough cancer pain with doses ranging from 100 to 800 mcg. The tablet is placed behind a rear molar tooth between the cheek and gums and adheres to the buccal mucosa and slowly dissolves on its own.

f. **Neuraxial route.** Some patients suffering from localized pain syndromes might benefit from epidural or intrathecal administration of opioids. The advantage of the neuraxial route is the potential to spare side effects of opioids as a relatively small dose of opioid may be effective for the pain problem. The disadvantage is the need for the insertion of catheters into the epidural or intrathecal space, the need for expensive infusion pumps, and, in some patients, the rapid development of tolerance to the analgesic effect of different opioids. To overcome this rapid development of tolerance, some clinicians have used a combined infusion of opioids and local anesthetic. Another issue that has become recognized is catheter tip granuloma formation. This may present as gradual loss of pain control or new back pain, sometimes associated with neurologic deficits. This complication can be diagnosed by MRI and is most common with high concentrations of intrathecal opioids (such as morphine >25 mg/mL). Because of the complexity associated with this route, it should only be considered for selected patients and after an adequate trial of systemic opioids and adjuvant drugs. The insertion of the catheter and the maintenance of the spinal analgesic regimen should be under the control of an interventional pain specialist.

10. **Adverse effects of opioids.** Concerns about opioid side effects are one of the main reasons cited by both patients and oncologists for limiting their use of opioids or the upward titration of these agents to achieve optimal pain control. It is important to understand the side-effect spectrum of these analgesics and be prepared to deal with side effects prophylactically or promptly when they do occur, as well as to educate patients and family members about side effects. Most patients develop tolerance for side effects much more rapidly than they develop tolerance for the analgesic effects of the opioids.

The analgesic and side effects of opioid agonists are not identical for all patients. Some patients may require a higher equivalent dose of a certain opioid agonist to achieve adequate analgesia. This higher equivalent dose may result in a higher incidence of side effects such as nausea or sedation. Therefore, when significant toxicity occurs in a patient treated with a certain opioid agonist such as morphine, it may be appropriate to change to another opioid. In addition, after prolonged treatment, high dosages, or renal failure, patients may experience the accumulation of active metabolites of opioid agonists. Active metabolites have been identified for morphine, hydromorphone, oxycodone, and fentanyl. This accumulation results in CNS side effects such as sedation, generalized myoclonus, confusion, and, in some patients, agitated delirium or grand mal seizures. In these patients, it is also useful to change from one opioid to another.

This so-called opioid rotation (or "opioid switching") can produce improved analgesia and fewer adverse effects. Most often, such a switch occurs from morphine to a more potent opioid such as methadone, hydromorphone, fentanyl, or oxycodone. The dose guidelines for switching to methadone are shown in Table 31.4. When switching from morphine to hydromorphone or oxycodone, the initial calculated equianalgesic dose should be reduced by 25% to 50% to account for incomplete cross-tolerance. When switching from morphine to transdermal fentanyl, dose reduction is not needed because the dosing guidelines already incorporated the safety factor necessary for opioid rotation.

a. **Sedation.** This occurs in most patients during the beginning of opioid treatment or after a major increase in dose. Most patients develop rapid tolerance to this side effect, and while the sedation disappears within 3 to 5 days, the analgesic effect persists. When sedation occurs in patients with cancer receiving a stable dose of opioid, one should suspect the potential accumulation of active opioid metabolites such as morphine-6-glucuronide. This occurs most frequently in patients who are receiving high doses of opioids or who present with renal failure. It is also important to consider non–opioid-related causes such as hypercalcemia, because these patients are frequently very ill and metabolic problems or comorbidity may contribute to sedation. Opioid-induced sedation can be managed by opioid rotation (some opioids have a higher ratio of analgesic effects to sedation than others) or by the addition of psychostimulants such as methylphenidate or modafinil.

b. **Nausea and vomiting.** Most patients present with these symptoms after initial administration or a major increase in dose. Some authors propose the use of prophylactic antiemetics on a regular basis during the first days of treatment because in most patients, nausea disappears after that period. These side effects can be well managed with a prokinetic agent such as metoclopramide (10 mg by mouth once a day). Dexamethasone 2 to 4 mg by mouth once a day is also a useful antiemetic that potentiates metoclopramide in these patients, but it is prudent to taper this corticosteroid within

1 or 2 weeks. Another reasonable option is to consider low-dose haloperidol as the antidopaminergic properties often play a key role in opioid-induced nausea. As with sedation, nausea is a syndrome with multiple possible etiologies in patients with cancer who are receiving opioids: severe constipation, cancer-induced autonomic dysfunction, gastritis, increased intracranial pressure, and opioid metabolite accumulation are all possible causes of nausea.

c. **Constipation.** This is probably the most common adverse effect of opioids, and it is necessary to anticipate constipation when opioid therapy is started. Opioids act at multiple sites in the gastrointestinal tract and spinal cord. The result is decreased intestinal secretions and peristalsis. Although tolerance to both sedation and nausea develops quickly, it develops very slowly to the smooth muscle effects of opioids, so that constipation persists when these drugs are used for chronic pain. At the same time that the use of opioid analgesics is initiated, provision for a regular bowel regimen, including stimulants and stool softeners, should be instituted to diminish this adverse effect (see Chapter 26). Methylnaltrexone has been recently approved for opioid-induced constipation. This agent is a peripheral opioid receptor antagonist, a quaternary derivative of naltrexone that does not cross the blood-brain barrier. In studies, methylnaltrexone is able to reverse constipation without affecting analgesia or precipitating the opioid withdrawal symptoms.

d. **Respiratory depression.** This is the most serious adverse effect of opioid analgesics. Opioids can cause increasing respiratory depression to the point of apnea. In humans, death due to overdose of opioids is nearly always due to respiratory arrest. At equianalgesic doses, the morphinelike agonists produce an equivalent degree of respiratory depression. When respiratory depression occurs, it is usually in opioid-naive patients after acute administration of an opioid and is associated with other signs of CNS depression including sedation and mental clouding. Tolerance quickly develops to this effect with repeated drug administration, allowing the opioid analgesics to be used in the management of chronic cancer pain without significant risk of respiratory depression.

If respiratory depression occurs, it can be reversed by the administration of the specific opioid antagonist naloxone. In patients chronically receiving opioids who develop respiratory depression, naloxone in a 1:10 dilution should be titrated carefully to prevent the precipitation of severe withdrawal syndromes while reversing the respiratory depression. Long-acting drugs such as methadone, fentanyl patches, or slow-release morphine or hydromorphone carry a greater risk of respiratory depression compared to short-acting opioids.

The simultaneous use of other depressants such as benzodiazepines or alcohol are also risk factors for respiratory depression. Preliminary evidence also indicates a history of obstructive sleep apnea may also increase the risk of respiratory complications. Although this is the most feared side effect of opioid analgesics, it seldom occurs in patients receiving chronic opioid therapy for the treatment of cancer pain.

e. **Allergic reactions.** These occur infrequently with opioids. However, patients are commonly described as being "allergic" to a number of opioid analgesics. This descriptor generally results from a misinterpretation by the patient or clinician of some of the common side effects of opioids, such as nausea, sedation, vomiting, diaphoresis, or pruritus. In most instances, a simple discussion with the patient is enough to clarify this issue.

f. **Urinary retention.** The increase in the tone of smooth muscle of the bladder induced by opioids results in increased sphincter tone, leading to urinary retention. This is most common in elderly patients. Attention should be directed to this potential transient side effect, and catheterization may be necessary, transiently, for management. Patients do accommodate this side effect, and it is seldom a barrier to effective pain management.

g. **"Newer" side effects.** During recent years, as a result of increased education in the assessment and management of cancer pain, patients have been receiving higher doses of opioids for longer periods of time than ever before. This more aggressive use of opioids is associated with additional side effects, usually seen only in patients with late-stage disease receiving high doses of opioids.

(1) **Cognitive failure.** Patients can experience a transient decrease in concentration and psychomotor coordination after starting opioids or after a sudden increase in the opioid dose. In some patients, opioid-induced cognitive failure can be permanent. Some of the cognitive effects can be reversed by the administration of amphetamine derivatives such as methylphenidate. Cognitive screening tools (such as the Mini-Mental State Examination and other similar bedside assessments) are useful in patients receiving high doses of opioids.

(2) **Other central effects.** Organic hallucinations, myoclonus, grand mal seizures, and even hyperalgesia have been observed in patients receiving high doses of opioids for

long periods. These effects are likely due to the accumulation of active opioid metabolites. Sometimes, the development of these problems in a previously stable patient heralds the onset of renal insufficiency or renal failure. Improvement is frequently seen after renal function improves and/or there is an opioid rotation. Hallucinations may be treated symptomatically with low doses of haloperidol 0.5 to 2 mg twice a day while the underlying problem is being addressed. Myoclonus can be treated with clonazepam 0.5 mg by mouth twice a day to start, with titration every 3 days up to a maximum daily dose of 20 mg.

(3) **Severe sedation and coma.** When coma occurs in patients receiving a stable dose of opioids for a long period of time, it should be suspected that accumulation of active opioid metabolites has occurred. These patients usually improve quickly after discontinuation of opioids.

(4) **Pulmonary edema.** Although noncardiogenic pulmonary edema is a well-recognized complication of opioid overdose in addicts, it had not been recognized until recently as a potential complication of cancer pain treatment. Pulmonary edema usually occurs when patients have undergone rapid increases in dose, usually as a result of severe neuropathic pain. Even though the mortality of the syndrome is very low among patients presenting with acute opioid overdoses, because of the conservative nature of the treatment of terminally ill patients with cancer, the mortality of pulmonary edema is much higher within this population.

V. ADJUVANT DRUGS

Opioid analgesics are the most important drugs for the treatment of cancer pain. Although these drugs can, in most patients, control severe pain even when they are used appropriately, they may produce new symptoms or exacerbate pre-existing symptoms, most notably nausea and somnolence. This aspect of treatment with opioid compounds is particularly problematic in patients with advanced cancer. The combination of severe pain, anorexia, chronic nausea, asthenia, and somnolence is a frequent finding in patients with advanced cancer. The term *adjuvant drug* has been used in a variety of ways, even in the context of cancer pain management. For the purposes of the following paragraphs, an adjuvant drug meets one or more of the following criteria:

- Increases the analgesic effect of opioids (adjuvant analgesia)
- Decreases the toxicity of opioids
- Improves other symptoms associated with terminal cancer.

Most symptomatic patients with cancer receive more than one or two adjuvant drugs. Unfortunately, there is still limited consensus on the type and dose of the most appropriate adjuvant drugs.

Claims have been made for the adjuvant analgesic effect of many drugs, but unfortunately, most of the evidence for these effects is anecdotal. Controlled clinical trials are needed to define more clearly the indications and risk-to-benefit ratios. These agents, some of which have the potential to produce significant toxicity, can aggravate the toxicity of opioids.

A. Acetaminophen is a peripherally acting analgesic that does not inhibit peripheral prostaglandin synthesis. Therefore, it does not have anti-inflammatory effects or the side effects associated with the use of NSAIDs. Acetaminophen may be safely combined with opioids, and there is evidence that adding acetaminophen produces meaningful improvement in analgesic efficacy. Commercial preparations containing codeine or oxycodone and acetaminophen or aspirin are among the most widely prescribed scheduled analgesics and are frequently administered to patients with cancer.

Hepatotoxicity remains the major side effect to be cognizant of as patients are often unaware of this, especially when used in combined products. For patients with normal liver function, 6 to 8 g per day is reasonable, but if individuals have compromised liver function, acetaminophen should be limited to 3 to 4 g per day.

B. Antidepressants

Tricyclic antidepressants have been found to be useful for various neuropathic pain syndromes, especially when pain has a prominent dysesthetic or burning character. Both amitriptyline and desipramine have been found to be effective in the management of postherpetic neuralgia, diabetic neuropathy, and other neurologic conditions.

Amitriptyline or imipramine (25 mg at bedtime) may be started at low doses; if the drug is not overly sedating and the patient does not experience bothersome anticholinergic side effects, the dose may be increased every 3 days to a total daily dose of 150 mg. The toxic effects of these drugs are mainly autonomic (dry mouth, postural hypotension) and centrally mediated (somnolence, confusion). Cardiovascular side effects are also possible at therapeutic dosing levels, including increased heart rate, prolonged PR interval, intraventricular conduction delays, increased corrected QT interval, and flattened T waves. Because their use may contribute to symptoms already present in debilitated patients, they should be administered cautiously in those who are very ill.

Duloxetine is a serotonin/norepinephrine reuptake inhibitor indicated for the treatment of diabetic neuropathy. The appropriate dose for this indication is 60 mg once daily. Adults treated with any antidepressant medication should be watched closely for worsening of depression and/or suicidal behavior or suicidal ideation. Monitoring should be particularly vigilant during initiation of therapy and during any change in dosage. Overall, clinical experience and expert consensus suggest that tricyclic antidepressants or duloxetine may be tried for the management of pain that is of central, deafferentation, or neuropathic origin.

C. Anticonvulsants

Carbamazepine, phenytoin, valproic acid, lamotrigine, gabapentin, pregabelin, and clonazepam, alone or in combination with the tricyclic antidepressants, have been used successfully to treat neuropathic pain. Based on the well-documented efficacy for the treatment of trigeminal neuralgia, considerable experience and expert consensus suggest these agents may be useful adjuvants for neuropathic cancer pain syndromes, including neural invasion by tumor, radiation fibrosis or surgical scarring, herpes zoster, and deafferentation. Some clinical improvement can be expected in half to two-thirds of patients whose predominant complaint is pain of a shooting, lancinating, burning, or hyperesthetic nature. Effective doses in the treatment of neuropathic pain in patients with cancer are not well established, and there is no clear-cut standard of care for use of these agents to guide the choice of agent or sequence of agents used in therapeutic trials. A common mistake is reporting that a patient failed to respond to this class of agents without either dose titration or adequate period of time to evaluate for response. For instance, clinical trials indicate a dose of 900 to 1200 mg per day before most patients begin to report relief of neuropathic symptoms. Because many of the side effects such as drowsiness occur when increasing the dose of neurontin, this should be done slowly over several weeks.

D. Corticosteroids

Controlled studies suggest that the administration of corticosteroids to selected patients with advanced cancer results in decreased pain and improved appetite and activity. Unfortunately, the duration of the effects is probably short-lasting. The mechanism by which corticosteroids appear to produce beneficial symptom effects in patients with terminal cancer is unclear but may involve their euphoric effects or the inhibition of prostaglandin metabolism. The optimal drug and dosing regimens have not been established. For the treatment of painful conditions, prednisone or dexamethasone is often administered in doses totaling 30 to 60 mg by mouth daily and 8 to 16 mg by mouth daily, respectively. As soon as symptomatic relief is obtained, attempts should be made to decrease the dose progressively to the minimally effective dose. Although long-term side effects are not an important consideration in many patients with advanced cancer, treatment may produce limiting side effects in these patients, particularly immunosuppression (candidiasis occurs in most patients), proximal myopathy, and psychiatric symptoms. The incidence of psychological disturbances ranges from 3% to 50%, with severe symptoms occurring in about 5% of patients. The spectrum of disturbances ranges from mild to severe affective disorders, psychotic reactions, and global cognitive impairment.

E. Clonidine, an α_2-adrenergic agonist developed for treatment of hypertension, can be administered orally or as part of an epidural regimen for control of cancer-related pain, especially neuropathic pain.

F. Approaches to metastatic bone pain

1. **Radioisotope therapy.** Strontium-89 and samarium-153 are isotopes that have been found to be useful in providing systemic radiotherapy for palliation of pain in patients with bony metastases. These agents can be useful in patients with adequate bone marrow reserve who have multiple pain locations that limit the feasibility of external beam radiation therapy. The main limitations of radioisotope therapy are its high cost and the potential for hematologic toxicity (mainly thrombocytopenia).

2. **Bisphosphonates.** These agents have been found to be significantly better than placebo in patients with bone pain due to a variety of primary tumors. Pamidronate, clodronate, and zoledronate are the agents that have been most frequently studied. Because of their poor oral bioavailability, these drugs are most useful when given intravenously. In addition to pain control, these drugs can significantly reduce a number of other complications of osteolysis, such as hypercalcemia, fractures, and need for radiation therapy. Osteonecrosis of the jaw is a serious but rare complication. Dental evaluation should be done prior to initiation of long-term therapy, and dental work completed as soon as possible, preferably when not actively receiving bisphosphonate therapy.

3. **External-beam radiotherapy.** Radiation therapy can effectively control bone pain in about 70% of patients within 2 to 4 weeks. This treatment is most useful in patients with a single or small number of painful areas. A single administration may be as effective as multiple smaller fractions, reducing the cost and discomfort of transportation back and forth associated with multiple doses.

VI. ADJUVANT PROCEDURES AND THERAPIES
A. Invasive procedures

Evaluation of the physical basis of the pain may indicate that a neuroablative procedure, in which the pain pathway is destroyed, would be of benefit for pain control. As aggressive opioid analgesia becomes more accepted, most patients with cancer do not require these neuroablative interventions. Destruction of the pain pathway can be accomplished surgically or through destructive nerve blocks using an agent such as phenol. The major barrier to the more widespread application of these techniques is the limited number of practitioners with expertise in their use. The most frequently used neurosurgical procedure is the anterolateral or spinothalamic cordotomy. This is often performed as closed percutaneous cordotomy by placing a radiofrequency needle in the anterolateral quadrant of the cervical spinal cord. Unilateral interventions for pain control can unmask significant pain on the contralateral side of the body. Most often, performance of such interventional pain procedures does not eliminate the need to administer and monitor the effectiveness of systemic analgesics. Because of afferent regeneration, destructive procedures have had their greatest application in patients whose expected life span is only a few months.

Destructive anesthetic block of the celiac plexus has been used for several decades in the management of pain in the abdominal region. This block, which can be preceded by reversible diagnostic block, is a boon to many patients suffering from the severe pain accompanying cancer of the pancreas and may also be helpful for pain from cancers of the liver, gallbladder, or stomach. If success is achieved with the diagnostic block, lasting disruption of the pain pathway can be achieved using alcohol or phenol. Pain from rib metastases or tumors of the chest wall can be relieved with intercostal nerve blocks.

Patients with bone metastases sometimes develop pathologic vertebral compression fractures. Percutaneous vertebroplasty is a surgical procedure that involves use of polymethylmethacrylate as bone cement that is injected at high pressure through a needle into the collapsed vertebral body in order to stabilize it and relieve pain. Another interventional technique with similar goals is called kyphoplasty. This procedure involves percutaneous insertion of a needle with an inflatable balloon placed into the fractured vertebra using fluoroscopic guidance. The balloon is inflated so that the vertebral endplates are elevated and bone height is restored. The resulting bone cavity is then filled with acrylic bone cement.

Finally, patients with painful metastatic lesions involving bone that have failed conventional treatments such as external beam radiation therapy and chemotherapy may benefit from percutaneous radiofrequency ablation as a salvage procedure. This is an image-guided procedure, and a single ablation procedure is effective in most patients and well tolerated.

B. Coping or behavioral skill techniques

Teaching specific skills to manage pain can be helpful to many patients, especially those who face pain for months to years. Evaluation and prescription of the specific skills most beneficial to the individual can often be obtained through consultation with a behavioral psychologist, psychiatrist, or nurse pain specialist. Such techniques should never be used as a substitute for appropriate analgesia. The skills include relaxation, self-hypnosis, and other distraction and cognitive control techniques. These measures can affect the sensation of pain by reducing muscle tension on pain-generating lesions as well as by maximizing the patient's ability to cope with the pain and remain as active as the disease permits. All patients need education about the nature of their pain, the methods that can be used to relieve it, and how they can cooperate with their healthcare providers to achieve good pain control.

C. Acupuncture

This ancient traditional Chinese medicine technique is based on qi, the body's vital energy. Needles are placed along qi meridians in order to help treat symptoms such as pain. For some patients, acupressure may be used, which involves applying heat or pressure to meridian points instead of puncturing the skin. Stainless steel or gold (semipermanent) needles, seeds, or "studs" are also sometimes placed at specific points on the ears and left in place for several days. Several acupuncture trials for pain have shown a beneficial effect including among cancer patients. Appropriate training and a strong working relationship are a prerequisite when considering the use of acupuncture for cancer patients. Patients at risk for infection (e.g., neutropenia) or bleeding (e.g., thrombocytopenia or on anticoagulation) may need to avoid acupuncture.

Selected Readings

Breivik H, Cherny N, Collett B, et al. Cancer-related pain: a pan-European survey of prevalence, treatment, and patient attitudes. *Ann Oncol.* 2009;20(8):1420–1433.

Burton AW, Fanciullo GJ, Beasley RD, Fisch MJ. Chronic pain in the cancer survivor: a new frontier. *Pain Med.* 2007;8(2):189–198.

Bruera E, Palmer JL, Bosnjak S, et al. Methadone versus morphine as a first-line strong opioid for cancer pain: a randomized, double-blind study. *J Clin Oncol.* 2004;22:185–192.

Bruera E, Kim HN. Cancer pain. *JAMA.* 2003;290:2476–2479.

Carr DB, Goudas LC, Balk EM, Bloch R, Ioannidis JP, Lau J. Evidence report on the treatment of pain in cancer patients. *J Natl Cancer Instit Monogr.* 2004;32:23–31.

Cherney N, Ripamonti C, Pereira J, et al. Strategies to manage the adverse effects of oral morphine: an evidence-based report. *J Clin Oncol.* 2001;19:2542–2554.

Cleeland CS, Gonin R, Hatfield AK, et al. Pain and its treatment in outpatients with metastatic cancer. *N Engl J Med.* 1994;330:592–596.

Davis MP, Weissman DE, Arnold RM. Opioid dose titration for severe cancer pain: a systematic, evidence-based review. *J Palliat Med.* 2004;7:462–468.

Davis MP. What is new in neuropathic pain? *Support Care Cancer.* 2007;15(4):363–372.

de Leon-Casasola OA. Interventional procedures for cancer pain management: when are they indicated? *Cancer Invest.* 2004;22:630–642.

Foley KM. Treatment of cancer-related pain. *J Natl Cancer Instit Monogr.* 2004;32:103–104.

Fourney DR, Schomer DF, Nader R, et al. Percutaneous vertebroplasty and kypho-plasty for painful vertebral body fractures in cancer patients. *J Neurosurg.* 2003; 98:21–30.

Goetz MP, Callstrom MR, Charboneau JW, et al. Percutaneous, image-guided radio-frequency ablation of painful metastases involving bone: a multicenter study. *J Clin Oncol.* 2004;22(2):300–306.

Lawlor PG. The panorama of opioid-related cognitive dysfunction in patients with cancer. *Cancer.* 2002;94:1836–1853.

Manfredi PL, Houde RW. Prescribing methadone, a unique analgesic. *J Support Oncol.* 2003;1:216–220.

Mercadante S, Bruera E. Opioid switching: a systematic and critical review. *Cancer Treat Rev.* 2006;32(4):304–315.

Moryl N, Coyle N, Foley KM. Managing an acute pain crisis in a patient with advanced cancer: "this is as much of a crisis as a code." *JAMA.* 2008;299(12):1457–1467.

Pereira J, Lawlor P, Vigano A, Dorgan M, Bruera E. Equianalgesic dose ratios for opi-oids: a critical review and proposals for long-term dosing. *J Pain Symptom Manage.* 2001;22:672–677.

Quigley C. Opioid switching to improve pain relief and drug tolerability. *Cochrane Da-tabase Syst Rev.* 2004;25:169–178.

Smith HS. Opioid metabolism. *Mayo Clin Proc.* 2009;84(7):613–624.

Stockler M, Vardy J, Pillai A, Warr D. Acetaminophen (paracetamol) improves pain and well-being in people with advanced cancer already receiving a strong opioid regimen: a randomized, double-blind, placebo-controlled cross-over trial. *J Clin Oncol.* 2004;22(16):3389–3394.

Strouse TB. Pharmacokinetic drug interactions in palliative care: focus on opioids. *J Palliat Med.* 2009;12(11):1043–1050.

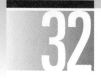

Emotional and Psychiatric Problems in Patients With Cancer
Kristi Skeel Williams and Kathleen S.N. Franco-Bronson

I. GENERAL PRINCIPLES

Clinical psychiatric disorders occur in up to half of patients with cancer at some point during their treatment. Delirium, depression, and anxiety are most frequently seen and may coexist in the same patient. Vigilant monitoring for early symptoms of psychiatric distress is important in the care of these patients. The clinician should inquire regularly about symptoms in affective and cognitive domains. Symptom clusters help differentiate anxiety, depression, and acute confusional states from other psychiatric disorders. Once an accurate diagnosis is made, safety, tolerability, efficacy, and price influence choice of medication. More than one psychiatric diagnosis may be present, requiring a hierarchical approach. For example, if both delirium and depression are present, the cause of the delirium should be determined and treated before starting antidepressant therapy (which could worsen the delirium). Once the delirium has improved, treatment for the depression can be considered. When major depression and an anxiety disorder coexist, treatment for the depression is started first and may adequately manage both disorders.

II. ACUTE CONFUSIONAL STATES

Approximately 15% of hospitalized patients with cancer experience delirium, but this can increase to 80% to 85% in those receiving palliative care.

A. Precepts

Attempting to treat delirium with psychotropic drugs, but without understanding the cause of the patient's confusion, can have serious consequences. Delirium is characterized by fluctuating levels of alertness and consciousness, shortened attention and concentration, rapidly changing moods, irregular sleep–wake cycles, garbled or slurred speech, hypervigilance, and behavior not consistent with good judgment. The delirious patient may also have delusional ideas or hallucinations or appear depressed. Visual, auditory, tactile, and occasionally olfactory hallucinations can be present. The more sensory modalities that are involved in the hallucinations, the greater the likelihood that the patient is experiencing a medically induced confusional state.

B. Etiologies

1. **Medications** remain the most common reason for acute confusional states. The most frequently identified medications to cause delirium are sedatives, narcotic analgesics, anxiolytics, anticholinergic drugs, and corticosteroids. Antineoplastic and immunotherapeutic agents can cause delirium: cytarabine, methotrexate, asparaginase, fluorouracil, interferon, and interleukin. Even histamine blockage from agents like diphenhydramine or famotidine can lead to delirium.

2. **Metabolic causes** are often seen in patients with cancer and include hypernatremia and hyponatremia, hyperthyroidism and hypothyroidism, poorly controlled diabetes mellitus, vitamin deficiencies (B_{12}, folate, thiamine), and hypercalcemia.

3. **Infections** of the respiratory, urinary, central nervous, and other systems are common, especially in immunosuppressed patients.

4. **Chemical withdrawal** from benzodiazepines, alcohol, and other drugs can induce delirium.

5. **Medical illness** such as tumors, particularly primary brain tumors and brain metastases, cardiac arrhythmias, congestive heart failure, liver disease, trauma, strokes, and renal failure. Hyperviscosity syndrome with lymphoma, myeloma, and Waldenström macroglobulinemia are unusual causes. After radiation to the brain, confusional states can occur, especially if the patient received a small amount of steroid. An acute confusional state can occur secondary to a paraneoplastic syndrome frequently associated with lymphoma. In addition to the original illness, postoperative head and neck surgery, often for malignancy, carries a higher risk than many other surgical procedures for delirium.

C. Therapeutic approach

Once an acute confusional state is identified, the primary therapeutic approach is to treat the cause. The key is to determine when symptoms of delirium first occurred and to look for preceding changes in medications, vital signs, laboratory studies, or imagery/radiology. This helps to determine how to best proceed with treatment (e.g., withdrawing a medication or treating a urinary tract infection found on a urinalysis). When hypoactive delirium occurs, inclining the head to 30% reduces the risk for aspiration. Moving the patient frequently may prevent bed sores. Hyperactive patients with delirium are at high risk for falls and subsequent fractures. Research has demonstrated that a combined protocol of physical mobilization, cognitive exercise through conversation and reorientation, appropriate hydration, use of glasses or hearing aids from home, and minimizing sedatives at night can reduce the number, severity, and cost of delirium episodes. Antipsychotic medications may be helpful for managing symptoms such as hallucinations, delusions, and extreme agitation, but they do not treat the cause of the delirium.

1. **Orientation (frequent reconnection)** of the patient aids in reduction of confusion.

   a. **It is helpful to orient the patient frequently** to place, time, and why they are at the hospital and to give current explanations of procedures. This routine should be done once or more per shift when the delirious patient is awake. Because the patient's attention, concentration, and recent memory are frequently impaired, the patient often does not recall instructions given earlier. Leaving a large, legibly written note card with the patient's name, date, hospital name, and other data is beneficial in some instances.

   b. **A large calendar, a clock, and family pictures or mementos** can assist the patient in feeling less estranged from his or her environment. It can be very reassuring to a patient if a family member can stay with them overnight.

   c. **Some patients are reassured by a small night light in their room,** which cuts down on illusions or misinterpretations. Patients with compromised vision or hearing are particularly distraught when they are even less able to discern what is happening around them, and they should be provided with their regular hearing aids and glasses.

2. **Medication** helps to control hallucinations, delusions, and psychotic agitation. The lowest dose to control symptoms is usually preferable.

   a. **Haloperidol** (Haldol; Table 32.1) is a butyrophenone, an antipsychotic agent with potent dopamine-blocking action. It is less likely to produce cardiovascular, respiratory, gastrointestinal, and general anticholinergic side effects than many of the other antipsychotic medications. However, moderate doses may cause extrapyramidal symptoms. The starting dose in a patient with an acute confusional state is 0.25 to 2 mg by mouth or intramuscularly, on an as-needed or regular dosing schedule every 4 to 6 hours. A marked advantage of haloperidol is that sedation is minimized while controlling agitation. There are exceptions to the usually preferred low doses of antipsychotic medications. For example, if patients tolerate higher doses with few side effects, they may benefit by having improved pain control. Intravenous (IV) haloperidol has not been approved by the U.S. Food and Drug Administration, although it is commonly used in the seriously agitated patient. There are fewer extrapyramidal symptoms with IV haloperidol, but the half-life in this form is much shorter, requiring more frequent administration. Avoid very high doses in patients

Agent	Starting Dose (mg)*	Characteristics
Phenothiazines		
Chlorpromazine (Thorazine)	10–25	Significant hypotension risk, lowers seizure threshold, highly sedating, anticholinergic
Thioridazine (Mellaril)	10–25	Similar to chlorpromazine but more likely to alter electrocardiogram, not available IM
Perphenazine (Trilafon)	4	Moderate sedation and hypotension
Trifluoperazine (Stelazine)	2	High frequency of extrapyramidal side effects
Others		
Haloperidol (Haldol)	0.5–2.0	Good for acute delirium, high frequency of extrapyramidal side effects, available IV, IM, or PO; short-acting; IV haloperidol has a very short half-life and must be given frequently, but there is much less extrapyramidal side-effect; IM depot every 2–4 weeks
Risperidone (Risperdal)	0.5–1.0	Some α-adrenergic effects, mild extrapyramidal side effects as dose increases, PO form for daily use; IM depot (2 week) form
Olanzapine (Zyprexa)	5	More sedation; weight gain; fewer extrapyramidal side effects; PO form regular capsule, liquid, and tablet that dissolves on tongue; IM for acute use up to two times per day
Quetiapine (Seroquel)	25–50	More sedation, fewer extrapyramidal effects
Ziprasidone (Geodon)	20	Less weight gain, fewer extrapyramidal effects, IM for acute use up to two times per day
Aripiprazole (Abilify)	5–20	Less weight gain and extrapyramidal effects, can elevate mood, occasionally to hypomania
Asenapine (Saphris)	5	Sublingual tablets, avoid eating or drinking for 10 minutes after administration

IM, intramuscularly; IV, intravenously; PO, by mouth.
*Dose generally can be repeated every 4–6 hours (other than risperidone, olanzapine, quetiapine, ziprasidone, asenapine), on either an as needed or a regular schedule (e.g., twice a day).

with alcoholic cardiomyopathy, those prone to torsades de pointes or similar arrhythmias, and those with an excessively long corrected QT interval.

b. **Risperidone, olanzapine, ziprasidone, quetiapine, and aripiprazole.** Risperidone (Risperdal, Risperdal M-Tab) is less likely to produce extrapyramidal side effects, but is available only in oral form for acute (nondepot) use. Olanzapine (Zyprexa, Zydis) is sedating and can be given in a tablet that dissolves on the tongue or in an intramuscular form. Ziprasidone (Geodon) can also be given in a rapid onset intramuscular preparation. Quetiapine (Seroquel) is only available orally, as is aripiprazole (Abilify, Abilify Discmelt). Aripiprazole acts slowly and would not help reduce symptoms quickly. Some immediate antipsychotic preparations can be crushed and put in a feeding tube.

c. **A delirious patient** with vision or hearing impairment is likely to hallucinate during periods of excessive sedation, especially if there is pulmonary compromise or a tendency toward hypoxia.

d. **If the patient demonstrates a predictable period of confusion,** such as during the early evening ("sun-downing") when there is less environmental activity, a small once-a-day dose at that time may be adequate.

e. **When increasing the dose of antipsychotic drugs,** muscle spasms, restlessness, or pseudoparkinsonian symptoms may occur with older first-generation antipsychotics and some second-generation agents like risperidone or ziprasidone. Adding a small amount of trihexyphenidyl (Artane) 1 to 2 mg twice a day, benztropine (Cogentin) 1 mg twice a day, or diphenhydramine (Benadryl) 25 mg twice a day can often reduce the side effects. However, increasing the level of anticholinergic activity with these choices may cause an atropenic-like psychosis. Constipation, urinary retention, dry mouth, tachycardia, and increasing confusion are warnings of this potential problem, especially when multiple anticholinergic medications (e.g., antiemetics, analgesics) are being prescribed. Therefore, antiparkinsonian drugs are not prescribed prophylactically but only if clearly indicated. Ondansetron (Zofran), granisetron (Kytril), or dolasetron (Anzemet) may be substituted for other antiemetics, reducing extrapyramidal symptoms and avoiding the need for an antiparkinsonian medication. Some antiemetics (e.g., droperidol) are also antipsychotics, but these, like metoclopramide, can lead to extrapyramidal symptoms like akathisia or dystonias.

f. **Benzodiazepines** such as lorazepam (Ativan) can be given 0.5 to 2.0 mg every 8 hours. They can be administered in small doses to a patient who needs some sedation without added anticholinergic activity or those whose cardiac status is at risk (i.e., heart block) if some antipsychotic medications were increased. Using both benzodiazepines and antipsychotics is sometimes helpful.

g. **Increasing delirium.** Too much medication may have been given if the patient's agitation increases with higher doses. Secondary hypoxia and akathisia should be excluded. High blood levels of longer-acting medications can accumulate, particularly if serum albumin and protein is low and hepatic and renal functioning are compromised.

h. **Hypotension.** Avoid adding a second antipsychotic (e.g., chlorpromazine), as it may predispose to hypotension and shock. If the blood pressure does drop significantly, norepinephrine bitartrate (Levophed) or a similar choice may be necessary as antipsychotic medications like haloperidol also block some peripheral actions of dopamine.

III. DEPRESSION

Depression is roughly four times more common in patients with cancer than in age-matched controls. Oropharyngeal, pancreatic, lung, and breast cancer are associated with the highest rates of depression. Earlier studies indicated that patients with both cancer and depression had a higher risk of death, but larger meta-analysis did not find this to be true. However, patients who are depressed report poorer pain control, poorer compliance, and more often choose to discontinue treatment.

Patients with cancer have various emotional responses to their diagnoses. The mourning period for some is brief, does not inhibit their ability to interact with family and friends, and does not hinder participation in their own treatment. Support from others, acceptance of their feelings, and time may be all that is necessary for them to continue the emotional work ahead. However, about one-fourth of patients with cancer develop longer, more severe depression. The greatest risk of depression is at the time of first relapse. There are many variables that influence this process, including emotional conflicts with loved ones, disproportionate guilt, previous losses that were never resolved, long-standing debilitating illness, individual personality characteristics such as dependency, and inadequate support systems. Any of these factors, along with a family history of depression, are warnings for the physician to heed.

Besides emotional response to the stress of having cancer and undergoing treatment, other causes of depression should be considered. Folate or vitamin B_{12} deficiencies, thyroid or parathyroid disorders, adrenal insufficiency, leptomeningeal disease, and brain metastases can induce depression. Interferon can sometimes precipitate sadness to suicidal proportions in patients who have never previously experienced depression. Some recommend an antidepressant be started 2 weeks prior to starting interferon if a patient has a prior history of major depression.

Passive suicidal thoughts with depression are common. Patients who actually do commit suicide are more likely to be male, have advanced disease, and a history of psychiatric illness, substance abuse, and prior attempts. Good pain control and efforts to reduce isolation can lessen suicidal thoughts and behavior.

A. Therapeutic approach

1. **Emotional support** at frequent intervals from the physician is generally needed. Some patients explore old emotional conflicts, whereas others just need a safe person to whom they can express their feelings. It is important for patients to be able to hold on to hope. A degree of denial is acceptable, normal, and upheld. Only when this denial makes it impossible for a patient to make informed treatment decisions is it necessary to probe into the denial.

   Psychotherapy of a supportive nature is often provided by the primary care physician, oncologist, psychiatrist, clergy, nurse, family, or friend individually or in any combination. For patients who wish to explore ambivalence, a professional psychotherapist trained in psychodynamic or interpersonal therapy is a good option. Cognitive therapy is helpful in letting go of detrimental interpretations while increasing one's ability to deal with emotional pain.

2. **Psychiatric care** may be particularly instrumental when the patient's pre-existing personality style is interfering with treatment. Anniversary responses to previous losses, important family events, or past hospitalizations may have a great impact on the presentation of the depression and deserve exploration by a psychotherapist if a pattern is found. If there is a designated psychiatric consultant, this individual must work closely with the rest of the oncology team, communicating in a helpful way to the patient, family, and staff.

   If a patient has felt depressed, distressed, or irritable for some time or describes a loss of pleasure from formerly enjoyable relationships or activities, inquiry about the following symptoms is necessary: insomnia or hypersomnia; alteration in appetite with expected weight change; reduced interest in family, sexuality, work, or hobbies; increased guilt; low energy level; poor concentration; thoughts of death or suicide; frequent crying episodes; and psychomotor hypoactivity or hyperactivity. When the diagnosis of depression in the medically ill patient is being made, the emphasis is placed on psychological features as opposed to physical ones. These include rumination or repetitive negative thoughts, increased tearfulness, hopeless–helpless feelings, withdrawal from family or friends, and anhedonia. These symptoms are characteristic of a major depressive disorder for which antidepressant medications in addition to psychotherapy are recommended. In some studies, group therapy for patients with breast cancer has improved quality of life and may prolong survival.

   It is important to screen for a past history of mania and hypomania in individuals with depression, as well as a family history of bipolar disorder, as antidepressants must be used with extreme caution, if used at all, for patients with a positive personal or family history.

3. **Medications.** In the past, patients with cancer were often undertreated for major depression that was mistaken as an "understandable" consequence of their illness or as simple grief. Now, evidence exists that psychosocial adjustment and improved life adaptation, in general, occur when patients with cancer and major depression are treated with antidepressant medications.

   a. **Selection of agents and their side effects.** In addition to efficacy, an antidepressant medication should be selected on the basis of its safety and tolerability, including any tendency to sedate or activate, cause orthostatic changes, or produce anticholinergic effects. Medication selection should also be tailored to the patient's symptom cluster such as the need for sedation or weight gain versus the need for activation (Tables 32.2 and 32.3). The route of metabolism and elimination, as well as any increased risk for seizures, should affect the choice. Agents like venlafaxine and duloxetine can reduce depression in patients with or without anxiety and improve pain control. Starting with lower doses and titrating up can lessen the risk of added nausea.

   There is increasing evidence that selective serotonin reuptake inhibitors (SSRIs) inhibit platelet aggregation and prolong bleeding. Although this might be helpful to patients who also have cardiovascular disease, these agents should

Antidepressant	Sedation*	Anticholinergic Actions[†]	Other Characteristics
Amitriptyline (Elavil, Endep)	+4 to +5[‡]	+4 to +5	Also available IM, orthostasis, quinidine-like, good for neuropathic pain
Doxepin (Sinequan, Adapin, Silenor)	+4	+3 to +4	Highest appetite increase, orthostasis, good for neuropathic pain
Nortriptyline (Pamelor, Aventyl)	+3	+3	Less likely to cause orthostasis than other tricyclic antidepressants

IM, intramuscularly.
Note: Do not use tricyclic if corrected QT interval >450. Tricyclics can also suppress respiratory drive and reduce seizure threshold.
*Associated with histaminergic blockade; appetite increase follows somewhat similar trends.
[†]Constipation, dry mouth, and urinary retention.
[‡]Scale of 1–5, where 1 is least and 5 is most.

TABLE 32.3 Characteristics of Commonly Used Nonheterocyclic Antidepressants

Antidepressant	Sedation*	Anticholinergic Actions[†]	Other Characteristics
Bupropion (Wellbutrin)	+1[‡]	+1	Associated with increased seizure risk especially if organic brain pathology or eating disorder is present, more activating, less weight gain
Fluoxetine (Prozac)**	+1	+1	May cause restlessness and gastrointestinal upset, more activating, less weight gain, safe in patients with renal disease but may accumulate in those with liver disease, self-tapers when discontinued
Sertraline (Zoloft)**	+1	+1	Similar to fluoxetine, more diarrhea, few drug interactions, short half-life, should be tapered if discontinued
Paroxetine (Paxil)**	+1	+2	Similar to fluoxetine, more anticholinergic than other SSRIs, should be tapered if discontinued
Citalopram (Celexa)	+1	+1	Similar to sertraline, few drug interactions
Escitalopram (Lexapro)	+1–2	+1	Similar to sertraline, few drug interactions
Venlafaxine (Effexor)	+1–2	+1	Both SSRI and norepinephrine reuptake inhibitor, increases blood pressure at higher doses, augments pain relief
Duloxetine (Cymbalta)	+1–2	+1	Similar to venlafaxine
Mirtazapine (Remeron)	+4	+2	Weight gain, potential increase in cholesterol, sedation, available as tablet that dissolves on tongue

SSRI, selective serotonin reuptake inhibitor.
*Associated with histaminergic blockade; appetite increase follows somewhat similar trends.
[†]Constipation, dry mouth, and urinary retention.
[‡]Scale of 1–5, where 1 is least and 5 is most.
**May interfere with conversion of tamoxifen to its metabolites due to inhibition of CYP450 2D6.

be discontinued when there is observed evidence of acute bleeding as indicated by rapid falls in hemoglobin and hematocrit. There is also some evidence that SSRIs inhibit CYP2D6 (see Table 32.3) and may interfere with the effectiveness of tamoxifen.

Highly anticholinergic medications frequently produce dry mouth, blurred vision, tachycardia, and constipation. They can also produce urinary retention, ileus, and acute confusion. Antihistaminergic drugs can increase sedation and appetite and worsen hypotension. Both H_1- and H_2-blocking agents can cause delirium, while a proton pump inhibitor will not. Medications that produce α-adrenergic receptor blockade are associated with increased orthostatic hypotension, dizziness, and reflex tachycardia. Stimulants such as methylphenidate and modafinil may be beneficial to treat depression and lethargy in the medically ill patient. Caution is advised in patients with cardiovascular disease or hepatic impairment.

b. **Dosages (Table 32.4).** Weak, debilitated, or elderly patients need protection from the side effects of psychotropic agents. Starting out with small doses and gradually increasing the dose is prudent. Splitting doses may also be helpful for minimizing side effects and maximizing pain relief from antidepressant medications.

   If a patient has a personal history, family history, or previous response to medication (e.g., steroids) that reflects manic or hypomanic symptoms, proceed carefully. A mood stabilizer such as lithium or an anticonvulsant should be considered, as should consultation with a psychiatrist.

c. **Monoamine oxidase inhibitors (MAOIs)** may be used to treat major depression or panic disorder but are somewhat inconvenient owing to tyramine dietary restrictions and medication interactions requiring much attention. They are sometimes tried when other choices have failed. There is a transdermal form of selegiline (Emsam) available that does not require dietary modification at the lowest dose of 6 mg/24 h.

TABLE 32.4	Dosages for Antidepressant Therapy	

Drug	Starting Daily Dose (mg)	Average Daily Dose for Patients With Cancer (mg)
Amitriptyline	10–25	75–150
Bupropion	75–150	300
Citalopram	10–20	20–40
Doxepin	25	75–150
Duloxetine	20 mg twice a day	30–40 mg twice a day
Escitalopram	10 mg	20 mg
Fluoxetine	10–20	20
Mirtazapine	7.5–15	30+
Nortriptyline	10–25	50–100
Paroxetine	10–20	20
Sertraline	25–50	100
Venlafaxine	25 or 37.5 (extended-release form)	75 mg (37.5 mg twice a day)

IV. ANXIETY

A. Approach to the problem

As grieving is described as normal, so is anxiety in patients with cancer. However, anxiety varies in its cause, severity, and treatment. A detailed history of the onset, characteristics, and length of distress is important. Knowledge of the patient's previous symptoms, current and past physical illness, substance abuse, and medication usage is essential to the evaluation process. Like depression, anxiety also amplifies pain. Antianxiety agents may be helpful for alleviating patients' distress and helping them cope with other problems associated with their cancer (Table 32.5).

B. Problems that present as anxiety

The duration of the symptoms is one of the first factors to assess in the anxious patient.

1. **Suspect an adjustment disorder** when maladaptive anxious symptoms have persisted less than 6 months and apparently represent an adjustment to learning the diagnosis or reactions to the treatment. This kind of anxiety may benefit from supportive therapy, relaxation therapy, or benzodiazepines.

2. **Generalized anxiety.** If the anxiety has been present for more than 6 months, continuing no matter what environmental alterations occur, and is accompanied by signs of physical tension or poor attention to conversation or other daily activities, the patient is likely to have generalized anxiety. Supportive therapy, relaxation tapes, biofeedback, buspirone, gabapentin, and benzodiazepines such as clonazepam are useful.

3. **Brief, isolated episodes of anxiety** that come and go lead the examiner to consider other diagnoses.

   a. **Panic attacks.** If the patient has repeated "attacks" that have a rapid onset and last 20 minutes to a few hours and if they are accompanied by tachycardia, palpitations, shortness of breath, hyperventilation, choking, sweating, dizziness, and the wish to flee, without a physical or chemical explanation, they are most likely panic attacks. They may be treated with benzodiazepines such as clonazepam and alprazolam; however, antidepressants such as tricyclics, SSRIs, MAOIs, or mirtazapine are also effective. Antidepressants must be started at a very low dose (e.g., sertraline 12.5 mg, paroxetine 5 mg, or imipramine 10 mg) and increased slowly every 1 to 2 days to avoid increased anxiety. While the dose is brought up to that typically used in depression, benzodiazepines may be added if needed. Benzodiazepines with a short half-life, like alprazolam, can induce breakthrough panic if tolerance develops, so those with longer half-lives, like clonazepam, may be preferred if tolerated. β-Blockers to block autonomic symptoms may be tried if performance anxiety around specific activities is identified, but they are less effective for panic disorder, as is buspirone.

TABLE 32.5 Antianxiety Agents and Nighttime Sedatives

Agent	Half-life (h)	Onset	Starting Dose (mg)*
Benzodiazepines			
Oxazepam (Serax)†	8–20	Moderate	10 (t.i.d.)
Lorazepam (Ativan)†	10–20	Rapid	0.5 (t.i.d.)
Temazepam (Restoril)†	12–24	Rapid	15 (qh.s.)
Alprazolam (Xanax)	12–24	Moderate	0.25 (t.i.d.)
Chlordiazepoxide (Librium)	12–48	Moderate	10 (b.i.d.)
Clonazepam (Klonopin)	20–30	Rapid	0.5 (b.i.d.)
Diazepam (Valium)	20–90	Rapid	2–5 (b.i.d.)
Clorazepate (Tranxene)	20–100	Rapid	7.5 (b.i.d.)
Flurazepam (Dalmane)	20–100	Rapid	15 (qh.s.)
Nonbenzodiazepine hypnotics			
Zolpidem (Ambien)†	1.5–4.5	Rapid	5 (qh.s.)
Zaleplon (Sonata)†	1.0	Rapid	5 (qh.s.)
Eszopiclone (Lunesta)	6	Rapid	1–2 (qh.s.)
Ramelteon (Rozerem)	1–2.5	Rapid	8 (qh.s.)

Other (for insomnia, pain, anxiety symptoms)
Gabapentin (Neurontin) 100–300 mg t.i.d. starting dose, can give larger dose qh.s.

Antidepressants (for panic disorder)
Start at lower doses than for depression (e.g., imipramine, starting dose of 10 mg t.i.d.).
  Some antidepressants, like bupropion, have no efficacy for panic disorder.

β-Blockers (for autonomic symptom control)
Propranolol (Inderal) 10–20 mg t.i.d.
Atenolol (Tenormin) 25–50 mg daily

Antipsychotics (for anxiety associated with delirium)

Antihistamines
May be safer in some cases when respiratory impairment is a complication; also used for insomnia.
Diphenhydramine (Benadryl) 25 mg; starting doses b.i.d. or t.i.d.
Hydroxyzine (Vistaril) 50 mg; starting doses t.i.d. or q.i.d.

b.i.d., twice daily; qh.s., at bedtime; q.i.d., four times daily; t.i.d., three times a day.
Note: Elderly or extremely debilitated patients should be given lower doses. Caution should be taken when prescribing long-acting sedating medications because they have been associated with a high incidence of falls and hip fracture.
*If chronic alcohol or benzodiazepine use exists, it is probable that the dose needed is at least double the starting doses listed.
†Preferred in the elderly.

  b. **Organic causes are often responsible for the anxiety**
    (1) **Hypoxia.** Repeating episodes of anxiety accompanied by alterations in intellectual functioning, poor orientation, reduced judgment, shortened attention, a rapidly fluctuating mood, and difficulty with memory suggest hypoxia. When anxiety is induced by hypoxia, it is wise to reduce

central nervous system (CNS) depressant medications and give small doses of an antipsychotic drug if the anxiety is accompanied by delirium. However, older antipsychotic and antiemetic medications as well as metoclopramide often produce akathisia, an extrapyramidal restlessness that mimics anxiety. Alternating the antipsychotic drug with small doses of a benzodiazepine with a short half-life is one option for organically induced anxiety, as long as respiratory status or arterial blood gas measurements do not worsen. Newer antipsychotic agents are less likely to produce extrapyramidal akathisia but still should be monitored with pulse oximetry measurements.

(2) Liver disease and other physical disorders. If anxiety is associated with liver disease, start by reducing CNS depressant medications. When needed, small infrequent doses of a short-acting benzodiazepine that requires conjugation but not oxidation in the liver are prescribed. These include lorazepam, oxazepam, and temazepam. Many other physical disorders can also produce anxious symptoms, including various brain tumors, pheochromocytoma, carcinoid, hyperthyroidism, cardiac arrhythmias, drug or alcohol withdrawal, and hyperparathyroidism. Gabapentin, which is renally cleared, may help with anxiety, sleep, and pain. It can also help augment other medications for mood stabilization and panic disorder.

(3) Medications such as theophylline, corticosteroids, antidepressants, and antipsychotic drugs can produce anxiety. Anxiety is frequently one of multiple symptoms associated with benzodiazepine or narcotic analgesic withdrawal. Akathisia mimics anxiety and often occurs with prochlorperazine, promethazine, perphenazine, and metoclopramide. It is generally wise to stop these medications to avoid prolonging this very uncomfortable, involuntary condition and find a suitable alternative.

c. Precipitating events that initiate the previously discussed adjustment disorder lasting generally no longer than 6 months can be identified in patients with cancer. Posttraumatic stress disorder (PTSD), less often seen in patients with cancer, follows a distressing event beyond what would be expected. Younger women with breast cancer are at higher risk for PTSD, especially if they have less education and lower income. More advanced disease, medical sequelae of treatments, and longer hospital admissions also contribute. More frequently observed, however, are patients who describe intense fears of needles, radiotherapy rooms, or confined-space scanning devices. Often, the history unfolds to describe previously existing phobias. These patients, like those with anticipatory anxiety about procedures or chemotherapy, may be assisted with relaxation or desensitization techniques, imagery, anti-anxiety medications, and assurance. If patients begin to experience procedures, treatments, or interpersonal situations as being particularly stressful, anticipatory anxiety intensifies the requirement for larger doses of as-needed medication to attain some relief. Therefore, regular scheduling of antianxiety medication similar to that of pain medication is in order.

V. INSOMNIA
A. Principles
Difficulty falling asleep may be associated with anxiety, whereas awakening in the middle of the night is generally more closely related to depression. In addition, there are a variety of physical disorders that cause sleeping irregularities. The sleep–wake cycle is almost always disturbed in a delirious patient, no matter what the cause. Pain often awakens a patient with cancer. Medications can awaken some patients directly (e.g., fluoxetine) or indirectly (e.g., diuretics). Aside from sorting out these influences, the physician must take into account the environment. Is the patient too hot or cold? Is the ward too brightly lit or too noisy? Do the patients awaken each time they are checked by the night staff? When any or several of these concerns are corrected, sleeping medication may not be necessary, although the need for sedatives remains in some patients.

B. Benzodiazepines (Table 32.5)
This class of drugs is most often prescribed if a patient needs nighttime sedation. The benzodiazepines with shorter half-lives (i.e., lorazepam or temazepam) with a rapid onset produce less daytime grogginess than those with a longer half-life. Short-acting agents tend to accumulate less and are safer for patients with liver disease. On the other hand, drugs with longer half-lives (i.e., diazepam or flurazepam) with a rapid onset produce less unwanted awakening during the very early morning.

C. Nonbenzodiazepine hypnotics (see Table 32.5)
The four medications in this class help patients fall asleep quickly and do not leave the patient groggy in the morning. Clinical experience shows tolerance can also develop to zolpidem, zaleplon, and eszopiclone. Ramelteon, a melatonin receptor agonist, is contraindicated in patients taking fluvoxamine.

D. Antihistamines (see Table 32.5)
These medications may be chosen if physicians are hesitant to prescribe benzodiazepines, such as for patients with severe respiratory disease. A disadvantage may be the higher anticholinergic potential of these drugs, compared with the benzodiazepine family, which can increase the risk of delirium.

E. Others

Chloral hydrate 500 to 1000 mg, an old standby hypnotic, is occasionally used as long as patients are free of gastrointestinal or liver disease. Barbiturates such as amobarbital sodium are occasionally used to treat some refractory sleeping disturbances for a short time but are not routinely used because they induce respiratory depression and have addictive potential. Gabapentin, which is renally cleared and has few drug interactions, has become increasingly popular. Doses may vary from 300 to 1200 mg at bedtime. It is always better to start with a lower dose.

Selected Readings

Breitbart W, Alici Y. Agitation and delirium at the end of life: "we couldn't manage him." *JAMA.* 2008;300:2898–2910.

Breitbart W, Alici Y. Pharmacologic treatments for cancer related fatigue: current state of clinical research. *Clin J Oncol Nurs.* 2008;12:27S–36S.

Breitbart W, Rosenfeld B, Gibson C, et al. Meaning-centered group psychotherapy for patients with advanced cancer; a pilot randomized control trial. *Psychooncology.* 2009;8:424–432.

Bush SH, Bruera E. The assessment and management of delirium in cancer patients. *Oncologist.* 2009;14:1039–1049.

Compton MT, Nemeroff CB. Depression and bipolar disorder. In: Dale D, Federman K, Antman, KH, et al., eds. *ACP Medicine (Annual).* New York: WebMD Professional; 2006:2608–2619.

Davidson JR, Feldman-Stewart D, Brennenstuhl S, Ram S. How to provide insomnia interventions to people with cancer: insights from patients. *Psychooncology.* 2007;16:1028–1038.

Foley E, Baillie A, Huxter M, Price M, Sinclair E. Mindfulness-based cognitive therapy for individuals whose lives have been affected by cancer: a randomized controlled trial. *J Consult Clin Psychol.* 2010;78:72–79.

Henry NL, Stearns, V, Flockhart D, et al. Drug interactions and pharmacogenomics in the treatment of breast cancer and depression. *Am J Psychiatry.* 2008;165:1251–1255.

Holland JC. *Psycho-oncology.* New York: Oxford University Press; 1998.

Homsi J, Walsh D, Nelson KA. Psychostimulants in supportive care. *Support Care Cancer* 2000;8:385–397.

Jacobsen PB, Jim HS. Psychosocial interventions for anxiety and depression in adult cancer patients: achievements and challenges. *CA Cancer J Clin.* 2008;58:214–230.

Jacobson SA, Pies RW, Katz IR. *Clinical Manual of Geriatric Psychopharmacology.* Washington, DC: American Psychiatric Press; 2009.

Kangas M, Bovbjerg DH, Montgomery GH. Cancer-related fatigue: a systematic and meta-analytic review of non-pharmacological therapies for cancer patients. *Psychol Bull.* 2008;134:700–741.

Massie MJ, Greenberg DB. Oncology. In: Levinson J, ed. *Textbook of Psychosomatic Medicine.* Washington, DC: American Psychiatry Press; 2005:517–530.

Miovic M, Block S. Psychiatric disorders in advanced cancer. *Cancer.* 2007;110:1665–1676.

Nasrallah H. CATIE'S surprises: in antipsychotics square-off, were there winners or losers? *Curr Psychiatr.* 2006;5:49–65.

Olin J, Massand P. Psychostimulants for depression in hospitalized cancer patients. *Psychosomatics.* 1996;37:57.

Patenaude AF, Last B. Cancer and children: where are we coming from? Where are we going? *Psychooncology.* 2001;10:281–283.

Potter WZ, Hollister LE. Antidepressant agents. In: Katzung B, ed. *Basic and Clinical Pharmacology.* 10th ed. New York: McGraw-Hill Medical; 2007:475–488.

Potter WZ, Hollister LE. Antipsychotic agents and lithium. In: Katzung B, ed. *Basic and Clinical Pharmacology.* 10th ed. New York: McGraw-Hill Medical; 2007:457–474.

Rasic DT, Belik SL, Bolton JM, Chochinov HM, Sareen J. Cancer, mental disorders, suicidal ideation and attempts in a large community sample. *Psychooncology.* 2008;17:660–667.

Roth AJ, McClear KZ, Massie MJ. Oncology. In: Stoudemire A, Fogel BS, Greenberg DB, eds. *Psychiatric Care of the Medical Patient.* Oxford: Oxford University Press; 2000:733–756.

Shear MK. Anxiety disorders. In: Dale D, Federman K, Antman, KH, et al., eds. *ACP Medicine (Annual).* New York: WebMD Professional; 2006:2651–2659.

Virani AS, Bizchlibnyk-Butler KZ, Jeffries JJ, eds. *Clinical Handbook of Psychotropic Drugs.* 18th ed. Seattle: Hogrefe and Huber Publications; 2009.

Zwahlen D, Hagenbuch N, Carley M, Jenewein J, Buchi S. Posttraumatic growth in cancer patients and partners – effects of role, gender and the dyad on couples' posttraumatic growth experience. *Psychooncology.* 2010;19:12–20.

SECTION IV: CHEMOTHERAPEUTIC AND MOLECULAR TARGETED AGENTS AND THEIR USE

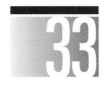

Classification, Use, and Toxicity of Clinically Useful Chemotherapy and Molecular Targeted Therapy

Roland T. Skeel

I. CLASSES OF DRUGS

Chemotherapeutic agents are customarily divided into several classes. For two of the classes, the *alkylating agents* and the *antimetabolites*, the names indicate the mechanism of cytotoxic action of the drugs in their class. For the *hormonal agents*, the name designates the physiologic action of the drug, and for the *natural products*, the name reflects the source of the agents. The *biologic response modifiers* include agents that mimic, stimulate, enhance, inhibit, or otherwise alter the host responses to the cancer. *Molecular targeted agents* affect defined and putative abnormalities in the cancer cell and its environment. Drugs that do not fit easily into other categories are grouped together as *miscellaneous agents*. Data for individual agents are given in Section III of this chapter.

Within each class are several types of agents (Table 33.1). As with the criteria for separating into class, the types are also grouped according to the mechanism of action, biochemical structure or derivation, and physiologic action. In some instances, these groupings into classes and types are arbitrary, and some drugs seem to fit into either more than one category or none. However, the classification of chemotherapeutic agents in this fashion is helpful in several respects. For example, because the antimetabolites interfere with purine and pyrimidine metabolism and the formation of DNA and RNA, they are all at least cell cycle–specific and in some instances primarily cell cycle phase–specific. The nitrosourea group of alkylating agents, on the other hand, contains drugs that are predominantly or entirely cell cycle–nonspecific. Such knowledge can be helpful in planning therapy for tumors when sufficient kinetic information permits a rational selection of agents and when drugs are selected for use in combination.

The classification scheme also may help to predict cross-resistance between drugs. Tumors that are resistant to one of the nitrogen mustard types of alkylating agents thus would be likely to be resistant to another of that same type, but not necessarily to one of the other types of alkylating agents such as the nitrosoureas or the metal salts (e.g., cisplatin). The classification system does not help in predicting multidrug resistance, which may have several phenotypes.

A. Alkylating agents

1. **General description.** The alkylating agents are a diverse group of chemical compounds capable of forming molecular bonds with nucleic acids, proteins, and many molecules of low molecular weight. The compounds either are electrophiles or generate electrophiles in vivo to produce polarized molecules with positively charged regions. These polarized molecules then can interact with electron-rich regions of most cellular molecules. The cytotoxic effect of the alkylating agents appears to relate primarily to the interaction between the electrophiles and DNA. This interaction may result in substitution reactions, cross-linking reactions, or strand-breaking reactions. The net effect of the alkylating agent's interaction with DNA is to alter the information coded in the DNA molecule. This alteration results in inhibition or inaccurate replication of DNA, with resultant mutation or cell death. One implication of the mutagenic capability of alkylating agents is the possibility that they are teratogenic and carcinogenic. Because they interact with preformed DNA, RNA, and protein, the alkylating agents are not phase-specific, and at least some are cell cycle–nonspecific.

Classification of Classical and Molecular Targeted Agents

Class and Type	Agents
Alkylating agents	
Alkyl sulfonate	Busulfan
Ethylenimine derivative	Thiotepa (triethylenethiophosphoramide)
Metal salt	Carboplatin, cisplatin, oxaliplatin
Nitrogen mustard	Bendamustine, chlorambucil, cyclophosphamide, estramustine, ifosfamide, mechlorethamine, melphalan
Nitrosourea	Carmustine, lomustine, streptozocin
Triazene–imidazole carboxamide	Dacarbazine, temozolamide
Antimetabolites	
Antifolates	Methotrexate, pemetrexed, pralatrexate
Purine analogs	Cladribine, fludarabine, mercaptopurine, nelarabine, pentostatin, thioguanine
Pyrimidine analogs	Azacitidine, capecitabine, cytarabine, decitabine, floxuridine, fluorouracil, gemcitabine
Natural products	
Antibiotics	Bleomycin, dactinomycin, daunorubicin, doxorubicin, epirubicin, idarubicin, mitomycin, mitoxantrone, valrubicin
Enzyme	Asparaginase
Microtubule polymer stabilizer	Cabazitaxel, docetaxel, paclitaxel
Mitotic inhibitor	Eribulin, ixabepilone, vinblastine, vincristine, vindesine, vinorelbine
Topoisomerase I inhibitors	Irinotecan, topotecan
Topoisomerase II inhibitors	Etoposide, teniposide
Hormones and hormone antagonists	
Androgen	Fluoxymesterone and others
Androgen antagonist	Bicalutamide, flutamide, nilutamide
Aromatase inhibitor	Aminoglutethimide, anastrozole, letrozole, exemestane
Corticosteroid	Dexamethasone, prednisone
Estrogen	Diethylstilbestrol
GNRH receptor antagonist	Degarelix
LHRH agonist	Goserelin, leuprolide, triptorelin
Polypeptide hormone release suppression	Octreotide
Progestin	Megestrol acetate, medroxyprogesterone acetate
Selective estrogen-receptor–modulator (estrogen antagonist)	Fulvestrant, raloxifene, tamoxifen, toremifene
Somatostatin analog	Octreotide
Thyroid hormones	Levothyroxine, liothyronine
Molecularly targeted agents	
Cyclin-dependent kinase inhibitor	Flavopiridol
Gene expression modulators	Retinoids, rexinoids, romidepsin

(continued)

TABLE 33.1	Useful Chemotherapeutic Agents *(continued)*

Class and Type	Agents
IL-2 receptor toxin	Denileukin diftitox
Monoclonal antibody	Alemtuzumab, cetuximab, gemtuzumab, ibritumomab tiuxetan, ipilimumab, ofatumumab, panitumumab, trastuzumab, rituximab, iodine-131 tositumomab
mTOR kinase inhibitor	Everolimus, temsirolimus
PARP1 inhibitor	Olaparib
Proteosome inhibitor	Bortezomib
Receptor tyrosine kinase inhibitors, multikinase inhibitors	Dasatinib, erlotinib, gefitinib, imatinib mesylate, lapatinib, midostaurin, pazopanib, semaxanib, sorafenib, sunitinib, vandetanib
Retinoic acid receptor expression modification	Tretinoin (all-*trans*-retinoic acid)
Biologic response modifiers	
Interferons	Interferon-α_{2a}, interferon-α_{2b}
Interleukins	Aldesleukin (IL-2), oprelvekin, denileukin diftitox
Myeloid- and erythroid-stimulating factors	Epoetin, filgrastim, sargramostim
Nonspecific immunomodulation	Thalidomide, lenalidomide
Vaccine (autologous)	Sipuleucel-T
Miscellaneous agents	
Adrenocortical suppressant	Mitotane
Bisphosphonates	Pamidronate, zoledronic acid
Cytoprotector (reactive species antagonists)	Amifostine, dexrazoxane, mesna
Methylhydrazine derivative	Procarbazine
Photosensitizing agents	Porfimer
Platelet-reducing agent	Anagrelide
Salt	Arsenic trioxide
Substituted melamine	Altretamine (hexamethylmelamine)
Substituted urea	Hydroxycarbamide (hydroxyurea)

GNRH, gonadotropin-releasing hormone; IL, interleukin; LHRH, luteinizing hormone-releasing hormone; mTOR, mammalian target of rapamycin; PARP, poly(ADP-ribose) polymerase.

2. **Types of alkylating agents**
    a. **Nitrogen mustards.** These compounds produce highly reactive carbonium ions that react with the electron-rich areas of susceptible molecules. They vary in reactivity from mechlorethamine, which is highly unstable in aqueous form, to cyclophosphamide, which must be biochemically activated in the liver. Bendamustine, a mechlorethamine derivative, contains a purinelike benzimidazole ring, and the exact mechanism of action of this unique agent is unknown.

　　b. **Ethylenimine derivatives.** Triethylenethiophosphoramide (thio-
　　　　tepa) is the only compound in this group that has much clinical
　　　　use. Ethylenimine derivatives are capable of the same kinds of
　　　　reactions as the nitrogen mustards.

　　c. **Alkyl sulfonates.** Busulfan is the only clinically active com-
　　　　pound in this group. It appears to interact more with cellular
　　　　thiol groups than with nucleic acids.

　　d. **Triazines.** Dacarbazine and its relative temozolomide are be-
　　　　lieved to act primarily as alkylators of DNA.

　　e. **Nitrosoureas.** The nitrosoureas undergo rapid, spontaneous
　　　　activation in aqueous solution to form products capable of
　　　　alkylation and carbamoylation. They are unique among the
　　　　alkylating agents with respect to not being cross-resistant
　　　　with other alkylating agents, being highly lipid soluble, and
　　　　having delayed myelosuppressive effects (6 to 8 weeks).

　　f. **Metal salts.** Cisplatin, carboplatin, and oxaliplatin inhibit DNA
　　　　synthesis probably through the formation of intrastrand cross-
　　　　links in DNA and formation of DNA adducts. They also react
　　　　with DNA through chelation or binding to the cell membrane.

B. Antimetabolites

　1. **General description.** The antimetabolites are a group of low-
　　　molecular-weight compounds that exert their effect by virtue
　　　of their structural or functional similarity to naturally occurring
　　　metabolites involved in nucleic acid synthesis. Because they are
　　　mistaken by the cell for normal metabolites, they either inhibit
　　　critical enzymes involved in nucleic acid synthesis or become
　　　incorporated into the nucleic acid and produce incorrect codes.
　　　Both mechanisms result in inhibition of DNA synthesis and ulti-
　　　mate cell death. Because of their primary effect on DNA synthe-
　　　sis, the antimetabolites are most active in cells that are actively
　　　growing and are largely cell cycle phase–specific.

　2. **Types of antimetabolites**

　　a. **Folic acid analogs.** Methotrexate, the earliest member of this
　　　　group and until recently, the only one in wide clinical use,
　　　　inhibits the enzyme dihydrofolate reductase. This inhibition
　　　　blocks the production of the reduced N-methylenetetra-
　　　　hydrofolate, the coenzyme in the synthesis of thymidylic
　　　　acid. Other metabolic processes in which there is one-carbon
　　　　unit transfer are also affected but are probably of less impor-
　　　　tance in the cytotoxic action of methotrexate. Pemetrexed
　　　　is a multitargeted pyrrolopyrimidine-based antifolate that,
　　　　when polyglutamated, inhibits dihydrofolate reductase,
　　　　thymidylate synthase, and glycinamide ribonucleotide form-
　　　　yltransferase. Pralatrexate is a folate analogue that competi-
　　　　tively inhibits dihydrofolate reductase. It is also an inhibitor
　　　　for polyglutamylation by folylpolyglutamyl synthetase.

b. **Pyrimidine analogs.** These compounds inhibit critical enzymes necessary for nucleic acid synthesis and may become incorporated into DNA and RNA.

c. **Purine analogs.** The specific site of action for the purine analogs is less well defined than for most pyrimidine analogs, although it is well demonstrated that they interfere with normal purine interconversions and thus with DNA and RNA synthesis. Some of the analogs also are incorporated into the nucleic acids. The adenosine deaminase inhibitor pentostatin increases the intracellular concentration of deoxyadenosine triphosphates in lymphoid cells and inhibits DNA synthesis, probably by blocking ribonucleotide reductase. Among the metabolic alterations is nicotinamide adenine dinucleotide depletion, which may result in cell death. Cladribine accumulates in cells as the triphosphate, is incorporated into DNA, and inhibits DNA repair enzymes and RNA synthesis. As with pentostatin, nicotinamide adenine dinucleotide levels are also depleted. Fludarabine is a purine analog that causes inhibition of DNA polymerase alpha, ribonucleotide reductase, and DNA primase, thus inhibiting DNA synthesis, though the primary mechanism is not known.

C. **Natural products**

1. **General description.** The natural products are grouped together not on the basis of activity but because they are derived from natural sources. The clinically useful drugs include plant products, fermentation products of various species of the soil fungus *Streptomyces*, and bacterial products.

2. **Types of natural products**

a. **Mitotic inhibitors.** Vincristine, vinblastine, and their semisynthetic derivatives vindesine and vinorelbine are derived from the periwinkle plant (*Catharanthus roseus*), a species of myrtle. They appear to act primarily through their effect on microtubular protein with a resultant metaphase arrest and inhibition of mitosis. Ixabepilone is an analog of epothilone B (produced by the myxobacterium *Sorangium cellulosum*) that binds to β-tubulin subunits on microtubules, causes suppression of microtubule dynamics, and blocks the cell in mitosis, which leads to cell death.

b. ***Podophyllum* derivatives.** Etoposide and teniposide, semisynthetic podophyllotoxins derived from the root of the Mayapple plant (*Podophyllum peltatum*), form a complex with topoisomerase II, an enzyme that is necessary for the completion of DNA replication. This interaction results in DNA strand breakage and arrest of cells in late S and early G_2 phases of the cell cycle.

c. **Camptothecins.** These agents are analogs of camptothecin, a derivative of the Chinese tree *Camptotheca accuminata*. The primary target of the two clinically active agents, irinotecan and topotecan, is DNA topoisomerase I.

d. **Antibiotics.** The antitumor antibiotics are a group of related antimicrobial compounds produced by *Streptomyces* species in culture. Their cytotoxicity, which limits their antimicrobial usefulness, has proved to be of great value in treating a wide range of cancers. All of the clinically useful antibiotics affect the function and synthesis of nucleic acids.

(1) **Dactinomycin, the anthracyclines (doxorubicin, daunorubicin, epirubicin, and idarubicin), and the anthracenedione mitoxantrone** cause topoisomerase II–dependent DNA cleavage and intercalate with the DNA double helix.

(2) **Bleomycins** cause DNA strand scission. The resulting fragmentation is believed to underlie the drug's cytotoxic activity.

(3) **Mitomycin** causes cross-links between complementary strands of DNA that impair replication.

e. **Enzymes.** Asparaginase, the one example of this type of agent, catalyzes the hydrolysis of asparagine to aspartic acid and ammonia and deprives selected malignant cells of an amino acid essential to their survival.

D. **Hormones and hormone antagonists**

1. **General description.** The hormones and hormone antagonists that are clinically active against cancer include steroid estrogens, progestins, androgens, corticoids and their synthetic derivatives, nonsteroidal synthetic compounds with steroid or steroid-antagonist activity, aromatase inhibitors, hypothalamic–pituitary analogs, and thyroid hormones. Each agent has diverse effects. Some effects are mediated directly at the cellular level by the drug binding to specific cytoplasmic receptors or by inhibition or stimulation of the production or action of the hormones. These agents may also act by stimulating or inhibiting natural autocrine and paracrine growth factors (e.g., epidermal growth factor, transforming growth factors [TGFs]-α and -β). The relative roles of the various actions of hormones and hormone antagonists are only partially understood and probably vary among tumor types. For selective estrogen receptor modulators such as tamoxifen, which, when bound to the estrogen receptor, ultimately controls the promoter region of genes that affect cell growth, there are a host of modulating factors including some 20 receptor-interacting proteins and 50 transcription-activating factors as well as many response elements. Other effects are mediated through indirect effects on the hypothalamus and its anterior pituitary–regulating hormones. The final

common pathway in most circumstances appears to lead to the malignant cell, which retains some sensitivity to direct or indirect hormonal control of its growth. An exception to this mechanism is the effect of corticosteroids on leukemias and lymphomas, in which the steroids appear to have direct lytic effects on abnormal lymphoid cells that have high numbers of glucocorticoid receptors.

2. **Types of hormones and hormone antagonists**
   a. **Androgens** may exert their antineoplastic effect by altering pituitary function or directly affecting the neoplastic cell.
   b. **Antiandrogens** inhibit nuclear androgen binding.
   c. **Corticosteroids** cause lysis of lymphoid tumors that are rich in specific cytoplasmic receptors and may have other indirect effects as well.
   d. **Estrogens** suppress testosterone production (through the hypothalamus) in males and alter breast cancer cell response to prolactin.
   e. **Progestins** appear to act directly at the level of the malignant cell receptor to promote differentiation.
   f. **Selective estrogen receptor modulators** (acting as estrogen antagonists) compete with estrogen for binding on the cytosol estrogen receptor protein in cancer cells. The receptor/hormone complex ultimately controls the promoter region of genes that affect cell growth.
   g. **Aromatase inhibitors** are nonsteroidal inhibitors of the aromatization of androgens to estrogens. Aminoglutethimide is relatively nonselective, having many biochemical sites of inhibition of steroidogenesis. Its use requires corticosteroid replacement. In contrast, the selective aromatase inhibitors such as anastrozole or letrozole primarily block the conversion of adrenally generated androstenedione to estrone by aromatase in peripheral tissues without inhibition of progesterone or corticosteroid synthesis.
   h. **Hypothalamic hormone analogs,** such as the luteinizing hormone–releasing hormone agonists leuprolide or goserelin, can inhibit luteinizing hormone (LH) and follicle-stimulating hormone (FSH; after initial stimulation) and the production of testosterone or estrogen by the gonads.
   i. **Thyroid hormones** inhibit the release of thyroid-stimulating hormone, thus inhibiting growth of well-differentiated thyroid tumors.

E. **Molecularly targeted agents**
   1. **General.** This classification is a relatively recent one in oncology that has become possible because of maturation of knowledge about the molecular events that are responsible for the development of cancer. Understanding of the genetic changes in the

cancer cell, the downstream molecular events that follow as a consequence, and the mechanisms by which these events regulate cell growth and death has led to a host of possibilities for the control of cancer growth.

2. **Tyrosine kinase and multikinase inhibitors.** The first clinical example of this was the signal transduction inhibitor imatinib mesylate, which inactivates the constitutively active fusion product tyrosine kinase arising from the Philadelphia chromosome (Ph) found in chronic myelogenous leukemia (CML), Bcr-Abl, as well as c-kit kinase, which is overexpressed in gastrointestinal stromal tumors. There are now a large number of small molecule inhibitors of intracellular kinase activity (receptor and nonreceptor molecules) in clinical use, with demonstrated clinical efficacy in breast cancer, colon cancer, renal cell carcinoma, lung cancer, pancreatic cancer, and hepatoma.

3. **Monoclonal antibodies** have emerged over the last 10 to 15 years as useful adjuncts to the medical oncologist's armamentarium. These agents, which may be directed at growth factors or their receptors, are derived from murine antibodies, may have varying levels of humanization (chimerism), and may be unconjugated (alemtuzumab, bevacizumab, cetuximab, ofatumumab, rituximab, trastuzumab) or conjugated with radionuclides (ibritumomab tiuxetan, tositumomab) or another toxic moiety (gemtuzumab).

4. **Other agents.** Other agents affect nuclear activity, such as the binding of all-*trans*-retinoic acid with cytoplasmic proteins, which in turn interact with nuclear retinoic acid receptors (RARs) that affect expression of genes that control cell growth and differentiation; inhibit proteosomes, which mediate protein degradation and play an essential role in intracellular protein regulation and consequent cellular signal transduction pathways and cellular homeostasis; or perturb other critical pathways.

F. **Miscellaneous agents**

These are listed in Table 33.1. Descriptions of specific agents are found in Section III.

II. CLINICALLY USEFUL CHEMOTHERAPEUTIC, BIOLOGIC, AND MOLECULAR TARGETED AGENTS

Section III of this chapter contains an alphabetically arranged compendium that contains a description of the chemotherapeutic, biologic, and molecular targeted agents that are recognized to be clinically useful. Each drug is listed by its generic name, with other common names or trade names included. A brief description is given of the probable mechanism of action, clinical uses, recommended doses and schedules, precautions, and side effects.

A. **Recommended doses: CAUTION**

Although every effort has been made to ensure that the drug dosages and schedules given here are accurate and in accord with published standards, readers are advised to check the product information sheet included in the package of each U.S. Food and Drug Administration (FDA)-approved drug. For drugs not yet approved for general use, active protocol guidelines and any current medical literature should be used to verify recommended dosages, contraindications, and precautions and to review potential toxicity.

B. **Dose selection and designation**

The doses are listed using body surface area (square meters) as the base for nearly all the agents included. Adult doses from the literature, which are expressed using a weight base, have been converted by multiplying the milligram-per-kilogram dose by 37 to give the milligram-per-square-meter dose. Doses using a weight base, which have been taken from the pediatric literature, have been converted using a factor of 25. Because many of the drugs are given in combination with other agents, doses most commonly used in popular combinations may also be indicated. These data should not be used as the sole source of information for any of the drugs but rather should be used as a guide to confirm and compare dose ranges and schedules and to identify potential problems. For some agents, the area under the curve (AUC) method of dose calculation seems to be most reliable for achieving the most accurate dosing and balance between efficacy and toxicity; when that is the standard, the AUC dose is used.

C. **Drug toxicity: frequency designation**

The designation of the frequency of toxic side effects is indicated as follows (probability of occurrence equals percentage of patients who may be expected to experience the toxic effect):

- Universal (90% to 100%)
- Common (15% to 90%)
- Occasional (5% to 15%)
- Uncommon (1% to 5%)
- Rare (<1%).

These designations are meant only to be guides, and the likelihood of a side effect in each patient depends on that patient's physical status, including comorbidities, treatment history, dose, schedule, and route of drug administration, as well as other concurrent treatment.

D. **Dose modification**

1. **Philosophy.** The optimal dose and schedule of a drug are those that give maximum benefit with tolerable toxicity. Most classical chemotherapeutic agents (and some of the targeted agents) have a steep dose–response curve; therefore, if no toxicity is seen, as a rule, a higher dose (dose escalation) of most of the classical

chemotherapeutic agents should be given to get the best possible therapeutic benefit. If toxicity is great, however, the patient's life may be threatened or the patient may decide that the treatment is worse than the disease and refuse further therapy. How much toxicity the patient and the physician are willing to tolerate depends on the likelihood that more intensive treatment will make a major therapeutic difference (e.g., cure versus no cure) and on the patient's physical and psychological tolerance for adverse effects.

The general grading scheme for all toxicity is as follows:

- 0: None
- 1: Mild
- 2: Moderate
- 3: Severe
- 4: Life-threatening.

2. Guidelines

a. Nonhematologic toxicity

(1) Acute effects. Acute drug toxicity that is limited to 1 to 2 days and is not cumulative is not usually a cause of dose modification unless it is of grade 3 or 4, that is, severe or life-threatening. (For individual toxicities, see the Common Terminology Criteria for Adverse Events v4.0, available on the Internet at http://ctep.cancer.gov/protocolDevelopment/electronic_applications/ctc.htm.) Occasionally, repeating a dose that caused intractable nausea and vomiting, a temperature higher than 40°C (104°F), or an acute infusion reaction is warranted, but for most other grade 3 or 4 toxicities, the subsequent doses should be reduced by 25% to 50%, assuming that the toxicity is believed to be dose-related. If the acute drug effects (e.g., severe paresthesias or abnormalities of renal or liver function) last longer than 48 hours, the subsequent doses should be reduced by 35% to 50%.

A recurrence of the grade 3 or 4 side effects at the reduced doses would be an indication either to reduce by another 25% to 50% or to discontinue the drug altogether. Non–dose-related toxicity such as anaphylaxis is an indication to discontinue the offending drug. Lesser degrees of hypersensitivity can often be dealt with effectively by increasing the dose of protective agents (like dexamethasone or diphenhydramine), desensitization (e.g., carboplatin), or slowing the rate of infusion (e.g., rituximab). For some biologic agents, such as trastuzumab, physiologic effects that look like immunologic hypersensitivity reactions are probably related to cytokine release, occur primarily on first or second infusions, and diminish with continued treatment.

(2) Chronic effects. Chronic or cumulative toxicity such as pulmonary function changes with bleomycin or decreased cardiac function with doxorubicin is nearly always an indication to discontinue the responsible agent. Chronic or cumulative neurotoxicity due to vincristine, cisplatin, paclitaxel, or other agents may require no dose change, reduction, or discontinuation, depending on the severity of the resultant neurologic dysfunction and the patient's ability to tolerate it.

b. Hematologic toxicity. The degree of myelosuppression and attendant risk of infection and bleeding that are acceptable depend on the cancer, the duration of the myelosuppression, the goals of therapy, and the general health of the patient. In addition, one must consider the relative benefit of less aggressive or more aggressive therapy. For example, with acute nonlymphocytic leukemia, remission is unlikely unless sufficient therapy is given to cause profound pancytopenia for at least 1 week. Because there is little benefit with lesser treatment, grade 4 leukopenia and thrombocytopenia are acceptable toxicities in this circumstance. Grade 4 myelosuppression is also acceptable when the goal is cure of a cancer that does not involve the marrow, such as testicular carcinoma. With breast cancer, on the other hand, responses are seen with less aggressive treatment, and prolonged pancytopenia may not be acceptable, particularly if chemotherapy is being used palliatively or in an adjuvant setting in which the proportion of patients expected to benefit from chemotherapy is relatively small and excessive toxicity would pose an unacceptable risk.

With these caveats in mind, the dose modification schemes shown in Tables 33.2 and 33.3 can serve as a guide to reasonable dose changes for drugs whose major toxicity is myelosuppression. Separate schemes are given for drugs with relatively short myelosuppression and for drugs such as the nitrosoureas that have more prolonged myelosuppression.

c. Dosing for the obese patient. In general, patients who are overweight (body mass index [BMI] 25–29.9) and those who are obese (BMI 30–34.9) should be treated with full doses of chemotherapy, based on the body surface area calculated from their actual weight. Whether this is true for those who are very obese (BMI 35–39.9) or extremely obese (BMI >40) is not clear, owing to a lack of sufficient data. Many clinicians would limit the dose, using a maximum weight based on a BMI of 35 (maximum treatment weight (kg) = 35 × [height (m)]^2).

TABLE 33.2 Dose Modifications for Myelosuppressive Drugs With a Nadir* at Less Than 3 Weeks

Degree of Suppression	ANC (WBC)/μL on Day of Scheduled Treatment†		Platelets/μL on Day of Scheduled Treatment	Dose as Percentage of Immediately Preceding Cycle
Minimal	≥1500 (≥3500)	and	≥100,000	100
Mild	1200–1500 (3000–3500)	or	75,000–100,000	75
Moderate	1000–1200 (2500–3000)	or	50,000–75,000	50
Severe	<1000 (<2500)	or	<50,000	0 (delay 1 week)

ANC, absolute neutrophil count; WBC, white blood cell count.
*If the nadir of ANC is <1000/μL and is associated with fever of >38.3°C (101°F) or the nadir of platelets is <40,000/μL, decrease dose by 25% in subsequent cycles. If the dose is already to be reduced on the basis of the ANC or platelet count on the day of treatment as per this table, do not reduce further because of the nadir count.
†ANC is the preferred parameter, if available. If counts are rising at the end of a treatment cycle, it is often appropriate to delay 1 week and then treat according to the dose modification scheme shown here.

III. DATA FOR CLINICALLY USEFUL CHEMOTHERAPEUTIC, BIOLOGIC, AND MOLECULAR TARGETED AGENTS

Note: Although every effort has been made to ensure that the drug dosage and schedules herein are accurate and in accordance with published standards, users are advised to check the product

TABLE 33.3 Dose Modifications for Myelosuppressive Drugs* With a Nadir at 3 Weeks or Later

Point in Time	ANC (WBC)/μL		Platelets/μL	Dose as Percentage of Immediately Preceding Cycle
I. On day of scheduled treatment†	≥1800 (≥3500)	and	≥100,000	Dose modified for nadir only
	<1800 (<3500)	or	<100,000	0‡
II. At last nadir	>750	and	>75,000	100
	500–750	or	40,000–75,000	75
	<500	or	<40,000	50
III. After 2-week delay	≥1800 (≥3500)	and	≥100,000	Dose modified for nadir only
	1200–1800 (2500–3500)	or	75,000–100,000	75
	<1200	or	<75,000	Continue to hold

ANC, absolute neutrophil count; WBC, white blood cell count.
*Nitrosoureas or other agents with prolonged nadir.
†ANC is the preferred parameter to use.
‡Withhold treatment and repeat count in 2 weeks. At 2 weeks, treat on basis of lowest dose indicated by nadir (II) or delay (III) section of table.

information sheet included in the package of each FDA-approved drug and FDA-National Cancer Institute guidelines for drugs that are not yet approved for general use to verify recommended dosages, contraindications, and precautions.

Agents that have not yet been approved by the FDA may be included because they either have shown preliminary efficacy in clinical trials or are currently being investigated and show promise of benefit. As their efficacy and toxicity are more firmly established, it is expected that some will be approved by the FDA for general use, whereas others will remain investigational or be dropped from further study.

DRUG PROFILES

ALDESLEUKIN

Other names. Interleukin-2 (IL-2), Proleukin.

Mechanism of action. Enhances mitogenesis of T-cells, natural killer (NK) cells, and lymphokine-activated killer (LAK) cells; augments cytotoxicity of NK and LAK cells; induces interferon subcutanously weekly.

Primary indications

1. Renal cell carcinoma
2. Melanoma.

Usual dosage and schedule. A wide range of doses and routes (intravenous [IV] or subcutaneous [SC]) have been used. In any of the schedules, therapy may be stopped prematurely for severe constitutional symptoms or for cardiovascular, renal, hepatic, neurologic, pulmonary, or hematologic toxicity.

1. 600,000 IU/kg (22×10^6 IU/m^2) as a 15-minute IV infusion every 8 hours for up to 14 doses on days 1 to 5. Repeat on days 15 to 19. Repeat cycle in 6 to 12 weeks if stable or responding disease. This schedule has the most experience and is generally the recommended regimen.
2. 18×10^6 IU/m^2/24 hours as a continuous IV infusion (CIVI) daily for up to 5 days. Repeat in 4 weeks. Repeat cycle in 4 to 6 weeks if stable or responding disease.
3. 22×10^6 IU/m^2 as a 15-minute infusion for 5 consecutive days for 2 successive weeks. Repeat every 3 to 6 weeks as tolerated. In some regimens, it is preceded by 3 days with a single dose of low-dose cyclophosphamide, 350 mg/m^2 IV push.

Schedules 1 and 2 require hospitalization. Schedule 3 can be given in an outpatient setting but may require several hours of observation after treatment. Lower dose schedules and SC administration are generally not recommended.

Special precautions. Patients must be carefully monitored after treatment using any of the dosing regimens. Outpatient regimens require that patients have cardiovascular status observed for up to 5 hours, particularly after the first several doses. With higher doses, capillary leak syndrome resulting in hypotension, pulmonary edema, myocardial infarction, arrhythmias, azotemia, and alterations in mental status may occur. Administration of dopamine (1 to 5 μg/kg/min) to patients manifesting capillary leak syndrome, before the onset of hypotension, can help to maintain organ perfusion and thus preserve urine output. Weight and urine output should be carefully monitored. If organ perfusion and blood pressure are not sustained, increasing the dose of dopamine to 6 to 10 μg/kg/min or adding phenylephrine hydrochloride (1 to 5 μg/kg/min) to low-dose dopamine may be indicated. Administration of IV fluids, either colloids or crystalloids, is recommended for treatment of hypovolemia. Correction of hypovolemia may require large volumes of IV fluids, but caution is required because unrestrained fluid administration may exacerbate problems associated with edema formation or effusions.

Prolonged use of pressors, either in combination or as individual agents, at relatively high doses may be associated with cardiac rhythm disturbances. Intensive care and intubation may be required.

Toxicity. All are dose dependent.

1. *Myelosuppression and other hematologic effects.* Uncommon at lower doses; common but rarely serious at higher doses. Anemia requiring transfusion is common at higher doses. Thrombocytopenia is common at higher doses.
2. *Nausea, vomiting, and other gastrointestinal effects:*
   a. Anorexia, nausea, vomiting, and diarrhea are common.
   b. Transient liver function abnormalities, including hyperbilirubinemia and hypoalbuminemia and elevation of the prothrombin time (PT) and partial thromboplastin time, are common.
   c. Colonic perforations are rare.
3. *Mucocutaneous effects.* Mucositis is occasional to common. Alopecia is uncommon. Pruritic erythematous rash is common.
4. *Cardiovascular effects:*
   a. Arrhythmias are common and dose-related.
   b. Hypotension is dose-related but is occasionally seen at the lower dose schedules.
   c. Myocardial injury is seen primarily at the higher dose schedules.
   d. Pulmonary edema from capillary leak syndrome is common with intensive dose regimens.
   e. Weight gain is common from edema, particularly in more intensive dose regimens.
5. *Neuropsychiatric effects:*
   a. Mental status changes are common, with dose-related severity.
   b. Dizziness or light-headedness is common.

    c. Blurry vision and other visual disturbances are occasional.

    d. Seizures are uncommon to rare at lower dose regimens.

  6. *Renal function impairment.* Common but reversible. More frequent laboratory abnormalities include creatinine elevation, hypomagnesemia, acidosis, hypocalcemia, hypophosphatemia, hypokalemia, hypouricemia, and hypoalbuminemia.

  7. *Fever.* With or without chills, fever is common and may be severe.

  8. *Bacterial infection.* Occasional. Probably related to chemotactic defect induced in granulocytes.

  9. *Myalgias and arthralgias.* Occasional to common.

  10. *Malaise and fatigue.* Common and dose-related.

Prophylaxis of acute toxicity

  1. Acetaminophen 650 mg by mouth before therapy and every 6 hours for one or two doses for outpatient IL-2 dosing; every 6 hours for 3 doses for inpatient IL-2 regimens.

  2. Cimetidine 800 mg by mouth, or other histamine H_2-receptor antagonist before therapy and daily for duration of treatment.

  3. Antiemetics: granisetron, ondansetron, or other $5HT_3$ antagonist; metoclopramide, and prochlorperazine may be used. Do not use dexamethasone.

  4. Meperidine 25 to 50 mg IV when chills start after first dose. For subsequent doses, meperidine 50 mg by mouth 1.5 hours before chills are predicated to start, based on the first treatment.

  5. Hydromorphone 0.5 to 1 mg IV may be substituted for meperidine in patients who tolerate meperidine poorly.

  6. Diphenoxylate with atropine (Lomotil) 1 tablet up to six times daily for diarrhea.

  7. Hydroxyzine 25 to 50 mg every 6 hours for itching.

ALEMTUZUMAB

Other names. Campath, Campath-1H

Mechanism of action. Alemtuzumab is a chimeric (murine and human) monoclonal antibody directed against the CD-52 antigen found on the surface of 95% of B- and T-lymphocytes. It is also expressed in other normal cells found in the peripheral blood and marrow, as well as some other somatic cells. Cellular cytotoxicity is mediated through complement-mediated lysis, antibody dependent cellular cytotoxicity, and induction of apoptosis.

Primary indications

  1. B-cell chronic lymphocytic leukemia

  2. Nonmalignant conditions and graft-versus-host disease.

Usual dosage and schedule (malignant conditions only).

1. Initiation: 3 mg as a 2-hour IV infusion daily.
2. Escalation: When infusion related toxicities are lower than grade 2, the dose is escalated to 10 mg as a 2-hour IV infusion daily. When the 10-mg dose is tolerated, maintenance therapy is initiated.
3. Maintenance: 30 mg as a 2-hour IV infusion three times a week—on alternate days—for 12 weeks.

Infusion-related events (see subsequent discussions) are ameliorated by pretreatment with antihistamines, acetaminophen, and antiemetics, as well as incremental dose escalation.

Special precautions. Must not be administered as IV push or bolus dose. Single doses of greater than 30 mg and cumulative doses of greater than 90 mg/week should not be given. If therapy is interrupted for 7 or more days, the dose initiation and escalation scheme is required to avert toxicity. Alemtuzumab is contraindicated in patients who have active systemic infections, underlying immunodeficiency, or known type I hypersensitivity or anaphylactic reactions to the drug or any of its components. Reactivation of hepatitis B or other viruses is a risk.

Toxicity

1. *Myelosuppression and other hematologic effects.* Lymphopenia is universal. Neutropenia, anemia, and thrombocytopenia are common and often severe (grade 3) or greater. Opportunistic and other infections, including pneumonia and sepsis, are seen in 10% to 15% of patients. Autoimmune hemolytic anemia and thrombocytopenia are uncommon (1% to 2%). Pancytopenia and marrow hypoplasia are uncommon but may require permanent discontinuation of therapy. Because of the high incidence of opportunistic infections, prophylaxis against *Pneumocystis jiroveci* pneumonia and herpes virus infections during and at least 2 months after completion of treatment is recommended.*
2. *Nausea, vomiting, and other gastrointestinal effects.* Nausea and vomiting are common; diarrhea, abdominal pain, and dyspepsia are occasional.
3. *Mucocutaneous effects.* Rash, urticaria, pruritis, and increased sweating are common. Stomatitis is occasional.
4. *Infusion-related events.* Rigors, fever, nausea and vomiting, and rash—including urticaria—are common. Shortness of breath, hypotension, bronchospasm, headache, pruritis, and diarrhea are occasional. Angioedema is uncommon.

---

* For *Pneumocystis jiroveci* pneumonia prophylaxis: trimethoprim-sulfamethoxazole double strength, 1 tablet by mouth twice a day (on Monday, Wednesday, and Friday). If allergic, use dapsone 100 mg on Monday, Wednesday, and Friday. For herpes zoster prophylaxis, famciclovir 250 mg by mouth twice a day or valacyclovir 500 mg by mouth three times a day.

5. *Miscellaneous effects:*
   a. Respiratory: Dyspnea, cough, and bronchitis are common. Pneumonia, pharyngitis, bronchospasm, and rhinitis are occasional.
   b. Cardiovascular: Hypotension is common; hypertension occasional. Tachycardia and supraventricular tachycardia are occasional, but usually not severe. Syncope is uncommon.
   c. Hypersensitivity reactions to alemtuzumab may occur (2%) and result in hypersensitivity to other monoclonal antibodies.
   d. Neuropsychiatric: Insomnia, depression, and somnolence are occasional. Headache, dysthesias, dizziness, and tremor are occasional.
   e. Infections: Reactivation of hepatitis B and other viruses is uncommon to rare.

ALITRETINOIN

Other names. 9-cis-retinoic acid, Panretin Gel.

Mechanism of action. Binds to cytoplasmic retinoic acid-binding proteins and then is transported to the nucleus where it interacts with nuclear RARs. These then affect expression of the genes that control cell growth and differentiation.

Primary indication. AIDS-related cutaneous Kaposi sarcoma.

Usual dosage and schedule. Apply sufficient gel (0.1%) to cover lesion with a generous coating 2 to 4 times daily, according to individual lesion tolerance. Allow to dry for 3 to 5 minutes before covering with clothing.

Special precautions. Women are advised to avoid becoming pregnant because of potential fetal risk. Minimize exposure to ultraviolet rays from sun or sun lamps.

Toxicity

1. *Myelosuppression and other hematologic effects.* None.
2. *Nausea, vomiting, and other gastrointestinal effects.* None
3. *Mucocutaneous effects.* Skin reactions with erythema, scaling, irritation, redness, rash, or other dermatitis are common. Pruritis, exfoliative dermatitis, or other erosive or draining skin lesions are occasional.
4. *Miscellaneous effects:*
   a. Neurologic complaints of burning or pain are common.
   b. Edema is occasional.

ALTRETAMINE

Other names. Hexamethylmelamine, Hexalen, HXM.

Mechanism of action. Unknown. Although it structurally resembles the known alkylating agent triethylenemelamine, it has some antimetabolite characteristics.

Primary indication. Carcinoma of the ovary that is persistent or recurrent after first-line therapy.

Usual dosage and schedule

1. 260 mg/m^2 by mouth daily in three or four divided doses after meals and at bedtime for 14 or 21 days every 4 weeks when used as a single agent.
2. 150 to 200 mg/m^2 by mouth daily in three or four divided doses for 2 out of 3 or 4 weeks when used in combination.

Special precautions. Concurrent altretamine and antidepressants of the monoamine oxidase inhibitor class may cause severe orthostatic hypotension. Cimetidine may increase toxicity.

Toxicity

1. *Myelosuppression and other hematologic effects.* Dose-limiting leukopenia and thrombocytopenia are uncommon, though lesser degrees are common. Anemia is common.
2. *Nausea, vomiting, and other gastrointestinal effects.* Mild to moderate nausea, vomiting, and other gastrointestinal effects occur in about 30% of patients and are rarely severe. Diarrhea is occasional. Tolerance may develop.
3. *Mucocutaneous effects.* Alopecia, skin rash, and pruritus are rare.
4. *Miscellaneous effects:*
   a. Peripheral sensory neuropathies are common and may be ameliorated by pyridoxine, but tumor response may be compromised.
   b. Central nervous system (CNS) effects, including agitation, confusion, hallucinations, depression, and parkinsonian-like symptoms are uncommon with recommended intermittent schedule.
   c. Decreased renal function is occasional.
   d. Increased alkaline phosphatase level is occasional.

AMIFOSTINE

Other name. Ethyol.

Mechanism of action. The prodrug amifostine is dephosphorylated to an active free thiol metabolite that can reduce the toxic effects of cisplatin. The differential activity between normal and cancer tissue is thought to be related to higher capillary alkaline phosphatase activity and better vascularity of normal tissue. Pretreatment reduces cumulative renal toxicity from cisplatin.

Primary indications

1. For reduction of cumulative renal toxicity associated with repeated administration of cisplatin in patients with advanced cancer.
2. For reduction of moderate to severe xerostomia from radiation of the head and neck where the radiation port includes a substantial portion of the parotid glands.

Usual dosage and schedule

1. For reduction of cumulative renal toxicity with chemotherapy: 910 mg/m^2 IV over 15 minutes once daily, starting 30 minutes before chemotherapy.
2. For reduction of xerostomia from radiation of the head and neck: 200 mg/m^2 administered once daily as a 3-minute IV infusion, starting 15 to 30 minutes prior to standard fraction radiation therapy (1.8 to 2.0 Gy).

Special precautions. To minimize hypotension during the infusion, patients should be adequately hydrated prior to the amifostine infusion and kept in a supine position during the infusion. Blood pressure should be monitored every 5 minutes during the infusion and thereafter as clinically indicated. Interrupt the infusion if the decrease in systolic pressure is more than 20% to 25% of the baseline systolic pressure.

Toxicity

1. *Myelosuppression and other hematologic effects.* Not increased by amifostine.
2. *Nausea, vomiting, and other gastrointestinal effects.* Nausea and vomiting are common and may be severe.
3. *Mucocutaneous effects.* Rarely, serious cutaneous reactions have been associated with amifostine administration. They have included erythema multiforme, Stevens-Johnson syndrome, toxic epidermal necrolysis, and exfoliative dermatitis.
4. *Miscellaneous effects:*
   a. Transient hypotension during the infusion is common. Loss of consciousness may occur, but is usually easily reversed.
   b. Flushing and feeling of warmth are occasional.
   c. Chilling and feeling of coldness are occasional.
   d. Dizziness, somnolence, hiccups, and sneezing are occasional.
   e. Allergic reactions are rare but have included anaphylactic reactions.
   f. Hypocalcemia is rare.
   g. Seizures are rare.

AMINOGLUTETHIMIDE

Other names. Cytadren.

Mechanism of action. Inhibits aromatization and cytochrome P-450 hydroxylating enzymes, thereby blocking the conversion of androgens to estrogens and the biosynthesis of all steroid hormones. This drug causes, in effect, a reversible chemical adrenalectomy.

Primary indications. Adrenocortical carcinoma and ectopic Cushing syndrome.

Usual dosage and schedule. 1000 mg by mouth daily in four divided doses.

Special precautions. Hydrocortisone must be given concomitantly to prevent adrenal insufficiency. Suggested dose is 100 mg by mouth daily in divided doses for 2 weeks, then 40 mg by mouth daily in divided doses.

Toxicity

1. *Myelosuppression and other hematologic effects.* Leukopenia and thrombocytopenia are rare; if they occur, they resolve rapidly when the drug is stopped.
2. *Nausea, vomiting, and other gastrointestinal effects.* Occasional and usually mild.
3. *Mucocutaneous effects.* A morbilliform rash is commonly seen during the first week of treatment, but it usually disappears within 1 week.
4. *Hormonal effects:*
   a. Adrenal insufficiency is common without replacement hydrocortisone in patients with normal adrenal glands.
   b. Hypothyroidism is uncommon.
   c. Masculinization is possible.
5. *Neurologic effects:*
   a. Lethargy is common. Although usually mild and transient, it is occasionally severe.
   b. Vertigo, nystagmus, and ataxia are occasional.
   c. Headache is uncommon.
6. *Miscellaneous effects:*
   a. Facial flushing is uncommon.
   b. Periorbital edema is uncommon.
   c. Cholestatic jaundice is rare.
   d. Fever is uncommon.

ANAGRELIDE

Other names. Imidazo(2,1-b)quinazolin-2-one, Agrylin.

Mechanism of action. Mechanism for thrombocytopenia unknown but may be due to impaired megakaryocyte function. Inhibitor of platelet aggregation but not at usual therapeutic doses.

Primary indication. Uncontrolled thrombocytosis in chronic myeloproliferative disorders, such as essential thrombocythemia, chronic granulocytic leukemia, and polycythemia rubra vera.

Usual dosage and schedule

1. 0.5 mg by mouth four times a day or 1 mg by mouth twice a day. Increase by 0.5 mg/d every 5 to 7 days if no response. Maximum daily dose is 10 mg/day. Maximum single dose is 2.5 mg. Higher doses cause postural hypotension.
2. Alternate dosing schedules:
   a. Elderly: 0.5 mg by mouth daily, increase by 0.5 mg each week.
   b. Abnormal renal or hepatic function: 0.5 mg by mouth twice a day.

Special precautions. Contraindicated in patients who are pregnant and in patients with severe hepatic impairment. Use with caution in patients with heart disease. Tachycardia and forceful heartbeat may be exacerbated by caffeine; consumption of caffeine should be avoided for 1 hour before and 1 hour after anagrelide is taken. Use other drugs that inhibit platelet aggregation (such as nonsteroidal anti-inflammatory drugs [NSAIDs]) with caution. Monitor platelet count every few days during the first week, then weekly until the maintenance dose is reached.

Toxicity

1. *Myelosuppression and other hematologic effects.* Leukopenia is rare. Anemia is common but mild. Thrombocytopenic hemorrhage is uncommon.

2. *Nausea, vomiting, and other gastrointestinal effects.* Nausea and vomiting are occasional. Diarrhea, gas, and abdominal pain are common; pancreatitis is rare. Lactase supplementation eliminates diarrhea (anagrelide formulated with lactose). Hepatic enzyme elevation is rare, but caution is recommended when there is evidence of hepatic dysfunction.

3. *Mucocutaneous.* Rash, including urticaria, is occasional (8%). Hyperpigmentation is rare. Sun sensitivity is possible.

4. *Miscellaneous effects:*
   a. Cardiovascular: Palpitations, forceful heartbeat, and tachycardia are common. Congestive heart failure is uncommon, but fluid retention or edema is common. Tachyarrhythmias (including atrial fibrillation and premature atrial beats) are occasional. Angina, cardiomyopathy, or other severe cardiovascular effects are rare, although there are somewhat more frequent (8%) episodes of chest pain. Drinking alcoholic beverages may cause flushing. Higher than recommended single doses cause postural hypotension. Cardiovascular effects appear to result from vasodilation, positive inotropy, and decreased renal blood flow.
   b. Neurologic: Headaches are common and occasionally are severe; they usually diminish in about 2 weeks. Weakness (asthenia) is common. Dizziness is occasional.
   c. Pulmonary: Infiltrates are rare but are a reason to stop anagrelide and treat with steroids.

ANASTROZOLE

Other name. Arimidex.

Mechanism of action. Decreases estrogen biosynthesis by selective inhibition of aromatase (estrogen synthetase).

Primary indications

1. Carcinoma of the breast as adjuvant treatment in postmenopausal women with positive hormone receptors.
2. Carcinoma of the breast that is advanced or metastatic as first therapy in postmenopausal women with positive or unknown hormone receptors.
3. Carcinoma of the breast that is advanced or metastatic as second therapy in postmenopausal women with progression following initial response to tamoxifen.

Usual dosage and schedule. 1 mg by mouth daily.

Special precautions. Potential hazard to fetus if given during pregnancy. In women with pre-existing ischemic heart disease, an increased incidence of ischemic cardiovascular events occurred with anastrozole use compared to tamoxifen use. Consider obtaining bone mineral density testing prior to initiation of anastrozole and treating as clinically indicated.

Toxicity

1. *Myelosuppression and other hematologic effects.* No dose-related myelosuppression. Thromboembolic events are uncommon (3%).
2. *Nausea, vomiting, and other gastrointestinal effects.* Nausea, diarrhea, and constipation are occasional. Vomiting is uncommon.
3. *Mucocutaneous effects.* Rash is occasional. Hot flushes are common (35%). Vaginal dryness and leukorrhea are uncommon.
4. *Miscellaneous effects:*
   a. Asthenia is common. Headache and dizziness are occasional.
   b. Musculoskeletal pain is occasional. Arthralgia is occasional.
   c. Peripheral edema and weight gain are occasional (lower than with megestrol).
   d. Dyspnea and cough are occasional.
   e. Cataracts are occasional (6%).
   f. Decreased bone mineral density with osteoporosis is occasional (11%), and there is increased risk for fractures (10%).
   g. Vaginal bleeding is uncommon, and endometrial cancer is rare (0.2%).

ARSENIC TRIOXIDE

Other names. Trisenox.

Mechanism of action. Although the mechanism is incompletely understood, effects of arsenic trioxide include morphologic changes and DNA fragmentation characteristic of apoptosis and alteration of the fusion protein PML-RAR alpha.

Primary indication. Acute promyelocytic leukemia that is refractory to retinoid and anthracycline therapy and has t(15;17) translocation or PML-RAR alpha gene expression.

Usual dosage and schedule

1. Induction: 0.15 mg/kg IV daily until marrow remission. Maximum of 60 doses.
2. Consolidation: 0.15 mg/kg IV daily for 25 doses over a period of up to 5 weeks. Consolidation is started 3 to 6 weeks after completion of induction therapy.

Special precautions. Tachycardia and prolonged QT interval are common. This may lead to complete arteriovenous (AV) block with fatal ventricular arrhythmia. Electrolyte (including magnesium) abnormalities should be corrected prior to initiation of therapy, and patients with prolonged QT intervals should have measures taken to reduce this prolongation prior to treatment with arsenic trioxide. A QT value greater than 500 msec during therapy is an indication to suspend arsenic trioxide treatment and to initiate measures to correct other risk factors that may be contributing to the prolongation of the QT.

Acute promyelocytic leukemic differentiation syndrome, similar to that seen with retinoic acid, may be seen and is potentially fatal. This syndrome consists of fever, dyspnea, weight gain, pulmonary infiltrates, and pleural or pericardial effusions with or without leukocytosis. High-dose corticosteroids (e.g. dexamethasone 10 mg twice a day) should be started at the first signs of this syndrome and continued until it has subsided.

Toxicity

1. *Myelosuppression and other hematologic effects.* Anemia, thrombocytopenia, and neutropenia are occasional. Leukocytosis is common. Disseminated intravascular coagulation is occasional and may be severe. Infections and neutropenic fever are occasional.
2. *Nausea, vomiting, and other gastrointestinal effects.* Nausea, vomiting, diarrhea, and abdominal pain are common ($>50\%$). Gastrointestinal bleeding, with or without diarrhea, is occasional (8%). Constipation, anorexia, and other abdominal distress are occasional.
3. *Mucocutaneous effects.* Sore throat is common (40%). Dermatitis, pruritis, and ecchymosis are also common. More severe mucocutanous reactions including local exfoliation, urticaria, and oral blistering are occasional to uncommon. Epistaxis is common (25%). Eye irritation and injection are occasional.
4. *Miscellaneous effects:*
   a. Cardiovascular: Tachycardia and prolonged QT interval are common. This may lead to complete AV block with fatal ventricular arrhythmia.
   b. Acute promyelocytic leukemic differentiation syndrome, similar to that seen with retinoic acid, may be seen. This consists of fever, dyspnea, weight gain, pulmonary infiltrates, and pleural or pericardial effusions with or without leukocytosis. This syndrome may be fatal.

    c. General and administration site: Headache and insomnia are common. Edema and pleural effusion are common (though not commonly serious), and general weight gain is occasional. Drug hypersensitivity is uncommon. Injection site edema, erythema, and pain are occasional.

    d. Metabolic: Hypokalemia, hypomagnesemia, and hyperglycemia are common (45% to 50%). Hyperkalemia is occasional to common (18%), as are elevated transaminases, hypocalcemia, and hypoglycemia.

    e. Pulmonary: Cough and dyspnea are common (>50%). Pleural effusion, hypoxia, wheezing, and asymptomatic ascultatory findings are occasional to common (8% to 20%).

    f. Renal: Renal failure is occasional.

ASPARAGINASE

Other names. L-Asparaginase, Elspar, Kidrolase, pegaspargase, Oncaspar.

Mechanism of action. Hydrolysis of serum asparagine occurs, which deprives leukemia cells of the required amino acid and inhibits protein synthesis. Normal cells are spared because they generally have the ability to synthesize their own asparagine. Pegaspargase is a chemically modified formulation of asparaginase in which the L-asparaginase is covalently conjugated with monomethoxypolyethylene glycol (PEG). This modification increases its half-life in the plasma by a factor of 4 to about 5.7 days and reduces its recognition by the immune system, which allows the drug to be used in patients previously hypersensitive to native L-asparaginase.

Primary indication. Acute lymphocytic leukemia, primarily for induction therapy.

Usual dosage and schedule. All schedules are used in combination with other drugs. The schedules listed are only a few of many acceptable dosing schedules.

    1. L-asparaginase 6000 IU/m^2 SC on days 5, 8, 11, 15, and 22 of the treatment period.

    2. L-asparaginase 10,000 IU IV daily for 10 successive days beginning on day 17 of the treatment period.

    3. Pegaspargase 2500 IU/m^2 intramuscularly (IM; or IV) once every 14 days, either for first-line acute lymphocytic leukemia or in patients who have developed hypersensitivity to native forms of asparaginase. For IM use, limit volume at single injection site to 2 mL. For IV administration, give over 1 to 2 hours in saline or normal saline with 5% dextrose.

Special precautions. Asparaginase is contraindicated in patients with pancreatitis or a history of pancreatitis. Asparaginase is contraindicated in patients who have had significant hemorrhagic events associated with prior L-asparaginase therapy. Pegaspargase is also contraindicated in patients who have had previous serious allergic reactions, such as generalized urticaria, bronchospasm, laryngeal edema, hypotension, or other unacceptable adverse reactions to prior pegaspargase.

Be prepared to treat anaphylaxis at each administration of the drug. Epinephrine, antihistamines, corticosteroids, and life-support equipment should be readily available. Giving concurrently with or immediately before vincristine may increase vincristine toxicity. The IM route is preferred for pegaspargase because of a lower incidence of hepatotoxicity, coagulopathy, and gastrointestinal and renal disorders compared to the IV route of administration.

Toxicity

1. *Myelosuppression and other hematologic effects.* Occasional myelosuppression. CNS thrombosis and other coagulopathies are uncommon.
2. *Nausea, vomiting, and other gastrointestinal effects.* Occasional and usually mild (see subsequent discussion for liver and pancreas effects).
3. *Mucocutaneous effects.* No toxicity occurs except as a sign of hypersensitivity.
4. *Anaphylaxis.* Mild to severe hypersensitivity reactions, including anaphylaxis, occur in 20% to 30% of patients. Such reaction is less likely to occur during the first few days of treatment. It is particularly common with intermittent schedules or repeat cycles. If the patient develops hypersensitivity to the *Escherichia coli*-derived enzyme (Elspar), *Erwinia*-derived asparaginase may be safely substituted because the two enzyme preparations are not cross-reactive. Note that hypersensitivity may also develop to *Erwinia*-derived asparaginase, and continued preparedness to treat anaphylaxis must be maintained.

   If given via the IM route, asparaginase should be given in an extremity so that a tourniquet can be applied to slow the systemic release of asparaginase should anaphylaxis occur.

   Approximately 30% of patients previously sensitive to L-asparaginase will have a hypersensitivity reaction to pegaspargase, while only 10% of those who were not hypersensitive to the native form will have a hypersensitivity reaction to the PEG-modified drug.
5. *Miscellaneous effects:*
   a. Mild fever and malaise are common and occasionally progress to severe chills and malignant hyperthermia.
   b. Hepatotoxicity is common and occasionally severe. Abnormalities observed include elevations of serum glutamic-oxaloacetic transaminase (SGOT), alkaline phosphatase, and bilirubin; depressed levels of hepatic-derived clotting factors and albumin; and hepatocellular fatty metamorphosis.
   c. Renal failure is rare.
   d. Pancreatic endocrine and exocrine dysfunction, often with manifestations of pancreatitis, occasionally occurs. Nonketotic hyperglycemia is uncommon.

> **e.** CNS effects (depression, somnolence, fatigue, confusion, agitation, hallucinations, or coma) are seen occasionally. They are usually reversible following discontinuation of the drug.

AZACITIDINE

Other name. Vidaza.

Mechanism of action. Pyrimidine analog that inhibits methyltransferase, causing hypomethylation of DNA and thus, it is believed, results in cellular differentiation or apoptosis. May restore normal function of genes that are critical for the control of cellular differentiation and proliferation. Nonproliferating cells are relatively insensitive to azacitidine.

Primary indication. Myelodysplastic syndromes (MDSs).

Usual dosage and schedule. 75 mg/m^2 SC or IV daily for 7 days, repeated every 4 weeks. Dose may be increased to 100 mg/m^2 if no toxicity other than nausea and vomiting. Therapy may be continued as long as the patient has improved from the drug.

Toxicity

1. *Myelosuppression and other hematologic effects.* Neutropenia, thrombocytopenia, and anemia are common. Febrile neutropenia is four times as common as in patients receiving supportive care. Petechiae or ecchymosis are occasional.
2. *Nausea, vomiting, and other gastrointestinal effects.* Anorexia, nausea, vomiting, and diarrhea or constipation are common. Abdominal pain is occasional.
3. *Mucocutaneous effects.* Pharyngitis and stomatitis are occasional. Skin rash and urticaria are occasional. Injection site pain is common.
4. *Neurotoxicity.* Insomnia is common. Lethargy, dizziness, or confusional state are occasional.
5. *Miscellaneous effects:*
   a. Cardiorespiratory: Cough and dyspnea are common. Pulmonary edema is uncommon. Edema is occasional. Tachycardia or other more serious cardiac disorders are uncommon.
   b. Fever is common.
   c. Fatigue and weakness are common.
   d. Arthralgias and back pain are occasional.
   e. Hypokalemia is occasional.

BENDAMUSTINE

Other names. Treanda, bendamustine hydrochloride.

Mechanism of action. Bendamustine is an alkylating agent that is a bifunctional mechlorethamine derivative containing a purinelike benzimidazole ring. It forms interstrand DNA crosslinks that lead to cell death in both resting and dividing cells, though the exact mechanism of cell death is not clear.

Primary indications

1. Chronic lymphocytic leukemia
2. Indolent B-cell non-Hodgkin lymphoma.

Usual dosage and schedule

1. Chronic lymphocytic leukemia: 100 mg/m^2 IV over 30 minutes on days 1 and 2 of a 28-day cycle, up to 6 cycles.
2. Non-Hodgkin lymphoma: 120 mg/m^2 IV over 30 minutes on days 1 and 2 of a 21-day cycle, up to 8 cycles.

Initiation of successive cycles of therapy is usually delayed until there is an absolute neutrophil count (ANC) of at least 1×10^9/L and a platelet count of at least 75×10^9/L. Dose reductions of 50% to 75% should be initiated for grade 3 to 4 hematologic or nonhematologic toxicity.

Special precautions. Infusion reactions consisting of fever, chills, pruritis, and rash are common. Severe anaphylactic or anaphylactoid reactions, particularly in the second or subsequent cycles of therapy, may rarely occur. Antihistamines (e.g., diphenhydramine and cimetidine) and corticosteroids are commonly used to minimize the severity of infusion reactions. Tumor lysis syndrome has been observed, particularly in the first cycle of therapy. Toxic epidermal necrolysis has rarely occurred when bendamustine was given with rituximab. Stevens-Johnson syndrome has rarely occurred when bendamustine was administered concomitantly with allopurinol. The relationship of these severe reactions to bendamustine is not known. If severe skin reactions occur, bendamustine should be withheld or discontinued. Do not give if known hypersensitivity to bendamustine or mannitol. Bendamustine can cause fetal harm and must not be administered to pregnant women.

Toxicity

1. *Myelosuppression and other hematologic effects.* Myelosuppression is common and is universal in the higher dosage ranges. Grade 3 to 4 leukopenia (both neutrophils and lymphocytes) is common. Grade 3 to 4 anemia and thrombocytopenia are occasional. Infections overall are occasional. Pneumonia and neutropenic sepsis are uncommon but may be fatal.
2. *Nausea, vomiting, and other gastrointestinal effects.* Nausea, vomiting, and diarrhea are occasional to common and dose-dependent, but rarely severe. Anorexia, dyspepsia, gastroesophageal reflux, upper abdominal pain, and distention are occasional.
3. *Mucocutaneous effects.* Skin rash and pruritis are occasional, including toxic skin reactions and bullous exanthema.

4. *Immunologic effects and infusion reactions.* Infusion reactions consisting of fever, chills, pruritis, and rash are common. Severe anaphylactic or anaphylactoid reactions, particularly in the second or subsequent cycles of therapy, are rare. Preventive measures, including antihistamines and corticosteroids, should be given if grade 1 or 2 infusion reactions were experienced in a prior cycle. Bendamustine should generally not be repeated if patients have had a prior grade 3 or 4 infusion reaction.

5. *Miscellaneous effects:*
   a. Fever (occasionally with chills) and fatigue are common; weakness and weight loss are occasional.
   b. Tumor lysis syndrome, including hyperuricemia, may occur, primarily with the first cycle of therapy, and lead to acute renal failure. With concomitant allopurinol, watch closely for severe skin reactions.
   c. Hypokalemia is only occasional, but may be severe.
   d. Cough, dyspnea, throat pain, wheezing, and nasal congestion are occasional to common.
   e. Hypotension is occasional.

BEVACIZUMAB

Other name. Avastin.

Mechanism of action. Binds vascular endothelial growth factor (VEGF) and prevents interaction of VEGF with its receptors on the surface of endothelial cells. This in turn impairs endothelial cell proliferation and new blood vessel formation, impeding tumor growth and metastasis.

Primary indications

1. Breast, colon, kidney, rectum, and nonsquamous non–small-cell lung cancers, usually with other agents.
2. Glioblastoma, alone or with other agents.

Usual dosage and schedule

1. 5 to 10 mg/kg IV once every 2 weeks
2. 15 mg/kg IV once every 3 weeks.

Special precautions. Gastrointestinal perforation occurs in up to 4% of patients and may have a fatal outcome. Impaired wound healing may rarely lead to anastomotic dehiscence. Bevacizumab should not be initiated for at least 28 days following major surgery. The interval between termination of bevacizumab and subsequent surgery should take into account the accumulation ratio of 2.8 (with dosing every 2 weeks) and the half-life of approximately 20 days. Blood pressure monitoring is recommended every 2 to 3 weeks because of the risk of hypertension. Reversible posterior leukoencephalopathy syndrome (RPLS) has been reported rarely; if it occurs, therapy must be discontinued immediately and treatment for hypertension initiated if it is present. Urinary protein should be evaluated prior to each treatment with a urine dipstick, and if 2+ or greater, the patient should undergo further assessment to rule out severe proteinuria, such as with a urine protein-creatinine (UPC) ratio. Hold therapy if UPC is greater than 3.5.

Toxicity

1. *Myelosuppression and other hematologic effects.* Leukopenia is common but associated primarily with the cytotoxic agents used together with bevacizumab. Thrombocytopenia is uncommon. Minor bleeding, such as epistaxis, is common; severe hemorrhage is not common, except for hemoptysis in patients with squamous cell carcinomas of the lung. Serious, and in some cases fatal, hemoptysis has occurred in non–small-cell lung cancer, with the highest risk appearing in patients with squamous cell histology; other severe or fatal hemorrhage, including CNS bleeding, has occurred. Thromboembolic events are occasional and may be severe.

2. *Nausea, vomiting, and other gastrointestinal effects.* Anorexia, nausea, vomiting, and constipation are common. Diarrhea is common, particularly when used with fluorouracil and irinotecan chemotherapy. Abdominal pain is common. Gastrointestinal hemorrhage is occasional.

3. *Mucocutaneous effects.* Dry skin, skin discoloration, stomatitis, and exfoliative dermatitis are occasional to common. Alopecia, skin ulcers, and nail changes are uncommon.

4. *Immunologic effects and infusion reactions.* Infusion reactions with hypertension, wheezing, stridor, desaturation, chest pain, headaches, and diaphoresis are uncommon. Severe reactions are rare (0.2%).

5. *Miscellaneous effects:*
   a. Fatigue, weakness, and headache are common.
   b. Cardiovascular and respiratory: Hypertension is common and occasionally is severe (>200/110 mm Hg). Blood pressure greater than 160/100 or rise of greater than 30 mm Hg requires holding therapy, at least temporarily. Hypotension is occasional. Dyspnea is occasional. Congestive heart failure is uncommon, but risk with anthracyclines is increased (14%). Venous thromboembolic events are increased by about 15% compared with chemotherapy not containing bevacizumab.
   c. Neurologic: Dizziness is common. RPLS has been reported rarely (<0.1%); if it occurs, therapy must be discontinued immediately and treatment for hypertension initiated if it is present.
   d. Metabolic: Proteinuria is common, but severe proteinuria (>3.5 g/24 h) is uncommon and rarely leads to nephrotic syndrome (<1%), but requires holding bevacizumab and rechecking prior to next cycle.

BEXAROTENE (capsules)

Other name. Targretin.

Mechanism of action. A member of the subclass of retinoids (rexinoid) that selectively activates retinoid X receptors (RXRs). These receptors are distinct from RARs, but also act as transcription factors that regulate the expression of genes that control cellular differentiation and proliferation. The exact mechanism in cutaneous T-cell lymphoma (CTCL) is unknown.

Primary indication. Cutaneous manifestations of CTCL in patients refractory to at least one prior systemic therapy.

Usual dosage and schedule. 300 mg/m^2/day to start as a single oral daily dose taken with a meal. Dosage is adjusted downward by 100 mg/m^2/day decrements for toxicity, or upward to 400 mg/m^2/day if there has been no response and good tolerability after 8 weeks of treatment. Treatment may be continued for up to 2 years.

Special precautions. Avoid use in pregnant women because of marked teratogenic potential.

Toxicity

1. *Myelosuppression and other hematologic effects.* Mild to moderate leukopenia is occasional to common with a time of onset of 4 to 8 weeks. Severe or worse leukopenia is occasional.
2. *Nausea, vomiting, and other gastrointestinal effects.* Mild nausea, abdominal pain, and diarrhea are occasional. Vomiting and anorexia are uncommon. Inflammatory bowel disease and pancreatitis (associated with hypertriglyceridemia) are rare.
3. *Mucocutaneous effects.* Skin reactions are occasional to common. They include redness, dryness, and pruritus of the skin and mucous membranes; possible vesicle formation; exfoliative dermatitis; cheilitis; and conjunctivitis. There also may be increased skin photosensitivity (e.g., to sun) and the nails may become brittle. Alopecia is uncommon.
4. *Miscellaneous effects:*
   a. Cataracts and corneal ulcerations or opacities are uncommon.
   b. Systemic: Arthralgias, bone pain, muscle aches are occasional. Fever, chills, and headache (flu syndrome) are occasional.
   c. Hypertriglyceridemia (80%) and hypercholesterolemia (35% to 40%) are common. Hypertriglyceridemia is usually more severe. These are reversible with discontinuation of therapy and may be reduced by antilipemic therapy.
   d. Neurologic: Headache is common. Lethargy, fatigue, confusion, and mental depression are uncommon; pseudotumor cerebri is rare.
   e. Hepatotoxicity with increased lactate dehydrogenase (LDH), SGOT, serum glutamic-pyruvic transaminase (SGPT), gamma-glutamyl transpeptidase (GGTP), and alkaline phosphatase is occasional.
   f. Hypothyroidism is common, with decreased T$_4$ and thyroid-stimulating hormone (TSH).

g. Peripheral edema is occasional.

h. Hypernatremia is rare.

BEXAROTENE (gel)

Other name. Targretin Gel (1%).

Mechanism of action. A member of the subclass of retinoids (rexinoid) that selectively activates RXRs. These receptors are distinct from RARs, but also act as transcription factors that regulate the expression of genes that control cellular differentiation and proliferation. The exact mechanism in CTCL is unknown.

Primary indication. Cutaneous manifestations of CTCL in patients who have refractory or persistent disease after other therapies or who have not tolerated other therapies.

Usual dosage and schedule. The gel is applied once every other day for the first week. The frequency is then increased at weekly intervals as tolerated to once daily, twice daily, and up to four times daily, according to individual lesion tolerance. Treatment frequency should be reduced or treatment suspended for severe local irritation.

Special precautions. Avoid use in pregnant women because of marked teratogenic potential.

Toxicity

1. *Myelosuppression and other hematologic effects.* Uncommon.
2. *Nausea, vomiting, and other gastrointestinal effects.* Not expected.
3. *Mucocutaneous effects.* Skin reactions are occasional to common. They include pain, redness, dryness, and pruritus of the skin; possible vesicle formation; exfoliative dermatitis. There also may be increased skin photosensitivity (e.g., to sun).
4. *Miscellaneous effects:*
   a. Hypertriglyceridemia is occasional.
   b. Neurologic: Headache and paresthesias are occasional.
   c. Peripheral edema is occasional.

BICALUTAMIDE

Other name. Casodex.

Mechanism of action. A nonsteroidal antiandrogen that is a competitive inhibitor of androgens at the cellular androgen receptor in target tissues, such as the prostate.

Primary indication. Carcinoma of the prostate.

Usual dosage and schedule. 50 mg daily in combination with luteinizing hormone-releasing hormone (LHRH) analog.

Special precautions. Rare cases of severe liver injury have been reported. Bicalutamide should be used with caution in patients with moderate-to-severe hepatic impairment.

Toxicity

1. *Myelosuppression and other hematologic effects.* No myelosuppression. May interact with warfarin and increase International Normalized Ratio (INR).
2. *Nausea, vomiting, and other gastrointestinal effects.* Nausea, diarrhea, flatulence, and constipation are occasional; vomiting is uncommon.
3. *Mucocutaneous effects.* Mild skin rash is occasional.
4. *Miscellaneous effects:*
   a. Secondary pharmacologic effects, including breast tenderness, breast swelling, hot flashes, impotence, and loss of libido, are common but reversible after cessation of therapy.
   b. Elevated liver function tests are uncommon, but severe hepatic failure has been observed only rarely.
   c. Dyspnea and cough are seen occasionally.
   d. Adverse cardiovascular events are similar to those seen with orchiectomy.
   e. Dizziness or vertigo is occasional.

BLEOMYCIN

Other name. Blenoxane.

Mechanism of action. Bleomycin binds to DNA, causes single- and double-strand scission, and inhibits further DNA, RNA, and protein synthesis.

Primary indications

- Testis, head and neck, penis, cervix, vulva, anus, and skin carcinomas
- Hodgkin and non-Hodgkin lymphomas
- Pleural effusions—used as sclerosing agent.

Usual dosage and schedule

1. 10 to 20 units/m^2 IV or IM once or twice a week, *or*
2. 30 units IV push weekly for 9 to 12 weeks in combination with other drugs for cancer of the testis.
3. 60 units in 50 mL of normal saline instilled intrapleurally.

Special precautions

1. In patients with lymphoma, a test dose of one or two units should be given IM prior to the first dose of bleomycin because of the possibility of anaphylactoid, acute pulmonary, or severe hyperpyretic responses. If no acute reaction occurs within 4 hours, regular dosing may begin.
2. Reduce dose for renal failure.

Serum Creatinine	Percent of Full Dose
2.5–4.0	25
4.0–6.0	20
6.0–10.0	10

3. The cumulative lifetime dose should not exceed 400 units because of the dose-related incidence of severe pulmonary fibrosis. Smaller limits may be appropriate for older patients or those with pre-existing pulmonary disease. Frequent evaluation of pulmonary status, including symptoms of cough or dyspnea, rales, infiltrates on chest x-ray film, and pulmonary function studies are recommended to avert serious pulmonary sequelae.

4. Glass containers are recommended for continuous infusion to minimize drug instability.

5. High fraction of inspired oxygen (such as might be used during surgery) should be avoided as it exacerbates lung injury, sometimes acutely.

Toxicity

1. *Myelosuppression and other hematologic effects.* Significant depression of counts is uncommon. This factor permits bleomycin to be used in full doses with myelosuppressive drugs.

2. *Nausea, vomiting, and other gastrointestinal effects.* Occasional and self-limiting.

3. *Mucocutaneous effects.* Alopecia, stomatitis, erythema, edema, thickening of nail bed, and hyperpigmentation and desquamation of skin are common.

4. *Pulmonary effects:*
   a. Acute anaphylactoid or pulmonary edema–like response is occasional in patients with lymphoma (see special precautions discussed previously).
   b. Dose-related pneumonitis with cough, dyspnea, rales, and infiltrates, progressing to pulmonary fibrosis.

5. *Fever.* Common. Occasionally, severe hyperpyrexia, diaphoresis, dehydration, and hypotension have occurred and resulted in renal failure and death. Antipyretics help control fever.

6. *Miscellaneous effects:*
   a. Lethargy, headache, and joint swelling are rare.
   b. IM or SQ injection may cause pain at injection site.

BORTEZOMIB

Other name. Velcade.

Mechanism of action. A reversible inhibitor of the chymotrypsin-like activity of the 26S proteasome, which mediates ubiquitinated protein degradation and plays an essential role in intracellular protein regulation, and consequent cellular signal transduction pathways and cellular homeostasis. Disruption of these homeostatic mechanisms can lead to cell death. Bortezomib is metabolized by liver enzymes.

Primary indications

1. Multiple myeloma
2. Mantle cell lymphoma.

Usual dosage and schedule

1. Multiple myeloma: 1.3 mg/m^2 IV bolus twice weekly (days 1, 4, 8, 11, 22, 25, 29, and 32), often together with oral melphalan and oral prednisone (days 1 to 4 every 6 weeks) for four 6-week treatment cycles. Then once weekly (days 1, 8, 22, and 29) together with oral melphalan and oral prednisone (days 1 to 4 every 6 weeks) for five more 6-week treatment cycles. The intensity may be modified by giving the twice weekly component for one cycle only followed by eight cycles of the weekly schedule, or by using the weekly schedule for all nine cycles. Similar schedule used in combination with other agents.
2. Mantle cell lymphoma: 1.3 mg/m^2 IV bolus twice weekly (days 1, 4, 8, and 11 every 3 weeks) for up to eight cycles. Frequency may be reduced to weekly for 3 out of 4 weeks for maintenance.
3. Reduce each dose to 0.7 mg/m^2 in the first cycle for patients with moderate or severe liver function impairment (bilirubin >1.5 upper limit of normal [ULN]). Consider dose escalation to 1.0 mg/m^2 or further dose reduction to 0.5 mg/m^2 in subsequent cycles based on patient tolerability.

Special precautions. Cardiogenic shock, congestive heart failure, and respiratory insufficiency have rarely been observed. Anaphylaxis has also been observed. Patients with hepatic impairment should be monitored closely, as bortezomib is metabolized by liver enzymes. Consider acyclovir 400 mg twice a day for herpes zoster prophylaxis.

Toxicity

1. *Myelosuppression and other hematologic effects.* Anemia, neutropenia, and thrombocytopenia are common; neutropenia is only occasionally severe (grade 3 or 4). Thrombocytopenia is severe in 30% of patients. Disseminated intravascular coagulation has been observed (rare to uncommon).
2. *Nausea, vomiting, and other gastrointestinal effects.* Anorexia, nausea, vomiting, diarrhea, and constipation are common. Dehydration is a concern because of vomiting and diarrhea and may be seen occasionally.
3. *Mucocutaneous effects.* Rash is common (20%).
4. *Neurotoxicity.* Peripheral neuropathy is common and occasionally (7%) severe. This is frequently manifest by paresthesias and dysesthesias. Headache is common.
5. *Immunologic effects and infusion reactions.* Hypersensitivity reactions have been seen, including anaphylactic reactions and immune complex mediated hypersensitivity (rare). Tumor lysis syndrome may be seen in patients with a high tumor burden. The incidence of herpes zoster is increased compared with controls and is occasional.

6. *Miscellaneous effects:*
    a. Fatigue and weakness are common.
    b. Arthralgias, muscle cramps, and back pain are occasional.
    c. Fever is common.
    d. Cardiovascular: Hypotension is occasional, is seen throughout therapy, and may or may not be orthostatic. Peripheral edema is common. Other cardiovascular events during treatment have included severe congestive heart failure, AV block, angina, atrial fibrillation, and flutter—these are probably uncommon to rare as a consequence of the drug.
    e. Infiltrative pulmonary disease is rare, but may be severe or fatal.
    f. Hepatitis and pancreatitis have been observed and are probably rare.

BUSULFAN

Other names. Myleran, Busulfex.

Mechanism of action. Bifunctional alkylating agent. Its effect may be greater on cellular thiol groups than on nucleic acids.

Primary indications

1. Standard doses: CML
2. High doses with stem cell rescue: Acute leukemia, lymphoma, chronic granulocytic leukemia.

Usual dosage and schedule

1. 3 to 4 mg/m^2 by mouth daily for remission induction in adults until the leukocyte count is 50% of the original level, then 1 to 2 mg/m^2 by mouth daily. Busulfan may be given continuously or intermittently for maintenance.
2. High doses with stem cell rescue—consult specific protocols. Not recommended outside of research setting. High-dose therapy requires pretreatment with phenytoin.

Special precautions. Obtain complete blood count weekly while patient is on therapy. If leukocyte count falls rapidly to less than 15,000/μL, discontinue therapy until nadir is reached and rising counts indicate a need for further treatment.

Toxicity

1. *Myelosuppression and other hematologic effects.* Dose-limiting. A fall in the leukocyte count may not begin for 2 weeks after starting therapy, and it is likely to continue for 2 weeks after therapy has been stopped. Recovery of marrow function may be delayed for 3 to 6 weeks after the drug has been discontinued. High-dose therapy requires stem cell rescue (e.g., bone marrow transplantation).

2. *Nausea, vomiting, and other gastrointestinal effects.* Rare at standard doses.
3. *Mucocutaneous effects.* Hyperpigmentation occurs occasionally, particularly in skin creases.
4. *Miscellaneous effects*
   a. Pulmonary effects: Interstitial pulmonary fibrosis is rare and is an indication to discontinue drug. Corticosteroids may improve symptoms and minimize permanent lung damage.
   b. Metabolic effects: Adrenal insufficiency syndrome is rare. Hyperuricemia may occur when the leukemia cell count is rapidly reduced. Ovarian suppression and amenorrhea are common.
   c. Secondary neoplasia is possible.
   d. Fatal hepatic veno-occlusive disease with high-dose therapy is occasional.
   e. Seizures after high-dose therapy are occasional.

CABAZITAXEL

Other name. Jevtana.

Mechanism of action. Microtubule inhibitor that binds to tubulin, which leads to the stabilization of microtubules and the inhibition of mitotic and interphase cellular functions.

Primary indication. Carcinoma of the prostate, metastatic, previously treated with a docetaxel-containing regimen.

Usual dosage and schedule. 25 mg/m^2 IV over 1 hour every 3 weeks in combination with prednisone 10 mg daily. Reduce dose to 20 mg/m^2 if the patient experiences prolonged grade 3 or higher neutropenia, febrile neutropenia, or severe or persistent diarrhea.

Special precautions. Hypersensitivity reactions can occur, and therefore patients should be premedicated with corticosteroids and histamine H_1 and H_2 antagonists. Should not be given to patients with hepatic impairment. Patients age 65 and older are more likely to experience adverse effects from cabazitaxel treatment. Because cabazitaxel is metabolized primarily through CYP3A, coadministration with strong CYP3A inhibitors should be avoided.

Toxicity

1. *Myelosuppression and other hematologic effects.* Neutropenia, anemia, and thrombocytopenia are common. Grade 3 to 4 febrile neutropenia is occasional but may be fatal.
2. *Nausea, vomiting, and other gastrointestinal effects.* Nausea, vomiting, anorexia, diarrhea, and constipation are common, but infrequently (2% to 6%) severe.
3. *Mucocutaneous effects.* Alopecia is occasional.
4. *Immunologic effects and infusion reactions.* Hypersensitivity reactions are uncommon but may occur within a few minutes following

initiation of therapy; they may be associated with rash, erythema, hypotension, and bronchospasm.

5. *Miscellaneous effects:*
   a. Fatigue and weakness are common. Fever is occasional.
   b. Renal failure is uncommon, but may be fatal (rare). Hematuria is occasional.
   c. Peripheral edema is occasional.
   d. Cardiac arrythmias and hypotension are uncommon.
   e. Back pain and arthralgias are occasional.
   f. Peripheral neuropathy and headache are occasional.
   g. Dyspnea and cough are occasional.

CAPECITABINE

Other name. Xeloda.

Mechanism of action. An orally administered prodrug that is converted to fluorouracil intracellularly. When this is converted to the active nucleotide, 5-fluoro-2-deoxyuridine monophosphate, it inhibits the enzyme thymidylate synthetase and blocks DNA synthesis. The triphosphate may also be mistakenly incorporated into RNA, which interferes with RNA processing and protein synthesis.

Primary indications

1. Metastatic breast cancer that is resistant to anthracycline- and paclitaxel-containing chemotherapy regimens. May also be used in patients in whom anthracyclines are contraindicated.
2. Colorectal (adjuvant or metastatic), small bowel, stomach, pancreas, and biliary carcinomas.

Usual dosage and schedule. Generally taken with water, twice daily (about 12 hours between doses) within 30 minutes after a meal. Dose reductions are commonly required by reducing the daily dose, the number of consecutive daily treatments, or both.

1. 1000 to 1250 mg/m^2 orally twice daily for 2 weeks as a single agent, followed by a 1-week rest, given as 3-week cycles.
2. 850 to 1250 mg/m^2 orally twice daily for 2 weeks when used in combination with other drugs, followed by a 1-week rest, given as 3-week cycles.
3. 800 mg/m^2 orally twice daily 5 days per week during radiotherapy as a radiosensitizer.

Special precautions. Increase in PT and INR may be seen in patients previously stable on oral anticoagulants. Monitor PT/INR more frequently when patient is on capecitabine. Patients with moderate renal impairment (C_{Cr} 30–50 mL/min) require a 25% dosage reduction: Diarrhea may be severe and require fluid and electrolyte replacement. Incidence and severity may be worse in patients 80 years of age or older. Therapy may need to be interrupted and subsequent doses decreased for severe or repeated toxicity. Phenytoin levels should be monitored, as elevated levels may occur.

Toxicity

1. *Myelosuppression and other hematologic effects.* Common, but when used as a single agent, these usually are mild to moderate with anemia predominating. Neutropenia is common when used in combination and may be associated with neutropenic fever.

2. *Nausea, vomiting, and other gastrointestinal effects.* Both nausea (45%) and vomiting (35%) are common, but usually not severe. Diarrhea is common (55%); in up to 15% of patients, it is severe to life-threatening. Gastrointestinal motility disorders, including ileus, may be seen, and necrotizing enterocolitis has been reported. Abdominal pain is occasional to common. Anorexia is occasional to common (26%). Hyperbilirubinemia is common (48%) but only occasionally severe or life-threatening.

3. *Mucocutaneous effects.* Hand-foot syndrome is common (54%) and may be severe. Dermatitis is also common (27%), as is stomatitis, but it is uncommon that these are severe. Eye irritation and increased lacrimation are occasional.

4. *Miscellaneous effects:*
   a. Fatigue is common.
   b. Paresthesias are occasional.
   c. Fever is occasional.
   d. Headache or dizziness is occasional.
   e. Cardiotoxicity is possible as with any fluorinated pyrimidine.

CARBOPLATIN

Other names. Paraplatin, CBDCA.

Mechanism of action. Covalent binding to DNA.

Primary indications. Ovarian, endometrial, breast, bladder, and lung cancers, and other cancers in which cisplatin is active.

Usual dosage and schedule. AUC dosing (Calvert formula) is generally preferred.

1. Target AUC is commonly 4 to 6, depending on previous treatment and other drugs to be used. Administration dose (mg) = (target AUC) × ([creatinine clearance] + 25). Administration dose is given by IV infusion over 15 to 60 minutes and repeated every 4 weeks.

2. Higher doses up to 1600 mg/m^2 divided over several days have been used followed by stem cell rescue (e.g., bone marrow transplantation).

Special precautions. Much less renal toxicity than cisplatin, so there is no need for a vigorous hydration schedule or forced diuresis. If AUC dosing is not used, reduce dose to 250 mg/m^2 for creatinine clearance of 41 to 59 mL/minute, reduce to 200 mg/m^2 for clearance of 16 to 40 mL/minute.

Anaphylactic-like reactions to carboplatin have been reported and may occur within minutes of carboplatin administration. Infusion reactions generally develop after several months of drug tolerance. Epinephrine, corticosteroids, antihistamines, and fluid administration for hypotension have been employed to alleviate symptoms. Skin testing for hypersensitivity (see Table 26.2) may be helpful.

Toxicity

1. *Myelosuppression and other hematologic effects.* Anemia, granulocytopenia, and thrombocytopenia are common and dose-limiting. Red blood cell transfusions or epoetin may be required. Thrombocytopenia may be delayed (days 18 to 28).

2. *Nausea, vomiting, and other gastrointestinal effects.* Nausea and vomiting are common, but vomiting (65%) is not as frequent or as severe as with cisplatin and can be controlled with combination antiemetic regimens. Liver function abnormalities are common. Gastrointestinal pain is occasional.

3. *Mucocutaneous effects.* Alopecia is uncommon. Mucositis is rare.

4. *Immunologic effects and infusion reactions.* Infusion reactions are occasional but may be severe. These may include rash, urticaria, pruritus, and rarely bronchospasm and hypotension. Desensitization protocols may allow continued therapy with carboplatin, but should be carried out under close observation (see Special precautions).

5. *Miscellaneous effects:*
   a. Peripheral neuropathies or central neurotoxicity are uncommon.
   b. Cardiovascular (cardiac failure, embolism, cerebrovascular accidents) complications are uncommon.
   c. Hemolytic uremic syndrome is rare.
   d. Renal tubular abnormalities: Elevation in serum creatinine or blood urea nitrogen occurs occasionally. More common is electrolyte loss with decreases in serum sodium, potassium, calcium, and magnesium.

CARMUSTINE

Other names. BCNU, BiCNU, Gliadel wafer (surgically implantable, biodegradable polymer wafer that releases impregnated carmustine from the hydrophobic matrix after implantation).

Mechanism of action. Alkylation and carbamoylation by carmustine metabolites interfere with the synthesis and function of DNA, RNA, and proteins. Carmustine is lipid soluble and easily enters the brain.

Primary indications

1. Systemic therapy:
   a. Brain tumors
   b. Hodgkin and non-Hodgkin lymphomas
   c. Melanoma.
2. Implantable carmustine-impregnated wafer: glioblastoma multiforme.

Usual dosage and schedule

1. Systemic therapy:
   a. 200 to 240 mg/m^2 IV as a 30- to 45-minute infusion every 6 to 8 weeks. Dose often is divided and given over 2 to 3 days. Some recommend limiting the cumulative dose to 1000 mg/m^2 to limit pulmonary and renal toxicity.
   b. Higher doses of up to 600 mg/m^2 have been used with stem cell rescue (e.g., bone marrow or peripheral blood stem cell transplantation).
2. Implantable carmustine-impregnated wafer: Up to eight wafers, each containing 7.7 mg of carmustine, are applied to the resection cavity surface after removal of the tumor.

Special precautions (systemic therapy). Because of delayed myelosuppression (3 to 6 weeks), do not administer drug more often than every 6 weeks. Await a return of normal platelet and granulocyte counts before repeating therapy. Amphotericin B may enhance the potential for renal toxicity, bronchospasm, and hypotension.

Toxicity

1. Systemic therapy:
   a. *Myelosuppression and other hematologic effects.* Delayed and often biphasic, with the nadir at 3 to 6 weeks; it may be cumulative with successive doses. Recovery may be protracted for several months. High-dose therapy requires stem cell rescue.
   b. *Nausea, vomiting, and other gastrointestinal effects.* Begins 2 hours after therapy and lasts 4 to 6 hours; it is common.
   c. *Mucocutaneous effects:*
      (1) Facial flushing and a burning sensation at the IV site may be due to alcohol used to reconstitute the drug; this is common with rapid injection.
      (2) Hyperpigmentation of skin after accidental contact is common.
   d. *Miscellaneous effects:*
      (1) Hepatotoxicity is uncommon but can be severe.
      (2) Pulmonary fibrosis is uncommon at low doses, but its frequency increases at doses higher than 1000 mg/m^2.
      (3) Secondary neoplasia is possible.
      (4) Renal toxicity is uncommon at doses of less than 1000 mg/m^2.
      (5) With high-dose therapy, encephalopathy, hepatotoxicity, and pulmonary toxicity are common and dose-limiting. Hepatic veno-occlusive disease also occurs (occasional).
2. Implantable carmustine-impregnated wafer. Limited toxicity beyond that expected from craniotomy is seen. Serious intracranial infection was seen in 4% of patients, compared with 1% of placebo-treated patients. Brain edema not responsive to steroids may also

be seen in a similar percentage of patients. Abnormal wound healing may occur. Remnants of the wafer may be seen for many months after implantation.

CETUXIMAB

Other names. Epidermal growth factor receptor (EGFR) antibody, C225, Erbitux.

Mechanism of action. EGFR antibody that blocks the ligand-binding site and inhibits proliferation of cells. It is thought potentially most useful in those tumors that overexpress EGFR, but correlation with percent of positive cells or intensity of EGFR expression is weak.

Primary indications

1. Carcinoma of head and neck, in combination with radiation therapy or after failure of platinum-based therapy.
2. Colon cancer when KRAS is wild type, after failure of irinotecan- and oxaliplatin-based regimens. Often in combination with irinotecan or other cytotoxic regimens.
3. Lung cancer if EGFR amplification.

Usual dosage and schedule. 400 mg/m^2 IV loading dose administered over 2 hours on day 1. Then 250 mg/m^2 IV maintenance doses administered over 1 hour weekly thereafter. May be administered in combination with other agents.

Special precautions. Sersious infusion reactions, some fatal, may occur (3% of patients). A 1-hour observation period is recommended following a cetuximab infusion. Cardiopulmonary arrest or sudden death has occurred in 2% of patients receiving cetuximab in combination with radiation therapy. Severe hypomagnesemia is seen in 10% to 15% of patients, and all patients should have magnesium levels monitored throughout the persistence of cetuximab (8 weeks).

All patients with metastatic colorectal cancer who might be candidates for cetuximab should have their tumor tested for KRAS and BRAF mutations. If KRAS mutation in codon 12 or 13 or BRAF V600E mutation is detected, cetuximab should not be given, as the patient is unlikely to benefit.

Toxicity

1. *Myelosuppression and other hematologic effects.* Leukopenia and anemia are occasional.
2. *Nausea, vomiting, and other gastrointestinal effects.* Anorexia, nausea, vomiting, diarrhea, and constipation are occasional. Abdominal pain is common.
3. *Mucocutaneous effects.* Acnelike rash is common (76%). Stomatitis is occasional when used alone, but universal when used in combination with radiation therapy. Severe radiation dermatitis may be seen when used concurrently with radiation therapy.

4. *Miscellaneous effects:*
 a. Asthenia is common; headache and back pain are occasional.
 b. Weight loss, peripheral edema, and dehydration are occasional.
 c. Infusion reactions with allergic or hypersensitivity reactions, fever, chills, or dyspnea are occasional to common (~20%) but may be severe.
 d. Human antichimeric antibodies (HACAs) are uncommon.
 e. Electrolyte depletion, particularly hypomagnesemia, occurs commonly. Hypomagnesemia is occasionally severe.

CHLORAMBUCIL

Other name. Leukeran.

Mechanism of action. Classic alkylating agent, with primary effect on preformed DNA.

Primary indications

1. Chronic lymphocytic leukemia
2. Low-grade non-Hodgkin lymphoma.

Usual dosage and schedule

1. 3 to 4 mg/m^2 by mouth daily until a response is seen or cytopenias occur; then, if necessary, maintain with 1 to 2 mg/m^2 by mouth daily.
2. 30 mg/m^2 by mouth once every 2 weeks (with or without prednisone 80 mg/m^2 by mouth on days 1 to 5).

Special precautions. Increased toxicity may occur with prior barbiturate use.

Toxicity

1. *Myelosuppression and other hematologic effects.* Dose-limiting and may be prolonged.
2. *Nausea, vomiting, and other gastrointestinal effects.* May be seen with higher doses but are uncommon.
3. *Mucocutaneous effects.* Rash is uncommon.
4. *Miscellaneous effects:*
 a. Liver function abnormalities are rare.
 b. Secondary neoplasia is possible.
 c. Amenorrhea and azoospermia are common.
 d. Drug fever is uncommon.
 e. Pulmonary fibrosis is rare.
 f. CNS effects including seizure and coma may be seen at very high doses (>100 mg/m^2).

CISPLATIN

Other names. *cis*-Diamminedichloroplatinum (II), DDP, CDDP, Platinol.

Mechanism of action. Similar to alkylating agents with respect to binding and cross-linking strands of DNA.

Primary indications. Usually used in combination with other cytotoxic drugs.

1. Testis, ovary, endometrial, cervical, bladder, head and neck, gastrointestinal, and lung carcinomas
2. Soft-tissue and bone sarcomas
3. Non-Hodgkin lymphoma.

Usual dosage and schedule

1. 40 to 120 mg/m^2 IV on day 1 as infusion every 3 weeks
2. 15 to 20 mg/m^2 IV on days 1 to 5 as infusion every 3 to 4 weeks.

Special precautions. Do not administer if serum creatinine level is more than 1.5 mg/dL. Irreversible renal tubular damage may occur if vigorous diuresis is not maintained, particularly with higher doses (>40 mg/m^2) and with additional concurrent nephrotoxic drugs, such as the aminoglycosides. At higher doses, diuresis with mannitol with or without furosemide plus vigorous hydration is mandatory.

1. An acceptable method for hydration in patients without cardiovascular impairment for cisplatin doses up to 80 mg/m^2 is as follows:
   a. Have patient void and begin infusion of 5% dextrose in half-normal saline with potassium chloride (KCl) 20 mEq/liter and magnesium sulfate (MgSO$_4$) 1 g/liter (8 mEq/liter); run at 500 mL/hour for 1.5 to 2.0 L.
   b. After 1 hour of infusion, give 12.5 gm of mannitol by IV push.
   c. Immediately thereafter, start the cisplatin (mixed in normal saline at 1 mg/mL) and infuse over 1 hour through the sidearm of the IV, while continuing the hydration.
   d. Give additional mannitol (12.5 to 50.0 gm) by IV push if necessary to maintain urinary output of 250 mL/hour over the duration of the hydration. If patient gets more than 1 L behind on urinary output or signs or symptoms of congestive heart failure develop, 40 mg of furosemide may be given.
2. For doses more than 80 mg/m^2 a more vigorous hydration is recommended:
   a. Have patient void and begin infusion of 5% dextrose in half-normal saline with KCl 20 mEq/liter and MgSO$_4$ 1 gm/liter (8 mEq/liter); run at 500 mL/hour for 2.5 to 3.0 L.
   b. After 1 hour of infusion, give 25 g of mannitol by IV push.
   c. Continue hydration.
   d. After 2 hours of hydration, if urinary output is at least 250 mL/hour, start the cisplatin (mixed in normal saline at 1 mg/mL) and infuse over 1 to 2 hours (1 mg/m^2/minute) through the sidearm of the IV, while continuing the hydration.
   e. Give additional mannitol (12.5 to 50 g by IV push) if necessary to maintain urinary output of 250 mL/hour over the duration of the hydration. If patient gets more than 1 L behind on urinary

output or signs or symptoms of congestive heart failure develop, 40 mg of furosemide may be given.

3. For patients with known or suspected cardiovascular impairment (ejection fraction <45%), a less vigorous rate of hydration may be used, provided the dose of cisplatin is limited (e.g., <60 mg/m²). An alternative is to give carboplatin.

Toxicity

1. *Myelosuppression and other hematologic effects.* Mild to moderate, depending on the dose. Relative lack of myelosuppression and other hematologic effects allows cisplatin to be used in full doses with more myelosuppressive drugs. Anemia is common and may have a hemolytic component. Anemia often is amenable to epoetin therapy.

2. *Nausea, vomiting, and other gastrointestinal effects.* Severe and often intractable vomiting regularly begins within 1 hour of starting cisplatin and lasts 8 to 12 hours. Prolonged nausea, vomiting, and other gastrointestinal effects occur occasionally. Nausea, vomiting, and other gastrointestinal effects may be minimized by the use of a combination antiemetic regimen (see Chapter 26).

3. *Mucocutaneous effects.* None.

4. *Renal tubular damage.* Acute reversible and occasionally irreversible nephrotoxicity may occur, particularly if adequate attention is not given to achieving sufficient hydration and diuresis. Nephrotoxic antibiotics increase risk of acute renal failure.

5. *Ototoxicity.* High-tone hearing loss is common, but significant hearing loss at vocal frequencies occurs only occasionally. Tinnitus is uncommon.

6. *Severe electrolyte abnormalities.* Marked hyponatremia, hypomagnesemia, hypocalcemia, and hypokalemia may be seen up to several days after treatment.

7. *Anaphylaxis.* May occur after several doses. Responds to epinephrine, antihistamines, and corticosteroids.

8. *Miscellaneous effects:*
   a. Peripheral neuropathies are clinically significant; signs and symptoms are common at cumulative doses more than 300 mg/m².
   b. Hyperuricemia is uncommon and parallels renal failure.
   c. Autonomic dysfunction with symptomatic postural hypotension is occasional.

CLADRIBINE

Other names. 2-Chlorodeoxyadenosine, Leustatin.

Mechanism of action. Deoxyadenosine analog with high cellular specificity for lymphoid cells. Resistant to effect of adenosine deaminase. Accumulates in cells as triphosphate, is incorporated into DNA, and inhibits DNA repair enzymes and RNA synthesis. Also results in nicotinamide adenine dinucleotide depletion. Effect is independent of cell division.

Primary indications. Hairy-cell leukemia, chronic lymphocytic leukemia, Waldenström macroglobulinemia, and possibly other lymphoid neoplasms.

Usual dosage and schedule

1. 0.09 mg/kg (3.33 mg/m^2) IV daily as a continuous 7-day infusion
2. 0.14 mg/kg (5.2 mg/m^2) IV as a 2-hour infusion daily for 5 days
3. 0.14 mg/kg (5.2 mg/m^2) SC daily for 5 days
4. 0.12 mg/kg IV daily × 3 together with cyclophosphamide 250 mg/m^2 IV daily × 3 every 28 days up to 6 cycles (for chronic lymphocytic leukemia [CLL] with TP53 [17p13] gene deletion).

Special precautions. Give allopurinol, 300 mg daily, as prophylaxis against hyperuricemia. Opportunistic infections occur occasionally and should be watched for closely.

Toxicity

1. *Myelosuppression and other hematologic effects.* Moderate granulocyte suppression is common. Marrow suppression with leukopenia and thrombocytopenia may be prolonged for over a year. Serious infection is common. Profound suppression of cluster of differentiation (CD) 4 and CD8 counts is common and often prolonged for over 1 year. Opportunistic infections, including herpes, fungus, and pneumocystis infection, may occur and should be monitored. Some routinely use prophylaxis against one or more of these infections, including acyclovir 400 mg twice a day and trimethoprim-sulfamethoxazole one double-strength tablet twice daily on 2 or 3 days a week. Autoimmune hemolytic anemia and immune thrombocytopenic purpura occur occasionally; pure red cell aplasia rarely.
2. *Nausea, vomiting, and other gastrointestinal effects.* Mild nausea with decrease in appetite is common, but no vomiting is expected. Mild reversible increase in liver function tests may be seen.
3. *Mucocutaneous effects.* Rash is common. Injection site reactions are occasional.
4. *Miscellaneous effects:*
   a. Fever, possibly due to release of pyrogens from tumor cells, is common.
   b. Fatigue is common. Headache, dizziness, insomnia, myalgia, and arthralgia are occasional.
   c. Edema and tachycardia are occasional.
   d. Cough, shortness of breath, and abnormal breath sounds are occasional.

CLOFARABINE

Other name. Clolar.

Mechanism of action. Clofarabine is a nucleoside analog (an adenine derivative) that is a potent inhibitor of ribonucleotide reductase. It also inhibits DNA polymerases and DNA synthesis. Increases intracellular arabinosylcytosine triphosphate (ara-CTP) when used with cytarabine.

Primary indications

1. Acute lymphoblastic leukemia (ALL) in children (age 1 to 21 years) who have relapsed or are refractory to other therapy
2. Acute lymphoblastic or acute myeloid leukemia (AML) in adults.

Usual dosage and schedule

1. 52 mg/m^2 IV over 2 hours daily for 5 consecutive days. May be repeated in 2 to 6 weeks.
2. 40 mg/m^2 IV over 1 hour (days 2 to 6), followed in 4 hours by cytarabine 1 g/m^2 IV as a 2-hour infusion (days 1 to 5) in adults with AML.
3. 30 mg/m^2 IV over 1 hour daily for 5 days in older adults with AML and unfavorable prognostic factors. For reinduction (day 29) or consolidation (on recovery of counts), dose reduced to 20 mg/m^2 IV daily for 5 days (6 cycles maximum).

Special precautions. Capillary leak syndrome or systemic inflammatory response syndrome have been observed with clofarabine administration.

Toxicity

1. *Myelosuppression and other hematologic effects.* Pancytopenia is common. Febrile neutropenia and documented infections are common.
2. *Nausea, vomiting, and other gastrointestinal effects.* Nausea, vomiting, diarrhea, and abdominal pain are common. Elevation of transaminases is common and may be severe (grade 3 to 4); jaundice is occasional. Anorexia is common.
3. *Mucocutaneous effects.* Nonspecific dermatitis and pruritis are common. Palmar-plantar erythrodysesthesia is occasional.
4. *Miscellaneous effects:*
   a. Arthralgia and back pain are occasional.
   b. Creatinine elevations are uncommon to occasional.
   c. Fatigue is common. Lethargy is occasional.
   d. Flushing and hypotension are occasional to common.

CORTICOSTEROIDS

Other names. Prednisone, dexamethasone (Decadron), and others.

Mechanism of action. Unknown but apparently related to the presence of glucocorticoid receptors in tumor cells. Mediated in part by bcl-2 gene and promotion of apoptotic cell death.

Primary indications

1. Acute and chronic lymphocytic leukemia
2. Hodgkin and non-Hodgkin lymphomas
3. Multiple myeloma
4. Carcinoma of the breast
5. Cerebral edema or spinal cord injury (compression)
6. Nausea and vomiting from chemotherapy.

Usual dosage and schedule

1. Prednisone: dose varies with neoplasm and combination. Typical regimen, except for acute lymphocytic leukemia, is as follows:
   a. 40 mg/m^2 by mouth days 1 to 14 every 4 weeks, *or*
   b. 100 mg/m^2 by mouth days 1 to 5 every 4 weeks.
2. Prednisone: for acute lymphocytic leukemia, 40 to 50 mg/m^2 by mouth daily for 28 days.
3. Dexamethasone: for cerebral edema or spinal cord injury, 10 mg IV push, then 16 to 32 mg by mouth daily in four divided doses. As signs and symptoms are controlled, gradually reduce to lowest effective dose.

Special precautions. Monitor for hyperglycemia.

Toxicity

1. *Myelosuppression and other hematologic effects.* No myelosuppression but may exacerbate hypercoagulability when given together with thalidomide or lenolidamide.
2. *Nausea, vomiting, and other gastrointestinal effects.* No acute nausea and vomiting. Epigastric pain, extreme hunger, and occasional peptic ulceration with bleeding may occur even with short courses. Antacids or inhibitors of acid secretion are recommended as prophylaxis.
3. *Mucocutaneous effects.* Acne; increased risk for oral, rectal, and vaginal yeast infections. Thinning of skin and striae develop with continuous use.
4. *Suppression of adrenal-pituitary axis.* May lead to adrenal insufficiency when corticosteroids are withdrawn. This problem is not common with intermittent schedules.
5. *Metabolic effects.* Potassium depletion, sodium and fluid retention, diabetes, increased appetite, loss of muscle mass, myopathy, weight gain, osteoporosis, and development of Cushingoid features. Their frequency depends on dose and duration of therapy.
6. *Miscellaneous effects:*
   a. CNS effects, including euphoria, depression, and sleeplessness, are common and may progress to dementia or frank psychosis.
   b. Increased susceptibility to infection is common.
   c. Subcapsular cataracts in patients are uncommon but have been seen even when used for prophylaxis and treatment of drug-induced emesis.

CYCLOPHOSPHAMIDE

Other names. CTX, Cytoxan, Neosar.

Mechanism of action. Metabolism of cyclophosphamide by hepatic microsomal enzymes produces active alkylating metabolites. Cyclophosphamide's primary effect is probably on DNA.

Primary indications

1. Breast, lung, ovary, testis, and bladder carcinomas
2. Bone and soft-tissue sarcomas
3. Hodgkin and non-Hodgkin lymphomas
4. Acute and chronic lymphocytic leukemias
5. Waldenström macroglobulinemia
6. Neuroblastoma and Wilms tumor of childhood
7. Gestational trophoblastic neoplasms
8. Multiple myeloma.

Usual dosage and schedule

1. 1000 to 1500 mg/m^2 IV every 3 to 4 weeks, *or*
2. 400 mg/m^2 by mouth days 1 to 5 every 3 to 4 weeks, *or*
3. 60 to 120 mg/m^2 by mouth daily.
4. High-dose regimens (4 to 7 g/m^2 divided over 4 days) are investigational and should only be used with some kind of stem cell rescue (e.g., bone marrow transplantation) and mesna bladder protection.

Special precautions. Give dose in the morning, maintain ample fluid intake, and have patient empty bladder several times daily to diminish the likelihood of cystitis.

Toxicity

1. *Myelosuppression and other hematologic effects.* Dose-limiting. Platelets are relatively spared. Nadir is reached approximately 10 to 14 days after IV dose with recovery by day 21.
2. *Nausea, vomiting, and other gastrointestinal effects.* Frequent with large IV doses; less common after oral doses. Symptoms begin several hours after treatment and are usually over by the next day.
3. *Mucocutaneous effects.* Reversible alopecia is common, usually starting after 2 to 3 weeks. Skin and nails may become darker. Mucositis is uncommon.
4. *Bladder damage.* Hemorrhagic or nonhemorrhagic cystitis may occur in 5% to 10% of patients treated. It is usually reversible with discontinuation of the drug, but it may persist and lead to fibrosis or death. Frequency is diminished by ample fluid intake and morning administration of the drug. Mesna will protect from this effect.
5. *Miscellaneous effects:*
   a. Immunosuppression is common.
   b. Amenorrhea and azoospermia are common.

   c. Inhibition of antidiuretic hormone is only of significance with very large doses.

   d. Interstitial pulmonary fibrosis is rare.

   e. Secondary neoplasia is possible.

   f. Acute and potentially fatal cardiotoxicity occurs with high-dose therapy. Abnormalities include pericardial effusion, congestive heart failure, decreased voltage on electrocardiogram (ECG), and fibrin microthrombi in cardiac capillaries with endothelial injury and hemorrhagic necrosis.

CYTARABINE

Other names. Cytosine arabinoside, ara-C, Cytosar-U, DepoCyt (cytarabine, liposomal for intrathecal use only).

Mechanism of action. A pyrimidine analog antimetabolite that, when phosphorylated to ara-CTP, is a competitive inhibitor of DNA polymerase.

Primary indications

   1. Acute nonlymphocytic leukemia

   2. Meningeal lymphoma or leukemia.

Usual dosage and schedule

   1. Induction: 100 to 200 mg/m^2 IV daily as a continuous infusion for 5 to 7 days (in combination with other drugs).

   2. Maintenance: 100 mg/m^2 SC every 12 hours for 4 or 5 days every 4 weeks (with other drugs).

   3. Intrathecally:

      a. 40 to 50 mg/m^2 of cytarabine, unencapsulated, every 4 days in preservative-free buffered isotonic diluent

      b. 50 mg of cytarabine, liposomal, repeated in 14 to 28 days.

   4. High dose:

      a. Induction: 2 to 3 g/m^2 IV over 1 to 2 hours every 12 hours for up to 12 doses.

      b. Consolidation: 3 g/m^2 IV over 3 hours every 12 hours on days 1, 3, and 5.

Special precautions. None for standard doses. High dose, give in 1- to 3-hour infusion. Longer infusion enhances toxicity. CNS toxicity is increased in patients with a decreased creatinine clearance. Cytarabine (liposomal [DepoCyt]) should be used only intrathecally.

Toxicity (standard dose only).

   1. *Myelosuppression and other hematologic effects.* Dose-limiting leukopenia and thrombocytopenia occur, with nadir at 7 to 10 days after treatment has ended and with recovery during the following 2 weeks, depending on the degree of suppression. Megaloblastosis is common.

   2. *Nausea, vomiting, and other gastrointestinal effects.* Common, particularly if the drug is given as a push or rapid infusion.

   3. *Mucocutaneous effects.* Stomatitis is seen occasionally.
   4. *Miscellaneous effects:*
      a. Flulike syndrome with fever, arthralgia, and sometimes a rash is occasional.
      b. Transient mild hepatic dysfunction is occasional.

Toxicity (high dose).

   1. *Myelosuppression and other hematologic effects.* Universal.
   2. *Nausea, vomiting, and other gastrointestinal effects.* Nausea, vomiting, and diarrhea are common.
   3. *Mucocutaneous effects.* Occasional to common mucositis. Keratoconjunctivitis is common; glucocorticoid eye drops may ameliorate or prevent this effect in some patients.
   4. *Neurotoxicity.* Cerebellar toxicity is common, particularly in the elderly, but is usually mild and reversible. However, on occasion it has been severe and permanent or fatal.
   5. *Hepatic toxicity with cholestatic jaundice.* Uncommon.

DACARBAZINE

Other names. Imidazole carboxamide, DIC, DTIC-Dome.

Mechanism of action. Uncertain but probably interacts with preformed macromolecules by alkylation. Inhibits DNA, RNA, and protein synthesis.

Primary indications

   1. Melanoma
   2. Soft-tissue sarcomas
   3. Hodgkin lymphoma.

Usual dosage and schedule

   1. 150 to 250 mg/m^2 IV push or rapid infusion on days 1 to 5 every 3 to 4 weeks, *or*
   2. 400 to 500 mg/m^2 IV push or rapid infusion on days 1 and 2 every 3 to 4 weeks, *or*
   3. 200 mg/m^2 IV daily as a continuous 96-hour infusion.

Special precautions

   1. Administer cautiously to avoid extravasation as tissue damage may occur.
   2. Venous pain along the injection site may be reduced by diluting dacarbazine in 100 to 200 mL of 5% dextrose in water and infusing over 30 minutes rather than injecting rapidly. Ice application may also reduce pain.

Toxicity

   1. *Myelosuppression and other hematologic effects.* Mild to moderate. This factor allows dacarbazine to be used in full doses with other myelosuppressive drugs.

2. *Nausea, vomiting, and other gastrointestinal effects.* Common and severe but decrease in intensity with each subsequent daily dose. Onset is within 1 to 3 hours, with duration up to 12 hours.
3. *Mucocutaneous effects.* Moderately severe tissue damage if extravasation occurs. Alopecia is uncommon. Erythematous or urticarial rash is uncommon.
4. *Miscellaneous effects:*
   a. Flulike syndrome with fever, myalgia, and malaise lasting several days is uncommon.
   b. Hepatic toxicity is uncommon.

DACTINOMYCIN

Other names. Actinomycin D, ACT-D, Cosmegen.

Mechanism of action. Binds to DNA and inhibits DNA-dependent RNA synthesis. Inhibition of topoisomerase II.

Primary indications

1. Gestational trophoblastic neoplasms
2. Wilms tumor, childhood rhabdomyosarcoma, and Ewing sarcoma.

Usual dosage and schedule

1. Children: 0.40 to 0.45 mg/m^2 (up to a maximum of 0.5 mg) IV daily for 5 days every 3 to 5 weeks
2. Adults:
   a. 0.40 to 0.45 mg/m^2 IV on days 1 to 5 every 2 to 3 weeks
   b. 0.5 mg IV daily for 5 days every 3 to 5 weeks
   c. 0.5 mg IV daily for 2 days every 2 weeks (in combination therapy).

Special precautions

1. Administer by slow IV push through the sidearm of a running IV infusion, being careful to avoid extravasation, which causes severe soft-tissue damage.
2. If given at or about the time of infection with chickenpox or herpes zoster, a severe generalized disease may occur that sometimes results in death.

Toxicity

1. *Myelosuppression and other hematologic effects.* Cytopenias may be dose-limiting and severe. They begin within the first week of treatment, but the nadir may not be reached for 21 days.
2. *Nausea, vomiting, and other gastrointestinal effects.* Severe vomiting often occurs during the first few hours after drug administration and lasts up to 24 hours.
3. *Mucocutaneous effects.* Erythema, hyperpigmentation, and desquamation of the skin with potentiation by previous or concurrent

radiotherapy are common. Oropharyngeal mucositis is potentiated by previous or concurrent radiotherapy. Alopecia is common. Moderately severe tissue damage occurs with extravasation.

4. *Miscellaneous effects:*
   a. Mental depression is rare.
   b. Hepatic veno-occlusive disease, worse with higher doses and shorter schedules (e.g., single dose of 2.5 mg versus 5 days at 0.5 mg/day).

DARBEPOETIN

Other names. Aranesp, darbepoetin alfa.

Mechanism of action. Darbepoetin is an erythropoiesis-stimulating protein, closely related to erythropoietin, that is produced in Chinese hamster ovary cells by recombinant DNA technology. It has the same biologic activity as endogenous erythropoietin, inducing erythropoiesis by stimulating the division and differentiation of committed erythroid progenitor cells.

Primary indications

1. Anemia from concomitant chemotherapy in patients with nonmyeloid malignancies, when cure is not the anticipated outcome
2. Anemia from low-risk MDS
3. Anemia associated with chronic renal failure.

Usual dosage and schedule

1. Patients with anemia during chemotherapy, if the hemoglobin is less than 10 or with low-risk MDS:
   a. 500 μg by SC injection every 3 weeks (schedule used in MDS), *or*
   b. 2.25 μg/kg/week by SC injection.
2. Adult patients with chronic renal failure: Starting dose of 0.45 μg/kg/week by IV or SC injection. Dose adjustments of 2% to 40% upward or downward are recommended to keep the hemoglobin below 12.

Special precautions. There is a greater risk for death, serious cardiovascular events, and stroke when erythropoiesis-stimulating agents (ESAs) are administered to target hemoglobin levels of 13 g/dL and above in chronic renal failure. ESAs shorten survival or increase tumor progression in some studies, and to decrease these risks, as well as the risk of serious cardio- and thrombovascular events, use the lowest dose needed to avoid red blood cell transfusion. Because of these risks, prescribers and hospitals must enroll in and comply with the ESA APPRISE Oncology Program (www.esa-apprise.com) to prescribe and/or dispense ESAs to patients with cancer. Contraindicated in patients with uncontrolled hypertension or known hypersensitivity to albumin or mammalian cell-derived products. Potential for serious allergic or anaphylactic reaction. Rare cases of pure red cell aplasia have been reported.

Toxicity

1. *Myelosuppression and other hematologic effects.* Myelosuppression is not seen, except for rare cases of pure red cell aplasia. Thromboembolic complications are uncommon but serious cardiovascular events and stroke may be seen.
2. *Nausea, vomiting, and other gastrointestinal effects.* Diarrhea is occasional.
3. *Mucocutaneous effects.* Uncommon rashes or urticaria. Pruritis is occasional.
4. *Miscellaneous effects:*
   a. Cardiovascular: Hypertension may occasionally occur in association with a significant increase in hematocrit; the risk is greatest in patients with pre-existing hypertension. Chest pain is uncommon and myocardial infarction is uncommon to rare; edema is occasional.
   b. Neurologic: Seizures, stroke, and transient ischemic attacks are all rare.
   c. Influenza-like syndrome is rare to uncommon. Fever alone is occasional.

DASATINIB

Other name. Sprycel.

Mechanism of action. Inhibition of multiple receptor tyrosine kinases (RTKs), including Bcr-Abl and the SRC family. Believed to bind to multiple conformations of the ABL kinase.

Primary indications

1. CML, chronic phase, newly diagnosed
2. CML in the chronic, accelerated, or blast phase (myeloid or lymphoid) with resistance or intolerance to prior therapy including imatinib
3. ALL that is Ph+ and refractory to prior therapy
4. ALL that is Ph+, newly diagnosed, in combination with chemotherapy (investigational).

Usual dosage and schedule

1. Chronic-phase CML 100 mg by mouth daily. Doses are adjusted up or down in 20 mg increments as needed.
2. Accelerated-phase CML, blast-phase CML, or Ph+ ALL: 140 mg by mouth daily.

Special precautions. Should not be administered to patients who have or are at risk for prolonged QT interval.

Toxicity

1. *Myelosuppression and other hematologic effects.* Neutropenia, thrombocytopenia, and anemia are common in all patients. Bleeding is

common and occasionally is severe, but is seen primarily in the accelerated or blastic phases. Use with caution in patients requiring platelet inhibitors or anticoagulants. Febrile neutropenia is uncommon.

2. *Nausea, vomiting, and other gastrointestinal effects.* Nausea and vomiting are occasional but rarely severe. Diarrhea is common, but severe diarrhea uncommon. Abdominal pain is common. Constipation is occasional.

3. *Mucocutaneous effects.* Stomatitis is occasional. Various skin maladies are occasional.

4. *Miscellaneous effects:*
   a. Cardiovascular: Fluid retention is common and occasionally severe. Pleural effusions are occasional. Pericardial effusions are uncommon. Severe pulmonary edema is rare. Prolonged cardiac ventricular repolarization (QT prolongation) is uncommon and rarely severe.
   b. Respiratory: Dyspnea, cough, and upper respiratory infections are common.
   c. Neurologic: Peripheral neuropathy is occasional. Headache is common.
   d. Musculoskeletal pain and myalagia are occasional to common.
   e. Fever is uncommon; fatigue is common.
   f. Hypophosphatemia is occasional. Hypokalemia and hypocalcemia are uncommon. Abnormal transaminases or elevated bilirubin are rare.

DAUNORUBICIN

Other names. Daunomycin, rubidomycin, DNR, Cerubidine.

Mechanism of action. DNA strand breakage mediated by anthracycline effects on topoisomerase II; DNA intercalation; DNA polymerase inhibition.

Primary indications. AML, ALL.

Usual dosage and schedule

1. 60 to 90 mg/m^2 IV push on days 1, 2, and 3 in combination with other drugs as induction therapy AML. Second cycle may be given at same or lower dose if blasts are not gone by day 15.

2. 45 to 60 mg/m^2 IV push in various schedules in combination with other drugs as induction therapy in ALL.

Special precautions

1. Administer over several minutes into the sidearm of a running IV infusion, taking precautions to avoid extravasation. Severe local tissue damage may progress to skin ulceration, and necrosis may occur with subcutaneous extravasation.

2. Do not give if patient has significantly impaired cardiac function (ejection fraction <45%), angina pectoris, cardiac arrhythmia, or recent myocardial infarction.

3. Do not exceed cumulative dosage of 550 mg/m^2 (400 mg/m^2 if given previous radiation therapy that has encompassed the heart).

4. Reduce dose if patient has impaired liver or renal function.

Serum Bilirubin (mg/dL)	Serum Creatinine (mg/dL)	Percent of Full Dose
1.2–3.0	—	75
>3.0 *or*	>3.0	50

Toxicity

1. *Myelosuppression and other hematologic effects.* Dose-limiting pancytopenia with nadir at 1 to 2 weeks.

2. *Nausea, vomiting, and other gastrointestinal effects.* Nausea and vomiting occur on the day of administration in 50% of patients.

3. *Mucocutaneous effects.* Alopecia is common, but stomatitis is rare. Severe local tissue damage may progress to skin ulceration, and necrosis may occur with subcutaneous extravasation.

4. *Cardiac effects.* Potentially irreversible congestive heart failure may occur owing to cardiomyopathy. The incidence is highly dependent on the lifetime cumulative dose, which should not exceed 550 mg/m^2 (400 mg/m^2 if patient was given previous radiotherapy that encompassed the heart). Discontinue drug if there is clinical congestive heart failure or if the ejection fraction falls on the radionuclide angiogram to:
   a. Less than 45%, *or*
   b. Less than 50% if the total decrease is 10% or more (e.g., falls from 59% to 49%).

   If repeat ejection fraction determination shows return of function, drug may be cautiously restarted, but ejection fraction should be measured before each dose. Transient ECG changes are common and are not usually serious.

5. *Miscellaneous effects:*
   a. Red urine caused by the drug and its metabolites is common.
   b. Chemical phlebitis and phlebothrombosis of veins used for injection is common.

DAUNORUBICIN, LIPOSOMAL

Other name. DaunoXome.

Mechanism of action. Daunorubicin, liposomal, which is designed to be protected from removal by the reticuloendothelial system, has a prolonged circulation time compared with the unprotected drug. The agent penetrates tumor tissue and releases the active ingredient daunorubicin.

Primary indication. Kaposi sarcoma, advanced, HIV-associated.

Usual dosage and schedule. 40 mg/m^2 IV over 60 minutes every 2 weeks.

Special precautions

1. Must be diluted to a concentration of 1 mg/mL with 5% dextrose for injection. Liposomal daunorubicin should be considered an irritant, and care should be taken to avoid extravasation.
2. Do not give if the patient has significantly impaired cardiac function.
3. Do not exceed a lifetime cumulative dose of 550 mg/m^2 (400 mg/m^2 if the patient was given prior chest radiotherapy). Patients with HIV may experience a decrease in left ventricular ejection fraction and congestive heart failure at lower doses than those without.
4. Reduce or hold dose in patients with impairment of liver function. A 25% dose reduction is recommended if the serum bilirubin is 1.2 to 3 mg/dL. One half the normal dose is recommended in patients with serum bilirubin concentration greater than 3 mg/dL.

Toxicity. Effects that are a result of the liposomal daunorubicin have been somewhat difficult to determine with certainty, because most patients have been on several other agents that can result in other drugs that may cause marrow or other toxicity.

1. *Myelosuppression and other hematologic effects.* Common and dose-related. May be severe.
2. *Nausea, vomiting, and other gastrointestinal effects.* Nausea, vomiting, and diarrhea are common.
3. *Mucocutaneous effects.* Alopecia is occasional. Stomatitis is occasional.
4. *Immunologic effects and infusion reactions.* Acute infusion-associated reactions with back pain, flushing, and tightness in the chest and throat, alone or in combination, occur occasionally. They usually occur with the first infusion and are not likely to occur later if the first infusion is given without a reaction. Generally occur during first 5 minutes of the infusion and subside with interruption of the infusion. Some patients tolerate restarting at a lower rate of infusion. Most patients are able to continue therapy.
5. *Miscellaneous effects:*
   a. Cardiac events, including cardiomyopathy or congestive heart failure, may occur and are dose dependent.
   b. Fatigue, fever, and headache are common.
   c. Pain at the injection site is likely after extravasation.
   d. Neuropathy is occasional.

DECITABINE

Other name. Dacogen.

Mechanism of action. Pyrimidine analog that inhibits methyltransferase, causing hypomethylation of DNA and thus, it is believed, results in cellular differentiation or apoptosis. May restore normal function of genes that are critical for the control of cellular differentiation and proliferation.

Primary indications

1. MDSs
2. AML in the elderly.

Usual dosage and schedule

1. MDS:
   a. 20 mg/m^2 IV over 1 hour daily for 5 days every 4 weeks
   b. 15 mg/m^2 CIVI over 3 hours, repeated every 8 hours for 3 days. This cycle is repeated every 6 weeks for a minimum of four cycles (older schedule).

   Therapy may be continued as long as the patient is improved from the drug.
2. AML: 20 mg/m^2 IV on days 1 to 10 of a 4-week cycle for induction. May be repeated if persistent AML. 20 mg/m^2 daily for 3 to 5 days for maintenance.

Toxicity

1. *Myelosuppression and other hematologic effects.* Neutropenia, thrombocytopenia, and anemia are common. Febrile neutropenia is five times as common as in patients receiving supportive care.
2. *Nausea, vomiting, and other gastrointestinal effects.* Nausea, vomiting, and diarrhea or constipation occurs in about one-third of patients. Abdominal pain may be associated.
3. *Mucocutaneous effects.* Stomatitis is occasional. Skin rash and alopecia are occasional. Urticaria is uncommon.
4. *Neurotoxicity.* Insomnia is common. Lethargy or confusional state are occasional.
5. *Miscellaneous effects:*
   a. Cardiovascular: Pulmonary edema is uncommon. Peripheral edema is occasional.
   b. Blurred vision is uncommon.
   c. Fever is common; infections are occasional.
   d. Arthralgias and back pain are occasional.
   e. Hypomagnesemia, hypokalemia, hyperglycemia, hyponatremia, and hypoalbuminemia occur in 20% to 25% of patients.
   f. Abnormal liver function tests are occasional.

DEGARELIX

Other name. Firmagon.

Mechanism of action. Gonadotropin-releasing hormone receptor antagonist that causes a decrease in LH and FSH and subsequently testosterone.

Primary indication. Carcinoma of the prostate.

Usual dosage and schedule. 240 mg as two 120-mg SC injections in the abdominal region, followed by a single injection of 80 mg every 28 days.

Special precautions. May prolong QT interval, as does other androgen depletion.

Toxicity

1. *Myelosuppression and other hematologic effects.* None.
2. *Nausea, vomiting, and other gastrointestinal effects.* Nausea, diarrhea, and constipation are uncommon.
3. *Mucocutaneous effects.* Injection site erythema, swelling, and induration are common.
4. *Miscellaneous effects:*
   a. Weight increase, fatigue, chills, and asthenia are occasional to uncommon.
   b. Hot flushes are common.
   c. Hypertension is occasional.
   d. Musculoskeletal: Occasional arthralgias.
   e. Increase in transaminases is occasional.
   f. Dizziness, headache, and insomnia are uncommon.
   g. Erectile dysfunction, gynecomastia, and testicular atrophy are reported, but the frequency above baseline is not established.

DENILEUKIN DIFTITOX

Other name. Ontak.

Mechanism of action. Denileukin diftitox is produced by genetically fusing protein from the diphtheria toxin to IL-2. This stable, fusion protein targets cells with receptors for IL-2 on their surfaces, including malignant cells and some normal lymphocytes, resulting in cell death. Efficacy in patients without the CD25 receptor is not known.

Primary indication. Persistent or recurrent CTCL that expresses the CD25 component of IL-2 receptor. (Confirm that the patient's malignant cells express CD25 prior to treatment.)

Usual dosage and schedule. 9 or 18 μg/kg/day (350 to 700 mg/m^2/day) IV over 30 to 60 minutes for 5 consecutive days every 21 days for eight cycles.

Special precautions. Acute hypersensitivity reactions occur commonly. Loss of visual acuity, usually with loss of color vision, usually resulting in permanent visual impairment.

Toxicity

1. *Myelosuppression and other hematologic effects.* Anemia and lymphopenia are common. Thrombocytopenia is occasional. Thrombotic events are occasional.
2. *Nausea, vomiting, and other gastrointestinal effects.* Nausea, vomiting, and diarrhea are common. Dehydration as a consequence is occasional.

3. *Mucocutaneous effects.* Rashes, including generalized macropapular, petechial, vesicular bullous, urticarial, and eczematous, may be seen, with both acute and delayed onset.

4. *Immunologic effects and infusion reactions.* Mild infusion reactions are common. Severe acute infusion reactions occur occasionally (8%), including hypotension, back pain, dyspnea, vasodilation, rash, chest pain or tightness, and tachycardia. Syncope is uncommon; anaphylaxis is rare. Fever is common. Neutralizing antibodies develop in most patients by three cycles of treatment.

5. *Miscellaneous effects:*
   a. Cardiovascular effects, including hypotension, vasodilation, fluid retention, and tachycardia, are occasional.
   b. Respiratory reactions of dyspnea, increase in cough, and pharyngitis are occasional.
   c. Capillary leak syndrome is common and is often delayed.
   d. Metabolic changes that include hypoalbuminemia, transaminase increase, and hypocalcemia are common.
   e. Arterial and venous thromboses are uncommon.
   f. Flulike symptoms with chills, fever, headache, and weakness are common. Myalgias and arthralgias are occasional.
   g. Visual changes, including loss of visual acuity, which may be persistent, are uncommon.

DEXRAZOXANE

Other names. Zinecard, ICRF-187.

Mechanism of action. Probably by means of conversion of dexrazoxane intracellularly to a chelating agent that interferes with iron-mediated free radical generation, which is thought to be responsible, in part, for anthracycline-related cardiomyopathy. Appears to protect against myocardial toxicity without impairment of tumor response.

Primary indication. Prophylaxis of cardiomyopathy in patients who have received a cumulative dose of doxorubicin of 300 mg/m^2 or greater and who are believed would benefit from continued therapy with this drug.

Usual dosage and schedule. 10 mg of dexrazoxane for every 1 mg of doxorubicin (e.g, 600 mg/m^2 of dexrazoxane for 60 mg/m^2 of doxorubicin). Repeat whenever doxorubicin is to be repeated. Administered as a slow injection or rapid infusion over 15 to 30 minutes.

Special precautions. None.

Toxicity. Most side effects encountered with dexrazoxane administration are likely to be from the concurrent chemotherapy regimen.

1. *Myelosuppression and other hematologic effects.* Nadir granulocyte and platelet counts lower than with chemotherapy alone, but duration not prolonged.

   2. *Nausea, vomiting, and other gastrointestinal effects.* No increase observed.
   3. *Mucocutaneous effects.* No increase observed.
   4. *Miscellaneous effects:*
       a. Pain at the injection site is occasional.
       b. Hepatic toxicity is possible.

DOCETAXEL

Other name. Taxotere.

Mechanism of action. Enhanced formation and stabilization of microtubules. Antineoplastic effect may result from nonfunctional tubules or altered tubulin–microtubule equilibrium. Mitotic arrest is seen and is associated with accumulated polymerized microtubules.

Primary indications. Carcinomas of the breast, stomach, head and neck, lung, ovary, and prostate.

Usual dosage and schedule. 75 mg/m^2 as a 1-hour infusion every 3 weeks, alone or in combination with other agents. Dose from 60 to 100 mg/m^2 may be used depending on tolerance. Dexamethasone, 8 mg by mouth twice a day for 3 days starting 1 day before docetaxel, should be given before each course of docetaxel to limit the frequency and severity of hypersensitivity reactions and to reduce the severity of fluid retention.

Special precautions. Severe hypersensitivity reactions with flushing and hypotension with or without dyspnea occur in about 1% of patients (even when premedication is used). Should be used with caution in patients with bilirubin above ULN or other abnormal liver function tests ($>$1.5 ULN), because of more profound neutropenia.

Toxicity

   1. *Myelosuppression and other hematologic effects.* Severe (grade 4) neutropenia is common and dose-related. Many patients have neutropenic fever.
   2. *Nausea, vomiting, and other gastrointestinal effects.* Common, but brief; severe episodes are uncommon.
   3. *Mucocutaneous effects.* Mild mucositis is common; severe mucositis is uncommon. Alopecia is common. Mild to moderate cutaneous reactions such as maculopapular eruptions are common; severe reactions that may be associated with desquamation or bullous eruptions occur only occasionally if systemic prophylaxis is used. Mild to moderate nail changes are common, but severe oncholysis is uncommon.
   4. *Immunologic effects and infusion reactions.* Mild to moderate hypersensitivity reactions with flushing, hypotension (or rarely hypertension) with or without dyspnea and drug fever are occasional with use of the prophylactic regimen recommended. Severe hypersensitivity reactions are uncommon.

5. *Miscellaneous effects:*
  a. Fluid retention syndrome is common and cumulative (more commonly after four courses); can be reduced to occasional frequency (6%) by prophylactic steroids; may limit continuing therapy. May be associated with both pleural and pericardial effusions.
  b. Neurologic: Mild and reversible dysesthesias or paresthesias are common; more severe sensory neuropathies are uncommon.
  c. Hepatic: Reversible increases in transaminase, alkaline phosphatase, and bilirubin
  d. Local reactions: Reversible peripheral phlebitis
  e. Mild diarrhea is common; severe diarrhea is rare.
  f. Fatigue, weakness (asthenia), and myalgia are common; arthralgia is occasional.

DOXORUBICIN

Other names. ADR, Adriamycin, Rubex, hydroxyldaunorubicin.

Mechanism of action. DNA strand breakage mediated by anthracycline effects on topoisomerase II; DNA intercalation; DNA polymerase inhibition.

Primary indications

  1. Breast, bladder, liver, lung, prostate, stomach, and thyroid carcinomas
  2. Bone and soft-tissue sarcomas
  3. Hodgkin and non-Hodgkin lymphomas
  4. Multiple myeloma
  5. Wilms tumor, neuroblastoma, and rhabdomyosarcoma of childhood.

Usual dosage and schedule

  1. 60 to 75 mg/m^2 IV every 3 weeks (or as 72- to 96-hour continuous infusion)
  2. 30 mg/m^2 IV on days 1 and 8 every 4 weeks (in combination with other drugs)
  3. 9 mg/m^2 IV daily for 4 days as a continuous infusion (in myeloma)
  4. 15 to 20 mg/m^2 IV weekly
  5. 50 to 60 mg instilled into the bladder weekly for 4 weeks, then every 4 weeks for six cycles.

Special precautions

  1. Administer over several minutes into the sidearm of a running IV infusion (except when given as a continuous infusion), taking care to avoid extravasation.
  2. Do not give if patient has significantly impaired cardiac function (ejection fraction <45%), angina pectoris, cardiac arrhythmia, or recent myocardial infarction.
  3. Do not exceed a lifetime cumulative dose of 550 mg/m^2 (450 mg/m^2 if patient was given prior chest radiotherapy or concomitant cyclophos-

phamide) unless there are known risk modifiers, such as continuous infusion, weekly dosing, or cardioprotective dexrazoxane, and serial measurements of cardiac ejection fraction show minimal change and adequate function.

4. Reduce or hold dose if patient has impaired liver function.
   a. For serum bilirubin of 1.2 to 3.0 mg/dL, give half the normal dose.
   b. For serum bilirubin of more than 3.0 mg/dL, give one-fourth the normal dose.

Toxicity

1. *Myelosuppression and other hematologic effects.* Dose-limiting for most patients. Nadir white blood cell (WBC) and platelet counts occur at 10 to 14 days; recovery by day 21.

2. *Nausea, vomiting, and other gastrointestinal effects.* Mild to moderate in about half of patients.

3. *Mucocutaneous effects.* Stomatitis that is dose-dependent. Alopecia beginning 2 to 5 weeks from start of therapy with recovery following completion of therapy is common. Recall of skin reaction due to prior radiotherapy is common. Severe local tissue damage possibly progressing to skin ulceration and necrosis if subcutaneous extravasation occurs is common. Hyperpigmentation of skin overlying veins used for drug injection in which chemical phlebitis has occurred is common.

4. *Cardiac effects.* Potentially irreversible congestive heart failure may occur owing to cardiomyopathy. The incidence is highly dependent on the lifetime cumulative dose, which should not exceed 550 mg/m². This limit is lower (450 mg/m²) if patient has received prior chest radiotherapy or is taking cyclophosphamide concomitantly. Weekly schedule and 96-hour infusions are less cardiotoxic and higher cumulative doses may be tolerable. Congestive heart failure may be predicted by serial measurement of left ventricular function or endomyocardial biopsy. Discontinue drug if there is clinical congestive heart failure or if the ejection fraction falls on the radionuclide angiogram to:
   a. Less than 45%, *or*
   b. Less than 50% if the total decrease is 10% or more (e.g., falls from 59% to 49%).

   If repeat ejection fraction determination shows return of function, drug may be cautiously restarted, but ejection fraction determination should be done before each dose. Transient ECG changes are common and are not usually serious.

5. *Miscellaneous effects:*
   a. Red urine caused by drug and its metabolites is common.
   b. Chemical phlebitis and phlebosclerosis of veins used for injection are common, particularly if a vein is used repeatedly.
   c. Fever, chills, and urticaria are uncommon.

DOXORUBICIN, LIPOSOMAL

Other name. Doxil.

Mechanism of action. Liposomal doxorubicin, which is designed to be protected from removal by the reticuloendothelial system, has a prolonged circulation time compared with unprotected drug. The agent penetrates tumor tissue and releases the active ingredient doxorubicin.

Primary indications

1. Kaposi sarcoma, advanced, HIV-associated
2. Ovarian and breast carcinomas
3. Multiple myeloma.

Usual dosage and schedule

1. 20 mg/m^2 IV infusion at a rate of 1 mg/min for the first dose, then over 30 minutes for subsequent doses every 3 weeks for Kaposi sarcoma
2. 40 to 50 mg/m^2 IV infusion at a rate of 1 mg/min for the first dose, then over 1 hour every 4 weeks for ovarian or breast carcinoma when used as a single agent
3. 40 mg/m^2 IV infusion at a rate of 1 mg/min for the first dose, then over 1 hour every 4 weeks for multiple myeloma, together with vincristine and dexamethasone
4. 30 mg/m^2 IV infusion on day 1 *or* 4 in combination with bortezomib in relapsed and refractory multiple myeloma.

Special precautions. Must be diluted in 250 mL of 5% dextrose for injection. Liposomal doxorubicin is not a vesicant but should be considered an irritant. Initial doses should be given at a rate of 1 mg/min to avoid infusion reactions.

Toxicity. Effects that are a result of the liposomal doxorubicin have been somewhat difficult to determine with certainty because most patients have been on several other agents that can result in marrow or other toxicity.

1. *Myelosuppression and other hematologic effects.* Common and dose-related. May be severe.
2. *Nausea, vomiting, and other gastrointestinal effects.* Nausea and vomiting are common at the higher doses. Constipation is occasional. Diarrhea is occasional. Anorexia is occasional.
3. *Mucocutaneous effects.* Palmar-plantar erythrodysesthesia is common at the higher doses and is occasionally severe. Stomatitis is common. Alopecia is occasional. Rash is occasional to common.
4. *Immunologic effects and infusion reactions.* Acute infusion-associated reactions with flushing, shortness of breath, facial swelling, headache, chills, back pain, tightness in the chest and throat, or hypotension, alone or in combination, have occurred in approximately 7% of patients treated with liposomal doxorubicin. They usually occur

with the first infusion and are not likely to occur later if the first infusion is given without a reaction. Most resolve over the course of several hours to a day.

5. *Miscellaneous effects:*
   a. Cardiac events, including cardiomyopathy or congestive heart failure, occur in 5% to 10% of patients treated. This is dose-dependent and not really adequately tested with liposomal doxorubicin.
   b. Asthenia is occasional.
   c. Fever is occasional.
   d. Pain at the injection site is likely after extravasation.

EPIRUBICIN

Other names. Ellence, 4′epi-doxorubicin, EPI.

Mechanism of action. DNA-strand breakage, mediated by anthracycline effects on topoisomerase II.

Primary indications

1. Carcinomas of the breast, esophagus, and stomach
2. Hodgkin and non-Hodgkin lymphoma.

Usual dosage and schedule

1. 100 mg/m^2 IV through the sidearm of a freely flowing IV infusion, repeated every 3 weeks administered, *or*
2. 60 mg/m^2 IV on days 1 and 8 repeated every 3 weeks.

Special precautions

1. Take care to avoid extravasation.
2. Do not exceed a lifetime cumulative dose of 900 mg/m^2. (Use a lesser dose for patients with prior chest radiotherapy or prior anthracycline or anthracenedione therapy. 720 mg/m^2 was the maximum cumulative dose in adjuvant studies.)
3. Reduce or hold dose if patient has impaired liver function.
   a. For serum bilirubin of 1.2 to 3.0 mg/dL, give half the normal dose.
   b. For serum bilirubin of more than 3.0 mg/dL, give one-fourth the normal dose.

Toxicity

1. *Myelosuppression and other hematologic effects.* Dose-limiting leukopenia with recovery by day 21.
2. *Nausea, vomiting, and other gastrointestinal effects.* Nausea and vomiting are common. Diarrhea and abdominal pain are occasional.
3. *Mucocutaneous effects:*
   a. Stomatitis that is dose-dependent.
   b. Alopecia beginning approximately 10 days after the first treatment with regrowth when cessation of drug treatment occurs is common but not universal (25% to 50%).

    c. Flushes, skin and nail hyperpigmentation, photosensitivity, and hypersensitivity to irradiated skin (radiation-recall reaction) have been observed.

    d. Severe local-tissue damage possibly progressing to skin ulceration and necrosis if subcutaneous extravasation occurs is common.

4. *Cardiac effects.* Potentially irreversible congestive heart failure may occur owing to cardiomyopathy. The incidence depends on the lifetime dose, which should not exceed 900 mg/m^2. This limit is lower if the patient has received prior chest radiotherapy or prior anthracycline or anthracenedione therapy. Congestive heart failure may be predicted by serial measurement of left ventricular function or endomyocardial biopsy. Transient ECG changes are similar in type and frequency to those observed after doxorubicin.

5. *Miscellaneous effects:*

    a. Red-orange urine for 24 hours after injection owing to drugs and its metabolites is common.

    b. Urticaria and anaphylaxis have been reported in patients treated with epirubicin; signs and symptoms of these reactions may vary from skin rash and pruritus to fever, chills, and shock.

    c. Secondary AML and MDS are rare.

EPOETIN

Other names. Recombinant human erythropoietin (rHuEPO), EPO, epoetin-alfa, Epogen, Procrit.

Mechanism of action. Epoetin-alfa is a recombinant glycoprotein that contains 165 amino acids in a sequence identical to that of endogenous human erythropoietin. It has the same biologic activity, inducing erythropoiesis by stimulating the division and differentiation of committed erythroid progenitor cells.

Primary indications

1. Anemia from concomitant chemotherapy in patients with nonmyeloid malignancies, when cure is not the anticipated outcome

2. Anemia from low-risk MDS

3. Anemia associated with chronic renal failure

4. Anemia associated with zidovudine therapy in HIV-infected patients.

Usual dosage and schedule (in malignancy). 40,000 units SC once weekly. If there is no response after 4 to 8 weeks, the dose may be increased to 60,000 units SC once weekly. If no response to this dose, it should be discontinued.

Special precautions. There is a greater risk for death, serious cardiovascular events, and stroke when ESAs are administered to target hemoglobin levels of 13 g/dL and above in chronic renal failure. ESAs shorten survival or cause increase of tumor progression in some studies, and to decrease these risks, as well as the risk of serious cardio- and thrombovascular events, use the lowest dose needed to avoid red blood cell transfusion. Because of these risks, prescribers and hospitals must enroll in and comply with the ESA APPRISE Oncology Program (www.esa-apprise.com) to prescribe and/or dispense ESAs to patients with cancer. Contraindicated in patients with uncontrolled hypertension or known hypersensitivity to albumin or mammalian cell–derived products. Potential for serious allergic or anaphylactic reaction. Rare cases of pure red cell aplasia have been reported. Iron supplementation is beneficial if there is any question of body iron stores.

Toxicity

1. *Myelosuppression and other hematologic effects.* Myelosuppression is not seen, except for rare cases of pure red cell aplasia. Thromboembolic complications are uncommon but serious cardiovascular events and stroke may be seen.
2. *Nausea, vomiting, and other gastrointestinal effects.* Diarrhea is occasional.
3. *Mucocutaneous effects.* Rare rashes or hives.
4. *Miscellaneous effects:*
   a. Edema is occasional.
   b. A rise in blood pressure occurs in about 25% of patients. Hypertension may rarely occur in association with a significant increase in hematocrit; the risk is greatest in patients with preexisting hypertension.
   c. Chest pain is uncommon.
   d. Edema is occasional.
   e. Seizures are rare.
   f. Influenzalike syndrome is rare to uncommon. Fever alone is occasional.

ERIBULIN MESYLATE

Other name. Halaven.

Mechanism of action. Eribulin is a nontaxane microtubule dynamics inhibitor that is a synthetic analog of halichondrin B, a product isolated from the marine sponge *Halichondria okadai.*

Primary indication. Carcinoma of the breast, metastatic, in patients who have previously received an anthracycline and a taxane (either adjuvant or metastatic) and at least two chemotherapeutic regimens for metastatic disease.

Usual dosage and schedule. 1.4 mg/m^2 IV over 2 to 5 minutes days 1 and 8 of a 21-day cycle.

Special precautions. Reduce dose by 20% to 50% in patients with mild (Child-Pugh class A) to moderate (Child-Pugh class B) hepatic impairment or moderate renal impairment. Monitor for prolonged QT intervals in patients with congestive heart failure, bradyarrhythmias, drugs known to prolong the QT interval, and electrolyte abnormalities. Avoid in patients with congenital long QT syndrome.

Toxicity

1. *Myelosuppression and other hematologic effects.* Neutropenia is common and often (57%) grade 3 or higher but febrile neutropenia is uncommon (4%). Anemia is common but not usually severe.
2. *Nausea, vomiting, and other gastrointestinal effects.* Nausea and anorexia are common, but vomiting is only occasional. Constipation is common. Diarrhea is occasional.
3. *Mucocutaneous effects.* Alopecia is common. Stomatitis or mucosal inflammation is occasional. Rash is occasional. Increased lacrimation is occasional.
4. *Miscellaneous effects:*
   a. Asthenia and fatigue are common and occasionally severe; insomnia and depression are occasional.
   b. Peripheral neuropathy is common and occasionally high grade (8%).
   c. Headache is common; dizziness is occasional.
   d. Myalgias and bone pain are occasional; muscle spasms and weakness are occasional.
   e. Weight loss is common; peripheral edema is occasional.
   f. Cough and dyspnea are occasional.
   g. Hypokalemia is occasional.

ERLOTINIB

Other name. Tarceva.

Mechanism of action. Inhibits intracellular phosphorylation of the tyrosine kinase associated with EGFR.

Primary indications

1. Non–small-cell lung cancer:
   a. Locally advanced after failure of one prior regimen
   b. Maintenance treatment after four cycles of platinum-based chemotherapy.
2. Pancreatic cancer (with gemcitabine).

Usual dosage and schedule. Give at least 1 hour before or 2 hours after food.

1. 150 mg by mouth daily for lung cancer
2. 100 mg daily for pancreatic cancer.

Special precautions. May be associated with interstitial lung disease–like events, manifest by unexplained dyspnea, cough, and fever. If this occurs, erlotinib therapy should be discontinued and management of the pulmonary condition instituted. Gastrointestinal perforation; bullous, blistering, and exfoliative skin conditions, suggestive of toxic epidermal necrolysis; and ocular disorders including corneal perforation or ulceration have been reported.

CYP3A4 inhibitors such as ketoconazole increase erlotinib AUC while inducers such as rifampicin decrease erlotinib AUC, resulting in potential increase in toxicity or reduction in efficacy respectively. Monitor closely for INR elevation in patients taking concomitant warfarin. Give with extreme caution if liver impairment (bilirubin $>3 \times$ ULN); monitor those with less liver impairment closely.

Toxicity

1. *Myelosuppression and other hematologic effects.* Myelosuppression is not an effect of erlotinib. Deep venous thrombosis is uncommon. Unexpected INR elevation may occur in patients taking warfarin. Microangiopathic hemolytic anemia with thrombocytopenia is rare.
2. *Nausea, vomiting, and other gastrointestinal effects.* Anorexia, dyspepsia, nausea, vomiting, diarrhea (second most common reason for dose interruption), constipation, and abdominal pain are common. Transaminase elevations are common and occasionally associated with increased bilirubin, but they are rarely life-threatening.
3. *Mucocutaneous effects.* Rash is common (75%) and the most common reason for dose interruption; stomatitis is occasional to common (17%). Keratoconjunctivitis is occasional.
4. *Miscellaneous effects:*
   a. Systemic: Fatigue, weight loss, and edema are common; fever is common, occasionally with rigors.
   b. Bone pain and myalgia are common.
   c. Dyspnea is common; cough is occasional.
   d. Anxiety, depression, headache, and neuropathy are occasional
   e. Myocardial ischemia or infarction is uncommon
   f. Cerebrovascular accidents are uncommon.

ETOPOSIDE

Other names. Epipodophyllotoxin, VP-16, VP-16-213, VePesid, Etopophos (etoposide phosphate).

Mechanism of action. Interaction with topoisomerase II produces single-strand breaks in DNA. Arrests cells in late S phase or G_2 phase.

Primary indications

1. Small cell anaplastic and non–small-cell lung carcinomas
2. Stomach carcinoma
3. Germ cell cancers
4. Lymphomas
5. Acute leukemia
6. Neuroblastoma.

Usual dosage and schedule

1. 120 mg/m^2 IV on days 1 to 3 every 3 weeks
2. 50 to 100 mg/m^2 IV on days 1 to 5 every 2 to 4 weeks
3. 50 mg/m^2 by mouth (rounded to nearest 50 mg) on days 1 to 5 every 3 weeks
4. 125 to 140 mg/m^2 IV on days 1, 3, and 5 every 3 to 5 weeks
5. High-dose therapy (750 to 2400 mg/m^2) is investigational and should only be used with progenitor cell rescue (e.g., bone marrow or peripheral blood stem cell transplantation).

Special precautions

1. Administer etoposide as a 30- to 60-minute infusion to avoid severe hypotension. Monitor blood pressure during infusion. Etoposide phosphate may be administered as a 5-minute bolus infusion.
2. Take care to avoid extravasation.
3. Etoposide must be diluted in 20 to 50 volumes (100 to 250 mL) of isotonic saline before use. Etoposide phosphate vials (100 mg) may be reconstituted in 5 to 10 mL (water, saline, or dextrose) to a concentration of 10 or 20 mg/mL.
4. Decrease dose by 50% for bilirubin levels of 1.5 to 3 mg/dL; decrease by 75% for bilirubin levels of 3 to 5 mg/dL; discontinue drug if bilirubin level is more than 5 mg/dL.
5. Decrease dose by 25% for creatinine clearance rate of less than 30 mL/min.

Toxicity

1. *Myelosuppression and other hematologic effects.* Dose-limiting leukopenia and less severe thrombocytopenia have a nadir at 16 days with recovery by days 20 to 22.
2. *Nausea, vomiting, and other gastrointestinal effects.* Usually mild to moderate nausea and vomiting in about one-third of patients receiving standard doses; common with high-dose therapy. Anorexia is common. Diarrhea is uncommon.
3. *Mucocutaneous effects:*
   a. Alopecia is common.
   b. Stomatitis is uncommon with standard doses; common with high-dose therapy.
   c. Painful rash may occur with high-dose therapy.
   d. Chemical phlebitis is occasional.
4. *Miscellaneous effects:*
   a. Hepatotoxicity is rare.
   b. Peripheral neurotoxicity is rare.
   c. Allergic reaction is rare.
   d. Hemorrhagic cystitis may occur with high-dose therapy.

EVEROLIMUS

Other name. Afinitor.

Mechanism of action. Everolimus, after complexing with an intracellular protein, FKBP-12, is an inhibitor of the mammalian target of rapamycin (mTOR), a serine threonine kinase, the pathway of which is dysregulated in several human cancers. It also inhibits the expression of hypoxia-inducible factor-1 and the expression of VEGF. Mechanism is similar, if not identical, to temsirolimus.

Primary indication. Advanced renal cell carcinoma.

Usual dosage and schedule

1. 10 mg by mouth once daily
2. Reduce dose to 5 mg by mouth once daily for patients with Child-Pugh class B hepatic impairment or as needed to manage adverse drug reactions.
3. If strong inducers of CYP3A4 are required, increase daily dose in 5 mg increments to a maximum of 20 mg once daily.

Special precautions. Coadministration of everolimus with strong or moderate inhibitors of CYP3A4 or the multidrug efflux pump P-glycoprotein, such as ketoconazole, increases the AUC of everolimus by up to 15-fold and should be avoided. CYP3A4 inducers may decrease everolimus AUC, and increased doses may be required.

Toxicity

1. *Myelosuppression and other hematologic effects.* Anemia and lymphopenia are common and occasionally severe. Thrombocytopenia and neutropenia occur only occasionally and are rarely grade 3 or 4. Hemorrhage is uncommon.
2. *Nausea, vomiting, and other gastrointestinal effects.* Diarrhea, nausea, and vomiting are common but rarely severe. Abdominal pain is occasional.
3. *Mucocutaneous effects.* Mucositis is common (44%), but grade 3 or 4 ulceration is uncommon. Rash is common; pruritis and dry skin are occasional. Hand-foot syndrome is uncommon, as are nail disorders and acneiform dermatitis.
4. *Miscellaneous effects:*
   a. Noninfectious pneumonitis (a class effect of rapamycin derivatives) is occasional, but grade 3 or 4 reaction is uncommon.
   b. Infections, particularly with opportunistic infections, are common and may occasionally be severe.
   c. Metabolic changes: Elevations in lipids, glucose, creatinine, transaminases, and decreased phosphate are common. Except for glucose elevation, which is occasional, severe (grade 3 or 4) abnormalities of the other changes are uncommon to rare.

   d. Asthenia, fatigue, peripheral edema, fever, headache, cough, and dyspnea are common (15% to 30%), but severe episodes are uncommon to rare. Decreased weight is occasional.
   e. Cardiovascular: Hypertension, tachycardia, and chest pain are uncommon, and congestive heart failure is rare.
   f. Nervous system: Insomnia, dizziness, and paresthesias are occasional to uncommon.
   g. Acute renal failure is rare.

EXEMESTANE

Other name. Aromasin.

Mechanism of action. Exemestane is an irreversible, steroidal aromatase inactivator that decreases estrogen biosynthesis by selective inhibition of aromatase (estrogen synthetase) in peripheral tissues.

Primary indications

1. Carcinoma of the breast in postmenopausal women that has progressed following tamoxifen therapy
2. Carcinoma of the breast as adjuvant treatment in postmenopausal women with estrogen-receptor–positive breast cancer.

Usual dosage and schedule. 25 mg by mouth once daily after meal.

Special precautions. Potential hazard to fetus if given during pregnancy.

Toxicity

1. *Myelosuppression and other hematologic effects.* No dose-related effect. Thromboembolic events are uncommon to rare.
2. *Nausea, vomiting, and other gastrointestinal effects.* Nausea, vomiting, constipation, and diarrhea are uncommon to occasional.
3. *Mucocutaneous effects.* Rash is uncommon.
4. *Miscellaneous effects:*
   a. Fatigue is occasional.
   b. Musculoskeletal pain (arthralgia or bone) is occasional to common.
   c. Headache is occasional.
   d. Peripheral edema and weight gain are occasional (lower than with megestrol).
   e. Dyspnea and cough are uncommon to occasional.
   f. Hot flushes are occasional.
   g. Decreased bone mineral density with osteoporosis is occasional and there is increased risk for fractures.
   h. Hypertension is occasional.

FILGRASTIM

Other names. Granulocyte colony-stimulating factor (G-CSF), Neupogen.

Mechanism of action. Promotes growth and differentiation of myeloid progenitor cells. May improve survival and function of granulocytes.

Primary indications

1. Prophylaxis of granulocytopenia secondary to intensive chemotherapy with febrile neutropenia rate of greater than 20% or in patients with previous episode of febrile neutropenia.
2. Treatment of granulocytopenia secondary to chemotherapy.
3. Granulocytopenia from primary marrow disorders, such as idiopathic neutropenia and aplastic anemia, and MDS.
4. Granulocytopenia associated with AIDS and its therapy.

Usual dosage and schedule

1. Adjunct to chemotherapy: commonly 200 to 400 $\mu g/m^2$ (5 to 10 $\mu g/kg$) SC daily, starting no sooner than 24 hours and no later than 4 days after the last dose of chemotherapy, for 10 to 20 days until the neutrophil count exceeds 10,000/μL after the expected nadir. Because of cost factors, vial size, and comparability of effect with "ballpark" doses, some physicians choose to treat patients weighing less than 75 kg with 300 μg daily and patients weighing more than 75 kg with 480 μg daily.
2. Other purposes: 40 to 500 $\mu g/m^2$ SC, IM, or IV daily. Dose and duration are dependent on the purpose of administration.

Special precautions. Use with caution in disorders of myeloid stem cells, as it may promote growth of leukemic cells.

Toxicity

1. *Myelosuppression and other hematologic effects.* None (leukocytosis).
2. *Nausea, vomiting, and other gastrointestinal effects.* Rare.
3. *Mucocutaneous effects.* Exacerbation of pre-existing dermatologic conditions are occasional; pyoderma gangrenosum is rare.
4. *Miscellaneous effects:*
   a. Bone pain, musculoskeletal symptoms such as cramps, and back or leg pain are common but are usually mild and short-lived.
   b. Splenomegaly occurs with prolonged use.
   c. Exacerbation of pre-existing inflammatory or autoimmune disorders is rare.
   d. Mild elevation of LDH and alkaline phosphatase.

FLAVOPIRIDOL

Other name. Alvocidib.

Mechanism of action. Cyclin-dependent kinase inhibitor that induces apoptosis. Also induces apoptosis independent of p53.

Primary indication. CLL with high-risk genetic features, including del(17p13.1) and del(11q22.3), that has previously been treated.

Usual dosage and schedule. 30 mg/m^2 by 30-minute IV bolus infusion followed by 30 mg/m^2 as a CIVI for dose 1. The CIVI dose could be escalated to 50 mg/m^2 if dose 1 was tolerated well without tumor lysis syndrome. Treatments are repeated days 1, 8, and 15 every 28 days.

Special precautions. Tumor lysis syndrome occurs commonly during the first and second cycles of treatment. Rasburicase, 2 hours before the first and second doses of flavopiridol, should be considered and plans made for urgent dialysis if needed. Treatment requires prophylactic dexamethasone 20 mg IV on each treatment day to modify the cytokine release syndrome, allopurinol daily, and valcyclovir 100 mg daily for the duration of the treatment. Prophylactic pegfilgrastim should be given on day 16 of each cycle, and ciprofloxacin 500 mg twice a day for the duration of the flavopiridol therapy. Pneumocystis pneumonia prophylaxis is frequently used.

Toxicity

1. *Myelosuppression and other hematologic effects.* Neutropenia is universal and commonly grade 3 to 4. Anemia and thrombocytopenia are common and only occasionally severe.
2. *Nausea, vomiting, and other gastrointestinal effects.* Nausea and vomiting are common and only occasionally severe. Diarrhea is universal and commonly severe. Anorexia is common.
3. *Mucocutaneous effects.* Not reported.
4. *Immunologic effects and infusion reactions.* Cytokine release syndrome is common; clinical tumor lysis syndrome is common (20% to 25%) and may be severe.
5. *Miscellaneous effects:*
   a. Infection is common and severe in about 25% of patients.
   b. Fatigue is universal.
   c. Anxiety and depression are occasional.
   d. Transaminase elevations are universal and commonly are grade 3 to 4. Bilirubin elevations are common, but grade 3 to 4 is uncommon.

FLUDARABINE

Other names. FAMP, Fludara, Oforta.

Mechanism of action. A purine analog that causes inhibition of DNA polymerase alpha, ribonucleotide reductase, and DNA primase, thus inhibiting DNA synthesis.

Primary indications

1. CLL (B-cell)
2. Macroglobulinemia
3. Indolent lymphomas
4. Acute leukemia (in combination).

Usual dosage and schedule

1. 25 mg/m^2 IV as a 30-minute infusion daily for 5 days (Fludara). Other dose schedules, usually less intensive, have been used, often in combinations with other drugs. Repeat every 4 weeks.
2. 40 mg/m^2 by mouth daily for 5 days. Repeat every 4 weeks (Oforta).

Special precautions. If there is the potential for tumor lysis syndrome, administer allopurinol and ensure good hydration and close clinical monitoring. Transfusion-associated graft-versus-host disease may be seen. Therefore, prior irradiation of blood products for transfusion in patients at risk is recommended. Fatal cases of autoimmune hemolytic anemia have been reported, and patients should be closely monitored for hemolysis, particularly if there is a prior history of autoimmune hemolysis or immune thrombocytopenia related to the chronic lymphocytic leukemia. Not recommended for use in combination with pentostatin because of high incidence of pulmonary toxicity. Adult patients with moderate impairment of renal function (creatinine clearance 30 to 70 mL/min/1.73 m^2 should have a 20% dose reduction of fludarabine). It should not be given to patients with severely impaired renal function (creatinine clearance less than 30 mL/min/1.73 m^2).

Toxicity

1. *Myelosuppression and other hematologic effects.* Granulocytopenia and thrombocytopenia are common but appear to become less common in patients whose disease is responding. May progress to trilineage marrow hypoplasia. Infection, particularly pneumonia, is common during early courses and uncommon after the sixth course. Autoimmune hemolytic anemia and immune thrombocytopenia have been observed (probably rare).
2. *Nausea, vomiting, and other gastrointestinal effects.* Nausea is occasional to common but not usually severe. Diarrhea is occasional.
3. *Mucocutaneous effects.* Occasional mucositis and rash; no alopecia.
4. *Neurotoxicity.* Uncommon at usual dosage. Somnolence or fatigue, paresthesias, and twitching of extremities may be seen. Severe neurologic symptoms, including visual disturbances, have been common at higher doses than those recommended.
5. *Immune suppression.* Common. Usually seen as a depression in CD4 and CD8 lymphocyte counts. Opportunistic infections may result, and many recommend *Pneumocystis* pneumonia prophylaxis with trimethoprim-sulfamethoxazole until the CD4 lymphopenia resolves.
6. *Miscellaneous effects:*
   a. Abnormal liver or renal function is rare.
   b. Cough, dyspnea, are upper respiratory infections are occasional.
   c. Fever, infection, diaphoresis, are headache are occasional.
   d. Allergic pneumonitis is occasional to uncommon.
   e. Edema is occasional.
   f. Tumor lysis syndrome is uncommon.

FLUOROURACIL

Other names. 5-FU, Adrucil, Efudex, Fluoroplex, 5-fluorouracil.

Mechanism of action. A pyrimidine antimetabolite that, when converted to the active nucleotide, inhibits the enzyme thymidylate synthetase and thereby blocks DNA synthesis.

Primary indications

1. Breast, colorectal, anal, stomach, pancreas, esophagus, liver, head and neck, and bladder carcinomas
2. Actinic keratosis; basal and squamous cell carcinomas of skin (topically).

Usual dosage and schedule

1. Systemic options (alternatives). Other schedules when in combinations.
   a. 500 mg/m^2 IV on days 1 to 5 every 4 weeks
   b. 450 to 600 mg/m^2 IV weekly
   c. 200 to 400 mg/m^2 daily as a CIVI
   d. 1000 mg/m^2 daily for 4 days as a CIVI every 3 to 4 weeks
   e. Leucovorin 20 mg/m^2 IV is followed by fluorouracil 425 mg/m^2 IV. The combination is given daily for 5 days. Courses are repeated every 4 weeks.
2. Intracavitary: 500 to 1000 mg for pericardial effusion; 2000 to 3000 mg for pleural or peritoneal effusions
3. Topically: Apply solution or cream twice daily. Use only 5% strength for carcinomas.

Special precautions

1. Reduce the dose in patients with compromised liver function.
2. Precipitation may occur if leucovorin and fluorouracil are mixed in the same bag.

Toxicity

1. *Myelosuppression and other hematologic effects.* Dose-limiting with a nadir at 10 to 14 days after the last dose and recovery by 21 days.
2. *Nausea, vomiting, and other gastrointestinal effects.* Nausea and vomiting may occur but are not usually severe. Diarrhea is common with higher doses, continuous infusion, or when used in combination with leucovorin and irinotecan. Esophagitis and proctitis may also occur.
3. *Mucocutaneous effects:*
   a. Stomatitis is an early sign of severe toxicity. It progresses from soreness and erythema to frank ulceration, which becomes hemorrhagic in a small number of patients.
   b. Partial alopecia is uncommon.
   c. Hyperpigmentation of skin over face, hands, and the veins used for infusion is occasional.
   d. Maculopapular rash is uncommon.
   e. Sun exposure tends to increase skin reactions.
   f. Hand-foot syndrome with painful, erythematous desquamation and fissures of palms and soles is common with continuous infusion and occasional with other schedules or combinations.

4. *Miscellaneous effects:*
   a. Neurotoxicity, including headache, minor visual disturbances, and cerebellar ataxia, is rare.
   b. Increased lacrimation is uncommon.
   c. Cardiac toxicity, including arrhythmias, angina, ischemia, and sudden death, is rare. May be more common with continuous infusion and previous history of coronary artery disease.

FLUTAMIDE

Other name. Eulexin.

Mechanism of action. Competitive inhibitor of androgens at the cellular androgen receptor in prostate cancer cells.

Primary indication. Carcinoma of the prostate, most often in combination with LHRH agonists.

Usual dosage and schedule. 250 mg by mouth every 8 hours.

Special precautions. Serum transaminase levels should be measured prior to starting treatment with flutamide. Flutamide is not recommended in patients whose serum transaminase values exceed twice the ULN.

Toxicity

1. *Myelosuppression and other hematologic effects.* None.
2. *Nausea, vomiting, and other gastrointestinal effects.* Nausea and vomiting are uncommon to occasional. Diarrhea, flatulence, and mild abdominal pain are occasional.
3. *Mucocutaneous effects.* Mild skin rash is occasional.
4. *Miscellaneous effects:*
   a. Secondary pharmacologic effects, including breast tenderness, breast swelling, hot flashes, impotence, and loss of libido, are common but reversible after cessation of therapy.
   b. Elevated liver function tests are uncommon; liver failure is rare but may be preceded by flulike symptoms or right upper quadrant pain and tenderness.
   c. Hypertension is occasional.
   d. Adverse cardiovascular events are similar to those seen with orchiectomy.

FULVESTRANT

Other name. Faslodex.

Mechanism of action. An estrogen receptor antagonist that binds to the estrogen receptor in a competitive manner. It downregulates the estrogen receptor protein in human breast cancer cells. In vitro, there is reversible inhibition in the growth of tamoxifen-resistant as well as estrogen-sensitive human breast cancer cell lines.

Primary indications

1. Hormone receptor–positive metastatic breast cancer in postmenopausal women with disease progression following antiestrogen therapy. (There are no efficacy data for premenopausal women with advanced breast cancer.)
2. Hormone receptor–positive metastatic breast cancer in postmenopausal women with disease progression following therapy with a third generation aromatase inhibitor.

Usual dosage and schedule

1. 500 mg IM over 1 to 2 minutes as two concurrent 5-mL injections (50 mg/mL) into each buttock, repeated once monthly after loading on days 1, 15, and 29.
2. Reduce dose to 250 mg in patients with moderate hepatic impairment (Child-Pugh class B), using the same schedule as previously discussed.

Special precautions. Safety has not been evaluated in patients with severe hepatic impairment.

Toxicity

1. *Myelosuppression and other hematologic effects.* Anemia is rare.
2. *Nausea, vomiting, and other gastrointestinal effects.* Nausea is common; vomiting, constipation, diarrhea, and anorexia are occasional.
3. *Mucocutaneous effects.* Rash and increased sweating are occasional.
4. *Miscellaneous effects:*
   a. For the body as a whole, headache, back pain, abdominal pain, injection site pain, and pelvic pain are occasional. Occasional patients also experience a flulike syndrome or fever.
   b. Vasodilation and edema are occasional.
   c. Dizziness, insomnia, paresthesias, depression, and anxiety are uncommon to occasional.
   d. Pharyngitis, dyspnea, and increased cough are occasional.

GEFITINIB

Other names. Iressa, ZD1839.

Mechanism of action. Selectively inhibits tyrosine kinase activity of the EGFR. EGFR tyrosine kinase inhibition by gefitinib impairs epidermal growth factor–stimulated autophosphorylation and thus blocks growth signals within the cell.

Primary indication. Carcinoma of the lung as monotherapy for the continued treatment of patients with locally advanced or metastatic non–small-cell lung cancer after failure of both platinum-based and docetaxel chemotherapies who are benefiting or have benefited from its use.

Usual dosage and schedule. 250 mg daily (may require interruption for diarrhea or skin reactions).

Special precautions. Diarrhea may be dose-limiting and require discontinuation of the drug.

Toxicity

1. *Myelosuppression and other hematologic effects.* Uncommon, except for anemia, which is occasional and not dose-related.
2. *Nausea, vomiting, and other gastrointestinal effects.* Nausea, vomiting, and diarrhea are common. Diarrhea may be dose-limiting. Anorexia, constipation, and abdominal pain are also common but usually not severe.
3. *Mucocutaneous effects.* Acnelike or folliculitis-type rash is common, usually appearing by day 14; frequency and severity are dose-related. May be associated with dry skin and itching. Rash usually does not worsen with continued treatment and resolves within a week of discontinuation of the drug. Dry mouth and conjunctivitis are occasional.
4. *Miscellaneous effects:*
   a. Dyspnea is occasional to common.
   b. Asthenia is common.
   c. Headache is occasional.
   d. Somnolence is occasional.
   e. Elevated hepatic transaminases are occasional but may be severe (grade 3 or 4).

GEMCITABINE

Other name. Gemzar.

Mechanism of action. After being metabolized intracellularly to the active diphosphate and triphosphate nucleotides, gemcitabine, a cytidine analog, inhibits ribonucleotide reductase and competes with deoxycytidine triphosphate for incorporation into DNA.

Primary indications

1. Carcinoma of the pancreas, locally advanced or metastatic
2. Non–small-cell carcinomas of the lung
3. Carcinomas of the breast, biliary tract, bladder, and ovary
4. Non-Hodgkin lymphoma
5. Soft-tissue sarcoma.

Usual dosage and schedule

1. 1000 mg/m^2 IV over 30 minutes once weekly for up to 7 weeks when used as a single agent. After 1 week of rest, subsequent cycles are given once weekly for 3 consecutive weeks out of 4.
2. 1000 to 1250 mg/m^2 IV over 30 minutes once weekly for 2 or 3 successive weeks during each 3- or 4-week cycle, when used in combination regimens.

Special precautions. Prolongation of infusion time beyond 60 minutes increases toxicity.

Toxicity

1. *Myelosuppression and other hematologic effects.* Dose-related and common. Overt hemolytic-uremic syndrome is rare, but milder cases with renal insufficiency may be more common.
2. *Nausea, vomiting, and other gastrointestinal effects.* Nausea and vomiting are common, but only occasionally severe. Diarrhea and constipation are occasional to common.
3. *Mucocutaneous effects.* Rash, alopecia, and mucositis are occasional.
4. *Miscellaneous effects:*
   a. Transient elevations of serum transaminases and alkaline phosphatase are common. Serious hepatotoxicity is rare.
   b. Mild proteinuria and hematuria are common.
   c. Fever without documented infection is common.
   d. Neurotoxicity: Mild paresthesias are occasional.
   e. Dyspnea is occasional.

GEMTUZUMAB OZOGAMICIN

Other name. Mylotarg.

Mechanism of action. Gemtuzumab ozogamicin is a humanized recombinant monoclonal antibody against the CD33 antigen that is conjugated with the cytotoxic antitumor antibiotic calicheamicin. Once bound to the CD33 antigen, the agent is internalized, calicheamicin is released, and its reactive intermediate binds to DNA and causes DNA double-strand breaks and cell death.

Primary indication. Patients with CD33-positive AML who are older than 60 years and are not considered candidates for other cytotoxic chemotherapy.

Usual dosage and schedule

1. 9 mg/m^2 as a 2-hour IV infusion on days 1 and 15
2. In combination therapy, 6 mg/m^2 as a 2-hour infusion for induction and 3 mg/m^2 for maintenance.

Special precautions

1. Infusion-related events may include fever, nausea, chills, hypotension, shortness of breath, and anaphylaxis. Pretreatment with acetaminophen and diphenhydramine should be given prior to treatment to lessen these effects, and prior methylprednisolone may also be of benefit.
2. If dyspnea or significant hypotension occurs, the infusion should be interrupted. Anaphylaxis, pulmonary edema, and acute respiratory distress syndrome usually necessitate discontinuation of therapy.
3. Hepatotoxicity, including veno-occlusive disease may occur, even in patients without a history of liver disease or hematopoietic stem cell transplant.

    4. Tumor lysis syndrome may occur, particularly when the WBC count is higher than $30,000/\mu L$.

Toxicity

1. *Myelosuppression and other hematologic effects.* Severe to life-threatening granulocytopenia and thrombocytopenia are universal. Severe or worse anemia is common.
2. *Nausea, vomiting, and other gastrointestinal effects.* Anorexia, nausea, vomiting, abdominal pain, and diarrhea are common but only occasionally severe.
3. *Mucocutaneous effects.* Rash, local reaction, petechiae, stomatitis, pharyngitis, and rhinitis are occasional to common. Herpes simplex is common. Alopecia is not seen.
4. *Immunologic effects and infusion reactions.* Chills, fever, headache, nausea, and vomiting are common but usually resolve within 4 hours of end of infusion. Fewer after second dose.
5. *Miscellaneous effects:*
   a. Hyperglycemia and dyspnea are occasional. Hypoxia is uncommon (about 5%).
   b. Increased cough, dyspnea, and epistaxis are common. Severe dyspnea or pneumonia is occasional. Pleural effusions, noncardiogenic pulmonary edema, and acute respiratory distress syndrome are rare.
   c. Severe or life-threatening infections are common. These include sepsis, pneumonia, and opportunistic infections.
   d. Hypertension, hypotension, and tachycardia are occasional.
   e. Reversible abnormalities in liver function are common and occasionally severe or life-threatening. Fatal liver abnormalities including veno-occlusive disease are rare. Findings that may indicate severe hepatotoxicity include rapid weight gain, right upper quadrant pain, hepatomegaly, ascites, and elevations in liver function tests.

GONADOTROPIN-RELEASING HORMONE ANALOGS

Other names. LHRH analogs, Leuprolide (Lupron, Lupron depot, Viadur), goserelin (Zoladex depot), triptorelin pamoate (Trelstar depot).

Mechanism of action. Initial release of FSH and LH from the anterior pituitary, followed by diminution of gonadotropin secretion owing to desensitization of the pituitary to gonadotropin-releasing hormone (GnRH) and consequent decrease in the respective gonadal hormones. May also have direct effects on cancer cells, at least in cancer of the breast, in which GnRH-binding sites have been demonstrated.

Primary indications

1. Metastatic prostate carcinoma
2. Breast carcinoma in premenopausal and perimenopausal women with metastatic disease (goserelin).

Usual dosage and schedule

1. Leuprolide depot 7.5 mg IM monthly, 22.5 mg IM every 3 months, or 30 mg IM every 4 months
2. Goserelin depot 3.6 mg SC every 4 weeks or 10.8 mg SC every 12 weeks. Use only 3.6 mg implant for breast carcinoma.
3. Triptorelin depot 3.75 mg IM monthly; triptorelin depot 22.5 mg IM every 6 months.

Special precautions. Worsening of symptoms may occur during the first few weeks.

Toxicity

1. *Myelosuppression and other hematologic effects.* Rare, if at all.
2. *Nausea, vomiting, and other gastrointestinal effects.* Anorexia, nausea, vomiting, and constipation are uncommon.
3. *Mucocutaneous effects.* Erythema and ecchymosis at the injection site, rash, hair loss, and itching are uncommon.
4. *Cardiovascular effects.* Congestive heart failure, hypertension, and thrombotic episodes are uncommon. Peripheral edema is occasional.
5. *Miscellaneous effects:*
   a. CNS: Dizziness, pain, headache, and paresthesias are uncommon.
   b. Endocrine: Hot flashes are common; decreased libido is common; gynecomastia with or without tenderness is uncommon; impotence is occasional to common.
   c. Bone pain, or "flare," is common on initiation of therapy in patients with bony metastasis. This can be minimized by pretreating with flutamide or another androgen antagonist in men with prostate cancer.
   d. Hypersensitivity reactions with rare angioneurotic edema and anaphylaxis have been reported.

HYDROXYUREA

Other names. Hydroxycarbamide, Hydrea, Droxia.

Mechanism of action. Interferes with DNA synthesis, at least in part by inhibiting the enzymatic conversion of ribonucleotides to deoxyribonucleotides.

Primary indications

1. Head and neck carcinomas
2. CML; ALL and acute nonlymphocytic leukemia with high blast counts
3. Essential thrombocythemia
4. Polycythemia rubra vera
5. Prevention of retinoic acid syndrome in acute promyelocytic leukemia
6. Sickle cell anemia with frequent painful crises.

Usual dosage and schedule

1. 800 to 2000 mg/m^2 by mouth as a single or divided daily dose. Dose is adjusted up or down, depending on efficacy and tolerability.
2. 3200 mg/m^2 by mouth as a single dose every third day (not for leukemias).
3. Starting dose in sickle cell anemia is 15 mg/kg/day, with increments of 5 mg/kg every 12 weeks, as long as ANC is greater than 2000 cells/μL and platelets are greater than 80,000/μL.

Special precautions. The daily dose must be adjusted for blood count trends. Be careful not to change dose too often, because there is a delay in response. Severe cutaneous vasculitic toxicities, including ulcers and gangrene, have been seen, particularly in association with current or prior interferon therapy. Toxic reactions may be greater in patients with impaired renal function, such as may be seen in elderly patients. Reduce doses by 50% if creatinine clearance less than 60.

Toxicity

1. *Myelosuppression and other hematologic effects.* Occurs at doses of more than 1600 mg/m^2 daily by day 10. Recovery is usually prompt. Increased red cell mean corpuscular volume is common.
2. *Nausea, vomiting, and other gastrointestinal effects.* Nausea is common at high doses. Other gastrointestinal symptoms are uncommon. Pancreatitis may be seen in patients with HIV disease being treated with didanosine and other antiviral agents.
3. *Mucocutaneous effects.* Stomatitis is rare. Maculopapular rash may be seen. Inflammation of mucous membranes caused by radiation may be exaggerated.
4. *Miscellaneous effects:*
   a. Temporary renal function impairment or dysuria is uncommon.
   b. CNS disturbances are rare.
   c. May be leukemogenic or teratogenic.

IBRITUMOMAB TIUXETAN

Other names. Zevalin, IDEC-Y2B8.

Mechanism of action. Ibritumomab is a murine monoclonal anti-CD20 antibody conjugated to tiuxetan that chelates to the pure beta-emitting yttrium-90 (90Y). The mechanism of action includes antibody-mediated cytotoxicity and cellularly targeted radiotherapy (radioimmunotherapy).

Primary indications

1. Non-Hodgkin lymphoma, low-grade or follicular B-cell, CD20-positive, rituximab refractory
2. Previously untreated patients with follicular non-Hodgkin lymphoma who achieve a partial or complete response to first-line chemotherapy.

Usual dosage and schedule

Day 1: Administer rituximab 250 mg/m^2 by IV infusion. Within 4 hours after rituximab infusion, administer 5 mCi indium-111 Zevalin IV. Assess biodistribution by radionuclide scan 48 to 72 hours after In-111 Zevalin. Only if biodistribution is acceptable, proceed to day 7 (or 8 or 9).

Day 7, 8, or 9: Administer rituximab 250 mg/m^2 by IV infusion.

1. If platelets are at least 150,000/mm^4: Within 4 hours after rituximab infusion, administer 0.4 mCi/kg (14.8 MBq per kg) 90Y Zevalin IV. Maximum allowable dose of 90Y Zevalin is 32 mCi.
2. If platelets are at least 100,000 but no more than 149,000/mm^3 in relapsed or refractory patients: Within 4 hours after rituximab infusion, administer 0.3 mCi/kg (11.1 MBq per kg) 90Y Zevalin IV.
3. Do not treat if platelets are less than 100,000.

Special precautions. Use with caution in patients with at least 25% marrow involvement with lymphoma, prior external beam radiotherapy to at least 25% of the bone marrow, or a history of human antimouse antibodies (HAMAs) or HACAs. Because the drug does not emit gamma radiation, hospitalization is not required.

Toxicity

1. *Myelosuppression and other hematologic effects.* Neutropenia, lymphopenia, anemia, and thrombocytopenia are common and related to the radionuclide dose. At the higher end of the dosing, 25% will develop nadir neutrophil counts of less than 500/µL. Cytopenias are prolonged in most patients.
2. *Nausea, vomiting, and other gastrointestinal effects.* Low-grade nausea and vomiting are common. Diarrhea is occasional.
3. *Mucocutaneous effects.* Severe cutaneous and mucocutaneous reactions, some fatal, can occur but are rare. Urticaria and pruritis are occasional.
4. *Immunologic effects and infusion reactions.* Infusion-related fever, chills, dizziness, asthenia, headache, back pain, arthralgia, and hypotension are occasional and may be severe. HAMA or HACA may develop.
5. *Miscellaneous effects:* Leukemia and MDS have been seen in 1% to 5% of patients treated.

IDARUBICIN

Other names. 4-Demethoxydaunorubicin, IDA, Idamycin.

Mechanism of action. DNA-strand breakage mediated by anthracycline effects on topoisomerase II or free radicals; DNA intercalation; DNA polymerase inhibition.

Primary indications

1. Acute nonlymphocytic leukemia

2. Blast crisis of CML
3. ALL.

Usual dosage and schedule. 12 to 13 mg/m² IV daily for 3 days (usually in a combination with cytarabine) during induction; 10 to 12 mg/m² IV daily for 2 days during consolidation.

Special precautions. Administer over several minutes into the sidearm of a running IV infusion, taking care to avoid extravasation. Cardiac toxicity may be less than that with daunorubicin. Maximum dose not yet established. Cumulative doses greater than 150 mg/m² have been associated with decreased cardiac ejection fraction.

Toxicity

1. *Myelosuppression and other hematologic effects.* Universal and dose-limiting.
2. *Nausea, vomiting, and other gastrointestinal effects.* Nausea, vomiting, and anorexia are common. Diarrhea is occasional to common.
3. *Mucocutaneous effects.* Alopecia is common; mucositis is common but usually not severe.
4. *Miscellaneous effects:*
   a. Hepatic dysfunction is common but usually not severe and not clearly due to the idarubicin.
   b. Renal effects are common but usually not clinically significant.
   c. Cardiac effects are uncommon during induction and consolidation (1% to 5%).
   d. Tissue damage is probable if infiltration occurs.
   e. Neurologic effects are occasional.

IFOSFAMIDE

Other name. Ifex.

Mechanism of action. Metabolic activation by microsomal liver enzymes produces biologically active intermediates that attack nucleophilic sites, particularly on DNA.

Primary indications

1. Testicular and lung cancers
2. Bone and soft-tissue sarcomas
3. Lymphoma.

Usual dosage and schedule

1. 1.2 g/m² IV over 30 minutes or more daily for 5 consecutive days every 3 or 4 weeks, usually with other agents. Mesna 120 mg/m² is given just before ifosfamide, then mesna 1200 mg/m² as a daily continuous infusion is given until 16 hours after the last dose of ifosfamide.

2. 3.6 g/m^2 IV daily as a 4-hour infusion for 2 consecutive days, usually with other agents. Mesna is given at a dose of 750 mg/m^2 IV just prior to and at 4 and 8 hours after the start of the ifosfamide.

Higher dosage schedules have been used experimentally with up to 14 g/m^2 being used per course over a 6-day period, with equal or greater doses of mesna.

Special precautions. Must be used with mesna to prevent hemorrhagic cystitis. Mesna dose is at least 20% of the ifosfamide dose (on a weight basis), administered just prior to (or mixed with) the ifosfamide dose and again at 4 and 8 hours after the ifosfamide to detoxify the urinary metabolites that cause the hemorrhagic cystitis. Higher doses of ifosfamide may require higher doses and longer durations of mesna. Neither mesna nor its only metabolite, mesna disulfide, affect ifosfamide or its antineoplastic metabolites. Mesna disulfide is reduced in the kidney to a free thiol compound, which then reacts chemically with urotoxic metabolites, resulting in their detoxification. Vigorous hydration is also required with a minimum of 2 L of oral or IV hydration daily. Administer as a slow IV infusion over a period of at least 30 minutes.

Toxicity

1. *Myelosuppression and other hematologic effects.* Myelosuppression is dose-limiting. Platelets are relatively spared. Granulocyte nadirs are commonly reached at 10 to 14 days, and recovery is seen by day 21. Thrombocytopenia may be seen with higher doses.
2. *Nausea, vomiting, and other gastrointestinal effects.* Nausea and vomiting are common without standard antiemetics.
3. *Mucocutaneous effects.* Alopecia is common; mucositis is rarely seen at standard doses; dermatitis is rare.
4. *Hemorrhagic cystitis.* Common and dose-limiting unless a uroprotective agent such as mesna is used. With mesna, the incidence of hemorrhagic cystitis is 5% to 10%, and gross hematuria is uncommon. Increasing the duration of mesna may alleviate the problem during subsequent cycles.
5. *Miscellaneous effects:*
   a. CNS toxicity (somnolence, confusion, depressive psychosis, hallucinations, disorientation, and uncommonly seizures, cranial nerve dysfunction, or coma) is occasional with doses in the lower range; it is more common with larger doses.
   b. Infertility is common in men and women, as with other alkylating agents.
   c. Renal impairment is occasional to common. Fanconi syndrome dependent on dose. May be severe acidosis.
   d. Liver dysfunction is uncommon.
   e. Phlebitis is uncommon.
   f. Fever is rare.
   g. Peripheral neuropathy with high-dose therapy is uncommon.

IMATINIB MESYLATE

Other names. Gleevec, signal transduction inhibitor 571.

Mechanism of action. Inhibitor of the constitutively activated Bcr-Abl tyrosine kinase that is created as a consequence of the (9;22) chromosomal translocation and is required for the transforming function and excess proliferation seen in CML. It also inhibits the RTKs for platelet-derived growth factor (PDGF), stem cell factor, and c-Kit, the latter of which is activated in gastrointestinal stromal tumors (GISTs).

Primary indications

1. CML in chronic, accelerated, or blast phase of the disease
2. ALL, Ph+
3. GIST that is Kit+ (CD117), adjuvant and metastatic disease
4. MDS or myeloproliferative diseases (MPD) with PDGF receptor gene rearrangements
5. Aggressive systemic mastocytosis (ASM) without D816V c-Kit mutation or with cKit mutation status unknown
6. Hypereosinophilic syndrome (HES) or chronic eosinophilic leukemia (CEL) with the FIP1L1-PDGFRα fusion kinase (CHIC2 deletion; and also if fusion kinase negative or unknown)
7. Dermatofibrosarcoma protuberans (DFSP).

Usual dosage and schedule

1. 400 mg by mouth daily in the chronic phase of CML, MDS or MPD, or GISTs. Reduce to 300 mg/day with severe liver impairment or moderate renal impairment.
2. 600 mg by mouth daily in the accelerated phase or blast crisis of CML or Ph+ ALL
3. 100 to 400 mg by mouth daily in ASM, HES, or CEL
4. 800 mg by mouth daily in DFSP.

Special precautions. Use caution when giving to patients with cardiac disease, who have an increased likelihood of developing severe congestive heart failure, edema, and severe fluid retention. Risk is particularly high in patients with high eosinophil counts who may develop cardiogenic shock. Gastrointestinal perforations have been reported, as have bullous dermatologic reactions. Patients who require anticoagulation should not receive warfarin. Imatinib is an inhibitor of and primarily metabolized by CYP3A4.

Toxicity

1. *Myelosuppression and other hematologic effects.* Moderate neutropenia and thrombocytopenia are common in all phases, but severe neutropenia or thrombocytopenia is uncommon unless patients are in the accelerated phase or blast crisis of CML.

2. *Nausea, vomiting, and other gastrointestinal effects.* Nausea, vomiting, abdominal pain, and diarrhea are common, but it is uncommon that they are severe.
3. *Mucocutaneous effects.* Skin rash and nasopharyngitis are common; pruritis and petechiae are occasional. Erythema multiforme and Stevens-Johnson syndrome have been reported.
4. *Miscellaneous effects:*
   a. Fluid retention and edema are common. Pleural effusion and ascites are occasional.
   b. Musculoskeletal pain or cramps, arthralgia, headache, fever, and fatigue are common, but it is uncommon that they are severe or life-threatening.
   c. Dyspnea and cough are occasional.
   d. Elevated liver function tests are occasional. Rare cases of severe hepatotoxicity have been seen.
   e. Rise in serum creatinine and hypokalemia are occasional but rarely severe.
   f. Congestive heart failure is uncommon but may lead to pulmonary edema and rarely pericardial effusion. It may be related to imatinib inhibition of Abl, which in turn may be related to mitochondrial function in the heart.
   g. Monitor TSH levels during imatinib treatment in patients who have had thyroidectomy and are on levothyroxine.

INTERFERON ALPHA

Other names. Roferon-A (interferon alfa-2a, recombinant alpha-A interferon), Intron A (interferon alfa-2b, recombinant alpha-2 interferon).

Mechanism of action. Believed to involve direct inhibition of tumor cell growth and modulation of the immune response of the host, including activation of NK cells, modulation of antibody production, and induction of major histocompatibility antigens.

Primary indications

1. Melanoma (both as adjuvant and metastatic disease therapy)
2. Renal cell carcinoma
3. Multiple myeloma
4. Kaposi sarcoma, HIV-associated
5. CML
6. Non-Hodgkin lymphoma (low-grade), mycosis fungoides
7. Condyloma acuminatum (intralesional)
8. Chronic hepatitis B and C.

Usual dosage and schedule

1. 3 to 10 million IU, IM or SC in various schedules. Daily dosing is often used for several weeks or months, followed by three times a week dosing.

2. As adjuvant therapy for high-risk melanoma, 20 million IU/m^2 IV 5 consecutive days weekly for 4 weeks, then 10 million IU/m^2 SC three times weekly for 48 weeks

3. For HIV-related Kaposi sarcoma, 1 to 5 million IU SC daily, with dose modifications based on toxicity

4. Investigationally, doses have been higher (up to 50 million IU/m^2 per dose), usually IV at doses higher than 10 million IU/m^2.

Special precautions. May cause or aggravate life-threatening or fatal neuropsychiatric, autoimmune, ischemic, and infectious disorders. Patients with persistently severe or worsening signs or symptoms of these conditions should be withdrawn from therapy.

Toxicity

1. *Myelosuppression and other hematologic effects.* Common but usually mild to moderate and transient, even with continued therapy. Higher doses may be associated (25% of patients receiving the recommended adjuvant therapy for melanoma) with granulocyte counts of less than $750/\mu L$ and consequent increased risk for infection.

2. *Nausea, vomiting, and other gastrointestinal effects.* Anorexia and nausea are common, occurring in up to two-thirds of all patients, but vomiting is only occasional. Diarrhea or loose stools are occasional to common.

3. *Mucocutaneous effects.* Rash, dryness, inflammation of the oropharynx, dry skin or pruritus, and partial alopecia are occasional to common.

4. *Miscellaneous effects:*
   a. Flulike syndrome with fatigue, fever, chills, sweating, myalgias, arthralgias, and headache is common to universal with greater severity at higher doses. Tends to diminish with continuing therapy and acetaminophen.
   b. Neurologic effects:
      (1) Peripheral nervous system: Occasional paresthesias or numbness
      (2) CNS toxicity is uncommon at lower doses, but with higher doses there is an increased likelihood of problems, including headache, dizziness, somnolence, anxiety, depression (including suicidal behavior), confusion, hallucinations, cerebellar dysfunction, and emotional lability.
   c. General systemic effects: Fatigue, anorexia, and weight loss are common with chronic administration.
   d. Cardiovascular effects: Mild hypotension is common but rarely symptomatic. Rarely to uncommonly seen are hypertension, chest pain, arrhythmias, or other cardiovascular disorders.
   e. Respiratory effects: Dyspnea and cough are occasional at higher doses.
   f. Infectious effects: Exacerbation of herpetic eruptions and nonherpetic cold sores is uncommon.

    g. Miscellaneous effects: Leg cramps, insomnia, urticaria, hot flashes, and coagulation disorders are uncommon. Visual problems, including blurring, diplopia, dry eyes, nystagmus, and photophobia are uncommon.

    h. Metabolic effects and laboratory abnormalities:

       (1) Elevated liver enzymes are common.

       (2) Mild proteinuria and increase in serum creatinine is occasional.

       (3) Hypercalcemia is occasional.

       (4) Hypothyroidism and hyperthyroidism with or without antithyroid antibodies.

       (5) Hypertriglyceridemia is rare.

       (6) Antibody development (binding and neutralizing) occurs more readily with interferon alfa-2a than with interferon alfa-2b. The significance of this is not clear, though it may be associated with the development of clinical resistance in some patients.

IPILIMUMAB

Other names. MDX 010, MDX-CTLA 4.

Mechanism of action. Ipilimumab is a monoclonal antibody that antagonizes cytotoxic T-lymphocyte–associated antigen-4 (CTLA-4), a negative regulator of the immune system, thus potentiating antitumor T-cell response.

Primary indication. Melanoma that is advanced or metastatic.

Usual dosage and schedule. 3 to 10 mg/kg over 90 minutes every 3 weeks for four doses. Treatment is repeated every 12 weeks in responders (complete or partial response or stable disease).

Special precautions. Diarrhea progressing to severe colitis, including abdominal perforation, has been seen, appears to be immunologic in etiology, and requires emergent therapy following standardized diarrhea treatment guidelines, including corticosteroids when evidence for severe diarrhea or documented colitis is present.

Toxicity

    1. *Myelosuppression and other hematologic effects.* Anemia, leukopenia, and lymphopenia are common, but only occasionally grade 3 or more. Venous thrombosis is uncommon.

    2. *Nausea, vomiting, and other gastrointestinal effects.* Nausea and vomiting are common, but usually not severe. Diarrhea is also common and occasionally severe (grade 3) and may be associated with colitis.

    3. *Mucocutaneous effects.* Pruritis is common (>40%), as is skin rash.

    4. *Immunologic effects and infusion reactions.* Many of the nonhematologic effects, particularly skin and gastrointestinal, may be immunologic in etiology and require emergent treatment.

    5. *Miscellaneous effects:*

      a. Fatigue is common and occasionally severe.

   b. Increased transaminases are common and occasionally (8%) grade 3 to 4. Significant rise in bilirubin may also be seen as well as pancreatitis.

   c. Endocrine: Adrenal insufficiency, hypothyroidism, and hypopituitarism are rare to uncommon.

   d. Dyspnea is common.

   e. Pain is common.

   f. Confusion is occasional.

IRINOTECAN

Other names. Camptosar, CPT-11.

Mechanism of action. Irinotecan, a semisynthetic water-soluble derivative of camptothecin, is a prodrug for the lipophilic metabolite SN38, a potent inhibitor of topoisomerase I, an enzyme essential for effective replication and transcription. It binds to the topoisomerase I–DNA cleavable complex, preventing religation after cleavage by topoisomerase I.

Primary indications

1. Carcinoma of the colon or rectum, esophagus, or stomach
2. Carcinoma of the lung
3. Glioblastoma multiforme.

Usual dosage and schedule

1. 80 to 125 mg/m^2 IV over 90 minutes weekly for 4 weeks followed by a 2-week rest to complete one cycle when used either as a single agent or in combination with fluorouracil and leucovorin.
2. 180 mg/m^2 IV over 90 minutes every 2 weeks when used with leucovorin (over 2 hours) plus bolus fluorouracil followed by a 22-hour infusion of fluorouracil. In patients being concurrently treated with enzyme-inducing antiepileptic drugs, doses must be increased approximately fourfold.

For severe or worse diarrhea (at least seven stools over pretreatment), doses should be held. When the diarrhea has improved (no more than 7 stools over pretreatment) treatment may be restarted with doses modified downward by 25 to 30 mg/m^2 during the current and subsequent cycles if there was an increase in stools of 7 to 9 per day, and by 50 to 60 mg/m^2 if there was an increase in stools of 10 or more. Doses are also held during treatment and reduced in the same and subsequent cycles for severe neutropenia (ANC <1000).

Special precautions. Both early and late diarrhea may occur. That which occurs within 24 hours (a cholinergic effect) should be treated with atropine 0.25 to 1 mg IV. Late diarrhea should be treated promptly with loperamide (up to 2 mg every 2 hours until the patient is free of diarrhea for 12 hours) and prompt fluid and electrolyte replacement as indicated, if the diarrhea becomes severe (increase of seven or more stools per day) or there is dehydration or postural hypotension. Consideration should be given to antibiotic therapy, such as with an oral fluoroquinolone, particularly if the patient is neutropenic. A vascular syndrome characterized by sudden unexpected thromboembolic events has also been described.

Dose must be reduced in patients who are homozygous for the UGT1A1*28 allele, a variation of a uridine diphosphate glucuronosyltransferase gene and its corresponding enzyme (UGT1A1), which is responsible for glucuronidation of bilirubin and involved in deactivation of irinotecan's toxic active metabolite SN-38. Testing may be done by the Invader UGT1A1 Molecular Assay (Hologic, Bedford, MA).

Toxicity

1. *Myelosuppression and other hematologic effects.* Neutropenia is common and often severe, particularly in combination therapy; anemia and thrombocytopenia are common, but uncommonly severe, unless homozygous for UGT1A1*28.
2. *Nausea, vomiting, and other gastrointestinal effects.* Nausea and vomiting are common and are occasionally severe. Early diarrhea is common but is uncommonly severe. Late diarrhea is common (85%) and is occasionally severe (15%) to life-threatening (5% to 10%). Severe diarrhea may be more common if homozygous for UGT1A1*28. Abdominal cramping is common and occasionally severe. Anorexia is common. Constipation and dyspepsia are occasional. Ileus, colitis, or toxic megacolon are seen rarely.
3. *Mucocutaneous effects.* Alopecia and mucositis are common. Rash and sweating occur occasionally.
4. *Miscellaneous effects:*
   a. Fever is common and rarely severe.
   b. Headache, back pain, chills, and edema are occasional.
   c. Grade 1 to 2 increases in liver function tests are common; it is uncommon for liver function abnormalities to be severe, except in patients with known liver metastasis.
   d. Dyspnea, cough, or rhinitis is occasional to common but usually not severe.
   e. Insomnia or dizziness is occasional.
   f. Flushing is occasional.
   g. Anaphylactic reactions are rare.

IXABEPILONE

Other name. Ixempra.

Mechanism of action. Ixabepilone is an analog of epothilone B that binds to β-tubulin subunits on microtubules, leading to suppression of microtubule dynamics, which blocks the cell in mitosis, leading to cell death.

Primary indication. Carcinoma of the breast, usually after failure with anthracyclines and taxanes. Often given in combination with capecitabine.

Usual dosage and schedule. 40 mg/m^2 IV over 3 hours every 3 weeks. All patients should be pretreated with both an H$_1$- and H$_2$-histamine–receptor antagonist.

Special precautions. Patients with a history of hypersensitivity reactions to ixabepilone or other agents containing polyoxyethylated castor oil must be pretreated with dexamethasone. If the reactions were severe, do not treat. Coadministration with potent inhibitors of CYP3A4, such as ketoconazole, increases ixabepilone AUC, and dose reduction should be considered. Strong inducers of CYP3A4, such as dexamethasone or phenytoin, may decrease ixabepilone concentrations. Do not give in combination with capecitabine in patients with aspartate aminotransferase (AST) or alanine aminotranferease (ALT) greater than 2.5 ULN or bilirubin greater than 1 × ULN. Dose reductions are required in patients with moderate hepatic impairment (AST or ALT >2.5 ULN or bilirubin >1.5 ULN).

Toxicity

1. *Myelosuppression and other hematologic effects.* Severe (grade 3 to 4) neutropenia is common. Severe anemia and thrombocytopenia are only occasional.
2. *Nausea, vomiting, and other gastrointestinal effects.* Anorexia, nausea, vomiting, and diarrhea are common, but it is uncommon that they are severe. Constipation and abdominal pain are occasional but rarely severe.
3. *Mucocutaneous effects.* Mucositis is common, but it is uncommon that it is severe. Alopecia is common. Skin rash, nail disorders, palmar-plantar erythrodysesthesia, and pruritis are occasional. Hyperpigmentation and skin exfoliation are uncommon.
4. *Immunologic effects and infusion reactions.* One percent of patients may have hypersensitivity reactions.
5. *Miscellaneous effects:*
   a. Neurologic: Peripheral neuropathy is common and cumulative and occasionally severe (grade 3 to 4). It is the most frequent toxicity responsible for drug discontinuation. Headache, dizziness, insomnia, and altered taste are occasional.
   b. Musculoskeletal: Myalagia and arthralgia are common.
   c. Fatigue and asthenia are common. Edema and fever are occasional.
   d. Cardiorespiratory: Use of ixabepilone in combination with capecitabine may increase cardiac adverse reactions such as myocardial ischemia or ventricular dysfunction (1.9%). Cough and dyspnea are occasional.

LAPATINIB

Other name. Tykerb.

Mechanism of action. Lapatinib is a dual tyrosine kinase inhibitor with specificity for EGFR and human epidermal receptor type 2 (HER2).

Primary indication. Advanced or metastatic carcinoma of breast that over-expresses the HER2 receptor in combination with the following:

- Capecitabine in women who have received prior therapy including an anthracycline, a taxane, and trastuzumab
- Letrozole in postmenopausal women with receptor-positive metastatic breast cancer
- Trastuzumab in women who have progressed on this drug (may be effective because of different mechanism of action on HER2).

Usual dosage and schedule. 1250 mg by mouth daily with capecitabine. 1500 mg by mouth daily with letrozole.

Special precautions. Confirm left ventricular ejection fraction before starting therapy. Monitor liver function tests before and every 4 to 6 weeks during therapy. Reduce dose for severe hepatic impairment (Child-Pugh class C). Discontinue therapy for severe pulmonary symptoms. Avoid strong CYP3A4 inhibitors, which will increase plasma concentrations of lapatinib.

Toxicity

1. *Myelosuppression and other hematologic effects.* Myelosuppression is not an effect of lapatinib. Other EGFR inhibitors may potentiate warfarin and cause unexpected rise in INR.
2. *Nausea, vomiting, and other gastrointestinal effects.* Nausea and diarrhea are common; diarrhea may be severe; vomiting and anorexia are occasional. Other EGFR inhibitors are associated with transaminase elevations and occasionally with increased bilirubin.
3. *Mucocutaneous effects.* Palmar-plantar erythrodysesthesia (with capecitabine) and rash (with letrozole) are common. Dry skin, alopecia, pruritis, and nail disorders are occasional. Epistaxis is occasional.
4. *Miscellaneous effects:*
   a. Left ventricular ejection fraction decrease is uncommon and rarely severe. Prolongation of QT interval is uncommon.
   b. Interstitial lung disease is rare to uncommon.
   c. Asthenia, fatigue, and headache are occasional to common
   d. Elevated liver enzymes or bilirubin is common, but severe (grade 3 to 4) is uncommon.

LENALIDOMIDE

Other name. Revlimid.

Mechanism of action. Multiple potential mechanisms, including immuno-modulatory and antiangiogenic effects. Precise mechanism not delineated.

Primary indications

1. MDS, low- or intermediate-risk, associated with deletion of 5q31 (del 5q). Also effective in some patients without 5q deletion.
2. Multiple myeloma.

Usual dosage and schedule

1. MDS: 10 mg by mouth daily, with dosing interruptions and subsequent dose reduction to 5 mg daily as determined by cytopenias or other toxicity.
2. Multiple myeloma: 25 mg by mouth daily for 21 of 28 days. Renal insufficiency is associated with decreased clearance and need for reduced starting doses.

Special precautions. Severe and life-threatening birth defects, primarily phocomelia, may be caused by this analog of thalidomide, a known human teratogen. For this reason, special precautions must be taken to assure that female patients are not pregnant when the drug is started, and that both female and male patients practice strict birth control measures.

Toxicity

1. *Myelosuppression and other hematologic effects.* Neutropenia and thrombocytopenia are common and dose-limiting. Febrile neutropenia is uncommon. Anemia is occasional and may be autoimmune in nature (uncommon). Hypercoagulability with thromboembolic events, including pulmonary emboli (2% to 3%), have been seen in patients treated with lenalidomide combination therapy but are uncommon to occasional. The relative benefit of prophylactic anticoagulation or antiplatelet therapy is uncertain, but some form of prophylaxis is generally recommended, particularly in patients with myeloma or others receiving concurrent corticosteroids.
2. *Nausea, vomiting, and other gastrointestinal effects.* Diarrhea is common; constipation is common but less often than diarrhea. Nausea is common, but vomiting only occasional. Abdominal pain is occasional.
3. *Mucocutaneous effects.* Macular rash, dryness of the skin, increased sweating, and pruritis are common. Urticaria is occasional.
4. *Miscellaneous effects:*
   a. Cough, nasopharyngitis, dyspnea, and bronchitis are occasional.
   b. Myalgia, arthralgia, muscle cramps, or limb pain are occasional.
   c. Fatigue and fever are common, but rigors are uncommon.
   d. Headache and dizziness are occasional. Peripheral neuropathy is uncommon (5%). Insomnia and depression are occasional.
   e. Hypothyroidism is occasional.
   f. Palpitations, hypertension, chest pain, and peripheral edema are occasional.
   g. Hypokalemia and hypomagnesemia are occasional.
   h. Birth defects (see Special precautions).

LETROZOLE

Other name. Femara.

Mechanism of action. Decreases estrogen biosynthesis by selective, competitive inhibition of the aromatase enzyme in peripheral tissues, thereby reducing the conversion of the adrenal androgens testosterone and androstenedione to estradiol and estrone respectively.

Primary indications

1. Carcinoma of the breast, advanced or metastatic, that is hormone-receptor–positive or unknown in postmenopausal women as first-line treatment, or in hormone-responsive postmenopausal women with progression following antiestrogen therapy.
2. Carcinoma of the breast as adjuvant therapy in hormone-receptor–positive postmenopausal women.

Usual dosage and schedule. 2.5 mg by mouth daily.

Special precautions. Potential hazard to fetus if given during pregnancy. Because of the potential fracture risk, calcium and vitamin D with or without bisphosphonates are often used.

Toxicity

1. *Myelosuppression and other hematologic effects.* No dose-related effect. Thromboembolic events are uncommon to rare and less than with tamoxifen.
2. *Nausea, vomiting, and other gastrointestinal effects.* Nausea, vomiting, constipation, and diarrhea are uncommon to occasional.
3. *Mucocutaneous effects.* Rash is uncommon.
4. *Miscellaneous effects:*
   a. Hot flushes are common, and night sweats are occasional.
   b. Musculoskeletal pain (arthralgia or bone) is occasional to common.
   c. Weight increase is occasional (lower than with megestrol).
   d. Fatigue is occasional.
   e. Acceleration of osteoporosis is occasional; increase in fracture risk is uncommon.
   f. Headache is uncommon.
   g. Peripheral edema is occasional (lower than with megestrol).
   h. Dyspnea and cough are uncommon to occasional.
   i. Hypercalcemia is rare.
   j. Endometrial cancer is rare (0.2%) and less likely than with tamoxifen.

LOMUSTINE

Other names. CCNU, CeeNU.

Mechanism of action. Alkylation and carbamoylation by lomustine metabolites interfere with the synthesis and function of DNA, RNA, and proteins. Lomustine is lipid-soluble and easily enters the brain.

Primary indication. Malignant brain tumors.

Usual dosage and schedule. 100 to 130 mg/m² by mouth once every 6 to 8 weeks (lower dose used for patients with compromised bone marrow function). Limit cumulative dose to 1000 mg/m² to limit pulmonary and renal toxicity.

Special precautions. Because of delayed myelosuppression (3 to 6 weeks), do not treat more often than every 6 weeks. Await a return of normal platelet and granulocyte counts before repeating therapy.

Toxicity

1. *Myelosuppression and other hematologic effects.* Universal and dose-limiting. Leukopenia and thrombocytopenia are delayed 3 to 6 weeks after therapy begins and may be cumulative with successive doses.
2. *Nausea, vomiting, and other gastrointestinal effects.* Nausea and vomiting may begin 3 to 6 hours after therapy and last up to 24 hours.
3. *Mucocutaneous effects.* Stomatitis and alopecia are rare.
4. *Miscellaneous effects:*
   a. Confusion, lethargy, and ataxia are rare.
   b. Mild hepatotoxicity is infrequent.
   c. Secondary neoplasia is possible.
   d. Pulmonary fibrosis is uncommon at doses of less than 1000 mg/m².
   e. Renal toxicity is uncommon at doses of less than 1000 mg/m².

MECHLORETHAMINE

Other names. Nitrogen mustard, HN2, Mustargen.

Mechanism of action. Mechlorethamine is a prototype alkylating agent. Its action involves transfer of the alkyl group to amino, carboxyl, hydroxyl, imidazole, phosphate, and sulfhydryl groups within the cell, altering structure and function of DNA (primarily), RNA, and proteins.

Primary indications

1. Hodgkin lymphoma
2. Malignant pleural and, less commonly, peritoneal or pericardial effusions
3. CTCLs (topically).

Usual dosage and schedule

1. 6 mg/m² IV on days 1 and 8 every 4 weeks (in mechlorethamine, Oncovin [vincristine], procarbazine, and prednisone [MOPP] regimen for Hodgkin disease)
2. 8 to 16 mg/m² by intracavitary injection
3. 10 mg in 60 mL of tap water applied to entire body surface (avoid eyes).

Special precautions

1. Administer over several minutes into the sidearm of a running IV infusion, taking care to avoid extravasation.

2. Because mechlorethamine is a potent vesicant, extreme care must be exercised while preparing and administering the drug. Gloves and eyeglasses are recommended to protect the preparer. If accidental eye contact should occur, institute copious irrigation with normal saline and follow by prompt ophthalmologic consultation. If accidental skin contact occurs, irrigate the affected part immediately with water for at least 15 minutes and follow by 2.6% sodium thiosulfate solution (1/6 M).
3. Mechlorethamine should be used soon after preparation (15 to 30 minutes) as it decomposes on standing. It *must not* be mixed in the same syringe with any other drug.

Toxicity

1. *Myelosuppression and other hematologic effects.* Dose-limiting, with the nadir at about 1 week and recovery by 3 weeks.
2. *Nausea, vomiting, and other gastrointestinal effects.* Universal. They usually begin within the first 3 hours and last 4 to 8 hours.
3. *Mucocutaneous effects.* Severe painful inflammation and necrosis are likely if extravasation occurs. May be ameliorated with sodium thiosulfate (see Table 26.1). Maculopapular rash is uncommon.
4. *Miscellaneous effects:*
   a. Phlebitis, thrombosis, or both of the vein used for the injection are common.
   b. Amenorrhea and azoospermia are common.
   c. Hyperuricemia with rapid tumor destruction.
   d. Weakness, sleepiness, and headache are uncommon.
   e. Severe allergic reactions, including anaphylaxis, are rare.
   f. Secondary neoplasms, including myelodysplasia, acute leukemia, and carcinomas, are possible.

MELPHALAN

Other names. Phenylalanine mustard, L-sarcolysin, L-PAM, Alkeran.

Mechanism of action. Alkylating agent with primary effect on DNA. Amino acid–type structure may result in cellular transport that is different from other alkylating agents.

Primary indications

1. Multiple myeloma
2. Stem cell transplant preparative regimens.

Usual dosage and schedule

1. 8 mg/m^2 by mouth on days 1 to 4 every 4 weeks, *or*
2. 10 mg/m^2 by mouth on days 1 to 4 every 6 weeks, *or*
3. 3 to 4 mg/m^2 by mouth daily for 2 to 3 weeks, then 1 to 2 mg/m^2 by mouth daily for maintenance.

4. High-dose regimens of 140 to 200 mg/m^2 IV have been used, followed by stem cell rescue (e.g., bone marrow transplantation).

Special precautions

1. Myelosuppression and other hematologic effects may be delayed and prolonged to 4 to 6 weeks. Reduce IV dose by 50% for creatinine that is greater than 1.5 × normal.
2. Use in early myeloma may preclude harvest of sufficient numbers of peripheral stem cells for autologous transplantation.

Toxicity

1. *Myelosuppression and other hematologic effects.* Dose-limiting; nadir at days 14 to 21.
2. *Nausea, vomiting, and other gastrointestinal effects.* Nausea, vomiting, and diarrhea are uncommon at standard doses, but common with high-dose regimens.
3. *Mucocutaneous effects.* Alopecia, dermatitis, and stomatitis are uncommon at standard doses; alopecia and mucositis are common with high-dose regimens.
4. *Miscellaneous effects:*
   a. Acute nonlymphocytic leukemia and myelodysplasia are rare but well documented.
   b. Pulmonary fibrosis is rare.

MERCAPTOPURINE

Other names. 6-Mercaptopurine, 6-MP, Purinethol.

Mechanism of action. A purine antimetabolite that, when converted to the nucleotide, inhibits the formation of nucleotides necessary for DNA and RNA synthesis.

Primary indication. ALL.

Usual dosage and schedule

1. 100 mg/m^2 by mouth daily if used alone
2. 50 to 90 mg/m^2 by mouth daily if used with methotrexate or other cytotoxic drugs.

Special precautions

1. Decrease dose by 75% when used concurrently with allopurinol.
2. Increase interval between doses or reduce dose in patients with renal failure.

Toxicity

1. *Myelosuppression and other hematologic effects.* Common but mild at recommended doses.

2. *Nausea, vomiting, and other gastrointestinal effects.* Nausea and vomiting are uncommon. Diarrhea is rare.
3. *Mucocutaneous effects.* Stomatitis may be seen with very large doses. Dry, scaling rash is uncommon.
4. *Miscellaneous effects:*
   a. Intrahepatic cholestasis and mild focal centrolobular necrosis with jaundice are uncommon.
   b. Hyperuricemia with rapid leukemia cell lysis is common.
   c. Fever is uncommon.

MESNA

Other name. Mesnex.

Mechanism of action. Mesna disulfide is reduced in the kidney to a free thiol compound, which then reacts chemically with urotoxic metabolites of ifosfamide or cyclophosphamide, resulting in their detoxification.

Primary indication. Prophylaxis for ifosfamide- or high-dose cyclophosphamide–induced hemorrhagic cystitis.

Usual dosage and schedule. Mesna dose is at least 20% of the ifosfamide dose (on a weight [mg] basis), administered just prior to (or mixed with) the ifosfamide dose, and again at 4 and 8 hours after the ifosfamide dose to detoxify the urinary metabolites that cause the hemorrhagic cystitis. Higher doses of ifosfamide may require higher doses and longer durations of mesna.

Special precautions. Contraindicated if patient is sensitive to thiol compounds. Does not prevent or ameliorate any adverse effects of ifosfamide or cyclophosphamide other than hemorrhagic cystitis. Neither mesna nor its only metabolite, mesna disulfide, affect ifosfamide, cyclophosphamide, or their antineoplastic metabolites.

Toxicity

1. *Myelosuppression and other hematologic effects.* None.
2. *Nausea, vomiting, and other gastrointestinal effects.* Nausea, vomiting, and diarrhea are occasional. Nausea and vomiting more commonly from ifosfamide.
3. *Mucocutaneous effects.* Bad taste in the mouth is common.
4. *Miscellaneous effects:*
   a. Headache, fatigue, and limb pain are occasional.
   b. Hypotension or allergic reactions are uncommon to rare.
   c. Gives false positive test for urinary ketones.

METHOTREXATE

Other names. Amethopterin, MTX, Mexate, Folex, Trexall.

Mechanism of action. Inhibition of dihydrofolate reductase, which results in a block of the reduction of dihydrofolate to tetrahydrofolate. This blockage in turn inhibits the formation of thymidylate and purines, and arrests DNA (predominantly), RNA, and protein synthesis.

Primary indications

1. Breast, head and neck, gastric, and gestational trophoblastic carcinomas
2. Osteosarcomas (high-dose methotrexate)
3. ALL
4. Meningeal leukemia or carcinomatosis
5. Non-Hodgkin lymphoma.

Usual dosage and schedule

1. Gestational trophoblastic carcinoma: 15–30 mg by mouth or IM on days 1 to 5 every 2 weeks
2. Other carcinomas: 40 to 80 mg/m^2 IV or by mouth 2 to 4 times monthly with a 7- to 14-day interval between doses
3. ALL: 15 to 20 mg/m^2 by mouth or IV weekly (together with mercaptopurine)
4. Osteosarcoma: Up to 12 g/m^2 with leucovorin rescue (high-dose methotrexate). This usage requires on-site monitoring of methotrexate levels and a high degree of expertise to administer safely.
5. Intrathecally: 12 mg/m^2 (not >20 mg) twice weekly.

Special precautions

1. High-dose methotrexate (>80 mg/m^2) should be administered only by individuals experienced in its use and at institutions where serum methotrexate levels can be readily measured.
2. Intrathecal methotrexate must be mixed in buffered physiologic solution containing no preservative.
3. Avoid aspirin, sulfonamides, tetracycline, phenytoin, and other protein-bound drugs that may displace methotrexate and cause an increase in free drug.
4. Oral anticoagulants (e.g., warfarin) may be potentiated by methotrexate; therefore, PTs/INRs should be followed carefully.
5. Oral antibiotics may decrease methotrexate absorption; penicillin and NSAIDs decrease clearance of methotrexate.
6. Monitor use with theophylline.
7. In patients with renal insufficiency, it may be necessary to markedly reduce the dose or discontinue methotrexate therapy.
8. Do not give if patient has a significant effusion because of "reservoir" effect.

Toxicity

1. *Myelosuppression and other hematologic effects.* Occurs commonly, with nadir at 6 to 10 days after a single IV dose. Recovery is rapid.
2. *Nausea, vomiting, and other gastrointestinal effects.* Occasional at standard doses.

3. *Mucocutaneous effects:*
   a. Mild stomatitis is common and is a sign that a maximum tolerated dose has been reached. Higher doses may result in confluent or hemorrhagic stomal ulcers and bloody diarrhea. This requires prompt leucovorin therapy to limit duration and severity.
   b. Erythematous rashes, urticaria, and skin pigment changes are uncommon.
   c. Mild alopecia is frequent.
4. *Miscellaneous effects:*
   a. Acute hepatocellular injury is uncommon at standard doses. Hepatic fibrosis is uncommon but seen at low chronic doses.
   b. Pneumonitis is rare. Polyserositis is rare.
   c. Renal tubular necrosis is rare at standard doses.
   d. Convulsions and a Guillain-Barré–like syndrome following intrathecal therapy are uncommon.

MIDOSTAURIN

Other name. PKC412.

Mechanism of action. A multikinase agent that inhibits *fms*-like tyrosine kinase 3 (FLT3), which is mutated in about 35% of patients with AML. Also directly or indirectly inhibits other molecular targets, including VEGF receptor 1, c-kit, H- and KRAS, and the multidrug resistance gene MDR.

Primary indications (all currently investigational)

1. AML with FLT3 mutation
2. Systemic mastocytosis and mast cell leukemia
3. MDS.

Usual dosage and schedule

1. 50 mg twice daily for 14 days of each 28-day cycle with cytotoxic agents for induction or consolidation therapy
2. 50 mg twice daily continuously when used as a single agent, as for maintenance.

Special precautions. CYP3A4 inhibitors increase midostaurin blood levels and increase toxicity.

Toxicity

1. *Myelosuppression and other hematologic effects.* Generally mild and not dose-limiting, but anemia and leukopenia may be seen.
2. *Nausea, vomiting, and other gastrointestinal effects.* Anorexia, nausea, vomiting, and diarrhea are common.
3. *Mucocutaneous effects.* Rash is occasional.
4. *Miscellaneous effects:*
   a. Laboratory: Transitory elevations of glucose, AST, ALT, and bilirubin are occasional; decreases in potassium, phosphate, and calcium are occasional.

    b. Pulmonary edema and pulmonary infiltrates are uncommon and possibly related to coadministration of azole antifungal drugs (CYP3A4 inhibitors).

    c. Headache and fatigue are occasional.

MITOMYCIN

Other names. Mitomycin C, Mutamycin.

Mechanism of action. Alkylation and cross-linking by mitomycin metabolites interfere with structure and function of DNA.

Primary indications. Bladder (intravesical), esophagus, stomach, anal, and pancreas carcinomas.

Usual dosage and schedule

1. 20 mg/m^2 IV on day 1 every 4 to 6 weeks, *or*
2. 2 mg/m^2 IV on days 1 to 5 and 8 to 12 every 4 to 6 weeks
3. 10 mg/m^2 IV on day 1 every 8 weeks in combination with fluorouracil and doxorubicin for stomach and pancreatic carcinomas
4. 30 to 40 mg instilled into the bladder weekly for 4 to 8 weeks, then monthly for 6 months.

Special precautions. Administer as slow push or rapid infusion through the sidearm of a rapidly running IV infusion, taking care to avoid extravasation. Pulmonary, renal, and hematologic toxicity (microangiopathic anemia and thrombocytopenia) may result from endothelial cell damage.

Toxicity

1. *Myelosuppression and other hematologic effects.* Myelosuppression is serious, cumulative, and dose-limiting. Nadir is reached usually by 4 weeks but may be delayed. Recovery is often prolonged over many weeks, and occasionally the cytopenia never disappears. Hemolytic-uremic syndrome is rare, but when it occurs, it may be poorly responsive to plasmapheresis and other therapies.
2. *Nausea, vomiting, and other gastrointestinal effects.* Nausea and vomiting are common at higher doses, but severity is usually mild to moderate.
3. *Mucocutaneous effects.* Stomatitis and alopecia are common.
4. *Miscellaneous effects:*
       a. Renal toxicity is uncommon. Hemolytic-uremic syndrome is rare.
       b. Pulmonary toxicity is uncommon but may be severe.
       c. Fever is uncommon.
       d. Cellulitis at injection site is common if extravasation occurs.
       e. Secondary neoplasia is possible.

MITOTANE

Other names. *o,p*'-DDD, Lysodren.

Mechanism of action. Suppresses adrenal steroid production, modifies peripheral steroid metabolism, and is cytotoxic to adrenal cortical cells.

Primary indications. Adrenocortical carcinoma.

Usual dosage and schedule. Begin with 2 to 6 g by mouth daily in three or four divided doses and build to a maximum tolerated daily dose that is usually 8 to 10 g, although it may range from 2 to 16 g. Glucocorticoid and mineralocorticoid replacements during mitotane therapy are necessary to prevent hypoadrenalism. Cortisone acetate (25 mg by mouth in the morning and 12.5 mg by mouth in the evening) and fludrocortisone acetate (0.1 mg by mouth in the morning) are recommended.

Special precautions. Patients who experience severe trauma, infection, or shock should be treated with supplemental corticosteroids. Because of the effect of mitotane on peripheral steroid metabolism, larger than usual replacement doses may be necessary.

Toxicity

1. *Myelosuppression and other hematologic effects.* None.
2. *Nausea, vomiting, and other gastrointestinal effects.* Nausea, vomiting, and anorexia are common and may be dose-limiting. Diarrhea is occasional.
3. *Mucocutaneous effects.* Skin rash occurs occasionally.
4. *CNS effects.* Lethargy, sedation, vertigo, or dizziness in up to 40% of patients; may be dose-limiting.
5. *Miscellaneous effects.* Albuminuria, hemorrhagic cystitis, hypertension, orthostatic hypotension, and visual disturbances are uncommon.

MITOXANTRONE

Other names. Novantrone, dihydroxyanthracenedione, DHAD, DHAQ.

Mechanism of action. DNA-strand breakage mediated by anthracenedione effects on topoisomerase II.

Primary indications

1. Acute nonlymphocytic leukemia
2. Carcinoma of the breast or ovary
3. Non-Hodgkin and Hodgkin lymphoma.

Usual dosage and schedule

1. 12 to 14 mg/m^2 IV as a 5- to 30-minute infusion once every 3 weeks for solid tumors
2. 12 mg/m^2 IV as a 5- to 30-minute infusion daily for 3 days for acute nonlymphocytic leukemia.

Special precautions. Rarely causes extravasation injury if infiltrated. Cardiotoxicity probably less than with doxorubicin; prior anthracycline, chest irradiation, or underlying cardiac disease increases the risk of cardiotoxicity.

Toxicity

1. *Myelosuppression and other hematologic effects.* Universal.
2. *Nausea, vomiting, and other gastrointestinal effects.* Nausea and vomiting are common but less frequent and less severe than with doxorubicin. Diarrhea is uncommon.
3. *Mucocutaneous effects.* Alopecia is common, but its frequency and severity is less than with doxorubicin. Mucositis is occasional.
4. *Miscellaneous effects:*
   a. Cardiac toxicity: Probably less than with doxorubicin; there is no clear maximum dose, though the risk appears to increase at 125 mg/m^2 cumulative dose.
   b. Local erythema and swelling with transient blue discoloration if extravasated, but rarely leads to severe skin damage.
   c. Green or blue discoloration of urine.
   d. Phlebitis is uncommon.

NELARABINE

Other name. Arranon.

Mechanism of action. Nelarabine is a prodrug of arabinofuranosylguanine (ara-G), a cytotoxic analog of deoxyguanosine. When converted to triphosphorylated ara-G, it is incorporated into DNA (preferentially into T-cells), inducing fragmentation and apoptosis.

Primary indications. T-cell ALL and T-cell lymphoblastic lymphoma that have relapsed or are refractory to at least two prior chemotherapy regimens.

Usual dosage and schedule

1. Adults: 1500 mg/m^2 IV over 2 hours on days 1, 3, and 5; repeated every 21 days
2. Children: 650 mg/m^2 IV over 1 hour daily for 5 consecutive days; repeated every 21 days.

Special precautions. Close monitoring for neurologic events is recommended, owing to the possibility of severe neurologic complications of therapy. Prophylaxis against tumor lysis syndrome recommended.

Toxicity

1. *Myelosuppression and other hematologic effects.* Anemia, neutropenia, and thrombocytopenia are common. Febrile neutropenia is occasional.
2. *Nausea, vomiting, and other gastrointestinal effects.* Nausea, vomiting, diarrhea, and constipation are common but usually low-grade. Abdominal pain is occasional.
3. *Mucocutaneous effects.* Stomatitis is occasional.

4. *Neurologic effects:*
   a. Headache is occasional.
   b. Somnolence and confusion are occasional.
   c. Peripheral neuropathy is occasional. May range from numbness and paresthesias to motor weakness and paralysis.
   d. Ataxia is occasional.
   e. Insomnia is occasional.
   f. Convulsions and coma are rare.
   g. Leukoencephalopathy and demyelination and ascending peripheral neuropathy are rare.
5. *Miscellaneous effects:*
   a. Fatigue, weakness, and fever (occasionally with rigors) are common.
   b. Cough, dyspnea, and pleural effusion are common to occasional.
   c. Abnormal liver function tests are occasional.
   d. Hypokalemia, hypomagnesemia, hypocalcemia, and increased creatinine are occasional.
   e. Edema is occasional.
   f. Sinus tachycardia is occasional.
   g. Musculoskeletal pain is occasional.

NILOTINIB

Other names. Tasigna, AMNI07.

Mechanism of action. Selective inhibitor of the constitutively activated Bcr-Abl tyrosine kinase that is created as a consequence of the (9;22) chromosomal translocation and is required for the transforming function and excess proliferation seen in CML. In vitro, nilotinib is active against many Bcr-Abl mutations associated with imatinib resistance.

Primary indications

1. CML, chronic phase, newly diagnosed
2. CML in chronic or accelerated phase in patients resistant or intolerant to imatinib
3. Investigational:
   a. Ph+ ALL
   b. GIST.

Usual dosage and schedule

1. Newly diagnosed chronic-phase CML: 300 mg orally twice daily
2. Resistant or intolerant chronic-phase CML and accelerated-phase CML: 400 mg orally twice daily
3. Lower doses recommended for hepatic impairment or for toxicity.

Special precautions. Do not use in patients with hypokalemia, hypomagnesemia, or long QT syndrome. Drugs known to prolong the QT interval and strong CYP3A4 inhibitors should be avoided. ECGs should be obtained to monitor the corrected QT (QTc) at baseline, 7 days after initiation, and periodically thereafter. Do not give if QTc is greater than 480 msec.

Toxicity

1. *Myelosuppression and other hematologic effects.* Thrombocytopenia and neutropenia are common. Anemia is occasional.
2. *Nausea, vomiting, and other gastrointestinal effects.* Nausea and vomiting are occasional.
3. *Mucocutaneous effects.* Skin rash is common; alopecia, dry skin, and pruritis are occasional.
4. *Miscellaneous effects:*
   a. Abnormal liver function tests, including elevations in bilirubin (primarily unconjugated), are occasional.
   b. Increase in the QTC interval by 5 to 15 msec is rare but has been seen and may result in sudden death.
   c. Increase in lipase and amylase are uncommon.
   d. Grade 3 or 4 hypophosphatemia, hypokalemia, hyperkalemia, hypocalcemia, and hyponatremia are occasional to uncommon.
   e. Arthralgia, myalagia, muscle spasms, and bone pain are occasional.
   f. Fatigue and insomnia are common; fever and weakness are occasional.
   g. Peripheral edema is occasional.
   h. Cough and dyspnea are occasional.

NILUTAMIDE

Other name. Nilandron.

Mechanism of action. Competitive inhibitor of androgens at the cellular androgen receptor in prostate cancer cells. Complements surgical castration.

Primary indication. Metastatic carcinoma of the prostate, in combination with surgical castration or LHRH agonist.

Usual dosage and schedule. 300 mg by mouth once daily for 30 days, followed by 150 mg by mouth once daily thereafter.

Special precautions. Should be restricted to patients with normal liver function test values. A routine chest radiograph should be obtained before therapy and any time that the patient reports new exertional dyspnea or worsening of pre-existing dyspnea. Inhibits activity of liver cytochrome P450 isoenzymes and may delay elimination of drugs such as warfarin, phenytoin, and theophylline.

Toxicity

1. *Myelosuppression and other hematologic effects.* None.
2. *Nausea, vomiting, and other gastrointestinal effects.* Nausea, constipation, and anorexia are occasional to common. Vomiting is uncommon.

3. *Mucocutaneous effects.* Rash, dry skin, and sweating are uncommon.
4. *Miscellaneous effects:*
   a. Hepatitis is rare (1%). Increased liver function test values are uncommon.
   b. Interstitial pneumonitis with dyspnea is uncommon (2%). May be higher in patients with Asian ancestry.
   c. Inhibits activity of liver cytochrome P450 isoenzymes and may delay elimination of drugs such as warfarin, phenytoin, and theophylline.
   d. Hot flashes are common.
   e. Impaired adaptation to dark is common (57%).
   f. Cardiac and other lung disorders are uncommon.

OFATUMUMAB

Other name. Arzerra.

Mechanism of action. Ofatumumab is a recombinant human monoclonal antibody that binds to extracellular loops of the CD20 molecule, resulting in B-cell lysis, possibly through both complement-dependent and cell-mediated cytotoxicity.

Primary indication. CLL, refractory to fludarabine and alemtuzumab.

Usual dosage and schedule. 12 doses administered as follows:

- 300 mg initial dose, followed 1 week later by
- 2000 mg weekly for seven doses, followed 4 weeks later by
- 2000 mg every 4 weeks for four doses.

Special precautions. Dose 1 should be infused at an initial rate of 3.6 mg/hr, dose 2 at an initial rate of 24 mg/hr, and doses 3 to 12 at an initial rate of 50 mg/hr. In the absence of infusion reactions, the infusion rate may be doubled every 30 minutes for a maximum of four doublings. Premedication with acetaminophen, an H_1-histamine–receptor antagonist, and corticosteroid is required.

Toxicity

1. *Myelosuppression and other hematologic effects.* Grade 3 or 4 neutropenia is common and may persist for over 1 week. Anemia is occasional to common. Seventy percent of patients in one trial developed bacterial, viral, or fungal infections, which were fatal in 12% of patients treated.
2. *Nausea, vomiting, and other gastrointestinal effects.* Nausea and diarrhea are occasional.
3. *Mucocutaneous effects.* Rash and urticaria are occasional.
4. *Immunologic effects and infusion reactions.* Infusion reactions occur in 44% on the first day of infusion, 29% on the second day, and less frequently during subsequent infusions.

5. *Miscellaneous effects:*
   a. Neurologic: Progressive multifocal leukoencephalopathy, including a fatal case, has occurred with ofatumumab, but is rare. Insomnia is occasional. Headache is occasional.
   b. Infections: Hepatitis B reactivation is possible as with other anti-CD20 antibodies. Pneumonia is occasional to common; bronchitis, sepsis, nasopharyngitis, and herpes zoster are occasional.
   c. Fever and chills, fatigue, headache, and peripheral edema are occasional.
   d. Respiratory: Cough and dyspnea are occasional.
   e. Cardiovascular: Hypertension, hypotension, and tachycardia are uncommon.

OLAPARIB and other PARP1 inhibitors

Other names. AZ2281, iniparib (BSI-201), veliparib (ABT888).

Mechanism of action. Inhibition of PARP1, one of a large family of poly(ADP-ribose) polymerases, which inhibits repair of DNA single-strand breaks.

Primary indications

1. Metastatic carcinoma of the breast with BRCA1 or BRCA2 mutation (olaparib)
2. Triple negative (estrogen receptor–/progesterone receptor–/HER2–negative) metastatic carcinoma of the breast (BSI-201)
3. BRCA-deficient ovarian cancer.

Usual dosage and schedule

1. Olaparib 100 to 400 mg by mouth twice daily, alone or with other agents
2. Iniparib 5.6 mg/kg IV on days 1, 4, 8, and 11 every 21 days, together with gemcitabine and carboplatin on days 1 and 8.

Special precautions. Too early in development to have complete information.

Toxicity

1. *Myelosuppression and other hematologic effects.* Occasionally low-grade.
2. *Nausea, vomiting, and other gastrointestinal effects.* Nausea and vomiting are common, but low-grade. Diarrhea is occasional.
3. *Mucocutaneous effects.* None reported.
4. *Miscellaneous effects.* Fatigue and dizziness are occasional.

OPRELVEKIN

Other names. Neumega, IL-11.

Mechanism of action. Stimulates proliferation of hematopoietic stem cells and megakaryocyte progenitor cells and induces megakaryocyte maturation, resulting in increased platelet production.

Primary indication. Prevention of severe thrombocytopenia after chemotherapy in patients with nonmyeloid malignancies. *Not* indicated after myeloablative therapy.

Usual dosage and schedule. 50 μg/kg SC once daily, starting 6 to 24 hours after completion of chemotherapy. Continue until the postnadir count is at least 50,000/μL. (Treatment for more than 21 days in a row is not recommended.) The next planned cycle of chemotherapy should begin at least 2 days after discontinuation of oprelvekin.

Special precautions. Use with caution in patients with history of atrial arrhythmia or congestive heart failure. Allergic and anaphylactic hypersensitivity reactions have occurred.

Toxicity

1. *Myelosuppression and other hematologic effects.* None. Mild decrease in hemoglobin concentration (10% to 15%), predominantly due to increase in plasma volume.
2. *Nausea, vomiting, and other gastrointestinal effects.* None.
3. *Mucocutaneous effects.* Occasional rash, particularly at injection site.
4. *Miscellaneous effects:*
   a. Cardiovascular: Atrial arrhythmia (flutter or fibrillation) and palpitations are occasional (about 10%), but usually transient. Syncope is occasional.
   b. Fluid retention with edema (renal sodium and water retention) or dyspnea on exertion is common, but usually mild to moderate. Not associated with capillary leak syndrome.
   c. Conjunctival injection and mild visual blurring is occasional. Papilledema is uncommon, but may be more common in children. Caution should be exerted in patients with pre-existing papilledema or tumors of the CNS.
   d. Asthenia is occasional.

OXALIPLATIN

Other name. Eloxatin.

Mechanism of action. Similar to alkylating agents with respect to binding and cross-linking strands of DNA, forming DNA adducts, and thereby inhibiting DNA replication and transcription.

Primary indications

1. Carcinoma of the colon and rectum
2. Carcinoma of the stomach
3. Carcinomas of the pancreas and biliary tract.

Usual dosage and schedule

1. Combination therapy: 85 to 100 mg/m^2 as a 2-hour infusion every 2 weeks in combination with fluorouracil (often as a continuous infusion)

   2. Single agent: 130 mg/m^2 as a 2-hour infusion every 3 weeks or 85 mg/m^2 as a 3-hour infusion every 2 weeks.

Special precautions. Acute neurosensory and neuromotor symptoms may develop with the infusion. Laryngospasm may be minimized by avoiding cold drinks or food for a few days following treatment. Chronic neurosensory symptoms are dose-limiting. Must never be diluted with or administered with sodium chloride or other chloride-containing solutions.

Toxicity

   1. *Myelosuppression and other hematologic effects.* Low-grade myelosuppression is common, but grade 3 or 4 neutropenia, thrombocytopenia, or anemia is uncommon (about 5%) when used as single agent. Its use with fluorouracil and leucovorin increases the neutropenia and its severity. Hemolytic anemia is rare.
   2. *Nausea, vomiting, and other gastrointestinal effects.* Nausea, vomiting, and diarrhea are common. Severe diarrhea may lead to hypokalemia. May be worsening of cholinergic syndrome when given with irinotecan. Hepatotoxicity is common with oxaliplatin, in some cases associated with fibrosis or severe veno-occlusive lesions, but grade 3 to 4 toxicity is uncommon.
   3. *Mucocutaneous effects.* Alopecia is uncommon. Stomatitis is increased when used with fluorouracil.
   4. *Miscellaneous effects:*
   a. Neurotoxicity, consisting of paresthesias and cold-induced dysesthesias in the stocking glove or perioral distribution, are common as acute transient changes that begin with the infusion and last for less than 1 week. Chronic sensory neuropathy, fine motor disturbance, or ataxia is occasional to common with cumulative dosing (cumulative dose-dependent) and may last for months. It is occasionally grade 3 to 4. Neurotoxicity incidence and severity can be reduced by giving 1 g magnesium sulfate and 1 g calcium gluconate both before and after the oxaliplatin infusion.
   b. Laryngospasm may develop during or within 2 hours of the infusion and can last up to 5 days. Cold temperatures may induce; warm liquids or a hot-pack may ameliorate.
   c. Fever is common.
   d. Nephrotoxicity is uncommon.
   e. Ototoxicity is rare.
   f. Allergic reactions are occasional. High-grade reactions or anaphylaxis are uncommon to rare.

PACLITAXEL

Other names. Taxol, Onxol.

Mechanism of action. Enhanced formation and stabilization of microtubules. Antineoplastic effect may result from nonfunctional tubules or altered tubulin–microtubule equilibrium. Mitotic arrest is seen and is associated with accumulated polymerized microtubules.

Primary indications

1. Carcinomas of the ovary, breast, lung, head and neck, bladder, and cervix
2. Melanoma
3. Kaposi sarcoma, AIDS-related.

Usual dosage and schedule

1. 135 to 225 mg/m^2 as a 3-hour infusion every 3 weeks
2. 135 to 200 mg/m^2 as a 24-hour infusion every 3 weeks
3. 100 to 135 mg/m^2 as a 3-hour infusion every 2 to 3 weeks for the treatment of AIDS-related Kaposi sarcoma
4. 80 to 100 mg/m^2 as a 1-hour weekly infusion
5. 200 mg/m^2 as a 1-hour infusion every 3 weeks.

Special precautions. Anaphylactoid reactions with dyspnea, hypotension (or occasionally hypertension), bronchospasm, urticaria, and erythematous rashes may occur as a result of the paclitaxel itself or the polyoxyethylated castor oil vehicle required to make paclitaxel water-soluble. Such reaction is minimized but not totally prevented by pretreatment with antihistamines and corticosteroids and by prolonging the infusion rate (to 24 hours). Paclitaxel must be filtered with a 0.2-μm in-line filter.

Standard pretreatment regimen

1. Dexamethasone 20 mg IV for doses greater than 100 mg/m^2 and 10 mg IV for doses no more than 100 mg/m^2 30 to 60 minutes prior to treatment.
2. Diphenhydramine 50 mg IV 30 to 60 minutes before treatment.
3. Histamine H_2-receptor–antagonist IV 30 to 60 minutes before treatment (e.g., cimetidine 300 mg).

Toxicity

1. *Myelosuppression and other hematologic effects.* Granulocytopenia is universal and dose-limiting; thrombocytopenia is common; anemia is occasional.
2. *Nausea, vomiting, and other gastrointestinal effects.* Common but usually not severe.
3. *Mucocutaneous effects.* Alopecia is universal; mucositis is occasional at recommended doses.
4. *Immunologic effects and infusion reactions.* Dyspnea, hypotension (or occasionally hypertension), bronchospasm, urticaria, and erythematous rashes are occasionally seen, despite precautions.
5. *Miscellaneous effects:*
   a. Sensory neuropathy is common (30% to 35%) and may be progressively worse with time. Recovery may take months to years.
   b. Hepatic dysfunction is uncommon.

   c. Diarrhea is occasional and mild.

   d. Myalgias and arthralgias are common (25%).

   e. Seizures are rare.

   f. Abnormal electrocardiogram is occasional. If clinically significant bradycardia, stop drug. Restart at slower rate when stable.

PACLITAXEL, PROTEIN-BOUND

Other names. Nanometer albumin bound paclitaxel (nab-paclitaxel), Abraxane.

Mechanism of action. Albumin binding circumvents the requirement for polyoxyethylated castor oil vehicle for paclitaxel and its associated toxicity; it also exploits albumin-receptor–mediated endothelial transport. As with parent compound, intratumor paclitaxel results in enhanced formation and stabilization of microtubules. An antineoplastic effect may result from nonfunctional tubules or altered tubulin–microtubule equilibrium. Mitotic arrest is seen and is associated with accumulated polymerized microtubules.

Primary indications

   1. Metastatic carcinoma of the breast

   2. Non–small-cell carcinoma of the lung.

Usual dosage and schedule. 260 mg/m^2 IV over 30 minutes every 3 weeks.

Special precautions. Hypersensitivity reactions may occur during the infusion of nab-paclitaxel, but are rare. Premedication, as is used with paclitaxel with polyoxyethylated castor oil, is not required.

Toxicity

   1. *Myelosuppression and other hematologic effects.* Granulocytopenia is common and dose-limiting; anemia is common as well but is rarely severe. Thrombocytopenia is uncommon. Febrile neutropenia is rare.

   2. *Nausea, vomiting, and other gastrointestinal effects.* Nausea and vomiting are occasional to common but usually not severe. Diarrhea is common but rarely severe.

   3. *Mucocutaneous effects.* Alopecia is universal; mucositis is occasional.

   4. *Hypersensitivity reactions.* Uncommon and rarely severe.

   5. *Miscellaneous effects:*

      a. Cardiovascular events during the infusion, including hypotension or bradycardia, are uncommon to rare. Late cardiovascular effects are also uncommon. Abnormal ECGs are common but not associated with symptoms and usually require no intervention. Edema is occasional.

      b. Sensory neuropathy is common and may be progressively worse with time. Recovery may take months to years.

      c. Asthenia is common.

      d. Ocular or visual disturbances are occasional.

      e. Cough and dyspnea are occasional.

      f. Abnormal liver function tests are common and occasionally severe.

g. Myalgias and arthralgias are common.

h. Seizures are rare.

PAMIDRONATE

Other name. Aredia.

Mechanism of action. A bisphosphonate that inhibits osteoclastic resorption of bone and calcium release induced by tumor cytokines.

Primary indications

1. Hypercalcemia associated with malignancy
2. Osteolytic bone metastases of breast cancer
3. Osteolytic and osteoporotic bone lesions of multiple myeloma
4. Paget disease.

Usual dosage and schedule

1. Multiple myeloma: 90 mg IV as a 4-hour infusion every month
2. Breast cancer: 90 mg IV as a 2-hour infusion every 3 to 4 weeks
3. Hypercalcemia of malignancy: 60 to 90 mg IV as a 4- to 24-hour infusion. May be repeated every 1 to 8 weeks, as needed.
4. Paget disease: 30 mg IV daily as a 4-hour infusion on 3 consecutive days.

Special precautions

1. Potential for renal tubular damage, particularly if infused more rapidly. Renal clearance parallels creatinine clearance, but adverse effects do not appear to be worse with decreased clearance when given on a monthly basis. Older patients (>75 years) may be more susceptible. Serum electrolytes and renal function should be monitored closely.
2. Osteonecrosis of the jaw has been reported, primarily in association with dental procedures such as tooth extraction; such procedures should be avoided during and following bisphosphonate treatment, if possible.

Toxicity

1. *Myelosuppression and other hematologic effects.* Rare.
2. *Nausea, vomiting, and other gastrointestinal effects.* Abdominal pain, anorexia, constipation, nausea, and vomiting are uncommon to occasional.
3. *Mucocutaneous effects.* Infusion site reaction is occasional.
4. *Miscellaneous effects:*
   a. Fatigue is occasional.
   b. Laboratory abnormalities are occasional (hypocalcemia, hypokalemia, hypomagnesemia, and hypophosphatemia, particularly at the 90-mg dose).
   c. Uveitis, iritis, scleritis, and episcleritis are rare.
   d. Bone pain or generalized pain is occasional.
   e. Osteonecrosis of the jaw is uncommon to rare.

PANITUMUMAB

Other names. Vectibix, EGFR antibody, rHuMAb-EGFR.

Mechanism of action. Fully humanized EGFR antibody that blocks the ligand-binding site and inhibits proliferation of cells. It is thought potentially most useful in those tumors that overexpress EGFR, but correlation with percent of positive cells or intensity of EGFR expression is lacking.

Primary indication. Colorectal cancer.

Usual dosage and schedule. 6 mg/kg (220 mg/m^2) IV over 60 to 90 minutes every 14 days.

Special precautions. Antipanitumumab antibodies have not been seen but are possible. Severe hypomagnesemia may be seen, and all patients should have magnesium levels monitored throughout the persistence of cetuximab (8 weeks).

All patients with metastatic colorectal cancer who might be candidates for panitumumab should have their tumor tested for KRAS or BRAF mutations. If KRAS mutation in codon 12 or 13 or BRAF V600E mutation is detected, panitumumab should not be given, as the patient is unlikely to benefit.

Toxicity

1. *Myelosuppression and other hematologic effects.* Leukopenia and anemia are occasional.
2. *Nausea, vomiting, and other gastrointestinal effects.* Anorexia, nausea, vomiting, and diarrhea are occasional to common, but high-grade effects are uncommon. Abdominal pain is common.
3. *Mucocutaneous effects.* Acnelike rash and other skin changes are universal and occasionally high-grade. Exposure to sunlight may exacerbate. Pruritis, erythema, nail changes, and fissures are common. Irritation of the eyes is occasional. Growth of the eyelashes is occasional. Stomatitis is occasional.
4. *Immunologic effects and infusion reactions.* Infusion reactions with allergic or hypersensitivity reactions, fever, chills, or dyspnea are uncommon and rarely high-grade (1%). Binding antibodies develop in 1% to 5% of patients, but there has been no effect on the pharmacokinetic or toxicity profile.
5. *Miscellaneous effects:*
   a. Fatigue, headache, and back pain are common to occasional.
   b. Weight loss, peripheral edema, and dehydration are occasional.
   c. Electrolyte depletion, particularly hypomagnesemia, occurs commonly. Hypomagnesemia is occasionally severe.
   d. Pulmonary fibrosis is rare.

PAZOPANIB

Other name. Votrient.

Mechanism of action. An oral multitargeted receptor tyrosine kinase inhibitor of VEGF receptor, PDGF receptor, fibroblast growth factor receptor, and c-kit that blocks tumor growth and inhibits angiogenesis. Metabolized primarily by CYP3A4 and excreted in the stool.

Primary indication. Advanced renal cell carcinoma.

Usual dosage and schedule

1. 800 mg by mouth daily without food
2. 200 mg by mouth daily without food, if moderate hepatic impairment
3. 400 mg or less by mouth if strong inhibitors of CYP3A4 cannot be avoided.

Special precautions. May cause severe liver toxicity; therefore, liver function tests should be monitored closely before and during treatment. Do not give pazopanib if severe hepatic impairment is present. Fatal hemorrhagic events have been seen, and use in patients with history of gastrointestinal hemorrhage, hemoptysis, or cerebral hemorrhage should be avoided. If possible, avoid use of strong inhibitors of CYP3A4, which may increase concentration of pazopanib. CYP3A4 inducers may decrease pazopanib concentrations.

Toxicity

1. *Myelosuppression and other hematologic effects.* Neutropenia, thrombocytopenia, and lymphocytopenia are common but rarely severe. Arterial thrombotic events have been observed and can be fatal. Fatal hemorrhagic events have also been observed.
2. *Nausea, vomiting, and other gastrointestinal effects.* Diarrhea is common, as are nausea, vomiting, and anorexia. Gastrointestinal perforation has been observed but is probably rare. Abdominal pain is occasional.
3. *Mucocutaneous effects.* Hair color change (depigmentation) is common. Hand-foot syndrome is occasional. Skin depigmentation is uncommon.
4. *Immunologic effects and infusion reactions.* None.
5. *Miscellaneous effects:*
   a. Systemic effects: Fatigue, asthenia, and headache are occasional to common.
   b. Hepatotoxicity: ALT and AST elevations are common and occasionally (12%) severe.
   c. Cardiovascular: Hypertension is common, but grade 3 or 4 hypertension is uncommon. Prolonged QT intervals and torsades de pointes have been observed but are rare. Chest pain is uncommon.
   d. Hyponatremia, hypomagnesemia, and hypophosphatemia are occasional.
   e. Hypothyroidism is occasional.
   f. Proteinuria is occasional but rarely severe.

PEGFILGRASTIM

Other names. Neulasta, pegylated G-CSF.

Mechanism of action. Pegfilgrastim is recombinant G-CSF that is conjugated to polyethylene glycol. This delays renal clearance and increases the serum half-life from about 3.5 to about 15 to 80 hours after a single SC injection. Promotes growth and differentiation of myeloid progenitor cells. May improve survival and function of granulocytes.

Primary indication. Prophylaxis of granulocytopenia and associated infection in patients who are at high risk from chemotherapy for nonmyeloid malignancies.

Usual dosage and schedule. 6 mg SC once (usually on day 2) for each 21- or 28-day chemotherapy cycle. Should not be given between 14 days before or 24 hours after each chemotherapy cycle.

Special precautions

1. Use with caution in disorders of myeloid stem cells as it may promote growth of leukemic cells.
2. The fixed-dose formulation should not be used in infants, children, and others weighing less than 45 kg.

Toxicity

1. *Myelosuppression and other hematologic effects.* None (leukocytosis with immature forms in the peripheral blood is common).
2. *Nausea, vomiting, and other gastrointestinal effects.* Rare to uncommon.
3. *Mucocutaneous effects.* Exacerbation of pre-existing dermatologic conditions is occasional; pyoderma gangrenosum is possible.
4. *Miscellaneous effects.* Usually mild and short-lived.
   a. Bone pain, musculoskeletal symptoms such as cramps, and back or leg pain are common, but uncommonly greater than in placebo-treated patients.
   b. Splenomegaly with prolonged use is possible. Splenic rupture has been reported with the parent compound filgrastim.
   c. Exacerbation of pre-existing inflammatory or autoimmune disorders is rare.
   d. Mild elevation of LDH and alkaline phosphatase.
   e. Allergic-type reactions may occur, as they have been seen with the parent compound filgrastim.
   f. Adult respiratory distress syndrome has been reported in neutropenic patients receiving filgrastim and is possible with pegfilgrastim.

PEMETREXED

Other name. Alimta.

Mechanism of action. Interference with folate-dependent metabolic processes, including inhibition of thymidylate synthase, dihydrofolate reductase, and glycinamide ribonucleotide formyltransferase, largely after being converted to polyglutamate forms.

Primary indications

1. Malignant pleural mesothelioma that is unresectable or not amenable to curative surgery. Given in combination with cisplatin.
2. Nonsquamous, non–small-cell lung cancer, as first- or second-line therapy and as maintenance after remission induction
3. Carcinoma of the ovary.

Usual dosage and schedule. 500 mg/m^2 IV over 10 minutes on day 1 of each 21-day cycle. For mesothelioma, it is followed in 30 minutes by cisplatin 75 mg/m^2 over 2 hours.

Special precautions

1. Folic acid 1 to 2 mg by mouth daily in divided doses, starting 7 days prior to pemetrexed and continuing for 21 days after the last dose, and vitamin B$_{12}$ 1000 μg IM during the week prior to pemetrexed and every three cycles thereafter must be taken as a prophylactic measure to reduce treatment-related hematologic and gastrointestinal toxicity.
2. Dexamethasone 4 mg by mouth twice daily the day before, the day of, and the day after pemetrexed should be given to reduce skin rash.
3. If creatinine clearance is less than 45 mL/min, give with caution and avoid NSAIDs.

Toxicity

1. *Myelosuppression and other hematologic effects.* Anemia and neutropenia are common when used with cisplatin and only occasional when used as a single agent; severe episodes are only occasional; thrombocytopenia is occasional.
2. *Nausea, vomiting, and other gastrointestinal effects.* Anorexia, nausea, vomiting, and diarrhea are occasional. Liver function abnormalities are occasional.
3. *Mucocutaneous effects.* Rash and pruritis are occasional. Stomatitis and pharyngitis are common. Alopecia is occasional. Taste disturbances are occasional. Conjunctivitis is uncommon.
4. *Immune suppression can occur.*
5. *Miscellaneous effects:*
   a. Fever is uncommon.
   b. Serum creatinine elevation is occasional; renal failure is rare.
   c. Fatigue is common. Myalgia and arthralgia are occasional. Sensory neuropathy is occasional.
   d. Hypersensitivity reactions are occasional but rarely severe.
   e. Supraventricular arrythmias are rare.

PENTOSTATIN

Other names. 2′-deoxycoformycin, Nipent.

Mechanism of action. Inhibition of adenosine deaminase, particularly in the presence of adenosine or deoxyadenosine, leads to cytotoxicity. Is associated with block of DNA synthesis through inhibition of ribonucleotide reductase. Other effects that may contribute to cytotoxicity include inhibition of RNA synthesis and increased DNA damage.

Primary indication. Hairy-cell leukemia.

Usual dosage and schedule. 4 mg/m^2 IV push over 1 to 2 minutes or diluted in a larger volume over 20 to 30 minutes. Patients should be given hydration with 500 to 1000 mL of 5% dextrose in 0.5 N saline or equivalent before pentostatin administration and 500 mL after the drug is given. Repeat every 2 weeks.

Special precautions. Hydration is required to ensure urine output of 2 L daily on the day pentostatin is administered. Patients often are hospitalized for their first drug administration. Allopurinol 300 mg twice a day is recommended in patients with a large tumor mass. Sedative and hypnotic drugs should be used with caution or not at all because CNS toxicity may be potentiated. Dose reduction or discontinuation needed for renal impairment (creatinine clearance <50 mL/minute).

Should not be used in combination with fludarabine because of a high probability of severe or fatal pulmonary toxicity.

Toxicity

1. *Myelosuppression and other hematologic effects.* Common but severity variable.
2. *Nausea, vomiting, and other gastrointestinal effects.* Nausea and vomiting are common but usually not severe. Diarrhea is occasional. Hepatic dysfunction is occasional at recommended doses.
3. *Mucocutaneous effects.* Mucositis is rare; skin rashes and pruritis are occasional to common.
4. *Miscellaneous effects.*
   a. Fatigue is common.
   b. Cough is common and dyspnea is occasional. Higher doses or use in combination with fludarabine may lead to severe pulmonary toxicity.
   c. Chills and fever are common.
   d. Infections, probably related both to myelosuppression and lymphocytopenia, are occasional.
   e. Renal insufficiency is rare at usual doses.
   f. Neuropsychiatric effects: High doses may cause serious neurologic and psychiatric symptoms, including seizures, mental confusion, irritability, and coma.

PRALATREXATE

Other name. Folotyn.

Mechanism of action. Pralatrexate is a folate analog that competitively inhibits dihydrofolate reductase. It is also an inhibitor for polyglutamylation by folylpolyglutamyl synthetase.

Primary indication. Relapsed or refractory peripheral T-cell lymphoma.

Usual dosage and schedule. 30 mg/m^2 IV push over 3 to 5 minutes weekly for 6 weeks in 7-week cycles.

Patients should take 1 to 1.25 mg oral folic acid daily starting 10 days prior to the first dose of pralatrexate as well as 1 mg of vitamin B$_{12}$ IM, which should be administered every 8 to 10 weeks during treatment.

Special precautions. Omitting a dose, with or without subsequent dose modifications, is required for mucositis that is greater than grade 1 and significant cytopenias (ANC <1000/μL; platelets <50,000/μL).

Toxicity

1. *Myelosuppression and other hematologic effects.* Thrombocytopenia, anemia, and neutropenia are common. Grade 3 or 4 thrombocytopenia is common, but grade 3 or 4 neutropenia is less frequent (~20%).
2. *Nausea, vomiting, and other gastrointestinal effects.* Nausea, vomiting, and diarrhea are common, but it is rare to uncommon that they are severe. Constipation is common. Anorexia and abdominal pain are occasional.
3. *Mucocutaneous effects.* Mucositis is very common (70%) and may be associated with a sore throat; grade 3 to 4 mucositis occurs about 20% of the time. Epistaxis is common. Rash and pruritis are occasional.
4. *Immunologic effects and infusion reactions.* Not reported.
5. *Miscellaneous effects:*
   a. Fatigue and fever are common.
   b. Cardiorespiratory effects: Cough, dyspnea, and edema are common. Tachycardia is occasional.
   c. Hypokalemia and elevated transaminases are occasional.

PROCARBAZINE

Other names. Matulane, Natulan.

Mechanism of action. Uncertain but appears to affect preformed DNA, RNA, and protein.

Primary indications

1. Hodgkin and non-Hodgkin lymphomas
2. Brain tumors
3. Melanoma.

Usual dosage and schedule. 60 to 100 mg/m^2 by mouth daily for 7 to 14 days every 4 weeks (in combination with other drugs).

Special precautions. Many food and drug interactions are possible, although their clinical significance may be low.

Drug or Food	Possible Result
Ethanol	Disulfiram-like reactions: nausea, vomiting, visual disturbances, headache
Sympathomimetics, tricyclic antidepressants, tyramine-rich foods (cheese, wine, bananas)	Hypertensive crisis, tremors, excitation, angina, cardiac palpitations
CNS depressants	Additive depression

Toxicity

1. *Myelosuppression and other hematologic effects.* Pancytopenia is dose-limiting. Recovery may be delayed.
2. *Nausea, vomiting, and other gastrointestinal effects.* Nausea is frequent during first few days until tolerance develops. Diarrhea is uncommon.
3. *Mucocutaneous effects.* Stomatitis is uncommon. Alopecia, pruritus, and drug rash are uncommon.
4. *CNS effects.* Paresthesias, neuropathies, headache, dizziness, depression, apprehension, nervousness, insomnia, nightmares, hallucinations, ataxia, confusion, convulsions, and coma have been reported with varying frequency.
5. *Miscellaneous effects:*
   a. Secondary neoplasia is possible.
   b. Visual disturbances are rare.
   c. Postural hypotension is rare.
   d. Hypersensitivity reactions are rare.
   e. Teratogenesis is strong potential.

PROGESTINS

Other names. Medroxyprogesterone acetate (Provera, Depo-Provera), hydroxyprogesterone caproate (Delalutin), megestrol acetate (Megace).

Mechanism of action. Mechanisms of antitumor effects or for appetite stimulation are not clear.

Primary indications

1. Endometrial carcinoma
2. Appetite stimulation.

Usual dosage and schedule

1. Megestrol acetate 80 to 320 mg by mouth daily
2. Medroxyprogesterone acetate 1000 to 1500 mg IM weekly or 400 to 800 mg by mouth twice weekly
3. Hydroxyprogesterone caproate 1000 to 1500 mg IM weekly.

Special precautions. Acute local hypersensitivity or dyspnea due to oil in IM preparations is uncommon. Hypercalcemia with initial therapy is occasional, particularly in patients with bone metastasis.

Toxicity

1. *Myelosuppression and other hematologic effects.* None.
2. *Nausea, vomiting, and other gastrointestinal effects.* Rare; is an appetite stimulant (800 mg by mouth daily).
3. *Mucocutaneous effects.* Mild alopecia or skin rash are uncommon.
4. *Miscellaneous effects:*
   a. Mild fluid retention is occasional to common.
   b. Mild liver function abnormalities are occasional; intrahepatic cholestasis may occur.
   c. Menstrual irregularities are common.
   d. Increased appetite and weight gain are common.

RALOXIFENE

Other name. Evista.

Mechanism of action. A selective estrogen-receptor modulator that inhibits estrogen effects by competing with estrogen for binding on the cytosol estrogen-receptor protein in normal and cancer cells. The receptor-hormone complex ultimately controls the promoter region of genes that affect cell growth. Effects may manifest as estrogen agonistic (bone) or antagonistic (breast and uterus), depending on the tissue and other modifying factors.

Primary indications

1. Prevention of osteoporosis in postmenopausal women
2. Prevention of invasive breast cancer in postmenopausal women at increased risk. (No apparent decrease in ductal or lobular in situ carcinomas.)

Usual dosage and schedule. 60 mg by mouth daily.

Special precautions. Contraindicated in women with active or past history of venous thromboembolic events, including deep vein thrombosis, pulmonary embolism, and retinal vein thrombosis. May cause fetal harm if administered to a pregnant woman.

Toxicity

1. *Myelosuppression and other hematologic effects.* Uncommon and mild.
2. *Nausea, vomiting, and other gastrointestinal effects.* Uncommon.
3. *Mucocutaneous effects.* Rash, sweating, and vaginitis are uncommon.
4. *Miscellaneous effects:*
   a. Thromboembolic events, including deep vein thrombosis, pulmonary embolism, and retinal vein thrombosis, are rare. Lower risk than with tamoxifen.

   b. Leg cramps are uncommon to occasional.

   c. Hot flashes are common.

   d. Lowers total cholesterol and low-density lipoprotein cholesterol.

5. *Carcinogenesis.* Risk for endometrial carcinoma is rare (0.5%) and lower than with tamoxifen (0.75%).

RITUXIMAB

Other name. Rituxan.

Mechanism of action. Rituximab is a genetically engineered chimeric (murine and human) monoclonal antibody directed against the CD20 antigen found on the surface of normal cells and in high copy number on malignant B-lymphocytes (but not stem cells). The F_{ab} domain of rituximab binds to the CD20 antigen on B-lymphocytes and B-cell non-Hodgkin lymphomas, and the F_c domain recruits immune effector functions to mediate B-cell lysis.

Primary indications

1. Non-Hodgkin B-cell lymphoma that is low-grade or follicular, and CD20-positive, as a single agent or in combination or sequence with cytotoxic chemotherapy

2. Non-Hodgkin lymphoma, diffuse large B-cell and CD20-positive, in combination or sequence with cytotoxic chemotherapy

3. Other B-cell Non-Hodgkin lymphomas

4. CLL, usually in combination or sequence with fludarabine, cyclophosphamide, or both.

Usual dosage and schedule

1. 375 mg/m^2 given as a slow IV infusion, initially at a rate of 50 mg/hr. If hypersensitivity or other infusion-related events do not occur, escalate in 50-mg/hr increments to a maximum of 400 mg/hr. Usually takes 4 to 6 hours to infuse initial therapy. Interrupt or slow the infusion rate for infusion-related events. As a single agent, often given once weekly for four to eight doses; in combination with cytotoxic chemotherapy, often given on day 1 or 2 of each cycle of chemotherapy. Premedication with acetaminophen and diphenhydramine may attenuate infusion-related symptoms. Corticosteroids should not be used for premedication.

2. For CLL when used with fludarabine and cyclophosphamide: 375 mg/m^2 given as a slow IV infusion (as in *1*) on the day prior to the first cycle of fludarabine and cyclophosphamide, then 500 mg/m^2 as an IV infusion on day 1 of each subsequent 28-day cycle.

Special precautions

1. An infusion-related set of symptoms consisting of fever and chills, with or without true rigors, occurs commonly during the first infusion.

Other hypersensitivity symptoms including nausea, urticaria, fatigue, headache, pruritus, bronchospasm, dyspnea, sensation of tongue or throat swelling, rhinitis, vomiting, hypotension, flushing, and pain at disease sites may also be seen. Rarely, infusion-related events result in a fatal outcome. Fatal reactions have followed a symptom complex that includes hypoxia, pulmonary infiltrates, acute respiratory distress syndrome, myocardial infarction, ventricular fibrillation, and cardiogenic shock. Hypersensitivity reactions generally start within 30 to 120 minutes of starting the infusion. Most will resolve with slowing or interruption of the infusion and with supportive care, including IV saline, diphenhydramine, and acetaminophen. Severe reactions will additionally require aggressive cardiorespiratory support including oxygen, epinephrine, vasopressors, corticosteroids, and bronchodilators and may preclude additional treatment with rituximab. The rate of infusion events decreases from 80% during the first infusion to 40% during subsequent infusions.

2. Abdominal pain, bowel obstruction, and perforation have been seen in patients receiving rituximab in combination with chemotherapy.

3. Hepatitis B reactivation with related fulminant hepatitis and other viral infections, including parvovirus B19, varicella-zoster, cytomegalovirus, and herpes simplex virus, have been reported. Obtaining a hepatitis panel (A, B, and C) is recommended. Hepatitis B surface antigen is a particular reason to monitor liver function closely. If HBsAG positive, consider monitoring serum viral load and administering antiviral prophylaxis.

Toxicity

1. *Myelosuppression and other hematologic effects.* Uncommon. However, B-cell depletion occurs in 70% to 80% of patients, with decreased immunoglobulins in a minority of patients. Infectious events occur in about 30% of patients treated with rituximab, but only uncommonly are they severe.

2. *Nausea, vomiting, and other gastrointestinal effects.* Nausea is common (23%) but rarely severe. Vomiting and diarrhea are occasional. Bowel obstruction and perforation is rare.

3. *Mucocutaneous effects.* Pruritus, rash, urticaria, and night sweats are occasional. Severe mucocutaneous reactions including Stevens-Johnson syndrome, lichenoid dermatitis, vesiculobullous dermatitis, and toxic epidermal necrolysis are rare but have been reported from 1 to 13 weeks following rituximab exposure.

4. *Immunologic effects and infusion reactions.* Infusion-related hypersensitivity reaction (may include fever, chills, headache, myalgia, weakness, nausea, urticaria, pruritus, throat irritation, rhinitis, dizziness, and hypertension) is common but usually resolves with interrupting or slowing the rate of the infusion and administration of supportive therapy (see Special precautions).

5. *Miscellaneous effects:*
   a. Myalgia and arthralgia are occasional. Rarely, a serum sickness–like reaction may be seen that requires corticosteroid therapy.
   b. Hypotension is occasional but rarely severe. Chest pain, bronchospasm, tachycardia, increased cough, edema, and postural hypotension are uncommon. Severe though potentially fatal cardiac events, including angioedema, arrhythmia, and angina, are rare.
   c. Renal failure, possibly requiring dialysis, has been seen, particularly in association with tumor lysis syndrome in patients with high tumor cell burden. Also may be seen if used in combination with cisplatin.
   d. Hepatitis B reactivation with related fulminant hepatitis is rare.
   e. Dizziness and anxiety are occasional.
   f. Progressive multifocal leukoencephalopathy has been observed in patients with rheumatoid arthritis treated with rituximab.

ROMIDEPSIN

Other name. Istodax.

Mechanism of action. Inhibits histone deacetylases (HDACs), enzymes that catalyze the removal of acetyl groups from lysine residues in histone and thereby modulate gene expression. In some cancer cell lines, this inhibition allows the accumulation of acetylated histones and induces cell cycle arrest and apoptosis.

Primary indication. CTCL in patients who have received at least one prior systemic therapy.

Usual dosage and schedule. 14 mg/m^2 IV over 4 hours on days 1, 8, and 15 of a 28-day cycle.

Special precautions. There is a risk of QT prolongation; be sure that potassium and magnesium are within the normal range before administration. Because romidepsin is metabolized by CYP3A4, avoid coadministration with strong inhibitors or inducers of CYP3A4 if possible.

Toxicity

1. *Myelosuppression and other hematologic effects.* Anemia, neutropenia, lymphopenia, and thrombocytopenia are common. Infections are common and may be fatal.
2. *Nausea, vomiting, and other gastrointestinal effects.* Nausea, vomiting, and anorexia are common. Constipation is occasional to common.
3. *Mucocutaneous effects.* Dermatitis, including exfoliative dermatitis and pruritis, are occasional to common.

4. *Miscellaneous effects:*
   a. Fatigue and fever are common.
   b. ECG T-wave and ST-segment changes are common but of uncertain significance. Supraventricular arrythmias and ventricular arrythmias have been observed. There is risk of QT prolongation, particularly in those with a history of congenital long QT syndrome, significant cardiovascular disease, or taking medications that lead to significant QT prolongation. Monitoring of electrolytes and ECG at baseline and during treatment is recommended. Hypotension is occasional.
   c. Hypomagnesemia, hypokalemia, hypocalcemia, and hyperuricemia are occasional to common but only rarely severe.
   d. Elevated transaminases are occasional to common but only rarely severe. However, use caution when using warfarin (Coumadin) or warfarin derivatives.

SARGRAMOSTIM

Other names. Granulocyte-macrophage colony-stimulating factor (GM-CSF), Leukine.

Mechanism of action. Promotes growth and differentiation of myeloid progenitor cells. May improve survival and function of granulocytes, eosinophils, monocytes, and macrophages. Induces release of secondary cytokines (IL-1 and tumor necrosis factor).

Primary indications

1. Myeloid reconstitution after peripheral blood or bone marrow progenitor cell transplantation
2. Neutrophil recovery following chemotherapy in AML
3. Mobilization of peripheral blood progenitor cells
4. Granulocytopenia from primary marrow disorders, such as MDS or aplastic anemia
5. Granulocytopenia associated with AIDS and its therapy.

Usual dosage and schedule

1. Myeloid reconstitution after autologous stem cell transplantation: 250 μg/m^2 IV daily as a 2-hour infusion beginning 2 to 4 hours after the autologous stem cell infusion and not less than 24 hours after the last dose of chemotherapy or less than 12 hours after the last dose of radiotherapy. Continue for 21 days or until the ANC reaches 20,000/μL.
2. Bone marrow transplantation failure or engraftment delay: 250 μg/m^2 daily for 14 days as 2-hour IV infusion. If no marrow recovery, may be repeated in 7 days at same or higher dose (500 μg/m^2). Dose and duration are dependent on the response.
3. Mobilization of peripheral blood progenitor cells: The recommended dose is 250 μg/m^2/day administered IV over 24 hours or

SC once daily. Dosing should continue at the same dose through the period of peripheral blood progenitor cell collection.

4. Neutrophil recovery following chemotherapy in AML: 250 $\mu g/m^2/$ day administered IV over a 4-hour period starting 4 days following the completion of induction chemotherapy and continuing until the ANC is greater than 1500 cells/μL for 3 consecutive days or a maximum of 42 days.

5. Aplastic anemia, MDS, and AIDS: Doses may be much lower (50 to 100 $\mu g/m^2$ SC or IM daily).

Special precautions. Flushing, tachycardia, dyspnea, and nausea occur commonly with the first dose of IV therapy; do not infuse over less than 2 hours; longer infusion may help.

Toxicity

1. *Myelosuppression and other hematologic effects.* None (leukocytosis).
2. *Nausea, vomiting, and other gastrointestinal effects.* Occasional.
3. *Mucocutaneous effects.* Rash is uncommon; exacerbation of pre-existing dermatologic conditions is occasional; mild local reactions at injection site are common.
4. *Miscellaneous effects.* Usually mild and short-lived at standard doses, but with increasing dose, may be more severe.
   a. Bone pain, musculoskeletal symptoms such as cramps and back or leg pain are common.
   b. Pericarditis, fluid retention, and venous thrombosis are dose-related and uncommon at standard doses.
   c. Flulike symptoms (fever, chills, aches, headache) are occasional at standard doses and common at higher doses.

SIPULEUCEL-T

Other name. Provenge.

Mechanism of action. The drug is a patient-specific (autologous) vaccine consisting of peripheral blood mononuclear cells, including antigen presenting cells (APCs), that have been collected by leukapheresis, sent to the manufacturing center, activated during a defined culture period with a recombinant human protein (prostatic acid phosphatase [PAP]-GM-CSF), and returned to the treating center for infusion. During ex vivo culture with PAP-GM-CSF, APCs take up and process the recombinant target antigen into small peptides that are then displayed on the APC surface and returned to the patient, stimulating an immune response by the patient's T-cells against tumor cells expressing PAP.

Primary indication. Hormone refractory carcinoma of the prostate.

Usual dosage and schedule. Each dose of sipuleucel-T contains a minimum of 50 million autologous CD54+ cells activated with PAP-GM-CSF.

The recommended course of therapy is three complete doses, given IV at approximately 2-week intervals. In controlled clinical trials, the median dosing interval between infusions was 2 weeks (range 1 to 15 weeks); the maximum dosing interval has not been established.

If, for any reason, the patient is unable to receive a scheduled infusion of sipuleucel-T, the patient will need to undergo an additional leukapheresis procedure if the course of treatment is to be continued. Patients should be advised of this possibility prior to initiating treatment.

Special precautions. Severe infusion reactions are uncommon but are greater after the second than the first infusion.

Toxicity

1. *Myelosuppression and other hematologic effects.* None reported.
2. *Nausea, vomiting, and other gastrointestinal effects.* Occasional to common.
3. *Mucocutaneous effects.* Rash and sweating are uncommon.
4. *Immunologic effects and infusion reactions.* Chills, fever, fatigue, dyspnea, hypoxia, bronchospasm, back pain, nausea, vomiting, hypertension, tachycardia, joint ache, and headache are common. For most patients, these reactions are mild or moderate.
5. *Miscellaneous effects:*
   a. Weakness and influenza-like illness are occasional.
   b. Both hemorrhagic and ischemic strokes have been observed uncommonly.

SOMATOSTATIN ANALOGS

Other names. Octreotide, Sandostatin, Sandostatin LAR depot (other related analogs are pasireotide and lanreotide).

Mechanism of action. Somatostatin analog that inhibits release of polypeptide hormones, particularly in the pancreas and gut. Slows gastrointestinal transit time. Promotes water and electrolyte absorption, reflecting change from overall secretory to absorptive state.

Primary indications

1. Carcinoid tumors
2. Vasoactive intestinal peptide tumors and other amine precursor uptake and decarboxylation tumors
3. Chemotherapy-induced diarrhea
4. Acromegaly.

Usual dosage and schedule. 100 to 1500 μg/day SC of the nondepot prepration, in two to four divided doses. Doses are usually started at the lower end and titrated upward to the best symptomatic improvement. If patients respond favorably to the rapid acting SC injections, they may be maintained on 20 mg IM of the depot preparation by intragluteal injection every 4 weeks. Caution should be used in treating for more than 3 months.

Special precautions. Lower doses indicated if severe renal dysfunction (creatinine >5 mg/dL).

Toxicity

1. *Myelosuppression and other hematologic effects.* None.
2. *Nausea, vomiting, and other gastrointestinal effects.* Nausea, abdominal discomfort, bloating, and diarrhea are common, particularly in early therapy. Vomiting is only occasionally seen. Decreased gallbladder contractility and decreased bile secretion may result in biliary abnormalities. Gallstones develop in less than 2% if treatment is for 1 month or less but can be 25% if treatment is for 1 year or more. Ascending cholangitis and pancreatitis are uncommon to rare.
3. *Mucocutaneous effects.* Local site reactions are occasional; other effects are rare.
4. *Miscellaneous effects:*
   a. Hypoglycemia or hyperglycemia is uncommon; hypothalamic pituitary dysfunction is rare.
   b. Bradycardia and other conduction abnormalities occur in up to 25% of patients with acromegaly who are treated with octreotide.

SORAFENIB

Other name. Nexavar.

Mechanism of action. Inhibition of multiple tyrosine kinases and serine/threonine kinases within tumor cells and tumor vasculature, resulting in decreased tumor cell proliferation and reduction of tumor angiogenesis.

Primary indications

1. Renal cell carcinoma
2. Angiosarcoma, GISTs
3. Hepatocellular carcinoma
4. Metastatic papillary, medullary, follicular, and Hürthle cell thyroid carcinoma.

Usual dosage and schedule. 400 mg by mouth twice daily either without food or with a moderate fat meal.

Special precautions. Increased risk of bleeding compared with placebo. In patients also taking warfarin, sorafenib may increase the PT and INR, resulting in increased risk of bleeding. May increase AUC of compounds metabolized by UGT1A1 pathway (e.g., irinotecan). Also increases AUC of docetaxel, doxorubicin, and in some patients, fluorouracil.

Toxicity

1. *Myelosuppression and other hematologic effects.* Lymphopenia is common; anemia, neutropenia, and thrombocytopenia are occasional;

various bleeding events (including epistaxis, gastrointestinal hemorrhage, respiratory tract hemorrhage, hematomas) are common but only rarely life-threatening.

2. *Nausea, vomiting, and other gastrointestinal effects.* Diarrhea is common (33%); nausea and vomiting are occasional to common (10% to 20%); anorexia and constipation are occasional. Increased amylase and lipase are common, and transient increases in transaminases are occasional. Clinical pancreatitis is uncommon. Gastrointestinal perforation is rare.

3. *Mucocutaneous effects.* Hand-foot skin reaction is common (27%). Alopecia is common (23%). Pruritis is occasional to common (17%). Other skin changes are rare to uncommon.

4. *Miscellaneous effects:*
  a. Hypertension, usually mild to moderate, is occasional. Hypertensive crisis is rare.
  b. Fatigue is common.
  c. Sensory neuropathy is occasional (10%).
  d. Hypophosphatemia is common (41%; unknown etiology).
  e. Cardiac ischemia or infarction are uncommon.

STREPTOZOCIN

Other name. Zanosar.

Mechanism of action. Inhibition of DNA synthesis, possibly by interference with pyridine nucleotide synthesis. Streptozocin appears to have some specificity for neoplastic pancreatic endocrine cells. Glucose moiety attached to nitrosourea appears to diminish myelotoxicity.

Primary indications

  1. Pancreatic islet cell and pancreatic exocrine carcinomas
  2. Carcinoid tumors.

Usual dosage and schedule

  1. 1.0 to 1.5 g/m^2 IV weekly for 6 weeks followed by 4 weeks of observation
  2. 1 g/m^2 IV on days 1 and 8 in combination with fluorouracil and mitomycin. Repeat every 4 weeks.
  3. 500 mg/m^2 IV on days 1 to 5 every 6 weeks.

Special precautions

  1. A 30- to 60-minute infusion is recommended to reduce local pain and burning around the vein during treatment.
  2. Avoid extravasation.
  3. Have 50% glucose available to treat sudden hypoglycemia.

Toxicity

1. *Myelosuppression and other hematologic effects.* Uncommon and mild.
2. *Nausea, vomiting, and other gastrointestinal effects.* Nausea and vomiting are common and severe. May become progressively worse over 5-day course of therapy.
3. *Mucocutaneous effects.* Uncommon.
4. *Miscellaneous effects:*
   a. Renal toxicity is common. Although it is not clearly dose-related, it may limit continued drug use in individual patients. Proteinuria, glucosuria, azotemia, and hypophosphatemia, if persistent or severe, are indications to discontinue therapy. Hydration may ameliorate the problem.
   b. Hypoglycemia: In patients with insulinoma, hypoglycemia may be severe (although transient), owing to a burst of insulin release.
   c. Hyperglycemia is uncommon in normal or diabetic patients, as normal β cells are usually insensitive to the effects of streptozocin.
   d. Transient mild hepatotoxicity is occasional.
   e. Second malignancies are possible.

SUNITINIB

Other names. Sutent, Sunitinib malate.

Mechanism of action. Inhibition of multiple RTKs, including PDGF receptors, VEGF receptors, and several forms of the mutation-activated stem cell factor receptor (KIT), with consequent inhibition of tumor cells expressing dysregulated target RTKs and tumor angiogenesis. Metabolized primarily by the cytochrome P450 enzyme allele, CYP34A.

Primary indications

1. GIST that has shown progression during prior treatment with imatinib or in patients who are intolerant to imatinib
2. Advanced renal cell carcinoma
3. Neuroendocrine tumors of the pancreas
4. Angiosarcoma
5. Metastatic papillary, medullary, follicular, and Hürthle cell thyroid carcinoma.

Usual dosage and schedule. 50 mg by mouth daily for 4 weeks followed by a 2-week rest, with incremental dose reductions or increase (12.5 mg/day) based on tolerability.

Special precautions. Dose reduction should be considered when administered concurrently with strong CYP3A4 inhibitors. Dose increase should be considered when administered concurrently with strong CYP3A4 inducers. Prolonged QT intervals and torsade de pointes have been observed. Use with caution in patients at higher risk for developing QT interval prolongation.

Toxicity

1. *Myelosuppression and other hematologic effects.* Myelosuppression and lymphopenia are common, but it is uncommon to rare for them to be high grade (3 or 4). Bleeding is occasional, with possible tumor-related hemorrhage. Venous thromboembolic events are uncommon.

2. *Nausea, vomiting, and other gastrointestinal effects.* Diarrhea, nausea, vomiting, anorexia, and abdominal pain are common. Rare fatal gastrointestinal complications, including perforation, have been seen. Hepatic and pancreatic enzyme elevations and other liver function abnormalities are occasional to common.

3. *Mucocutaneous effects.* Stomatitis is common. Skin discoloration is common. Rash and hand-foot syndrome are occasional. Alopecia is uncommon.

4. *Miscellaneous effects:*
   a. Congestive heart failure with decrease in left ventricular ejection fraction to below the lower limit of normal is occasional (15%).
   b. Hypertension is occasional, but severe hypertension is uncommon.
   c. Adrenal insufficiency is possible, based on animal studies.
   d. Asthenia, headache, arthralgia, myalgia, oral pain, and back pain are occasional.
   e. Cough and dyspnea are occasional.
   f. Renal function abnormalities (low-grade) are occasional. Hypo- and hyperkalemia, hypo- and hypernatremia, and hypophosphatemia are occasional.
   g. Hypothyroidism is uncommon.
   h. Edema is occasional.

TAMOXIFEN

Other name. Nolvadex.

Mechanism of action. Tamoxifen is a selective estrogen-receptor modulator that inhibits estrogen effects by competing with estrogen for binding on the cytosol estrogen-receptor protein in cancer cells. This complex is probably transported into the nucleus, where it affects nucleic acid function. It also has effects on cellular growth factors, epidermal growth factors, and TGF-α and TGF-β.

Primary indications

1. Breast carcinoma
   a. Metastatic tumors in postmenopausal or premenopausal women with estrogen-receptor–positive (or unknown) tumors.
   b. Adjuvant therapy in premenopausal women with estrogen-receptor–positive (or progesterone-receptor–positive) tumors after primary therapy. Optimal duration of therapy for most premenopausal women is 5 years. For postmenopausal women,

aromatase inhibitors are substituted after 2 to 3 years of tamoxifen or given instead of tamoxifen.

c. Breast cancer prevention in very high-risk women, including women with carcinoma in situ of the breast after primary therapy.

Usual dosage and schedule. 20 mg by mouth as single daily dose.

Special precautions. Hypercalcemia may be seen during initial therapy. Use of selective serotonin reuptake inhibitors (except citalopram, escitalopram, and the serotonin-norepinephrine reuptake inhibitor venlafaxine) with tamoxifen decreases formation of endoxifen, the active metabolite of tamoxifen, by inhibition of CYP2D6, and should be avoided, if possible.

Toxicity

1. *Myelosuppression and other hematologic effects.* Myelosuppression is uncommon and mild. Thromboembolic phenomena are rare.
2. *Nausea, vomiting, and other gastrointestinal effects.* Nausea occurs early in the course of therapy in up to 20% of patients but abates rapidly as therapy is continued. Diarrhea is occasional.
3. *Mucocutaneous effects.* Cataracts and other eye toxicities have been observed, but effects due to drug are uncommon. Skin rash and pruritus vulvae are uncommon. May cause increase or marked decrease in vaginal secretions and result in difficult or painful intercourse.
4. *Miscellaneous effects:*
   a. Thromboembolism and strokes are rare but increased among women taking tamoxifen.
   b. Hot flashes are common.
   c. Vaginal bleeding and menstrual irregularity are uncommon to occasional.
   d. Lassitude, headache, leg cramps, and dizziness are uncommon.
   e. Peripheral edema is occasional.
   f. Increased bone pain, tumor pain, and local disease flare (associated both with good tumor response as well as with tumor progression) are occasional.
   g. Slowed progression of osteoporosis.
   h. Reduction in serum cholesterol with favorable changes in lipid profile.
   i. Liver function test abnormalities are occasional.
5. Uterine carcinomas are rare (two to four times the predicted incidence in adjuvant trials).

TEMOZOLOMIDE

Other name. Temodar.

Mechanism of action. Undergoes rapid conversion to the reactive substituted imidazole carboxamide, MTIC. This compound is believed to be active primarily through alkyation (methylation) of DNA at the O^6 and N^7 positions of guanine.

Primary indications

1. Glioblastoma, concurrently with radiotherapy and as maintenance after radiotherapy
2. Anaplastic astrocytoma that is refractory to nitrosoureas
3. Melanoma
4. Metastatic carcinomas to the brain.

Usual dosage and schedule

1. 150 to 200 mg/m^2 by mouth on an empty stomach daily for 5 days every 28 days
2. 75 mg/m^2 by mouth on an empty stomach daily during radiation therapy for up to 7 weeks.

Special precautions. Contraindicated in patients with a hypersensitivity to dacarbazine, since both drugs are metabolized to MTIC. Preventive treatment for *Pneumocystis jiroveci* pneumonia is required when temozolomide is administered with radiotherapy.

Toxicity

1. *Myelosuppression and other hematologic effects.* Myelosuppression with anemia, thrombocytopenia, and neutropenia is common and dose-dependent, but only occasionally is it severe.
2. *Nausea, vomiting, and other gastrointestinal effects.* Nausea and constipation are common, but usually not severe. Vomiting is occasional as is anorexia. Abdominal pain is uncommon.
3. *Mucocutaneous effects.* Rash and pruritis are occasional. Alopecia is common.
4. *Miscellaneous effects:*
   a. Headache, fatigue, asthenia, and fever are common (20% to 65%).
   b. Peripheral edema is occasional.
   c. Neurologic symptoms are common on temozolomide, but it is difficult to distinguish whether the symptoms are from the drug or the disease. Common findings are convulsions, hemiparesis, dizziness, abnormal coordination, amnesia, or insomnia. Occasional findings are paresthesias, somnolence, paresis, incontinence, ataxia, dysphasia, gait abnormality, myalgias, and confusion. Diplopia or other visual abnormalities are occasional.
   d. Anxiety and depression are occasional.
   e. Upper respiratory and urinary tract infections are occasional.
   f. MDS, acute leukemia, and other secondary malignancies have been observed.

TEMSIROLIMUS

Other names. Torisel, CCI-779.

Mechanism of action. After temsirolimus complexes with the immunophilin FKBP12, the complex inhibits mTOR kinase activity. mTOR, as a master regulator of cell physiology, is involved in regulation of cell growth and angiogenesis, and changes that are induced downstream from mTOR as a consequence of the temsirolimus inhibition lead to cell cycle arrest at the G_1 phase.

Primary indication. Renal cell carcinoma.

Usual dosage and schedule

1. 25 mg IV over a 30- to 60-minute period weekly
2. Reduce dose to 12.5 mg/week if patients must be coadministered a strong CYP3A4 inhibitor
3. An increase from 25 mg/week up to 50 mg/week should be considered if patients must be coadministered a strong CYP3A4 inducer.

Special precautions. The concomitant use of strong CYP3A4 inhibitors or inducers should be avoided, if possible. Not recommended in combination with sunitinib. Avoid live vaccines.

Toxicity

1. *Myelosuppression and other hematologic effects.* Anemia and thrombocytopenia are common. Venous thrombosis and embolism are uncommon.
2. *Nausea, vomiting, and other gastrointestinal effects.* Anorexia, nausea, and vomiting are common. Diarrhea and abdominal pain are common. Bowel perforation may occur rarely.
3. *Mucocutaneous effects.* Mucositis is common. Maculopapular rash or acne are common. Nail disorders are common. Wound healing may be impaired.
4. *Immunologic effects and infusion reactions.* Hypersensitivity reactions manifested by symptoms including, but not limited to, anaphylaxis, dyspnea, flushing, and chest pain have been observed are are occasional.
5. *Miscellaneous effects:*
   a. Asthenia, edema, and fever are common.
   b. Dyspnea and cough are common.
   c. Increased liver transaminases and alkaline phosphatase is common; increased bilirubin is occasional.
   d. Back pain, arthralgia, and myalagia are occasional.
   e. Headache, chills, and chest pain are occasional.
   f. Hyperglycemia is common and occasionally severe.
   g. Hypophosphatemia is occasional and may be severe.
   h. Hypertriglyceridemia is common and may be severe.
   i. Interstitial lung disease is uncommon.
   j. Creatinine is commonly increased, but renal failure is rare.
   k. Taste perversion is common.

TENIPOSIDE

Other names. VM-26, Vumon.

Mechanism of action. Topoisomerase II-mediated double-strand DNA breaks. Causes cell cycle transit delay through S phase and arrest at late S/G_2.

Primary indications

1. ALL
2. Neuroblastoma
3. Non-Hodgkin lymphomas.

Usual dosage and schedule

1. 165 mg/m^2 IV over 30 to 60 minutes twice weekly for eight to nine doses (with cytarabine)
2. 250 mg/m^2 IV over 30 to 60 minutes weekly for 4 to 8 weeks (with vincristine and prednisone).

Special precautions

1. Hypersensitivity reactions usually resolve with interruption of the infusion and often can be prevented with diphenhydramine and hydrocortisone pretreatment. Hypotension is alleviated by prolonging the infusion time. It is a possible vesicant.
2. See package insert for IV preparation and administration equipment requirements.

Toxicity

1. *Myelosuppression and other hematologic effects.* Common and dose-limiting.
2. *Nausea, vomiting, and other gastrointestinal effects.* Nausea, vomiting, and diarrhea are common.
3. *Mucocutaneous effects.* Alopecia and mucositis are common.
4. *Miscellaneous effects:*
   a. Hepatic and renal dysfunction is rare.
   b. Hypersensitivity reactions with urticaria and flushing are occasional. Anaphylaxis is uncommon.
   c. Hypotension is related to drug infusion rate but should be seen only occasionally at the recommended dose schedules.
   d. Secondary leukemias are uncommon.
   e. Chemical phlebitis is uncommon.

THALIDOMIDE

Other name. Thalomid.

Mechanism of action. Multiple potential mechanisms, including inhibition of VEGF, inhibition of TNF-α, direct inhibition of G_1 growth and promotion of apoptosis, expansion of NK cells, and costimulation of T-cells.

Primary indications

1. Multiple myeloma

2. MDS

3. Primary myelofibrosis.

Usual dosage and schedule. A starting dose of 50 to 100 mg by mouth once daily in the evening. The dose is escalated weekly by 50 to 100 mg until the maximum dose specified, commonly 400 mg daily.

Special precautions. Severe and life-threatening birth defects, primarily phocomelia, can be caused by taking even a single 50-mg dose. For this reason, special precautions must be taken to assure that female patients are not pregnant when the drug is started, and that both female and male patients practice strict birth control measures. Prophylactic anticoagulation or aspirin may diminish frequency of thromboembolism.

Toxicity

1. *Myelosuppression and other hematologic effects.* Minimal myelosuppression in most patients. Hypercoagulability with deep venous thrombosis is common (22%) in patients receiving the drug in combination with dexamethasone.

2. *Nausea, vomiting, and other gastrointestinal effects.* Constipation is common.

3. *Mucocutaneous effects.* Macular rash, usually involving the trunk, is common. Alopecia is uncommon. Severe or life-threatening epidermal damage is rare.

4. *Miscellaneous effects:*
   a. Dose-dependent somnolence and dizziness is common. Tolerance usually develops to the sedative effects. Dizziness may be related to hypotension and can be minimized by adequate hydration and avoidance of rapid postural changes.
   b. Peripheral neuropathy is common (25%) with chronic therapy. Occasional patients develop myalagia, tremor, or muscle spasms.
   c. Fatigue is common.
   d. Headache is occasional.
   e. Edema is occasional to common.
   f. Hypothyroidism is occasional.
   g. Birth defects (see Special precautions).

THIOTEPA

Other names. Triethylenethiophosphoramide, Thioplex.

Mechanism of action. Alkylating agent similar to mechlorethamine.

Primary indications

1. Superficial papillary carcinoma of urinary bladder
2. Malignant peritoneal, pleural, or pericardial effusions
3. Neoplastic meningeal infiltrates.

Usual dosage and schedule

1. 30 to 60 mg in 40 to 50 mL water instilled into the bladder and retained for 1 hour. Dose is repeated weekly for 3 to 6 weeks, then every 3 weeks for five cycles.
2. 25 to 30 mg/m^2 in 50 to 100 mL saline solution as a single intracavitary injection. Dose may be repeated as tolerated by blood counts.
3. 10 to 15 mg intrathecally.

Special precautions. Dose should be reduced in patients with impaired renal function, as the drug is primarily excreted in the urine.

Toxicity

1. *Myelosuppression and other hematologic effects.* Dose-limiting. Pancytopenia and sepsis may follow intravesical or intracavitary administration. Nadir counts are reached in 1 to 2 weeks; recovery by 4 weeks is usual.
2. *Nausea, vomiting, and other gastrointestinal effects.* Uncommon.
3. *Mucocutaneous effects.* Uncommon. Thiotepa is not a vesicant. Hyperpigmentation of skin occurs at high doses.
4. *Miscellaneous effects:*
   a. Local pain, dizziness, headache, and fever are uncommon.
   b. Secondary neoplasms are possible.
   c. Amenorrhea and azoospermia are common.

TOPOTECAN

Other name. Hycamtin.

Mechanism of action. Topotecan, a semisynthetic derivative of camptothecin, is a potent inhibitor of topoisomerase I, an enzyme essential for effective replication and transcription. It binds to the topoisomerase I–DNA cleavable complex, preventing religation after cleavage by topoisomerase I.

Primary indications

1. Ovarian carcinoma
2. Carcinoma of the cervix
3. Small-cell and non–small-cell carcinoma of the lung.

Usual dosage and schedule

1. As a single agent, 1.5 mg/m^2 IV as a 30-minute infusion daily times five every 3 weeks.
2. In combination with cisplatin, 0.75 mg/m^2 IV as a 30-minute infusion daily times three every 3 weeks.

Special precautions. None.

Toxicity

1. *Myelosuppression and other hematologic effects.* Leukopenia is universal and dose-limiting. Anemia and thrombocytopenia are common and occasionally severe. Febrile neutropenia is occasional to common.
2. *Nausea, vomiting, and other gastrointestinal effects.* Nausea, vomiting, and diarrhea are common but usually mild. Other gastrointestinal symptoms, including constipation and abdominal pain, occur occasionally.
3. *Mucocutaneous effects.* Alopecia is common; stomatitis is occasional but usually mild; skin rash is rare.
4. *Miscellaneous effects:*
   a. Fever, headache, fatigue, and weakness are common (15% to 25%) but rarely severe.
   b. Microscopic hematuria is occasional.
   c. Dyspnea occurs occasionally, but it is uncommon for it to be severe.
   d. Infection as a consequence of severe leukopenia is common.

TOREMIFENE

Other name. Fareston.

Mechanism of action. A selective estrogen-receptor modulator that inhibits estrogen effects by competing with estrogen for binding on the cytosol estrogen-receptor protein in cancer cells. The receptor-hormone complex ultimately controls the promoter region of genes that affect cell growth.

Primary indication. Metastatic carcinoma of the breast in postmenopausal women with estrogen-receptor–positive (or unknown) tumors.

Usual dosage and schedule. 60 mg by mouth daily.

Special precautions. Uncertain whether it has any carcinogenic effect on endometrium, as has been observed with tamoxifen. May result in increased PT in patients taking warfarin (Coumadin). Cytochrome P450 3A4 enzyme inhibitors, such as phenobarbital, phenytoin, and carbamazepine, increase the rate of toremifene metabolism, lowering the concentration in the serum.

Toxicity

1. *Myelosuppression and other hematologic effects.* Uncommon and mild. Thromboembolic phenomena are rare.
2. *Nausea, vomiting, and other gastrointestinal effects.* Minimal nausea is common early in treatment; vomiting is uncommon.
3. *Mucocutaneous effects.* Dry eyes and cataracts are rare. May cause an increase or decrease in vaginal secretions, which may result in difficult or painful intercourse.

4. *Miscellaneous effects:*
   a. Hot flashes are common.
   b. Dizziness is occasional.
   c. Sweating is occasional.
   d. Vaginal discharge, bleeding, and menstrual irregularity are occasional.
   e. Hypercalcemia is uncommon.
   f. Occasional elevation of liver function tests.

TOSITUMOMAB, IODINE-131

Other name. Bexxar.

Mechanism of action. I-131 tositumomab is a murine Ig2a monoclonal anti-CD20 antibody radiolabeled with I-131, an emitter of both beta and gamma radiation. The mechanism of action includes antibody-mediated cytotoxicity and cellularly targeted radiotherapy (radioimmunotherapy).

Primary indication. Non-Hodgkin lymphoma, chemotherapy-refractory, CD20-positive, low-grade or transformed low-grade.

Usual dosage and schedule

1. Before dosimetric and therapeutic doses, patients are premedicated with acetaminophen 650 mg and diphenhydramine 50 mg. A saturated solution of potassium iodide, two to three drops orally three times daily, is given beginning 24 hours before the dosimetric dose and continuing for 14 days after the therapeutic dose to prevent uptake of I-131 by the thyroid.
2. Dosimetric dose of 450 mg of unlabeled tositumomab is given as a 1-hour infusion followed by a 20-minute infusion of 5 mCi (35 mg) of I-131 tositumomab to determine the patient-specific activity (millicuries) of radiolabeled tositumomab to deliver a therapeutic dose of 65 to 75 cGy 7 to 15 days later.
3. Assessment of biodistribution of I-131 tositumomab: Do not administer therapeutic step if biodistribution is altered.
4. Therapeutic dose: 450 mg of unlabeled tositumomab is given as a 1-hour infusion followed by a 20-minute infusion of calculated patient-specific (in millicuries) activity labeled to 35 mg of tositumomab (median 90 mCi, range is approximately 50 to 200 mCi).

Special precautions. Use with caution in patients with at least 25% marrow involvement with lymphoma, prior external beam radiotherapy to at least 25% of the bone marrow, or a history of HAMAs or HACAs. A saturated solution of potassium iodide, two to three drops orally three times daily, is given beginning 24 hours before the dosimetric dose and continuing for 14 days after the therapeutic dose to prevent uptake of I-131 by the thyroid.

Toxicity

1. *Myelosuppression and other hematologic effects.* Myelosuppression is universal, with about 35% to 65% of patients having grade 3 or 4 thrombocytopenia or neutropenia. The nadir counts occur at a median of 4 to 7 weeks and last 3 weeks, with recovery to baseline by 10 to 12 weeks after drug administration. Febrile neutropenia is common in previously treated patients but not when used as initial therapy.

2. *Nausea, vomiting, and other gastrointestinal effects.* Nausea is common; vomiting, abdominal pain, and anorexia are occasional.

3. *Mucocutaneous effects.* Pruritis, rash, and sweating are occasional.

4. *Miscellaneous effects:*
   a. Immunologic: HAMAs or HACAs are common and associated with influenza-like syndrome. Hypersensitivity reactions are occasional and may range from mild allergic reactions or injection site reactions to anaphylaxis and serum sickness.
   b. Infusion-related fever, chills, dizziness, asthenia, wheezing or coughing, nasal congestion, headache, back pain, arthralgia, and hypotension are common, more with dosimetric than therapeutic dose. Most commonly, these are self-limited and mild to moderate in severity.
   c. Fatigue or asthenia is common.
   d. Cardiorespiratory: Cough, dyspnea, and edema are occasional; hypotension and vasodilatation are uncommon.
   e. Thyroid suppression is occasional despite prophylaxis with potassium iodide.
   f. Myelodysplasia and secondary leukemia are uncommon.

TRASTUZUMAB

Other names. Humanized anti-HER2 antibody, Herceptin.

Mechanism of action. A recombinant humanized monoclonal antibody that targets the extracellular domain of the human EGFR protein, HER2 (p185^{HER2}).

Primary indications

1. Carcinoma of the breast that has overexpression of HER2 (c-erbB-2), either in advanced disease or as adjuvant therapy
2. Metastatic gastric or gastroesophageal junction adenocarcinoma and other carcinomas that exhibit overexpression of HER2.

Usual dosage and schedule

1. Initial dose of 4 mg/kg IV over 90 minutes, then 2 mg/kg IV over 30 minutes weekly
2. Initial dose of 8 mg/kg over 90 minutes IV infusion, then 6 mg/kg over 30 to 90 minutes IV infusion every 3 weeks for 52 weeks (adjuvant

breast cancer) until disease progression or intolerable toxicity (advanced breast cancer or other cancers).

Special precautions

1. During the first infusion, and occasionally during later infusions, a systemic symptom complex similar to that seen with other human monoclonal antibodies is common. Severe hypersensitivity reactions and pulmonary adverse events have been reported but are uncommon to rare. These events include anaphylaxis, angioedema, bronchospasm, hypotension, hypoxia, dyspnea, pulmonary infiltrates, pleural effusions, noncardiogenic pulmonary edema, and acute respiratory distress syndrome. A more common symptom complex consists of mild to moderate chills, fever, asthenia, pain, nausea, vomiting, and headache. These latter symptoms are generally well managed by temporary slowing or interruption of the infusion and administration of acetaminophen, diphenhydramine, and meperidine.

2. Cardiac dysfunction (cardiac symptoms or an asymptomatic decrease in ejection fraction of 10% or greater) occurs in about 7% of patients treated with trastuzumab alone but in 28% of patients treated with trastuzumab plus anthracycline and in 11% of patients treated with trastuzumab plus paclitaxel. In most cases, this improves with symptomatic therapy. Severe disability or death from cardiac dysfunction occurs in about 1% of patients. Extreme caution should be exercised in treating patients with pre-existing cardiac dysfunction.

Toxicity

1. *Myelosuppression and other hematologic effects.* Uncommon.
2. *Nausea, vomiting, and other gastrointestinal effects.* Nausea and vomiting are common with the first infusion. Diarrhea is also common.
3. *Mucocutaneous effects.* A rash is occasional to common and may be associated with urticaria or pruritus.
4. *Miscellaneous effects:*
   a. Mild to moderate chills, fever, asthenia, pain, and headache are common, primarily during the first infusion.
   b. Cardiac dysfunction occurs in about 7% of patients treated with trastuzumab alone, but in 28% of patients treated with trastuzumab plus anthracycline and in 11% of patients treated with trastuzumab plus paclitaxel. In most cases, this improves with symptomatic therapy.
   c. Chest pain, back pain, dyspnea, and cough are occasional to common.
   d. Peripheral edema is occasional.

TRETINOIN

Other names. All-*trans*-retinoic acid, t-RNA, ATRA, Vesanoid, Retin-A.

Mechanism of action. Binds to cytoplasmic retinoic acid-binding proteins and then is transported to the nucleus where it interacts with nuclear RARs. These then affect expression of the genes that control cell growth and differentiation. In acute promyelocytic leukemia, which characteristically has a chromosomal translocation, t(15:17), abnormal mRNA transcripts are seen for RAR-α, the gene for which is on chromosome 17.

Primary indication. Acute promyelocytic leukemia for induction of remission.

Usual dosage and schedule. 45 mg/m^2 by mouth daily (divided into two doses in the morning and 6 hours later) until 30 days after complete remission is documented, up to a maximum of 90 days. Therapy usually initiated concurrently with anthracycline.

Special precautions. Avoid use in pregnant women because of marked teratogenic potential. Advise patients to avoid pregnancy by using two reliable contraceptive methods simultaneously. Retinoic acid acute promyelocytic (RA-APL) syndrome (see subsequent discussion) may require mechanical ventilation and dexamethasone 10 mg every 12 hours at the first signs of fever with respiratory distress until resolution of the acute symptoms (often several days). Continuation of retinoid therapy is controversial.

Toxicity

1. *Myelosuppression and other hematologic effects.* Myelosuppression is rare. Forty percent of patients develop leukocytosis, which increases the risk of RA-APL syndrome. Disseminated intravascular coagulation is common (26%).
2. *Nausea, vomiting, and other gastrointestinal effects.* Nausea and vomiting, abdominal pain, diarrhea, anorexia, and constipation are common but usually not severe. Gastrointestinal hemorrhage is occasional to common and may be severe. Inflammatory bowel disease is rare.
3. *Mucocutaneous effects.* Universal, particularly at doses at higher end of range. They include redness, dryness, and pruritus of the skin and mucous membranes; increased sweating; possible vesicle formation; peeling of the skin of the palms and soles; cheilitis; and conjunctivitis. There also may be increased skin photosensitivity (e.g., to sun) and the nails may become brittle. Alopecia is uncommon.
4. *Retinoic acid syndrome.* High fever, respiratory distress, weight gain, diffuse pulmonary infiltrates, pleural or pericardial effusions with the possibility of impaired myocardial contractility, and hypotension, with or without concomitant leukocytosis, are common in patients with acute promyelocytic leukemia (25%; see Chapter 18).

5. *Miscellaneous effects:*
   a. Cardiovascular: Arrythmias, flushing, hypotension, hypertension, and phlebitis are occasional. Cardiac failure, cardiac arrest, pulmonary hypertension, and other more severe cardiovascular problems are uncommon.
   b. Cataracts and corneal ulcerations or opacities are uncommon.
   c. Musculoskeletal: Arthralgias, bone pain, and muscle aches are occasional to common; skeletal hyperostosis is common at higher doses (80 mg/m^2/day).
   d. Hypertriglyceridemia: Mild to moderate elevations are common; marked elevations (more than five times normal) are uncommon; hypercholesterolemia occurs to lesser degree.
   e. Neurologic: Headache is common; paresthesias, dizziness, and visual disturbances are occasional; lethargy, fatigue, and mental depression are uncommon; pseudotumor cerebri is rare.
   f. Hepatotoxicity with increased LDH, SGOT, SGPT, GGTP, and alkaline phosphatase is common.
   g. Hyperhistaminemia with shock is rare.
   h. Renal insufficiency is occasional.
   i. Fever, malaise, shivering, and edema are common.

VALRUBICIN

Other name. Valstar.

Mechanism of action. Valrubicin, a semisynthetic analog of doxorubicin, penetrates into cells where its metabolites inhibit the incorporation of nucleosides into nucleic acids, cause chromosomal damage, and arrest cell cycle in G$_2$. A principal mechanism of valrubicin metabolites is DNA-strand breakage mediated by anthracycline effects on topoisomerase II.

Primary indication. Intravesical therapy of BCG-refractory carcinoma in situ of the urinary bladder in patients for whom immediate cystectomy would be associated with unacceptable morbidity or mortality.

Usual dosage and schedule. 800 mg, diluted in 75 mL of normal saline, intravesically once a week for 6 weeks. Retain in bladder for 2 hours before voiding.

Special precautions. Should not be administered if there is any question about perforation of the bladder or integrity of bladder mucosa.

Toxicity

1. *Myelosuppression and other hematologic effects.* Uncommon, unless bladder rupture or perforation occurs, in which case severe neutropenia can be expected 2 weeks after administration.
2. *Nausea, vomiting, and other gastrointestinal effects.* Uncommon.
3. *Mucocutaneous effects.* Rash is uncommon.

4. *Miscellaneous effects:*
   a. Local reactions: Frequency, dysuria, urgency, bladder spasm, hematuria, and bladder pain are common. Urinary incontinency and cystitis are occasional. Local burning symptoms associated with the procedure, urethral pain, pelvic pain, and gross hematuria are uncommon to rare.
   b. Body as a whole: Abdominal pain, asthenia, back pain, chest pain, fever, headache, and malaise are uncommon.

VANDETANIB

Other names. Zactima, ZD6474.

Mechanism of action. An oral multitargeted RTK inhibitor of EGFR and VEGF receptor, and the RET proto-oncogene RTK, which is associated with both hereditary and sporadic medullary thyroid cancer, blocking both tumor growth and inhibiting tumor angiogenesis.

Primary indications

1. Non–small-cell carcinoma of the lung
2. Medullary thyroid carcinoma.

Usual dosage and schedule. 300 mg by mouth daily.

Special precautions. Do not use in patients with hypokalemia, hypomagnesemia, or long QT syndrome. Drugs known to prolong the QT interval and strong CYP3A4 inhibitors should be avoided. ECGs should be obtained to monitor the QTc at baseline, 7 days after initiation, and periodically thereafter. Do not give if QTc is greater than 480 msec.

Toxicity

1. *Myelosuppression and other hematologic effects.* None reported.
2. *Nausea, vomiting, and other gastrointestinal effects.* Diarrhea is common and occasionally grade 3 to 4. Nausea is common, but vomiting is only occasional and usually not severe. Constipation is occasional to common. Anorexia is common, but usually only grade 1 to 2.
3. *Mucocutaneous effects.* Rash is common, but high-grade dermatologic abnormalities are uncommon.
4. *Miscellaneous effects:*
   a. Fatigue is common and occasionally grade 3 to 4. Weight loss is occasional.
   b. Headache is common.
   c. QTc interval prolongation is occasional (about 15%).
   d. Hypertension is occasional and may be high-grade (rise of >30 mm Hg systolic) but usually easily controlled.
   e. Dyspnea is common in patients receiving vandetanib for lung cancer.

VINBLASTINE

Other names. VLB, Velban.

Mechanism of action. Mitotic inhibition with reversible metaphase arrest due to action on microtubular and spindle contractile proteins.

Primary indications

1. Hodgkin and non-Hodgkin lymphomas
2. Testicular, gestational trophoblastic carcinomas.

Usual dosage and schedule

1. 6 mg/m^2 IV on days 1 and 15 in combination with doxorubicin, bleomycin, and dacarbazine for lymphomas
2. 4 to 18 mg/m^2 IV weekly.

Special precautions. Administer as a slow push, taking care to avoid extravasation.

Toxicity

1. *Myelosuppression and other hematologic effects.* Dose-related leukopenia occurs with a nadir at 4 to 10 days and recovery in 7 to 10 days. Severe thrombocytopenia is uncommon.
2. *Nausea, vomiting, and other gastrointestinal effects.* Common but not usually severe.
3. *Mucocutaneous effects.* Extravasation may lead to severe inflammation, pain, and tissue damage. Local infiltration with 1 to 6 mL of hyaluronidase (150 units/mL) may help (see Table 26.1). Mild alopecia is common. Stomatitis is occasionally severe.
4. *Miscellaneous effects:*
   a. Neurotoxicity manifested by (1) constipation, adynamic ileus, and abdominal pain if very high doses are used; or (2) paresthesias, peripheral neuropathy, and jaw pain with lower doses. Neurotoxicity is less frequent with vinblastine than with vincristine.
   b. Transient hepatitis is uncommon.
   c. Depression, headache, convulsions, and orthostatic hypotension are rare.

VINCRISTINE

Other names. VCR, Oncovin, Vincasar.

Mechanism of action. Mitotic inhibition with reversible metaphase arrest due to drug action on microtubular and spindle contractile proteins.

Primary indications

1. Hodgkin and non-Hodgkin lymphomas
2. ALL
3. Multiple myeloma

4. Wilms tumor, neuroblastoma, rhabdomyosarcoma, and Ewing sarcoma of childhood.

Usual dosage and schedule

1. 1 to 2 mg/m^2 (maximum 2.0 to 2.4 mg, except in Hodgkin lymphoma) IV weekly
2. 0.4 mg/day as a continuous IV infusion on days 1 to 4.

Special precautions

1. Administer as a slow IV push, taking care to avoid extravasation.
2. Because neurotoxicity is cumulative, neurologic evaluation should be done before each dose and therapy withheld if severe paresthesias, motor weakness, or other severe abnormalities occur. Underlying neurologic problems accentuate the effect of vincristine.
3. Reduce dose if liver disease is significant.
4. Stool softeners or high-fiber or bulk diets may avert severe constipation.

Toxicity

1. *Myelosuppression and other hematologic effects.* Mild and rarely of clinical significance.
2. *Nausea, vomiting, and other gastrointestinal effects.* Nausea and vomiting are not seen unless paralytic ileus occurs. Constipation is common.
3. *Mucocutaneous effects.* Severe local inflammation if extravasation occurs. Alopecia is common.
4. *Miscellaneous effects:*
   a. Neurotoxicity: Dose-dependent and dose-limiting. Mild paresthesias and decreased deep tendon reflexes are to be expected. More extensive peripheral neuropathies, severe constipation, or ileus are indications to reduce or hold therapy. Autonomic dysfunction with orthostatic hypotension or urinary retention may be seen.
   b. Uric acid nephropathy due to rapid tumor cell lysis and release of uric acid is always a potential problem when therapy is first given.
   c. Syndrome of inappropriate antidiuretic hormone is rare.
   d. Jaw pain is uncommon.

VINORELBINE

Other name. Navelbine.

Mechanism of action. Binds to tubulin, depolymerizes microtubules causing mitotic inhibition, similar to other vinca alkaloids. Lower affinity for axonal microtubules associated with lower neurotoxicity.

Primary indications

1. Metastatic carcinoma of the breast
2. Non–small-cell carcinoma of the lung.

Usual dosage and schedule

1. 30 mg/m^2 IV as 6- to 10-minute rapid infusion weekly when used with a single agent or with cisplatin
2. 20 to 25 mg/m^2 IV as a 6- to 10-minute rapid infusion in various schedules, when used with other myelotoxic agents.

Special precautions. Administer infusion through the side arm of a freely flowing IV, taking care to avoid extravasation. Reduce dose by 50% for serum bilirubin levels of 2.1 to 3 mg/dL; by 75% for bilirubin levels of more than 3 mg/dL.

Toxicity

1. *Myelosuppression and other hematologic effects.* Granulocytopenia is common and dose-limiting, with nadir at 7 to 10 days. Thrombocytopenia is uncommon. Anemia is occasional to common.
2. *Nausea, vomiting, and other gastrointestinal effects.* Nausea and vomiting are common but usually mild to moderate. Diarrhea occurs occasionally.
3. *Mucocutaneous effects.* Alopecia, mild diarrhea, and stomatitis are occasional. Severe local inflammation can occur with extravasation.
4. *Miscellaneous effects:*
   a. Neurotoxicity: Cumulative but reversible constipation and decreased deep tendon reflexes are occasional; paresthesias are uncommon.
   b. Erythema, pain, and skin discoloration at injection site are common; phlebitis at injection site is occasional.

VORINOSTAT

Other name. Zolinza.

Mechanism of action. Inhibits HDACs, which are overexpressed in some cancer cells. Accumulation of acetylated histones following vorinostat exposure induces cell cycle arrest or apoptosis in some transformed cells in vitro.

Primary indication. CTCL with progressive, persistent, or recurrent skin disease after two other systemic therapies.

Usual dosage and schedule. 400 mg by mouth daily with food. May be reduced to 300 mg daily or 5 days weekly if the higher dose is not tolerated.

Special precautions. Patients should drink at least 2 L of fluid daily to prevent dehydration from vomiting and diarrhea. Deep venous thrombosis and pulmonary embolism (5%) have been reported. Serum chemistries (including potassium, magnesium, calcium, glucose, and creatinine) and platelets should be monitored every 2 weeks during the first 2 months of treatment. Severe thrombocytopenia and gastrointestinal bleeding may occur with concomitant use with other HDAC inhibitors, such as valproic acid.

Toxicity

1. *Myelosuppression and other hematologic effects.* Thrombocytopenia is common; anemia and neutropenia are occasional. Increased PT and INR may be seen with concomitant use of warfarin with vorinostat.
2. *Nausea, vomiting, and other gastrointestinal effects.* Anorexia, nausea, and diarrhea are common. Vomiting, constipation, and weight loss are occasional.
3. *Mucocutaneous effects.* Alopecia is occasional to common.
4. *Miscellaneous effects:*
   a. Blood chemistry abnormalities: Hypercholesterolemia, hypertriglyceridemia, hyperglycemia, and increased creatinine are common and may be severe (grade 3 or higher).
   b. Cardiovascular: QTc prolongation on the electrocardiogram is uncommon. Pulmonary embolism and deep venous thrombosis are uncommon.
   c. Edema is occasional.
   d. Neuromuscular: Fatigue is common. Headache, muscle spasms, and dizziness are occasional.
   e. Neoplastic: Squamous cell carcinoma is uncommon.

ZOLEDRONIC ACID

Other name. Zometa.

Mechanism of action. A bisphosphonate that inhibits osteoclastic resorption of bone and calcium release induced by tumor cytokines.

Primary indications

1. Hypercalcemia associated with malignancy
2. Bone metastases, breast cancer, prostate cancer (after progression on hormonal therapy), and from other solid tumors in conjunction with standard antineoplastic therapy
3. Osteolytic and osteoporotic bone lesions of multiple myeloma.

Usual dosage and schedule

1. Hypercalcemia of malignancy: 4 mg IV as a 15-minute infusion. May be repeated every 1 to 8 weeks, as needed.
2. Multiple myeloma or metastatic bone lesions: 4 mg IV as a 15-minute infusion every 3 to 4 weeks.

Special precautions. Do not infuse over less than 15 minutes. Potential for renal tubular damage, particularly if infused more rapidly. The risk of adverse reactions, particularly renal adverse reactions, may be greater in patients with impaired renal function. Dose adjustments are not necessary when treating for hypercalcemia, as long as serum creatinine is less than 4.5 mg/dL. In patients with multiple myeloma or metastatic bone lesions of solid tumors, the dose should be progressively reduced for baseline creatinine clearance of 30 to 60 mL/min. Do not give if clearance less than 30 mL/min. Hold therapy if creatinine increases during therapy. Use caution when administered concurrently with aminoglycosides. Serum creatinine should be monitored before each treatment.

Osteonecrosis of the jaw has been reported, primarily in association with dental procedures such as tooth extraction; such procedures should be avoided during and following bisphosphonate treatment, if possible.

Toxicity

1. *Myelosuppression and other hematologic effects.* Rare.
2. *Nausea, vomiting, and other gastrointestinal effects.* Abdominal pain, anorexia, constipation, nausea, and vomiting are uncommon to occasional.
3. *Mucocutaneous effects.* Infusion site reaction is occasional.
4. *Miscellaneous effects:*
   a. Flulike syndrome with fever, chills, skeletal aches, and pains is occasional.
   b. Hypocalcemia and hypomagnesemia are occasional, but grade 3 or 4 abnormalities are uncommon to rare.
   c. Increase of the serum creatinine of 0.5 mg/dL above baseline is occasional, but elevation to greater than three times ULN is uncommon.
   d. Hypophosphatemia less than 2 mg/dL is occasional but does not appear to have serious consequences or require treatment.
   e. Osteonecrosis of the jaw is uncommon to rare.
   f. Conjunctivitis or other ocular abnormalities are rare.
   g. There is potential for bronchoconstriction in aspirin-sensitive patients.

Selected Readings

Chabner B, Longo DL. *Cancer Chemotherapy and Biotherapy: Principles and Practice.* 4th ed. Philadelphia: Lippincott Williams & Wilkins; 2006.

Dorr RT, Van Hoff DD, eds. *Cancer Chemotherapy Handbook.* Norwalk: Appleton & Lange; 1994.

National Cancer Institute Cancer Therapy Evaluation Program. Common terminology criteria for adverse events v4.0. Retrieved from http://ctep.cancer.gov/reporting/ctc.html.

Perry MC. *The Chemotherapy Source Book.* Philadelphia: Lippincott Williams & Wilkins; 2008.

Rosner GL, Hargis JB, Hollis DR, et al. Relationship between toxicity and obesity in women receiving adjuvant chemotherapy for breast cancer: results from cancer and leukemia group B study 8541. *J Clin Oncol.* 1996;14:3000–3008.

Sparreboom A, Wolff AC, Mathijssen RH, et al. Evaluation of alternate size descriptors for dose calculation of anticancer drugs in the obese. *J Clin Oncol.* 2007;25: 4707–4713.

Tannock IF, Hill RP, eds. *The Basic Science of Oncology.* New York: McGraw-Hill; 1998.

A
Nomogram for Determining Body Surface Area of Adults from Height and Mass*

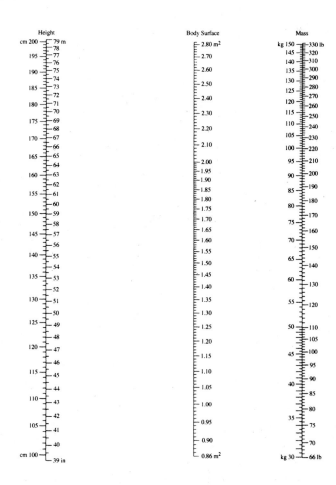

Height	Body Surface	Mass

---

*From the formula of Du Bois and Du Bois (*Arch Intern Med.* 1916;17:863): $S = M^{0.425} \times H^{0.725} \times 71.84$, or $S = \log M \times 0.425 + \log H \times 0.725 + 1.8564$, where S is body surface (cm²), M is mass (kg), and H is height (cm). (From Lenter C, ed. *Geigy Scientific Tables,* Vol 1. 8th ed. Basel: Ciba-Geigy; 1981:227.)

B) Nomogram for Determining Body Surface Area of Children from Height and Mass*

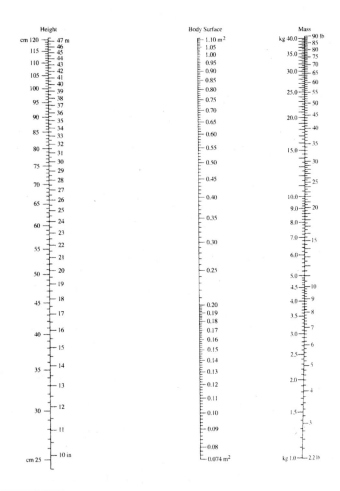

Height	Body Surface	Mass

*From the formula of Du Bois and Du Bois (*Arch Intern Med.* 1916;17:863): $S = M^{0.425} \times H^{0.725} \times 71.84$, or $S = \log M \times 0.425 + \log H + 0.725 + 1.8564$, where S is body surface (cm^2), M is mass (kg), and H is height (cm). (From Lenter C, ed. *Geigy Scientific Tables*, Vol 1. 8th ed. Basel: Ciba-Geigy; 1981:226.)

Note: Page numbers followed by *f* indicate figures; those followed by *t* indicate tables.

A

absolute neutrophil count (ANC), 350, 527, 567, 720
ABVD regimen, Hodgkin lymphoma, 443*t*, 446–448
AC regimen, breast cancer, 188
ACC. *See* adrenal cortical carcinoma
accelerated phase (AP), chronic myelogenous leukemia, 397, 397*t*
acetaminophen, 672
acetazolamide, tumor lysis syndrome, 628–629
acetylsalicylic acid. *See* aspirin
aclarubicin, acute leukemias, 351
acquired immune deficiency syndrome (AIDS). *See* HIV-associated malignancies
   lymphomas and, 485
   malignancies, diagnosis and, 523
acquired resistance, 13
actinomycin D. *See* dactinomycin
Actinomycosis, 573
activated partial thromboplastin time (aPTT), 598
acupuncture, 676
acute confusional states
   etiologies, 679
   precepts, 678
   therapeutic approach, 679–683, 681*t*
acute leukemias, 337–394
   of ambiguous lineage, 344–345
   general features
      clinical, laboratory features, 339*t*
      epidemiology, 337
      etiology, risk factors, 337–338
   initial support
      birth control, fertility and, 349
      blood product support, 347–348
      coagulopathy correction, 347
      fever, infection, 348
      HLA typing, 348
      hydration, electrolyte imbalance, 346
      hyperleukocytosis, leukostasis, leukaphere-sis, 345–346
      menses suppression, 348–349
      uric acid nephropathy prevention, 346–347
      vascular access, 348
   therapy
      aim of, 349
      definition of response, 350–351

      induction chemotherapy, 349–350
      postremission chemotherapy, 350
acute lymphoblastic leukemia (ALL)
   adult, therapy and, 374
      CNS disease, 381–383
      consolidation (intensification) therapy, 375
      induction, 374–375
      maintenance, 375
      mature (Burkitt) B-Cell, 380–381
      minimal residual disease (MRD), 381
      pre-B–, T-cell lineage, 375–380
   classification, 343, 343*t*
   clinical, laboratory features, 339*t*
   epidemiology, 337
   etiology, risk factors, 337–338
   hematopoietic stem cell transplantation, 389–391
   immunophenotypes of, 343*t*
   novel, investigational strategies, therapy, 388–389, 389*t*
   older adults, CNS disease, 383–384
   Ph1+ and, therapy for
      background, 385–386
      recommendations for, 386
   prognostic factors, 344
   salvage therapy, 386–387
acute myelogenous leukemia, 60
acute myeloid leukemia (AML)
   adult AML therapy, 351
      common HDAC toxicities, 354
      induction therapy, 351–353, 352*t*
      postremission therapy, 354–357, 355*t*
      primary refractory AML, 357
      relapsed AML, 357–361, 358*t*
      residual disease, 354
   classification, 338–341, 340*t*
   clinical, laboratory features, 339*t*
   common HDAC toxicities, 354
   cytarabine dose intensification, 352–353
   epidemiology, 337
   etiology, risk factors, 337–338
   induction therapy, 351–352, 352*t*
   myeloma and, 509
   older adults and
      background, 361–362
      gemutuzumab ozogamicin (GO), 364
      induction therapy, 362–363

acute myeloid leukemia (AML) *(continued)*
    postremission therapy, 363–364
      RIC (mini)-HCST, 364–365
  postremission therapy, 354–357, 355*t*
  pregnancy and, 366
  primary refractory, 357
  prognostic factors, 341, 342*t*
  regimens, 353
  relapsed, 357–361, 358*t*
  residual disease, 354
  therapy-related
    background, 365
    therapy, 365
acute promyelocytic leukemia (APL), 366
  APL differentiation syndrome, 371–372
  clinical, laboratory features, 339*t*
  coagulopathy, 347, 367, 367*t*
  cytogenetic abnormalities, prognostic factors
    and, 366, 366*t*
  epidemiology, 337
  postremission chemotherapy, 350
  relapsed, 372
    ATO, 372
    GO, 372–373
    HSCT in, 373, 373*t*
  therapy, 367, 368–369*t*
    consolidation, 370–371
    HSCT, 371
    induction, 367–369
    maintenance, 371
  vascular access, 348
acute undifferentiated leukemia (AUL), 345
acyclovir
  herpes zoster prophylaxis, 727
  secondary oral infections, 556
  varicella zoster prophylaxis, 503
  viral prophylaxis, 593
adalimumab, 572
adenocarcinoma of unknown origin, 514–515,
  517, 519
adenocarcinomas
  esophageal, 121
  small intestine cancer, 137
ADIC regimen, soft tissue sarcomas, 318
adjuvant drugs, 671–674
adrenal cortical carcinoma (ACC)
  clinical manifestations, 269
  incidence and etiology, 268
  pathology and diagnosis, 269–270
  staging prognosis, 270
  treatment
    alternative modalities, 273–274
    radiotherapy, 271
    surgery, 270–271
    systemic therapy, 271–273
adrenal cortical suppressants, 271–272
Adriamycin. *See* doxorubicin
adverse-risk AML, postremission therapy, 356–357
aerodigestive anatomy, 69, 70*t*
a-fetoprotein (AFP), 224
Afinitor. *See* everolimus
AIDS. *See* acquired immune deficiency syndrome
AIDS clinical trials group staging system, 526, 526*t*

AIN. *See* anal intraepithelial neoplasia
AI regimen, soft tissue sarcomas, 317
albuterol, anaphylaxis, 625
ALCLs. *See* anaplastic large cell lymphomas
aldesleukin (Proleukin). *See* Interleukin-2
alemtuzumab (Campath), 40–41
  CLL, 411–412
  dosage, schedule, 709
  MDS, 430, 434
  mechanism of action, 708
  primary indications, 708
  special precautions, 709–710
alitretinoin
  dosage, schedule, 710
  KS, 527
  mechanism of action, 710
  primary indications, 710
  toxicity, 710
alkyl sulfonates, 697
alkylating agents
  general description, 694, 695*t*
  types of, 696–697
ALL. *See* acute lymphoblastic leukemia
allogeneic (allo-) HSCT
  ALL, 385–387, 389–391
  AML, 356–357, 360, 365
  APL, 365, 371, 373
allogeneic stem cell transplantation (ASCT)
  CML, 402–404, 403*t*
  MDS, 433
  PMF, 425, 426
allogeneic transplantation
  CML, 402–404, 403*t*
  non-Hodgkin lymphoma, 484
allopurinol
  acute leukemias, 346–347
  hyperuricemia, 421, 738
  Stevens-Johnson syndrome, 720
  tumor lysis syndrome, 628–629, 721
  uric acid nephropathy, 346–347
all-trans retinoic acid (ATRA), 366–373, 367*t*,
  368*t*, 369*t*, 373*t*
altretamine
  dosage, schedule, 711
  mechanism of action, 710
  primary indications, 710
  special precautions, 711
  toxicity, 711
alveolar soft-part sarcomas, 316
amifostine
  dosage, schedule, 712
  mechanism of action, 711
  primary indications, 711
  special precautions, 712
  toxicity, 712
aminocaproic acid, 435, 615
aminoglutethimide
  ACC, 272–273
  dosage, schedule, 712
  mechanism of action, 712
  primary indications, 712
  special precautions, 712–713
  toxicity, 713

aminoglycosides, 59, 498
amitriptyline
  cancer pain, 672
  patient psychiatric problems, 685*f*, 687*f*
AML. *See* acute myeloid leukemia
amoxicillin, 581*t*, 588*t*, 589
amphotericin, 588*t*, 589, 733
ampicillin, 587
amsacrine, acute leukemias, 351
amyloidosis, 512
anagrelide
  dosage, schedule, 713
  EV, 423
  mechanism of action, 713
  primary indications, 713
  PV, 421
  special precautions, 714
  toxicity, 714
anal cancer, 147–148, 539
  local disease, 148–149
  metastatic disease, 149
  staging, 148*t*
anal intraepithelial neoplasia (AIN), 538
anaphylaxis
  causes, 624
  clinical manifestations, 624–625
  management, 625
Anaplasma phagocytophilum, 570
anaplastic large cell lymphomas (ALCLs), 480
anaplastic thyroid cancer (ATC), 260
  diagnosis and staging, 262–263
  treatment, 262–263, 266–268
anastrozole
  breast cancer, 193, 195
  dosage, schedule, 715
  mechanism of action, 714
  primary indications, 715
  special precautions, 715
  toxicity, 715
ANC. *See* absolute neutrophil count
androgen ablation, 240
  estrogens, 241
  LHRH analogs, 240–241
  LHRH analogs and antiandrogens, 241
  orchiectomy, 240
  second-line hormonal therapies, 241
androgens, 700
anemia
  MDS, 434
  MM, 509
  PMF, 425
angiogenesis, 108
angiogenesis-targeted therapy, 36
Ann Arbor staging, 465*t*
  PET/CT imaging, 464–465
  workup, imaging, 463–464, 464*t*
anthracenedione, acute leukemias, 351, 353
anthracenedione mitoxantrone, 699
anthracycline, 699
  AML, 351, 353, 359
  breast cancer, 188
  HNC therapy, 82–83
antiandrogens, 700

antibiotics
  directed therapy, specific pathogens, 588*t*
  dosages, 581–582*t*
  empiric use, 580, 585–587
  prophylactic use, 591–593
anti-CD20 radioimmunoconjugates, 471
anticonvulsants
  cancer pain, 673
  cytochrome P-450 induction, 308
antidepressants, 685*t*, 686*t*, 687*t*
antiemetic drugs, 550–552, 552*t*
antifibrinolytic agents, 615
antifungal prophylaxis, 592
antihistamines, 689*t*, 691
antimetabolites
  general description, 697
  types of, 697
antineoplastic agents
  resistance to, 12–13
    biochemical causes, 13–14
    cell kinetics and, 13
    nonselectivity, 15
    pharmacologic causes, 14–15
antipsychotic medications, 681*t*, 682
antithrombotic therapy, 420–421
antithymocyte globulin (ATG), 430, 433–434
antiviral prophylaxis, 593
anxiety, 688–691, 689*t*
Anzemet. *See* dolasetron
APL. *See* acute promyelocytic leukemia
apoptosis, 4
aprepitant (Emend), 553*t*, 554*t*
aPTT. *See* activated partial thromboplastin time
aromatase inhibitors, 700
arsenic trioxide (ATO), 366
  APL therapy, 369–371
  dosage, schedule, 716
  mechanism of action, 715
  primary indications, 715
  relapsed APL, 372
  special precautions, 716
  toxicity, 716–717
arterial embolization, 273–274
Arzerra. *See* ofatumumab
asparaginase, 599
  dosage, schedule, 717
  mechanism of action, 717
  primary indications, 717
  special precautions, 717–718
  toxicity, 718–719
Aspergillus species, 409, 567, 575, 590
aspiration pneumonia, 90
aspirin (acetylsalicylic acid)
  cancer pain, 658, 658*t*
  ET, 423
  MM, 500
  PV, 419
  side effects, 659
  thrombosis, neoplasia and, 602
Astler-Coller modifications, 138
ATC. *See* anaplastic thyroid cancer
ATG. *See* antithymocyte globulin
Ativan. *See* lorazepam

ATO. *See* arsenic trioxide
atorvastatin, 605
ATRA. *See* all-trans retinoic acid
atropine, 559*t*
AUL. *See* acute undifferentiated leukemia
autologous bone marrow transplantation
    (ABMT), 441
autologous hematopoietic stem cell transplanta-
    tion (auto-HSCT)
  ALL, 385, 389
  AML
    adult, 354
    adverse-risk, 356
    older adults, 364
    relapsed, 360
    therapy-related, 365
  APL, 371, 373
azacitidine
  AML, in older adults, 365
  MDS, 429, 431, 434
  mechanism of action, 719
  primary indications, 719
  toxicity, 719
AZD8055 inhibitor, 35
azithromycin, 531
azoospermia, 61
aztreonam, 581*t*, 582

B

β₂-microglobulin, multiple myeloma, 493, 495*t*
Babesia microti, 570
Bacillus Calmette-Guérin (BCG) vaccine,
    233, 288
Barrett esophagitis, 121
basal cell carcinoma (BCC), 290
  diagnosis, 290–291
  local treatment, 291–292
  metastatic disease treatment, 292
β-blockers, 274–275
BCG vaccine. *See* Bacillus Calmette-Guérin
    vaccine
BCNU. *See* carmustine
Bcr-Abl tyrosine kinase, 2, 31–32
BEACOPP regimen, Hodgkin lymphoma, 443*t*,
    446–448
BEAM regimen, Hodgkin lymphoma, 449*t*
Beckwith-Wiedemann syndrome, 268
Benadryl. *See* diphenhydramine
bendamustine
  CLL, 412
  dosage, schedule, 720
  indolent lymphoma, 470
  mechanism of action, 719–720
  primary indication, 720
  toxicity, 720–721
benzodiazepines
  acute confusional states, 682
  insomnia, 689*t*, 691
benztropine (Cogentin), acute confusional
    states, 682
Berlin-Frankfurt-Muenster (BFM)-like regimens
    (MRC/ECOG), 376–377
bevacizumab

biliary tract cancer, 166
breast cancer, 191–192
carcinoid tumors, 137
colorectal cancer, 140, 143
dosage, schedule, 721
GBM, recurrent, 301
kidney cancer, 254–255
mechanism of action, 721
NSCLC, 107*t*, 108
ovarian cancer, 216*t*, 217–218
primary indications, 721
special precautions, 721–722
toxicity, 722
bexarotene (capsules), 294
CTCL, 473
dosage, schedule, 723
mechanism of action, 723
primary indications, 723
special precautions, 723
toxicity, 723–724
bexarotene (gel)
dosage, schedule, 724
mechanism of action, 724
primary indications, 724
special precautions, 724
toxicity, 724
Bexxar. *See* tositumomab, iodine-131
BHD syndrome. *See* Birt-Hogg-Dubé syndrome
β-human chorionic gonadotropin
    (β-hCG), 348
bicalutamide
dosage, schedule, 724
mechanism of action, 724
primary indications, 724
special precautions, 724
toxicity, 725
bile duct carcinoma, 163
chemotherapy, 165–166
current recommendations, 166
epidemiology, 164
natural history, 164–165
pathogenesis, 164–165
presentation, 164
biochemotherapy, melanoma, 287–288, 287*t*
biologic response modifiers, 4, 66
classification, 693–694, 696*t*
KS, 527*t*
birth control, acute leukemias, 349
Birt-Hogg-Dubé (BHD) syndrome, 251
bisphosphonates
bone metastasis, 635
breast cancer, 196
hypercalcemia, 631–632
metastatic bone pain, 674–675
MM, 498, 507
BL. *See* Burkitt lymphoma
bladder cancer
approach to therapy, 233–234
bladder-sparing therapy, 236
combinations chemotherapy, active single
    agents and, 237*t*
general considerations, 233
intravesical chemotherapy, 234–236

neoadjuvant chemotherapy, 236
systemic chemotherapy, advanced disease, 236–238
TNM staging, 234*t*
bladder-sparing therapy, 236
blastic phase (BP), 395, 397–398, 397*t*
bleeding
  and hemostatic abnormalities, 603–605
  MDS, 435
  screening tests, 606–608
  tumor invasion, 603
bleomycin, 699
  dosage, schedule, 725
  head and neck cancer therapy, 82
  mechanism of action, 725
  metastatic cancer of unknown origin, 521
  osteosarcoma, 332
  ovarian germ cell tumors, 224
  penile cancer, 248
  peritoneal effusions, 643
  pleural effusion treatment, 638–639
  primary indications, 725
  special precautions, 725–726
  testicular cancer, 246
  toxicity, 726
blood product support, 347–348
body surface area, nomogram
  adults, 843*t*
  children, 844*t*
bone marrow biopsy
  Hodgkin lymphoma, 441
  non-Hodgkin lymphoma, 530
bone marrow function, head and neck cancer, 75
bone marrow transplantation
  Ewing sarcoma, 330–331
  MM, 505–506
bone metastasis, 632
  clinical findings, 632–633
  radiologic findings, 633
  treatment, 633–635
bone sarcomas, 324, 335
  Ewing sarcoma
    chemotherapy, 328–331
    general considerations, therapy aims, 325–328, 326–327*t*
  malignant fibrous histiocytoma of bone, 335
  osteosarcoma
    administration, special precautions, 332–333
    chemotherapy, role of, 331
    complications, 333–334
    effective agents, 331
    general considerations, 331
    high-dose chemotherapy, 334–335
    recommended regimen, 331–332
    recurrence, treatment of refractory disease, 334
  staging
    AJCC staging system, 324–325
    evaluation of, 325
    musculoskeletal tumor society staging system, 325

bortezomib, 36–37
  dosage, schedule, 727
  mechanism of action, 726
  MM, 502–504
  primary indications, 726
  special precautions, 727
  toxicity, 727–728
brain metastases
  incidence, 304
  treatment, 304–305
brain tumors, primary
  gliomas, 297
    grades I and II astrocytoma, 298
    grades III and IV astrocytoma, 298–301
    oligodendroglioma, 301–304
  incidence, 297
  medulloblastoma, 302–303
  PCNSL, 303–304
breast cancer
  cytotoxic therapy, 186
    advanced disease treatment, 191–193
    early disease treatment, 187–191, 188*t*
    response to, 186
  diagnostic evaluation, 176–180
  endocrine therapy, 193
    advanced disease treatment, 194–195
    early disease treatment, 193–194
  epidemiology, risk factors, 172–174
  histology, 179–180
  prevention, 174
  prognosis, 184, 187*t*
    estrogen, progesterone receptors, 185
    gene profiling, 185–186
    Her-2/neu gene, 185
    online tools, 186
    other factors, 186
    stage, 184–185
  screening, 175
  signs, symptoms, 175–176
  staging, 176, 179*t*
  therapy, approach to, 180
    consultation, 180
    endocrine therapy, 184
    radiation therapy, 182–183
    surgery, 182
    systemic therapy, 183–184
    therapy goals, 180–181
  therapy complications, 195–196
  TNM classification, 177–178*t*
bronchioloalveolar cancer, 100
bronchoscopy
  esophageal carcinoma, 122
  infection, sputum and, 577–578
  pneumonia, 579
Burkitt lymphoma (BL), 474, 482*t*, 535
busulfan
  dosage, schedule, 728
  EV, 423
  mechanism of action, 728
  primary indications, 728
  PV, 421
  special precautions, 728
  toxicity, 728–729

C

C225. *See* cetuximab
cabazitaxel
    dosage, schedule, 729
    mechanism of action, 729
    primary indications, 729
    special precautions, 729
    toxicity, 729–730
calcitonin
    hypercalcemia, 507, 632
    MM, 507
Campath. *See* alemtuzumab
Camptotheca accuminata, 699
camptothecins, 699
cancer of the large intestine, 137–138
    adjuvant chemotherapy
        colon cancer, 144–145
        rectal cancer, 146–147
        resected hepatic metastases, 145
    complications, 146–147
    follow-up, 146
    serum CEA, 140
    staging, 138–140, 139*t*
    treatment, advanced disease, 140–143
cancer of the small intestine
    adenocarcinomas, 137
    NETs, 134
        carcinoid syndrome, 135–136
        TNM stages, 135*t*
        treatment, 136–137
    TNM stages, 138*t*
cancer treatment
    choice of modality
        biologic response modifiers, MTT and, 66
        chemotherapy, 65–66
        combined-modality therapy, 67
        radiotherapy, 65
        surgery, 64–65
    goals, setting
        medical perspective, 64
        patient perspective, 63
    palliative care, 67–68
cancer treatment, late physical effects
    late organ toxicities
        cardiac toxicity, 58
        hematologic, immunologic impairment, 59–60
        nephrotoxicity, 59
        neurotoxicity, 59
        pulmonary toxicity, 58
    other sequelae
        endocrine problems, 61
        gonadal failure, dysfunction, 61
        musculoskeletal system, 61
        premature menopause, 61
        psychological, social concerns, 61
    second malignancies
        acute myelogenous leukemia, 60
        solid tumors, other malignancies, 60
cancer vaccines, 43–44
Candida species, 409
    dissemination, 567, 570, 575
    therapy, 580, 588*t*, 589
capecitabine
    biliary tract cancer, 166

breast cancer, 191–192
colorectal cancer, 142–143, 145
dosage, schedule, 730
gastric carcinoma, 131–132
mechanism of action, 730
pancreatic cancer, 156, 159
primary indications, 730
rectal cancer, 146
special precautions, 730–731
toxicity, 731
Capnocytophaga canimorsus, 570
carbamazepine
    cancer pain, 673
    seizures, 307
carboplatin
    cervical cancer, 204
    dosage, schedule, 731
    endometrial cancer, 208–209, 209*t*
    esophageal carcinoma, 126
    HL, 448
    head and neck cancer therapy, 81, 84–85
    lung cancer
        NCLC, 105, 107*t*, 110
        SCLC, 115, 115*t*
    mechanism of action, 731
    melanoma, 286
    metastatic cancer of unknown origin, 521
    ovarian cancer, 215–219, 216*t*
    ovarian germ cell tumors, 224
    peritoneal effusions, 643
    primary indications, 731
    skin testing protocol, 547*t*
    special precautions, 731–732
    toxicity, 732
carcinoid syndrome, 135–136
cardiac toxicity, 58
carfilzomib, 37
carmustine
    dosage, schedule, 733
    mechanism of action, 732
    primary indications, 732
    special precautions, 733
    toxicity, 733–734
cART. *See* combination antiretroviral therapy
Catharanthus roseus, 698
CBC. *See* complete blood cell count
CBTRUS. *See* Central Brain Tumor Registry
        of the United States
CBV regimen, Hodgkin lymphoma, 449*t*
CD4. *See* cluster of differentiation 4
cell cycle, 5–6, 5*f*
cell cycle-nonspecific drugs, 8, 8*t*
cell cycle-specific drugs, 8, 8*t*
cell death, 2–3, 3*f*
cell signaling targeted therapy, 21
    intracellular signaling proteins, inhibition
        of, 30–35
    ligand-receptor binding, blocking, 21–22
        EGFR family, 22–25
        IGF1R, 26–27
        VEGF, 25–26
    RTKs, inhibition of, 27–30
cell-mediated immunity (CMI), 566–567
cellular immune system suppression, 571–572

cellular therapy, melanoma, 289–290
cellular toxin conjugated antibodies, 41
Central Brain Tumor Registry of the United States (CBTRUS), 297
central nervous system (CNS), 15
  DLBCL, 476
  NSCLC, 99
cerebral edema
  clinical evaluation, 620–621
  refractory
    treatment, 307
  treatment, 306–307, 621–622
cervical cancer, 199, 538
  clinical presentation, 200
  diagnosis, 200–201
  histology, 199
  prognostic factors, 201
  screening, 199–200
  staging, 201, 201*t*
  treatment
    adenocarcinoma, 204
    advanced stage disease, 203–204
    dysplasia, in situ carcinoma, 202
    early stage disease, 202–203
    neoadjuvant chemotherapy, 204
    novel biologics, 204
    palliative care, 204–205
    palliative chemotherapy, 204
cervical intraepithelial neoplasia (CIN), 538
cetuximab
  colorectal cancer, 143
  dosage, schedule, 734
  esophageal carcinoma, 126
  head and neck cancer therapy
    radiation sensitizer, 85
    single agent activity, 82, 84
  mechanism of action, 734
  primary indications, 734
  special precautions, 734
  toxicity, 734–735
  vulvar cancer, 223
chelation therapy, iron overload and, 434
chemotherapeutic agents, 701
  dose modification, 702–705, 705*t*
  dose recommendation, 702
  dose selection and designation, 702
  drug toxicity, 702
  drugs, classes of, 693–694, 695–696*t*
    alkylating agents, 694–697
    antimetabolites, 697–698
    hormones, hormone antagonists, 699–700
    molecularly target agents, 700–701
    natural products, 698–699
chemotherapy, 65–66
chlorambucil
  CLL, 409–410, 410
  dosage, schedule, 735
  mechanism of action, 735
  primary indications, 735
  special precautions, 735
  toxicity, 735
  WM, 510
cholangiocarcinoma
  chemotherapy, 165–166

current recommendations, 166
  epidemiology, 164
  natural history, 164–165
  pathogenesis, 164–165
  presentation, 164
chondrosarcoma, 335
CHOP regimen
  DLBCL, 474
  NHL, in elderly, 487
  phenotype directed-targeted therapy, 40
chronic lymphocytic leukemia (CLL), 394, 405, 468
  complications of
    autoimmunity, 408
    malignancies, 408
    recurrent infections, 409
  diagnosis and staging, 405–408, 407*t*
  therapy, 409
    bendamustine, 412
    initial, 409–410
    monoclonal antibody-based, 410–412, 413*t*
    other agents, 412–413
    response assessment, 413*t*, 414
    stem cell transplantation, 413–414
chronic myelogenous leukemia (CML), 395
  classification
    accelerated phase (AP), 397, 397*t*
    blast phase (BP), 397–398, 397*t*
    chronic phase (CP), 397
  diagnosis, 395–396
  prognosis, 398
  therapy, 398–399
    advanced-phase, 404–405
    allogeneic stem cell transplant, 402–404, 403*t*
    conclusion, 405
    dasatinib, 401–402
    imatinib, 399–401, 400*t*
    interferon-α, cytarabine, 404
    nilotinib, 402
chronic phase (CP), 395, 397
cimetidine, anaphylaxis, 625
CIN. *See* cervical intraepithelial neoplasia
circulating immunoglobulins (IVIGs), 566–567
circulating phagocytic cells, 567
cisplatin
  ACC, 273
  anal cancer, 149
  biliary tract cancer, 165–166
  cervical cancer, 203–205
  dosage, schedule, 736
  endometrial cancer, 208–209, 209*t*
  esophageal carcinoma, 126
  Ewing sarcoma, 330
  gastric carcinoma, 128, 130–132
  GTN, 227*t*, 228
  HL, 448
  head and neck cancer chemotherapy
    combination, metastatic disease, 84–85
    radiation sensitizer, 85
    single agent activity, 80–81
  lung cancer
    NCLC, 100, 101*t*, 102–103, 107*t*, 109
    SCLC, 115, 115*t*
  mechanism of action, 735

cisplatin *(continued)*
melanoma, 286
metastatic cancer of unknown origin, 520
neuroendocrine carcinoma, 521
osteosarcoma, 331–332, 334
ovarian cancer, 215–217, 216*t*
ovarian germ cell tumors, 224
penile cancer, 248
peritoneal effusions, 643
primary indications, 736
special precautions, 736–737
testicular cancer, 246–247
thyroid cancer, 268
toxicity, 737
uterine sarcomas, 210
vulvar cancer, 223
cladribine
dosage, schedule, 738
HCL, 415
mechanism of action, 737–738
primary indications, 738
special precautions, 738
toxicity, 738
classic chemotherapy agents, 2–3
CLL. *See* chronic lymphocytic leukemia
clofarabine
ALL, 388–389
AML, in older adults, 365
dosage, schedule, 739
mechanism of action, 739
primary indications, 739
relapsed AML, 361
special precautions, 739
toxicity, 739
clonazepam, 673
clonidine, 674
cloretazine, 365
Clostridium difficile, 570, 587–588
cluster of differentiation 4 (CD4), 571–572
CMF regime, breast cancer, 188
CMI. *See* cell-mediated immunity
CML. *See* chronic myelogenous leukemia
CMV. *See* cytomegalovirus (CMV)
CMV-seronegative cellular blood products, 614
CNS. *See* central nervous system
CNS toxicity, of ifosfamide, 321, 778
coagulation factors and bleeding
cryoprecipitated antihemophilic factor, 613
factor IX concentrates, 613
FFP, 612
plasma, 612
coagulopathy, acute leukemias, 347, 367, 367*t*
CODOX-M/IVAC regimen, 481, 481*t*, 535
Cogentin. *See* benztropine
colon cancer, 139*t*, 144–145
colorectal cancer, 137–138
adjuvant chemotherapy
colon cancer, 144–145
rectal cancer, 145–146
resected hepatic metastases, 145
complications, 146–147
follow-up, 146
serum CEA, 140

staging, 138–140, 139*t*
treatment, advanced disease, 140–144
combination antiretroviral therapy (cART), 523
combination chemotherapy
agent selection, principles of, 11–12
clinical effectiveness, 12
effectiveness, reasons for, 10–11
head and neck cancer
adjuvant therapy, 86
induction therapy, 86–87
metastatic disease, 83–85, 83*t*
combined-modality therapy, 67
combretastatin, thyroid cancer, 267
Common Toxicity Criteria, 57
Compazine. *See* prochlorperazine
complete blood cell count (CBC), 233
complete response (CR)
acute leukemias, 349–351
definition, 52
computed tomography (CT)
bladder cancer, 233
brain tumor, 298
esophageal carcinoma, 121
head and neck cancer, 73
lung cancer screening, 95
melanoma, 280
metastatic cancer of unknown origin, 516
pancreatic cancer, 152–153
soft-tissue sarcomas, 315
spinal cord compression, 618–619
thyroid cancer, 262
tumor size, baseline, 51
concomitant drugs, 76
conjugated antibodies, 41–42
consolidation therapy
acute leukemia, 350
ALL, adult, 355*t*, 377, 384
APL, 368*t*
constipation, 558–559, 669
corticosteroids, 700
anaphylaxis, 625
cancer pain, 673–674
cerebral edema, 306–307
dosage, schedule, 740
mechanism of action, 739
PMF, 425
primary indications, 740
special precautions, 740
spinal cord compression, 619
toxicity, 740
Cotswold staging system, 438–439, 439*t*
CPT-11. *See* topoisomerase I inhibitor
irinotecan
CR. *See* complete response
CT. *See* computed tomography
CTLA-4 inhibitors, 37–38
cutaneous T-cell lymphomas (CTCL; mycosis
fungoides), 472, 472*t*
CyADIC regimen, soft-tissue sarcomas, 317–318
cyclophosphamide
ALL, 376
breast cancer, 188–191
DLBCL, 475*t*

dosage, schedule, 741
Ewing sarcoma, 328–330
indolent lymphoma, 471*t*
GTN, 227, 227*t*
mechanism of action, 741
melanoma, 287*t*, 294
MM, 503
osteosarcoma, 332
primary indications, 741
relapsed AML, 359
soft-tissue sarcomas, 317–319, 322
special precautions, 741
thyroid and adrenal carcinomas, 275
toxicity, 741–742
WM, 510
cytarabine, 7–8
ALL, 368*t*, 375–380, 382–383, 386–387, 388*t*
AML, in adults, 351–354, 352*t*, 361–362
AML, in older adults, 363–364
AML, relapsed, 357–359
APL, 368*t*, 369–370
CML, 404
dosage, schedule, 742
leptomeningeal metastases, 306
malignant subarachnoid infiltrates, 646
mechanism of action, 742
primary indications, 742
special precautions, 742
t-AML, 365
toxicity, 742–743
cytokine, suppression, 572
cytokine-release syndrome, 547–548
cytomegalovirus (CMV), 409, 590, 593
cytopenias, 510
cytoreductive surgery, 213–214
cytosine arabinoside, 643
cytotoxic therapy, 186
ACC, 273
advanced disease treatment, 191–193
early disease treatment, 187–191, 188*t*
favorable-risk AML, 355–356
kidney cancer, 255
prostate cancer, 241–242
response to, 186–187
thyroid cancer, 266
cytotoxicity, 10
CyVADIC regimen, Ewing sarcoma, 328–329

D

dacarbazine
carcinoid tumors, 137
dosage, schedule, 743
Ewing sarcoma, 329–330
melanoma, 286
osteosarcoma, 334
primary indications, 743
soft-tissue sarcomas, 317, 322
special precautions, 743
toxicity, 743–744
dactinomycin, 699
dosage, schedule, 744
GTN, 227
mechanism of action, 744

osteosarcoma, 332, 334
primary indications, 744
soft-tissue sarcomas, 319
special precautions, 744
toxicity, 744–745
DA-EPOCH regimen. *See* dose-adjusted EPOCH
regimen
darbepoetin
dosage, schedule, 745
MDS, 431
mechanism of action, 745
primary indications, 745
special precautions, 745
toxicity, 746
dasatinib (Sprycel), 32
CML, 401–402
dosage, schedule, 746
mechanism of action, 746
primary indications, 746
special precautions, 746
toxicity, 746–747
DAT. *See* direct antiglobulin test
daunorubicin, 699
adult ALL, 376–379
adult AML, 351–353, 352*t*
ALL, salvage therapy, 386
AML, in older adults, 362–363
AML, pregnancy and, 366
APL, 368*t*
dosage, schedule, 747
mechanism of action, 747
primary indications, 747
special precautions, 747–748
toxicity, 748
daunorubicin, liposomal
dosage, schedule, 749
mechanism of action, 748
primary indication, 749
special precautions, 749
toxicity, 749
decitabine
AML, in older adults, 365
dosage, schedule, 750
MDS, 429, 432, 434
mechanism of action, 749–750
primary indications, 750
relapsed AML, 361
toxicity, 750
deferasirox (Exjade), 435
deferoxamine (Desferal), 434
degarelix
dosage, schedule, 751
mechanism of action, 750
primary indications, 750
special precautions, 751
toxicity, 751
dendritic (DC) cell vaccine, prostate cancer, 242
denileukin diftitox (Ontak), 42–43
CTCL, 473
dosage, schedule, 751
mechanism of action, 751
MF, 295
primary indications, 751

denileukin diftitox (Ontak) *(continued)*
  special precautions, 751
  toxicity, 751–752
Depo-Provera. *See* medroxyprogesterone
depression, 683–687, 685*t*, 686*t*, 687*t*
DES (diethylstilbestrol), 241
desmopressin, 615
dexamethasone
  DLBCL, 475
  gastric carcinoma, 128
  melanoma, 288
  MM, 499–500
  refractory cerebral edema, 307
dexrazoxane
  dosage, schedule, 752
  mechanism of action, 752
  primary indication, 752
  toxicity, 752–753
DFS. *See* disease-free survival
DHAP regimen, non-Hodgkin lymphoma, 483*t*
diagnosis
  clinical and, 46
  pathologic, 45–46
  treatment, without pathologic diagnosis,
    46–47
diarrhea, 557–558, 559*t*, 587–588
DIC. *See* disseminated intravascular coagulation
differentiated thyroid cancer (DTC), 259
  diagnosis and staging, 261–263
  prognosis, 260–261
  treatment
    radiotherapy, 265–266
    RAI, 264–265
    surgery, 263
    TSH suppression, 263–264
diffuse large B-cell lymphoma (DLBCL),
    472–473, 475*t*, 476–477
diphenhydramine (Benadryl)
  acute confusional states, 682
  anaphylaxis, 625
direct antiglobulin test (DAT), 406
discrete vascular thrombosis, 600–602
disease-free survival (DFS), 50, 437
disseminated intravascular coagulation (DIC)
  discrete vascular thrombosis, 602–603
  laboratory diagnosis of, 597–598, 597*t*
DLBCL. *See* diffuse large B-cell lymphoma
DNP-VACC. *See* M-Vax
docetaxel
  breast cancer, 190–191
  dosage, schedule, 753
  gastric carcinoma, 130, 132
  head and neck cancer therapy, 81, 84–85
  mechanism of action, 753
  NSCLC, 107*t*, 110–111
  ovarian cancer, 219
  primary indications, 753
  prostate cancer, 242
  soft-tissue sarcomas, 320, 322
  special precautions, 753
  toxicity, 753–754
dolasetron (Anzemet), acute confusional
    states, 682

dose-adjusted (DA-EPOCH) regimen,
    HIV-associated NHL, 531–534, 533*t*
doxorubicin (Adriamycin), 699
  ACC, 273
  ALL, 378, 380, 386
  breast cancer, 188–191
  cardiac damage, 321
  DLBCL, 475*t*
  dosage, schedule, 754
  endometrial cancer, 208–209, 209*t*
  Ewing sarcoma, 328–329
  gastric carcinoma, 128
  HL, 448
  mechanism of action, 754
  MF, 294
  MM, 504
  osteosarcoma, 331–332
  primary effusion lymphoma, 529–530
  peritoneal effusions, 643
  PNETs, 162
  primary indications, 754
  soft-tissue sarcomas, 317–319, 322
  special precautions, 754–755
  thyroid cancer, 267–268
  toxicity, 755
doxorubicin, liposomal
  dosage, schedule, 756
  mechanism of action, 756
  MM, 504
  primary indications, 756
  special precautions, 756
  toxicity, 756–757
doxycycline, pleural effusion treatment, 638, 640
DTC. *See* differentiated thyroid cancer
Dukes staging system, 138
duloxetine, cancer pain, 672–673
dysphasia, aspiration and, 89–90

E

EAC. *See* esophageal adenocarcinoma
Early Lung Cancer Action Project, 95
Eastern Cooperative Oncology Group (ECOG)
  kidney cancer, 252–253
  melanoma, 283
  Eastern Cooperative Oncology Group (ECOG)/
    World Health Organization (WHO)/
    Zubrod Performance Status Scale, 49, 49*t*
EATCL. *See* enteropathy-associated T-cell
    lymphoma
EBV. *See* Epstein-Barr virus
EGFR. *See* epidermal growth factor receptor
EGFR TKIs. *See* epidermal growth factor recep-
    tor tyrosine kinase inhibitors
Ehrlichia chaffeensis, 570
elderly patients
  AML
    auto-HSCT, 364
    azacitidine, 365
    background, 361–362
    clofarabine, 365
    cytarabine, 363–364
    daunorubicin, 362–363
    decitabine, 365

GO, 364
HDAC, 363–364
idarubicin, 363
induction therapy, 362–363
postremission therapy, 363–364
RIC (mini)-HCST, 364–365
NHL, 487–488
CHOP regimen, 487
EMA-CO regimen, GTN, 227*t*, 228
EMA-EP regimen, GTN, 227*t*
Emend. *See* aprepitant
emetic potential, 550, 551*t*
endocrine problems, 60
endocrine therapy, breast cancer, 184
endometrial cancer, 205
clinical presentation, 205–206
diagnosis, 206
histology, 205
prognostic factors, 206
screening, 205
staging, 206, 207*t*
treatment
chemotherapy, 208–209, 209*t*
follow-up, 209
hormonal therapy, 208
multimodality therapy, 209
novel biologics, 209
radiation, 207–208
surgery, 206–207
uterine papillary serous carcinoma, 209
endometrial stromal sarcoma (ESS), 209–210
endoscopic esophageal ultrasound (EUS)
carcinoma of esophagus, 122
pancreatic cancer, 153
endoscopic retrograde cholangiopancreatography, 153
Enterobacteriaceae, 576
Enterococcus, 588*t*, 589
enteropathy-associated T-cell lymphoma
(EATCL), 455
enzymes, 699
epidermal growth factor receptor (EGFR),
22, 564
EGFR1-targeted therapy, 22–24
HER2, erbB2-targeted therapy, 24–25
lung cancer, 94–95, 108–109
epidermal growth factor receptor (EGFR)
tyrosine kinase inhibitors (TKIs),
109–110, 112–114
epinephrine, anaphylaxis, 625
epirubicin, 699
breast cancer, 190
dosage, schedule, 757
gastric carcinoma, 128, 130–131
mechanism of action, 757
primary indications, 757
special precautions, 757
toxicity, 757–758
EPOCH regimen, DLBCL, 475
epoetin
dosage, schedule, 758
mechanism of action, 758
primary indications, 758

special precautions, 758–759
toxicity, 759
epratuzumab, 41
Epstein-Barr virus (EBV), NPC and, 72
eribulin mesylate
dosage, schedule, 759
mechanism of action, 759
primary indications, 759
special precautions, 759–760
toxicity, 760
erlotinib (Tarceva), 27–28
dosage, schedule, 760
mechanism of action, 760
NSCLC, 112, 112–113
pancreatic cancer, 159
primary indications, 760
special precautions, 760–761
toxicity, 761
vulvar cancer, 223
erythropoietin
MDS, 430–431
PMF, 425
ESCC. *See* esophageal squamous cell
carcinoma
Escherichia coli, 570
ESHAP regimen
Hodgkin lymphoma, 448
non-Hodgkin lymphoma, 483*t*
esophageal adenocarcinoma (EAC), 121
esophageal squamous cell carcinoma
(ESCC), 121
esophagus carcinoma
advanced disease treatment, 125–127
clinical manifestations, 121–122
combined-modality treatment, 122
epidemiology, 121
follow-up studies, 127
preoperative chemotherapy, 124
pretreatment evaluation, 121–122
radiation therapy, 124–125
supportive care, 127
TNM stages, 123–124*t*
treatment, prognosis, 122
ESS. *See* endometrial stromal sarcoma
essential thrombocythemia (ET)
diagnosis, 421–422
evolution, outcome, 423
treatment regimens, 422–423
estrogen receptors, breast cancer, 185
estrogens, 700
prostate cancer, 241
thromboembolism in cancer, 600
ET. *See* essential thrombocythemia
ethyleneimine derivatives, 697
etoposide
ACC, 273
acute leukemias, 353
DLBCL, 475*t*
dosage, schedule, 762
Ewing sarcoma, 329–330
gastric carcinoma, 128
GTN, 227, 227*t*
HL, 448, 449*t*

etoposide *(continued)*
  KS, 528
  mechanism of action, 761
  metastatic cancer of unknown origin, 520–521
  neuroendocrine carcinoma, 521
  ovarian cancer, 216*t*
  ovarian germ cell tumors, 224
  peritoneal effusions, 643
  primary indications, 761–762
  relapsed AML, 358–360
  SCLC, 115*t*
  special precautions, 762
  testicular cancer, 246
  toxicity, 762
EUS. *See* endoscopic esophageal ultrasound
evaluable disease, 53–54
everolimus (Afinitor), 34
  dosage, schedule, 763
  kidney cancer, 255
  mechanism of action, 763
  primary indication, 763
  special precautions, 763
  toxicity, 763–764
Ewing Family of Tumors (EFT), 325
Ewing sarcoma
  chemotherapy, 328
    alternative regimens, 329
    CyVADIC regimen, 328–329
    dose modifications, 329
    high-dose, 330–331
    high-dose VAI regimen, 328
    responses, 329–330
    secondary, 330
  primary treatment, 328
  tumor characteristics, 325–328, 326–327*t*
exemestane
  breast cancer, 193, 195
  dosage, schedule, 764
  mechanism of action, 764
  primary indications, 764
  special precautions, 764
  toxicity, 764
external-beam therapy
  bone metastasis, 634
  metastatic bone pain, 674
EXTREME trial, 83

F

FAB classification. *See* French-American-British
      classification
familial MTC (FMTC) syndrome, 259
Fanconi syndrome, 334
fatigue, 557
favorable-risk AML, postremission therapy,
      355–356
FDA. *See* Food and Drug Administration
FDG-PET. *See* fluorodeoxyglucose-positron
      emission tomography
FEC regimen, breast cancer, 190
fertility
  acute leukemias, 349
  head and neck cancer and, 76
fever, 348, 580–584

fibrin glue, 615
fibrinolytic therapy, 601–602
fibrosis, head and neck cancer and, 90–91
filgrastim
  dosage, schedule, 765
  Ewing sarcoma, 328
  HL, 450
  MDS, 431
  mechanism of action, 764
  primary indications, 765
  SCLC, 118
  soft-tissue sarcomas, 318, 320
  special precautions, 765
  toxicity, 765
fine needle aspiration (FNA)
  pancreatic cancer, 153
  thyroid cancer, 261
FISH analysis. *See* fluorescence in-situ hybridiza-
      tion analysis
5-azacitidine, 361
5-fluorouracil, 188
5-FU
  biliary tract cancer, 165–166
  PNETs, 162
FLAG-IDA regimen, acute myeloid leukemia, 359
flavopiridol
  CLL, 413
  dosage, schedule, 765–766
  mechanism of action, 765
  primary indication, 765
  special precautions, 766
  toxicity, 766
FLIPI. *See* follicular lymphoma international
      prognostic index
FLO regimen, colorectal cancer, 145
floxuridine, peritoneal effusions, 643
FLT-3 gene, 341–342
FLT-3-ITD gene, 341–342
fludarabine
  CLL, 409–410
  dosage, schedule, 766
  mechanism of action, 766
  MF, 294
  primary indication, 766
  relapsed AML, 358–359
  special precautions, 767
  toxicity, 767
  WM, 511
fluorescence in-situ hybridization (FISH)
      analysis, 396
fluorodeoxyglucose (FDG)-positron emission
      tomography (PET), 52, 464–467, 530
fluoroquinolones, 592
fluorouracil
  anal cancer, 148–149
  breast cancer, 190–191
  carcinoid tumors, 136
  colorectal cancer, 141–143, 145
  dosage, schedule, 766
  esophageal carcinoma, 125–126
  gastric carcinoma, 128, 130–134
  head and neck cancer chemotherapy
      combination, metastatic disease, 83–85

radiation sensitizer, 85–86
single agent activity, 82
mechanism of action, 767
nonmelanoma skin cancer, 291
pericardial effusions, 645
peritoneal effusions, 643
pleural effusion treatment, 640
primary indications, 768
rectal cancer, 145–146
special precautions, 768–769
flutamide
dosage, schedule, 769
mechanism of action, 769
primary indications, 769
toxicity, 769
FMTC syndrome. *See* familial MTC syndrome
FNA. *See* fine needle aspiration
Foley catheter/UTIs, 587
FOLFIRI regimen, colorectal cancer, 142–143
FOLFOX4 regimen, colorectal cancer, 142, 145
FOLFOXIRI regimen, colorectal cancer, 143
folic acid analogs, 697
follicular lymphoma (FL), 467
pathology, 467
prognostic scoring systems, 467–468, 468*t*
Follicular Lymphoma International Prognostic
Index (FLIPI), 468–469, 469*t*
Food and Drug Administration (FDA), 16
fractionated radiotherapy, 100
French-American-British (FAB) classification, 338
Fuhrman Nuclear Grade, 250
fulvestrant
breast cancer, 195
dosage, schedule, 770
mechanism of action, 769
primary indications, 770
special precautions, 770
toxicity, 770
function-directed therapy, 17
angiogenesis-targeted therapy, 36
cell signaling targeted therapy, 21
intracellular signaling proteins, inhibition
of, 30–35
ligand-receptor binding, blocking, 21–27
RTKs, inhibition of, 27–30
immune modulation-targeted therapy, 37–39
protein degradation-targeted therapy, 36–37

G

gabapentin
anxiety, 688
cancer pain, 673
insomnia, 692
gallbladder carcinoma, 163
chemotherapy, 165–166
current recommendations, 166
epidemiology, 164
natural history, 164–165
pathogenesis, 164–165
presentation, 164
gastric acid suppression, 161
gastric carcinoma
adjuvant chemotherapy, 133

clinical manifestations, 127–128
combined-modality therapy, 133
complications, 134
epidemiology, 127
follow-up studies, 134
postoperative adjuvant combined modality
regimen, 133–134
refractory disease treatment, 134
TNM states, 129*t*
treatment, advanced disease, 128–132
treatment, prognosis, 128
gastroesophageal reflux disease (GERD), 121
gastrointestinal stromal tumors (GISTs), 311
gastrointestinal (GI) tract carcinomas, 120–149
Gastrointestinal Tumor Study Group
(GITSG), 155
GCTs. *See* germ cell tumors; granulosa cell
tumors
GDC-0941 inhibitor, 35
gefitinib (Iressa), 28
dosage, schedule, 770
mechanism of action, 770
NSCLC, 109, 112
primary indications, 770
special precautions, 770
toxicity, 771
gemcitabine
biliary tract cancer, 165–166
breast cancer, 192
cervical cancer, 204
dosage, schedule, 771
HL, 448
head and neck cancer therapy, 82
mechanism of action, 771
metastatic cancer of unknown origin, 521
MF, 295
NCLC, 107*t*, 110
ovarian cancer, 216*t*
pancreatic cancer, 156–159
primary indications, 771
soft-tissue sarcomas, 317, 320, 322
special precautions, 771
toxicity, 772
uterine sarcomas, 210
GemOx. *See* oxaliplatin
Gem-Tax regimen, soft-tissue sarcomas,
320, 322
gemtuzumab ozogamicin (Mylotarg), 41
dosage, schedule, 772
mechanism of action, 772
primary indications, 772
special precautions, 772–773
toxicity, 773
gemtuzumab ozogamicin (GO), AML, in older
adults, 364
gene expression profiling (GEP), 460–463, 467
GERD. *See* gastroesophageal reflux disease
germ cell tumors (GCTs), 243
gestational trophoblastic neoplasm (GTN)
clinical presentation, 226
diagnosis, 226
histology, 225
prognostic factors, 226

gestational trophoblastic neoplasm *(continued)*
 screening, 226
 staging, 226, 227t
 treatment, 226–228, 227t
GI tract carcinomas. *See* gastrointestinal tract
  carcinomas
GITSG. *See* Gastrointestinal Tumor Study Group
Gleevec. *See* imatinib
gliomas, 297
 grades I and II astrocytoma, 298
 grades III and IV astrocytoma, 298–299
  chemotherapy, 299–300
  regimens, newly diagnosed malignant,
   300–301
  regimens, recurrent GBM, 301
glucocorticoids, hypercalcemia, 632
GO. *See* gemtuzumab ozogamicin
gonadal failure, dysfunction, 61
gonadotropin-releasing hormone analogs
 dosage, schedule, 774
 mechanism of action, 773
 primary indication, 773
 special precautions, 774
 toxicity, 774
graft-versus-host disease (GVHD), 347–348, 604
granisetron (Kytril), 682
granulocytopenia, 321
granulosa cell tumors (GCTs), 225
 clinical presentation, 225
 histology, 225
 prognostic factors, 225
 staging, 225
 treatment, 225
GSK2141795 inhibitor, 35
GTN. *See* gestational trophoblastic neoplasm
GVHD. *See* graft-versus-host disease
gynecologic cancer, 199–228. *See also* specific
  cancers

H

Haemophilus influenzae, 409, 567, 570
hairy cell leukemia (HCL), 406, 414–415
Haldol. *See* haloperidol
haloperidol (Haldol), 680–681
HBV. *See* hepatitis B virus
HCC. *See* hepatocellular carcinoma
hCG. *See* human chorionic gonadotropin
HCL. *See* hairy cell leukemia
HCV. *See* hepatitis C virus
HDAC. *See* high-dose cytarabine
HDAC regimens, acute leukemias, 359–360
head and neck cancer (HNC)
 anatomy, 69, 70t, 71f
 epidemiology, 69–71
  HPV-associated oropharyngeal
   carcinomas, 72
  NPC, 71–72
  SCA, traditional risk factors, 71
 initial work-up, 73
 natural history, 76–77
 patient assessment, 74–75
  bone marrow function, 75
  concomitant drugs, 76

 fertility, 76
 hepatic function, 76
 neuropathy, 76
 pulmonary function, 75
 renal function, 75
 presenting symptoms, 72–73
 secondary cancer prevention, 91
 staging, 73–74, 74t, 75t
 supportive care
  dysphasia, aspiration, 89–90
  lymphedema, fibrosis, 90–91
  metabolic abnormalities, 91
  mucositis, 89
  nutrition, 87–88, 88t
  support systems, 87
  xerostomia, oral care, 90
 treatment, chemotherapy
  combination, adjuvant therapy, 86
  combination, induction therapy, 86–87
  combination, metastatic disease, 83–85, 83t
  radiation sensitizer, 85–86
  single agent activity, 80–83, 81t
 treatment, general considerations
  HPV-associated oropharyngeal
   carcinomas, 80
  NPC, 79
  SCA, 77–79
hematologic impairment, 59–60
hematologic toxicity, dose modification, 704
hematopoietic stem cell transplantation
  (HSCT). *See also* allogeneic (allo-) HSCT;
   autologous bone marrow transplantation
   (ABMT)
 ALL, 389–391
 infections, 590–591
 prophylaxis of infection, 593–594
hemorrhagic cystitis
 cyclophosphamide therapy and, 321, 741
 ifosfamide and, 778
hemorrhagic syndromes
 other therapies, 615–616
 transfusion therapy, 608–615, 611t
heparin, discrete vascular thrombosis,
  601–602
hepatic function, head and neck cancer and, 76
hepatic toxicity, 321
hepatitis B virus (HBV), 524
hepatitis C virus (HCV), 524
hepatocellular carcinoma (HCC)
 advanced therapy, 170–171
 diagnostic evaluation, screening, 168
 epidemiology, 166–167
 etiology, 167
 laboratory tests, 168
 preoperative evaluation, 169
 primary therapy, 169–170
 risk factors, 167
 signs, symptoms, 167
 staging, 168–169
 TNM staging, 169t
hepatosplenic T-cell lymphoma (HSTCL), 455
Her-2/neu gene, breast cancer, 185
herpes simplex virus (HSV), 576

high-dose cytarabine (HDAC)
  acute leukemias, 352–356, 355*t*
  AML, in older adults, 363–364
  relapsed AML, 358–360
high-dose therapy (HDT), HIV-associated NHL, 535–536
HIV. *See* human immunodeficiency virus
HIV-associated malignancies, 523–524
  HPV, associated cancers, 537–539
  KS
    epidemiology, 524–525
    presentation, patient evaluation, 525
    staging, 526, 526*t*
    treatment, 526–528, 527*t*
  KSHV, 524
  KSHV-MCD, 528–529
  NADMS, 539–540
  NHL, 530–536, 532*t*, 533*t*
  PCNSL, 536–537
  PEL, 529–530
HLA typing, acute leukemias, 348
HNC. *See* head and neck cancer
Hodgkin lymphoma (HL), 60, 437
  diagnosis, pathology, 438
  follow-up, 449–450
  staging
    Cotswold staging system, 438–439, 439*t*
    prognostic score, advanced HL, 439
    tests, 439–441
  therapy, 441–442, 441*t*
    ABVD, 446–448
    chemotherapy, 443*t*, 445–446
    RT, 442–443, 442*t*
    salvage, 447–448, 448*t*
    treatment, by stage, 443–445
    treatment, of symptoms, 450
hormone antagonists, 698–699
  general description, 699–700
  types of, 700
hormone replacement therapy (HRT), 173–174
hormones, 698–699
  general description, 699–700
  types of, 700
hospice, 67–68
HPV. *See* human papillomavirus
HPV-associated cancers. *See* human papillomavirus–associated cancers
HRT. *See* hormone replacement therapy
HSCT. *See* hematopoietic stem cell transplantation
HSTCL. *See* hepatosplenic T-cell lymphoma
HSV. *See* herpes simplex virus
human chorionic gonadotropin (hCG), 224, 243
human immunodeficiency virus (HIV), 485
human papillomavirus (HPV)
  cervical cancer, 199–200
  epidemiology, 72
  natural history, 76
  secondary cancer prevention, 91
  treatment, 80, 87
human papillomavirus (HPV)–associated cancers, 537–539
hydroxycarbamide, 399–400, 774

hydroxyurea
  dosage, schedule, 775
  EV, 423
  gastric carcinoma, 128
  head and neck cancer chemotherapy radiation sensitizer, 85–86
  mechanism of action, 774
  primary indications, 774
  PV, 420
  special precautions, 775
  toxicity, 775
hypercalcemia
  associated tumors, 629
  humoral mediators, 629
  laboratory findings, 629–630
  MM, 507
  rehydration, 630
  symptoms and signs, 629–630
  treatment, 629–632
hyperkalemia
  acute leukemias, 346
  tumor lysis syndrome, 628
hyperleukocytosis, 345–346
hyperphosphatemia, 346
hyperuricemia
  acute leukemias, 346–347
  tumor lysis syndrome, 627
  uric acid nephropathy, 346
hyperviscosity, 508
hypocalcemia
  acute leukemias, 346
  osteosarcoma, 334
hypogammaglobulinemia, 409
hypomethylating agents
  PMF, 426
  relapsed AML, 361
hypotension, 683
hypothalamic hormone analogs, 700
hypoxia, 689–690

I

ibritumomab tiuxetan (Zevalin), 41–42
  dosage, schedule, 776
  indolent lymphoma, 471
  mechanism of action, 775
  non-Hodgkin lymphoma, 485
  primary indications, 775
  special precautions, 776
  toxicity, 776
ICE regimen
  Hodgkin lymphoma, 448, 449*t*
  non-Hodgkin lymphoma, 483*t*
idarubicin, 699
  ALL, 387
  AML
    adult, 351, 352*t*
    in older adults, 363
    in pregnancy, 366
    relapsed, 358–360
  APL, 368*t*, 369
  dosage, schedule, 777
  mechanism of action, 776
  primary indications, 776–777

idarubicin *(continued)*
  relapsed AML, 359
  special precautions, 777
  toxicity, 777
IFN. *See* interferon
ifosfamide
  cervical cancer, 204
  dosage, schedule, 777–778
  Ewing sarcoma, 328–330
  HL, 448
  head and neck cancer therapy, 82, 85
  mechanism of action, 777
  osteosarcoma, 332–334
  primary indications, 777
  soft-tissue sarcomas, 317, 322
  special precautions, 778
  testicular cancer, 247
  toxicity, 778
  uterine sarcomas, 210
IGF. *See* insulinlike growth factor
IGF1R. *See* insulinlike growth factor type 1
      receptor
IGFR. *See* insulinlike growth factor receptor
IHC techniques. *See* immunohistochemical
      techniques
IL-2-diphtheria toxin fusion protein, 284
imatinib (Gleevec), 399–401, 400*t*
imatinib mesylate, 31
  dosage, schedule, 779
  mechanism of action, 779
  primary indications, 779
  special precautions, 779
  stromal or granulosa cell tumors, 225
  toxicity, 779–780
IMiDs. *See* immunomodulatory agents
imipramine, 672
immune modulation-targeted therapy, 37–39
immunohistochemical (IHC) techniques, breast
      cancer, 176
immunologic impairment, 59–60
immunomodulatory agents (IMiDs), 426
immunotherapy
  kidney cancer, 254
  MDS, 433–434
immunotoxins, 42–43
indolent lymphoma. *See* indolent non-Hodgkin
      lymphoma (NHL)
indolent non-Hodgkin lymphoma (NHL),
      466–467
  FL pathology, 467
  FL, prognostic scoring systems, 467–468, 468*t*
  front-line treatment principles, 469–471, 470*t*
  maintenance therapy, 471
induction therapy
  acute leukemias, 351–353, 352*t*
  AML, in older adults, 362–363
  head and neck cancer, 86–87
infections
  acute leukemias, 348
  clinical evaluation, 572–577, 574–575*t*
  clinical history of patient, 571–572
  CLL, 409
  diagnostic imaging, 578–579

etiology, 566–570, 568–569*t*
  HSCT recipients, 590–591
  invasive diagnostic procedures, 579
  MDS, 435
  microbiologic evaluation, 577–578
  MM, 507
  oral, secondary, 556–557
  prophylaxis, 591–594
  treatment, 579–590, 581–582*t*
insomnia, 691–692
insulin suppression, 161
insulinlike growth factor (IGF), 26
insulinlike growth factor receptor (IGFR), 162–163
insulinlike growth factor type 1 receptor
      (IGF1R), 26–27
insulinomas, 160
interferon (IFN)
  carcinoid tumors, 137
  kidney cancer, 254
  melanoma, 284–285
interferon alpha
  dosage, schedule, 780–781
  mechanism of action, 780
  primary indications, 780
  special precautions, 781
  toxicity, 781–782
interferon-α
  CML, 404
  EV, 423
  indolent lymphoma, 472
  KS, 528
  peritoneal effusions, 643
  pleural effusion treatment, 640
  PV, 420–421
Interleukin-2
  dosage, schedule, 706–707
  kidney cancer, 254
  mechanism of action, 706
  primary indications, 706
  prophylaxis, of acute toxicity, 708
  special precautions, 707
  toxicity, 707–708
interleukin-11. *See* oprelvekin
intermediate-risk AML, postremission
      therapy, 356
internal tandem duplication (ITD), 341
International Prognostic Index (IPI),
      465–466, 466*t*
International Prognostic Score (IPS), 439
International Union Against Cancer (UICC), 311
International Workshop on CLL (IWCLL), 409
intraperitoneal chemotherapy, 217–218
intravesical chemotherapy
  administration and follow-up, 234–235
  complications of therapy, 235–236
  response to therapy, 235
  selection of patients, 235
  selection of therapy, 235
  therapeutic regimens, 235
iodine-131, tositumomab (Bexxar), 42
  dosage, schedule, 832
  indolent lymphoma, 470
  mechanism of action, 832

non-Hodgkin lymphoma, 485
primary indications, 832
special precautions, 832
toxicity, 833
ipilimumab, 37–38, 285
dosage, schedule, 782
mechanism of action, 782
primary indications, 782
special precautions, 782
toxicity, 782–783
IPS. *See* International Prognostic Score
Iressa. *See* gefitinib
irinotecan
colorectal cancer, 142–144
dosage, schedule, 783
esophageal carcinoma, 126
Ewing sarcoma, 330
gastric carcinoma, 128, 132
mechanism of action, 783
primary indications, 783
rectal cancer, 147
special precautions, 783–784
toxicity, 784
islet cell tumors, 159–163
ITD. *See* internal tandem duplication
IWCLL. *See* International Workshop on CLL
ixabepilone
breast cancer, 191
dosage, schedule, 785
mechanism of action, 784
primary indications, 784
special precautions, 785
toxicity, 785

J

JAK2 inhibitors, 426

K

Kaposi sarcoma (KS)
epidemiology, 524–525
presentation, patient evaluation, 525–526
staging, 526, 526*t*
treatment, 526–528, 527*t*
Kaposi Sarcoma (KS)-associated herpesvirus
(KSHV), 524
Karnofsky Performance Status Scale, 48, 48*t*
kidney cancer
clinical characteristics, 251–252
epidemiology, 250–251
histopathology, 250
risk factors, 251, 253*t*
staging, 252–253, 252*t*
treatment considerations, 253
treatment regimens, 254–256
Klebsiella pneumoniae, 570
Klinefelter syndrome, 247
KS. *See* Kaposi sarcoma
KSHV. *See* Kaposi Sarcoma-associated
herpesvirus
KSHV-associated MCD (KSHV-MCD), 528–529
KSHV-MCD. *See* KSHV-associated MCD
Kytril. *See* granisetron

L

lactate dehydrogenase (LDH), 353
lamotrigine (Lamictal)
antiepileptic drugs, 308*t*
cancer pain, 673
LAP score. *See* leukocyte alkaline phosphatase
score
laparoscopy
esophageal carcinoma, 122
gastric carcinoma, 128
lapatinib ditosylate (Tykerb), 29–30
breast cancer, 192
dosage, schedule, 786
mechanism of action, 785
primary indications, 786
special precautions, 786
toxicity, 786
large intestine cancer, 137–138
adjuvant chemotherapy
colon cancer, 144–145
rectal cancer, 146–147
resected hepatic metastases, 146
advanced disease treatment, 140–144
complications, 146–147
follow-up, 146
serum CEA, 140
staging, 138–140, 139*t*
LBL. *See* lymphoblastic lymphoma
LDH. *See* lactate dehydrogenase
lenalidomide (Revlimid), 39
CLL, 412–413
dosage, schedule, 787
MDS, 429, 432–433, 434
mechanism of action, 786
MM, 500–501, 503–506
PMF, 425
primary indications, 786
special precautions, 787
toxicity, 787
leptomeningeal metastases, 305
administration, 306
chemotherapy regimens, 305–306
complications, 306
lesions, melanoma, 278–279
letrozole
breast cancer, 193–195
dosage, schedule, 788
mechanism of action, 787–788
primary indications, 788
special precautions, 788
toxicity, 788
leucovorin
ALL, 377
colorectal cancer, 140–146
esophageal carcinoma, 126
gastric carcinoma, 132–134
GTN, 227*t*
osteosarcoma, 332
leucovorin rescue, osteosarcoma, 333
leukapheresis, 345–346
leukocyte alkaline phosphatase (LAP) score,
395–396
leukocyte reduced blood products, 613–614

leukostasis, 345–346
levetiracetam, seizures and, 307
LHRH. *See* luteinizing hormone-releasing hormone
lidocaine (Xylocaine), 644–645
Li-Fraumeni syndrome, 268
ligand-receptor binding, blocking, 21–22
    EGFR family, 22–25
    IGF1R, 26–27
    VEGF, 25–26
liposomal cytarabine, 646
Listeria, 409
LMWH. *See* low-dose low-molecular-weight heparin
lobectomy, 100
lomustine, 301
    dosage, schedule, 789
    mechanism of action, 788
    primary indication, 788
    special precautions, 789
    toxicity, 789
lorazepam (Ativan)
    acute confusional states, 682
    nausea, vomiting, 554*t*
low-dose low-molecular-weight heparin (LMWH), 599
lung carcinoma, 94
    etiology, 94
    molecular biology, 94–95
    NSCLC. *See* Non–small-cell lung cancer (NSCLC)
    palliation
        colony-stimulating factors, 117–118
        pleural effusions, 117
        radiotherapy, 117
    SCLC. *See* Small-cell lung cancer (SCLC)
    screening, 95
Lung Screening Study, 95
lupus anticoagulant, 598
luteinizing hormone-releasing hormone (LHRH), 240–241
lymphedema, fibrosis and, 90–91
lymphoblastic lymphoma (LBL), 480
Lyrica. *See* pregabalin

M

MACOP-B regimen, non-Hodgkin lymphoma, 475
macromolecular synthesis or function, 2
MAGIC trial, 133
magnetic resonance imaging (MRI)
    breast cancer screening, 174
    cervical cancer, 201
    NHL, 530
    NSCLC, 99
    soft-tissue sarcomas, 315
    spinal cord compression, 618–619
    thyroid and adrenal cancer, 269
MAID regimen, 318
malignant fibrous histiocytoma (MFH), 310–311, 335
malignant mixed müllerian tumor (MMMT), 209–210

malignant subarachnoid infiltrates
    causes, 645
    complications, 647
    diagnosis, 645–646
    response to treatment, 647
    treatment, 646–647
MALT lymphoma, 471
mammalian target of rapamycin (mTOR) pathway, 163, 255
MammaPrint test, 185
mammography, 175
mannitol
    cerebral edema, 307, 622
    Hodgkin lymphoma, 448
mantle cell lymphoma (MCL), 477, 478*t*, 479*t*
MAOIs. *See* monoamine oxidase inhibitors
m-BACOD regimen, non-Hodgkin lymphoma, 475
MCL. *See* mantle cell lymphoma
MCL 2 regimen, 479*t*
MDR. *See* multidrug resistance
MDS. *See* myelodysplastic syndrome
MEC regimen, acute myeloid leukemia, 359
mechlorethamine, 8
    CTCL, 473
    dosage, schedule, 789
    EV, 423
    mechanism of action, 789
    primary indications, 789
    special precautions, 789–790
    toxicity, 790
median survival time, 50
medroxyprogesterone (Depo-Provera), 348–349
medullary thyroid cancer (MTC), 259–260
    diagnosis and staging, 262
    treatment, 266
medulloblastoma (WHO grade IV)
    characteristics, 302–303
    treatment, 303
megestrol acetate, endometrial cancer, 209*t*
megestrol, breast cancer, 195–196
melanoma
    adjuvant therapy, 283
    experimental and future therapies, 289–290
    natural history
        etiology and epidemiology, 277–278
        metastases, patterns of, 279–280
        ocular melanoma, 280
        precursor lesions, genetics, familial melanoma, 278
        primary lesions, 278–279
    regional therapy, 288–289
    staging, 280, 281*t*
    surgical treatment, 280–282
    survival, 282*t*
    therapy of metastases
        biochemotherapy, 287–288
        biologic agents, 284–286
        chemotherapy, 286–287
        systemic therapy, 283–284
    TNM classification, 281*t*
melphalan
    dosage, schedule, 790–791

mechanism of action, 790
MM, 501–503
PMF, 425–426
primary indications, 790
special precautions, 791
toxicity, 791
Memorial Sloan-Kettering Cancer Center (MSKCC), 252
MEN syndrome. *See* multiple endocrine neoplasia type syndrome
MEN-I syndrome. *See* multiple endocrine neoplasia type I syndrome
MEN-IIa syndrome. *See* multiple endocrine neoplasia type I syndrome
MEN-IIb syndrome. *See* multiple endocrine neoplasia type I syndrome
menses suppression, acute leukemias, 348–349
mercaptopurine
    ALL, 376
    dosage, schedule, 791
    mechanism of action, 791
    primary indication, 791
    special precautions, 791
    toxicity, 791–792
Merkel cell carcinoma
    clinical features, 292
    etiology and epidemiology, 292
    treatment, 292–293
mesna
    dosage, schedule, 792
    Ewing sarcoma, 328
    mechanism of action, 792
    primary indications, 792
    soft-tissue sarcomas, 317–318
    special precautions, 792
    toxicity, 792
metaiodobenzylguanidine (MIBG), 274
metal salts, 697
metaproterenol aerosol treatments, 625
metastatic bone pain, 674–675
metastatic cancer of unknown origin, 514
    diagnostic evaluation
        adenocarcinoma, poorly differentiated carcinoma, 519
        biopsy specimen analysis, 517–518
        initial workup, 516–517
        malignant melanoma, 519
        SCC, 518–519
    future directions, 522
    general considerations, 514–516
    malignant, 519
    treatment
        adenocarcinoma, poorly differentiated carcinoma, 520–521
        general strategy, 519
        malignant melanoma, 521
        neuroendocrine carcinoma, 521
        SCC, 520
metastatic disease
    androgen ablation and, 240–241
    complications of therapy, 242–243
    cytotoxic chemotherapy and, 241–242
    evaluation of response, 242
    follow-up, 243
    vaccine therapy, 242
methadone, 662–664, 663*t*, 664*t*
methotrexate
    breast cancer, 188, 191
    DLBCL, 475*t*
    dosage, schedule, 793
    GTN, 227–228, 227*t*
    head and neck cancer therapy, 82
    leptomeningeal metastases, 305
    malignant subarachnoid infiltrates, 646
    mechanism of action, 792–793
    osteosarcoma, 332–334
    PCNSL, 304
    penile cancer, 248
    peritoneal effusions, 643
    primary indications, 793
    relapsed AML, 358
    special precautions, 793
    toxicity, 793–794
methylprednisolone acetate, pleural effusion treatment, 640
metyrosine, 275
MFH. *See* malignant fibrous histiocytoma
mFOLFOX6 regimen. *See* modified FOLFOX6 regimen
MGUS. *See* monoclonal gammopathy of undetermined significance
MIBG. *See* metaiodobenzylguanidine
midostaurin
    dosage, schedule, 794
    mechanism of action, 794
    primary indications, 794
    special precautions, 794
    toxicity, 794–795
minimal residual disease (MRD), 344, 381
mitomycin, 699
    anal cancer, 148–149
    dosage, schedule, 795
    gastric carcinoma, 128
    mechanism of action, 795
    primary indications, 795
    special precautions, 795
    toxicity, 795
mitotane (Lysodren)
    ACC, 271–273
    dosage, schedule, 796
    mechanism of action, 796
    primary indications, 796
    special precautions, 796
    toxicity, 796
mitotic inhibitors, 698
mitoxantrone
    ALL, 375, 387
    AML, adult, 351, 352*t*, 353
    AML, relapsed, 358–360
    APL, 368*t*
    dosage, schedule, 796
    mechanism of action, 796
    peritoneal effusions, 643
    primary indications, 796
    prostate cancer, 242

mitoxantrone *(continued)*
  special precautions, 796–797
  toxicity, 797
MM. *See* multiple myeloma
MMMT. *See* malignant mixed müllerian tumor
modified FOLFOX6 (mFOLFOX6) regimen, 142, 145–146
Mohs micrographic surgery, 291
molecular targeted therapy (MTT), 66
  angiogenesis-targeted therapy, 36
  cell signaling targeted therapy
    intracellular signaling proteins, 30–35
    ligand-receptor binding, blocking, 21–27
    RTKs, inhibition of, 27–30
  characteristics of, 16–17
  classification and type of, 17, 18–20*t*
  immune modulation-targeted therapy, 37–39
  phenotype directed-targeted therapy, 40
    cancer vaccines, 43–44
    immunotoxins, 42–43
    nonreceptor protein-directed MoAbs, 40–42
  protein degradation-targeted therapy, 36–37
  side effects
    altered nutritional status, 560–561
    anaphylaxis, 546–550
    carboplatin skin testing, 547*t*
    constipation, 558–559
    cytokine-release syndrome, 546–550
    diarrhea, 557–558, 559*t*
    extravasation, 544–546, 545*t*
    fatigue, 557
    hypersensitivity, 546–550, 548*t*
    infusion reactions, 546–550, 549*t*
    nausea and vomiting, 550–555, 551*t*, 552–553*t*, 554*t*
    neurotoxicity, 561–562
    oral complications, 555–557
    PPE, 562–564, 563*t*
    skin reactions, 564–565
molecularly targeted agents
  dose modification, 702–705, 705*t*
  dose recommendation, 702
  dose selection and designation, 702
  drug toxicity, 702
  general description, 700–701
  monoclonal antibodies, 701
  other agents, 701
  tyrosine kinase and multikinase inhibitors, 701
monoamine oxidase inhibitors (MAOIs), 687
monoclonal antibodies, 701
monoclonal gammopathy of undetermined significance (MGUS), 491–493
monoclonal protein (M-protein), 491–492
MOPP regimen, Hodgkin lymphoma, 443*t*, 445
morphine, 661–662
MPNs. *See* myeloproliferative neoplasms
M-protein. *See* monoclonal protein
MRC/ECOG. *See* Berlin-Frankfurt-Muenster (BFM)-like regimens
MRD. *See* minimal residual disease
MRI. *See* magnetic resonance imaging

MSKCC. *See* Memorial Sloan-Kettering Cancer Center
MTC. *See* medullary thyroid cancer
mTOR pathway. *See* mammalian target of rapamycin pathway
MTT. *See* molecular targeted therapy
mucositis
  head and neck cancer therapy and, 89
  soft-tissue sarcomas, chemotherapy and, 321
multidrug resistance (MDR), 11, 14
multikinase inhibitors, 701
multiple endocrine neoplasia type I (MEN-I) syndrome, 160
multiple endocrine neoplasia type I (MEN-IIa) syndrome, 274
multiple endocrine neoplasia type I (MEN-IIb) syndrome, 274
multiple endocrine neoplasia type (MEN) syndrome, 259
multiple myeloma (MM)
  complications, 507–509
  diagnosis, 493–495, 493*t*
  epidemiology, 495
  initial treatment, 496–506
  MGUS, 492–493
  M-protein, 491–492
  prognostic factors, 496
  radiotherapy, 506
  staging, 494*t*, 495*t*
  stem cell transplantation, 505–506
  therapy, goals of, 495–496, 497*t*
musculoskeletal system toxicity, 61
Musculoskeletal Tumor Society staging system, 311–312
M-Vax (DNP-VACC), 44
Mycobacterium avium, 531
Mycobacterium tuberculosis, 573
mycosis fungoides (MF), 472
  clinical features, 293–294, 294*t*
  etiology and epidemiology, 293
  TNMB classes, 293*t*
  treatment, 294–295
myelodysplastic syndrome (MDS), 426–427
  classification, 428, 428*t*, 429*t*
  diagnosis, 427–428
  prognosis, 428–429
  therapy
    general approach, 429–430, 430*t*
    growth factors, 430–431, 431*t*
    other agents, 434
    specific agents, 431–434
    supportive care, 434–435
myeloproliferative neoplasms (MPNs), 418
  ET
    diagnosis, 421–422
    treatment regimens, 422–423
  MDSs, 426–427
    classification, 428, 428*t*, 429*t*
    diagnosis, 427–428
    prognosis, 428–429
    therapy, 429–435, 430*t*, 431*t*
  PMF
    diagnosis, 423–424

novel therapies, 426
treatment regimens, 425–426
PV
  ancillary treatments, 421
  antithrombotic therapy, 420
  diagnosis, 418–419
  evolution, outcome, 421
  myelosuppressive agents, 420–421
  phlebotomy, 419–420
  therapy, aims of, 419
myelosuppressive agents, 420–421
Mylotarg. *See* gemtuzumab ozogamicin

N

nab-paclitaxel, breast cancer, 192
NADM. *See* non-AIDS-defining malignancies
nasopharyngeal carcinoma (NPC)
  epidemiology, 69–72
  natural history, 76
  staging, 73
  treatment
    chemotherapy, radiation sensitizer, 85
    chemotherapy, single agent activity, 81*t*,
      82–83
    combination chemotherapy, adjuvant
      therapy, 86
    combination chemotherapy, metastatic
      disease, 83*t*
    general considerations, 79
National Cancer Institute (NCI), 57, 95
natural killer (NK) cell, 452
natural products, 698–699
natural resistance, 13
nausea, 550–555, 551*t*, 552–553*t*, 554*t*,
  668–669
NCI. *See* National Cancer Institute
Neisseria meningitidis, 567
nelarabine
  dosage, schedule, 797
  mechanism of action, 797
  primary indications, 797
  special precautions, 797
  toxicity, 797–798
neoadjuvant therapy, 50, 236
neoplasms, SVCS, 624
nephrotoxicity, 59, 334
neuroendocrine carcinoma, 521
neuroendocrine tumors (NETs), 135
  carcinoid syndrome, 135–136
  TNM stages, 135*t*
  treatment, 136–137
neurogenic pain, 650
neuropathic pain, 650
neurotoxicity, 59
  acute leukemias, 354
  side effects, cancer chemotherapy, 561–562
neutropenia
  fever and, 580–584
  infection role, 571
Nexavar. *See* sorafenib
nilotinib (Tasigna), 32
  CML, 402
  dosage, schedule, 798

mechanism of action, 798
primary indications, 798
special precautions, 798–799
toxicity, 799
nilutamide
  dosage, schedule, 799
  mechanism of action, 799
  primary indications, 799
  special precautions, 799
  toxicity, 799–800
nitrogen mustards, 294, 423, 696. *See also*
  mechlorethamine
nitrosoureas, 8, 697
  gastric carcinoma, 128
  melanoma, 286
NK cell. *See* natural killer cell
nociceptive pain, 650
nodular lymphocyte predominant HL
  (NLPHL), 438
nomogram, body surface area
  adults, 843*t*
  children, 844*t*
non–AIDS-defining malignancies (NADM),
  523–524, 539–540
nonbacterial thrombotic endocarditis, 598
nonbenzodiazepine hypnotics, 689*t*, 691
nonhematologic toxicity, dose modification,
  703–704
non-Hodgkin lymphoma (NHL), 60, 451–452
  epidemiology, 452–453, 453*t*
  high-grade form
    BL, 480–481, 481*t*
    LBL, 480
    tumor lysis prophylaxis, 481
  and HIV infection, 530–536, 532*t*, 533*t*
  intermediate-grade form
    CNS prophylaxis, 476
    DLBCL, 472–473, 476–477
    initial treatment, advanced stage, 474–475
    initial treatment, localized form, 475–476
    MCL, 477, 478*t*, 479*t*
    PMBL, 476
    PTCLs, 477–478
    rare, extranodal T-cell lymphoma,
      479–480
  pathologic classification, 455–459, 457*t*, 458*t*,
    459*t*, 460*t*, 461–462*t*
  radiation therapy, 484–485
  relapsed, therapy of
    allogeneic transplantation, 483
    novel/targeted agents, 483–484
    salvage chemotherapy, 482–483, 482*t*
  risk factors, 453–455, 453*t*, 454*t*, 455*t*
  staging, prognosis and
    Ann Arbor staging, 460–463, 463*t*, 464*t*
    diagnosis, 459–460
    functional biomarkers, 466
    GEP, prognostic marker, 465–466
    IPI, 465, 465*t*
  subgroups, special considerations
    AIDS-related lymphomas, 485
    elderly patients, 487–488
    PCNSL, 486–487

non-Hodgkin lymphoma (NHL) *(continued)*
    PTLDs, 485–486, 485*t*
    testicular lymphomas, 487
nonmelanoma skin cancer
    diagnosis and clinical features, 290–292
    etiology and epidemiology, 290
nonseminoma
    follow-up, 246
    recommended therapy, 246
    stage I disease, 245
    stage II disease, 245
    stage III disease, 245–246
    surgery, residual disease and, 246
non–small-cell lung cancer (NSCLC), 94
    histology, 96
    locally advanced disease, 103
        bulky stage IIIA (N2), no pleural effusion,
            104–106, 105*t*
        bulky stage IIIB, no pleural effusion,
            104–106, 105*t*
        nonbulky stage IIIA, 103–104
    pretreatment evaluation, 96–100
    second-line chemotherapy, 111–113
    stage I disease, 100–102, 101*t*
    stage II disease, 102–103
    stage IV disease, 106
        angiogenesis inhibition, 108
        chemotherapy, choice of, 106–108, 107*t*
        EGFR inhibition, 108–109
        first-line chemotherapy, 106
        non-platinum-based regimens, 110
        oligometastatic disease, 111
        poor performance status, patients and, 111
        therapy/maintenance duration, 109–110
    staging, 96, 97*t*, 98*t*, 99*t*
nonspecific immunomodulators, 39
nonsteroidal anti-inflammatory drugs (NSAIDs)
    cancer pain, 658–659, 658*t*
    MM, 498
    osteosarcoma, 334
nosocomial infections, 584–588
NPC. *See* nasopharyngeal carcinoma
NSAIDs. *See* nonsteroidal anti-inflammatory
        drugs
NSCLC. *See* Non–small-cell lung cancer
nucleoside analog, 511
nutrition
    altered status, 560–561
    head and neck cancer therapy and, 87–88

O
obesity, dose modification, 704–705
objective response, measures
    evaluable disease, 53–54
    performance status changes, 54
    tumor products, 53
    tumor size, 51–53
octreotide acetate (Sandostatin)
    carcinoid tumors, 136
    PNETs, 161
ocular melanoma, 280
ofatumumab (Arzerra), 41
    CLL, 412

    dosage, schedule, 800
    mechanism of action, 800
    primary indications, 800
    special precautions, 800
    toxicity, 800–801
olaparib
    dosage, schedule, 801
    mechanism of action, 801
    primary indications, 801
    special precautions, 801
    toxicity, 801
oligodendroglioma (WHO grades II and III)
    characteristics, 301–302
    treatment, 302
oligometastatic disease, 111
Onco Vax, 44
OncotypeDx, 185–186
ondansetron (Zofran), 682
Ontak. *See* denileukin diftitox
oophorectomy, breast cancer, 195–196
opioid analgesics
    adverse effects, 667–671
    alternative routes, 664–667
    chronic cancer pain, 662
    long-acting preparations, 662
    methadone, 662–664, 663*t*, 664*t*
    oral morphine, 661–662
    potent opioid alternatives, 664
    therapy, starting, 659–660
    treatment schedule, dose selection, 660, 661*t*
    weak opioids, 660–661
oprelvekin, 615–616
    dosage, schedule, 802
    MDS, 435
    mechanism of action, 801
    primary indications, 802
    special precautions, 802
    toxicity, 802
oral infections, secondary, 556–557
oral phosphate supplements, 632
orchiectomy, metastatic disease, 240
osmotic diuretic, cerebral edema, 307
osteosarcoma
    administration, special precautions, 332–333
    chemotherapy, 331
    complication, 333–334
    effective agents, 331
    general considerations, 331
    high-dose chemotherapy, 334–335
    recommended regimen, 331–332
ovarian cancer, 210–211
    clinical presentation, diagnosis, 212
    histology, 211
    prognostic factors, 212–213
    screening, 211–212
    staging, 213, 214*t*
    treatment
        advanced-stage disease, 215, 216*t*
        cytoreductive surgery, 213–214
        early-stage disease, 214–215
        intraperitoneal chemotherapy, 217–218
        maintenance, 218
        palliative care, 220

PARP inhibition, 218–219
platinum-based first-line chemotherapy, 215–216
platinum-resistant disease, 220
platinum-sensitive disease, 219
promising strategies, 217
recurrent disease, 219
ovarian germ cell tumors, 223
clinical presentation, diagnosis, 223–224
histology, 223
prognostic factors, 224
screening, 223
staging, 214t, 224
treatment, 224
overall survival rate, 50
overdiagnosis, 95
oxaliplatin
biliary tract cancer, 165–166
colorectal cancer, 143
dosage, schedule, 802–803
gastric carcinoma, 131–132
mechanism of action, 802
pancreatic cancer, 159
primary indications, 802
special precautions, 803
toxicity, 803
oxcarbazepine, 307

P

paclitaxel
breast cancer, 189–192
cervical cancer, 204
dosage, schedule, 804
endometrial cancer, 208t, 209
esophageal carcinoma, 126
gastric carcinoma, 132
head and neck cancer chemotherapy
combination, metastatic disease, 84–85
radiation sensitizer, 85–86
single agent activity, 81
KS, 528
mechanism of action, 803–804
metastatic cancer of unknown origin, 521
NCLC, 105, 105t, 107t
ovarian cancer, 215–220, 216t
peritoneal effusions, 643
primary indications, 804
side effects, cancer chemotherapy, 548–549
special precautions, 804
standard pretreatment regimen, 804
testicular cancer, 247
toxicity, 804–805
uterine sarcomas, 210
paclitaxel, protein-bound
dosage, schedule, 805
mechanism of action, 805
primary indications, 805
special precautions, 805
toxicity, 805–806
pain, 649
adjuvant drugs, 671–674
adjuvant procedures and therapies, 675–676
assessment, 651–655

etiology, 650–651
prevalence, severity, and risk, 649–650
severity, 651–653
treatment, 651–655
general aspects, 655–658, 656–657t
NSAIDs, 658–659, 658t
opioid analgesics, 659–671, 661t, 663t, 664t
pain attacks, 688
pain expression, 650
pain perception, 650
palliative care, 67–68
palmar-plantar erythrodysesthesia (PPE), 562–564, 563t
palonosetron, 552t, 554t
pamidronate
bone metastasis, 635
dosage, schedule, 806
hypercalcemia, 631
mechanism of action, 806
MM, 507
primary indications, 806
special precautions, 806
toxicity, 806
Pancoast tumors, 103
pancreatic cancer
diagnostic evaluation, 152–153
epidemiology, 151
etiology, 151–152
laboratory tests, 153
metastases, chemotherapy, 157
combination, 157–158
current recommendations, 159
novel targeted agents, 158
second-line, 159
single agents, 157
preoperative evaluation, 154
primary therapy
combined-modality therapy, 155–157
radiation therapy, 154
surgery, 154
signs, symptoms, 152
staging, 153
TNM staging, 154t
pancreatic neuroendocrine tumors (PNETs)
epidemiology, 159–160
islet cell tumor management, 161–163
presentation, 160
primary treatment, 161
panitumumab
cancer, of large intestine, 143
dosage, schedule, 807
mechanism of action, 807
primary indications, 807
special precautions, 807
toxicity, 807
Pap test, 200
papillary thyroid cancer (PTC), 259–260
paracentesis, 641
paraganglioma
description and diagnosis, 274
treatment
chemotherapy, 275

paraganglioma *(continued)*
    radiation therapy, 275–276
    surgery, 274–275
paroxetine, 421, 686*t*, 687*t*
PARP inhibition, ovarian cancer, 218–219
PARP1 inhibitors
    dosage, schedule, 801
    mechanism of action, 801
    primary indications, 801
    special precautions, 801
    toxicity, 801
partial response
    acute leukemias, 351
    definition, 52
pasireotide, 162, 820
pazopanib (Votrient), 30
    dosage, schedule, 808
    kidney cancer, 255
    mechanism of action, 808
    primary indications, 808
    special precautions, 808
    toxicity, 808
PBL. *See* plasmablastic lymphoma
PBSCT. *See* peripheral blood stem cell
    transplantation
PCNSL. *See* primary central nervous system
    lymphoma
PCTs. *See* proximal convoluted tubules
PCV regimen, 301
PD. *See* progressive disease
PD1 inhibitors, 38–39
pegfilgrastim
    dosage, schedule, 809
    mechanism of action, 809
    primary indications, 809
    soft-tissue sarcomas, 320
    special precautions, 809
    toxicity, 809
peginterferon, 283
pegylated liposomal doxorubicin, 504
PEL. *See* primary effusion lymphoma
pemetrexed
    dosage, schedule, 810
    lung cancer
      NSCLC, 107*t*, 111–112
    mechanism of action, 809–810
    primary indications, 810
    special precautions, 810
    toxicity, 810
penicillamine, 605
penicillin, 589, 605
penicillin allergy, 582–583
penile cancer, 248
pentamidine, 590
pentostatin
    dosage, schedule, 811
    HCL, 415
    mechanism of action, 811
    MF, 295
    primary indications, 811
    special precautions, 811
    toxicity, 811
percutaneous hepatic perfusion (PHP), 163

performance status
    quality of life, 49
    treatment and, 49
    types of scales, 48–49, 48*t*, 49*t*
pericardial effusions, 644
    causes, 644
    diagnosis, 644
    treatment, 644–645
perifosine, 35
peripheral blood stem cell transplantation
    (PBSCT)
    HIV-associated malignancies, 535–536
    MM, 505–506
peripheral T-cell lymphomas (PTCLs),
    477–478
peritoneal effusions
    causes, 640–641
    diagnosis, 641
    therapy, 642–643
peritoneal-venous shunts, 643
pertuzumab, 25
PFS. *See* progression-free survival
P-glycoprotein, 14
phase and cell cycle specificity, 6–8, 6*t*, 8*t*
phase-nonspecific drugs, 8
phase-specific drugs, 6, 6*t*
    cytarabine, 7–8
    implications of, 6–7
phenacetin, 251
phenazopyridine, 146–147
phenobarbital, 308, 308*t*
phenotype directed-targeted therapy, 40
    cancer vaccines, 43–44
    immunotoxins, 42–43
    nonreceptor protein–directed MoAbs, 40–42
phenoxybenzamine, 274
phenytoin
    cancer pain, 673
    seizures, 307
pheochromocytoma
    description and diagnosis, 274
    treatment, 275
phlebotomy, 419–420
PHP. *See* percutaneous hepatic perfusion
PI3K/Akt/mTOR pathway inhibitors, 34–36
pilocarpine, 556
pimecrolimus, 565
piperacillin-tazobactam, 581*t*, 582, 585, 587
plasmablastic lymphoma (PBL), 535
Plasmodium falciparum, 570
platelet transfusions, 609–612, 611*t*
pleiotropic drug resistance, 14. *See also* multi-
    drug resistance (MDR)
plerixafor, 505
pleural effusion
    causes, 636–637
    diagnosis, 637–638
    SCLC, 117
    treatment, 638–640
PLL. *See* prolymphocytic leukemia
PMBL. *See* primary mediastinal B-cell lymphoma
PMF. *See* primary myelofibrosis
PNETs. *See* pancreatic neuroendocrine tumors

Pneumocystis carinii pneumonia
  CLL complications, 409
  dissemination, 576
  prophylaxis, 531
Pneumocystis jiroveci (carinii), 411
Podophyllum peltatum, 698
polycythemia vera (PV), 418
  diagnosis, 418–419
  evolution, outcome, 421
  therapy, aims of, 419
  treatment regimes
    ancillary treatments, 421
    antithrombotic therapy, 420
    myelosuppressive agents, 420–421
    phlebotomy, 419–420
polyglutamated paclitaxel (Xyotax), 218
pomalidomide, 426, 505
posaconazole, 589, 592
positron emission tomography (PET)
  cervical cancer, 201
  esophageal carcinoma, 121
  HL, 440, 444
  head and neck cancer, 73
  metastatic cancer of unknown origin, 516, 518
  NHL, 464–465
  NSCLC, 99
  thyroid and adrenal cancer, 262, 269
posttransplant lymphoproliferative disorders
    (PTLDs), 455, 485–486, 485t
posttraumatic stress disorder (PTSD), 690–691
PPE. *See* palmar-plantar erythrodysesthesia
PR. *See* partial response
pralatrexate
  dosage, schedule, 812
  mechanism of action, 812
  primary indications, 812
  special precautions, 812
  toxicity, 812
prazosin, 275
prednisolone
  FL, 471t
  WM, 510
prednisone
  ALL, 376
  DLBCL, 475t
  MF, 294
  MM, 501–503
  PMF, 425
  prostate cancer, 242
pregabalin (Lyrica), 673
pregnancy, acute myeloid leukemia, 366
premature menopause, 61
primary central nervous system lymphoma
    (PCNSL), 303–304, 486–487, 536–537
primary effusion lymphoma (PEL), 524,
    529–530
primary mediastinal B-cell lymphoma (PMBL),
    467, 476
primary myelofibrosis (PMF)
  diagnosis, 423–424
  novel therapies, 426
  treatment regimens, 425
    anemia, 425

curative intent, 426
splenomegaly, 425–426
primary refractory AML, 357
primary testicular lymphoma (PTL), 487
primidone, 308t
procarbazine, 301
  dosage, schedule, 813
  mechanism of action, 812
  primary indications, 812
  special precautions, 813
  toxicity, 813
prochlorperazine (Compazine), 147, 552t, 554t,
    690, 708
progesterone receptors, breast cancer, 185
progestins, 700
  dosage, schedule, 813
  mechanism of action, 813
  primary indications, 813
  special precautions, 814
  toxicity, 814
progression-free survival (PFS), 50
progressive disease (PD), 52
prolymphocytic leukemia (PLL), 406, 414
Pro-MACE-CytaBOM regimen, 475
prophylactic cranial irradiation, 117
prostate cancer
  androgen ablation, 240–241
  background, 238
  complications of therapy, 242–243
  cytotoxic chemotherapy, 241–242
  evaluation of response, 242
  follow-up, 243
  general considerations, therapy, 239–240
  staging, 238–239
  TNM staging, 239t
  vaccine therapy, 242
protein degradation-targeted therapy, 36–37
proteins, intracellular signaling, inhibition of, 30
  Bcr-Abl tyrosine kinase, 31–32
  PI3K, AKT, and mTOR pathway inhibitors, 34–35
  Raf/MAP kinase pathway, 32–34
Provenge. *See* sipuleucel-T
proximal convoluted tubules (PCTs), 250
Pseudomonas, 576, 588t
Pseudomonas aeruginosa, 589
psoralen, 294
psoralen and ultraviolet radiation (PUVA), 294
psychiatric problems, 678
  acute confusional states, 678–683, 681t
  anxiety, 688–691, 689t
  depression, 683–687, 685t, 686t, 687t
  insomnia, 691–692
PTC. *See* papillary thyroid cancer
PTCLs. *See* peripheral T-cell lymphomas
PTL. *See* primary testicular lymphoma
PTLDs. *See* posttransplant lymphoproliferative
    disorders
PTSD. *See* posttraumatic stress disorder
pulmonary function
  head and neck cancer and, 75
  NSCLC and, 99–100
pulmonary toxicity, 58, 321
purine analogs, 698

PUVA. *See* psoralen and ultraviolet radiation
PV. *See* polycythemia vera
pyridoxine, 434
pyrimidine analogs, 698

Q

quality of life (QOL), 49, 54–55
quinupristin-dalfopristin, 581*t*, 589

R

radiation therapy
  brain metastases, 305
  breast cancer, 182–183
  esophagus carcinoma, 124–125
  NHL, 484–485
  pancreatic cancer, 154
  paraganglioma, 275–276
  PMF, 425–426
  spinal cord compression, 619–620
  thyroid and adrenal carcinomas, 275
radioactive phosphorus, 420–421
radioactive remnant ablation (RRA), 264–265
radiofrequency ablation (RFA), 163
radioimmunoconjugate antibodies, 41–42
radioisotope therapy
  bone metastases, 634
  malignant ascites, 642
  metastatic bone pain, 674
  pericardial effusions, 645
radiotherapy (RT), 65
  ACC, 271
  anal cancer, 148
  ATC, 267
  DTC, 264–266
  HL, 439*t*, 442–443
  KS, 527
  melanoma, 288–289
  MM, 506
  MTC, 266
  pericardial effusions, 645
  pheochromocytoma, paraganglioma, 275–276
  SCLC, 117
Raf/MAP kinase pathway, 32–34
RAI therapy, 264–265
raloxifene
  breast cancer, 193
  dosage, schedule, 814
  mechanism of action, 814
  primary indications, 814
  special precautions, 814
  toxicity, 814–815
rasburicase
  acute leukemias, 347
  tumor lysis syndrome, 628–629
RCC. *See* renal cell carcinoma
R-CDE regimen, 532, 532*t*
R-CHOP regimen
  DLBCL, 475–476
  indolent lymphoma, 470
  MCL, 478
  NHL, 531
receptor tyrosine kinases (RTKs), 22, 27–30

RECIST. *See* Response Evaluation Criteria in
    Solid Tumors
rectal cancer
  postoperative chemotherapy, 146
  preoperative chemoradiation, 145–146
  TNM stages, 139*t*
reduced intensity conditioning (RIC) (mini)-
    HCST, 364–365
relapsed AML
  interventions on relapse
    CNS prophylaxis, 361
    investigational strategies, novel agents,
      360–361
    non-HDAC regimens, 360
    standard chemotherapy, 357–360
  prognostic factors, 357
renal cell carcinoma (RCC)
  clinical characteristics, 251–252
  epidemiology, 250–251
  histopathology, 250
  risk factors, 251, 253*t*
  staging, 252–253, 252*t*
  treatment considerations, 253
  treatment regimens, 254–256
renal dysfunction
  AML, 354
  HDAC consolidation regimes, 355*t*
  MM, 508
renal insufficiency, soft-tissue sarcomas, 321
RES. *See* reticuloendothelial system
resectable disease, 153
resistance
  antineoplastic agents, 12–13
    biochemical causes, 13–14
    cell kinetics and, 13
    nonselectivity, 15
    pharmacologic causes, 14–15
respiratory depression and opioids, 669–670
respiratory failure
  causes, 626
  management, 626
  prevention, 626–627
Response Evaluation Criteria in Solid Tumors
    (RECIST), 315
response to therapy
  considerations, 50–51
  definitions, 50
  objective response, 51–54
  subjective change, QOL considerations and,
    54–55
  survival, 50
reticuloendothelial system (RES), 566, 570
retroperitoneal lymph node dissection
    (RPLND), 245
Revlimid. *See* lenalidomide
RFA. *See* radiofrequency ablation
R-HyperCVAD/MA cycles regimen
  BL, 480–481
  mantle cell lymphoma, 479*t*
RIC (mini)-HCST. *See* reduced intensity
    conditioning (mini)-HCST
ridaforolimus, 35
Rituxan. *See* rituximab

rituximab (Rituxan), 40
  CLL, 410–411
  DLBCL, 474
  dosage, schedule, 815
  FL, 469, 471*t*
  HCL, 415
  indolent lymphoma, 472
  mechanism of action, 815
  NHL, 532*t*
  primary indications, 815
  special precautions, 815–816
  toxicity, 816–817
  WM, 511
romidepsin
  dosage, schedule, 817
  mechanism of action, 817
  primary indications, 817
  special precautions, 817
  toxicity, 817–818
RPLND. *See* retroperitoneal lymph node
      dissection
RT. *See* radiotherapy
RTKs. *See* receptor tyrosine kinases
RVD regimen, 503–504

S

saline diuresis, in hypercalcemia, 630–631
salmon calcitonin, hypercalcemia, 632
Sandostatin. *See* octreotide acetate
sargramostim
  dosage, schedule, 818–819
  HL, 450
  mechanism of action, 818
  primary indications, 818
  SCLC, 118
  special precautions, 819
  toxicity, 819
SCA. *See* squamous cell carcinoma
SC-EPOCH-RR regimen, non-Hodgkin lym-
      phoma, 531, 532*t*
SCLC. *See* Small-cell lung cancer
SCT. *See* stem cell transplantation
SD. *See* stable disease
second malignancies
  acute myelogenous leukemia, 60
  solid tumors, 60
secondary cancer prevention, head and neck
      cancer, 91
sedation, opioid-induced, 668
seizures
  treatment of, 308*t*
    common side effects, 307–308
    cytochrome P-450 induction, 308
    presenting feature, 307
selective estrogen receptor modulators (SERMs),
      174, 700
seminoma
  clinical stage I, 244
  clinical stage II, 244
serum carcinoembryonic antigen (CEA), 140
serum CEA. *See* serum carcinoembryonic
      antigen
serum methotrexate levels, 333

side effects, chemotherapy, molecular targeted
      therapy and
  altered nutritional status, 560–561
  anaphylaxis, 546–550
  carboplatin skin testing, 547*t*
  constipation, 558–559
  cytokine-release syndrome, 546–550
  diarrhea, 557–558, 559*t*
  extravasation, 544–546, 545*t*
  fatigue, 557
  hypersensitivity, 546–550, 548*t*
  infusion reactions, 546–550, 549*t*
  nausea and vomiting, 550–555, 551*t*,
      52–553*t*, 554*t*
  neurotoxicity, 561–562
  oral complications, 555–557
  PPE, 562–564, 563*t*
  skin reactions, 564–565
sipuleucel-T
  dosage, schedule, 819–820
  mechanism of action, 819
  primary indications, 819
  prostate cancer, 242
  special precautions, 820
  toxicity, 820
sipuleucel-T (Provenge), 43–44
skeletal destruction, multiple myeloma, 508–509
SLL. *See* small lymphocytic lymphoma
sLV5FU2 regimen
  colon cancer, 145
  rectal cancer, 146
small intestine cancer
  adenocarcinomas, 137
  NETs, 134
    carcinoid syndrome, 135–136
    TNM stages, 135*t*
    treatment, 136–137
  TNM stages, 138*t*
small lymphocytic lymphoma (SLL),
      405–406, 468
small-cell lung cancer (SCLC), 94, 114
  chemotherapy, chest irradiation, 116–117
  pretreatment evaluation, 114
  prognostic factors, 114–115
  prophylactic cranial irradiation, 117
  staging, 114
  therapy
    combination chemotherapeutic regimens,
      115, 115*t*
    dose intensity, 115–116
    duration, 116
    second-line, 116
soft-tissue sarcomas
  chemotherapy
    complications of, 320–322
    effective drugs, 317
    general considerations, therapy aims, 316
    secondary, 319–320
    special precautions, 322
  evaluation, 313–314*t*
  metastases, 311
  primary treatment, 314–315
  prognosis, 315

soft-tissue sarcomas *(continued)*
  treatment response, 315–316
  types of, 310–311
somatostatin analogs
  dosage, schedule, 820
  mechanism of action, 820
  primary indications, 820
  special precautions, 821
  toxicity, 821
sorafenib (Nexavar), 33
  dosage, schedule, 821
  HCC, 170–171
  kidney cancer, 254
  mechanism of action, 821
  primary indications, 821
  special precautions, 821
  toxicity, 821–822
Sorangium cellulosum, 698
specific immune modulators, 37
  CTLA-4 inhibitors, 37–38
  PD1 inhibitors, 38–39
  TGF-b antibodies, 39
spinal cord compression
  diagnosis, 618–619
  symptoms, signs, 618
  treatment, 618–619
  tumors, 618
spiral computed tomography (CT), 95
splenectomy, PMF, 425
splenomegaly, 425–426
Sprycel. *See* dasatinib
squamous cell carcinoma (SCA). *See also* head
        and neck cancer (HNC)
  diagnosis, 290–291
  etiology and epidemiology, 290
  head and neck cancer
    chemotherapy, 80–87
    epidemiology, 69–71
    natural history, 76–77
    presenting symptoms, 72–73
    secondary cancer prevention, 91
    staging and work-up, 73–76
    supportive care, 87–91
    treatment, 77–79
  local treatment, 291–292
  of thyroid, 260
  treatment, 292
squamous cell carcinoma (SCC), 514
  diagnostic evaluation, 518–519
  histology, 515
  sites of origin, 515
  treatment, 520
stable disease (SD), 52
staging
  system criteria, 47
  therapy decisions and, 47–48
Stanford V regimen, Hodgkin lymphoma, 443*t*
Staphylococcus aureus, 409, 575, 588–589, 588*t*
Staphylococcus epidermidis, 588*t*, 589
stem cell transplantation (SCT)
  CLL, 413–414
  testicular cancer, 247
  WM, 511

Stevens-Johnson syndrome, 307
stomatitis, 555–556
Streptococcus pneumoniae, 409, 567, 570, 575
streptozocin
  adrenal cortical carcinoma (ACC), 273
  carcinoid tumors, 136
  dosage, schedule, 822
  mechanism of action, 822
  PNETs, 162
  primary indications, 822
  special precautions, 822
  thyroid and adrenal carcinomas, 275
  toxicity, 823
stromal or granulosa cell tumors (GCTs), 225
  clinical presentation, 225
  histology, 225
  prognostic factors, 225
  staging, 225
  treatment, 225
strontium-89 therapy, 634
subjective change, 54–55
sunitinib (Sutent), 29
  carcinoid tumors, 137
  dosage, schedule, 823
  kidney cancer, 254
  mechanism of action, 823
  primary indications, 823
  special precautions, 823
  toxicity, 824
superior vena cava syndrome (SVCS),
        617, 622
  neoplasms, 624
  radiologic evaluation, 623
  symptoms, signs, 622–623
  thrombi, 624
  tissue diagnosis, 623
  treatment, 623
surgery, 64–65
Surveillance, Epidemiology and End Results
        database, 138
survival curves, 53
Sutent. *See* sunitinib
SVCS. *See* superior vena cava syndrome
systemic chemotherapy
  complications of, 238
  drugs and regimens, 236, 237*t*
  follow-up, 238
  response to therapy, 236–238

T

TAC regimen, breast cancer, 190
TAD-HAM regimen, acute myeloid leukemia, 353
TAD-TAD regimen, acute myeloid leukemia, 353
talc, pleural effusion treatment, 638, 639
t-AML. *See* therapy-related AML
tamoxifen
  breast cancer, 193–195
  dosage, schedule, 825
  mechanism of action, 824
  primary indications, 824–825
  special precautions, 825
  thromboembolism, 600
  toxicity, 825

Tarceva. *See* erlotinib
Tasigna. *See* nilotinib
taxanes
  breast cancer, 188–189
  gastric carcinoma, 128
  melanoma, 286
  stromal or granulosa cell tumors, 225
  thyroid cancer, 267
TCC. *See* transitional cell carcinoma
T-cell lymphoma, 479–480
temozolomide
  dosage, schedule, 826
  glioma, 300
  mechanism of action, 825
  melanoma, 286
  primary indications, 826
  special precautions, 826
  toxicity, 826
temsirolimus (Torisel), 34
  dosage, schedule, 87, 827
  kidney cancer, 255
  mechanism of action, 826–827
  primary indications, 827
  special precautions, 827
  toxicity, 827
teniposide
  dosage, schedule, 828
  mechanism of action, 828
  primary indications, 828
  special precautions, 828
  toxicity, 828
testicular cancer (germ cell tumors)
  complications of therapy, 247
  histology, 243
  mediastinal, other midline germ cell tumors,
    247–248
  overview, 243
  prognosis, 247
  salvage chemotherapy, 247
  staging, 244
  treatment strategies
    nonseminoma, 245–246
    seminoma, 244
testicular lymphomas, 487
TGF-β antibodies, 39
thalidomide
  dosage, schedule, 829
  mechanism of action, 828
  MM, 500, 501–502
  PMF, 425
  primary indications, 828–829
  special precautions, 829
  toxicity, 829
therapy-related AML (t-AML), 365
thioguanine, acute leukemias, 353
thiotepa
  dosage, schedule, 830
  leptomeningeal metastases, 306
  malignant subarachnoid infiltrates, 647
  mechanism of action, 829
  pericardial effusions, 645
  peritoneal effusions, 643
  primary indications, 829

special precautions, 830
toxicity, 830
^{32}P, alkylating agents, 423
thrombi, SVCS, 624
thromboembolism
  clinical syndromes, 597–600
  pathophysiology, 596–597
  risk factors, 596
  therapy, 600–603
thrombotic thrombocytopenic purpura (TTP),
  598–599
thyroid carcinoma
  diagnosis and staging, 261–263, 261*t*
  etiology and prevention, 259–260
  histologic types, 259–260
  incidence, 259
  prognosis, 260–261
  TNM staging, 263*t*
  treatment, ATC
    radiotherapy, 267
    surgery, 266–267
    systemic therapies, 267–268
  treatment, DTC
    RAI, 264–266
    surgery, 263
    systemic therapies, 266
    TSH suppression, 263–264
  treatment, MTC
    radiotherapy, 266
    surgery, 266
    systemic therapies, 266
thyroid lymphoma, 260
thyroid sarcoma, 260
thyroid-stimulating hormone (TSH), 259, 442
time to progression, 52
TKI. *See* tyrosine kinase inhibitor
TNM Committee of the International Union
    Against Cancer, 47
topoisomerase I inhibitor irinotecan
    (CPT-11), 308
topotecan
  cervical cancer, 204
  dosage, schedule, 830
  endometrial cancer, 208*t*, 209
  mechanism of action, 830
  ovarian cancer, 216*t*
  primary indications, 830
  relapsed AML, 359
  toxicity, 831
toremifene
  breast cancer, 193
  dosage, schedule, 831
  mechanism of action, 831
  primary indications, 831
  special precautions, 831
  toxicity, 831–832
Torisel. *See* temsirolimus
tositumomab, iodine-131 (Bexxar)
  dosage, schedule, 832
  indolent lymphoma, 471
  mechanism of action, 832
  non-Hodgkin lymphoma, 485
  primary indications, 832

tositumomab, iodine-131 (Bexxar) *(continued)*
  special precautions, 832
  toxicity, 833
total parenteral nutrition (TPN), 561
toxicity
  acute management, 57–58
  common acute toxicities, 56
  drugs for, clinical testing of, 56
  factors affecting, 55
  recognition, evaluation, 57
  selective toxicities, 56–57
Toxoplasma, 537
TPN. *See* total parenteral nutrition
trabectedin, soft-tissue sarcomas, 317, 320, 322
transfusion therapy
  blood component therapy, 608–613
  CMV-seronegative cellular blood products, 614
  general guidelines, 608
  irradiated blood products, 614–615
  leukocyte reduction, 613–614
transitional cell carcinoma (TCC), 233
transurethral resection (TUR), bladder
        cancer, 233
trastuzumab
  breast cancer, 189–192
  dosage, schedule, 833–834
  gastric carcinoma, 131–132
  mechanism of action, 833
  primary indications, 833
  special precautions, 834
  toxicity, 834
tremelimumab, 37–38
tretinoin
  dosage, schedule, 835
  mechanism of action, 835
  primary indication, 835
  primary indications, 835
  special precautions, 835
  toxicity, 835–836
triazines, 697
trihexyphenidyl (Artane), 682
Trousseau syndrome, 598
TroVax, 44
TSH. *See* thyroid-stimulating hormone
TTP. *See* thrombotic thrombocytopenic purpura
tumor cell kinetics, chemotherapy and, 4
  cell cycle, 5–6, 5f
  phase and cell cycle specificity, 6–8, 6t, 8t
  tumor cell kinetics, therapy implications and,
        8–10
  tumor growth, 4–5
tumor growth
  chemotherapy, effectiveness, 9–10
  stages of
    lag phase, 9
    log phase, 9
    plateau phase, 9
tumor lysis prophylaxis, 481
tumor lysis syndrome, 627
  monitoring, 628
  prevention, 627–628
  treatment, 628–629
tumor products, 53

tumor size, 51
  baseline lesions, 51
  response categories, 52
  survival curves, 53
  time to progression, 52
TUR. *See* transurethral resection
Tykerb. *See* lapatinib ditosylate
typhlitis, 588
tyrosine kinase, 701
tyrosine kinase inhibitor (TKI), 108–109, 285–286

U

UICC. *See* International Union Against Cancer
UISS. *See* University of California, Los Angeles,
        integrated staging system
unclassified sarcomas, 310
unconjugated antibodies, 40–41
University of California, Los Angeles, integrated
        staging system (UISS), 252
uric acid nephropathy, 346–347
U.S. Gastrointestinal Intergroup, 133
uterine sarcomas
  clinical presentation, diagnosis, 209–210
  histology, 209
  prognostic factors, 210
  staging, 210
  treatment, 210

V

vaccination
  melanoma, 289
  prostate cancer, 242
VAdCA regimen, Ewing sarcoma, 329
VAdriaC regimen, Ewing sarcoma, 328
VAI regimen, Ewing sarcoma, 328
valproic acid
  cancer pain, 673
  seizures, 307
valrubicin
  dosage, schedule, 836
  mechanism of action, 836
  primary indications, 836
  special precautions, 836
  toxicity, 836–837
vancomycin, 581t, 582, 583
vancomycin-resistant enterococcus (VRE), 587
vandetanib, 30
  dosage, schedule, 837
  mechanism of action, 837
  primary indications, 837
  special precautions, 837
  toxicity, 837
vascular access, acute leukemias, 348
vascular endothelial growth factor (VEGF),
        25–26, 162–163, 250, 259
vascular endothelial growth factor receptor
        (VEGFR), 162–163
VEGF. *See* vascular endothelial growth factor
VEGFR. *See* vascular endothelial growth factor
        receptor
venlafaxine, 195
VHL gene. *See* Von Hippel-Lindau gene

vinblastine
  dosage, schedule, 838
  mechanism of action, 838
  primary indications, 838
  special precautions, 838
  testicular cancer, 247
  toxicity, 838
vinca alkaloids, melanoma, 286
vincristine, 301
  ALL, 376–379, 384, 386
  DLBCL, 475t
  dosage, schedule, 839
  Ewing sarcoma, 328–330
  FL, 471t
  GTN, 227, 227t
  mechanism of action, 838
  MF, 294
  primary indications, 838–839
  soft-tissue sarcomas, 317–319
  special precautions, 839
  toxicity, 838, 839
vinorelbine
  breast cancer, 191–192
  cervical cancer, 204
  dosage, schedule, 840
  HL, 448
  lung cancer
    NCLC, 107t, 109
  mechanism of action, 839
  primary indications, 839
  special precautions, 840
  toxicity, 840
VMP regimen, 502–503
vomiting, 550–555, 551t, 552–553t, 554t, 668–669
Von Hippel-Lindau (VHL) gene, 250
vorinostat
  dosage, schedule, 840
  mechanism of action, 840
  primary indication, 840
  special precautions, 840
  toxicity, 841
Votrient. See pazopanib
VRE. See vancomycin-resistant enterococcus
vulvar cancer, 220
  clinical presentation, diagnosis, 221
  histology, 220
  prognostic factors, 221
  screening, 220–221

  staging, 221, 222t
  treatment
    advanced-stage disease, 222–223
    early-stage disease, 221–222

W

Waldenström macroglobulinemia (WM), 491
  diagnosis, presentation, 509
  general considerations, therapy, 509–510
  general considerations, therapy aims, 509–510
  treatment, 510–511
warfarin therapy, 601–602
WBRT. See whole-brain radiation therapy
WHO classification. See World Health Organiza-
    tion classification
whole-brain radiation therapy (WBRT),
    303–304, 487, 537
WM. See Waldenström macroglobulinemia
World Health Organization (WHO) classifica-
    tion, 338–339

X

XELOX regimen, 143
xerostomia, 90, 556
XL147 inhibitor, 35
XL765 inhibitor, 35
Xylocaine. See lidocaine
Xyotax. See polyglutamated paclitaxel

Z

Zevalin. See ibritumomab tiuxetan
Zofran. See ondansetron
zoledronic acid
  bone metastasis, 635
  breast cancer, 196
  dosage, schedule, 841
  hypercalcemia, 631
  me chanism of action, 841
  MM, 507
  primary indications, 841
  special precautions, 841–842
  toxicity, 842breast cancer
        (continued)hepatocellular car-
        cinoma (continued) progestins
        (continued)aspirin (acetylsalicylic
        acid) (continued)esophagus carcinoma
        (continued)letrozole (continued)